the calorie carb and fat bible

The UK's Most Comprehensive Calorie Counter

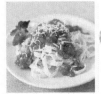

Juliette Kellow BSc RD, Lyndel Costain BSc RD & Rebecca Walton

The Calorie, Carb & Fat Bible

© Weight Loss Resources 2022
Lyndel Costain's contributions © Lyndel Costain

Published by:
Weight Loss Resources Ltd
2C Flag Business Exchange
Vicarage Farm Road
Peterborough
PE1 5TX.

Tel: 01733 345592
www.weightlossresources.co.uk

Companies and other organisations wishing to make bulk purchases of the Calorie, Carb and Fat Bible should contact their local bookstore or Weight Loss Resources direct.

ISBN 978-1-1904512-28-8

Authors: Lyndel Costain BSc RD
                Juliette Kellow BSc RD
                Rebecca Walton, Weight Loss Resources

Database Editor: Sam Holt
Design and Layout: Joanne Putney

Printed and bound in the UK by Bonacia Ltd
www.bookprintinguk.com

Contents

Losing weight – the easy way

Juliette Kellow BSc RD

PIZZA, curries, chocolate, chips and the odd glass of wine! Imagine being told the best diet to help you lose weight can include all these foods and more. It sounds too good to be true, doesn't it? But the truth is, these are exactly the types of foods you can still enjoy if you opt to lose weight by counting calories.

But you'd be forgiven for not knowing you can still eat all your favourite foods and lose weight. In recent years, endless trendy diets have helped to make dieting a complicated business. Added to this, an increasing number of celebrities and so-called nutrition experts have helped mislead us into thinking that dieting is all about restriction and denial. Is it any wonder then that most of us have been left feeling downright confused and miserable about what we should and shouldn't be eating to shift those pounds?

Dieting doesn't have to be a complicated or unhappy experience. In fact, there's really only one word you need to remember if you want to shift those pounds healthily and still eat all your favourite foods. And that's CALORIE!

It's calories that count

When it comes to losing weight, there's no getting away from the fact that it's calories that count. Ask any qualified nutrition expert or dietitian for advice on dropping pounds and you'll receive the same reply: quite simply you need to create a calorie deficit or shortfall. In other words, you need to take in fewer calories than you use up so that your body has to draw on its fat stores to provide it with the energy it needs to function properly. The result: you start losing fat and the pounds start to drop off!

Fortunately, it couldn't be easier to create this calorie deficit. Regardless of your age, weight, sex, genetic make up, lifestyle or eating habits, losing weight is as simple as reducing your daily calorie intake slightly by modifying your diet and using up a few more calories by being slightly more active each day.

Better still, it's a complete myth that you need to change your eating and exercise habits dramatically. You'll notice I've said you need to reduce your calorie intake 'slightly' and be 'slightly' more active. It really is just LITTLE differences between the amount of calories we take in and the amount we use up that make BIG differences to our waistline over time. For example, you only need to consume one can of cola more than you need each day to gain a stone in a year. It's no wonder then that people say excess weight tends to 'creep up on them'.

The good news is the reverse is also true. You only need to swap that daily can of cola for the diet version or a glass of sparking water and you'll lose a stone in a year – it really is as easy as that!

10 simple food swaps you can make every day (*and won't even notice!*)

Make these simple swaps every day and in just 4 weeks you'll lose 7lb!

SWAP THIS...	FOR THIS...	SAVE...
300ml full-fat milk (*195 calories*)	300ml skimmed milk (*100 calories*)	*95 calories*
1tsp butter (*35 calories*)	1tsp low-fat spread (*20 calories*)	*15 calories*
1tbsp vegetable oil (*100 calories*)	10 sprays of a spray oil (*10 calories*)	*90 calories*
1tsp sugar (*16 calories*)	Artificial sweetener (*2 calories*)	*14 calories*
1tbsp mayonnaise (*105 calories*)	1tbsp fat-free dressing (*10 calories*)	*95 calories*
Regular sandwich (*600 calories*)	Low-fat sandwich (*350 calories*)	*250 calories*
Can of cola (*135 calories*)	Can of diet cola (*1 calorie*)	*134 calories*
Large (50g) packet of crisps (*250 calories*)	Small (25g) packet of crisps (*125 calories*)	*125 calories*
1 chocolate digestive (*85 calories*)	1 small chocolate chip cookie (*55 calories*)	*30 calories*
1 slice thick-cut wholemeal bread (*95 calories*)	1 slice medium-cut wholemeal bread (*75 calories*)	*20 calories*
	TOTAL CALORIE SAVING:	***868 calories***

Of course, most people don't want to wait a year to shift a stone. But there's more good news. To lose 1lb of fat each week you need to create a calorie deficit of just 500 calories a day. That might sound like a lot, but you can achieve this by simply swapping a croissant for a wholemeal fruit scone, a regular sandwich for a low-fat variety, a glass of dry white wine for a gin and slimline tonic and using low-fat spread on two slices of toast instead of butter. It is also important to become more active and increase your level of exercise; simply walking a little more will help. Losing 1lb a week, amounts to a stone under 4 stone in a year!

...ories

...really is calories that count when it comes to shifting

...lled diet is one of the few that allows you to include ...pizza, wine or chocolate. A healthy diet means including ...see 'Healthy Eating Made Easy' page 32).

...this book can really help. Gone are the days when it was ...obtain information about the calorie contents of foods. ...rie information for more than 20,000 different branded ...ds so that counting calories has never been easier.

...e easy

Forget weird and wacky science, complicated diet rules and endless lists of foods to fill up on ...d every day! Counting calories to lose weight couldn't

The benefits of cou... ...alories

- *It's guaranteed to help you lose weight providing you stick to your daily calorie allowan...*
- *You can include... ...foods*
- *No foods are banned*
- *It's a great way to lose weight slowly and steadily*
- *Nutrition experts agree that it's a proven way to lose weight*

be easier. Quite simply, you set yourself a daily calorie allowance to help you lose between ½-2lb (¼-1kg) a week and then add up the calories of everything you eat and drink each day, making sure you don't go over your limit.

To prevent hunger from kicking in, it's best to spread your daily calorie allowance evenly throughout the day, allowing a certain amount of calories for breakfast, lunch, dinner and one or two snacks. For example, if you are allowed 1,500 calories a day, you could have 300 calories for breakfast, 400 calories for lunch, 500 calories for dinner and two snacks or treats of 150 calories each. You'll find more detailed information on p26-31 (Your step-by-step guide to using this book and shifting those pounds).

Eat for good health

While calories might be the buzz word when it comes to shifting those pounds, it's nevertheless important to make sure your diet is healthy, balanced and contains all the nutrients you need for good health. Yes, you can still lose

QUESTION
What affects the calorie content of a food?

ANSWER:
Fat, protein, carbohydrate and alcohol all provide the body with calories, but in varying amounts:

- *1g fat provides 9 calories*

- *1g alcohol provides 7 calories*

- *1g protein provides 4 calories*

- *1g carbohydrate provides 3.75 calories*

The calorie content of a food depends on the amount of fat, protein and carbohydrate it contains. Because fat provides more than twice as many calories as an equal quantity of protein or carbohydrate, in general, foods that are high in fat tend to contain more calories. This explains why 100g of chips (189 calories) contains more than twice as many calories as 100g of boiled potato (72 calories).

DIET MYTH:
Food eaten late at night stops you losing weight

DIET FACT:

It's not eating in the evening that stops you losing weight. It's consuming too many calories throughout the day that will be your dieting downfall! Providing you stick to your daily calorie allowance you'll lose weight, regardless of when you consume those calories.

Nevertheless, it's a good idea to spread your calorie allowance throughout the day to prevent hunger from kicking in, which leaves you reaching for high-calorie snack foods.

weight by eating nothing but chocolate, crisps and biscuits providing you stick to your calorie allowance, but you'll never find a nutrition expert or dietitian recommending this. And there are plenty of good reasons why.

To start with, an unbalanced diet is likely to be lacking in essential nutrients such as protein, vitamins, minerals and fibre, in the long term putting you at risk of nutritional deficiencies. Secondly, research proves that filling up on foods that are high in saturated fat and/or salt and sugar can lead to many different health problems. But most importantly, when it comes to losing weight, it's almost impossible to stick to a daily calorie allowance if you're only eating high-calorie foods.

Filling up on lower-calorie foods also means you'll be able to eat far more with the result that you're not constantly left feeling unsatisfied. For example, six chocolates from a selection box contain around 300 calories, a lot of saturated fat and sugar, few nutrients – and are eaten in just six mouthfuls! For 300 calories, you could have a grilled skinless chicken breast (packed with protein and zinc), a large salad with fat-free dressing (a great source of fibre, vitamins and minerals), a slice of wholemeal bread with low-fat spread (rich in fibre and B vitamins) and a satsuma (an excellent source of vitamin C). That's a lot more food that will take you a lot more time to eat! Not convinced? Then put six chocolates on one plate, and the chicken, salad, bread and fruit on another!

Bottom line: while slightly reducing your calorie intake is the key to losing weight, you'll be healthier and far more likely to keep those pounds off if you do it by eating a healthy diet *(see 'Healthy Eating Made Easy' page 32)*.

Eight steps to a healthy diet
1 *Base your meals on starchy foods.*
2 *Eat lots of fruit and vegetables.*
3 *Eat more fish.*
4 *Cut down on saturated fat and sugar.*
5 *Try to eat less salt - no more than 6g a day.*
6 *Get active and try to be a healthy weight.*
7 *Drink plenty of water.*
8 *Don't skip breakfast.*

SOURCE: www.nhs.uk/live-well/eat-well/eight-tips-for-healthy-eating/

Fat facts

Generally speaking, opting for foods that are low in fat can help slash your calorie intake considerably, for example, swapping full-fat milk for skimmed, switching from butter to a low-fat spread, not frying food in oil and chopping the fat off meat and poultry. But don't be fooled into believing that all foods described as 'low-fat' or 'fat-free' are automatically low in calories or calorie-free.

In fact, some low-fat products may actually be higher in calories than standard products, thanks to them containing extra sugars and thickeners to boost the flavour and texture.

The solution: always check the calorie content of low-fat foods, especially for things like cakes, biscuits, crisps, ice creams and ready meals. You might be surprised to find there's little difference in the calorie content when compared to the standard product.

Uncovering fat claims on food labels

Many products may lure you into believing they're a great choice if you're trying to cut fat, but you need to read between the lines on the labels if you want to be sure you're making the best choice. Here's the lowdown on what to look for:

LOW FAT	by law the food must contain less than 3g of fat per 100g for solids. These foods are generally a good choice if you're trying to lose weight.
REDUCED FAT	by law the food must contain 30 percent less fat than a similar standard product. This doesn't mean the product is low-fat (or low-calorie) though! For example, reduced-fat cheese may still contain 14g fat per 100g.
FAT FREE	the food must contain no more than 0.5g of fat per 100g or 100ml. Foods labelled as Virtually Fat Free must contain less than 0.3g fat per 100g. These foods are generally a good choice if you're trying to lose weight.
LESS THAN 8% FAT	this means the product contains less than 8g fat per 100g. It's only foods labelled 'less than 3% fat' that are a true low-fat choice.
X% FAT FREE	claims expressed as X% Fat Free shall be prohibited.
LIGHT OR LITE	claims stating a product is 'light' or 'lite' follows the same conditions as those set for the term 'reduced'.

10 easy ways to slash fat (and calories)

1   Eat fewer fried foods – grill, boil, bake, poach, steam, roast without added fat or microwave instead.

2   Don't add butter, lard, margarine or oil to food during preparation or cooking.

3   Use spreads sparingly. Butter and margarine contain the same amount of calories and fat – only low fat spreads contain less.

4   Choose boiled or jacket potatoes instead of chips or roast potatoes.

5   Cut off all visible fat from meat and remove the skin from chicken before cooking.

6   Don't eat too many fatty meat products such as sausages, burgers, pies and pastry products.

7   Use semi-skimmed or skimmed milk instead of full-fat milk.

8   Try low-fat or reduced-fat varieties of cheese such as reduced-fat Cheddar, low-fat soft cheese or cottage cheese.

9   Eat fewer high-fat foods such as crisps, chocolates, cakes, pastries and biscuits.

10   Don't add cream to puddings, sauces or coffee.

Getting Ready for Weight Loss Success

Lyndel Costain BSc RD

THIS BOOK not only provides tools to help you understand more about what you eat and how active you are, but guidance on how to use this information to develop a weight loss plan to suit your needs. Getting in the right frame of mind will also be a key part of your weight control journey, especially if you've lost weight before, only to watch the pounds pile back on.

The fact is that most people who want to lose weight know what to do. But often there is something that keeps stopping them from keeping up healthier habits. The same may be true for you. So what's going on? For many it's a lack of readiness. When the next diet comes along with its tempting promises it's so easy to just jump on board. But if you have struggled with your weight for a while, will that diet actually help you to recognise and change the thoughts and actions that have stopped you shifting the pounds for good?

Check out your attitude to weight loss programmes

Before starting any new weight loss programme, including the Weight Loss Resources approach, ask yourself:

Am I starting out thinking that I like myself as a person right now?	(YES or NO)
OR I feel I can only like myself once I lose weight?	(YES or NO)
Do I want to stop overeating, but at the same time find myself justifying it – in other words I want to be able to eat what I want, but with no consequences?	(YES or NO)
Do I believe that I need to take long-term responsibility for my weight?	(YES or NO)
OR Am I relying on 'it' (the diet) to do it for me?	(YES or NO)

Keep these questions, and your replies, in mind as you read through this chapter.

Next Steps

You may have already assessed the healthiness of your weight using the BMI guide on page 37. If not, why not do it now, remembering that the tools are a guide only. The important thing is to consider a weight at which you are healthy and comfortable – and which is realistic for the life you lead *(see opposite - What is a healthy weight?)*.

The next step is to have a long hard think about why you want to lose weight. Consider all the possible benefits, not just those related to how you look. Psychologists have found that if we focus only on appearance we are less likely to succeed in the long-term. This is because it so often reflects low self-esteem or self-worth – which can sabotage success – as it saps confidence and keeps us stuck in destructive thought patterns. Identifying key motivations other than simply how you look - such as health and other aspects of physical and emotional well being - is like saying that you're an OK person right now, and worth making changes for. Making healthy lifestyle choices also has the knock on effect of boosting self-esteem further.

Write down your reasons for wanting to lose weight in your Personal Plan *(see page 42)* – so you can refer back to them. This can be especially helpful when the going gets tough. It may help to think of it in terms of what your weight is stopping you from doing now. Here's some examples: to feel more confident; so I can play more comfortably with my kids; my healthier diet will give me more energy; to improve my fertility.

What is a Healthy Weight?

With all the mixed messages in the media it can be easy to get a distorted view about whether your weight is healthy or not. However, as the BMI charts suggest, there is no single 'ideal' weight for anybody. Research also shows that modest amounts of weight loss can be very beneficial to health and are easier to keep off. Therefore, health professionals now encourage us to aim for a weight loss of 5-10%. The ideal rate of weight loss is no more than 1-2 pounds (0.5-1kg) per week – so averaging a pound a week is great, and realistic progress.

The health benefits of modest weight loss include:

- *Reduced risk of developing heart disease, stroke and certain cancers*

- *Reduced risk of developing diabetes and helping to manage diabetes*

- *Improvements in blood pressure*

- *Improvements in mobility, back pain and joint pain*

- *Improvements with fertility problems and polycystic ovarian syndrome*

- *Less breathlessness and sleep/snoring problems*

- *Increased self esteem and control over eating*

- *Feeling fitter and have more energy*

Are You Really Ready to Lose Weight?

When you think of losing weight, it's easy just to think of what weight you'd like to get to. But weight loss only happens as a result of making changes to your usual eating and activity patterns – which allow you to consume fewer calories than you burn *(see 'It's calories that count' page 5).*

So here comes the next big question. Are you really ready to do it? Have you thought about the implications of your decision? If you have lost weight in the past, and put it all back on - have you thought about why that was? And how confident do you feel about being successful this time?

To help you answer these questions, try these short exercises.

Where would you place yourself on the following scales?

Importance

How important is it to you, to make the changes that will allow you to lose weight?

0 1 2 3 4 5 6 7 8 9 10

| | | | | | | | | | | |

Not at all important   *Extremely important*

If you ranked yourself over half way along the scale then move on to the next question. If you were half way or less along the scale, you may not be mentally ready to make the required changes to lose weight. To further explore this, go to '*The Pros and Cons of Weight Loss*' *(page 17)*.

Confidence

How confident are you in your ability to make the changes that will allow you to lose weight?

0 1 2 3 4 5 6 7 8 9 10

| | | | | | | | | | | |

Not at all confident   *Extremely confident*

Now ask yourself (regarding your confidence ratings):

1. Why did I place myself here?

2. What is stopping me moving further up the scale (if anything)?

3. What things, information, support would help me move further up the scale? (if not near 10)

If you aren't sure about answers to question 3, then keep reading for some pointers.

The Pros and Cons of Weight Loss

Making lifestyle changes to lose weight is simpler if there are lots of clear benefits or pros, for example, clothes fit again, more energy, helps back pain - but there will also be associated downsides or cons. For example, some may feel it interferes with their social life, or don't have the time to plan meals or check food labels. Or overeating can help, if only temporarily, as a way of coping with unwanted feelings. Being overweight allows some people to feel strong and assertive, or to control their partner's jealousy. So in these cases there are downsides to losing weight, even if the person says they are desperate to do it.

If you are aware of the possible downsides, as well as the pros, you will be better prepared to deal with potential conflicts. Understanding what could be (or were with past weight loss efforts) barriers to success gives you the chance to address them. This boosts confidence in your ability to succeed this time, which in turn maintains your motivation.

Have a go at weighing up the pros and cons using the charts below and on page 18. Some examples are included. If you decide that the pros outweigh the cons, then great. You can also use the cons as potential barriers to plan strategies for (see page 42). If you find it's the other way around, this may not be the best time to actively lose weight. Try the exercise again in a month or so.

Making Lifestyle Changes to Lose Weight Now

| CONS
e.g. Must limit eating out, take aways | PROS
e.g. Feel more energetic, slimmer |
|---|---|
| | |
| | |
| | |
| | |

Not Making Changes Now – how would I feel in 6 months time?

PROS *e.g. Haven't had to worry about failing;* *Still able to eat take aways a lot*	CONS *e.g. Perhaps gained more weight;* *Still don't like how I look and feel*

To change your weight, first change your mind

To lose weight you may already have a list of things to change, such as eating more fruit and veg, calculating your daily calorie intake, going for a walk each morning or buying low fat options. Others could also give you tips to try. But knowing what to do isn't the same as feeling motivated or able to do it. To be effective, you have to believe the changes are relevant, do-able and worth it.

What you think, affects how you feel, and in turn the actions you take.

Self-efficacy

In fact, research is telling us that one of the most important factors that influences weight loss success are your feelings of 'self-efficacy'.

Self-efficacy is a term used in psychology to describe a person's belief that any action they take will have an effect on the outcome. It reflects our inner expectation that what we do will lead to the results we want. Not surprisingly, high levels of self-efficacy can enhance motivation, and allow us to deal better with uncertainty and conflict, and recovery from setbacks. But low levels, can reduce our motivation.

We fear that whatever we do will not bring about our desired goal. This can lead self-defeating thoughts or 'self-talk', which make it hard to deal with set-backs, meaning we are more likely to give up. Here's some examples.

Examples: Low self-efficacy

'No matter how carefully I diet, I don't lose weight . . .'

'I have eaten that chocolate and as usual blown my diet, so I may as well give up now.'

'I had a rich dessert – I have no willpower to say no. I can't stand not being able to eat what I want.'

If you have a strong sense of self-efficacy, your mindset and 'self-talk' will be more like:

Examples: High self-efficacy

' I know from previous weight loss attempts, that if I stay focussed on what I am doing I do lose weight. I have always expected to lose too much too quickly which frustrates me. I know that I will lose weight if I keep making the right changes, and this time it is important to me.'

' The chocolate bar won't ruin my diet, but if I think it has and keep on eating, then my negative self-talk will. So I will get back on track.'

*' Losing weight is very important to me, so I **can** make better food choices. After all, the world won't stop if I say no to dessert, and I will feel great afterwards. If I think about it, I am not hungry so would just feel bloated and guilty if I ate it.'*

Willpower is a Skill

Many people feel that they just need plenty of willpower or a good telling off to lose weight. But willpower isn't something you have or you don't have. Willpower is a skill. Like the dessert example on page 19, it's a sign that you've made a conscious choice to do something, because you believe the benefits outweigh any downsides. In reality everything we do is preceded by a thought. This includes everything we eat. It just may not seem like it because our actions often feel automatic *(see 'Look out for trigger eating' page 21).*

When it comes to weight loss, developing a range of skills – including choosing lower calorie options, coping with negative self-talk and managing things that don't go to plan - will boost your sense of self-efficacy to make the changes you want. This is especially important because we live in such a weight-promoting environment.

Our weight-promoting environment

We are constantly surrounded by tempting food, stresses that can trigger comfort eating and labour-saving devices that make it easy not to be physically active. In other words, the environment we live in makes it easy to gain weight, unless we stop and think about the food choices we make and how much exercise we do. In fact, to stay a healthy weight/maintain our weight, just about all of us need to make conscious lifestyle choices everyday. This isn't 'dieting' but just part of taking care of ourselves in the environment we live in.

It is also true that some people find it more of a challenge than others to manage their weight, thanks to genetic differences in factors such as appetite control, spontaneous activity level and emotional responses to food – rather than metabolic rate, as is often believed. The good news is that with a healthy diet and active lifestyle a healthier weight can still be achieved. But do talk to your doctor if you feel you need additional support.

Coping with Common Slimming Saboteurs

Lyndel Costain BSc RD

Look out for 'trigger' eating

Much of the overeating we do or cravings we have are actually down to unconscious, habitual, responses to a variety of triggers. These triggers can be external, such as the sight or smell of food, or internal and emotion-led, such as a response to stress, anger, boredom or emptiness. Your food diary (see page 43) helps you to recognise 'trigger' or 'non-hungry' eating which gives you the chance to think twice before you eat (see below).

Get some support

A big part of your success will be having someone to support you. It could be a friend, partner, health professional, health club or website. Let them know how they can help you most.

Make lapses your ally

Don't let a lapse throw you off course. You can't be, nor need to be perfect all the time. Doing well 80-90% of the time is great progress. Lapses are a normal part of change. Rather than feel you have failed and give up, look at what you can learn from a difficult day or week and use it to find helpful solutions for the future.

Understand why you eat

When I ask people what prompts them to eat, hunger usually comes down near the bottom of their list of reasons. Some people struggle to remember or appreciate what true hunger feels like. We are lucky that we have plenty of food to eat in our society. But its constant presence makes it harder to control what we eat, especially if it brings us comfort or joy.

If you ever find yourself in the fridge even though you've recently eaten, then you know hunger isn't the reason but some other trigger. The urge to eat can be so automatic that you feel you lack willpower or are out of control. But it is in fact a learned or conditioned response. A bit like Pavlov's dogs. He rang a bell every time he fed them, and from then on, whenever they heard the bell ring they were 'conditioned' to salivate in anticipation of food.

Because this 'non-hungry' eating is learned, you can reprogramme your response to the situations or feelings that trigger it. The first step is to identify when these urges strike. When you find yourself eating when you aren't hungry ask yourself 'why do I want to eat, what am I feeling?' If you aren't sure think back to what was happening before you ate. Then ask yourself if there is another way you can feel better without food. Or you could chat to your urge to eat in a friendly way, telling it that you don't want to give into it, you have a planned meal coming soon, and it's merely a learned response. Whatever strategy you choose, the more often you break into your urges to eat, the weaker their hold becomes.

Practise positive self-talk

Self-talk may be positive and constructive (like your guardian angel) or negative and irrational (like having a destructive devil on your shoulder).

If you've had on-off battles with your weight over the years, it's highly likely that the 'devil' is there more often. 'All or nothing' self-talk for example, 'I ate a "bad food" so have broken my diet', can make you feel like a failure which, can then trigger you into the action of overeating and/or totally giving up (see 'Diet-binge cycle' page 23). One of the most powerful things about it is that the last thoughts we have are what stays in our mind. So if we think 'I still look fat' or 'I will never be slim', these feelings stay with us.

To change your self-talk for the better, the trick is to first recognise it's happening (keeping a diary really helps, *see Keep a Food Diary, page 29*). Then turn it around into a positive version of the same events *(see Self-efficacy, page 18)* where the resulting action was to feel good and stay on track. Reshaping negative self-talk helps you to boost your self-esteem and feelings of self-efficacy, and with it change your self-definition - from someone who can't 'lose weight' or 'do this or that', to someone 'who can'. And when you believe you can...

The Diet – Binge Cycle

If this cycle looks familiar, use positive self-talk, and a more flexible dietary approach, to help you break free.

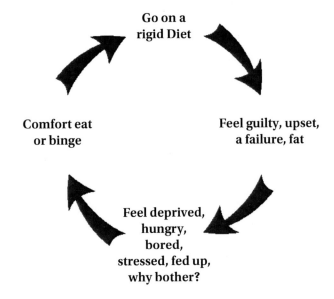

**Go on a
rigid Diet**

**Feel guilty, upset,
a failure, fat**

**Feel deprived,
hungry,
bored,
stressed, fed up,
why bother?**

**Comfort eat
or binge**

Really choose what you want to eat

This skill is like your personal brake. It also helps you to manage 'trigger/non-hungry' eating and weaken its hold. It legalises food and stops you feeling deprived. It helps you to regularly remind yourself why you are making changes to your eating habits, which keeps motivation high. But it doesn't just happen. Like all skills it requires practise. Sometimes it will work well for you, other times it won't – but overall it will help. Basically, ask yourself if you really want to eat that food in front of you. This becomes the prompt for you to make a conscious choice, weighing up the pros and cons or consequences of making that choice, and feeling free to have it, reject it or just eat some. Remembering all the while that you can eat this food another time if you want to.

Action Planning

Successful people don't just wait for things to happen. They believe in themselves, plan ahead, take action and then refine their plan until it gets, and keeps on getting the results they want. Successful slimmers use a very similar approach. They don't rely on quick-fixes or magic formulas, but glean information from reliable sources to develop a plan or approach that suits their needs, tastes and lifestyle. Thinking of weight management as a lifelong project, which has a weight loss phase and a weight maintenance phase, is also a route to success.

When the Going Gets Tough - Staying on Track

If things start to go off track, don't panic. Learning new habits takes time. And life is never straightforward so there will be times when it all seems too much, or negative 'self- talk' creeps in to try and drag you back into old ways. So if the going gets tough:

- Value what you've achieved so far, rather than only focus on what you plan to do.

- Look back at your reasons to lose weight and refer to the list often.

- Don't expect to change too much, too quickly. Take things a step at a time.

- Accept difficulties as part of the learning and skill building process.

- Enjoy a non-food reward for achieving your goals (including maintaining your weight).

- Use recipes and meal ideas to keep things interesting.

- Talk to your supporters and get plenty of encouragement. This is really vital!

Strategies of Successful Slimmers

Thanks to research conducted by large studies such as the US National Weight Control Registry and the German Lean Habits Study, we now know more about what works best for people who have lost weight and successfully kept it off. So be inspired!

The key elements of success are to:

- Believe that you can control your weight and the changes involved are really worth it.
- Stay realistic and value what you have achieved rather than dwell on a weight you 'dream' of being.
- Be more active – plan ways to fit activity into your daily life – aim for 1 hour of walking daily.
- Plan ahead for regular meals and snacks, starting with breakfast.
- Choose a balanced, low-fat diet with plenty of fruit and vegetables (see Healthy Eating Made Easy, page 32).
- Watch portion size and limit fast food.
- Sit down to eat and take time over meals, paying attention to what you are eating.
- Have a flexible approach – plan in and enjoy some favourite foods without guilt.
- Recognise and address 'all or nothing' thinking and other negative 'self-talk'.
- Keep making conscious choices.
- Learn to confront problems rather than eat, drink, sleep or wish they would go away.
- Enlist ongoing help and support from family, friends, professionals or websites.
- Regularly (at least once a week but not more than once daily) check your weight.
- Take action before your weight increases by more than 4-5lb (2kg).
- Accept that your weight management skills need to be kept up long-term.
- Take heart from successful slimmers, who say that it gets easier over time.

Your step-by-step guide to using this book and shifting those pounds

Juliette Kellow BSc RD and Rebecca Walton

1. Find your healthy weight

Use the weight charts, body mass index table and information on pages 36-43 to determine the right weight for you. Then set yourself a weight to aim for. Research shows it really helps if you make losing 10% of your weight your first overall target. It also brings important health benefits too (see 'What is a Healthy Weight?' page 15). You can break this down into smaller manageable steps, for example, 3kg/6.5lbs at a time. If 10% is too much, then go for a 5% loss – this has important health benefits too. In fact, just keeping your weight stable is a great achievement these days, because of our weight-promoting environment *(see page 20)*.

Waist Management

In addition to BMI, another important way to assess your weight is by measuring your waist just above belly button level. It is especially useful for men as they tend to carry more excess weight around their bellies, but women should test it out too. Having excess weight around your middle (known as being 'apple-shaped') increases your risk of heart disease and type 2 diabetes. A simple way to stay aware of your waist is according to how well, or otherwise, skirts and trousers fit. Talk to your doctor about any weight and health concerns.

WAIST MEASUREMENT

	Increased Health Risk	High Risk to Health
Women	32-35in (81-88cm)	more than 35in (88cm)
Men	37-40in (94-102cm)	more than 40in (102cm)

---

2. Set a realistic time scale

With today's hectic lifestyles, everything tends to happen at breakneck speed, so it's no wonder that when it comes to losing weight, most of us want to shift those pounds in an instant. But it's probably taken years to accumulate that extra weight, with the result that it's unrealistic to expect to lose the excess in just a few weeks! Instead, prepare yourself to lose weight slowly and steadily. It's far healthier to lose weight like this. But better still, research shows you'll be far more likely to maintain your new, lower weight.

If you only have a small amount of weight to lose, aim for a weight loss of around 1lb (½kg) a week. But if you have more than 2 stone (28kg) to lose, you may prefer to aim for 2lb (1kg) each week. Remember though, it's better to keep going at 1lb (½kg) a week than to give up because trying to lose 2lb (1kg) a week is making you miserable! The following words may help you to keep your goal in perspective:

**'Never give up on a goal because of the time it will take to
achieve it – the time will pass anyway.'**

Weight Fluctuations

Weight typically fluctuates on a day to day basis. You know that shock/horror feeling when you weigh yourself in the morning then later in the day, or after a meal out, and it looks like youve gained pounds in hours! But this is due to fluid not fat changes. Real changes in body fat can only happen more gradually (remember, to gain 1lb you need to eat 3500 calories more than you usually do). Don't be confused either by seemingly very rapid weight loss in the first week or so.

When calorie intake is initially cut back, the body's carbohydrate stores in the liver and muscles (known as glycogen) are used up. Glycogen is stored with three times its weight in water, meaning that rapid losses of 4.5- 6.6lb (2 -3 kg) are possible. These stores can be just as rapidly refilled if normal eating is resumed. True weight loss happens more gradually and this book helps you to lose weight at the steady and healthy rate of no more than 1-2 lbs per week.

3. Calculate your calorie allowance

Use the calorie tables on pages 39-40 to find out how many calories you need each day to maintain your current weight. Then use the table below to discover the amount of calories you need to subtract from this amount every day to lose weight at your chosen rate. For example, a 35 year-old woman who is moderately active and weighs 12 stone (76kg) needs 2,188 calories a day to keep her weight steady. If she wants to lose ½lb (¼kg) a week, she needs 250 calories less each day, giving her a daily calorie allowance of 1,938 calories. If she wants to lose 1lb (½kg) a week, she needs 500 calories less each day, giving her a daily calorie allowance of 1,688 calories, and so on.

TO LOSE...	Cut your daily calorie intake by	In three months you could lose...	In six months you could lose...	In one year you could lose...
½lb a week	250	6.5lb	13lb	1st 12lb
1lb a week	500	13lb	1st 12lb	3st 10lb
1½lb a week	750	1st 5.5lb	2st 11lb	5st 8lb
2lb a week	1,000	1st 12lb	3st 10lb	7st 6lb

TO LOSE...	Cut your daily calorie intake by	In three months you could lose...	In six months you could lose...	In one year you could lose...
¼kg a week	250	3.25kg	6.5kg	13kg
½kg a week	500	6.5kg	13kg	26kg
¾kg a week	750	9.75kg	19.5kg	39kg
1kg a week	1,000	13kg	26kg	52kg

4. Keep a food diary

Writing down what you eat and drink and any thoughts linked to that eating helps you become more aware of your eating habits. Recognising what is going on helps you feel in control and is a powerful way to start planning change. Keeping a food diary before you start to change your eating habits will also help you identify opportunities for cutting calories by substituting one food for another, cutting portion sizes of high-calorie foods or eating certain foods less often.

Simply write down every single item you eat or drink during the day and use this book to calculate the calories of each item. Then after a few days of eating normally, introduce some changes to your diet to achieve your daily calorie allowance. Remember to spread your daily calorie allowance fairly evenly throughout the day to prevent hunger. You'll find a template for a daily food and exercise diary on page 43.

Top Tip

If you only fill in your main food diary once a day, keep a pen and notepad with you to write down all those little extras you eat or drink during the day – that chocolate you ate in the office, the sliver of cheese you had while cooking dinner and the few chips you pinched from your husband's plate, for example!

It's easy to forget the little things if they're not written down, but they can make the difference between success and failure.

QUESTION: Why are heavier people allowed more calories than those who have smaller amounts of weight to lose?

ANSWER:

This confuses a lot of people but is easily explained. Someone who is 3 stone overweight, for example, is carrying the equivalent of 42 small packets of butter with them everywhere they go – up and down the stairs, to the local shops, into the kitchen. Obviously, it takes a lot more energy simply to move around when you're carrying that extra weight.

As a consequence, the heavier you are, the more calories you need just to keep your weight steady.

In turn, this means you'll lose weight on a higher calorie allowance. However, as you lose weight, you'll need to lower your calorie allowance slightly as you have less weight to carry around.

5. Control your portions

As well as making some smart food swaps to cut calories, it's likely you'll also need to reduce your serving sizes for some foods to help shift those pounds. Even 'healthy' foods such as brown rice, wholemeal bread, chicken, fish and low-fat dairy products contain calories so you may need to limit the amount you eat. When you first start out, weigh portions of foods like rice, pasta, cereal, cheese, butter, oil, meat, fish, and chicken rather than completing your food diary with a 'guesstimated' weight! That way you can calculate the calorie content accurately. Don't forget that drinks contain calories too, alcohol, milk, juices and sugary drinks all count.

6. Measure your success

Research has found that regular weight checks do help. Weighing yourself helps you assess how your eating and exercise habits affect your body weight. The important thing is to use the information in a positive way – to assess your progress - rather than as a stick to beat yourself up with. Remember that weight can fluctuate by a kilogram in a day, for example, due to fluid changes, premenstrually, after a big meal out, so weigh yourself at the same time of day and look at the trend over a week or two.

People who successfully lose weight and keep it off, also tend to continue weighing themselves at least once a week, and often daily (but not in an obsessive way), because they say it helps them stay 'on track'. Probably because they use it as an early warning system. People who weigh themselves regularly (or regularly try on a tight fitting item of clothing) will notice quickly if they have gained a few pounds - and can take action to stop gaining more. Checking your weight less often can mean that you might discover one day that you gained more than you thought. That can be pretty discouraging, and it might trigger you to just give up.

Top Tip

Don't just focus on what the bathroom scales say either – keep a record of your vital statistics, too. Many people find it doubly encouraging to see the inches dropping off, as well as the pounds!

7. Stay motivated

Each time you lose half a stone, or reach your own small goal – celebrate! Treat yourself to a little luxury – something new to wear, a little pampering or some other (non-food) treat. It also helps replace the comfort you once got from food and allows you to take care of yourself in other ways. Trying on an item of clothing that used to be tight can also help to keep you feeling motivated. Make sure you keep in touch with your supporters, and if the going gets tough take another look at the *'Coping with Common Slimming Saboteurs' section on page 21*. Once you've reviewed how well you've done, use this book to set yourself a new daily calorie allowance based on your new weight to help you lose the next half stone *(see point 3 - page 28 - Calculate your calorie allowance)*.

8. Keep it off

What you do to stay slim is just as important as what you did to get slim. Quite simply, if you return to your old ways, you are likely to return to your old weight. The great thing about calorie counting is that you will learn so much about what you eat, and make so many important changes to your eating and drinking habits, that you'll probably find it difficult to go back to your old ways – and won't want to anyway. It's still a good idea to weigh yourself at least once a week to keep a check on your weight. The key is to deal with any extra pounds immediately, rather than waiting until you have a stone to lose (see page 30). Simply go back to counting calories for as long as it takes to shift those pounds and enjoy the new slim you. Page 25 has more information about how successful slimmers keep it off.

QUESTION: Do I need to stick to exactly the same number of calories each day or is it OK to have a lower calorie intake during the week and slightly more at the weekend?

ANSWER:

The key to losing weight is to take in fewer calories than you need for as long as it takes to reach your target, aiming for a loss of no more than 2lb (1kg) a week. In general, most nutrition experts recommend a daily calorie allowance. However, it's just as valid to use other periods of time such as weeks.

If you prefer, simply multiply your daily allowance by seven to work out a weekly calorie allowance and then allocate more calories to some days than others. For example, a daily allowance of 1,500 calories is equivalent to 10,500 calories a week. This means you could have 1,300 calories a day during the week and 2,000 calories a day on Saturday and Sunday.

Healthy Eating Made Easy

Juliette Kellow BSc RD

HEALTHY EATING doesn't just mean eating salads and smoothies. Eating healthily means we're positively encouraged to eat a wide range of foods, including some of our favourites – it's just a question of making sure we don't eat high fat, high sugar or highly processed foods too often.

Eating a healthy diet, together with taking regular exercise and not smoking, has huge benefits to our health, both in the short and long term. As well as helping us to lose or maintain our weight, a healthy diet can boost energy levels, keep our immune system strong and give us healthy skin, nails and hair. Meanwhile, eating well throughout life also means we're far less likely to suffer from health problems such as constipation, anaemia and tooth decay, or set ourselves up for serious conditions in later life such as obesity, heart disease, stroke, diabetes, cancer or osteoporosis.

Fortunately, it couldn't be easier to eat a balanced diet. To start with, no single food provides all the calories and nutrients we need to stay healthy, so it's important to eat a variety of foods. Meanwhile, most nutrition experts also agree that mealtimes should be a pleasure rather than a penance. This means it's fine to eat small amounts of our favourite treats from time to time.

To help people eat healthily, the NHS recommends eating plenty of different foods from four main groups of foods and limiting the amount we eat from a smaller fifth group. Ultimately, we should eat more fruit, vegetables, starchy, fibre-rich foods and fresh products, and fewer fatty, sugary, salty and processed foods.

The following guidelines are all based on the healthy eating guidelines recommended by health professionals.

Bread, other cereals and potatoes

Eat these foods at each meal. They also make good snacks.

Foods in this group include bread, breakfast cereals, potatoes, rice, pasta, noodles, yams, oats and grains. Go for high-fibre varieties where available, such as wholegrain cereals, wholemeal bread and brown rice. These foods should fill roughly a third of your plate at mealtimes.

TYPICAL SERVING SIZES

* *2 slices bread in a sandwich or with a meal*

* *a tennis ball sized serving of pasta, potato, rice, noodles or couscous*

* *a bowl of porridge*

* *around 40g of breakfast cereal*

Fruit and vegetables

Eat at least five portions every day.

Foods in this group include all fruits and vegetables, including fresh, frozen, canned and dried products, and unsweetened fruit juice. Choose canned fruit in juice rather than syrup and go for veg canned in water without added salt or sugar.

TYPICAL PORTION SIZES

* *a piece of fruit eg: apple, banana, pear*

* *2 small fruits eg: satsumas, plums, apricots*

* *a bowl of fruit salad, canned or stewed fruit*

* *a small glass of unsweetened fruit juice*

* *a cereal bowl of salad*

* *3tbsp vegetables*

Milk, dairy and alternatives

Eat two or three servings a day.

Foods in this group include milk, cheese, yoghurt and fromage frais. Choose low-fat varieties where available such as skimmed milk, reduced-fat cheese and fat-free yoghurt.

TYPICAL SERVING SIZES

• *200ml milk*

• *a small pot of yoghurt or fromage frais*

• *a small matchbox-sized piece of cheese*

Meat, fish and alternatives

Eat two servings a day

Foods in this group include meat, poultry, fish, eggs, beans, nuts and seeds. Choose low-fat varieties where available such as extra-lean minced beef and skinless chicken and don't add extra fat or salt.

TYPICAL SERVING SIZES

• *a piece of meat, chicken or fish the size of a deck of cards*

• *1-2 eggs*

• *3 heaped tablespoons of beans*

• *a small handful of nuts or seeds*

Healthy Eating on a plate

A simple way to serve up both balance and healthy proportions is to fill one half of your plate with salad or vegetables and divide the other half between protein-rich meat, chicken, fish, eggs or beans, and healthy carbs (potatoes, rice, pasta, pulses, bread or noodles).

Fatty and sugary foods

Eat only small amounts of these foods

Foods in this group include oils, spreading fats, cream, mayonnaise, oily salad dressings, cakes, biscuits, puddings, crisps, savoury snacks, sugar, preserves, confectionery and sugary soft drinks.

TYPICAL SERVING SIZES:

* *a small packet of sweets or a small bar of chocolate*

* *a small slice of cake*

* *a couple of small biscuits*

* *1 level tbsp mayo, salad dressing or olive oil*

* *a small packet of crisps*

Useful Tools

Body Mass Index

The Body Mass Index (BMI) is the internationally accepted way of assessing how healthy our weight is for most people. It is calculated using height and weight. Use the BMI Chart to look up your BMI, and use this table to see which range you fall into.

BMI *Under 18.5*	*Underweight*
BMI *18.5-25*	*Healthy*
BMI *25-30*	*Overweight*
BMI *30-40*	*Obese*
BMI *Over 40*	*Severely Obese*

This is what different BMI ranges mean.

- **Underweight:** you probably need to gain weight for your health's sake. Talk to your doctor if you have any concerns, or if you feel frightened about gaining weight.

- **Healthy weight:** you are a healthy weight, so aim to stay in this range (note that most people in this range tend to have a BMI between 20-25).

- **Overweight:** aim to lose some weight for your health's sake, or at least prevent further weight gain.

- **Obese:** your health is at risk and losing weight will benefit your health.

- **Severely obese:** your health is definitely at risk. You should visit your doctor for a health check. Losing weight will improve your health.

Please note that BMI is not as accurate for athletes or very muscular people (muscle weighs more than fat), as it can push them into a higher BMI category despite having a healthy level of body fat. It is also not accurate for women who are pregnant or breastfeeding, or people who are frail.

Body Mass Index Table

HEIGHT IN FEET / INCHES

WEIGHT IN STONES / LBS	4'6	4'8	4'10	5'0	5'2	5'4	5'6	5'8	5'10	6'0	6'2	6'4	6'6	6'8	6'10
6st 7	22.0	20.5	19.1	17.8	16.7	15.7	14.7	13.9	13.1	12.4	11.7	11.1	10.6	10.0	9.5
7st 0	23.7	22.1	20.6	19.2	18.0	16.9	15.9	15.0	14.1	13.3	12.6	12.0	11.4	10.8	10.3
7st 7	25.4	23.6	22.0	20.6	19.3	18.1	17.0	16.0	15.1	14.3	13.5	12.8	12.2	11.6	11.0
8st 0	27.1	25.2	23.5	22.0	20.6	19.3	18.1	17.1	16.1	15.2	14.4	13.7	13.0	12.3	11.8
8st 7	28.8	26.8	25.0	23.3	21.8	20.5	19.3	18.2	17.1	16.2	15.3	14.5	13.8	13.1	12.5
9st 0	30.5	28.4	26.4	24.7	23.1	21.7	20.4	19.2	18.1	17.2	16.2	15.4	14.6	13.9	13.2
9st 7	32.2	29.9	27.9	26.1	24.4	22.9	21.5	20.3	19.2	18.1	17.1	16.2	15.4	14.7	14.0
10st 0	33.9	31.5	29.4	27.4	25.7	24.1	22.7	21.4	20.2	19.1	18.0	17.1	16.2	15.4	14.7
10st 7	35.6	33.1	30.8	28.8	27.0	25.3	23.8	22.4	21.2	20.0	18.9	18.0	17.0	16.2	15.4
11st 0	37.3	34.7	32.3	30.2	28.3	26.5	24.9	23.5	22.2	21.0	19.8	18.8	17.9	17.0	16.2
11st 7	39.0	36.2	33.8	31.6	29.6	27.7	26.1	24.6	23.2	21.9	20.7	19.7	18.7	17.8	16.9
12st 0	40.7	37.8	35.2	32.9	30.8	28.9	27.2	25.6	24.2	22.9	21.6	20.5	19.5	18.5	17.6
12st 7	42.3	39.4	36.7	34.3	32.1	30.1	28.3	26.7	25.2	23.8	22.5	21.4	20.3	19.3	18.4
13st 0	44.0	41.0	38.2	35.7	33.4	31.4	29.5	27.8	26.2	24.8	23.5	22.2	21.1	20.1	19.1
13st 7	45.7	42.5	39.6	37.0	34.7	32.6	30.6	28.8	27.2	25.7	24.4	23.1	21.9	20.8	19.8
14st 0	47.4	44.1	41.1	38.4	36.0	33.8	31.7	29.9	28.2	26.7	25.3	23.9	22.7	21.6	20.6
14st 7	49.1	45.7	42.6	39.8	37.3	35.0	32.9	31.0	29.2	27.6	26.2	24.8	23.5	22.4	21.3
15st 0	50.8	47.3	44.0	41.2	38.5	36.2	34.0	32.0	30.2	28.6	27.1	25.7	24.4	23.2	22.0
15st 7	52.5	48.8	45.5	42.5	39.8	37.4	35.2	33.1	31.2	29.5	28.0	26.5	25.2	23.9	22.8
16st 0	54.2	50.4	47.0	43.9	41.1	38.6	36.3	34.2	32.3	30.5	28.9	27.4	26.0	24.7	23.5
16st 7	55.9	52.0	48.5	45.3	42.4	39.8	37.4	35.2	33.3	31.4	29.8	28.2	26.8	25.5	24.2
17st 0	57.6	53.6	49.9	46.6	43.7	41.0	38.6	36.3	34.3	32.4	30.7	29.1	27.6	26.2	25.0
17st 7	59.3	55.1	51.4	48.0	45.0	42.2	39.7	37.4	35.3	33.3	31.6	29.9	28.4	27.0	25.7
18st 0	61.0	56.7	52.9	49.4	46.3	43.4	40.8	38.5	36.3	34.3	32.5	30.8	29.2	27.8	26.4
18st 7	62.7	58.3	54.3	50.8	47.5	44.6	42.0	39.5	37.3	35.3	33.4	31.6	30.0	28.6	27.2
19st 0	64.4	59.9	55.8	52.1	48.8	45.8	43.1	40.6	38.3	36.2	34.3	32.5	30.8	29.3	27.9
19st 7	66.1	61.4	57.3	53.5	50.1	47.0	44.2	41.7	39.3	37.2	35.2	33.3	31.7	30.1	28.6
20st 0	67.8	63.0	58.7	54.9	51.4	48.2	45.4	42.7	40.3	38.1	36.1	34.2	32.5	30.9	29.4
20st 7	69.4	64.6	60.2	56.3	52.7	49.4	46.5	43.8	41.3	39.1	37.0	35.1	33.3	31.6	30.1
21st 0	71.1	66.2	61.7	57.6	54.0	50.6	47.6	44.9	42.3	40.0	37.9	35.9	34.1	32.4	30.9
21st 7	72.8	67.7	63.1	59.0	55.3	51.9	48.8	45.9	43.3	41.0	38.8	36.8	34.9	33.2	31.6
22st 0	74.5	69.3	64.6	60.4	56.5	53.1	49.9	47.0	44.4	41.9	39.7	37.6	35.7	34.0	32.3
22st 7	76.2	70.9	66.1	61.7	57.8	54.3	51.0	48.1	45.4	42.9	40.6	38.5	36.5	34.7	33.1
23st 0	77.9	72.5	67.5	63.1	59.1	55.5	52.2	49.1	46.4	43.8	41.5	39.3	37.3	35.5	33.8
23st 7	79.6	74.0	69.0	64.5	60.4	56.7	53.3	50.2	47.4	44.8	42.4	40.2	38.2	36.3	34.5
24st 0	81.3	75.6	70.5	65.9	61.7	57.9	54.4	51.3	48.4	45.7	43.3	41.0	39.0	37.0	35.3
24st 7	83.0	77.2	71.9	67.2	63.0	59.1	55.6	52.3	49.4	46.7	44.2	41.9	39.8	37.8	36.0
25st 0	84.7	78.8	73.4	68.6	64.2	60.3	56.7	53.4	50.4	47.6	45.1	42.8	40.6	38.6	36.7
25st 7	86.4	80.3	74.9	70.0	65.5	61.5	57.8	54.5	51.4	48.6	46.0	43.6	41.4	39.4	37.5
26st 0	88.1	81.9	76.3	71.3	66.8	62.7	59.0	55.5	52.4	49.5	46.9	44.5	42.2	40.1	38.2
26st 7	89.8	83.5	77.8	72.7	68.1	63.9	60.1	56.6	53.4	50.5	47.8	45.3	43.0	40.9	38.9
27st 0	91.5	85.1	79.3	74.1	69.4	65.1	61.2	57.7	54.4	51.5	48.7	46.2	43.8	41.7	39.7
27st 7	93.2	86.6	80.8	75.5	70.7	66.3	62.4	58.7	55.4	52.4	49.6	47.0	44.7	42.4	40.4
28st 0	94.9	88.2	82.2	76.8	72.0	67.5	63.5	59.8	56.4	53.4	50.5	47.9	45.5	43.2	41.1
28st 7	96.5	89.8	83.7	78.2	73.2	68.7	64.6	60.9	57.5	54.3	51.4	48.7	46.3	44.0	41.9
29st 0	98.2	91.4	85.2	79.6	74.5	69.9	65.8	62.0	58.5	55.3	52.3	49.6	47.1	44.8	42.6
29st 7	99.9	92.9	86.6	80.9	75.8	71.1	66.9	63.0	59.5	56.2	53.2	50.5	47.9	45.5	43.3

Weight Chart

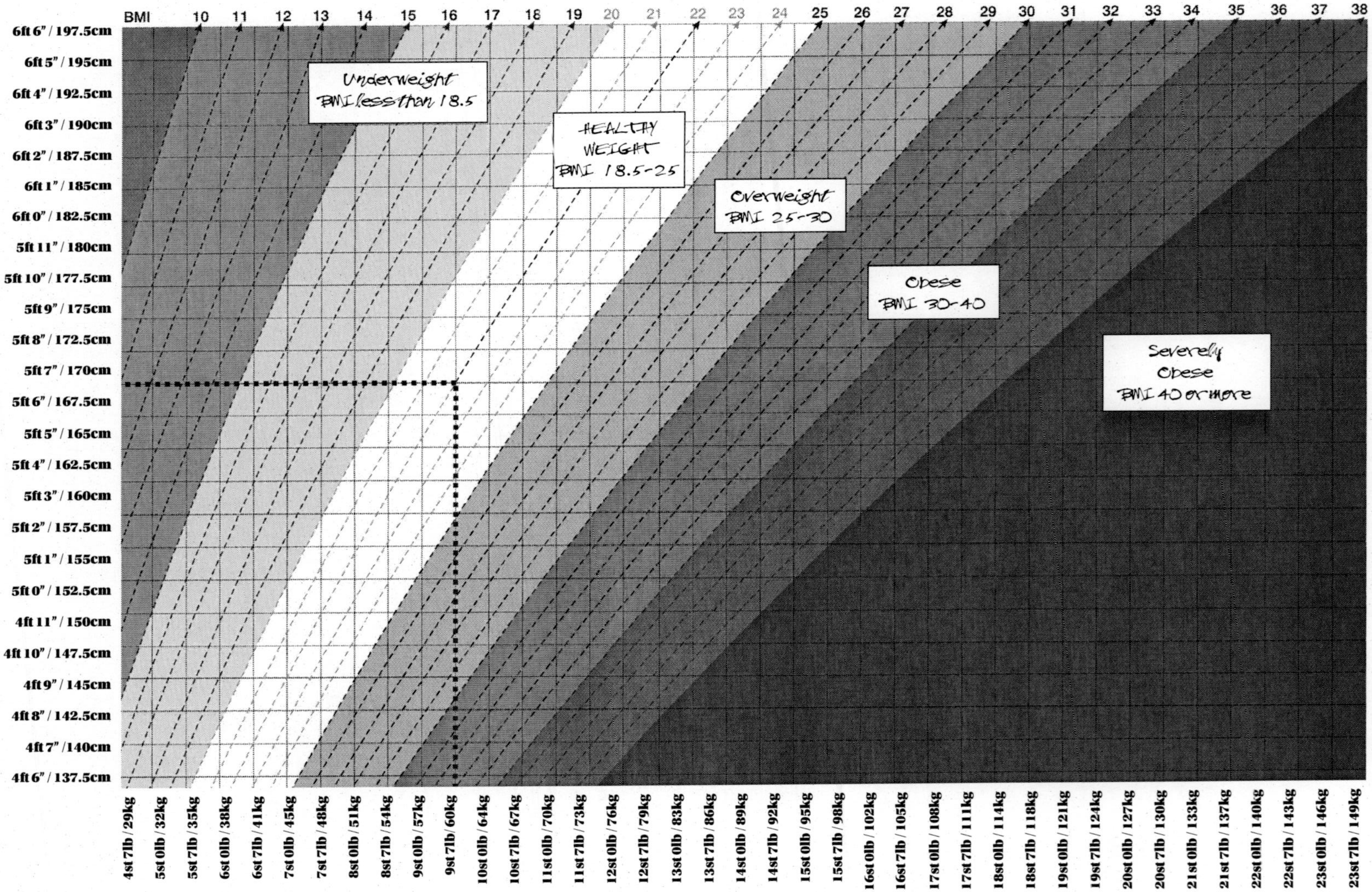

BMI scale (top): BMI, 10, 11, 12, 13, 14, 15, 16, 17, 18, 19, 20, 21, 22, 23, 24, 25, 26, 27, 28, 29, 30, 31, 32, 33, 34, 35, 36, 37, 38

Category labels:
- Underweight *BMI less than 18.5*
- HEALTHY WEIGHT *BMI 18.5-25*
- Overweight *BMI 25-30*
- Obese *BMI 30-40*
- Severely Obese *BMI 40 or more*

Height axis (left):
6ft 6"/197.5cm, 6ft 5"/195cm, 6ft 4"/192.5cm, 6ft 3"/190cm, 6ft 2"/187.5cm, 6ft 1"/185cm, 6ft 0"/182.5cm, 5ft 11"/180cm, 5ft 10"/177.5cm, 5ft 9"/175cm, 5ft 8"/172.5cm, 5ft 7"/170cm, 5ft 6"/167.5cm, 5ft 5"/165cm, 5ft 4"/162.5cm, 5ft 3"/160cm, 5ft 2"/157.5cm, 5ft 1"/155cm, 5ft 0"/152.5cm, 4ft 11"/150cm, 4ft 10"/147.5cm, 4ft 9"/145cm, 4ft 8"/142.5cm, 4ft 7"/140cm, 4ft 6"/137.5cm

Weight axis (bottom):
4st 7lb/29kg, 5st 0lb/32kg, 5st 7lb/35kg, 6st 0lb/38kg, 6st 7lb/41kg, 7st 0lb/45kg, 7st 7lb/48kg, 8st 0lb/51kg, 8st 7lb/54kg, 9st 0lb/57kg, 9st 7lb/60kg, 10st 0lb/64kg, 10st 7lb/67kg, 11st 0lb/70kg, 11st 7lb/73kg, 12st 0lb/76kg, 12st 7lb/79kg, 13st 0lb/83kg, 13st 7lb/86kg, 14st 0lb/89kg, 14st 7lb/92kg, 15st 0lb/95kg, 15st 7lb/98kg, 16st 0lb/102kg, 16st 7lb/105kg, 17st 0lb/108kg, 17st 7lb/111kg, 18st 0lb/114kg, 18st 7lb/118kg, 19st 0lb/121kg, 19st 7lb/124kg, 20st 0lb/127kg, 20st 7lb/130kg, 21st 0lb/133kg, 21st 7lb/137kg, 22st 0lb/140kg, 22st 7lb/143kg, 23st 0lb/146kg, 23st 7lb/149kg

Calories Required to Maintain Weight
Adult Females

ACTIVITY LEVEL / AGE

WEIGHT IN STONES / LBS	VERY SEDENTARY			MODERATELY SEDENTARY			MODERATELY ACTIVE			VERY ACTIVE		
	<30	30-60	60+	<30	30-60	60+	<30	30-60	60+	<30	30-60	60+
7st 7	1425	1473	1304	1544	1596	1412	1781	1841	1630	2138	2210	1956
8st 0	1481	1504	1338	1605	1629	1450	1852	1880	1673	2222	2256	2008
8st 7	1537	1535	1373	1666	1663	1487	1922	1919	1716	2306	2302	2059
9st 0	1594	1566	1407	1726	1696	1524	1992	1957	1759	2391	2349	2111
9st 7	1650	1596	1442	1787	1729	1562	2062	1996	1802	2475	2395	2163
10st 0	1706	1627	1476	1848	1763	1599	2133	2034	1845	2559	2441	2214
10st 7	1762	1658	1511	1909	1796	1637	2203	2073	1888	2644	2487	2266
11st 0	1819	1689	1545	1970	1830	1674	2273	2111	1931	2728	2534	2318
11st 7	1875	1720	1580	2031	1863	1711	2344	2150	1975	2813	2580	2370
12st 0	1931	1751	1614	2092	1897	1749	2414	2188	2018	2897	2626	2421
12st 7	1987	1781	1648	2153	1930	1786	2484	2227	2061	2981	2672	2473
13st 0	2044	1812	1683	2214	1963	1823	2555	2266	2104	3066	2719	2525
13st 7	2100	1843	1717	2275	1997	1861	2625	2304	2147	3150	2765	2576
14st 0	2156	1874	1752	2336	2030	1898	2695	2343	2190	3234	2811	2628
14st 7	2212	1905	1786	2397	2064	1935	2766	2381	2233	3319	2858	2680
15st 0	2269	1936	1821	2458	2097	1973	2836	2420	2276	3403	2904	2732
15st 7	2325	1967	1855	2519	2130	2010	2906	2458	2319	3488	2950	2783
16st 0	2381	1997	1890	2580	2164	2047	2976	2497	2362	3572	2996	2835
16st 7	2437	2028	1924	2640	2197	2085	3047	2535	2405	3656	3043	2887
17st 0	2494	2059	1959	2701	2231	2122	3117	2574	2449	3741	3089	2938
17st 7	2550	2090	1993	2762	2264	2159	3187	2613	2492	3825	3135	2990
18st 0	2606	2121	2028	2823	2298	2197	3258	2651	2535	3909	3181	3042
18st 7	2662	2152	2062	2884	2331	2234	3328	2690	2578	3994	3228	3093
19st 0	2719	2182	2097	2945	2364	2271	3398	2728	2621	4078	3274	3145
19st 7	2775	2213	2131	3006	2398	2309	3469	2767	2664	4162	3320	3197
20st 0	2831	2244	2166	3067	2431	2346	3539	2805	2707	4247	3366	3249
20st 7	2887	2275	2200	3128	2465	2383	3609	2844	2750	4331	3413	3300
21st 0	2944	2306	2235	3189	2498	2421	3680	2882	2793	4416	3459	3352
21st 7	3000	2337	2269	3250	2531	2458	3750	2921	2836	4500	3505	3404
22st 0	3056	2368	2303	3311	2565	2495	3820	2960	2879	4584	3552	3455
22st 7	3112	2398	2338	3372	2598	2533	3890	2998	2923	4669	3598	3507
23st 0	3169	2429	2372	3433	2632	2570	3961	3037	2966	4753	3644	3559
23st 7	3225	2460	2407	3494	2665	2608	4031	3075	3009	4837	3690	3611
24st 0	3281	2491	2441	3554	2699	2645	4101	3114	3052	4922	3737	3662
24st 7	3337	2522	2476	3615	2732	2682	4172	3152	3095	5006	3783	3714
25st 0	3394	2553	2510	3676	2765	2720	4242	3191	3138	5091	3829	3766
25st 7	3450	2583	2545	3737	2799	2757	4312	3229	3181	5175	3875	3817
26st 0	3506	2614	2579	3798	2832	2794	4383	3268	3224	5259	3922	3869
26st 7	3562	2645	2614	3859	2866	2832	4453	3307	3267	5344	3968	3921
27st 0	3618	2676	2648	3920	2899	2869	4523	3345	3310	5428	4014	3973
27st 7	3675	2707	2683	3981	2932	2906	4594	3384	3353	5512	4060	4024
28st 0	3731	2738	2717	4042	2966	2944	4664	3422	3397	5597	4107	4076
28st 7	3787	2768	2752	4103	2999	2981	4734	3461	3440	5681	4153	4128

Calories Required to Maintain Weight
Adult Males

ACTIVITY LEVEL / AGE

WEIGHT IN STONES / LBS	VERY SEDENTARY			MODERATELY SEDENTARY			MODERATELY ACTIVE			VERY ACTIVE		
	<30	30-60	60+	<30	30-60	60+	<30	30-60	60+	<30	30-60	60+
9st 0	1856	1827	1502	2010	1979	1627	2320	2284	1878	2784	2741	2254
9st 7	1913	1871	1547	2072	2026	1676	2391	2338	1933	2870	2806	2320
10st 0	1970	1914	1591	2134	2074	1724	2463	2393	1989	2955	2871	2387
10st 7	2027	1958	1636	2196	2121	1772	2534	2447	2045	3041	2937	2454
11st 0	2084	2001	1680	2258	2168	1820	2605	2502	2100	3127	3002	2520
11st 7	2141	2045	1724	2320	2215	1868	2677	2556	2156	3212	3067	2587
12st 0	2199	2088	1769	2382	2262	1916	2748	2611	2211	3298	3133	2654
12st 7	2256	2132	1813	2444	2310	1965	2820	2665	2267	3384	3198	2720
13st 0	2313	2175	1858	2506	2357	2013	2891	2719	2322	3470	3263	2787
13st 7	2370	2219	1902	2568	2404	2061	2963	2774	2378	3555	3329	2854
14st 0	2427	2262	1947	2630	2451	2109	3034	2828	2434	3641	3394	2920
14st 7	2484	2306	1991	2691	2498	2157	3106	2883	2489	3727	3459	2987
15st 0	2542	2350	2036	2753	2545	2205	3177	2937	2545	3813	3525	3054
15st 7	2599	2393	2080	2815	2593	2253	3248	2992	2600	3898	3590	3120
16st 0	2656	2437	2125	2877	2640	2302	3320	3046	2656	3984	3655	3187
16st 7	2713	2480	2169	2939	2687	2350	3391	3100	2711	4070	3721	3254
17st 0	2770	2524	2213	3001	2734	2398	3463	3155	2767	4155	3786	3320
17st 7	2827	2567	2258	3063	2781	2446	3534	3209	2823	4241	3851	3387
18st 0	2884	2611	2302	3125	2828	2494	3606	3264	2878	4327	3917	3454
18st 7	2942	2654	2347	3187	2876	2542	3677	3318	2934	4413	3982	3520
19st 0	2999	2698	2391	3249	2923	2591	3749	3373	2989	4498	4047	3587
19st 7	3056	2741	2436	3311	2970	2639	3820	3427	3045	4584	4112	3654
20st 0	3113	2785	2480	3373	3017	2687	3891	3481	3100	4670	4178	3721
20st 7	3170	2829	2525	3434	3064	2735	3963	3536	3156	4756	4243	3787
21st 0	3227	2872	2569	3496	3112	2783	4034	3590	3211	4841	4308	3854
21st 7	3285	2916	2614	3558	3159	2831	4106	3645	3267	4927	4374	3921
22st 0	3342	2959	2658	3620	3206	2880	4177	3699	3323	5013	4439	3987
22st 7	3399	3003	2702	3682	3253	2928	4249	3754	3378	5098	4504	4054
23st 0	3456	3046	2747	3744	3300	2976	4320	3808	3434	5184	4570	4121
23st 7	3513	3090	2791	3806	3347	3024	4392	3862	3489	5270	4635	4187
24st 0	3570	3133	2836	3868	3395	3072	4463	3917	3545	5356	4700	4254
24st 7	3627	3177	2880	3930	3442	3120	4534	3971	3600	5441	4766	4321
25st 0	3685	3220	2925	3992	3489	3168	4606	4026	3656	5527	4831	4387
25st 7	3742	3264	2969	4054	3536	3217	4677	4080	3712	5613	4896	4454
26st 0	3799	3308	3014	4116	3583	3265	4749	4135	3767	5699	4962	4521
26st 7	3856	3351	3058	4177	3630	3313	4820	4189	3823	5784	5027	4587
27st 0	3913	3395	3103	4239	3678	3361	4892	4243	3878	5870	5092	4654
27st 7	3970	3438	3147	4301	3725	3409	4963	4298	3934	5956	5158	4721
28st 0	4028	3482	3191	4363	3772	3457	5035	4352	3989	6042	5223	4787
28st 7	4085	3525	3236	4425	3819	3506	5106	4407	4045	6127	5288	4854
29st 0	4142	3569	3280	4487	3866	3554	5177	4461	4101	6213	5354	4921
29st 7	4199	3612	3325	4549	3913	3602	5249	4516	4156	6299	5419	4987
30st 0	4256	3656	3369	4611	3961	3650	5320	4570	4212	6384	5484	5054

Calories Burned in Exercise

This table shows the approximate number of extra* calories that would be burned in a five minute period of exercise activity.

ACTIVITY	CALORIES BURNED IN 5 MINUTES	ACTIVITY	CALORIES BURNED IN 5 MINUTES
Aerobics, Low Impact	25	Situps, Continuous	17
Badminton, Recreational	17	Skiing, Moderate	30
Cross Trainer	30	Skipping, Moderate	30
Cycling, Recreational, 5mph	17	Squash Playing	39
Dancing, Modern, Moderate	13	Tennis Playing, Recreational	26
Fencing	24	Toning Exercises	17
Gardening, Weeding	19	Trampolining	17
Hill Walking, Up and Down, Recreational	22	Volleyball, Recreational	10
Jogging	30	Walking, Uphill, 15% Gradient, Moderate	43
Kick Boxing	30	Walking Up and Down Stairs, Moderate	34
Netball Playing	23	Walking, 4mph	24
Rebounding	18	Weight Training, Moderate	12
Roller Skating	30	Yoga	13
Rowing Machine, Moderate	30		
Running, 7.5mph	48		

*Extra calories are those in addition to your normal daily calorie needs.

My Personal Plan

Date: _____

Body Mass Index: _____

Weight: _____

Waist Measurement: _____

Height: _____

Body Fat % (if known) _____

10% Weight Loss Goal:

Current weight	16stone (224lb)	100kg
- 10% weight	1stone 8½lb (22½lb)	10kg
= 10% loss goal	14stone 5½lb (201½lb)	90kg

My smaller weight targets on the way to achieving my 10% goal will be:

_____ _____ _____ _____

Reasons why I want to lose weight:

_____

Changes I will make to help me lose weight:
Diet:

_____

_____

Activity:

_____

_____

Potential saboteurs or barriers will be:

_____

_____

Ways I will overcome these:

_____

_____

My supporters will be:

_____

I will monitor my progress by:

_____   _____

I will reward my progress with:
In the short term:

_____

_____

In the long term:

_____

_____

Food and Exercise Diary

Date:

[/ /]

Daily Calorie Allowance: [ ] **Ⓐ**

Food/Drink Consumed	Serving Size	Calories
_____	_____	_____
_____	_____	_____
_____	_____	_____
_____	_____	_____
_____	_____	_____
_____	_____	_____
_____	_____	_____
_____	_____	_____
_____	_____	_____
_____	_____	_____
_____	_____	_____
_____	_____	_____
_____	_____	_____
_____	_____	_____
_____	_____	_____
_____	_____	_____

You are aiming for your Calorie Balance (Box D) to be as close to zero as possible - ie. you consume the number of calories you need.

Your Daily Calorie Allowance (Box A) should be set to lose ½-2lb (¼-1kg) a week, or maintain weight, depending on your goals.

Total calories consumed [ ] **Ⓑ**

Daily Calorie Allowance (A) <u>plus</u> Extra Calories used in Exercise (C) <u>minus</u> Total Calories Consumed (B) <u>equals</u> Calorie Balance (D)

$$A + C - B = D$$

Exercise/Activity	No. mins	Calories
_____	_____	_____
_____	_____	_____
_____	_____	_____
_____	_____	_____

Calories used in exercise [ ] **Ⓒ**

Calorie balance [ ] **Ⓓ**

You can also write down any comments or thoughts related to your eating if you want to.

Food Information

Nutritional Information

CALORIE AND FAT values are given per serving, plus calorie and nutrition values per 100g of product. This makes it easy to compare the proportions of fat, protein, carbohydrate and fibre in each food.

The values given are for uncooked, unprepared foods unless otherwise stated. Values are also for only the edible portion of the food unless otherwise stated. ie - weighed with bone.

Finding Foods

The Calorie, Carb & Fat Bible has an Eating Out section which is arranged alphabetically by brand. In the General Foods and Drinks A-Z most foods are grouped together by type, and then put in to alphabetical order. This makes it easy to compare different brands, and will help you to find lower calorie and/or fat alternatives where they are available.

This format also makes it easier to locate foods. Foods are categorised by their main characteristics so, for example, if it is bread, ciabatta or white sliced, you'll find it under "Bread".

Basic ingredients are highlighted to make them easier to find at a glance. You'll find all unbranded foods in bold - making the index easier to use, whether it's just an apple or all the components of a home cooked stew.

There are, however, some foods which are not so easy to categorise, especially combination foods like ready meals. The following pointers will help you to find your way around the book until you get to know it a little better.

FILLED ROLLS AND SANDWICHES - Bagels, baguettes, etc which are filled are listed as "Bagels (filled)" etc. Sandwiches are under "Sandwiches".

CURRIES - Popular types of curry, like Balti or Jalfrezi, are listed under their individual types. Unspecified or lesser known types are listed under their main ingredient.

BURGERS - All burgers from fast-food outlets are listed under "Burgers".

CHIPS & FRIES - Are listed separately, depending on the name of the particular brand. All other types of potato are listed under "Potatoes".

SWEETS & CHOCOLATES - Well-known brands, eg. Aero, Mars Bar, are listed under their brand names. Others are listed under "Chocolate" (for bars) and "Chocolates" (for individual sweets).

READY MEALS - Popular types of dishes are listed under their type, eg. "Chow Mein", "Casserole", "Hot Pot", etc. Others are listed by their main ingredient, eg. "Chicken With", "Chicken In", etc.

EATING OUT & FAST FOODS - By popular demand this edition has the major eating out and fast food brands listed separately, at the back of the book. They are alphabetised first by brand, then follow using the same format as the rest of the book, with calories provided per serving.

Serving Sizes

Many ready-meal type foods are given with calories for the full pack size, so that an individual serving can be worked out by estimating the proportion of the pack that has been consumed. For example, if you have eaten a quarter of a packaged pasta dish, divide the calorie value given for the whole pack by 4 to determine the number of calories you have consumed.

Where serving sizes are not appropriate, or unknown, values are given per 100g and per 1oz/28g. Serving sizes vary greatly from person to person and, if you are trying to lose weight, it's important to be accurate – especially with high calorie foods such as those that contain a fair amount of fat, sugar, cream, cheese, alcohol etc.

Food Data

Nutrition information for basic average foods has been compiled by the Weight Loss Resources food data team using many sources of information to calculate the most accurate values possible. Some nutrition information for non-branded food records is from The Composition of Foods 6th Edition. Reproduced under licence from The Controller of Her Majesty's Stationary Office. Where basic data is present for ordinary foodstuffs such as 'raw carrots'; branded records are not included.

Nutrition information for branded goods is from details supplied by retailers and manufacturers, and researched by Weight Loss Resources staff. The Calorie Carb & Fat Bible contains data for over 1400 UK brands, including major supermarkets and fast food outlets.

The publishers gratefully acknowledge all the manufacturers and retailers who have provided information on their products. All product names, trademarks or registered trademarks belong to their respective owners and are used only for the purpose of identifying products.

Calorie & nutrition data for all food and drink items are typical values.

Caution
The information in The Calorie, Carb and Fat Bible is intended as an aid to weight loss and weight maintenance, and is not medical advice. If you suffer from, or think you may suffer from a medical condition you should consult your doctor before starting a weight loss and/or exercise regime. If you start exercising after a period of relative inactivity, you should start slowly and consult your doctor if you experience pain, distress or other symptoms.

Weights, Measures & Abbreviations

ABBREVIATIONS

kcal	kilocalories / calories
prot	protein
carb	carbohydrate
sm	small
med	medium
av	average
reg	regular
lge	large
tsp	teaspoon
tbsp	tablespoon
dtsp	dessertspoon
gf	gluten free

BRAND ABBREVIATIONS USED

ASDA

Good for You	GFY
Chosen by You	CBY
Good & Counted	G&C

MARKS & SPENCER — M&S

Count on Us	COU
Balanced For You	BFY

MORRISONS

Better For You	BFY

SAINSBURY'S

Be Good to Yourself	BGTY
Way to Five	WTF
Taste the Difference	TTD

TESCO

Healthy Eating	HE
Healthy Living	HL
Hearty Food Co	HFC
Light Choices	LC

WAITROSE

Perfectly Balanced	PB
Cambridge Weight Plan	CWP

	Measure			Nutrition Values per 100g / 100ml				
	INFO/WEIGHT	KCAL	FAT	KCAL	PROT	CARB	FAT	FIBRE
ABSINTHE								
Average	**1 Pub Shot/35ml**	**127**	**0**	**363**	**0**	**38.8**	**0**	**0**
ACKEE								
Canned, Drained, Average	**1oz/28g**	**43**	**4.3**	**151**	**2.9**	**0.8**	**15.2**	**0**
ADVOCAAT								
Average	**1 Pub Shot/35ml**	**91**	**2.2**	**260**	**4.7**	**28.4**	**6.3**	**0**
AERO								
Bliss, Salted Caramel, Aero, Nestle*	1 Piece/8g	43	2.4	537	7.4	58	30.2	1.4
Creamy White Centre, Nestle*	1 Bar/46g	244	13.8	530	7.6	57.4	30	0
Milk, Medium, Bar, Nestle*	1 Bar/43g	232	13.3	539	6.6	57.7	30.9	2.2
Milk, Purely Chocolate, Aero*	1 Bar/37g	197	11.2	538	6.8	57.8	30.5	1.9
Milk, Snacksize, Bar, Nestle*	1 Bar/21g	110	6.5	537	6.6	55.9	31.9	2.2
Mint, Bubbles, Aero, Nestle*	1 Bubble/3g	16	0.9	533	4.4	62.7	29.1	0.8
Mint, Nestle*	1 Bar/41g	218	11.9	531	5.4	61.6	28.9	1.1
Mint, Standard, Aero, Nestle*	1 Bar/43g	233	13.2	542	5.2	60.5	30.8	0.9
Orange, Bubbles, Aero, Nestle*	1 Bubble/3g	16	0.9	538	5.4	60.5	30	1.4
Peppermint, Bar, Nestle*	1 Bar/37g	199	11.1	537	5.1	61	30	1
ALFALFA SPROUTS								
Raw, Average	**1 Serving/33g**	**8**	**0.3**	**24**	**3**	**3**	**0.9**	**3**
ALLSPICE								
Ground, Schwartz*	1 Tsp/3g	11	0.1	358	6.1	74.3	4	0
ALMONDS								
Blanched, Average	**1 Serving/100g**	**617**	**54.3**	**617**	**25.1**	**6.9**	**54.3**	**8.1**
Candied, Sugared	**1 Serving/100g**	**458**	**16.3**	**458**	**8.4**	**69.2**	**16.3**	**2.2**
Chocolate Covered, Milk, 40%, Hotel Chocolat*	1 Serving/26g	145	9.4	557	10.7	46.3	36.3	4.7
Flaked, Average	**1oz/28g**	**172**	**15.2**	**613**	**24.9**	**6.5**	**54.3**	**7.6**
Flaked, Toasted, Average	**1oz/28g**	**176**	**15.8**	**629**	**24.6**	**5.8**	**56.4**	**7.5**
Ground, Average	**1 Serving/10g**	**62**	**5.6**	**625**	**24**	**6.6**	**55.8**	**7.4**
Hickory, Smokey, Co-Op*	1 Pack/40g	254	22	634	24	7.7	55	6.2
Marcona, Average	**1 Serving/100g**	**608**	**53.7**	**608**	**22.1**	**13**	**53.7**	**9.7**
Roasted, Salted, Tesco*	1 Serving/25g	158	13.6	631	25.3	5	54.5	9.7
Salted, Chocolate Dipped, Deliciously Ella*	1 Pack/30g	176	14.2	585	14	28.4	47.2	12.1
Toasted, Average	**1oz/28g**	**178**	**15.8**	**634**	**25**	**6.6**	**56.4**	**6.6**
Whole, Average	**1 Serving/20g**	**122**	**11**	**612**	**23.4**	**6.9**	**54.8**	**8.4**
Yoghurt Coated, Holland & Barrett*	1 Pack/100g	536	37	536	10.9	45.3	37	2.8
ALOO								
Bombay, M&S*	1 Serving/100g	81	2.7	81	1.4	11.8	2.7	2
Bombay, Takeaway for One, M&S*	1 Pack/151g	110	2.6	73	1.5	12.3	1.7	1.1
Saag, Gobi, Side, Asda*	½ Pack/148g	114	5.3	77	2.4	7.6	3.6	2.4
Saag, Gobi, Takeaway, Microwaved, Morrisons*	½ Pack/105g	88	3.6	84	2	9.5	3.4	3.9
Saag, Gobi, Waitrose*	½ Pack/150g	129	8.2	86	2	6	5.5	2.4
Saag, Indian, Serves 2, Sainsbury's*	1 Pack/300g	216	10.5	72	2	7	3.5	2.2
Tikki, Average	**1 Serving/25g**	**48**	**2**	**191**	**4.5**	**25.2**	**8**	**3.5**
AMARANTH								
Seed, Holland & Barrett*	1 Tbsp/15g	56	1	371	14	55	7	6.5
ANCHOVIES								
in Oil, Canned, Drained	**1 Anchovy/4g**	**8**	**0.5**	**195**	**23.4**	**0**	**11.3**	**0**
Marinated, with Peppers, & Kalamata Olives, Tesco*	½ Pack/35g	84	6.7	239	15.1	1	19.2	0.8
ANGEL DELIGHT								
Chocolate Flavour, Kraft*	1 Sachet/67g	305	12.1	455	3.7	69.5	18	0.4
Strawberry Flavour, Kraft*	1 Sachet/59g	286	12.4	485	2.5	71	21	0
Vanilla Ice Cream Flavour, Kraft*	1 Sachet/59g	289	12.7	490	2.5	71.5	21.5	0
ANGEL HAIR								
Pasta, Dry	**1 Serving/50g**	**181**	**1.1**	**362**	**12.4**	**73.6**	**2.2**	**4.4**

A

A

ANTIPASTI	Measure INFO/WEIGHT	per Measure KCAL	FAT	Nutrition Values per 100g / 100ml KCAL	PROT	CARB	FAT	FIBRE
Mixed, in Olive Oil, Extra Virgin, Drained, M&S*	¼ Jar/40g	76	7	191	1.3	4.8	17.5	4.3
Roasted Aubergine, Mezze, Belazu*	1 Serving/55g	76	7.4	138	0.6	2.9	13.4	1
Sundried Tomato, Drained, Tesco*	1 Serving/34g	55	4	163	3	7	11.9	7.9
APPLE SAUCE								
Bramley, British, with Cider, Extra Special, Asda*	1 Serving/10g	14	0	145	0.4	35	0.4	1
Ocean Spray*	1 Tbsp/15g	17	0	111	0.2	27.1	0	2.4
APPLES								
Braeburn, Average	*1 Apple/123g*	*58*	*0*	*47*	*0.3*	*12.9*	*0*	*2.9*
Cooking, Baked with Sugar, Flesh Only, Average	*1 Serving/140g*	*104*	*0.1*	*74*	*0.5*	*19.2*	*0.1*	*1.7*
Cooking, Raw, Peeled, Average	*1oz/28g*	*10*	*0*	*35*	*0.3*	*8.9*	*0.1*	*1.6*
Cooking, Stewed with Sugar, Average	*1 Serving/140g*	*104*	*0.1*	*74*	*0.3*	*19.1*	*0.1*	*1.2*
Cooking, Stewed without Sugar, Average	*1 Serving/140g*	*46*	*0.1*	*33*	*0.3*	*8.1*	*0.1*	*1.5*
Cox, English, Average	*1 Apple/123g*	*53*	*0.1*	*43*	*0.4*	*10.2*	*0.1*	*1.8*
Discovery, Average	*1 Apple/182g*	*82*	*0.9*	*45*	*0.4*	*10.6*	*0.5*	*1*
Dried, Average	*1 Pack/250g*	*537*	*0.7*	*215*	*0.8*	*52.8*	*0.3*	*5.9*
Empire, Average	*1 Apple/120g*	*52*	*0.1*	*44*	*0.4*	*10.7*	*0.1*	*1.8*
Envy, Select Farms, M&S*	1 Apple/130g	66	0.6	51	0.6	11.6	0.5	1.2
Fuji	*1 Apple/132g*	*64*	*0.1*	*48*	*0.4*	*11.8*	*0.1*	*1.8*
Gala, Average	*1 Apple/152g*	*66*	*0.2*	*43*	*0.3*	*10.4*	*0.1*	*1.4*
Golden Delicious, Average	*1 Med/102g*	*44*	*0.1*	*43*	*0.3*	*10.1*	*0.1*	*1.6*
Granny Smith, Average	*1 Sm/125g*	*56*	*0.1*	*45*	*0.3*	*10.7*	*0.1*	*1.8*
Green, Raw, Average	*1 Med/182g*	*86*	*0.2*	*48*	*0.4*	*11.3*	*0.1*	*1.8*
Jazz, Tesco*	1 Apple/133g	70	0.1	53	0.4	11.8	0.1	1.8
Pink Lady, Average	*1 Apple/150g*	*67*	*0.1*	*45*	*0.4*	*10.6*	*0.1*	*1.9*
Red, Average	*1 Med/149g*	*71*	*0.2*	*48*	*0.3*	*11.8*	*0.1*	*2*
Sliced, Average	*1oz/28g*	*14*	*0*	*49*	*0.4*	*11.6*	*0.1*	*1.8*
APPLETISER*								
Juice Drink, Sparkling, Appletiser, Coca-Cola*	1 Glass/200ml	94	0	47	0	11	0	0.4
APRICOTS								
Canned, in Syrup, Average	*1oz/28g*	*18*	*0*	*63*	*0.4*	*16.1*	*0.1*	*0.9*
Dried, Average	*1 Apricot/10g*	*17*	*0.1*	*171*	*3.6*	*37.4*	*0.5*	*6.3*
Dried, Soft, Average	*1 Serving/30g*	*62*	*0.1*	*208*	*2.4*	*48.5*	*0.4*	*5.2*
Halves, in Fruit Juice, Average	*1 Can/221g*	*87*	*0.1*	*40*	*0.5*	*9.2*	*0.1*	*1*
Raw, Flesh Only, Average	*1 Apricot/37g*	*19*	*0.2*	*52*	*1.5*	*12*	*0.4*	*2.2*
Raw, Weighed with Stone, Average	*1 Apricot/40g*	*19*	*0.2*	*47*	*1.4*	*10.8*	*0.4*	*1.9*
AQUAFABA								
Average	*1 Tbsp/15ml*	*3*	*0*	*18*	*1*	*2.9*	*0.2*	*0*
ARTICHOKE								
Chargrilled, in Olive Oil, Cooks Ingredients, Waitrose*	1 Serving/30g	54	4.9	134	1.7	2.7	12.3	2.7
Fresh, Raw, Average	*1oz/28g*	*13*	*0*	*47*	*3.3*	*10.5*	*0.2*	*5.4*
Hearts, Canned, Drained, Average	*½ Can/117g*	*35*	*0.1*	*30*	*1.9*	*5.4*	*0*	*2.2*
in Oil, Tesco*	1 Piece/15g	17	1.5	115	1.9	2.4	10	4
Marinated, Roasted, M&S*	1 Pack/200g	300	26.6	150	1.9	5	13.3	2.3
ASPARAGUS								
Boiled, in Salted Water, Average	*5 Spears/125g*	*28*	*0.3*	*22*	*2.4*	*4.1*	*0.2*	*2*
Canned, Average	*1 Can/250g*	*41*	*0.4*	*16*	*2*	*1.8*	*0.2*	*1.4*
Trimmed, Raw, Average	*1 Serving/80g*	*20*	*0.4*	*24*	*2.9*	*1.9*	*0.6*	*1.7*
White, Raw, Average	*1 Spear/17g*	*3*	*0*	*17*	*1*	*2.5*	*0.3*	*1*
AUBERGINE								
Canned, in Tomato Sauce, Palirria*	¼ Can/140g	189	16.2	135	1.3	4.4	11.6	3.3
Fried, Average	*1oz/28g*	*85*	*8.9*	*302*	*1.2*	*2.8*	*31.9*	*2.3*
Glazed, Sweet & Spicy, Centrepieces, BOL Foods*	½ Pack/202g	204	13.7	101	1.6	6.7	6.8	2.5
Parmigiana di Melanzane, Cook*	1 Pack/310g	477	35.6	154	4.7	6.9	11.5	1.9

	Measure INFO/WEIGHT	per Measure KCAL	FAT	Nutrition Values per 100g / 100ml KCAL	PROT	CARB	FAT	FIBRE
AUBERGINE								
Parmigiana, M&S*	1 Pack/350g	332	18.6	95	4.6	7.6	5.3	1.1
Raw, Fresh, Average	***1 Sm/250g***	***36***	***1***	***14***	***0.9***	***2.1***	***0.4***	***1.9***
AVOCADO								
Breakfast, Holy Moly*	1 Serving/30g	45	4.5	151	2	9	15	7
Flesh Only, Average	***1 Med/145g***	***276***	***28.3***	***190***	***1.9***	***1.9***	***19.5***	***3.4***
Smash, Twist of Lemon, Waitrose*	1/3 Pack/50g	93	8.8	186	1.5	2.8	17.7	4.9
Smashed, Aldi*	1 Serving/50g	72	7	143	1.6	1.2	14	4.4
Smashed, M&S*	½ Pack/100g	140	9.7	140	2.5	9.8	9.7	1.8
Smashed, Pure, Holy Moly*	¼ Pot/40g	64	6.4	160	2	9	16	7
Smashed, Touch of Lime, Tesco*	½ Pot/100g	189	16.7	189	1.5	6.5	16.7	3.6

	Measure INFO/WEIGHT	KCAL	FAT	KCAL	PROT	CARB	FAT	FIBRE
		per Measure		Nutrition Values per 100g / 100ml				

BACARDI*

	Measure INFO/WEIGHT	KCAL	FAT	KCAL	PROT	CARB	FAT	FIBRE
37.5% Volume, Bacardi*	1 Pub Shot/35ml	72	0	207	0	0	0	0
40% Volume, Bacardi*	1 Pub Shot/35ml	78	0	222	0	0	0	0
Breezer, Cranberry, Bacardi*	1 Bottle/275ml	154	0	56	0	7.1	0	0
Breezer, Lime, Bacardi*	1 Bottle/275ml	182	0	66	0	9.1	0	0

BACON

	Measure INFO/WEIGHT	KCAL	FAT	KCAL	PROT	CARB	FAT	FIBRE
Back, Dry Cured, Average	1 Rasher/31g	77	4.7	250	28.1	0.3	15.1	0.3
Back, Dry Fried or Grilled, Average	1 Rasher/25g	72	5.4	287	23.2	0	21.6	0
Back, Lean, Average	1 Rasher/33g	57	4	174	16.3	0.1	12	0.5
Back, Smoked, Average	1 Rasher/25g	66	5	265	20.9	0	19.9	0
Back, Smoked, Lean, Average	1 Rasher/25g	41	1.2	163	28.2	1.1	5	0.2
Back, Smoked, Rindless, Average	1 Rasher/25g	60	4.3	241	21	0.1	17.4	0
Back, Unsmoked, Average	1 Rasher/32g	78	5.5	242	21.3	0.4	17.3	0
Back, Unsmoked, Rindless, Average	1 Rasher/23g	56	3.9	241	22.5	0	16.9	0
Bits, Average	1oz/28g	75	5.9	268	18.6	0.7	21.2	0.1
Chops, Average	1oz/28g	62	4.2	222	22.3	0	14.8	0
Collar Joint, Lean & Fat, Boiled	1oz/28g	91	7.6	325	20.4	0	27	0
Collar Joint, Lean & Fat, Raw	1oz/28g	81	7.4	290	13.3	0	26.3	0
Collar Joint, Lean Only, Boiled	1oz/28g	53	2.7	191	26	0	9.7	0
Fat Only, Cooked, Average	1oz/28g	194	20.4	692	9.3	0	72.8	0
Fat Only, Raw, Average	1oz/28g	209	22.7	747	4.8	0	80.9	0
Gammon Rasher, Lean Only, Grilled	1oz/28g	48	1.5	172	31.4	0	5.2	0
Lardons, Unsmoked, As Sold, Birchwood, Lidl*	¼ Pack/39g	98	8.2	252	15.2	0.2	21	0
Lean Only, Fried, Average	1 Rasher/25g	83	5.6	332	32.8	0	22.3	0
Lean Only, Grilled, Average	1 Rasher/25g	73	4.7	292	30.5	0	18.9	0
Lean, Average	1 Rasher/33g	47	2.2	142	19.6	0.9	6.7	0.2
Loin Steaks, Grilled, Average	1 Serving/120g	229	11.6	191	25.9	0	9.7	0
Meat Free, Rashers, Smoked, Richmond*	1 Rasher/38g	68	4.2	179	12	4.9	11	6.4
Medallions, Average	1 Rasher/18g	27	0.6	151	29.4	0.9	3.3	0.1
Middle, Fried	1 Rasher/40g	140	11.4	350	23.4	0	28.5	0
Middle, Grilled	1 Rasher/40g	123	9.2	307	24.8	0	23.1	0
Middle, Raw	1 Rasher/43g	95	7.9	222	14	0	18.4	0
Plant Based, Unsmoked, Naked , Finnebrogue*	2 Rashers/36g	72	4.6	200	10	6.8	12.7	8.9
Plant, Pieces, Vivera*	½ Pack/88g	76	0.5	87	17	1.4	0.6	4.6
Rashers, Lean Only, Trimmed, Average	1 Rasher/20g	24	0.8	119	20.6	0	4	0
Smoked, Crispy, Cooked, Average	1 Serving/10g	46	2.7	460	53	2.1	26.9	0
Streaky, Cooked, Average	1 Rasher/20g	68	5.6	342	22.4	0.3	27.8	0
Vegan, No Pork, Streaky, M&S*	2 Rashers/36g	72	4.6	199	10	6.8	12.7	8.9
Vegan, Pieces, Vivera*	½ Pack/88g	81	0.4	92	18	1.9	0.4	6
Vegan, Thick Cut, Pan Fried, V Taste, Morrisons*	1 Rasher/12g	40	2.3	339	27	13.1	19.2	2.7
Vegan, Vacon, Smoky, Plant Pioneers, Sainsbury's*	4 Rashers/44g	153	9.3	347	24.5	12.7	21.1	4.2
Vegetarian, Rashers	1 Rasher/16g	33	1.7	206	19.5	8.6	10.4	2.8

BAGUETTE

	Measure INFO/WEIGHT	KCAL	FAT	KCAL	PROT	CARB	FAT	FIBRE
Beef, & Horseradish, Freshly Prepared, M&S*	1 Baguette/274g	795	31	290	12.1	37.2	11.3	2
Brown, Bake At Home, Sainsbury's*	½ Baguette/73g	208	0.8	285	8.8	57.7	1.1	4.4
Cheese, & Ham, Average	1 Baguette/203g	593	20.8	292	14	35.9	10.3	1.4
Cheese, & Tomato, Tesco*	1 Baguette/108g	243	8.3	225	9.7	29.3	7.7	1.8
Cheese, Mixed, & Spring Onion, Asda*	1 Pack/190g	629	34.8	331	9.5	32.1	18.3	1.3
Chicken, & Salad, Asda*	1 Serving/158g	326	9.5	206	9	29	6	2.1
Chicken, Tikka, Asda*	1 Pack/190g	439	17.9	231	10.4	32.8	9.4	1.3
Garlic, Essential, Waitrose*	1 Baguette/210g	706	34.9	336	6.8	38.8	16.6	2.4
Ham, & Turkey, Asda*	1 Baguette/360g	774	18.4	215	11.6	30.7	5.1	1.3
Ham, & Cheese, Freshly Prepared, M&S*	1 Baguette/231g	555	11.3	240	13.4	35.9	4.9	2.4
Multi Grain, Rustic, Tesco*	1 Slice/35g	96	1.2	275	11.8	47.8	3.3	3.6

	Measure INFO/WEIGHT	per Measure KCAL	FAT	Nutrition Values per 100g / 100ml KCAL	PROT	CARB	FAT	FIBRE
BAGUETTE								
Pepperoni, Pizza, Morrisons*	1 Baguette/120g	272	8.8	227	10.2	28.8	7.3	2.7
Prawn Mayonnaise, Asda*	1 Pack/190g	399	9.3	210	9.1	32.5	4.9	1.3
Salmon, Smoked, & Egg, Freshly Prepared	**1 Baguette/178g**	**455**	**17.3**	**255**	**13.7**	**28.4**	**9.7**	**1.6**
Steak, & Onion, Snack 'n' Go, Sainsbury's*	1 Baguette/177g	398	8.8	225	14.3	30.6	5	2.2
BAILEYS*								
Almande, Dairy Free, Baileys*	1 Serving/25ml	10	0.2	38	0.6	3.1	0.8	0
Irish Cream, Original, Baileys*	1 Serving/50ml	164	6.5	327	3	25	13	0
BAKE								
3 Fish, Roast, Deluxe, Lidl*	¼ Pack/172g	249	12.7	145	12.5	6.8	7.4	0.6
Aubergine, & Grain, Moroccan Inspired, Waitrose*	½ Pack/189g	151	8.3	80	1.3	6.9	4.4	3.7
Broccoli, & Cheese, M&S*	1 Pack/400g	480	31.2	120	6.5	5.4	7.8	1.6
Cheese, & Onion, Greggs, Iceland*	1 Bake/141g	437	29.6	310	6.1	23	21	0
Cheese, & Onion, Tesco*	1 Bake/110g	332	17	302	7.8	31.8	15.5	2.3
Haddock, Average	**1 Serving/400g**	**312**	**9.2**	**78**	**6.4**	**8**	**2.3**	**0.9**
Lamb, Spiced, Indian Inspired, Finest, Tesco*	½ Pack/315g	369	13.2	117	4.9	13.8	4.2	2.1
Lentil, Spiced, Vegetarian, TTD, Sainsbury's*	1 Bake/132g	245	8.4	186	4.8	27.3	6.4	4.2
Mushroom, Rice, Vegetarian, Tesco*	1 Bake/133g	264	11.3	199	5.4	23.6	8.5	3
No Cheez, Plant Menu, Aldi*	1 Bake/134g	364	21.4	272	4.6	27	16	2.3
Steak, Tesco*	1 Bake/131g	296	10.5	226	9.5	28	8	2
Vegetable, Mediterranean, Cooked, CBY, Asda*	1 Bake/120g	279	13.2	232	8.4	22.8	11	4.2
BAKING POWDER								
Average	**1 Tsp/2g**	**3**	**0**	**163**	**5.2**	**37.8**	**0**	**0**
BAKLAVA								
Average	**2 Pieces/50g**	**239**	**14.2**	**478**	**8**	**47.4**	**28.4**	**2.8**
BALTI								
Chicken, Asda*	1 Pack/400g	400	19.6	100	11	2.5	4.9	1.7
Chicken, Canned, Sainsbury's*	½ Pack/200g	192	7.4	96	11	3.3	3.7	2.8
Chicken, Garlic, Chilli, Takeaway, Iceland*	1 Pack/343g	446	24	130	11.1	4.9	7	1.5
Chickpea & Spinach, Cauldron Foods*	1 Pack/400g	356	8	89	2.3	15.5	2	1
Prawn, Budgens*	1 Pack/350g	374	24.8	107	5.6	5.2	7.1	1.3
Vegetable, Average	**1 Serving/200g**	**182**	**8.3**	**91**	**1.9**	**11.3**	**4.1**	**1.7**
BAMBOO SHOOTS								
Canned, Average	**1 Sm Can/120g**	**10**	**0.1**	**8**	**1**	**0.8**	**0.1**	**0.8**
BANANA								
Chips, Average	**1oz/28g**	**143**	**8.8**	**511**	**1**	**59.9**	**31.4**	**1.7**
Green, Medium, Average	**1 Sm/101g**	**91**	**0**	**90**	**1**	**23**	**0**	**3**
Raw, Flesh Only, Average	**1 Med/118g**	**105**	**0.4**	**89**	**1.1**	**22.8**	**0.3**	**2.6**
BARLEY								
Canned, in Water, Drained, Napolina*	1 Can/240g	122	0.2	51	1.7	10	0.1	1.9
Flakes, Organic, BuyWholeFoodsOnline*	1 Serving/10g	31	0.2	314	9.8	65.1	1.6	11
Mix, Pearl, Peas, & Lentils, Cooked, Sainsbury's*	1 Serving/75g	83	0.4	110	6.9	17.3	0.5	5.8
Pot, Raw, Average	**1 Serving/60g**	**212**	**1.4**	**354**	**12.5**	**73.5**	**2.3**	**17.3**
BARS								
Almond Macaroon, Nak'd*	1 Bar/35g	134	5.2	383	6.9	52.3	14.9	6
Almond, & Cashew, Paleo, Aldi*	1 Bar/45g	203	10.8	451	13	40	24	8.9
Almond, Dark Chocolate, & Sea Salt, Deluxe, Lidl*	1 Bar/40g	219	14.8	548	15.5	34.2	37	6.8
Almond, Madagascan Vanilla, Kind*	1 Bar/40g	203	15.6	507	16	36	39	14
Almond, Peanut, & Double Choc, Yes!*	1 Bar/45g	231	15.2	514	22.9	24	33.8	11.2
Almond, Sweet & Nutty, Nature Valley*	1 Bar/30g	143	6.9	475	10	54.3	23	5.4
Apple, Fruit & Oat Bakes, Go Ahead*	1 Bar/35g	127	2.7	363	2.7	72.3	7.7	4.3
Apple, Fruit Bakes, Crownfield, Lidl*	1 Bar/33g	128	2.6	387	3.8	73.9	8	2
Apple, Granola, McVitie's*	1 Bar/35g	128	3.4	366	6.6	63.1	9.7	4.3
Apricot, & Almond, Eat Natural*	1 Bar/50g	238	13.4	476	6.6	49.7	26.7	5

BARS

	Measure INFO/WEIGHT	per Measure KCAL	FAT	KCAL	PROT	CARB	FAT	FIBRE
Apricot, & Almond, Yoghurt Coated, Eat Natural*	1 Bar/50g	233	13.1	476	6.6	49.7	26.7	5
Apricot, & Sultana, Special K, Kellogg's*	1 Bar/27g	104	1.7	385	5.6	74.1	6.3	7.8
Baked, Cranberry, & Hazelnut, Belvita*	1 Bar/40g	168	6.4	421	5.5	60	16	7.1
Baked, Dark Chocolate, & Hazelnut, Belvita*	1 Bar/40g	166	6.4	416	5.7	60	16	7.4
Banana, Oat Boosts, Graze*	1 Bar/30g	137	7.2	457	7.4	51	24	15
Banana, Oat, Nom*	1 Bar/40g	177	7.8	443	7.8	54.6	19.6	6.3
Banana, Oaty, Mamia Organic, Aldi*	1 Bar/25g	98	3.1	392	6.4	60	12.4	6.4
Banoffee Pie, Nakd*	1 Bar/35g	129	4.6	368	6.9	53.1	13.2	4.6
Beetroot, & Apple, Yes!*	1 Bar/32g	123	3.7	386	4.8	62.3	11.6	6.6
Berry Delight, The Foodie Market, Aldi*	1 Bar/35g	141	5.2	402	6.4	57	15	6.8
Berry, & Almond, Seed, Nine*	1 Bar/50g	228	12	456	18.1	39.3	23.9	6.7
Berry, & Yoghurt, Giant, Ma Baker*	1 Bar/100g	491	24.5	491	5.7	61.9	24.5	1
Berry, Delight, GF, Nak'd*	1 Bar/35g	135	5.2	385	9	52	15	6
Berry, Nut Free, Get Buzzing*	1 Bar/62g	173	8.7	279	3.2	50	14	2.9
Better Brownie, Cherry Bakewell, Vive*	1 Bar/35g	153	8.8	437	15	33	25	13
Better Brownie, Chocolate Berry, Vive*	1 Bar/35g	147	7.7	418	16	34	22	13
Better Brownie, Chocolate Orange, Vive*	1 Bar/35g	150	8.8	429	17	29	25	14
Better Brownie, Coconut Cashew, Vive*	1 Bar/35g	148	8.4	423	15	32	24	16
Birthday Cake, High Protein, Harvest Morn, Aldi*	1 Bar/60g	214	7.7	357	35.4	28.8	12.8	9.4
Birthday Cake, Protein, Battle Bites*	1 Bar/62g	220	8.1	355	33	26	13	13.9
Birthday Cake, Squares, Fibre One*	1 Bar/24g	84	1.5	350	2.8	47.6	6.2	25.1
Biscuit, Chocolate, Chunky, Belmont Biscuit Co, Aldi*	1 Bar/24g	126	6.7	526	6.6	61	28	1.8
Biscuit, Chocolate, Mint, Penguin, McVitie's*	1 Bar/25g	133	6.9	531	5.4	65	27.7	1.5
Biscuit, Chocolate, Orange, Penguin, McVitie's*	1 Bar/25g	133	6.9	531	5.4	65	27.7	1.5
Biscuit, Chocolate, Original, Penguin, McVitie's*	1 Bar/20g	106	5.6	515	5.1	61.4	27.1	2.4
Biscuit, Groovy, Aldi*	1 Bar/27g	123	5.3	457	4.9	64.2	19.7	1.8
Biscuit, M&M's, Mars*	1 Bar/20g	101	5.1	512	6	63	26	0
Biscuit, Milk Chocolate, M&S*	1 Bar/21g	107	5.5	509	6.4	60	26.4	2.8
Biscuit, Twin Twix, Caramel, Mister Choc, Lidl*	1 Bar/29g	146	7	505	5.3	66	24	0
Black Forest, Hi-Fi, Slimming World*	1 Bar/20g	71	2	355	3.3	53	10	19
Blondie, Chocolate Treat, Baileys*	1 Bar/32g	160	8.8	501	4.3	58.3	27.6	0
Blue Riband, Caramel, Nestle*	1 Bar/20g	99	4.5	495	4.9	66.9	22.7	1.5
Blueberry, Muffin, Fibre, Asda*	1 Bar/24g	86	2.3	359	3.6	54	9.5	22
Bon Gelati, Lidl*	1 Bar/84g	285	17.9	339	5.4	30.7	21.3	1.4
Breakfast, Almond Butter, Kind*	1 Bar/30g	134	6.6	445	8.5	54	22	7.2
Breakfast, Blueberry, & Almond, Kind*	1 Bar/30g	126	6	421	7	54	20	8.3
Breakfast, Golden Grahams, Nestle*	1 Bar/25g	101	3.2	403	7.4	65	13	4.4
Breakfast, Peanut Butter, Kind*	1 Bar/50g	230	11	460	10	44	22	10
Breakfast, Porridge to Go, Almond, & Honey, Quaker*	1 Bar/55g	221	4.6	401	7.2	68	8.4	12
Breakfast, Porridge to Go, Blueberry & Apple, Quaker*	1 Bar/55g	214	4.1	390	7.2	68	7.4	12
Breakfast, Porridge to Go, Cocoa, & Hazelnut, Quaker*	1 Bar/65g	268	8.4	413	8	62	13	9.5
Brownie, Chocolate Orange, Weight Watchers*	1 Bar/18g	63	1.8	346	21	29.6	9.8	27.8
Brownie, Chocolate, Fibre, Asda*	1 Bar/24g	89	2.9	369	5	49	12	23
Brownie, Double Dough, Myprotein*	1 Bar/60g	245	9.6	408	24	40	16	14
Brownie, Sticky Toffee, WW*	1 Bar/17g	60	1.4	351	16.4	41	8.2	23.9
Brunch, Peanut, Cadbury*	1 Bar/32g	151	7.7	473	15	50	24	4.3
Brunch, Raisin, Cadbury*	1 Bar/32g	133	4.8	417	5.4	66	15	4.5
Cacao Mint, Protein, Energy Ball, Bounce*	1 Ball/42g	176	7.1	422	23	41	17	6.4
Cacao, & Almond, Energy Ball, Deliciously Ella*	1 Ball/40g	173	11.1	433	12.5	35.3	27.8	7.2
Cacao, & Almond, Oat, Baked, Deliciously Ella*	1 Bar/50g	218	9.6	435	7.4	55.8	19.1	5.1
Cacao, Coffee, & Ameretto, Love Vegan*	1 Bar/33g	131	6.5	398	9.6	48.2	19.7	4.2
Cacao, Raw Fruit & Nut, Wild Trail*	1 Bar/30g	115	3.3	383	8.6	56	11	11
Cake, M&M's, Mars*	1 Bar/26g	126	6.7	485	5.2	59.4	25.6	0

B

	Measure INFO/WEIGHT	per Measure KCAL	FAT	Nutrition Values per 100g / 100ml KCAL	PROT	CARB	FAT	FIBRE

BARS

	Measure INFO/WEIGHT	KCAL	FAT	KCAL	PROT	CARB	FAT	FIBRE
Cake, Red Velvet, Fibre One*	1 Bar/25g	90	3.1	360	3.6	47.2	12.3	22.4
Caramel Crisp, Barebells Double Bite*	1 Bar/55g	196	7.7	357	31	34	14	13
Caramel, Almond, & Sea Salt, Kind*	1 Bar/40g	211	15.6	527	16	19	39	18
Caramel, Chewy, Mini, Sainsbury's*	1 Bar/18g	80	3.3	444	3.5	66.4	18.2	0.5
Caramel, Chocolate, Chewy, Sainsbury's*	1 Bar/36g	167	6.9	464	3.9	68.9	19.2	0
Caramel, Crazy, Tesco*	1 Bar/40g	192	9.2	480	3.9	64	23	1
Caramel, Crunchy, Tesco*	1 Bar/21g	98	5.2	467	4.6	56	25	1.4
Caramel, Nougat, WW*	1 Bar/19g	74	1.7	391	4.6	70	8.7	7
Caramel, Salted, Huel*	1 Bar/49g	200	7.8	408	24	36	16	9
Caramel, Salted, Protein, Ball, Bounce*	1 Ball/40g	170	7	425	1	30	17.5	25
Caramel, Skinny Whip*	1 Bar/25g	96	2.3	384	3.6	64	9.2	15.2
Caramel, Wafer, Chewy, Ms Mollys*	1 Bar/18g	88	3.9	489	6.2	66.5	21.6	2
Carrot, Cake, Fibre One*	1 Bar/25g	90	3.4	361	4.2	44	13.4	23.9
Cashew Crush, Raw, Fruit & Nut, Foodie Market, Aldi*	1 Bar/35g	158	8	451	11.7	45.7	22.9	7.7
Cashew, Cookie, Raw Fruit & Nut, GF, Nak'd*	1 Bar/35g	143	8	410	10	46	23	5
Cashew, Crush, Alesto, Aldi*	1 Bar/35g	155	8.2	444	10	46	23.4	4.7
Cereal, & Milk, Nesquik, Nestle*	1 Bar/25g	108	3.7	433	6.2	68.5	14.9	1
Cereal, Apple & Cinnamon, Chewy, Frusli, Jordans*	1 Bar/30g	114	2.1	380	5.7	71.6	6.9	4.3
Cereal, Apricot, Almond, & Yoghurt, Tesco*	1 Bar/35g	156	6.8	447	5.9	59.7	19.4	4.9
Cereal, Banana Bonanza, Tesco*	1 Bar/21g	82	1.8	390	6.6	69	8.8	4.3
Cereal, Banoffee, Light, Alpen, Weetabix*	1 Bar/19g	66	1.3	346	4.7	54	7	24
Cereal, Caramel, Boka*	1 Bar/30g	88	0.8	295	6	58	2.7	19
Cereal, Choc Chip, Brunch, Cadbury*	1 Bar/32g	137	5.1	427	6.1	65	16	4.7
Cereal, Choco Snaps, Asda*	1 Bar/20g	79	2.2	393	4.6	62	11	13
Cereal, Chocolate Chip, Ms Mollys*	1 Bar/21g	83	1.6	394	5.4	73.4	7.8	4.3
Cereal, Chocolate Chip, Special K, Kellogg's*	1 Bar/21g	84	1.5	401	9	76	7	1.5
Cereal, Chocolate Chunks, & Pecan, Special K, Kellogg's*	1 Bar/36g	170	9	472	25	44.4	25	11.1
Cereal, Chocolate Delight, Dark, Special K, Kellogg's*	1 Bar/24g	97	3.4	404	4.5	57	14	17
Cereal, Chocolate, & Fudge, Asda*	1 Bar/19g	66	1.3	347	4.5	53	6.9	28
Cereal, Chocolate, & Fudge, Light, Alpen*	1 Bar/19g	67	1.3	353	5.6	57	6.7	21
Cereal, Chocolate, Double, Asda*	1 Bar/19g	67	1.2	352	5.5	58	6.3	21
Cereal, Chocolate, Double, Benefit, Harvest Morn, Aldi*	1 Bar/19g	62	1	326	6.8	52	5.1	25
Cereal, Chocolate, Double, Light, Alpen*	1 Bar/19g	67	1.2	351	5.6	58	6.3	20
Cereal, Chocolate, Great Shape, Asda*	1 Bar/20g	72	2	361	4.7	54	10	18
Cereal, Chocolate, Milk, Double, Special K, Kellogg's*	1 Bar/20g	80	2	400	10	65	10	10
Cereal, Chocolate, Mint, Great Shape, Asda*	1 Bar/20g	72	2.2	361	4.6	51	11	20
Cereal, Chocolate, Orange, Great Shape, Asda*	1 Bar/20g	72	2	361	4.7	54	10	18
Cereal, Cornflake Crunch, Hi-Fi, Slimming World*	1 Bar/20g	70	1.7	351	2.3	59	8.3	16
Cereal, Cranberry & Orange, Weight Watchers*	1 Bar/28g	102	1.1	365	4.5	77.6	4.1	2.3
Cereal, Cranberry & Yoghurt, Harvest Morn, Aldi*	1 Bar/29g	117	2.6	403	6.5	71.9	9	4.1
Cereal, Crunchy Granola, Ginger Nut, Nature Valley*	1 Bar/42g	189	7.1	451	7.9	64.2	16.9	2.3
Cereal, Dark Chocolate, & Cranberries, Special K*	1 Bar/27g	100	2.5	372	5.9	68	9.1	10
Cereal, Dark Chocolate, Berry, WW*	1 Bar/18g	60	1.6	335	9.4	45.7	8.8	21.2
Cereal, Dark Chocolate, Coconut, WW*	1 Bar/18g	61	1.6	338	8.3	47	9.1	21
Cereal, Ecosize, Decathlon*	1 Bar/21g	83	1.8	393	5.8	70	8.8	5.5
Cereal, Fruit & Fibre, Asda*	1 Bar/29g	111	2.8	390	6	69	10	4.1
Cereal, Fruit, Average	*1 Bar/34g*	*130*	*3.9*	*382*	*5.9*	*64.7*	*11.5*	*6.5*
Cereal, Frusli, Blueberry, Jordans*	1 Bar/30g	113	2.1	375	5.2	70.1	7.1	4.9
Cereal, Frusli, Raisin & Hazelnut, Jordans*	1 Bar/30g	120	3.7	399	5.8	64.3	12.2	4.5
Cereal, Hazelnut, Brunch, Cadbury*	1 Bar/35g	160	7.4	460	7	60.5	21.4	2.2
Cereal, Milk Chocolate, WW*	1 Bar/18g	61	1.5	339	9.1	48	8.5	20
Cereal, Nut & Seed, Organic, Green & Black's*	1 Bar/50g	258	16.3	516	8.4	47.2	32.6	10
Cereal, Oat & Raisin, Basics, Sainsbury's*	1 Bar/25g	98	2.2	391	5.1	72.8	8.8	3.8

BARS

	Measure INFO/WEIGHT	per Measure		Nutrition Values per 100g / 100ml				
		KCAL	FAT	KCAL	PROT	CARB	FAT	FIBRE
Cereal, Oats, & Honey, M&S*	1 Bar/30g	110	1.9	367	7.3	63.5	6.3	13.5
Cereal, Red Berries, Frusli, Jordans*	1 Bar/30g	118	2.2	395	4.8	75.1	7.2	5.4
Cereal, Red Berry, Special K, Kellogg's*	1 Bar/22g	84	1.4	384	5.3	73	6.3	7.7
Cereal, Red Fruit, Chewy & Crispy, Sainsbury's*	1 Bar/20g	78	1.4	391	6.8	73.6	6.8	4.4
Cereal, Rice Snaps, Asda*	1 Bar/20g	77	2.1	385	3.5	60	10.5	15.5
Cereal, Strawberry with Yoghurt, Alpen*	1 Bar/29g	120	2.9	415	4.8	75	10	2.7
Cereal, Strawberry, Fruit 'n' Grain, Asda*	1 Bar/37g	126	2.6	340	4.2	65	7	4.5
Cereal, Strawberry, Raspberry, & Cranberry, Quaker*	1 Bar/55g	214	3.6	390	5.9	74	6.6	5.9
Cereal, Summer Fruits, Light, Alpen*	1 Bar/19g	65	0.8	341	5.3	60	4.3	20
Cereal, Summer Fruits, Tesco*	1 Bar/19g	65	0.8	343	4.2	61	4.3	21.8
Cherry Bakewell, CWP*	1 Bar/57g	207	6.3	363	23	44	11	4.4
Cherry Bakewell, Porridge Oat, Thins, Stoats*	1 Bar/22g	93	3.3	422	7.2	60.4	15	7.9
Chewy Oat, Toffee Apple, Graze*	1 Bar/23g	97	3.9	422	6.2	59	17	21
Choc Orange, Chunky, Macro Munch, Bulk*	1 Bar/62g	228	8.7	368	32.2	26	14	15
Choc Orange, Hi-Fi, Slimming World*	1 Bar/20g	69	1.6	343	3.4	55	8	19
Choc Peanut, Skinny dream*	1 Bar/24g	96	2.7	398	3.9	66.3	11.1	8.6
Choc, Coconut, & Cashew, Smart, PhD Nutrition*	1 Bar/64g	258	12.2	403	35	11	19	23
Choc, Salted Caramel, Tribe*	1 Bar/50g	236	12.5	472	11	48	25	5.6
Choco Trio, Milka*	1 Bar/30g	142	7.2	472	5.8	57	24	1.8
Chocolate Brownie, Misfits*	1 Bar/45g	184	9.7	410	34	16.6	21.5	19.4
Chocolate Fudge, Brownie, Fibre One*	1 Bar/24g	83	3.3	345	4.8	40.7	13.7	25.3
Chocolate Honeycomb, Macro Munch, Bulk*	1 Bar/62g	223	8.7	360	32	33	14	11
Chocolate Orange, Skinny Whip*	1 Bar/25g	98	2.8	392	4	60	11.2	17.2
Chocolate Raisin, Lighterlife*	1 Bar/60g	224	6.7	374	25.4	36.3	11.2	12.6
Chocolate, & Caramel, Rice Krispies Squares, Kellogg's*	1 Bar/36g	155	5	430	4.5	71	14	2
Chocolate, & Peanut, Tracker, Mars*	1 Bar/26g	112	5	432	6.6	50.6	19.1	15.5
Chocolate, Almond, Protein, Vegan, Foodspring*	1 Bar/60g	199	5.3	331	31	24	8.9	25
Chocolate, Brownie, Average	**1 Bar/68g**	**240**	**4**	**353**	**14.7**	**60.3**	**5.9**	**8.8**
Chocolate, Caramel, & Sea Salt, Nomo*	1 Bar/38g	212	13.7	559	1.9	55	36	0
Chocolate, Caramel, Mini, Mister Choc, Lidl*	1 Bar/22g	100	4.2	453	3.9	66	19	1.1
Chocolate, Caramel, Protein, Misfits*	1 Bar/45g	186	9.2	413	35.6	12.9	20.4	17.8
Chocolate, Caramel, Protein, Novo *	1 Bar/60g	220	9	366	33	28	15	11
Chocolate, Caramel, Wacko, Belmont, Aldi*	1 Bar/21g	102	4.6	485	5.3	65	22	1.7
Chocolate, Cosmic Whip, Tesco*	1 Bar/22g	100	3.7	452	3.6	72.4	16.6	0.8
Chocolate, Crispy Delight, Indulgent, Bliss*	1 Bar/20g	94	3.6	470	2.9	73	18	1.2
Chocolate, Dark, & Peanut Butter, Deluxe, Lidl*	1 Bar/40g	218	14.6	545	20.2	30.5	36.5	6.8
Chocolate, Dark, & Raspberry, Tesco*	1 Bar/23g	96	2.7	419	6.2	69.5	11.8	5
Chocolate, Dark, Chewy Delight, Special K, Kellogg's*	1 Bar/24g	97	3.4	404	4.5	57	14	17
Chocolate, Dark, Energy, Jungle*	1 Bar/48g	206	8.4	430	6.5	61	17.4	6.4
Chocolate, Dark, Intense, The Dark One, M&S*	1 Bar/32g	180	10.9	564	9.6	53.1	34.2	2.5
Chocolate, Dark, Mint, Hi-Fi, Slimming World*	1 Bar/20g	70	1.8	351	4	54	8.8	20
Chocolate, Dark, Nuts, & Sea Salt, Kind*	1 Bar/40g	198	14.8	495	14	23	37	17
Chocolate, Double, Snack, Skinny Whip*	1 Bar/25g	96	2.3	385	3.7	64	9.3	15
Chocolate, Free From, Co-Op*	1 Bar/30g	169	10.5	562	2.5	58	35	3.1
Chocolate, Fruit & Nut, M&S*	1 Bar/50g	235	12	470	6.5	57.1	24.1	2.5
Chocolate, Fruit & Crunch, NOMO*	1 Bar/32g	160	8	501	3.2	61	25	0
Chocolate, Fudge, Exante Diet*	1 Bar/60g	206	5.9	344	29	38	9.9	8.3
Chocolate, Golden Crunch, Vegan Store*	1 Bar/49g	211	4.8	431	1	83.3	9.7	4
Chocolate, Hazelnot Smooth, NOMO*	1 Bar/38g	190	9.9	500	2.6	63	26	0
Chocolate, Hazelnut Whip, Fulfil Nutrition*	1 Bar/55g	210	9.9	382	36	27	18	5.5
Chocolate, Hazelnut, High Protein, Misfits*	1 Bar/45g	199	10.8	442	34	15	24	17.7
Chocolate, Hazelnut, Tony's Chocolonely*	1 Bar/47g	262	17	558	8.4	47.8	36.1	0
Chocolate, Hazelnut, Wow Bakes, Graze*	1 Pack/20g	94	5.2	472	6.4	50	26	15

	Measure INFO/WEIGHT	per Measure KCAL	FAT	Nutrition Values per 100g / 100ml KCAL	PROT	CARB	FAT	FIBRE

BARS

	Measure INFO/WEIGHT	KCAL	FAT	KCAL	PROT	CARB	FAT	FIBRE
Chocolate, Honeycomb, Bunnycomb, Mini Moos*	1 Bar/25g	143	9.4	571	2.7	59.5	37.6	0
Chocolate, Honeycomb, Hi-Fi, Slimming World*	1 Bar/20g	70	1.8	348	3.6	54	9	1.8
Chocolate, Huel*	1 Bar/49g	200	7.9	406	24	36	16	10
Chocolate, Little, Tasting Set, Divine Chocolate*	1 Bar/15g	87	6.2	577	7.3	40.8	41.2	6.9
Chocolate, Maple, Triple Decker, Tribe*	1 Bar/40g	194	13.2	485	21	22	33	10
Chocolate, Marshmallow, Rice Krispie Squares, Kellogg's*	1 Bar/36g	158	5	438	3.1	75	14	0.8
Chocolate, Meal Replacement, Ultra Slim, Tesco*	1 Bar/60g	219	6.7	365	28.5	37.3	11.1	8.2
Chocolate, Milk, & Nut, Weight Watchers*	1 Bar/15g	80	5.7	533	13.3	22.7	38	24
Chocolate, Milk, Belgian, WW*	1 Bar/16g	80	5.6	502	12.3	22.4	34.9	24.4
Chocolate, Milk, Swiss, M&S*	1 Bar/50g	285	18.4	570	0.2	51	36.8	2
Chocolate, Mint, Club, Mcvitie's*	1 Bar/23g	117	6.1	510	5.7	61.2	26.4	2.3
Chocolate, Mint, Polar, Sainsbury's*	1 Bar/25g	135	7.6	534	4.9	59.9	29.9	2.6
Chocolate, Nutty Nougat, Sainsbury's*	1 Bar/36g	181	9.9	503	9.2	53.6	27.5	2.4
Chocolate, Orange, Huel*	1 Bar/49g	200	7.9	406	24	36	16	10
Chocolate, Orange, Skinny Crunch*	1 Bar/20g	74	2.2	368	4.8	50.2	10.9	24.9
Chocolate, Orange, Whip, Bliss*	1 Bar/25g	98	2.2	393	4.2	71	8.6	6.2
Chocolate, Peanut Butter, Fulfil*	1 Bar/40g	154	6.8	386	37	27	17	5.4
Chocolate, Peanut Butter, Smart, PhD Nutrition*	1 Bar/64g	239	10.2	373	31	38	16	1
Chocolate, Peanut, Protein, Misfits*	1 Bar/45g	189	9.9	420	40	13.6	22	17.8
Chocolate, Racer, Dairyfine, Aldi*	1 Bar/38g	185	9.5	486	8.6	54	25	4.2
Chocolate, Raspberry Cream, Frys*	1 Bar/49g	203	6.2	414	0	65.3	12.6	0
Chocolate, Reeses Sticks, Hershey*	1 Bar/42g	214	12.8	510	10.3	56	30.4	0
Chocolate, Salted Caramel, Protein, Fulfil Nutrition*	1 Bar/40g	148	6	371	37	28	15	6.2
Chocolate, Sandwich, Seal, Aldi*	1 Bar/25g	131	7	523	5.5	60.6	28.1	3.1
Chocolate, Soft, Noir, Farmer*	1 Bar/28g	134	5.9	479	6.4	64.3	21.1	6.1
Chocolate, Sour Cherry Chilli, Moser Roth, Aldi*	1 Bar/38g	202	13.7	532	7.6	40	36	9.8
Chocolate, Super Snackers, Graze*	1 Bar/23g	99	4.4	430	6.7	57	19	20
Chocolate, The Milk One, M&S*	1 Bar/32g	174	10.1	545	8.3	56	31.6	1.5
Chocolate, Titan, Aldi*	1 Bar/38g	169	6.8	444	3.5	66	18	0.5
Chocolate, Toffee Biscuit, Sainsbury's*	1 Bar/42g	194	9.7	463	4.6	58.5	23.2	0.9
Chocolate, Toffee Pecan, M&S*	1 Bar/36g	179	9.8	498	4.9	58.3	27.3	0.7
Chocolate, Toffee, Indulgent, Skinny Dream*	1 Bar/25g	93	2.8	372	3.6	50	11.2	27.6
Chocolate, Viennese, Sandwich, Fox's*	1 Bar/14g	76	4.4	542	6.9	57.4	31.6	1.6
Chocolate, Wafer, Blue Riband, Nestle*	1 Bar/18g	92	4.5	513	5	65.8	25.1	1.7
Chocolate, Wafer, Twin, Eat Me, Sondey, Lidl*	1 Bar/15g	85	5.7	568	4.5	51	38	1.9
Chocolate, White, Creamy, The White One, M&S*	1 Bar/32g	184	12	574	6.6	51.6	37.5	1.7
Chocolix, Schar*	1 Bar/22g	101	3.9	463	3.6	70	18	4.2
Cinnamon, & Apple, Fruit & Peanut, Asda*	1 Bar/35g	135	5.6	386	12	40	16	16
Club, Fruit, Jacob's*	1 Bar/24g	119	5.9	496	5.9	61.1	24.7	3
Club, Milk Chocolate, Jacob's*	1 Bar/24g	123	6.3	511	5.8	62.6	26.4	2
Club, Mint, Jacob's*	1 Bar/24g	124	6.5	517	5.6	62.5	27.2	1.7
Club, Orange, Crunchies, McVitie's*	1 Bar/24g	115	6.1	481	5.1	59	25.7	1.4
Club, Orange, McVitie's*	1 Bar/23g	116	6	512	5.7	61	26.6	2.3
Cocoa, Orange, & Hazelnut, M&S*	1 Bar/35g	129	3.8	368	5.5	59.8	10.9	4.1
Cocoa, Orange, GF, Nak'd*	1 Bar/35g	145	7	415	11	45.1	20	6.4
Cocoa, Orange, The Foodie Market, Aldi*	1 Bar/35g	151	6.6	432	8.4	52	19	7
Cocoa, Twist, Nak'd*	1 Bar/30g	99	1.7	329	7	59.9	5.6	6
Coconut, & Chocolate, Saint *	1 Bar/21g	97	3.8	460	4.8	66.7	18.1	7.1
Coffee, Espresso, Double, Protein, Primal Pantry*	1 Bar/55g	200	4.7	363	27	43	8.6	3.8
Cookie, Oaty, Maryland*	1 Bar/19g	94	4.6	493	6.8	58.5	24.2	6.1
Cookie, Triple Chocolate, Cream, New You Plan*	1 Bar/35g	139	4.6	397	31.4	40.9	13	2.5
Cranberry, & Dark Chocolate, Yes!*	1 Bar/35g	183	11.9	523	20.3	25.4	34.1	16.5
Crunch, Hazelnut Choc, Fitbakes*	1 Bar/19g	62	1.9	326	25	50	10	23

BARS

INFO/WEIGHT	per Measure KCAL	FAT	Nutrition Values per 100g / 100ml KCAL	PROT	CARB	FAT	FIBRE
Crunchy, Wafer, with Cocoa Creme, Kuljanka*	6 Wafers/32g	180	11.6	564	6.4	51.5	36.3	0
Crunchy, Wafer, with Milk Creme Filling, Kuljanka*	6 Wafers/32g	177	10.8	552	7.7	54.1	33.6	0
Dark Chocolate, & Coconut, Whip, Bliss*	1 Bar/98g	384	9.8	392	4	68	10	6.8
Dark Chocolate, Raspberry, Plant Based, Misfits*	1 Bar/45g	189	9.8	421	34.1	13.7	21.8	17
Digestive, Milk Chocolate, Ms Mollys*	1 Bar/19g	95	4.5	501	6.8	64	23.6	2.5
Double Chocolate, Whip, Bliss*	1 Bar/25g	98	2.3	393	3.8	71	9.1	6
Energy, Cacao & Raspberry, High Five*	1 Bar/50g	212	10	423	21	38	20	0
Energy, Cool Mint Chocolate, Cliff*	1 Bar/68g	268	5	394	14	65	7.3	5.9
Fibre Now, Birthday Cake, Harvest Morn, Aldi*	1 Square/24g	79	2.1	328	3.4	47.4	8.8	22.9
Fibre Now, Harvest Morn, Aldi*	1 Bar/24g	84	2.5	350	5.4	50	10.4	21.2
Fibre, Lemon Drizzle, Morrisons*	1 Bar/24g	85	2.6	353	3.5	48.7	10.9	23.5
Fibre, Mint Chocolate Chip, Mo Health*	1 Bar/24g	87	2.2	362	4.5	54	9	23.5
Flapjack , Co-Op*	1 Bar/34g	142	5.8	418	6.7	57	17	4
Flapjack, Buttery, Traditional, Organic, Dove's Farm*	1 Bar/40g	173	7.5	432	6.1	59.4	18.8	5.7
Flapjack, Salted Caramel, Protein, Trek*	1 Bar/50g	223	10.2	446	18.5	45.8	20.4	3.7
Flapjack, Slices, Morrisons*	1 Bar/35g	146	5.8	418	7	57	16.7	6
Flapjack, White Chocolate, & Raspberry, Trek*	1 Bar/40g	185	8.4	462	18.5	48.7	21.1	2.7
Frosties, & Milk, Kellogg's*	1 Bar/25g	102	2.8	408	7	71	11	1
Frosties, Snack Bar, Kellogg's*	1 Bar/25g	104	2.8	414	7	72	11	1
Fruit & Nut, Salted Caramel, & Peanuts, Eat Natural*	1 Bar/45g	223	12.8	496	26	31.3	28.4	5.4
Fruit & Nut, Simply Vegan, Eat Natural*	1 Bar/45g	223	13.5	496	12	40.4	30	7.8
Fruit & Nut, with Chocolate, & Orange, Eat Natural*	1 Bar/45g	224	12.8	498	26.1	31.1	28.5	6
Good Fibrations, Cocoa & Hazelnut, The Gut Stuff*	1 Bar/35g	151	5.3	431	5.8	54	15	29
Good Fibrations, Peanut Butter, The Gut Stuff*	1 Bar/35g	147	4.6	420	7.5	54	13	29
Granola, Chocolate & Nut, Crunchy Nut, Kellogg's*	1 Bar/32g	167	10.6	521	12	41	33	6.6
Granola, Coconut, & Chocolate, Tesco*	1 Bar/30g	150	8	500	6.8	54.6	26.8	6.5
Granola, Crunchy Nut, Cranberries & Nuts, Kellogg's*	1 Bar/32g	144	6.4	449	8.9	56	20	4.9
Granola, Crunchy, Canadian Maple Syrup, Nature Valley*	1 Bar/21g	98	3.7	465	8.7	64.3	17.8	6.4
Granola, Crunchy, Oats & Chocolate, Nature Valley*	1 Bar/21g	99	4.2	473	8.7	61.5	19.8	7
Granola, Crunchy, Oats & Honey, Nature Valley*	1 Bar/21g	98	3.8	467	8.7	64.3	18.1	6.4
Granola, Honey, Tesco*	1 Bar/30g	146	7.6	485	7.4	53.3	25.5	6.1
Granola, Maple Syrup, Crunchy, Harvest Morn, Aldi*	2 Bars/42g	189	6.7	450	8.2	65	16	5.9
Granola, Oat, & Honey, Tesco*	1 Bar/30g	145	7.6	485	7.4	53.3	25.5	6.1
Hazelnut Spirals, Dairyfine, Aldi*	1 Bar/21g	119	7.6	567	8.6	51	36	1.5
Hazelnut, Dark Chocolate Coated, Vive*	1 Bar/50g	227	14	453	21	26	28	13
Hazelnut, Wafer, Princessa, Nestle*	1 Bar/34g	188	11.3	552	5.6	57.1	33.1	1.7
Hi-Fi, Lemon Drizzle, Slimming World*	1 Bar/20g	70	1.8	351	4.4	55	9.1	18
High Protein, Aldi*	1 Bar/50g	175	4.6	350	50	23	9.3	0
Hobnob, Flapjack, Peanut Butter Fudge, McVitie's*	1 Bar/31g	136	5.2	444	5.8	64.5	17.1	4.6
Hobnobs, Choc & Golden Syrup, McVitie's*	1 Bar/31g	129	4	421	6.3	68.2	13.1	4.8
Honey, & Almond, Crunchy, Original, Jordans*	1 Bar/30g	139	6.8	463	8.3	56.7	22.7	6.7
Honey, Almond, & Greek Yoghurt, Atkins*	1 Bar/40g	160	9	400	30	37.5	22.5	22.5
Honeycomb, Caramel, Wow Bakes, Graze*	1 Bar/20g	94	5	470	6.4	52	25	16
Hype, Milk & Cookies, Oatein*	1 Bar/60g	187	4.8	311	29.8	35.1	8	7.6
Hype, Salty Caramel, Oatein*	1 Bar/60g	191	4.9	319	30.1	36.1	8.2	7.7
Jaffa Cake, Benefit, Harvest Morn, Aldi*	1 Bar/66g	228	3.6	346	5.2	58	5.5	22
Jive, Chocolate, Shortcake Finger, Dairyfine, Aldi*	1 Bar/42g	194	9.7	463	4.6	58	23	0.9
Lemon Drizzle, Nak'd*	1 Bar/35g	133	5.4	381	6.1	51.8	15.5	5.1
Lemon, & Poppy Seed, The Primal Pantry*	1 Bar/30g	126	5.7	421	11	48	19	7.9
Lemon, Meringue, Flower & White*	1 Bar/24g	99	3.1	421	4	72	13	0
Lemon, Yoghurt, New You Plan*	1 Bar/34g	124	3.6	365	25	41.7	10.6	6.6
Loaf, Chocolate, Soreen*	1 Bar/42g	141	2	336	8.2	62.9	4.7	3.4
Malt Loaf, Soreen*	1 Bar/42g	124	1	295	8.2	57.8	2.3	5.1

BARS

	Measure INFO/WEIGHT	per Measure KCAL	per Measure FAT	Nutrition Values per 100g / 100ml KCAL	PROT	CARB	FAT	FIBRE
Maple Pecan, Salted, The Yes Bar*	1 Bar/40g	220	17	550	12.5	32.5	42.5	7.5
Maple, Glazed Pecan, & Sea Salt, Kind*	1 Bar/40g	213	17.2	532	14	33	43	13
Marshmallow Bliss, Crispy, Lexi's Treats*	1 Bar/26g	99	1.7	381	2.7	79	6.5	0
Marshmallow, Rice Krispies Squares, Kellogg's*	1 Bar/28g	119	3.4	424	3	76	12	0.9
Marshmallow, Salted Caramel, Mallow & Marsh*	1 Bar/30g	79	0.4	262	2.6	63.1	1.2	0
Marshmallow, Vanilla Bean, Mallow Puffs*	1 Bar/30g	123	4.2	410	1.4	68	14	0
Marshmallow, Vanilla, Mallow & Marsh*	1 Bar/35g	134	3.7	383	7.1	68.9	10.6	0
Meal Replacement, Choc Chip, Slim Fast*	1 Bar/60g	211	5.4	351	24	38	9	11
Meal Replacement, Choc Orange, Slim Fast*	1 Bar/60g	218	5.6	364	24	40	9.4	12
Meal Replacement, Chocolate Crunch, Asda*	1 Bar/56g	220	6.7	393	25	44	12	4
Meal Replacement, Chocolate Orange, Profirst*	1 Bar/60g	202	6	337	24	42	10	9.2
Meal Replacement, Hazelnut, Lighter Life *	1 Bar/56g	203	6.7	362	32	29	12	11
Meal Replacement, Lemon, Shake That Weight*	1 Bar/56g	204	5.9	365	24.2	41.7	10.6	6.6
Meal Replacement, Pro First*	1 Bar/60g	202	6.1	337	23.3	41.7	10.2	9.2
Meal Replacement, Rocky Road, Slimfast*	1 Bar/60g	217	5.4	362	24	41	9	11
Meal Replacement, S'mores, One Brand*	1 Bar/60g	210	7	350	33.3	41.7	11.7	13.3
Meal Replacement, Strawberry, Choc, Slim Fast*	1 Bar/25g	99	2.2	396	3.2	64	8.8	18.8
Meal Replacement, Vanilla, & Caramel, Asda*	1 Bar/58g	200	6.4	344	36	29	11	4.7
Meal Replacement, Very Berry, Slim Fast*	1 Bar/60g	225	6.6	375	25	39	11	10
Melto, GF, Schar*	1 Bar/30g	165	9.9	549	6.8	55	33	0
Milk Chocolate, Double Take, Sainsbury's*	1 Bar/22g	115	6.3	534	5.8	61	29.3	1.7
Milk Chocolate, Guylian*	1 Bar/25g	136	8.2	546	9	51	33	0
Millionaire Crunch, Oatein*	1 Bar/58g	214	10.6	368	26.2	38.2	18.2	0.6
Millionaire, Salted Caramel, Hazelnut, M&S*	1 Bar/62g	285	12	459	2.2	67.1	19.4	3.4
Mint Truffle, M&S*	1 Bar/33g	189	13.1	574	4.4	47.9	39.7	3.5
Mint, & Dark Chocolate, Skinny Whip*	1 Bar/25g	98	2.8	390	2.6	63	11.2	14
Muesli, & Seeds, Bountiful, Aldi*	1 Bar/30g	98	1.4	328	3	53	4.8	18
Muesli, Chocolate, Crownfield, Lidl*	1 Bar/25g	101	2.4	404	7.4	69.1	9.5	6.1
Muesli, Chocolate, No Added Sugar, Crownfield, Lidl*	1 Bar/25g	91	2.2	364	7	68.8	8.7	5.9
Muesli, Fruit, Morning, Oat So Simple, Quaker*	1 Bar/35g	142	3.4	407	6.7	69.1	9.7	8.4
Muesli, Peanut, No Added Sugar, Crownfield, Lidl*	1 Bar/25g	98	3.3	391	7.9	65.7	13.2	4.7
Munchy, Peanut, Dairyfine, Aldi*	1 Bar/32g	137	6	428	8.1	50	18.8	10.6
Noisette, Creamy, Nucao*	1 Bar/41g	256	21.5	631	11	24	53	7.2
Nougat Whip, Morrisons*	1 Bar/22g	102	3.8	464	3.6	72.3	17.3	0.9
Nougat, Chewy, Barratt*	1 Bar/35g	133	1.5	380	4.6	79.2	4.2	2.1
Nougat, Cool Mint, & Dark Chocolate, Shapers, Boots*	1 Bar/25g	81	3.1	324	2.4	48	12.4	1.2
Nougat, Honeycomb, Shapers, Boots*	1 Bar/22g	96	2.9	435	2.8	76	13	1.2
Nougat, Nutty, Treat Size, Sainsbury's*	1 Bar/17g	88	4.6	518	10	57.6	27.1	2.9
Nougat, Summer Strawberry, Shapers, Boots*	1 Bar/23g	83	3	361	2.7	73	13	0.6
Nut Butter, Triple Decker, Choc Raspberry, Tribe*	1 Bar/40g	195	12.8	487	21	24	32	9.9
Nut Butter, Triple Decker, Doisy & Dam Special, Tribe*	1 Bar/40g	210	32	525	50	65	80	24
Nut, & Sea Salt, Dark Chocolate Coated, Morrisons*	1 Bar/40g	215	15.8	537	17.4	18.8	39.5	18.1
Nut, Dark Chocolate, Peanut Butter, Aldi*	1 Bar/40g	213	14.8	533	23	21	37	15
Nut, Feast, Mixed, Eat Natural*	1 Bar/50g	278	20.5	556	18.8	28	41	0
Nutri-Grain, Apple, Kellogg's*	1 Bar/37g	131	3.3	355	4	67	9	4
Nutri-Grain, Apple, Soft & Fruity, Kellogg's*	1 Bar/37g	133	3	359	4	70.3	8.1	4
Nutri-Grain, Blueberry, Kellogg's*	1 Bar/37g	133	3	359	3.5	69	8	3.5
Nutri-Grain, Cherry, Nutrigrain*	1 Bar/37g	130	3.5	351	5.4	67.6	9.5	2.7
Nutri-Grain, Elevenses, Choc Chip Bakes, Kellogg's*	1 Bar/45g	179	5.8	397	4	66	13	2
Nutri-Grain, Elevenses, Raisin Bakes, Kellogg's*	1 Bar/45g	168	4	374	4.5	68	9	2.5
Nutri-Grain, Strawberry, Kellogg's*	1 Bar/37g	133	3	359	3.5	69	8	3.5
Nutri-Grain, Strawberry, Soft & Fruity, Kellogg's*	1 Bar/37g	133	3	359	4	70.3	8.1	4
Nuts, Honey Roasted, & Sea Salted, Kind*	1 Bar/40g	218	16.4	544	17	23	41	8.7

BARS

	Measure INFO/WEIGHT	per Measure KCAL	FAT	Nutrition Values per 100g / 100ml KCAL	PROT	CARB	FAT	FIBRE
Nuts, Seeds, & Sea Salt, M&S*	1 Bar/40g	200	13.5	501	22.1	17.3	33.7	20.2
Nutter, Peanut & Almond, Cadbury*	1 Bar/40g	206	13.2	516	16	34	33	10
Nutty Nougat Caramel, Tesco*	1 Bar/40g	200	11.1	490	8.7	52.7	27.2	3.8
Nutty, Snack Size, Asda*	1 Bar/38g	182	9.5	479	9	54	25	0.9
Oat Boost, Cocoa & Orange , Graze*	1 Bar/30g	139	7.5	464	6.6	51	25	17
Oat Millionaire, Orange, & Dark Cacao, Graze*	1 Bar/50g	188	7	376	21	38	14	6.6
Oat, Apple & Cinnamon, Nairn's*	1 Bar/40g	169	7.1	422	7	54.7	17.7	8
Oat, Berry & Vanilla, Mini, Graze*	1 Bite/30g	136	6.3	452	12	51	21	5.3
Oat, Blueberry, & Yoghurt, Sainsbury's*	1 Bar/40g	161	5.8	404	7	56.8	14.5	9
Oat, Cacao, & Orange, Nairn's*	1 Bar/40g	171	7.5	427	7.2	53.5	18.7	7.9
Oat, Chewy, Strawberry, Super Snackers, Graze*	1 Bar/23g	97	3.9	423	6.1	59	17	20
Oat, Choc Chip & Raisin, Mini, Graze*	1 Bite/30g	140	7.6	477	11	53	26	6.2
Oat, Chocolate Chip, Freee, Dove's Farm*	1 Bar/35g	141	6.4	402	6.6	46	18.2	13.6
Oat, Peanut Butter, Deliciously Ella *	1 Bar/50g	230	11.8	460	10.2	50	23.6	5
Oats, Seeds, & Berries, M&S*	1 Bar/30g	128	5.3	427	14.5	47	17.6	11.1
Oaty, Carrot, Orange, Kellogg's*	1 Bar/22g	87	2.9	395	7.2	60	13	5.2
Orange, & Cacao, Dark, Millionaire, Graze*	1 Bar/50g	188	7	376	21	38	14	6.6
Original, Seed, Nine*	1 Bar/40g	221	16	552	16.6	26.7	40.1	9.3
Peach, & Apricot, Special K, Kellogg's*	1 Bar/23g	90	1.4	383	8	75	6	2.5
Peanut Butter Crunch, Power, Trek, Natural Balance Foods*	1 Bar/55g	229	10.4	416	28.3	27.1	18.9	12.1
Peanut Butter Crunch, Trek, Natural Balance Foods*	1 Bar/55g	229	10.4	416	28.3	27.1	18.9	12.1
Peanut Butter, Breakfast, Bounce*	1 Bar/45g	168	7.2	374	22	27	16	16
Peanut Butter, Dark Chocolate, Multipack, Kind*	1 Bar/30g	158	10.2	525	18	33	34	7.5
Peanut Butter, Hi-Fi, Slimming World*	1 Bar/20g	73	2.4	367	8	47	12	19
Peanut Butter, High Protein, Aldi*	1 Bar/60g	223	9.4	372	36	23.1	15.7	11.4
Peanut Chocolish, Nakd*	1 Bar/35g	141	6.9	403	7.5	49.8	19.7	6
Peanut Crunch, Organic, Rude Health*	1 Bar/25g	145	9.9	578	19.3	32.6	39.5	7.7
Peanut, & Almond, in Milk Chocolate, Nuttier, Cadbury*	1 Bar/40g	206	13.2	516	16	34	33	10
Peanut, & Caramel, Milka*	1 Bar/37g	200	12.2	540	9.2	51	33	2.3
Peanut, & Caramel, Tracker, Mars*	1 Bar/26g	113	4.9	436	8.6	51.3	18.9	13
Peanut, & Choco, Minis, Lidl*	1 Bar/22g	108	5.3	491	9.1	58.2	24.1	2.7
Peanut, & Choco, Mister Choc, Lidl*	1 Bar/38g	191	10.6	502	9.5	52	28	0
Peanut, & Dark Chocolate, Tesco*	1 Bar/35g	175	10.4	500	22.2	33	29.7	6
Peanut, & Date, Breakfast, M&S*	1 Bar/40g	171	9.5	428	22.8	19.5	23.8	21.8
Peanut, & Ginger, Snack, Love Vegan*	1 Bar/33g	150	8.9	456	14.3	38.6	26.9	5.4
Peanut, Caramel, Payday, Hershey*	1 Bar/19g	88	4.8	462	13.5	51.9	25	3.8
Peanut, Crispy, Lighter Life*	1 Bar/46g	154	4	334	27.5	35.3	8.6	12.4
Peanut, Crispy, Meal Replacement, CWP*	1 Bar/55g	206	6.9	374	24.3	40.5	12.6	7.8
Peanut, Crunchy, Foodspring*	1 Bar/65g	228	9.8	351	31	30	15	9
Peanut, Mr Toms*	1 Bar/40g	210	13	525	20	42.5	32.5	2.5
Peanut, Nature Bake*	1 Bar/30g	182	14	610	26	17	47	7
Peanut, Nutty Crunch, Go Ahead, McVitie's*	1 Bar/20g	94	4.8	483	11	52.8	24.6	3.6
Peanut, Protein, Energy Ball, Bounce*	1 Ball/35g	159	8.2	453	27.7	29.9	23.4	6
Peanut, Sweet & Salty Nut, Nature Valley*	1 Bar/30g	143	7.8	478	12.3	43.1	26.1	11
Peanuts, & Pumpkin Seeds, Harvest Morn, Aldi*	1 Bar/30g	136	7.2	452	27	25	24	16
Peanuts, Coconut, & Chocolate, Vegan, Eat Natural*	1 Bar/45g	223	13.5	496	11.9	40.4	30	7.8
Pecan, Hazelnut & Cocoa, Adonis*	1 Bar/35g	178	15.7	509	7.9	17	44.8	22.9
Pecan, Pie, GF, Nak'd*	1 Bar/35g	156	10.3	477	7.6	36.4	31.4	8.9
Pineapple, & Cashew Nut, Tropical Wholefoods*	1 Bar/40g	146	3.8	366	5.6	62	9.4	4.7
Popcorn, Milk chocolate, Fibre Now, Harvest Morn, Aldi*	1 Bar/21g	80	2.8	380	5.8	46.2	13.2	26.8
Popcorn, Peanut Butter, Fibre One*	1 Bar/21g	90	4.3	427	7.6	41.4	20.3	23.9
Popcorn, Peanut, & Sunflower, Asda*	1 Bar/20g	90	4.4	448	8.6	45	22	16
Popcorn, Salted Caramel, Almond, Pretzel, Aldi*	1 Bar/20g	93	4.7	465	8.5	47	23.5	14.5

BARS

INFO/WEIGHT	Measure	per Measure KCAL	FAT	Nutrition Values per 100g / 100ml KCAL	PROT	CARB	FAT	FIBRE
Porridge Oat, Merry Berry, Blackfriars*	1 Bar/50g	192	6	385	5.4	58	12	11
Protein, Caramel Chaos, Carb Killa, Grenade*	1 Bar/60g	214	7.9	357	38.7	22.5	13.2	11.1
Protein, Caramel, Protein One, Fibre One*	1 Bar/24g	87	2.4	363	41.8	17.9	10.1	16.8
Protein, Cherry Bakewell, Tribe*	1 Bar/46g	213	12.9	464	20	29	28	12
Protein, Chocolate Brownie, GF, Quest*	1 Bar/60g	191	7.2	318	33	12	12	25
Protein, Chocolate Caramel, Pas Nutrition *	1 Bar/65g	237	7.2	365	31	29	11	12
Protein, Chocolate, Coconut, Rxbar*	1 Bar/52g	211	9.2	406	23.1	34.6	17.7	7.7
Protein, Chocolate, Coconut, Vegan, Bulk*	1 Bar/75g	279	11	372	28	22.7	14.7	14.7
Protein, Chocolate, Peanut Butter, Rxbar*	1 Bar/52g	205	8	394	23.1	36.5	15.4	8.1
Protein, Chocolate, Peanut, Asda*	1 Bar/55g	212	10.4	386	33	25	19	6.2
Protein, Chocolate, Peanut, Vegan, The Protein Works*	1 Bar/48g	203	9.6	422	32	20	20	17
Protein, Chocolate, Sea Salt, Rxbar*	1 Bar/52g	207	8.8	398	23.1	34.6	16.9	7.5
Protein, Cinnamon Roll, GF, Quest*	1 Bar/60g	191	7.2	318	33	16	12	23
Protein, Coconut, Cocoa, & Cashew, Special K, Kellogg's*	1 Bar/28g	118	4.5	423	23	44	16	5.6
Protein, Cookies & Cream, Asda*	1 Bar/60g	221	7.2	368	49	24	12	0
Protein, Cookies & Cream, Barebells*	1 Bar/55g	199	6.7	358	36	30	12	6.1
Protein, Cookies & Cream, Fulfil*	1 Bar/55g	208	9.3	379	36.4	14.9	16.9	20.8
Protein, Cookies & Cream, GF, Quest*	1 Bar/60g	209	9	349	35	12	15	23
Protein, Crispy Coconut, Foodspring*	1 Bar/65g	225	9	346	30.9	30.7	13.9	8.2
Protein, Crunchy Fudge, Barebells*	1 Bar/55g	204	8.2	370	36	33	15	5.1
Protein, Dark Chocolate, & Mint, Carb Killa, Grenade*	1 Bar/60g	214	8.5	357	36.8	22.6	14.2	11.6
Protein, Dark Chocolate, & Raspberry, Grenade*	1 Bar/60g	233	10.2	388	33	31	17	5.6
Protein, Gooey, Salted Caramel, Pro2go*	1 Bar/60g	199	4.3	331	37	32	7.1	7.6
Protein, Lemon Curd, White Chocolate, Barebells*	1 Bar/55g	205	7.7	372	36	33	14	5.8
Protein, Millionaire Shortbread, Power, Trek*	1 Bar/55g	224	9.9	408	28.1	27.3	18	12.7
Protein, Oats & Honey, Soft Baked, Nature Valley*	1 Bar/38g	154	5.9	404	22	43.5	15.5	7.8
Protein, Peanut & Caramel, Protein, Nutramino*	1 Bar/60g	236	11.4	393	35	31	19	0
Protein, Peanut Butter, Crisp, Optimum Nutrition*	1 Bar/65g	215	7.2	330	31	24	11	20
Protein, Peanut Crunch, BSN*	1 Bar/60g	209	7.2	349	33	38	12	3.9
Protein, Salted Peanut, Caramel, Weider*	1 Bar/45g	167	4.6	372	60	16	10.2	0
Protein, Vegan, Smart, PhD Nutrition*	1 Bar/64g	259	13	405	32.8	11.9	20.3	21.9
Protien, Caramel Crunch Brownie, Awesom*	1 Bar/60g	259	11.2	432	31.2	26.1	18.6	17.7
Pumpkin Seed, & Almond, Tesco*	1 Bar/35g	204	15.8	582	20	21	45	6.6
Quinoa, Goji, & Cranberry, Perkier*	1 Bar/35g	129	3.9	370	12.7	51.1	11.2	10.1
Raisin, & Hazelnut, Protein, Asda*	1 Bar/28g	120	4.8	427	17	48	17	7.7
Raisin, Munch, Tesco*	1 Bar/32g	135	4.1	423	6.2	68	13	4.7
Raisin, Munchy, Dairyfine, Aldi*	1 Bar/32g	132	3.8	413	5.5	69	12	4.2
Raspberry Cheesecake, Macro Munch, Bulk*	1 Bar/62g	224	8.1	362	32	34	13	11
Raspberry Crisp, Nu+cao*	1 Bar/40g	248	20	621	12.1	27	50.1	6.7
Raspberry Crunch, Protein, Weight Watchers*	1 Bar/23g	68	2.5	297	21.9	49.8	10.9	9.7
Raspberry, & Almond Butter, M&S*	1 Bar/35g	130	3.9	372	8.7	56.9	11.2	4.2
Raspberry, & White Chocolate, Tesco*	1 Bar/60g	200	6.6	333	26	43.5	11	4.6
Raspberry, Chocolish, Nakd*	1 Bar/35g	137	6.4	392	6.2	53.9	18.4	5.3
Raspberry, Meringue, Flower & White*	1 Bar/24g	96	3.1	410	4	68	13	0
Raw Choc Brownie, Keto, Boostball *	1 Ball/25g	65	6	258	5.2	4.2	23.7	4.5
Rice Krispies, Snack, Kellogg's*	1 Bar/20g	83	2	415	7	70	10	0.5
Rice Krispies, Squares, Totally Chocolatey, Kellogg's*	1 Bar/36g	156	5.3	439	4.5	72	15	1.5
Rocky Road, M&S*	1 Bar/68g	330	18	486	4.1	56.7	26.5	1.9
Rocky Road, Skinny Dream*	1 Bar/20g	70	1.8	352	4.9	49	8.8	29
Rocky Road, Skinny Whip*	1 Bar/20g	70	1.8	350	24.5	49	9	145
Salted Caramel , Warrior Crunch*	1 Bar/64g	239	10.2	374	31	38	16	0
Salted Caramel Drizzle, Squares, Fibre One*	1 Square/24g	82	3.1	342	3.3	42.9	12.9	27.5
Salted Caramel, Dark Chocolate Coated, Vive*	1 Bar/50g	219	13	438	21	28	26	13

	Measure INFO/WEIGHT	per Measure KCAL	FAT	Nutrition Values per 100g / 100ml KCAL	PROT	CARB	FAT	FIBRE
BARS								
Salted Caramel, Exante Diet*	1 Bar/60g	207	6.1	345	26.7	38.3	10.2	9
Salted Caramel, Fruit & Nut, Protein, Deluxe, Lidl*	1 Bar/45g	231	14.3	514	26.7	28.3	31.7	4.2
Salted Caramel, Hi-Protein, Mars*	1 Bar/59g	209	4.9	355	33	39	8.3	0
Salted Caramel, High Protein, Musclefood*	1 Bar/45g	117	2.7	259	24.7	28.3	5.9	20.7
Salted Caramel, Lighter Life*	1 Bar/60g	210	6.3	350	24.2	34.2	10.5	16.5
Salted Caramel, Meringue, Flower & White*	1 Bar/24g	75	1.9	318	4	58	8	0
Salted Caramel, Munch, Tesco*	1 Bar/32g	133	3.8	416	6.8	68	12	4.2
Salted Caramel, Tru, The Foodie Market, Aldi*	1 Bar/35g	138	4.9	393	7.6	57	14	6.8
Salted Caramel, Whip, Bliss*	1 Bar/25g	97	2.2	389	3.4	66	8.8	18
Salted Caramel, Wow Bakes, Graze*	1 Bar/24g	86	1.9	360	6	62	7.8	18
Salted Peanut, Carb Killa, Grenade*	1 Bar/60g	242	12	403	33	32	20	4.1
Salty Caramel, Nut, Crunchy, Keto Bar*	1 Bar/35g	126	6	360	27.3	19.9	17.1	27.3
Seed, Salted Caramel, Nine*	1 Bar/49g	260	18.6	531	16.8	24.9	38	11.1
Sesame Crunch, Organic, Rude Health*	1 Bar/25g	156	11	622	18.4	28.8	43.7	8.7
Sesame Snaps, Anglo-Dal*	1 Bar/30g	157	8.8	522	12.2	49.4	29.4	0
Sesame Snaps, in Chocolate, Anglo-Dal*	1 Bar/40g	211	11.9	527	9.3	55.6	29.7	0
Shortcake, Caramel, Deluxe, Lidl*	1 Bar/40g	198	11.2	494	4.9	55	28	1.4
Snack, Dreamy Caramel, Tesco*	1 Bar/40g	185	7.8	462	4.3	66.9	19.5	1
Snack, Milk Chocolate, & Golden Syrup, McVitie's*	1 Bar/30g	128	4	420	6.2	68.1	13.2	4.7
Snack, Peanut Butter, Skinny Crunch*	1 Bar/20g	68	2.7	340	7	36	13.5	24.5
Sos Berry Boost, Juicemaster*	1 Bar/55g	210	8.2	381	8.2	50	15	6.3
Sticky Toffee, Snack, Skinny Crunch*	1 Bar/20g	63	1.8	316	3.8	52.9	8.9	24
Strawberry Sundae, Nakd*	1 Bar/35g	130	4.6	371	7.1	54.4	13	4
Strawberry, & Vanilla, Vitamin & Protein, Fulfil Nutrition*	1 Bar/60g	185	4.9	309	33.4	10.1	8.2	33.1
Strawberry, & Chocolate, Skinny Whip*	1 Bar/25g	96	2.3	385	3.7	64	9.3	15
Strawberry, & Coconut, Porridge Oat, Stoats*	1 Bar/22g	92	3	416	7.5	62.1	13.7	8.8
Strawberry, Fruit & Oat Bakes, Go Ahead*	1 Bar/35g	129	2.7	369	2.8	73.4	7.8	4.2
Strawberry, Fruit Bakes, Go Ahead, McVitie's*	1 Bar/35g	131	3	375	3.5	72	8.5	4
Tiffin, GF, Free From, Co-Op*	1 Bar/62g	321	19.8	518	3.2	53	32	4
Toffee Apple, Super Snackers, Graze*	1 Bar/23g	97	3.9	422	6.2	59	17	21
Toffee, & Chocolate, Snack, Skinny Whip*	1 Bar/25g	96	2.3	384	3.6	64	9.2	15.2
White Chocolate, & Lemon, Whip, Bliss*	1 Bar/25g	96	2.2	384	2.9	70	8.9	6
White Chocolate, & Raspberry, Whip, Bliss*	1 Bar/25g	96	2	386	2.1	73	8.2	6
BASA								
Fillet, Smoked, Fishmongers Selection, Asda*	1 Fillet/115g	133	3.1	116	23	0	2.7	0
Fillet, Tempura Battered, Lemon & Herb, Gastro, Youngs*	1 Fillet/145g	240	9.6	165	16.3	9.4	6.6	0.3
Fillets, Lemon & Herb, The Tasty Catch Co., Aldi*	1 Fillet/148g	237	9.8	160	16	8.8	6.6	1.2
Fillets, Sea Salt & Cracked Black Pepper, Gastro, Youngs*	1 Fillet/151g	261	12.1	173	14.7	10.5	8	0.3
Fillets, Skinless & Boneless, Aldi*	1 Fillet/120g	140	2.9	117	23.7	0.1	2.4	0
Fillets, Skinless, & Boneless, Raw, Tesco*	1 Fillet/133g	116	2.5	87	17.4	0	1.9	0
Fillets, Smoked, Skinless, Tesco*	1 Fillet/125g	112	2.8	90	17.5	0	2.2	0
Fillets, Tempura Battered, Lemon & Herb, Grilled, Iceland*	1 Fillet/155g	279	11.8	180	15.4	12	7.6	1
BATTER MIX								
As Sold, Sainsbury's*	½ Pack/128g	588	21.7	461	17	59.3	17	4.7
for Yorkshire Puddings & Pancakes, Tesco*	1 Serving/17g	34	0.3	200	2.3	43.3	1.5	2.5
for Yorkshire Puddings, Baked, Aunt Bessie's*	1 Pudding/13g	48	1.1	356	9.8	34	8.1	2.3
BAY LEAVES								
Dried, Average	*1 Tsp/0.6g*	*2*	*0.1*	*313*	*7.6*	*48.6*	*8.4*	*0*
BEAN SPROUTS								
Mung, Raw, Average	*1oz/28g*	*9*	*0.1*	*31*	*2.9*	*4*	*0.5*	*1.5*
Mung, Stir-Fried in Blended Oil, Average	*1 Serving/90g*	*65*	*5.5*	*72*	*1.9*	*2.5*	*6.1*	*0.9*
Raw, Average	*1 Serving/150g*	*55*	*2.6*	*37*	*2.2*	*3.2*	*1.8*	*1.2*

		per Measure		Nutrition Values per 100g / 100ml				
Measure INFO/WEIGHT		KCAL	FAT	KCAL	PROT	CARB	FAT	FIBRE
BEANS								
Aduki, Cooked in Unsalted Water, Average	1 Tbsp/30g	37	0.1	123	9.3	22.5	0.2	5.5
Aduki, Dried, Raw	1 Tbsp/30g	82	0.2	272	19.9	50.1	0.5	11.1
Baked, & Sausages, Canned, Morrisons*	1 Can/400g	460	15.6	115	5.5	12.9	3.9	3.1
Baked, & Sausages, Vegan, Suma*	½ Can/200g	224	6.6	112	8	10	3.3	5
Baked, Barbecue, Beanz, Heinz*	1 Can/390g	343	0.8	88	4.9	14.6	0.2	3.8
Baked, Curried, Average	½ Can/210g	203	1.9	96	4.8	17.2	0.9	3.6
Baked, Five, in Tomato Sauce, Heinz*	1 Can/415g	361	0.8	87	5.4	13.6	0.2	4.3
Baked, Giant, in Tomato Sauce, Cypressa*	1 Can/280g	398	18.8	142	6	10.8	6.7	7
Baked, in Tomato Sauce, Average	1 Can/400g	318	1.6	80	4.6	13.9	0.4	3.7
Baked, in Tomato Sauce, Reduced Sugar & Salt	½ Can/210g	159	0.7	76	4.6	13.6	0.3	3.8
Baked, with Sausages, in Tomato Sauce, Corale, Aldi*	1 Can/400g	412	11.6	103	5.2	12	2.9	3.5
Barbecue, Good Grains, Worldwide Foods, Aldi*	1 Pack/256g	264	3.1	103	5.5	15	1.2	5
Black, Cooked, Average	1 Cup/172g	227	0.9	132	8.8	23.7	0.5	8.7
Borlotti, Canned, Average	1oz/28g	29	0.1	103	7.6	16.9	0.5	4.7
Borlotti, Dried, Raw, Average	1 Serving/100g	335	1.2	335	23	60	1.2	24.7
Brazilian, Smoky, Protein By Nature, Whitworths*	1 Pouch/250g	252	1	101	8.3	13.2	0.4	5.6
Broad, Canned, Drained, Average	1 Can/195g	136	1.1	70	6.9	9.2	0.6	6.8
Broad, Dried, Raw, Average	1oz/28g	69	0.6	245	26.1	32.5	2.1	27.6
Broad, Fresh, without Pod, Boiled, Average	1 Serving/80g	78	0.5	97	7.9	11.7	0.6	6.5
Broad, Frozen, Average	1 Serving/80g	63	0.6	79	7.6	10.8	0.7	5.3
Butter, Canned, Drained, Average	1oz/28g	23	0.1	81	6	12.8	0.5	4.3
Butter, Dried, Boiled, Average	1oz/28g	30	0.2	106	7.2	18.6	0.6	5.2
Butter, Dried, Raw, Average	1oz/28g	81	0.2	290	19.1	52.9	1.7	16
Cannellini, Canned, Drained, Average	1 Portion/80g	75	0.4	94	8.7	15	0.5	5.7
Chilli, Canned, Average	1 Can/420g	381	3.1	91	5.2	15.8	0.7	4.4
Edamame, Lightly Salted, Taiko Foods*	1 Pack/150g	132	3.9	88	6.9	3.6	2.6	11.1
Edamame, Sainsbury's*	1 Serving/150g	212	9.6	141	12.3	6.8	6.4	4.2
Five, Canned, in Tomato Sauce, Sainsbury's*	½ Can/200g	168	1	84	4.9	12.4	0.5	5.4
Flageolet, Canned, Average	1 Can/265g	235	1.6	89	6.8	14	0.6	3.5
French, Boiled, Average	1 Serving/150g	38	0	25	2.3	3.8	0	3.7
French, Raw	1oz/28g	6	0.1	20	1.6	2.7	0.4	1.8
Green, Cut, Average	1oz/28g	7	0.1	24	1.7	3.6	0.2	2.7
Green, Fine, Average	1 Serving/75g	18	0.3	24	1.8	3.2	0.4	2.9
Green, Sliced, Average	1oz/28g	6	0.1	23	1.9	3.5	0.2	2.1
Green, Sliced, Frozen, Average	1 Serving/50g	13	0	26	1.8	4.4	0.1	4.1
Green, Whole, Average	1oz/28g	6	0.1	22	1.6	3	0.4	1.7
Haricot, Canned, Average	1 Can/400g	307	2	77	6.2	10.7	0.5	5.9
Haricot, Dried, Average	1 Serving/80g	281	1.2	351	22.3	60.8	1.5	24.4
Kidney, Red, Canned, Drained, Average	½ Can/120g	115	0.7	96	7.4	20.7	0.5	5.5
Kidney, Red, Dried, Boiled in Unsalted Water	1oz/28g	29	0.1	103	8.4	17.4	0.5	6.7
Kidney, Red, Dried, Raw	1oz/28g	74	0.4	266	22.1	44.1	1.4	15.7
Mixed, Canned, Average	1 Can/300g	300	3.5	100	6.8	15.6	1.2	4.1
Mixed, in Mild Chilli Sauce, Sainsbury's*	1 Can/420g	328	1.3	78	4.9	13.8	0.3	3.7
Mung, Whole, Dried, Boiled in Unsalted Water	1oz/28g	25	0.1	91	7.6	15.3	0.4	3
Mung, Whole, Dried, Raw	1oz/28g	78	0.3	279	23.9	46.3	1.1	10
Pinto, Dried, Boiled in Unsalted Water	1oz/28g	38	0.2	137	8.9	23.9	0.7	0
Pinto, Dried, Raw	1oz/28g	92	0.4	327	21.1	57.1	1.6	14
Refried, Average	1 Serving/215g	162	1.5	76	4.6	12.7	0.7	1.8
Runner, Average	1 Serving/80g	15	0.3	19	1.3	2.8	0.4	2.2
Soya, Dried, Boiled in Unsalted Water	1oz/28g	39	2	141	14	5.1	7.3	6.1
Soya, Shelled, Frozen, Raw, Average	1 Serving/80g	99	4.3	124	12.2	6.9	5.3	4.4
BEEF								
Brisket, Boiled, Lean	1 Serving/100g	225	11	225	31.4	0	11	0

B

BEEF

INFO/WEIGHT	Measure	per Measure KCAL	FAT	Nutrition Values per 100g / 100ml KCAL	PROT	CARB	FAT	FIBRE
Brisket, Boiled, Lean & Fat	1 Serving/100g	268	17.4	268	27.8	0	17.4	0
Brisket, Braised, Lean	1 Serving/100g	280	17.4	280	29	0	17.4	0
Brisket, Raw, Lean	1oz/28g	39	1.7	139	21.1	0	6.1	0
Brisket, Raw, Lean & Fat	1oz/28g	60	4.4	216	18.2	0	15.8	0
British, Slow Cooked, Peppery, Tender, M&S*	½ Pack/234g	250	6.8	107	17.8	2.3	2.9	0
Carpaccio, Parmesam, & Extra Virgin Olive Oil, Lidl*	1 Pack/120g	241	16.7	201	18.3	0.6	13.9	0
Cheeks, Ox, Aberdeen Angus, Waitrose*	1 Serving/100g	123	4.6	123	22	0	4.6	0
Diced, Casserole, Lean, Average	1oz/28g	35	1.1	126	23	0	3.8	0
Escalope, Healthy Range, Average	1 Serving/170g	233	6.7	137	24.2	1.2	4	0.4
Flank, Pot-Roasted, Lean	1oz/28g	71	3.9	253	31.8	0	14	0
Flank, Raw, Lean	1oz/28g	49	2.6	175	22.7	0	9.3	0
Fore Rib, Lean & Fat, Average	1oz/28g	40	1.8	144	21.7	0	6.2	0.2
Fore Rib, Raw, Lean	1oz/28g	41	1.8	145	21.5	0	6.5	0
Fore Rib, Roasted, Lean	1oz/28g	66	3.2	236	33.3	0	11.4	0
Fore Rib, Roasted, Lean & Fat	1oz/28g	84	5.7	300	29.1	0	20.4	0
Grill Steak, Average	1 Steak/170g	501	39.5	295	19.3	2.1	23.2	0.1
Grill Steak, Peppered, Average	1 Serving/172g	419	24.4	244	23.6	5.2	14.2	0.3
Joint, for Roasting, Average	1oz/28g	38	1	134	24.5	1.4	3.4	0.2
Joint, Sirloin, Roasted, Lean	1oz/28g	53	1.8	188	32.4	0	6.5	0
Joint, Sirloin, Roasted, Lean & Fat	1oz/28g	65	3.5	233	29.8	0	12.6	0
Mince, Cooked, Average	1 Serving/75g	214	15.3	286	24	0	20.3	0
Mince, Extra Lean, Raw, Average	1 Serving/100g	124	5	124	21.2	0.1	5	0
Mince, Extra Lean, Stewed	1oz/28g	50	2.4	177	24.7	0	8.7	0
Mince, Lean, Raw, Average	1oz/28g	48	2.8	172	20.8	0	10	0.1
Mince, Raw, Average	1oz/28g	68	5.1	242	19.6	0.2	18.1	0
Mince, Raw, Frozen, Average	1 Serving/100g	176	10	176	20.4	0	10	0
Mince, Steak, Extra Lean, Average	1oz/28g	37	1.6	131	20.5	0.4	5.6	0
Mince, Steak, Raw, Average	1 Serving/125g	318	25	254	17.2	0	20	0
Mince, Stewed	1oz/28g	59	3.8	209	21.8	0	13.5	0
Peppered, Sliced, Average	1 Slice/20g	26	1.1	129	18.2	1.3	5.6	1
Potted, Binghams*	1 Serving/30g	76	6.6	254	13.8	1	22	0.6
Roast, Sliced, Average	1 Slice/35g	48	1.3	136	26.1	0.4	3.6	0.2
Salt, Average	1 Serving/70g	80	1.7	114	21.7	1	2.5	0.1
Salted, Dried, Raw	1oz/28g	70	0.4	250	55.4	0	1.5	0
Silverside, Pot-Roasted, Lean	1oz/28g	54	1.8	193	34	0	6.3	0
Silverside, Pot-Roasted, Lean & Fat	1oz/28g	69	3.8	247	31	0	13.7	0
Silverside, Raw, Lean	1oz/28g	38	1.2	134	23.8	0	4.3	0
Silverside, Raw, Lean & Fat	1oz/28g	60	4.1	213	20.2	0	14.7	0
Silverside, Salted, Boiled, Lean	1oz/28g	52	1.9	184	30.4	0	6.9	0
Silverside, Salted, Raw, Lean	1oz/28g	39	2	140	19.2	0	7	0
Silverside, Salted, Raw, Lean & Fat	1oz/28g	64	5	227	16.3	0	18	0
Sliced, Cooked, From Supermarket, Average	1 Slice/35g	47	1.2	135	23.6	2	3.5	0.5
Steak, 8oz Rump & Chips	1 Serving/466g	870	41.1	187	10.7	16.2	8.8	0
Steak, Braising, Braised, Lean	1oz/28g	63	2.7	225	34.4	0	9.7	0
Steak, Braising, Lean, Raw, Average	1oz/28g	40	1.4	144	24.8	0	5	0
Steak, Braising, Raw, Lean & Fat	1oz/28g	44	2.4	158	20.5	0	8.5	0
Steak, Economy, Average	1oz/28g	53	2.4	190	26.9	1.2	8.7	0.4
Steak, Fillet, Cooked, Average	1oz/28g	54	2.4	191	28.6	0	8.5	0
Steak, Fillet, Lean, Average	1oz/28g	42	2	150	21	0	7.3	0
Steak, Fillet, Lean, Cooked, Average	1oz/28g	52	2.2	186	28.6	0	8	0
Steak, Frying, Average	1 Steak/110g	128	2.7	116	23.7	0	2.5	0
Steak, Rump, Cooked, Average	1oz/28g	69	4	246	29.1	0.5	14.1	0
Steak, Rump, Grilled, Rare, Lean	1 Steak/227g	381	15.6	168	26.5	0	6.9	0

	Measure INFO/WEIGHT	per Measure KCAL	FAT	Nutrition Values per 100g / 100ml KCAL	PROT	CARB	FAT	FIBRE
BEEF								
Steak, Rump, Lean, Cooked, Average	1oz/28g	50	1.7	179	31	0	6.1	0
Steak, Rump, Picanha, Cooked, Average	1 Serving/100g	225	14.7	225	22.5	0.5	14.7	0.5
Steak, Rump, Raw, Lean & Fat	1oz/28g	49	2.8	174	20.7	0	10.1	0
Steak, Rump, Raw, Lean, Average	1 Steak/175g	219	7.2	125	22	0	4.1	0
Steak, Sirloin, Fried, Rare, Lean	1oz/28g	53	2.3	189	28.8	0	8.2	0
Steak, Sirloin, Fried, Rare, Lean & Fat	1oz/28g	65	3.9	231	26.5	0	13.9	0
Steak, Sirloin, Grilled, Medium-Rare, Lean	1oz/28g	49	2.2	176	26.6	0	7.7	0
Steak, Sirloin, Grilled, Medium-Rare, Lean & Fat	1oz/28g	59	3.5	211	24.6	0	12.5	0
Steak, Sirloin, Grilled, Rare, Lean	1oz/28g	46	1.9	166	26.4	0	6.7	0
Steak, Sirloin, Grilled, Well-Done, Lean	1oz/28g	63	2.8	225	33.9	0	9.9	0
Steak, Sirloin, Grilled, Well-Done, Lean & Fat	1oz/28g	71	4	254	31.5	0	14.3	0
Steak, Sirloin, Raw, Lean & Fat	1oz/28g	56	3.6	201	21.6	0	12.7	0
Steak, Sirloin, Raw, Lean, Average	1 Steak/150g	202	6.8	135	23.5	0	4.5	0
Stewed Steak, Average	1 Serving/220g	258	10.1	117	15.8	3.3	4.6	0
Stewing Steak, Lean & Fat, Raw, Average	1 Serving/100g	136	4.3	136	24.2	0.1	4.3	0.1
Stewing Steak, Raw, Lean	1oz/28g	34	1	122	22.6	0	3.5	0
Stewing Steak, Stewed, Lean	1oz/28g	52	1.8	185	32	0	6.3	0
Stewing Steak, Stewed, Lean & Fat	1oz/28g	57	2.7	203	29.2	0	9.6	0
Stir Fry Strips, Raw, Average	1 Serving/125g	149	3.8	119	23	0	3	0.2
Topside, Lean & Fat, Raw, Average	1oz/28g	55	3.6	198	20.4	0	12.9	0
Topside, Raw, Lean	1oz/28g	32	0.8	116	23	0	2.7	0
Vegan, No Beef, Teriyaki, Strips, Plant Menu, Aldi*	½ Pack/90g	181	6.8	201	15.4	14.6	7.5	7.1
Vegan, Steak, Fillet, Vegan Butcherie*	1 Serving/100g	161	8.2	161	5	16.3	8.2	3.2
Vegetarian, Slices, Peppered Style, Quorn*	¼ Pack/25g	29	0.5	115	14.5	7.6	2.1	4
Wafer Thin Sliced, Cooked, Average	1 Slice/10g	13	0.3	129	24.5	0.5	3.2	0.2
BEEF BOURGUIGNON								
Finest, Tesco*	½ Pack/300g	247	7.8	82	9.9	4.8	2.6	0.5
Gastropub, M&S*	½ Pack/294g	315	12.9	107	13.3	3.3	4.4	0.7
No.1, Waitrose*	½ Pack/310g	375	19.5	121	11.2	3.7	6.3	2.5
Slow Cooked, Finest, Tesco*	½ Pack/249g	259	6.7	104	16	3.5	2.7	0.7
BEEF DINNER								
Microwaved, Asda*	1 Pack/364g	306	5.8	84	4.8	12	1.6	2.2
Roast with Trimmings, Average	1 Dinner/840g	1310	63	156	6.1	17.7	7.5	2.3
Roast, Chef Select, Lidl*	1 Pack/350g	322	11.6	92	6.5	7.6	3.3	3
Roast, Frozen, Tesco*	1 Serving/400g	340	6.4	85	5.9	10.8	1.6	2.3
Roast, Oven Cooked, Morrisons*	1 Pack/380g	361	8.7	95	8.5	9.4	2.3	1.4
Roast, What's Cooking?, Lidl*	1 Pack/400g	328	6.4	82	5.3	10.5	1.6	2.4
BEEF RAGU								
Superquick, with Penne Pasta, & Spinach, Hello Fresh*	1 Serving/650g	838	26	129	7.5	15.1	4	0
with Rigatoni Pasta, Chianti, BFY, M&S*	1 Pack/370g	492	15.9	133	10.2	12.6	4.3	1.4
BEEF VEGETARIAN								
Strips, No Beef, Taste & Glory*	½ Pack/83g	121	3.3	146	22	2.1	4	6.6
BEEF WELLINGTON								
Average	1 Serving/200g	530	33.3	265	12.4	17	16.6	1
BEER								
Ale, 1698, Kentish Strong, Shepherd Neame*	1 Bottle/500ml	285	0	57	0.4	4.8	0	0
Ale, American Pale, Low Tide, 0.5%, Shipyard*	1 Bottle/500ml	85	0	17	0.3	3.2	0	0
Ale, Bottled, Old Speckled Hen*	1 Bottle/330ml	124	0.3	38	0.2	1.8	0.1	0.2
Ale, Gem, 4.1%, Bath Ales*	1 Bottle/500ml	215	1	43	0.4	3.2	0.2	0.5
Ale, Hoppy, Nanny State, Alcohol Free, BrewDog*	1 Bottle/330ml	20	0.3	6	0.1	1.2	0.1	0
Ale, IPA, Punk AF, Alcohol Free, Brewdog *	1 Can/330ml	50	0	15	0	3	0	0
Ale, Low Alcohol, Nanny State, BrewDog*	1 Bottle/330ml	20	0.3	6	0.1	1	0.1	0
Ale, Low Alcohol, Old Speckled Hen*	1 Bottle/500ml	110	0.5	22	0.4	4.1	0.1	0

B

BEER

INFO/WEIGHT	Measure INFO/WEIGHT	per Measure KCAL	FAT	Nutrition Values per 100g / 100ml KCAL	PROT	CARB	FAT	FIBRE
Ale, Old Speckled Hen*	1 Pint/568ml	185	0.6	32	0.2	1.6	0.1	0.2
Ale, Pale, IPA, Greene King*	1 Pint/568ml	157	0.1	28	0.2	1.6	0	0.1
Ale, Pale, IPA, Innis & Gunn*	1 Bottle/330ml	162	0	49	0.3	4.6	0	0
Ale, Pale, IPA, TTD, Sainsbury's*	½ Bottle/250ml	128	0	51	0.5	4.4	0	0.5
Ale, Punk IPA, 5.4% ABV, BrewDog*	1 Bottle/330ml	158	0	48	0	4.7	0	0
Argus, Lidl*	1 Bottle/250ml	200	0	80	0	0	0	0
Becks Blue Lemon, No Alcohol, Beck & Co*	1 Bottle/1196ml	275	0.1	23	0.2	6	0	0
Bitter, Average	*1 Can/440ml*	*141*	*0*	*32*	*0.3*	*2.3*	*0*	*0*
Bitter, Draught, Average	*1 Pint/568ml*	*182*	*0*	*32*	*0.3*	*2.3*	*0*	*0*
Bitter, Keg, Average	*1 Pint/568ml*	*176*	*0*	*31*	*0.3*	*2.3*	*0*	*0*
Bitter, Low Alcohol, Average	*1 Pint/568ml*	*74*	*0*	*13*	*0.2*	*2.1*	*0*	*0*
Brown Ale, Bottled, Average	*1 Bottle/330ml*	*99*	*0*	*30*	*0.3*	*3*	*0*	*0*
Brune, Leffe*	1 Bottle/330ml	184	0	56	0.5	11.3	0	0
Craft, 3.5% ABV, (Calculated Estimate)	*1 Bottle/330ml*	*102*	*0*	*31*	*0*	*0*	*0*	*0*
Craft, 4% ABV, (Calculated Estimate)	*1 Bottle/330ml*	*116*	*0*	*35*	*0*	*0*	*0*	*0*
Craft, 4.5% ABV, (Calculated Estimate)	*1 Bottle/330ml*	*132*	*0*	*40*	*0*	*0*	*0*	*0*
Craft, 5% ABV, (Calculated Estimate)	*1 Bottle/330ml*	*146*	*0*	*44*	*0*	*0*	*0*	*0*
Craft, 5.5% ABV, (Calculated Estimate)	*1 Bottle/330ml*	*160*	*0*	*49*	*0*	*0*	*0*	*0*
Craft, 6% ABV, (Calculated Estimate)	*1 Bottle/330ml*	*175*	*0*	*53*	*0*	*0*	*0*	*0*
Craft, 6.5% ABV, (Calculated Estimate)	*1 Bottle/330ml*	*189*	*0*	*57*	*0*	*0*	*0*	*0*
Craft, 7% ABV, (Calculated Estimate)	*1 Bottle/330ml*	*204*	*0*	*62*	*0*	*0*	*0*	*0*
Craft, 7.5% ABV, (Calculated Estimate)	*1 Bottle/330ml*	*218*	*0*	*66*	*0*	*0*	*0*	*0*
Craft, 8% ABV, (Calculated Estimate)	*1 Bottle/330ml*	*233*	*0*	*71*	*0*	*0*	*0*	*0*
Craft, 8.5% ABV, (Calculated Estimate)	*1 Bottle/330ml*	*248*	*0*	*75*	*0*	*0*	*0*	*0*
Doom Bar, Ale, 0% Alcohol, Sharps Brewery*	1 Bottle/500ml	65	0.5	13	0.1	3.2	0.1	0
Guinness* Extra Stout, Bottled	1 Bottle/500ml	215	0	43	4	0	0	0
Guinness, Draught*	*1 Can/440ml*	*158*	*0.2*	*36*	*0.3*	*3*	*0*	*0*
Guinness, Stout*	*1 Pint/568ml*	*205*	*0*	*36*	*0.3*	*3*	*0*	*0*
Hophead, Dark Star*	1 Bottle/500ml	160	0	32	0	0	0	0
Lager, Alcohol Free, Erdinger*	1 Bottle/500ml	125	0.5	25	0.1	5.3	0.1	0
Lager, Alcohol Free, Lost AF, Brewdog *	1 Can/330ml	135	0.3	41	0.1	3	0.1	0
Lager, Premium, 4.3%, Thuringer*	1 Can/330ml	119	0	36	0	0	0	0
Lager, Unfiltered, 0.5%, Lucky Saint*	1 Bottle/330ml	53	0	16	0.6	3.5	0	0
Low Calorie, Low Carb, Cobra*	1 Bottle/330ml	96	0	29	0.1	1.3	0	0
Mackeson, Stout	*1 Pint/568ml*	*205*	*0*	*36*	*0.4*	*4.6*	*0*	*0*
Mild, Draught, Average	*1 Pint/568ml*	*136*	*0*	*24*	*0.2*	*1.6*	*0*	*0*
Non Alcoholic, Zero, Cobra*	1 Bottle/330ml	79	0	24	0.8	2	0	0
Oak Aged, Original, Innis & Gunn*	1 Bottle/330ml	182	0	55	0.3	4.7	0	0
Pale Ale, Dead Pony Club, Brewdog *	1 Bottle/330ml	116	0	35	0	0	0	0
Pale Ale, Ghost Ship, Adnams*	1 Bottle/500ml	195	0	39	0	0	0	0
Pale Ale, Landlord, Timothy Taylor*	1 Bottle/500ml	171	0	34	0	0.6	0	0
Patronus, Weissbier, Alcohol Free, Perlenbacher*	1 Bottle/500ml	125	0	25	0.5	5.4	0	0
Pilsner, Alcohol Free, Kromacher*	1 Bottle/330ml	89	0	27	0	6.4	0	0
Porter, Plum, St Peter's Brewery Co Ltd*	1 Bottle/500ml	230	0.5	46	0.5	4.1	0.1	0
Prohibition Brew, Alcohol Free, Budweiser *	1 Can/330ml	112	0	34	0.2	8	0	0
Raspberry, Non Alcoholic, Moussy*	1 Bottle/330ml	139	0	42	0.1	10.4	0	0
Skinny, GF, Skinny Brands*	1 Can/330g	89	0	27	0.2	0.9	0	0
Stout, Coopers*	1 Pint/375ml	191	0	51	0	2.9	0	0
Stout, Dark Matters, Aldi*	1 Bottle/328ml	128	0	39	0	0	0	0
Ultra, Kingfisher*	1 Bottle/330ml	140	0	42	0	0	0	0
Weissbier, Alcohol Free, Erdinger*	1 Bottle/500ml	125	0	25	0.4	5.3	0	0
Weissbier, Hefe, Franziskaner*	1 Bottle/500ml	225	0	45	0	0	0	0
Xoris, Non Alcoholic, Alfa*	1 Can/330ml	82	0.3	25	0.3	5.4	0.1	0

	Measure INFO/WEIGHT	per Measure KCAL	FAT	Nutrition Values per 100g / 100ml KCAL	PROT	CARB	FAT	FIBRE
BEETROOT								
Baby, Pickled, Average	1 Beetroot/12g	5	0	37	1.7	7.2	0.1	1.2
Cocktail, Sweet Chilli, M&S*	½ Pack/90g	58	0.3	65	1.5	12.3	0.3	3.6
Cooked, Boiled, Drained, Average	1 Serving/100g	44	0.2	44	1.7	10	0.2	2
Pickled, in Sweet Vinegar, Average	1oz/28g	16	0	57	1.2	12.8	0.1	1.5
Pickled, in Vinegar, Average	1 Serving/50g	18	0	36	1.6	7.3	0.1	1.2
Raw, Unprepared, Average	1oz/28g	8	0	29	1.4	5.4	0.1	1.7
Rosebud, Sweet Chilli Marinated, M&S*	1 Serving/80g	52	0.2	65	1.5	12.3	0.3	3.6
with Balsamic Vinaigrette, Side Salad, M&S*	1 Pack/225g	146	2.9	65	0.7	12.4	1.3	2.2
BERRIES								
Mix, Naturally Wonky, Frozen, Morrisons*	1 Serving/80g	23	0.2	29	0.9	5.6	0.3	0.3
Mixed, Fresh, Average	1 Serving/80g	29	0.2	37	0.9	8.3	0.2	3.4
Mixed, Summer Fruits, Frozen, Tesco*	1 Serving/80g	37	0.4	46	1.1	7.5	0.5	3.9
BHAJI								
Aubergine, & Potato, Fried in Vegetable Oil, Average	1oz/28g	36	2.5	130	2	12	8.8	1.7
Cabbage, & Pea, Fried in Vegetable Oil, Average	1oz/28g	50	4.1	178	3.3	9.2	14.7	3.4
Cauliflower, Fried in Vegetable Oil, Average	1oz/28g	60	5.7	214	4	4	20.5	2
Mushroom, Fried in Vegetable Oil, Average	1oz/28g	46	4.5	166	1.7	4.4	16.1	1.3
Okra, Bangladeshi, Fried in Butter Ghee, Average	1oz/28g	27	1.8	95	2.5	7.6	6.4	3.2
Onion, Fried in Vegetable Oil, Takeaway, Average	1 Bhaji/70g	190	10.3	270	9.8	24.6	14.7	5.6
Onion, Indian, Waitrose*	1 Bhaji/43g	103	5.5	240	5.8	22.4	12.8	5.6
Onion, Taste of India, Tesco*	1 Bhaji/46g	115	7.6	251	5.9	17	16.6	4.9
Onon, Indian Takeaway, Morrisons*	1 Bhaji/47g	119	7.3	254	5.7	20.4	15.6	4.6
Potato, & Onion, Fried in Vegetable Oil, Average	1oz/28g	45	2.8	160	2.1	16.6	10.1	1.6
Potato, Onion & Mushroom, Fried, Average	1oz/28g	58	4.9	208	2	12	17.5	1.5
Potato, Spinach & Cauliflower, Fried, Average	1oz/28g	47	4.2	169	2.2	7.1	15.1	1.4
Spinach, & Potato, Fried in Vegetable Oil, Average	1oz/28g	53	3.9	191	3.7	13.4	14.1	2.3
Spinach, Fried in Vegetable Oil, Average	1oz/28g	23	1.9	83	3.3	2.6	6.8	2.4
Sweet Potato, Oven Baked, Asda*	1 Bhaji/28g	63	2.8	224	4.6	25	10	7.2
Vegetable, Fried in Vegetable Oil, Average	1oz/28g	59	5.2	212	2.1	10.1	18.5	2.4
BHUNA								
Chicken, with Rice, Ready Meal, Average	1 Pack/350g	444	20.8	127	9.4	8.9	5.9	1.4
Lamb, 405, Oakhouse Foods Ltd*	1 Meal/400g	412	14	103	4.8	13	3.5	0.8
Prawn, King, M&S*	1 Pack/400g	308	15.2	77	6.7	3.3	3.8	1.5
Prawn, King, Specially Selected, Aldi*	½ Pack/169g	132	6.8	78	5.3	4.4	4	1.4
BILBERRIES								
Fresh, Raw	1oz/28g	8	0.1	29	0.6	6.8	0.2	1.8
BILTONG								
Average	1 Serving/25g	64	1	256	50	0	4	0
Original, GF, Cruga*	1 Serving/10g	24	0.6	242	42	5.8	5.6	0.4
BIRYANI								
Chicken, Ready Meal, Average	1 Pack/400g	521	17.1	130	7.5	15.2	4.3	1.6
Chicken, Tikka, Ready Meal, Average	1 Pack/400g	460	11.5	115	7.3	14.8	2.9	1.5
Chicken, Vegetarian, Linda McCartney*	½ Pack/180g	300	11.7	167	8.6	17	6.5	3.3
Lamb, Average	1 Serving/200g	390	19.4	195	7.3	20.9	9.7	0
Vegetable, Meal for 1, Sainsbury's*	1 Pack/376g	481	19.9	128	2.4	16.6	5.3	2.3
Vegetable, Slimming World*	1 Pack/550g	456	2.8	83	2.7	15.9	0.5	2.3
BISCUITS								
Abbey Crunch, McVitie's*	1 Biscuit/9g	43	1.6	477	6	72.8	17.9	2.5
Abernethy, Simmers*	1 Biscuit/12g	61	2.7	490	5.7	69.2	21.9	0
Ace Milk Chocolate, McVitie's*	1 Biscuit/24g	122	5.9	510	6.1	66.2	24.5	1.6
All Butter, M&S*	1 Biscuit/8g	42	2.1	505	5.8	63.1	25	2.2
Almond & Chocolate, Biscotti, TTD, Sainsbury's*	1 Biscuit/30g	132	4.8	440	8.4	65.6	16	3.1
Almond, M&S*	1 Biscuit/9g	46	2.4	512	6.9	60.5	26.4	2.3

B

BISCUITS

	Measure INFO/WEIGHT	per Measure KCAL	per Measure FAT	Nutrition Values per 100g / 100ml KCAL	PROT	CARB	FAT	FIBRE
Almond, Thins, TTD, Sainsbury's*	1 Biscuit/4g	16	0.5	450	6.7	72.8	14.7	3.1
Amaretti, Average	*1 Biscuit/5g*	*22*	*0.8*	*434*	*8.1*	*66.4*	*15.4*	*2.8*
Amaretti, Soft, TTD, Sainsbury's*	1 Biscuit/13g	58	2.4	450	9.7	58.9	18.7	3.5
Anzac, Bitesmart*	1 Biscuit/20g	84	4.6	420	5.1	46.8	23	0
Baileys Square, Bahlsen*	1 Square/10g	56	3.5	561	6.4	54	35	0
Baked Bites, Cheddar, Mini, Cathedral City*	1 Pack/22g	115	6.4	521	12.2	51.4	29.2	2.6
Belgian Milk Chocolate, M&S*	1 Biscuit/12g	60	2.5	490	6.2	70.1	20.3	2.5
Biscoff, Cream, Lotus*	1 Biscuit/10g	52	2.6	522	4.6	66	26	1.2
Bites, Choc Choc Chip, Doubly Delicious, Nibble Simply*	1 Pack/36g	175	15.8	486	13	26	44	9.7
Bites, Cookie Dough, Cheeky Choc Chip, Nibble Simply*	1 Pack/36g	172	15.5	479	14	26	43	9.1
Bourbon, Average	*1 Biscuit/13g*	*63*	*2.8*	*488*	*5.7*	*68.2*	*21.3*	*2.1*
Brandy Snaps, Average	*1 Biscuit/15g*	*69*	*2.2*	*460*	*2.7*	*79.8*	*14.4*	*0.5*
Breakfast, Blueberries, Soft Bakes, Belvita*	1 Biscuit/50g	194	6	388	5.5	63	12	7.5
Breakfast, Choc Chips, Soft Bakes, Belvita*	1 Pack/50g	202	7.5	405	5.7	61	15	6.9
Breakfast, Choco Hazlenut, Tops, Belvita*	1 Pack/50g	230	8	460	7.2	69	16	4.9
Breakfast, Cocoa, Chocolate Chip, Belvita*	1 Pack/50g	220	7.5	440	7.8	66	15	7.1
Breakfast, Honey & Nuts, Belvita*	1 Pack/50g	228	7.5	455	7.6	69	15	4.4
Breakfast, Milk & Cereals, Belvita*	1 Pack/50g	220	7.2	440	7.9	67	14.5	6.5
Breakfast, Oat, Golden, Asda*	1 Pack/45g	210	9	467	6	64	20	5.1
Breakfast, Red Berries, Soft Bakes, Belvita*	1 Pack/50g	190	5.5	380	5.5	65	11	6.6
Breakfast, Whole Grain, No Added Sugar, Gullon*	1 Biscuit/9g	37	1.3	410	6.8	65	14	9.8
Butter, Chocolate Brownie, Farmhouse Biscuits*	1 Biscuit/17g	88	5.1	528	5.3	56.1	30.6	0
Butter, Dark Chocolate, Tesco*	1 Biscuit/14g	72	3.7	511	6.9	58.3	26.7	4.9
Butter, Milk Chocolate, Belmont Biscuit Co, Aldi*	1 Biscuit/14g	69	3.2	492	7.3	63	23	2.8
Butter, Milk Chocolate, Ritter Sport*	1 Biscuit/25g	139	8.5	555	6.1	55	34	0
Butter, Milk Chocolate, Tesco*	1 Biscuit/14g	71	3.6	508	7.8	61	25.4	2.2
Butter, with Dark Chocolate, Belmont Biscuit Co, Aldi*	1 Biscuit/14g	71	3.6	509	6.4	61	26	4.5
Cafe Noir, with Coffee Flavour Icing, McVitie's*	1 Biscuit/6g	27	0.8	458	4.9	76	14	1.7
Cantuccini, with Almonds, Average	*1 Biscotti/30g*	*130*	*5*	*433*	*10*	*60*	*16.7*	*3.3*
Caramelised, Belmont Biscuit Co, Aldi*	1 Biscuit/8g	40	1.5	480	6.2	72	18	1.2
Caramelised, Biscoff, Lotus*	1 Biscuit/8g	38	1.5	484	4.9	72.7	19	1.3
Cheese Savouries , Crawfords*	1 Serving/25g	131	7.7	523	10.7	48.4	30.8	2.9
Cheese Savouries, Sainsbury's*	1 Serving/30g	159	9.4	531	11.3	50	31.3	2.1
Cheese, & Chutney, Delicious, Boots*	1 Pack/134g	290	14.7	217	9	19	11	2.3
Cheese, Baked, Cheddars, Jacob's*	1 Cheddar/4g	20	1.2	525	10.8	47	31.8	2.9
Choc Chip, Paterson's*	1 Biscuit/17g	79	3.6	474	5.6	64	21.6	3.1
Choco Leibniz, Dark Chocolate, Bahlsen*	1 Biscuit/14g	69	3.6	493	6.8	59	26	5.1
Choco Leibniz, Milk, Bahlsen*	1 Biscuit/14g	71	3.5	505	7.5	61	25	2.4
Choco Leibniz, Orange Flavour, Bahlsen*	1 Biscuit/14g	70	3.7	504	7.9	58.5	26.4	0
Chocolate Florentine, M&S*	1 Serving/39g	195	9.7	500	7.4	64.5	24.9	1.7
Chocolate Ginger, Organic, Duchy Originals*	1 Biscuit/12g	64	3.6	518	4.6	59.7	29	2.1
Chocolate Viennese, Fox's*	1 Biscuit/16g	85	4.9	530	6.7	56.6	30.7	1.7
Chocolate, Breakaway, Nestle*	1 Bar/19g	99	4.9	511	6.1	63.5	25.2	3
Chocolate, Fingers, Average	*1 Biscuit/6g*	*31*	*1.6*	*514*	*6.7*	*61.4*	*26.8*	*1.5*
Chocolatey Orange, Fox's*	1 Biscuit/17g	91	5	536	4.8	62.3	29.5	0.9
Classic, Milk Chocolate, Fox's*	1 Biscuit/13g	67	3.1	517	6.1	64.9	24	1.6
Coconut, Ring, Average	*1 Biscuit/9g*	*44*	*2*	*490*	*6.1*	*67.4*	*21.8*	*2.6*
Cookies & Cream, Belmont Biscuit Co, Aldi*	1 Biscuit/11g	52	2	469	4.9	72	18	2.2
Cookies & Cream, GF, Free From, Morrisons*	1 Biscuit/18g	87	4	490	7.2	63.1	22.4	3.5
Cookies & Cream, WW*	1 Biscuit/8g	38	2	475	7.7	53.1	24.4	6.1
Crispy Fruit Slices, Apple, Sultana, Go Ahead, McVitie's*	1 Biscuit/13g	50	0.9	388	5.4	74	7.1	2.9
Crispy Fruit Slices, Forest Fruit, Go Ahead, McVitie's*	1 Biscuit/13g	49	0.9	380	5.4	73.7	7	3
Crispy Slices, Raspberry, Crownfield, Lidl*	1 Biscuit/15g	58	1	399	9.5	73	7	2.8

	Measure	per Measure		Nutrition Values per 100g / 100ml				
	INFO/WEIGHT	KCAL	FAT	KCAL	PROT	CARB	FAT	FIBRE

BISCUITS

	INFO/WEIGHT	KCAL	FAT	KCAL	PROT	CARB	FAT	FIBRE
Crispy Slices, Raspberry, Go Ahead, McVitie's*	1 Biscuit/13g	50	0.9	385	5.3	74	7	2.8
Crunch Creams, Double Choc, Fox's*	1 Biscuit/15g	77	3.8	511	4.7	65	25	2.7
Crunchy Caramel, Tesco*	1 Bar/21g	98	5.2	467	4.6	56	25	1.4
Custard Cream, Savers, Morrisons*	1 Biscuit/13g	65	2.9	513	5.8	69.6	22.9	2.4
Custard Creams, Asda*	1 Biscuit/12g	59	2.7	495	5	67	23	2
Custard Creams, Co-Op*	1 Biscuit/12g	59	2.6	493	5.8	67	22	1.6
Custard Creams, M&S*	1 Biscuit/13g	63	2.8	494	5.5	67.2	22	2.4
Custard Creams, Sainsbury's*	1 Biscuit/12g	59	2.4	474	5.5	68.8	19	3
Custard Creams, Tesco*	1 Biscuit/12g	58	2.4	490	5.7	70.1	20.5	1.1
Dark Chocolate Gingers, & Orange, Border Biscuits Ltd*	1 Biscuit/17g	78	3.7	458	4.6	58.7	21.9	0
Dark Chocolate Gingers, Border*	1 Biscuit/17g	74	3.4	445	4.4	61.4	20.1	2.9
Diet Fibre, Gullon*	2 Biscuits/16g	65	2.6	405	6.5	48.7	16.4	23
Digestive with Wheatgerm, Hovis*	1 Biscuit/12g	57	2.4	475	8.3	65	20	3.3
Digestive, Caramels, Milk Chocolate, McVitie's*	1 Biscuit/17g	81	3.7	478	5.6	65.1	21.7	2.3
Digestive, Chocolate	*1 Biscuit/17g*	*84*	*4.1*	*493*	*6.8*	*66.5*	*24.1*	*2.2*
Digestive, Chocolate, Free From, Morrisons*	1 Biscuit/17g	83	4.2	497	8.8	55.6	25.4	5.4
Digestive, Dark Choc Chip, Sainsbury's*	1 Biscuit/12g	59	2.6	475	7.1	62.2	20.7	5.5
Digestive, Dark Chocolate, McVitie's*	1 Biscuit/17g	83	4.1	495	6	60.8	24.2	4.2
Digestive, Dark Chocolate, Thins, McVitie's*	1 Biscuit/6g	31	1.5	499	6	60.9	24.7	4.7
Digestive, Free From, Asda*	1 Biscuit/11g	55	2.7	485	11	53	24	7.5
Digestive, GF, Schar*	1 Biscuit/10g	48	2.2	483	6.1	62	22	6.2
Digestive, Lemon & Ginger, McVitie's*	1 Biscuit/15g	72	3.1	480	6.7	66.7	20.7	2.7
Digestive, Light, McVitie's*	1 Biscuit/15g	66	2.1	444	7.3	69.5	14.4	3.6
Digestive, Mcvitie's*	1 Biscuit/15g	72	3.2	483	7	63.6	21.3	3.7
Digestive, Milk Chocolate, McVitie's*	1 Biscuit/17g	83	3.9	496	6.7	62.5	23.6	3
Digestive, Plain Chocolate, Tesco*	1 Biscuit/17g	85	4.1	499	6.2	63.5	24.4	2.8
Digestive, Plain, Average	*1 Biscuit/14g*	*67*	*2.9*	*480*	*7.1*	*65.6*	*20.5*	*3.5*
Digestive, Sugar Free, Gullon*	1 Biscuit/13g	57	2.1	430	6.2	68	16	6.5
Digestives, Dark Chocolate, Sugar Free, Zeroh!, Gullon*	1 Biscuit/14g	61	2.9	449	7	63	21	6
Empire, Mathiesons*	1 Biscuit/17g	69	2.5	416	4.5	67.5	15.3	0
Extremely Chocolatey, Dark Chocolate Rounds, M&S*	1 Biscuit/19g	97	5.6	510	6.2	55.7	29.3	6.3
Extremely Chocolatey, Milk Chocolate, Rounds, M&S*	1 Pack/44g	227	11.7	517	6.4	61.6	26.7	2.3
Fig Roll, Tesco*	1 Biscuit/19g	70	1.6	375	4	69.3	8.8	3.1
Fig Rolls, Mcvitie's*	1 Biscuit/17g	65	1.5	383	3.4	71.7	8.6	3
Florentines, Milk Chocolate, & Orange, No.1, Waitrose*	1 Biscuit/19g	102	6.5	536	7.7	47.7	34.1	3.5
Forest Fruit, Yoghurt, Breaks, Go Ahead, McVitie's*	1 Slice/18g	72	1.8	402	5.4	72.6	10	2.2
Fruit Shortcake, McVitie's*	1 Biscuit/8g	37	1.5	462	5.6	65.9	18.9	3.1
Fruit Shortcake, Morrisons*	1 Biscuit/8g	38	1.5	469	6.2	68	18.7	1.9
Fruit Shortcake, Tesco*	1 Biscuit/9g	43	1.7	473	5.8	70.1	18.8	1.9
Fruit Shorties, Hill Biscuits Ltd*	1 Biscuit/7g	33	1.3	464	5.7	69	18	2.9
Garibaldi, Asda*	1 Biscuit/10g	39	0.9	375	4.7	68.5	9.1	2.2
Garibaldi, Sainsbury's*	1 Biscuit/9g	35	0.8	385	5.6	68.5	8.6	5.5
Garibaldi, Tesco*	1 Biscuit/10g	40	0.9	400	4.7	74	9.1	2.2
Ginger Crunch Creams, Fox's*	1 Biscuit/15g	77	3.5	501	4.1	68	23	1.6
Ginger, Belgian Dark Chocolate, Thins, Waitrose*	1 Biscuit/10g	48	2.2	481	6.2	61.2	22.5	4.6
Ginger, Thins, Heart Shaped, Ikea*	1 Biscuit/6g	28	1	462	5.4	72	17	0
Gingerbread, Glazed, Lambertz Pfeffernusse*	1 Biscuit/10g	35	0.1	346	5.1	77.7	0.7	4.3
Gingernut	*1 Biscuit/11g*	*50*	*1.7*	*456*	*5.6*	*79.1*	*15.2*	*1.4*
Gingers, Dark Chocolate, Deluxe, Lidl*	1 Biscuit/15g	78	4	517	5.2	62.7	26.8	2
Golden Crunch Creams, Fox's*	1 Biscuit/15g	75	3.8	515	4.7	64.8	26.3	1.2
Hobnob's, Milk Chocolate, Fully Coated, McVitie's*	1 Biscuit/25g	127	6.4	501	6.9	59.3	25.1	4.8
Hobnobs, Choc Chip, Mcvities*	1 Biscuit/15g	72	3.2	471	7.2	60.5	20.8	6.4
Hobnobs, Chocolate Creams, McVitie's*	1 Biscuit/12g	60	3.1	503	6.7	60.3	26.1	4

BISCUITS

	Measure INFO/WEIGHT	per Measure KCAL	per Measure FAT	Nutrition Values per 100g / 100ml KCAL	PROT	CARB	FAT	FIBRE
Hobnobs, McVitie's*	1 Biscuit/15g	72	3.2	473	7	61.8	20.7	5.4
Hobnobs, Milk Chocolate, McVitie's*	1 Biscuit/19g	92	4.5	479	6.8	60.7	23.3	4.5
Hobnobs, Plain Chocolate, McVitie's*	1 Biscuit/16g	81	3.9	498	6.7	63.3	24.3	4.2
Hobnobs, Vanilla Creams, McVitie's*	1 Biscuit/12g	60	3	501	6.1	62.3	25.2	3.6
Jaffa Cakes, Asda*	1 Cake/12g	43	1	368	4.7	67.5	8.8	1.9
Jaffa Cakes, Belmont Biscuit Co, Aldi*	1 Cake/13g	52	1.3	400	3.7	72.8	10.2	1
Jaffa Cakes, Cherry, McVitie's*	1 Cake /12g	46	1	375	5	69.6	8	2.1
Jaffa Cakes, Dark Chocolate, M&S*	1 Cake/11g	45	1.5	395	3.7	64.9	13.2	2.8
Jaffa Cakes, Dark Chocolate, Mini, M&S*	1 Cake/5g	20	0.8	410	3.9	62.8	15.8	1.9
Jaffa Cakes, McVitie's*	1 Cake/12g	46	1	380	4.9	70.8	8	2.2
Jam Sandwich Creams, M&S*	1 Biscuit/17g	80	3.7	485	5.7	64.5	22.6	1.8
Jam Sandwich Creams, Tesco*	1 Biscuit/15g	72	3.2	482	4.8	67.1	21.4	1.2
Jam, & Creams, Asda*	1 Biscuit/15g	74	3.3	493	5.1	69	22	1.6
Jammie Dodgers, Minis, Burton's*	4 Biscuits/20g	88	2.9	438	4.6	72.2	14.7	2.4
Jammie Dodgers, Minis, Lunchbox, Burton's*	1 Pack/20g	89	3	445	6	70	15.1	2.3
Jammie Dodgers, Original, Burton's*	1 Biscuit/18g	78	2.5	436	5.4	71.3	13.9	1.7
Jammy Wheels, GF, Prewett's*	1 Biscuit/24g	95	5.6	394	5	60.1	23.2	4.7
Lebkuchen, Chocolate, Weiss*	1 Biscuit/28g	109	2.7	393	0	68.9	9.9	0
Lemon, Farmhouse*	1 Biscuit/19g	104	5.7	545	4.6	63.3	29.9	0
Malted Milk, Average	**1 Biscuit/9g**	**42**	**1.9**	**490**	**7**	**65.6**	**22.2**	**1.8**
Malted Milk, Chocolate, Tesco*	1 Biscuit/10g	52	2.5	500	6.7	64.4	24	1.9
Malted Milk, Milk Chocolate, Sainsbury's*	1 Biscuit/11g	56	2.7	505	6.4	64.4	24.2	2.1
Maria, Gullon*	1 Biscuit/6g	24	0.7	408	7	75	11	4.5
Marie, Crawfords*	1 Biscuit/7g	33	1.1	475	7.5	76.3	15.5	2.3
Marie, Pingo Doce *	1 Biscuit/6g	26	0.6	430	7.8	76.9	9.6	2.8
Milk Chocolate, All Butter, M&S*	1 Biscuit/14g	70	3.6	490	7.9	57.4	25.5	1.4
Milk Chocolate, Squares, M&S*	1 Biscuit/14g	70	3.5	498	6.3	61.4	24.8	1.9
Milkshake, Belmont Biscuit Co, Aldi*	1 Biscuit/25g	134	7.5	536	6.4	59	30	1.7
Mint, Viscount*	1 Biscuit/14g	73	4	525	4.5	61.6	28.5	1.8
Moments, Chocolate, Special K, Kellogg's*	1 Bar/25g	96	2.3	383	5.5	72	9.1	2.3
Nice, Average	**1 Biscuit/8g**	**36**	**1.6**	**484**	**6.3**	**67.3**	**21**	**2.5**
Nut Butter Cups, Cocoa, & Hazelnut, Nature Valley*	2 Cups/35g	178	9.6	510	8.3	54.4	27.3	6.6
Nutella, Ferrero*	1 Biscuit/14g	71	3.4	513	8.4	63.3	24.5	0
Oat Crumbles, Border*	1 Biscuit/15g	66	3.1	443	5.3	58.9	20.7	1.8
Oat Crumbles, Chocolate, Border*	1 Biscuit/15g	71	3.7	475	5.7	56.4	24.7	0
Oat Crumbles, Golden, Border*	1 Biscuit/15g	63	2.9	422	4.9	56.2	19.2	0
Oat, & Chocolate Chip, GF, Breaks, Nairn's*	1 Biscuit/10g	47	2	470	7.6	61.8	20.1	5.5
Oat, & Fruit, GF, Breaks, Nairn's*	1 Biscuit/10g	46	1.9	460	8.4	61.8	18.6	6
Oat, & Stem Ginger, GF, Breaks, Nairn's*	1 Biscuit/10g	46	1.9	463	8.2	62.4	18.8	5.7
Oat, Apple, & cinnamon, Chunky, GF, Breaks, Nairn's*	1 Biscuit/13g	61	2.8	471	8	57	21.7	8
Oat, Dark Chocolate Chip, Nairn's*	1 Biscuit/10g	46	1.7	454	8.1	63.8	16.9	6.7
Oat, Mixed Berries, Nairn's*	1 Biscuit/10g	43	1.5	427	7.5	64.8	15.3	7.1
Oatie Crumbles, Milk Chocolate, Asda*	1 Biscuit/19g	93	4.4	489	7	62	23	4.6
Oaties, Belmont Biscuit Co, Aldi*	1 Biscuit/20g	95	4.2	476	7.8	62	21	4.8
Oaties, Chocolate, Milk, Aldi*	1 Biscuit/20g	95	4.2	476	7.8	62	21	4.8
Oaties, Chocolate, Orange, & Cranberry, Frank's*	1 Biscuit/38g	171	7.1	456	5	65	19	0
Oaties, GF, Nairn's*	1 Biscuit/10g	48	2.2	480	9	58	22	7
Oaties, Tower Gate, Lidl*	1 Biscuit/15g	74	3.2	491	8.9	63	21	7
Oatmeal Crunch, Jacob's*	1 Biscuit/8g	37	1.5	458	6.8	65.9	18.6	3.6
Oatmeal, Asda*	1 Biscuit/12g	54	2.5	470	6	62	22	6
Olive Oil, Savoury Ships, Brindisa*	1 Biscuit/8g	33	0.9	409	11.2	63.5	11.6	6
Oreo, Thins, Mondelez*	4 Biscuits/24g	118	5.1	490	4.8	69	21	2.6
Parmesan Cheese, Sainsbury's*	1 Biscuit/3g	18	1	553	14.7	56.4	29.9	1.8

BISCUITS

	Measure INFO/WEIGHT	per Measure KCAL	FAT	Nutrition Values per 100g / 100ml KCAL	PROT	CARB	FAT	FIBRE
Party Rings, Iced, Fox's*	1 Biscuit/6g	29	0.9	459	5.1	75.8	15	0
Peanut Butter, American Style, Sainsbury's*	1 Biscuit/13g	63	2.9	504	5.2	68.7	23.1	2.2
Petit Beurre, Stella Artois*	1 Biscuit/6g	26	0.9	440	9	73	15	0
Pink Wafers, Crawfords*	1 Biscuit/7g	36	1.9	521	2.5	68.6	26.5	1.1
Pink Wafers, Sainsbury's*	1 Biscuit/8g	36	1.8	486	4.6	64.2	23.4	1.7
Praline Squares, Bahlsen*	1 Biscuit/11g	62	4	561	7.7	50	36	0
Raspberry & Cream Viennese, Melts, Fox's*	1 Biscuit/16g	84	4.5	521	4	62.1	28.1	1.7
Redcurrant Puffs, Eat Well, M&S*	1 Biscuit/7g	32	1.4	470	5.6	67.7	19.8	2
Rhubarb & Custard Creams, Tesco*	1 Biscuit/13g	65	2.9	498	5.3	67.5	22.6	1.9
Rich Shorties, Asda*	1 Biscuit/10g	50	2.3	486	6	66	22	2
Rich Tea, Average	**1 Biscuit/10g**	**45**	**1.5**	**451**	**6.8**	**72.8**	**14.5**	**2.5**
Rich Tea, Light, McVitie's*	1 Biscuit/8g	36	0.9	436	7.6	75.3	10.7	3.1
Rich Tea, Reduced Fat, Tesco*	1 Biscuit/9g	40	0.8	424	8.1	76.7	8.7	3.4
Rocky, Chocolate, Fox's*	1 Biscuit/21g	106	5.4	505	5.7	62.4	25.7	2.4
Rose, Fortnum & Mason*	1 Biscuit/13g	71	3.7	543	6.5	63.2	28.8	0
Rounds, Chocolatey, Seriously, Tower Gate, Lidl*	1 Biscuit/17g	84	4	503	5.5	65	24.2	1.5
Sandwich Fingers, Raspberry Cream, M&S*	1 Biscuit/15g	77	4.2	512	4.8	58.8	28.1	2.2
Shortbread, Salted Toffee, GF, Free From, Sainsbury's*	1 Biscuit/20g	100	4.8	502	4.7	65.8	24.2	0.9
Shortbread, WW*	1 Biscuit/6g	30	1.3	503	6.4	63.9	21.9	1.6
Shortcake Snack, Cadbury*	2 Biscuits/20g	102	5.2	512	6.6	63	26	2.1
Shortcake with Real Milk Chocolate, Cadbury*	1 Biscuit/15g	75	3.5	500	6.3	65.8	23.5	0
Shortcake, Average	**1 Biscuit/11g**	**55**	**3**	**501**	**6.3**	**66.1**	**27.1**	**2.1**
Shortcake, Caramel, Mini, Thorntons*	1 Biscuit/15g	71	4.6	492	4.8	46.3	31.9	0.6
Shortcake, Caramel, Squares, Tesco*	1 Square/54g	274	16.4	507	4.6	54.1	30.4	0.4
Shortcake, Dairy Milk Chocolate, Cadbury*	1 Bar/49g	252	13.5	515	7.5	59.2	27.5	0
Shortcake, Fruit, Crawfords*	1 Biscuit/8g	34	1.5	419	5.4	55.9	19.3	2.4
Shorties, Rich, Tesco*	1 Biscuit/10g	48	2.2	484	6.4	65.6	21.8	2
Shorties, Sainsbury's*	1 Biscuit/10g	48	2.1	485	6.6	65.9	21.3	1.5
Soft Bakes, Choco Hazelnut, Harvest Morn, Aldi*	1 Bar/50g	200	6.5	401	5.5	60	13	8.9
Soft Bakes, Red Berries, Harvest Morn, Aldi*	1 Bar/50g	185	4.8	370	6.1	60	9.5	10
Speculaas, Sandwich, Fortnum & Mason*	1 Biscuit/22g	111	5.4	504	5.4	63.3	24.7	0
Spekulatius, Chocolate, Tesco*	1 Biscuit/2g	10	0.5	488	6.9	64	22	3.3
Spekulatius, Cinnamon, Tesco*	1 Biscuit/2g	7	0.2	455	6	71.1	15.7	2.5
Spiced, German, Christmas, Favorina, Lidl*	1 Biscuit/10g	47	1.9	472	5.8	70.2	18.7	0
Triple Chocolate, Fox's*	1 Biscuit/21g	100	5.2	478	5.7	57.3	25.1	2.5
Twix, Soft Centre, Mars*	1 Biscuit/18g	83	3.7	462	4.5	64.3	20.4	0
V.I.B, Heavenly Hazelnut, McVitie's*	1 Biscuit/17g	80	3.6	480	5.6	65.5	21.7	2.4
Viennese Finger, Belmont Biscuit Co, Aldi*	1 Biscuit/16g	84	4.7	521	4.8	61	29	1.5
Viennese Swirls, All Butter, Waitrose*	1 Biscuit/14g	76	4.7	548	4.9	55.2	33.7	2.1
Viennese, Fingers, Milk Chocolate Dipped, M&S*	1 Biscuit/13g	71	4	527	5.4	58.6	29.7	1.8
Viennese, Sandwich, Chocolate, M&S*	1 Biscuit/15g	80	4.6	535	7.2	58	30.6	1.7
Viennese, with Milk Chocolate Filling	**1 Biscuit/15g**	**81**	**4.5**	**533**	**6.5**	**59.6**	**29.4**	**2.1**
Wafer, Chocolate, Loacker*	1 Pack/90g	460	23.4	511	7.7	59	26	0
Water, Average	**1 Biscuit/6g**	**24**	**0.7**	**440**	**10.8**	**75.8**	**12.5**	**3.1**
Yoghurt Break, Red Cherry, Go Ahead, McVitie's*	1 Slice/18g	72	1.8	407	5.5	73.4	10.1	2.2
Yoghurt Break, Strawberry, Go Ahead, McVitie's*	1 Slice/18g	72	1.8	402	52	72.4	10.3	3.4
Yoghurt Slices, Forest Fruits, Crownfield, Lidl*	1 Slice/18g	80	2.3	430	7	71.8	12.2	2.6
Yoghurt, Crownfield, Lidl*	2 Slices/37g	160	5	433	6.2	70.6	13.4	2.4
Yorkie, Nestle*	1 Biscuit/25g	126	6.2	505	6.1	62.6	24.8	3.2

BISON

Raw	**1oz/28g**	**31**	**0.5**	**109**	**21.6**	**0**	**1.8**	**0**

BITES

Blueberry, & Lemon, Oat Squares, Superfood, Graze*	1 Bite/30g	138	7.2	460	6.5	51	24	16

	Measure INFO/WEIGHT	per Measure KCAL	FAT	Nutrition Values per 100g / 100ml KCAL	PROT	CARB	FAT	FIBRE
BITES								
Brownie, Chocolate, Tesco*	1 Bite/11g	43	1.6	394	5.3	58	15	30.7
Cake, Fruity, Orange & Lemon, Go Ahead*	1 Pack/27g	96	1.9	357	4.3	68.6	6.9	8
Caramel Shortcake, Mini, Bakers Selection, Asda*	1 Bite/12g	60	3.1	499	5.6	60	26	1.4
Caramel Shortcake, Thorntons*	1 Bite/12g	60	3.5	496	5	53	29	0
Cauliflower, Biryani, Asda*	1 Bite/10g	22	0.8	224	3.5	32	8.5	3.3
Cauliflower, Goan, Gosh!*	1 Bite/22g	44	2.6	199	4.8	22.6	11.6	7.3
Chicken, Breast, Tempura, Cooked, Tesco*	½ Pack/126g	239	8.7	189	17.9	13.7	6.9	0
Chicken, Katsu, Supermarket, Yo! Sushi*	1 Pack/90g	259	16.4	288	17.8	13.2	18.2	0
Chicken, Katsu, with Teri-Mayo, Taiko Foods*	1 Pack/98g	370	30.1	378	13.9	12	30.7	0
Chicken, Pep'd Up, Peperami*	1 Pack/50g	104	5.2	207	21	6.7	10.3	0
Chocolate Cornflake, Mini, M&S*	1 Bite/11.8g	55	2.4	470	6.2	66.3	20.1	3.6
Chocolate Orange, Mini, M&S*	1 Bite/22g	95	4.8	430	5.5	54.6	21.6	1.8
Chocolate, Double, Mini, M&S*	1 Mini Roll/18g	86	4.3	469	5.8	57.2	23.6	2.1
Cocoa, & Orange, Oat Bites, Superfood, Graze*	1 Bite/30g	139	7.5	464	6.6	51	25	17
Cornflake Clusters, Morrisons*	1 Cluster/10g	47	1.8	474	6.2	70.4	18.2	2.1
Cornflake, Cluster, Dairy Milk, Cadbury*	1 Bite/11g	54	2.4	493	7	65.6	22.1	2
Flapjack, Co-Op*	1 Bite/15g	66	2.8	426	6.1	56	18	6.3
Flapjack, Mini, M&S*	1 Bite/14g	64	3.1	458	6.1	56.7	21.9	5
Granola, & Yoghurt, Mini, M&S*	1 Piece/10g	49	2.3	492	7.1	62.3	23.4	2
Hash Brown, Oven Baked, Asda*	½ Pack/125g	285	13.8	228	2.4	29	11	2.7
Jaffa Cake, Nibbles, McVitie's*	1 Serving/25g	108	4.1	433	4.8	66	16.4	6.3
Lentil, The Foodie Market, Aldi*	1 Pack/20g	89	3.1	445	10	65	15.5	4
Meringue, Salted Caramel, Chocolate, Flower & White*	1 Bite/6g	27	0.8	449	5.8	75.7	13.9	0
Millionaire, Mini, Waitrose*	1 Bite/16g	76	4	484	5.4	57.2	25.6	1.5
Millionaires, Tesco*	1 Bites/12g	60	3.4	500	5.1	55.6	28	2.5
Mozzarella, & Pepperoni, Tesco *	1 Bite/21g	71	4.4	339	10.8	26	20.8	2.2
Nacho, Chicken, Tesco*	1 Bite/12g	27	1.1	225	18.3	16.7	9.2	3.3
Oat, Protein, Cocoa, & Vanilla, Graze*	1 Square/30g	138	7.2	459	15	44	24	15
Protein, Honey & Seed, Oat Squares, Graze*	1 Square/30g	143	7.8	474	16	42	26	14
Rocky Road, Mini, M&S*	1 Bite/12g	50	1.6	410	5.2	66.9	13.3	2.5
Rocky Road, Mini, Specially Selected, Aldi*	1 Bite/20g	108	6.2	538	5.8	58	31	3.1
Rocky Road, Mini, Waitrose*	1 Bite/14g	71	3.8	506	5.2	59	27.1	2.4
Rocky Road, Sainsbury's*	1 Bite/11g	52	2.5	477	2.9	64	22.5	3.3
Salted Caramel, CWP*	1 Serving/57g	203	5.9	356	23	43	10.4	6.3
Spinach, Oven Cooked, Strong Roots*	3 Bites/75g	202	10	269	4.3	30.5	13.3	5.1
Spinach, Strong Roots*	3 Bites/93g	202	11.2	218	3.4	20.8	12.1	6.4
Sweet Chilli, Quorn*	3 Bites/60g	146	5.9	244	14	24	9.9	3.5
Veggie, Mexican Heatwave, Fridge Raiders, Mattessons*	1 Sm Pack/50g	98	3.5	195	5.3	25	7	5.6
BLACK PUDDING								
Average, Uncooked	**1 Serving/40g**	**101**	**6**	**252**	**10.2**	**19**	**14.9**	**0.6**
BLACKBERRIES								
Fresh, Raw, Average	**1 Blackberry/8g**	**3**	**0**	**32**	**0.9**	**5.1**	**0.2**	**3.1**
Frozen, Average	**1 Serving/80g**	**26**	**0.2**	**32**	**0.9**	**5.1**	**0.2**	**3.1**
in Fruit Juice, Average	**½ Can/145g**	**52**	**0.3**	**36**	**0.6**	**7.9**	**0.2**	**1.3**
BLACKCURRANTS								
Dried, Graze*	1 Pack/30g	95	0.3	317	3.3	79	1	0
Fresh, Raw, Average	**1 Serving/80g**	**22**	**0**	**27**	**0.9**	**6.5**	**0**	**3.5**
Stewed with Sugar	**1oz/28g**	**16**	**0**	**58**	**0.7**	**15**	**0**	**2.8**
Stewed without Sugar	**1oz/28g**	**7**	**0**	**24**	**0.8**	**5.6**	**0**	**3.1**
BLUEBERRIES								
Dried, Love Life, Waitrose*	1 Serving/30g	107	0.2	358	1.1	80.1	0.8	3.6
Frozen, Average	**1 Serving/80g**	**41**	**0.2**	**51**	**0.6**	**13.8**	**0.2**	**4.4**
Raw, Average	**50 Berries/68g**	**39**	**0.2**	**57**	**0.7**	**14.5**	**0.3**	**2.4**

| | | Measure | | per Measure | | Nutrition Values per 100g / 100ml | | | | |
		INFO/WEIGHT		KCAL	FAT	KCAL	PROT	CARB	FAT	FIBRE
BOAR										
Wild, Raw, Average		**1 Serving/200g**		**244**	**6.7**	**122**	**21.5**	**0**	**3.3**	**0**
BOILED SWEETS										
Average		**1 Sweet/7g**		**21**	**0**	**327**	**0**	**87.1**	**0**	**0**
Blackcurrant & Liquorice, Co-Op*		1 Sweet/8g		32	0.4	405	0.9	91	5	0
Cherry Drops, Bassett's*		1 Sweet/5g		18	0	390	0	98.1	0	0
Clear Fruits, Sainsbury's*		1 Sweet/7g		26	0	372	0.1	92.9	0	0
Fruit Drops, Co-Op*		1 Sweet/6g		24	0	395	0.2	98	0	0
Fruit Sherbets, Assorted, M&S*		1 Sweet/9g		35	0.4	405	0.3	91.6	4.3	0.1
Lockets, Mars*		1 Pack/43g		165	0	383	0	95.8	0	0
Pear Drops, Bassett's*		1 Sweet/4g		16	0	390	0	96.4	0	0
Pear Drops, Sugar Free, Sula*		1 Sweet/3g		7	0	235	0.1	97	0.1	0
Soothers, Cherry, Hall's*		1 Pack/45g		165	0	365	0	91.3	0	0
Soothers, Strawberry Flavour, Hall's*		1 Sweet/5g		19	0	385	0	96	0	0
BOLOGNESE										
Mushroom, with Tagliatelle, Cooked, Plant Menu, Aldi*		1 Pack/377g		275	2.6	73	3.1	13	0.7	1.8
Rainbow, Microwaved, Slimming World*		1 Serving/550g		346	1.1	63	3.3	11.4	0.2	1.5
Rigatoni, Allplants*		1 Serving/380g		559	20.1	147	6.1	16	5.3	3.1
Soya, Vegan, Sauce, Fresh, Waitrose*		½ Pot/175g		163	9.4	93	6.2	3.5	5.4	3
Spaghetti, Calorie Controlled, Tesco*		1 Pack/380g		361	7.6	95	6.5	12	2	1.6
Spaghetti, Cook*		1 Serving/390g		491	14.8	126	8.9	14.8	3.8	1.6
Spaghetti, Italian, Microwaved, Morrisons*		1 Pack/396g		400	9.1	101	6.5	12.7	2.3	1.6
Spaghetti, Meal for One, M&S*		1 Pack/400g		612	31.6	153	7.4	12.3	7.9	1.6
Spaghetti, Microwaved, Iceland*		1 Pack/461g		530	18	115	4.4	14.2	3.9	2.4
Spaghetti, Mushroom, Plant Chef, Tesco*		1 Pack/426g		511	9.8	120	9.1	14.6	2.3	2.4
Vegetarian, Spaghetti, Quorn*		1 Pack/300g		255	1.8	85	4.4	14.8	0.6	1.5
BOMBAY MIX										
Average		**1oz/28g**		**141**	**9.2**	**503**	**18.8**	**35.1**	**32.9**	**6.2**
Hot, Philon*		1 Sm Bag/47g		228	15.3	485	17.6	43.2	32.6	0
BOOST										
Duo, Cadbury*		2 Bars/68g		391	19	575	5.6	59	28	1.9
Protein, Cadbury*		1 Bar/49g		249	13.3	507	25	42	27	1.2
Standard Bar, Cadbury*		1 Bar/49g		250	13.8	515	5.8	58.6	28.5	1.5
Treat Size, Cadbury*		1 Bar/24g		130	7.4	535	5.3	59.6	30.5	0
BOUILLABAISSE										
Average		**1 Serving/400g**		**556**	**38.8**	**139**	**11.2**	**2**	**9.7**	**0.4**
BOUILLON										
Powder, Miso, Marigold*		1 Tsp/5g		12	0.5	248	7	34	9.3	1.4
Powder, Swiss Vegetable, Green Tub, Marigold*		1 Tsp/5g		12	0.4	245	10.1	30.1	8.5	0
BOUNTY										
Dark, Mars*		1 Funsize/29g		141	7.9	493	3.6	55.8	27.5	0
Milk, Mars*		1 Funsize/29g		139	7.3	487	3.7	58.9	25.7	0
BOVRIL*										
Beef Extract, Drink, Made Up with Water, Bovril*		1 Serving/12g		22	0.1	184	38.9	4.6	1.2	0
Beef, Paste, High Protein, As Sold, Bovril*		1 Serving/12g		25	0.1	206	37	13	1.1	0.8
Chicken Savoury Drink, Bovril*		1 Serving/13g		16	0.2	129	9.7	19.4	1.4	2.1
BRANDY										
36% ABV, Average		**1 Pub Shot/35ml**		**88**	**0**	**250**	**0**	**0**	**0**	**0**
37.5% Volume, Average		**1 Pub Shot/35ml**		**91**	**0**	**260**	**0**	**0**	**0**	**0**
40% Volume, Average		**1 Pub Shot/35ml**		**98**	**0**	**280**	**0**	**0**	**0**	**0**
Cherry, Average		**1 Pub Shot/35ml**		**89**	**0**	**255**	**0**	**32.6**	**0**	**0**
BRAWN										
Average		**1 Serving/100g**		**153**	**11.5**	**153**	**12.4**	**0**	**11.5**	**0**

B

	Measure INFO/WEIGHT	per Measure KCAL	FAT	Nutrition Values per 100g / 100ml KCAL	PROT	CARB	FAT	FIBRE
BRAZIL NUTS								
Average	**6 Whole/20g**	**136**	**13.7**	**682**	**15.3**	**2.8**	**68.4**	**5.4**
Carob, Coated, Good Food*	1 Pack/125g	719	51.5	575	5.8	44.3	41.2	0
Milk Chocolate, Tesco*	1 Nut/8g	47	3.5	585	9.9	38	43.7	1.9
BREAD								
50/50, Little Loaf, Kingsmill*	1 Slice/29g	68	0.7	235	9.2	41.9	2.3	4.9
50/50, Multiseed, Kingsmill*	1 Slice/44g	125	3.7	283	11.5	37.3	8.3	6.4
50/50, No Crusts, Kingsmill*	1 Slice/23g	49	0.5	214	8.3	38.6	2	4.1
50/50, Wholegrain, No Bits, Medium, 400g, Kingsmill*	1 Slice/29g	68	0.6	233	9.2	42.2	2	4.9
50/50, Wonderloaf, Med Sliced, Warburton's*	1 Slice/43g	106	1.2	244	8.8	43.4	2.8	4.3
50/50, Wonderloaf, Thick Sliced, Warburton's*	1 Slice/50g	124	1.4	249	10	43.6	2.8	4.2
Ancient Grain, Pave, Bakery, Tesco*	1 Slice/80g	213	3.9	267	9.8	44.1	4.9	3.3
Bagel, Ancient Grain, Fitzgeralds*	1 Bagel/85g	241	3.7	283	11.8	46.6	4.3	5.4
Bagel, Cinnamon & Raisin, Tesco*	1 Bagel/85g	230	1.4	270	10.4	51.3	1.7	3.8
Bagel, Cinnamon & Raisin, Warburton's*	1 Bagel/80g	212	1.2	265	10.1	51	1.5	3.6
Bagel, GF, Schar*	1 Bagel/100g	278	3.7	278	4.4	53	3.7	7
Bagel, Multigrain, Sainsbury's*	1 Bagel/113g	293	3.5	259	10	49.6	3.1	2
Bagel, Multiseed, & Cereal, Fitzgeralds*	1 Bagel/85g	228	3.8	268	10.9	50.8	4.5	9.5
Bagel, Onion & Poppy Seed, Average	**1 Bagel/85g**	**225**	**2.8**	**264**	**9**	**50.5**	**3.3**	**3.2**
Bagel, Onion, New York Bagel Co*	1 Bagel/85g	222	1.6	261	10.6	50.4	1.9	3.1
Bagel, Plain, Average	**1 Bagel/78g**	**202**	**1.5**	**259**	**10.1**	**50.4**	**1.9**	**3.1**
Bagel, Plain, Sliced, Warburtons*	1 Bagel/80g	207	1.4	259	10.6	49	1.7	2.7
Bagel, Red Onion, & Chive, New York Bakery Co*	1 Bagel/90g	233	1	259	10.6	50.1	1.1	3.3
Bagel, Sesame Seed, Essential, Waitrose*	1 Bagel/85g	243	2.7	286	9.6	54.6	3.2	3.6
Bagel, Sesame, New York Bakery*	1 Bagel/90g	242	2.5	269	10.7	47.8	2.8	4.5
Bagel, Sesame, Sliced, Warburton's*	1 Bagel/80g	214	1.9	268	10.4	50	2.4	2.6
Bagel, Sesame, Sourdough, M&S*	1 Bagel/80g	219	1.8	274	11.1	49.9	2.3	4.4
Bagel, Sourdough, Deli Style, Fitzgeralds*	1 Bagel/85g	235	2.6	277	10.1	49.4	3	4.1
Bagel, Sourdough, M&S*	1 Bagel/75g	205	0.8	273	11	53.3	1	3.6
Bagel, Sourdough, New York Bagel Co*	1 Bagel/90g	245	1.2	272	10.1	53.9	1.3	2.8
Bagel, Thin, Connell*	1 Bagel/55g	157	0.8	286	10.7	55.7	1.4	3.8
Bagel, Thins, Plain, New York Bakery Co*	1 Thin/45g	122	0.5	271	11.3	55.5	1.1	3.3
Bagel, Thins, Seeded, Sliced, New York Bakery Co*	1 Thin/45g	129	1.5	286	10	52.1	3.4	3.9
Bagel, Wholemeal, & Rye, Thins, New York Bakery Co*	1 Bagel/45g	117	0.9	260	12.2	45.1	2	6.1
Bagel, Wholemeal, Average	**1 Bagel/90g**	**235**	**2.7**	**261**	**12.7**	**44.6**	**3**	**7.7**
Baguette, Bake At Home, Tesco*	½ Baguette/75g	216	0.9	289	8.6	59.1	1.2	3.5
Baguette, Brioche, Wholemeal, Waitrose*	1 Piece/85g	286	8.2	336	11	49	9.7	4.5
Baguette, French, Tesco*	1 Serving/60g	144	0.7	240	7.8	49.5	1.2	3.4
Baguette, Garlic, & Herb, Asda*	¼ Baguette/55g	189	8.2	345	7.5	44	15	2.1
Baguette, Garlic, Cheesy, Slices, M&S*	2 Slices/55g	202	9.7	368	10.1	40.8	17.7	2.5
Baguette, Garlic, Slices, Frozen, CBY, Asda*	1 Slice/26g	92	4.7	355	8.2	38.3	18.1	2.8
Baguette, Granary, Average	**1 Serving/100g**	**250**	**2.8**	**250**	**20**	**46**	**2.8**	**6**
Baguette, Multiseed, Mini, GF, Fria*	1 Baguette/70g	203	6	290	3.5	47	8.5	6
Baguette, Part Baked, H.W. Nevill's*	½ Baguette/75g	217	0.9	289	8.6	59.1	1.2	3.5
Baguette, Seeded, Stone Baked, Bakery, Tesco*	1 Baguette/280g	784	13.4	280	10.4	47.1	4.8	3.5
Baguette, Sourdough, la Brea Bakery*	1 Serving/60g	160	0.4	266	8.8	56.1	0.7	1.8
Baguette, Sourdough, Menissez*	½ Baguette/125g	304	1.2	243	7.9	50.3	1	0
Baguette, Tiger, Tesco*	¼ Baguette/50g	145	0.9	290	10.8	56.4	1.8	2.5
Baguette, White, Half, Crusty, M&S*	1 Baguette/162g	420	1.8	260	8.4	53.5	1.1	2.3
Baguette, White, Part Baked, Morrisons*	1 Baguette/150g	422	2	281	9	56.5	1.3	3.7
Baguette, White, Sainsbury's*	1 Serving/50g	136	0.3	273	10.3	55.2	0.6	2.8
Baguette, White, Sliced, Asda*	1 Baguette/85g	272	6.1	320	9.3	53	7.2	2.9
Baguette,Seeded, Sourdough, Part Baked, Aldi*	1 Baguette/112g	335	3.5	299	9.7	56	3.1	3.7
Bap, White, Large, Co-Op*	1 Bap/80g	202	3	253	8.1	45.2	3.8	2.6

BREAD

INFO/WEIGHT	Measure	per Measure		Nutrition Values per 100g / 100ml				
		KCAL	FAT	KCAL	PROT	CARB	FAT	FIBRE
Bap, Wholemeal, M&S*	1 Bap/56g	134	2.7	239	10.4	35.3	4.8	6.5
Baps, Brown, Large, Asda*	1 Bap/58g	140	0.9	242	10	47	1.6	0
Baps, Cheese Topped, Baker's Soft, Tesco*	1 Bap/65g	176	3.3	268	10.8	43.5	5.1	2.6
Baps, White, Average	**1 Bap/65g**	**167**	**2.3**	**257**	**9.5**	**47**	**3.5**	**1.9**
Baps, White, Giant, Sainsbury's*	1 Bap/86g	235	3.2	273	8.3	51.7	3.7	3.4
Baps, White, Large, Tesco*	1 Bap/95g	242	2.5	255	8.4	47.7	2.6	3.3
Baps, Wholemeal, Giant, Sainsbury's*	1 Bap/86g	230	3.5	268	9.7	48.1	4.1	7.7
Baps, Wholemeal, Tesco*	1 Bap/46g	104	2.4	227	9.6	41.4	5.3	5.6
Baps, Wholemeal, Waitrose*	1 Bap/80g	191	3.4	238	12	34.8	4.2	6.7
Best of Both, Med Sliced, Eat Well, M&S*	1 Slice/36g	83	0.8	229	9.4	41.2	2.2	3.5
Best of Both, Medium, Hovis*	1 Slice/38g	86	0.8	230	10.2	40.4	2.2	3.9
Best of Both, Thick Sliced, Hovis*	1 Slice/47g	108	1	230	10.2	40.4	2.2	3.9
Black Olive, Finest, Tesco*	1 Slice/72g	184	4.6	255	9.7	39.7	6.4	2.9
Bloomer, Brown, Slices, GF, Made Without Wheat, M&S*	1 Slice/53g	131	2.9	247	4.3	41.4	5.4	7.8
Bloomer, Multiseed, Average	**1 Slice/50g**	**120**	**2.4**	**240**	**11.8**	**37.2**	**4.9**	**7.7**
Bloomer, Sunflower Seeded, with Rye, TTD, Sainsbury's*	1 Slice/28g	90	3.4	317	12.6	36	12.1	6.8
Bloomer, White, Crusty, Bakery, Tesco*	1 Slice/50g	122	0.8	244	8.3	47.2	1.7	3.3
Bloomer, White, Sliced, Waitrose*	1 Slice/50g	130	0.9	259	8.5	52.1	1.8	2.6
Bloomer, White, Traditional, Village Bakery, Aldi*	1 Slice/37g	92	0.8	250	9.2	47	2.2	2.7
Both in One, Village Bakery, Aldi*	1 Slice/40g	95	1	237	8.5	43	2.5	4.3
Both Together, Med Sliced, Tesco*	1 Slice/40g	93	0.7	233	9.9	42.1	1.7	4.9
Breadcakes, Big Brown, Morrisons*	1 Cake/63g	154	2.1	245	9	44.6	3.4	4.3
Brioche, Bun, Gourmet, Bundy *	1 Bun/80g	206	2.6	257	9.6	46.2	3.2	2.9
Brioche, Burger Bun, Deluxe, Lidl*	1 Bun/50g	170	4.9	339	10.1	51.8	9.8	1.6
Brioche, Burger Bun, M&S*	1 Bun/72g	212	6.1	294	9	43.5	8.5	3.6
Brioche, Burger Buns, Luxury, Specially Selected, Aldi*	1 Bun/50g	159	3.7	317	9.5	52	7.3	3.1
Brioche, Burger Buns, Signature, Morrisons*	1 Bun/55g	156	2.3	284	9.4	51	4.2	2.2
Brioche, Burger Buns, Warburton's*	1 Roll/54g	159	3.2	294	10.2	49.1	6	1.2
Brioche, Raisin, Swirls, Sainsbury's*	1 Swirl/45g	130	3.4	288	6.9	47.3	7.5	2
Brioche, Swirl, Bon Appetit, Aldi*	1 Slice/50g	152	5	305	6.1	46	10	1.9
Brown, Bloomer, Organic, Bakery, Tesco*	1 Slice/80g	193	1.8	241	9	42.8	2.3	6.5
Brown, Crustless, Xrysos Milos, Wheat & Rye, Lidl*	1 Slice/24g	58	0.9	243	8.7	41.8	3.8	0
Brown, Danish, Weight Watchers, Warburton's*	1 Slice/20g	48	0.4	233	10.3	40.7	1.8	6.2
Brown, Farmhouse, GF, Newburn, Warburton's*	1 Slice/35g	82	1.9	234	7.8	35.8	5.4	5.7
Brown, Farmhouse, Soft, Sliced, GF, Genius *	1 Slice/36g	92	2.1	256	2.2	44	5.8	9.1
Brown, Malted, Bloomer, Rowan Hill Bakery, Lidl*	1 Slice/57g	155	2.3	272	9.7	46.7	4.1	4.9
Brown, Malted, Farmhouse Gold, Morrisons*	1 Slice/38g	94	0.5	248	8.2	49.6	1.4	3
Brown, Med Sliced	**1 Slice/34g**	**74**	**0.7**	**218**	**8.5**	**44.3**	**2**	**3.5**
Brown, Mixed Grain, Original, Vogel*	1 Slice/45g	102	0.6	227	9.8	47.1	1.2	6.4
Brown, Mixed Seed, Sliced, Free From, Waitrose*	2 Slices/67g	184	6.1	275	4.4	37	9.1	13.7
Brown, Oaty, Super, Sliced, Roberts*	1 Slice/33g	76	0.7	229	8.6	43.6	2.2	3.9
Brown, Premium, Med Sliced, Warburton's*	1 Slice/24g	61	0.9	258	10.6	43.2	3.7	4.3
Brown, Pumpkin & Sunflower, Aldi*	1 Slice/47g	151	4.4	322	10.7	41.3	9.3	4.8
Brown, Sainsbury's*	1 Slice/34g	81	0.7	239	8.4	46.8	2.1	4.2
Brown, Seeded, Free From, Co-Op*	1 Slice/38g	87	3.1	229	6.3	25	8.1	16
Brown, Seeded, GF, Loaf, Made Without Wheat, M&S*	1 Slice/33g	89	3.2	268	4.8	34.5	9.7	11.9
Brown, Seeded, GF, Sliced, Co-Op*	1 Slice/38g	87	3.1	229	6.3	25	8.1	16
Brown, Seeded, Sliced, Half Loaf , Morrisons*	1 Slcie/47g	133	5	283	3.2	39.8	10.7	7.2
Brown, Soda, M&S*	1 Slice/40g	92	1.4	229	9.2	43.6	3.6	4.9
Brown, Sourdough, 500g, Paul Rhodes Bakery*	1 Slice/50g	89	0.4	179	7.2	37.2	0.8	3.3
Brown, Sourdough, Boule, San Francisco Style, Waitrose*	1 Slice/50g	120	0.7	239	9.1	45.5	1.4	3.8
Brown, Super Seeded, Jacksons Of Yorkshire*	1 Slice/45g	130	4	290	13.3	35.5	9	6.9
Brown, Super Seeded, Sliced, Loaf, Extra Special, Asda*	1 Slice/44g	131	4.3	298	12	39	9.7	5.5

B

BREAD

INFO/WEIGHT	Measure	per Measure KCAL	per Measure FAT	Nutrition Values per 100g / 100ml KCAL	PROT	CARB	FAT	FIBRE
Brown, Super Seeds, Kingsmill*	1 Slice/47g	138	2	294	10.9	40	4.2	4.9
Brown, Toasted, Average	*1 Slice/24g*	*65*	*0.5*	*272*	*10.4*	*56.5*	*2.1*	*4.5*
Bun, Burger, Brioche, The Country Miller*	1 Bun/68g	249	5.4	366	7.3	48.8	7.9	2.8
Bun, Burger, Sesame Seeded, Sheldon's*	1 Bun/58g	154	2.7	266	10.5	44.7	4.6	1.7
Buns, Burger Seeded, Sliced, Warburton's*	1 Roll/60g	158	3.2	264	9	43.6	5.3	2.7
Buns, Burger, American Style, Sainsbury's*	1 Bun/50g	131	2.1	261	10.5	45.6	4.1	3.6
Buns, Burger, Brioche, TTD, Sainsbury's*	1 Bun/80g	257	8.2	322	7.8	48.1	10.3	2.6
Buns, Burger, GF, Made Without Wheat, M&S*	1 Bun/80g	201	5	251	4.8	38.9	6.2	10.4
Buns, Burger, Sainsbury's*	1 Bun/56g	154	2.9	275	9.2	47.8	5.2	4.1
Buns, Burger, Seeded, Large, Tesco*	1 Bun/90g	240	3.2	267	9.5	47.7	3.6	2.9
Buns, Burger, Sesame, American Style, Sainsbury's*	1 Bun/60g	162	3.8	270	7.3	46.2	6.3	2.2
Buns, Burger, Sesame, Sliced, Tesco*	1 Bun/60g	168	4	280	7.9	47.3	6.6	2.1
Buns, White, Burger, Waitrose*	1 Bun/64g	169	2.5	264	10	47.2	3.9	2.7
Buns, White, Stay Fresh, Tesco*	1 Bun/56g	152	3.7	271	7.5	45.5	6.6	0
Butterbread, Nature's Own*	1 Slice/30g	70	0.6	231	11.5	46.2	1.9	0
Challah, Average	*1 Slice/50g*	*143*	*3.6*	*286*	*8.9*	*53.6*	*7.1*	*3.6*
Chapatti, Sainsbury's*	1 Chapatti/99g	287	5	290	8.8	50.5	5	4.1
Cheese & Garlic, Pizza, Oven Cooked, Tesco*	½ Pizza/102g	304	11.7	298	9.2	38.1	11.5	2.4
Cheese, & Garlic, Pizza Style, Sainsbury's*	¼ Bread/63g	199	8.1	318	10.7	39.7	13	2.2
Cheese, & Onion, Toastie, Warburton's*	1 Slice/42g	120	5.8	286	7.5	33.1	13.7	0
Cheese, & Tomato, Tear & Share, Sainsbury's*	¼ Bread/72g	211	9.5	293	8	35.7	13.2	1.5
Cheese, & Garlic, Slices, Tesco*	1 Slice/32g	103	3.3	322	10.6	44.9	10.4	3.2
Cheese, Morrisons*	1 Serving/96g	297	13.6	311	9.9	35.9	14.2	3
Cheese, Three, Bloomer, Bakery, Tesco*	1 Slice/82g	214	5.3	261	13.1	36.7	6.4	2
Cholla, Average	*1/10 Loaf/154g*	*421*	*14.3*	*274*	*6.9*	*40.8*	*9.3*	*1*
Ciabatta, Black Olive, Bake At Home, Aldi*	¼ Baguette/75g	220	3.1	294	8.9	54	4.1	3.3
Ciabatta, Garlic, Slices, Tesco*	1 Slice/43g	129	3.2	301	9.6	46.9	7.5	3.6
Ciabatta, Half, Handcrafted, TTD, Sainsbury's*	1 Pack/270g	794	12.7	294	11.6	49.8	4.7	3.1
Ciabatta, Half, M&S*	1 Ciabatta/135g	354	5.5	262	10.3	48.1	4.1	2.1
Ciabatta, Mixed Olive, Waitrose*	1 Serving/35g	91	2.2	260	8.1	40.9	6.4	3.3
Ciabatta, Ready to Bake, Sainsbury's*	½ Ciabatta/66g	172	2.4	260	8.9	47.7	3.7	2.2
Ciabatta, Sun Dried Tomato & Basil, Tesco*	¼ Ciabatta/75g	193	4.3	257	8.9	42.4	5.7	2.4
Ciabatta, TTD, Sainsbury's*	¼ Pack/68g	185	4	274	10.4	44.8	5.9	2.7
Ciabatta. Sourdough, Bakery, Waitrose*	¼ Ciabatta/45g	111	0.9	247	12.8	42.5	2	3.8
Cinnamon, & Raisin, Toasty Loaf, Rankin*	1 Slice/40g	113	2	283	6.6	54.2	5	2.5
Cob, Cheese & Chutney, Bakery, Tesco*	1 Slice/50g	124	2.2	249	11.3	39.7	4.4	2.5
Corn, Soft, Old El Paso*	1 Tortilla/42g	121	2	289	8.5	51.8	4.8	2.4
Corn, with Sunflower Seed & Mixed Spice, Bakery, Tesco*	1 Slice/50g	131	2	262	9.9	45	4.1	2.6
Cottage Loaf, Stonebaked, Asda*	1 Serving/67g	155	0.9	232	10	45	1.3	3.2
Farl, Irish Soda, Irwin's Bakery*	1 Farl/150g	334	5.1	223	4	44	3.4	2.3
Farmhouse, Seeded, Sliced, Co-Op*	1 Slice/44g	112	2.5	254	13	34	5.6	7.5
Farmhouse, Wholemeal, Average	*1 Slice/43g*	*94*	*1.4*	*219*	*10.7*	*36.2*	*3.3*	*7.3*
Farmhouse, with Oatmeal, Batch, Finest, Tesco*	1 Slice/44g	110	1.4	240	9.8	43.2	3.1	5.2
Ficelle, Mixed Olive, Waitrose*	1/5 Stick/50g	133	1.4	267	7.5	51.1	2.8	3.4
Five Seed, Fully Loaded, Aldi*	1 Slice/50g	135	3.3	270	10.9	36.4	6.7	7.9
Flat, Italian, Piada Sfogliata, Italiamo, Lidl*	1 Piece/130g	402	12.5	309	7.9	45.9	9.6	2
Flatbread, Folded, Lge Plain, by, Sainsbury's*	1 Flatbread/65g	192	3.4	295	8.5	51.4	5.3	4.1
Flatbread, Folded, Plain, Sainsbury's*	1 Flatbread/33g	97	1.7	295	8.5	51.4	5.3	4.1
Flatbread, Garlic, & Cheese, Tesco*	¼ Flatbread/55g	150	4	273	9.9	40.6	7.2	3
Flatbread, Garlic, BGTY, Sainsbury's*	¼ Bread/56g	177	5.7	316	9.6	46.6	10.1	2.7
Flatbread, Greek Style, Deli Kitchen*	1 Bread/80g	204	3.4	255	11.3	39.7	4.2	6.7
Flatbread, Greek Style, Sainsburys*	1 Flat Bread/77g	212	4	275	12.3	40.9	5.2	7.6
Flatbread, Multiseed, Folded, Tesco*	1 Flatbread/35g	107	2.4	305	10.4	47.8	6.8	5.3

BREAD

INFO/WEIGHT	Measure	per Measure		Nutrition Values per 100g / 100ml				
		KCAL	FAT	KCAL	PROT	CARB	FAT	FIBRE
Flatbread, Piadina, Specially Selected, Aldi*	1 Flatbread/75g	220	6.2	294	11	42	8.3	4.1
Flatbread, Seeded, Folded, Rowan Hill Bakery, Lidl*	1 Bread/35g	121	3.3	346	10.9	52.6	9.4	4
Flatbread, Super Seeded, Folded, Village Bakery, Aldi*	1 Flatbread/35g	123	4.6	352	9.7	47	13	5.5
Flatbread, White, Folded, Village Bakery, Aldi*	1 Flatbread/35g	106	2.1	303	9.1	51.4	6	2.6
Flatbread, Wholemeal, Folded, Sainsbury's*	1 Flatbread/35g	102	2.4	292	9.5	44	7	7.4
Focaccia, Balsamic Onion, & Thyme, Co-Op*	1 Focaccia/60g	155	3.6	258	7.3	41	6	4.9
Focaccia, Mozzarella, & Krauter, Aldi*	1 Focaccia/150g	441	18	294	8	38	12	1.7
Focaccia, Rosemary & Sea Salt, TTD, Sainsbury's*	1/3 Loaf/125g	326	8.7	261	7.4	40.7	7	2.8
Focaccia, Rosemary, & Sea Salt, Tesco*	1 Focaccia/50g	151	4.2	301	9.4	45.5	8.3	3.4
Focaccia, Sliced, Deli Kitchen*	1 Slice/90g	219	5	243	8.7	38.5	5.5	2.3
French, Stick, Average	*1 Serving/60g*	*147*	*0.2*	*245*	*8.7*	*52.2*	*0.4*	*2.1*
Fried, Average	*1 Slice/28g*	*141*	*9*	*503*	*7.9*	*48.5*	*32.2*	*1.6*
Fruit Loaf, & Cinnamon, Finest, Tesco*	1 Slice/37g	134	4.9	363	6.4	54.6	13.2	1.5
Fruit Loaf, Apple & Cinnamon, Soreen*	1 Serving/10g	31	0.4	307	6.9	60.5	4.2	0
Fruit Loaf, Banana, Soreen*	1 Bar/42g	131	1.8	313	8.7	57.2	4.4	4.3
Fruit Loaf, Plum, Lincolnshire, Soreen*	1 Slice/25g	65	0.8	261	8.4	49.3	3.4	2.1
Fruit Loaf, Sliced, Bakers Selection, Asda*	1 Slice/36g	100	1.5	278	8.2	50	4.2	3.6
Fruit Loaf, Sliced, Sainsbury's*	1 Slice/40g	104	1.4	260	8.9	47.9	3.6	2.4
Fruit Loaf, Sliced, Tesco*	1 Slice/36g	101	1.3	281	7.9	52.6	3.6	3.2
Fruit Loaf, with Cinnamon, & Raisin, Warburton's*	1 Slice/36g	98	1.3	273	7.2	51.1	3.7	3.2
Fruit, Loaf, Banana, Lunchbox, Soreen*	1 Bar/30g	98	1.7	326	8.1	59.5	5.5	4.6
Fruit, Loaf, Toasted, Cafe Instore, Asda*	1 Slice/33g	89	1.2	269	8	51	3.7	2.9
Garlic, Average	*1 Serving/100g*	*327*	*13.8*	*327*	*8.1*	*43.7*	*13.8*	*1.4*
Garlic, Baguette, Average	*1 Slice/20g*	*66*	*2.8*	*330*	*7.8*	*43.1*	*14.2*	*1.8*
Garlic, Baguette, Free From, Tesco*	1/4 Baguette/39g	137	6.2	352	1.2	49.1	15.8	4.4
Garlic, Cheesy, Slices, M&S*	1 Slice/28g	103	5	368	10.1	40.8	17.7	2.5
Garlic, Ciabatta, & Herb Butter, Sainsbury's*	1/2 Ciabatta/105g	345	16.3	329	8.5	38.8	15.5	0
Garlic, Ciabatta, Finest, Tesco*	1 Serving/65g	205	8.9	316	8.1	40.1	13.7	2.4
Garlic, Ciabatta, Morrisons*	1/4 Pack/73g	241	9.6	330	9.6	42.1	13.1	2.7
Garlic, Focaccia, & Rosemary, Sainsbury's*	1/4 Focaccia/75g	219	7.4	292	8	43	9.8	2.8
Garlic, Focaccia, & Herb, Italian Style, Morrisons*	1/6 Focaccia/76g	259	10.9	341	8.5	44.7	14.3	2.5
Garlic, Reduced Fat, Slices, Inspired Cuisine, Aldi*	1 Slice/30g	84	1.6	279	7.4	49	5.5	2.8
Garlic, Slices, Asda*	1 Slice/26g	92	4.7	352	8.2	38	18	2.8
Garlic, Slices, BGTY, Sainsbury's*	1 Slice/33g	98	2.1	299	9.2	50.5	6.3	1.9
Garlic, Slices, Morrisons*	1 Slice/32g	109	4.1	341	8.5	46.9	12.9	1.7
Garlic, Slices, Sainsbury's*	1 Slice/30g	101	4.2	338	8.4	43	14	3.1
Garlic, Stonebaked, M&S*	1 Loaf/85g	314	14.4	369	8.6	44.4	16.9	2.4
Giraffe, Sainsbury's*	1 Slice/50g	119	0.2	238	8.9	48.1	0.5	2.7
Grained, Soft, Farmhouse, Warburton's*	1 Slice/42g	109	1.7	258	10.2	44.6	4	5
Granary, Average	*1 Slice/35g*	*85*	*1*	*242*	*9.8*	*44*	*2.8*	*4.8*
Granary, Baps, Large, Asda*	1 Bap/64g	143	1.4	224	10	41	2.2	4.3
Granary, Malted, Med Brown, Asda*	1 Slice/35g	81	0.9	231	9	43	2.6	3.3
Granary, Med Sliced, 800g, Hovis*	1 Slice/38g	97	0.9	256	10.3	46.4	2.4	3.7
Granary, Sliced, Sm Loaf, Hovis*	1 Slice/33g	84	0.8	256	10.3	46.4	2.4	3.7
Granary, Thick, Sliced, 800g, Hovis*	1 Slice/44g	112	1	256	10.3	46.4	2.4	3.7
Granary, Wholemeal, Average	*1 Slice/35g*	*80*	*0.9*	*228*	*10.8*	*38.4*	*2.6*	*6.6*
Half & Half, Medium, Warburton's*	1 Slice/40g	95	0.8	240	8.8	44.2	2	5
Half & Half, Thick Sliced, Warburtons *	1 Slice/47g	118	1.3	248	10	43.6	2.8	4.2
Irish, Barm Brack, Tesco*	1 Slice/75g	232	5.2	310	16	47.6	6.9	3
Irish, Brown Soda, Tesco*	1 Slice/50g	110	1.9	219	9.2	36.2	3.8	6.4
Irish, Cottage Wheaten, Loaf, Tesco*	1 Slice/50g	116	1.3	231	8.6	41.4	2.6	4.2
Kebab, Grilled, BFY, Asda*	1/2 Pack/83g	221	4	268	12	42	4.8	5
Lightly Seeded, Loaf, Sliced, Village Bakery, Aldi*	1 Slice/44g	112	1.6	255	9.3	44	3.7	4.5

BREAD

	Measure INFO/WEIGHT	per Measure KCAL	FAT	Nutrition Values per 100g / 100ml KCAL	PROT	CARB	FAT	FIBRE
Loaf, Sliced, Seriously Low-Carb Food*	1 Slice/23g	30	1.9	131	25	4.1	8.3	8.3
Malt Loaf, Fruity, Sliced, Soreen*	1 Slices/21g	64	0.6	300	8.2	58.2	3	3.9
Malt Loaf, Original, Low Fat, Soreen*	1 Slice/22g	63	0.4	288	7.5	60	1.6	2
Malt Loaf, Original, Sliced, Soreen*	1 Slice/26g	78	0.7	298	8.7	58.2	2.5	4.7
Malt Loaf, Rowan Hill Bakery, Lidl*	1 Slice/37g	107	1	289	8.4	55.4	2.6	5.4
Malt Loaf, Strawberry, Lunchbox, Soreen*	1 Loaf/30g	91	0.9	302	8	58.3	3	4.6
Malt Loaf, Tesco*	1 Slice/50g	146	1.4	291	8.6	58	2.7	4.8
Malted, & Seeded, Batch, Organic, Waitrose*	1 Slice/50g	118	2	236	10.9	39.5	3.9	6.2
Malted, Bloomer, Med Sliced, Iceland*	1 Slice/40g	108	1.5	270	9	48	3.8	3.8
Malted, Bloomer, Thick Sliced, Iceland*	1 Slice/51g	136	1.9	269	8.9	48	3.8	3.9
Malted, Danish, Weight Watchers, Warburton's*	1 Slice/20g	51	0.3	249	11.8	45.1	1.5	4.2
Malted, Grain, Loaf, Bakery, Tesco*	1 Slice/40g	100	0.4	250	10.5	47.6	0.9	5
Malted, Grain, Loaf, Sliced, Bakery, Tesco*	1 Slice/50g	122	0.7	244	9.1	46.6	1.4	4.3
Medium, 50/50, Kingsmill*	1 Slice/40g	94	0.9	234	9.4	41.9	2.2	4.7
Multi Seed, Thick Sliced, Loaf, Morrisons*	1 Slice/40g	119	2.8	297	12.3	37.9	7	7.5
Multi-Seeded, Farmhouse, Sliced, Loaf, Waitrose*	1 Slice/33g	96	2.9	291	11.2	38.5	8.8	6.7
Multigrain, Batch, Sliced, Tesco*	1 Slice/50g	120	0.9	241	9.3	43.7	1.8	6.2
Multigrain, Brown, Farmhouse Baker's, M&S*	1 Slice/51g	115	2.8	225	13	31.2	5.4	5.1
Multigrain, Crusty, Finest, Tesco*	1 Slice/40g	98	1.4	245	9	44.7	3.4	5
Multigrain, Farmhouse, Deluxe, Lidl*	1 Slice/40g	101	1.2	253	10.1	44.3	2.9	4.6
Multigrain, Farmhouse, Loaf, 400g, Waitrose*	1 Slice/33g	83	0.6	253	9.9	47.4	1.7	4.3
Multigrain, Thick Sliced, Tesco*	1 Slice/50g	112	1.2	225	8.4	42.2	2.5	3.9
Multiseed, Farmhouse Batch, Finest, Tesco*	1 Slice/44g	108	1.9	245	9.9	40.4	4.4	7.5
Naan, Average	**1 Naan/130g**	**344**	**5.6**	**264**	**8.3**	**48.5**	**4.3**	**2**
Naan, Chicken Tikka, Tandoori, Naanzza*	½ Naan/150g	337	9.6	225	10.9	30.7	6.4	1.3
Naan, Garlic & Coriander, Free From, Tesco*	1 Naan/90g	215	6	240	5.1	38.7	6.7	4.9
Naan, Garlic & Coriander, Tesco*	½ Naan/65g	184	3	283	7.5	51.2	4.6	3.3
Naan, Garlic & Coriander, TTD, Sainsbury's*	1 Naan/70g	219	8.4	313	7	44	12	2.9
Naan, Garlic & Coriander, Bilash, Aldi*	1 Naan/130g	333	6.5	256	7.4	44	5	2.2
Naan, Garlic & Coriander, Clay Oven Bakery*	1 Naan/120g	311	7.8	259	7.6	41.3	6.5	2.3
Naan, Garlic & Coriander, M&S*	1 Naan/75g	212	3.6	283	9.8	48.8	4.8	2.7
Naan, Garlic & Coriander, Mini, Asda*	1 Naan/47g	151	3.7	320	8.7	52	7.9	3.4
Naan, Garlic & Coriander, Mini, Sainsbury's*	1 Naan/48g	147	3.4	307	8.3	51.2	7	3
Naan, Garlic & Coriander, Mini, Sharwood's*	1 Naan/65g	196	4.2	302	8	51.5	6.5	2.8
Naan, Garlic & Coriander, Mini, Tesco*	1 Naan/50g	130	2.3	261	7.6	45.9	4.6	3
Naan, Garlic & Coriander, Weight Watchers*	1 Naan/60g	155	2.6	259	8.9	46	4.3	3.4
Naan, Garlic, Asda*	1 Naan/160g	410	6.6	256	8.3	46	4.1	1.8
Naan, Ocado*	½ Naan/75g	194	1.7	258	8.4	48.3	2.3	5.3
Naan, Peshwari, Apple & Coconut, Mini, Sharwood's*	1 Naan/65g	179	3.1	275	7.5	47.1	4.8	6.7
Naan, Peshwari, Sharwood's*	1 Naan/130g	334	6.9	257	7.2	45.1	5.3	2.5
Naan, Plain, Average	**1 Naan/160g**	**437**	**10.5**	**273**	**8**	**45.7**	**6.5**	**2.1**
Naan, Tandoori Baked, Waitrose*	1 Naan/140g	372	4.3	266	9.8	49.6	3.1	2.9
Naan, Tandoori, M&S*	1 Naan/150g	408	7.2	272	8.6	47.6	4.8	2.1
Naan, Tandoori, Mini, Indian, Waitrose*	1 Naan/73g	224	3.3	308	10.4	55.1	4.5	3.2
Naan, Tandoori, Sharwood's*	1 Naan/130g	330	6.5	254	7.3	45	5	2
Oat & Barley, Thick Sliced, Morrisons*	1 Slice/44g	111	1.6	252	8.9	43.2	3.7	5
Oat, Sunflower, & Pumpkin, Loaf, Irresistible, Co-Op*	1 Slice/50g	152	5.5	304	11	38	11	4.4
Olive, Kalamata, TTD, Sainsbury's*	1 Slice/50g	121	1.4	242	8.1	44.7	2.8	3
Parmesan, & Garlic, Rustic Wheel, M&S*	¼ Wheel/74g	230	8.7	311	10.4	40	11.7	2
Pave, Ancient Grain, TTD, Sainsbury's*	1 Slice/50g	128	1.7	256	9.6	44.6	3.4	4
Pave, Walnut, Sainsbury's*	1 Slice/50g	140	4.8	280	9	40	9.5	3.5
Pave, Walnut, TTD, Sainsbury's*	1 Slice/50g	138	3.6	277	9.5	41.5	7.3	3.7
Petit Pain, Bake at Home, Sainsbury's*	1 Roll/48g	137	0.5	285	8.5	58.8	1.1	2.9

	Measure INFO/WEIGHT	per Measure KCAL	FAT	Nutrition Values per 100g / 100ml KCAL	PROT	CARB	FAT	FIBRE
BREAD								
Petit Pain, Mini, Homebake, Tesco*	1 Roll/45g	110	0.6	245	7.8	49.7	1.3	2.5
Petit Pains, Bake at Home, Tesco*	1 Petit Pain/50g	144	0.6	289	8.8	59.1	1.2	3.5
Petit Pains, Part Baked, Morrisons*	1 Roll/45g	126	0.6	280	9.1	56.4	1.3	3.8
Pitta, Free From, Sainsbury's*	1 Pitta/65g	164	2.5	252	4.1	50	3.9	2.9
Pitta, Garlic, Morrisons*	1 Pitta/60g	149	1.1	249	9.7	51.1	1.8	0
Pitta, Grains & Goodness, The Food Doctor*	1 Pitta/60g	143	1.7	239	9.8	40.4	2.9	7
Pitta, Mediterranean Style, The Bakery, M&S*	1 Pitta/85g	247	3.7	291	6.7	54.9	4.3	2.8
Pitta, Multi Seed, & Cereal, The Food Doctor*	1 Pitta/60g	150	1.3	250	9.3	51.8	2.1	6.6
Pitta, Pocket, Stone Baked, GF, BFree*	1 Pitta/32g	68	0.6	214	4.9	39.6	1.8	9.8
Pitta, Pockets, Sainsbury's*	1 Pitta/75g	188	0.8	250	8.5	52	1	3.5
Pitta, Seeded, HL, Tesco*	1 Pitta/60g	153	3.6	255	10.8	39.4	6	12.8
Pitta, Soft, Warburton's*	1 Pitta/63g	164	1.5	260	10.5	48.5	2.4	1.5
Pitta, Stone Baked, Genius*	1 Pitta/62g	142	3.2	229	2.6	37.1	5.2	11.9
Pitta, Stonebaked, with Sourdough, The Best, Morrisons*	1 Pitta/64g	159	1.3	250	8.5	47.9	2	3
Pitta, White, Average	**1 Pitta/75g**	**191**	**1.1**	**255**	**9.2**	**50.8**	**1.5**	**2.7**
Pitta, White, Greek Style, Asda*	1 Pitta/50g	126	1	253	8	51	1.9	0
Pitta, White, Mini, Sainsbury's*	1 Pitta/20g	54	0.2	268	8.8	54.6	1.2	2
Pitta, White, Sainsbury's*	1 Pitta/58g	160	0.7	275	9.8	54.7	1.2	3.1
Pitta, Wholegrain, GF, BFree*	1 Pitta/55g	118	1.6	215	5.5	37.7	2.9	8.2
Pitta, Wholemeal, Average	**1 Pitta/64g**	**154**	**1.1**	**241**	**11**	**45.8**	**1.7**	**6.4**
Pitta, Wholemeal, Mini, M&S*	1 Pitta/18g	44	0.4	247	10.3	45.8	2.5	5.6
Pitta, Wholemeal, So Organic, Sainsbury's*	1 Pitta/60g	140	1	233	9.8	44.8	1.6	8.1
Potato, Farls, M&S*	1 Farl/55g	79	0.2	144	4.2	33.8	0.4	4.7
Potato, Farls, Slims, Rankin Selection*	1 Farl/60g	80	1.8	134	2.3	24.3	3	1.8
Potato, Farls, Sunblest*	1 Farl/100g	156	0.9	156	3.8	33.2	0.9	1.9
Pumpernickel, Average	**1 Slice/50g**	**96**	**0.6**	**191**	**5.5**	**37.9**	**1.1**	**7.8**
Roll, Brown, Deli Sub, Asda*	1 Roll/60g	142	1.9	236	0	35	3.2	0
Roll, Brown, Jackson's Bakery*	1 Roll/74g	203	3.6	274	9	46	4.8	5.1
Roll, Cheese & Onion, Bap, Market St, Morrisons*	1 Roll/40g	337	12	842	32.5	100	30	7.5
Roll, Cheese Topped, Rowan Hill Bakery, Lidl*	1 Roll/75g	208	6.2	278	11.1	38.2	8.3	2.8
Roll, Ciabatta, Asda*	1 Roll/90g	230	2.2	256	9.3	48	2.4	2.3
Roll, Cream Cheese, M&S*	1 Roll/48g	129	1.5	269	8.4	49.5	3.2	4.3
Roll, Crusty, Iceland*	1 Roll/50g	130	0.8	260	8.7	51.1	1.6	3.3
Roll, Malted Wheat, Bakery, Waitrose*	1 Roll/85g	222	1	262	7.9	52.2	1.2	5.5
Roll, Oatmeal, Deli, M&S*	1 Roll/75g	202	2.8	270	10.9	46.3	3.7	3.7
Roll, Scotch, Sainsbury's*	1 Roll/79g	200	1.9	253	9.2	47	2.4	3.4
Roll, Seeded, Bakers Selection, Asda*	1 Roll/88g	266	6.8	302	10.1	45.9	7.7	0
Roll, Seeded, Morrisons*	1 Roll/127g	338	5.8	266	10.2	44.2	4.6	3.2
Roll, Sourdough, White, Irresistible, Co-Op*	1 Roll/73g	176	0.4	241	9	49	0.6	2.6
Roll, Super Seeded, GF, Made Without Wheat, M&S*	1 Roll/75g	170	6.2	227	8	24	8.3	12
Roll, White, Large, Barm, Jones Village Bakery *	1 Roll/50g	135	2.2	270	8.2	52.5	4.5	2.9
Roll, White, Soft, Sainsbury's*	1 Roll/54g	138	1.6	255	8.5	47.3	2.9	2.8
Roll, White, Soft, Warburton's*	1 Roll/55g	146	2.1	265	9.7	46.6	3.9	2.4
Roll, Wholemeal, Bap, Bakers Selection, Asda*	1 Roll/54g	133	2	247	12	38	3.7	6.6
Roll, Wholemeal, Roberts Bakery*	1 Roll/50g	116	1.4	232	12.1	0	2.9	6.4
Roll, Wholemeal, Seeded, Love Life, Waitrose*	1 Roll/72g	192	6.3	266	12.6	34.1	8.8	6.4
Rolls, Ancient Grain, Tesco*	1 Roll/80g	231	6.7	289	14.7	34.4	8.4	8.6
Rolls, Best of Both, Hovis*	1 Roll/62g	148	2.9	239	9.8	39.7	4.6	5
Rolls, Brioche, Asda*	1 Roll/35g	127	4.2	362	7.8	55	12	1.9
Rolls, Brioche, Average	**1 Roll/49g**	**177**	**6.9**	**361**	**8.8**	**50.1**	**14.1**	**1.5**
Rolls, Brioche, Chocolate Chip, Tesco*	1 Roll/35g	131	4.4	374	7.6	56.3	12.7	2.1
Rolls, Brioche, French Milk, Bon Appetit, Aldi*	1 Roll/35g	116	2.7	330	8.3	56	7.8	2.2
Rolls, Brioche, Hot Dog, Specially Selected, Aldi*	1 Roll/45g	142	3.4	316	9.4	52	7.5	2

BREAD

	Measure INFO/WEIGHT	per Measure KCAL	FAT	Nutrition Values per 100g / 100ml KCAL	PROT	CARB	FAT	FIBRE
Rolls, Brioche, Hot Dog, TTD, Sainsbury's*	1 Roll/70g	229	7.3	327	8.3	48.6	10.4	2.8
Rolls, Brioche, Plain Chocolate Chip, Sainsbury's*	1 Roll/35g	126	4.5	361	8	52.1	12.9	2.1
Rolls, Brioche, Sweet, GF, Schar*	1 Roll/50g	146	3.6	293	3.4	52	7.3	3
Rolls, Brown, Ciabatta, Schar*	1 Roll/50g	138	4.1	274	5.8	40	8.1	8.9
Rolls, Brown, Crusty	*1 Roll/50g*	*128*	*1.4*	*255*	*10.3*	*50.4*	*2.8*	*3.5*
Rolls, Brown, Free From, Tesco*	1 Roll/65g	174	5.3	268	5.4	43.2	8.2	3.6
Rolls, Brown, Malted Grain, Tesco*	1 Roll/58g	144	1.9	248	8.7	46.2	3.2	1.9
Rolls, Brown, Morning, Farmfoods*	1 Roll/50g	134	1.8	269	12	47	3.7	4.2
Rolls, Brown, Old Fashioned, Waitrose*	1 Roll/63g	152	2.6	241	9.6	41.3	4.1	4.7
Rolls, Brown, Seeded, Organic, Sainsbury's*	1 Roll/70g	166	3.2	237	9.9	39.1	4.6	6.5
Rolls, Brown, Snack, Allinsons*	1 Roll/47g	128	2.5	272	10.2	43.5	5.3	4.9
Rolls, Brown, Soft, Average	*1 Roll/50g*	*134*	*1.9*	*268*	*10*	*51.8*	*3.8*	*3.5*
Rolls, Cheese, Rustique, Waitrose*	1 Roll/90g	255	3.4	283	11.3	49.7	3.8	2.6
Rolls, Chunky Cheese, Tesco*	1 Roll/80g	219	4.8	274	12.8	41.1	6	2
Rolls, Ciabatta, Crisp & Floury, Waitrose*	1 Roll/80g	206	2.8	258	8.4	46.5	3.5	3.4
Rolls, Ciabatta, GF, Schar*	1 Roll/50g	116	1.6	231	4.6	42	3.3	6.8
Rolls, Ciabatta, Sun Dried Tomato, Mini, Finest, Tesco*	1 Roll/30g	79	1.9	262	8.7	42.3	6.4	2.6
Rolls, Ciabatta, Tesco*	1 Roll/105g	274	4.4	261	9.2	45.3	4.2	2.4
Rolls, Crusty, French, M&S*	1 Roll/65g	159	0.8	245	8.1	50.5	1.2	3.3
Rolls, Deli, Maize Topped, Sainsbury's*	1 Roll/70g	187	2.4	267	10.9	46.7	3.4	3
Rolls, Finger, White, Sainsbury's*	1 Roll/40g	96	1	240	9	45.2	2.6	3.2
Rolls, Granary, Average	*1 Roll/70g*	*176*	*2.7*	*251*	*9.6*	*45.2*	*3.9*	*3.3*
Rolls, Hot Dog, Potato, Weis*	1 Roll/57g	160	2	281	8.8	52.6	3.5	1.8
Rolls, Hot Dog, Sliced, Sheldon's*	1 Roll/58g	147	1.4	255	9.8	47.2	2.5	1.9
Rolls, Hot Dog, Value, Tesco*	1 Roll/40g	93	0.8	232	8.7	45	1.9	2.2
Rolls, Hot Dog, White, Warburton's*	1 Roll/55g	142	2.1	259	8.8	46.4	3.9	1.6
Rolls, Large, Seriously Low-Carb Food*	1 Roll/65g	85	5.4	131	25	4.1	8.3	8.3
Rolls, Low Carb, Low Carb Food Company*	1 Roll/75g	173	11.1	231	22.4	1.9	14.8	16.1
Rolls, Low GI, Lidl*	1 Roll/60g	177	5.1	295	14	44.9	8.5	8.4
Rolls, Malted Grain, Sainsbury's*	1 Roll/68g	190	2.9	280	8.7	51.6	4.3	4.2
Rolls, Malted, Big Eat, Bakers Selection, Asda*	1 Roll/80g	207	2.5	259	9.7	46	3.1	4.6
Rolls, Mature Cheddar, with Black Pepper, Waitrose*	1 Roll/65g	189	5.7	291	11.3	40.2	8.7	3.1
Rolls, Mini Submarine, M&S*	1 Roll/23g	63	1.1	275	11.4	47.7	4.9	1.1
Rolls, Morning, Tesco*	1 Roll/48g	117	1.2	243	10.4	44.8	2.5	4.7
Rolls, Multi Seeded, GF, Promise*	1 Roll/50g	99	0.7	197	5.6	34.4	1.4	11.9
Rolls, Multigrain, Torpedo, Sainsbury's*	1 Roll/112g	328	7.5	293	10.5	47.7	6.7	6.3
Rolls, Multiseed, Deli, Tesco*	1 Roll/65g	188	4.6	289	10.5	40.7	7.1	10.3
Rolls, Oatmeal, Soft, M&S*	1 Roll/83g	224	3.9	270	12.3	43.4	4.7	3.4
Rolls, Olive, Mixed, Waitrose*	1 Roll/90g	240	2.5	267	8.8	50	2.8	3
Rolls, Panini, White, Tesco*	1 Roll/85g	232	4.1	273	10.7	44.9	4.8	3.4
Rolls, Part Baked, Iceland*	1 Roll/50g	130	0.8	260	8.7	51.1	1.6	3.3
Rolls, Part Baked, Mini, Tesco*	1 Roll/50g	120	0.6	240	7.8	49.5	1.2	3.4
Rolls, Posh Dog, The Grill, M&S*	1 Roll/64g	195	5.6	305	8.7	45.4	8.8	4.5
Rolls, Pumpkin Seed, Lidl*	1 Roll/80g	271	9	339	15	42.5	11.2	3.8
Rolls, Rustic, Ready to Bake, Paul Hollywood*	1 Roll/75g	199	0.8	265	8.5	54.7	1	1.7
Rolls, Rye, Toasting, Good & Hot*	1 Roll/65g	143	0.7	220	7.3	44.6	1.1	7.1
Rolls, Scotch, Morning, Tesco*	1 Roll/50g	136	0.6	273	11.8	52	1.3	3.2
Rolls, Scottish Morning, Mcghees*	1 Roll/48g	126	0.2	262	10.6	54.6	0.4	5.4
Rolls, Scottish Morning, Morrisons*	1 Roll/60g	157	1.3	261	11.3	51.4	2.2	2.4
Rolls, Seeded, Deli, Rowan Hill Bakery, Lidl*	1 Roll/75g	243	8.2	324	11.4	42.2	11	5.4
Rolls, Seeded, GF, Free From, Morrisons*	1 Roll/75g	166	6.4	222	7.1	20.9	8.5	16.7
Rolls, Seeded, Mixed Mini Loaf Pack, M&S*	1 Roll/76g	220	7.3	290	10.6	39.7	9.6	4
Rolls, Soft, White, Rowan Hill Bakery, Lidl*	1 Roll/66g	157	1.6	238	8.5	44	2.5	2.8

BREAD

INFO/WEIGHT	Measure	per Measure KCAL	per Measure FAT	Nutrition Values per 100g / 100ml KCAL	PROT	CARB	FAT	FIBRE
Rolls, Soft, Wholemeal, Finger, M&S*	1 Roll/66g	145	1.3	220	12.6	38	2	5.8
Rolls, Sourdough, White, No.1, Waitrose*	1 Roll/92g	229	1.7	249	9.8	47.1	1.9	2.2
Rolls, Square, Super Soft, GF, Warburton's*	1 Roll/58g	136	3.5	235	5.8	37.2	6	4.7
Rolls, Sub, White, Batch, Warburton's*	1 Roll/80g	215	3.5	269	11	45	4.4	2.4
Rolls, Sub, Wholemeal, Warburton's*	1 Roll/94g	231	4.1	246	10.9	40.6	4.4	6.3
Rolls, Tiger, Crusty, Baked by Us, Morrisons*	1 Roll/63g	143	1.8	227	6.3	46	2.9	2.5
Rolls, Tiger, Tesco*	1 Roll/73g	212	1.3	290	10.8	56.4	1.8	2.6
Rolls, Triple Seeded, Genius *	1 Roll/70g	209	7.8	299	3.9	40.6	11.2	10
Rolls, White, 50/50, Soft, Kingsmill*	1 Roll/63g	154	2.4	245	9.3	41.2	3.8	4.4
Rolls, White, Cheese Topped, Sainsbury's*	1 Roll/75g	218	6.4	291	12.1	41.6	8.5	2
Rolls, White, Crusty, Average	*1 Roll/50g*	*140*	*1.2*	*280*	*10.9*	*57.6*	*2.3*	*1.5*
Rolls, White, Feel Good, GF, Genius*	1 Roll/70g	158	3.1	225	4.6	36	4.4	12
Rolls, White, Finest, Tesco*	1 Roll/80g	198	2	247	9.3	45.3	2.5	3
Rolls, White, Finger, Tesco*	1 Roll/45g	112	0.4	250	9.2	49.7	1	2.6
Rolls, White, Floured, Batch, Tesco*	1 Roll/76g	193	2.5	254	8.8	47.3	3.3	2.2
Rolls, White, Floury Batch, Sainsbury's*	1 Roll/68g	168	1.9	247	8.3	47.2	2.8	2.2
Rolls, White, Floury, Roberts Bakery*	1 Roll/63g	160	1.6	254	8.4	49.5	2.5	2
Rolls, White, Hot Dog, Jumbo, Sainsbury's*	1 Roll/85g	239	5.2	281	7.5	49.1	6.1	2.9
Rolls, White, Hot Dog, Large, Asda *	1 Roll/86g	224	2.1	260	8.7	50	2.4	1.9
Rolls, White, Hot Dog, Tesco*	1 Roll/65g	162	0.6	250	9.2	49.7	1	2.6
Rolls, White, Hot Dog, Tesco*	1 Roll/70g	177	2.5	254	9	45.5	3.6	1.9
Rolls, White, Large, Warburton's*	1 Roll/88g	223	3.3	252	9.1	44.3	3.7	2.4
Rolls, White, Mini, Submarine, M&S*	1 Roll/30g	86	1.5	285	11.4	47.7	4.9	1.1
Rolls, White, Morning, Co-Op*	1 Roll/47g	134	1.4	285	12	53	3	2
Rolls, White, Morning, Sainsbury's*	1 Roll/79g	200	1.9	253	9.2	47	2.4	3.4
Rolls, White, Organic, Sainsbury's*	1 Roll/65g	170	2	262	8.7	49.9	3	1
Rolls, White, Sandwich, Sliced, Warburton's*	1 Roll/55g	146	2.1	265	9.7	46.6	3.9	2.4
Rolls, White, Seeded, Sainsbury's*	1 Roll/80g	217	4.7	271	10.9	43.4	5.9	4.8
Rolls, White, Seeded, Soft, M&S*	1 Roll/75g	214	4.3	285	11.7	46.2	5.7	2.8
Rolls, White, Sliced, Warburton's*	1 Roll/55g	146	2.2	265	9.7	46.6	3.9	2.4
Rolls, White, Soft, Average	*1 Roll/45g*	*114*	*1.5*	*253*	*9.2*	*46.5*	*3.3*	*2.2*
Rolls, White, Soft, GF, Promise*	1 Roll/50g	100	0.5	199	2.4	39	1	12.2
Rolls, White, Sourdough, Waitrose*	1 Roll/70g	161	0.8	230	9	44.4	1.1	3.1
Rolls, White, Submarine, M&S*	1 Roll/109g	300	5.4	275	11	47	5	1
Rolls, White, with Sourdough, Country Miller*	1 Roll/72g	189	0.8	262	9.3	52.3	1.1	2.9
Rolls, Wholemeal	*1 Roll/45g*	*108*	*1.3*	*241*	*9*	*48.3*	*2.9*	*5.9*
Rolls, Wholemeal, Deli, Tesco*	1 Roll/65g	156	3.1	240	9	40.2	4.8	5.7
Rolls, Wholemeal, Oat Topped, Deli, Tesco*	1 Roll/65g	170	3.5	260	10.9	38.3	5.3	6.7
Rolls, Wholemeal, Plaited, Morrisons*	1 Roll/100g	195	1	195	6	30	1	6
Rolls, Wholemeal, Rustic, Bakery, Sainsbury's*	1 Roll/76g	173	1.1	228	11.6	37.6	1.4	9.3
Rolls, Wholemeal, Soft, Average	*1 Roll/65g*	*151*	*2.7*	*233*	*10.8*	*37.3*	*4.1*	*6.3*
Rolls, Wholemeal, Sunflower & Honey, Sainsbury's*	1 Roll/100g	311	8.1	311	10.8	45.9	8.1	5.4
Rolls, Wholemeal, Tasty, Kingsmill*	1 Roll/68g	171	2.5	251	10.7	39.1	3.7	6.5
Rolls, Wholemeal, Tasty, Kingsmill*	1 Roll/68g	165	2.7	243	10.8	38.3	3.9	5.7
Rolls, Wholemeal, The Best, Morrisons*	1 Roll/72g	174	2.1	242	10.5	39.7	2.9	7.6
Rolls, Wholemeal, Village Bakery, Aldi*	1 Roll/63g	144	0.9	228	10	40	1.5	5.3
Rolls, York Baps, Adkins Bakery*	1 Roll/100g	264	2.2	264	10.7	53.7	2.2	2.4
Roti, Chakki, Nishaan*	1 Roti/58g	166	4	286	8.2	46.4	6.9	2.7
Roti, Tesco*	1 Roti/95g	256	5.2	269	8.4	46.4	5.5	3.2
Rye, & Flax, Organic, Profusion*	1 Slice/50g	120	4.4	241	20.1	14.4	8.9	11.4
Rye, 100% Organic, Sliced, Celtic Bakers*	1 Slice/42g	109	0.5	259	8.4	56.1	1.2	10.1
Rye, Average	*1 Slice/25g*	*55*	*0.4*	*219*	*8.3*	*45.8*	*1.7*	*4.4*
Rye, Bloomer, Co-Op*	1 Slice/45g	113	0.4	251	7.1	51	0.9	5.4

BREAD

	Measure INFO/WEIGHT	per Measure KCAL	FAT	Nutrition Values per 100g / 100ml KCAL	PROT	CARB	FAT	FIBRE
Rye, Bloomer, Dulcesol*	1 Slice/40g	102	1.2	255	9.4	45	3.1	4.8
Rye, German Style, Kelderman*	1 Slice/64g	113	0.6	177	6.1	34.4	1	8.3
Rye, German Style, Loaf, Bakery in Store, M&S*	1 Slice/25g	56	0.3	225	9.5	40.8	1.1	6.3
Rye, Half Wheat, The Polish Bakery, Tesco*	1 Slice/40g	93	0.6	233	5.7	51.1	1.5	6.6
Rye, Light, Boule, Bakery, Waitrose*	1 Slice/50g	132	2.1	264	8.5	45.6	4.2	5.2
Rye, Seeded, Walmart*	1 Slice/44g	110	1.5	250	9.1	45.4	3.4	4.6
Rye, Sourdough, Part Baked, TTD, Sainsbury's*	1 Slice/30g	70	0.4	233	6.5	45	1.3	7.8
Rye, Stone Baked, Dutch Style , Kelderman*	1 Slice/55g	128	0.5	233	8.1	46	0.9	5.1
Rye, Whole Grain, Schneiderbrot*	1 Slice/50g	100	0.5	201	5.2	38.9	1	7.7
Rye, Wholegrain , Sliced, Rowan Hill Bakery, Lidl*	1 Slice/56g	118	1	210	5.8	38	1.8	9.3
Rye, Wholegrain, with Sunflower Seeds, Rowan Hill*	1 Slice/56g	126	2.6	225	6.3	35	4.6	9.3
Rye, Wholemeal with Sunflower Seeds, Organic, Biona*	1 Slice/72g	150	2.9	210	7	36	4	6
Rye, Wholemeal, Mestemacher*	1 Slice/72g	165	0.6	229	4.9	44.6	0.9	11.5
Rye, with Sunflower Seeds, Organic, Schneider Brot*	1 Slice/72g	138	2.6	191	6.2	33.4	3.6	7.9
Sandwich Thins, Brown, Warburton's*	1 Thin/40g	100	1.1	252	9.9	45.2	2.8	3.5
Sandwich Thins, Half & Half, Warburtons *	1 Thin/40g	100	1.2	251	10	44.5	2.9	3.6
Sandwich Thins, Multiseed, GF, Warburton's*	1 Thin/50g	142	4	284	6.5	43.1	8.1	6.5
Sandwich Thins, Seeded, GF, Free From, Waitrose*	1 Thin/50g	132	5.1	263	9.3	24.5	10.2	18
Sandwich Thins, Seeded, GF, Warburton's*	1 Thin/43g	122	3.5	284	6.5	43.1	8.1	6.5
Sandwich Thins, White, GF, Warburton's*	1 Thin/50g	124	3.2	247	6	38.7	6.3	5.7
Sandwich, 12 Grain & Seed, Walmart*	1 Slice/46g	122	3.3	265	10.2	42.8	7.2	4.1
Seeded, Batch, Finest, Tesco*	1 Slice/65g	168	4	259	9.3	41.8	6.1	6.1
Seeded, Batch, Hovis*	1 Slice/50g	134	3.4	267	10.9	38.1	6.7	5.6
Seeded, Bloomer, Loaf, Rowan Hill Bakery, Lidl*	1 Slice/57g	166	4.5	292	10.3	42.3	7.9	5
Seeded, Bloomer, Sliced, Co-Op*	1 Slice/57g	153	3.8	268	12	40	6.7	0.5
Seeded, Cob, 450g, Hovis*	1 Slice/45g	126	3.3	280	10.7	40.7	7.4	4.3
Seeded, Farmhouse, GF, Warburton's*	1 Slice/35g	92	3.2	262	8.7	33	9.1	6.5
Seeded, Farmhouse, Loaf, Extra Special, Asda*	1 Slice/44g	92	0.5	207	11	38	1.2	8
Seeded, Free From, Gluten, Wheat, & Milk, Tesco*	1 Slice/37g	107	3.5	288	6.2	39.3	9.5	10.3
Seeded, GF, Sliced, Cob, Waitrose*	1 Slices/34g	93	2.4	278	5.8	42.7	7.3	9.2
Seeded, GF, Sliced, Free From, Morrisons*	1 Slice/42g	93	3.4	221	6	23.3	8.1	15.2
Seeded, Honey Soaked, Bloomer, Village Bakery, Aldi*	1 Slice/58g	154	3.2	266	11.2	39.7	5.5	6.4
Seeded, Loaf, Sliced, Village Bakery, Aldi*	1 Slice/33g	92	2.6	280	11	38	7.9	6.9
Seeded, Med Sliced, Average	**1 Slice/44g**	**116**	**2.9**	**262**	**11.3**	**38.6**	**6.5**	**5.6**
Seeded, Sliced, Low Carb Food Company*	1 Slice/26g	54	3.5	208	19.6	2.3	13.5	14.2
Seeded, Triple, Farmhouse, Loaf, GF, Genius*	1 Slice/36g	100	2.9	277	3.5	43.8	8	8
Slimbo, Sesame & Linseed, Pat The Baker*	1 Slimbo/35g	100	1.6	285	12.8	50.5	4.7	5.4
Soda	**1oz/28g**	**72**	**0.7**	**258**	**7.7**	**54.6**	**2.5**	**2.1**
Soda, Brown, Irish, Rankin Selection, Irwin's Bakery*	1 Slice/36g	86	1.2	238	8.2	41.8	3.4	4
Sourdough, Average	**1 Slice/50g**	**144**	**0.9**	**289**	**11.8**	**56.4**	**1.8**	**2.4**
Sourdough, Bloomer, Specially Selected, Aldi*	1 Slice/50g	117	1.1	234	9.4	42.5	2.2	3.4
Sourdough, Boule , Bertinet Bakery*	1 Slice/50g	114	0.4	228	6.9	47	0.8	2.4
Sourdough, Dark Rye, Specially Selected, Aldi*	1 Slice/58g	140	1	242	7.6	46.6	1.8	4.4
Sourdough, GF, Loaf, Made Without Wheat, M&S*	1 Slice/39g	86	1.9	223	4.7	36.8	4.9	6.6
Sourdough, Malted Wheat, Sliced, Bertinet Bakery*	1 Slice/80g	189	1	236	8.9	45.7	1.2	3.6
Sourdough, Mixed Olive, Bakery, Sainsbury's*	1 Slice/40g	90	3.8	224	6	27	9.5	2.8
Sourdough, Multigrain, Gallaghers Bakery*	2 Slices/67g	185	4.6	276	11.8	39.2	6.8	6.2
Sourdough, Pave, 400g, TTD, Bakery, Sainsbury's*	1 Serving/50g	126	0.5	252	9.4	50.1	1	2.5
Sourdough, Rye, & Mixed Seed, Finest, Tesco*	1 Slice/44g	106	1.6	241	9.1	40.3	3.7	5
Sourdough, Rye, Banneton, Sainsbury's*	1 Slice/50g	115	0.6	230	6.6	46.1	1.1	4.7
Sourdough, Rye, Bloomer, Tesco*	1 Slice/40g	97	0.5	243	8.3	47.2	1.2	4.9
Sourdough, San Francisco, Gail's*	1 Slice/63g	106	0.4	170	6.4	34.6	0.7	1.2
Sourdough, Seeded, Finest, Tesco*	1 Slice/44g	106	1.6	241	9.1	40.3	3.7	5

BREAD

INFO/WEIGHT	Measure	per Measure		Nutrition Values per 100g / 100ml				
		KCAL	FAT	KCAL	PROT	CARB	FAT	FIBRE
Sourdough, Seeded, Half Bloomer, TTD, Sainsbury's*	1 Slice/40g	113	2.2	283	10.7	46.1	5.4	3.8
Sourdough, Spelt, Organic, Sliced, Modern Baker*	1 Slice/45g	106	0.6	236	7.1	47	1.4	2.5
Sourdough, Three Cheese, Bloomer, Irresistible, Co-Op*	1 Slice/50g	137	3.8	274	13	38	7.7	1.9
Sourdough, Tiger Bay, Brace's*	1 Slice/44g	117	0.9	266	10.1	49.3	2	5
Sourdough, Tomato, Slow Roasted, Irresistible, Co-Op*	1 Slice/50g	110	0.7	219	8.2	41	1.4	4.4
Sourdough, White, Sliced, Bertinet Bakery*	1 Slice/42g	99	0.3	236	7.1	49	0.8	2.1
Sourdough, White, Sliced, Half Bloomer, TTD, Sainsbury's*	1 Slice/40g	102	1.2	256	9.6	46.7	2.9	2.1
Sourdough, White, Sliced, No.1, Waitrose*	1 Slice/50g	115	0.4	230	7.8	46.6	0.7	2.9
Soya & Linseed, Seeded Loaf, Burgen *	1 Slice/44g	126	4.8	287	15.2	26.9	11	9.8
Soya, & Linseed, Vogel*	1 Slice/42g	95	2.1	227	11.7	34.1	4.9	6.8
Soya, & Linseed, The Best, Morrisons*	1 Slice/44g	116	2.7	264	11.2	37.9	6.1	6.3
Spelt, Soul bakery*	1 Slice/45g	116	0.8	258	10.4	50	1.7	7.6
Sunflower, & Pumpkin, Cob, Sliced, Finest, Tesco*	1 Slice/40g	120	4.4	299	12.3	34.7	10.9	6.6
Super Seeded, 400g , M&S*	1 Slice/34g	103	3.5	304	12	38.2	10.3	5
Super Seeded, 800g, M&S*	1 Slice/50g	152	5.2	304	12	38.2	10.3	5
Super Seeded, Farmhouse, Loaf, Co-Op*	1 Slice/44g	136	4.8	309	11	39	11	5.3
Super Seeded, Farmhouse, Loaf, Finest, Tesco*	1 Slice/44g	129	4.2	294	11.2	37.9	9.6	5.8
Super Seeded, Only Half the Carbs, LivLife*	1 Slice/33g	80	2.7	243	25.9	10.2	8.3	12.2
Sweet Potato, with Pumpkin & Sunflower Seeds, BFree*	1 Slice/40g	93	2.5	232	3.5	30.6	6.3	9.2
Tea Loaf, Fruit & Walnut, Organic, Daylesford*	1 Slice/35g	102	2.4	290	4.5	50.2	6.9	0
Tiger, Artisan, Bloomer, GF, Warburton's*	1 Slice/50g	120	2.6	241	7.1	38.5	5.3	5.5
Tiger, Baton, Bakery, Tesco*	½ Baton/100g	288	2	288	9.1	57.4	2	2.2
Tiger, Bloomer, GF, Genius*	1 Slice/80g	242	7.8	302	2.5	48	9.7	6.5
Tiger, Bloomer, Med Sliced, Iceland*	1 Slice/40g	108	1.8	271	9	46.9	4.5	3.5
Tiger, Bloomer, Soft, Warburton's*	1 Slice/38g	94	0.9	251	10.1	46.2	2.4	2
Tiger, Bloomer, The Great, Village Bakery, Aldi*	1 Slice/58g	159	2.6	274	8.8	49	4.4	2.1
Tiger, Cob, Sliced, Free From, Waitrose*	1 Slice/34g	80	1.3	238	3.2	43.9	3.9	7.4
Tiger, Loaf, Bloomer, Bakery, Tesco*	1 Slice/50g	133	1.6	266	8.4	49.2	3.2	3.2
Tiger, White, Warburton's*	1 Slice/40g	106	1.3	266	8.4	49.2	3.2	3.2
Walnut, Cob, TTD, Bakery, Sainsbury's*	1 Slice/50g	139	3.7	277	9.5	41.5	7.3	3.7
Wheat, Spelt, & Rye, Loaf, Baked by Us, Morrisons*	1 Slice/35g	82	0.7	236	11.3	39.9	2	6.6
Wheaten, Big Slice	*1 Slice/65g*	*139*	*1.7*	*214*	*7.5*	*40.2*	*2.6*	*3.6*
White & Bran, Med Sliced, Co-Op*	1 Slice/40g	98	1.2	244	9.1	42	3	5.3
White, & Bran, Thick Sliced, Co-Op*	1 Slice/45g	110	1.4	244	9.1	42	3	5.3
White, & Wheat, Med Sliced, M&S*	1 Slice/38g	93	0.8	247	10.4	45	2	3.6
White, 50/50, Vitamin Boost, Sliced, Kingsmill*	1 Slice/38g	89	0.8	234	9.4	41.9	2.2	4.7
White, Average	*1 Slice/40g*	*94*	*0.8*	*235*	*8.4*	*49.3*	*1.9*	*1.5*
White, Bakers Bloomer, Warburtons *	1 Slice/62g	148	1.5	239	9.2	43.9	2.5	2.4
White, Batch Loaf, Extra Special, Asda*	1 Slice/47g	109	0.9	233	9	45	1.9	2.2
White, Batch, Warburton's*	1 Slice/42g	98	0.9	233	9.8	43.6	2.1	2.7
White, Baton, Bakery, Sainsbury's*	½ Baton/100g	273	0.6	273	10.3	55.2	0.6	2.8
White, Baton, Cheese, Bakery, Sainsbury's*	1 Serving/50g	159	2.6	318	12.1	54.3	5.3	2.5
White, Baton, Part-Baked, TTD, Sainsbury's*	1 Serving/50g	125	0.4	250	7.5	51.4	0.9	3
White, Bloomer, 400g, M&S*	1 Slice/40g	98	1.1	246	8.9	45	2.7	3.2
White, Classic, Med Sliced, Hovis*	1 Slice/38g	91	0.9	240	11.4	40.3	2.3	2.5
White, Commercially Prepared, Average	*1oz/28g*	*74*	*0.9*	*266*	*7.6*	*50.6*	*3.3*	*2.4*
White, Commercially Prepared, Toasted, Average	*1oz/28g*	*82*	*1.1*	*293*	*9*	*54.4*	*4*	*2.5*
White, Crusty, Fresh, Finest, Tesco*	1 Slice/52g	130	1	250	8.6	48.5	1.9	2.4
White, Crusty, Hovis*	1 Slice/44g	103	1	233	8.8	44.3	2.2	2.1
White, Crusty, Sliced Loaf, Tesco*	1 Slice/50g	127	0.6	254	9.2	50.1	1.2	3.2
White, Crusty, Split Tin, Bakery, Tesco*	1 Slice/50g	134	0.8	268	9.4	52.6	1.5	3.3
White, Danish, Lighter, Warburton's*	1 Slice/26g	63	0.3	243	10.5	45.8	1.2	2.6
White, Danish, Lighter, Warburtons*	1 Slice/26g	63	0.3	243	10.5	45.8	1.2	2.6

B

BREAD

	Measure INFO/WEIGHT	per Measure KCAL	FAT	Nutrition Values per 100g / 100ml KCAL	PROT	CARB	FAT	FIBRE
White, Danish, Med Sliced, Loaf, 400g, Tesco*	1 Slice/22g	57	0.4	258	9.6	48.6	2	3.6
White, Danish, Soft, Weight Watchers, Warburton's*	1 Slice/21g	50	0.3	243	9.8	46.5	1.3	2.9
White, Farmhouse Crusty, M&S*	1 Slice/34g	82	0.7	240	8.9	46.6	2.2	3
White, Farmhouse, 400g Loaf, Bakery, Sainsbury's*	1 Slice/50g	121	0.4	242	9.1	48.1	0.9	2.7
White, Farmhouse, Co-Op*	1 Slice/36g	85	0.6	237	8.6	46	1.7	1.9
White, Farmhouse, Extra Special, Asda*	1 Slice/44g	109	0.9	248	9.5	47	2	2.4
White, Farmhouse, GF, Newburn, Warburton's*	1 Slice/35g	83	2.1	236	6.8	35.6	6.1	5.5
White, Farmhouse, Hovis*	1 Slice/44g	103	1	234	8.7	44.6	2.3	2.4
White, Farmhouse, Sliced, Bakery, Tesco*	1 Slice/44g	106	1	240	7.9	46	2.3	2
White, Farmhouse, Sliced, Rowan Hill Bakery, Lidl*	1 Slice/44g	101	0.7	229	8.3	44.4	1.5	2.4
White, Farmhouse, Soft, 400g Loaf, Warburton's*	1 Slice/27g	66	0.7	245	10.1	43.7	2.6	2.8
White, Farmhouse, Soft, 800g Loaf, Warburton's*	1 Slice/43g	104	1.1	243	9	45	2.5	2.3
White, Farmhouse, Soft, Thick Sliced, Waitrose*	1 Slice/34g	86	0.7	253	8.7	47.9	2.2	3.4
White, Fried in Blended Oil	***1 Slice/28g***	***141***	***9***	***503***	***7.9***	***48.5***	***32.2***	***1.6***
White, GF, Sliced, Free From, Co-Op*	1 Slice/38g	70	1	183	4.2	30	2.7	10
White, GF, Sliced, Free From, Morrisons*	1 Slice/42g	84	1.7	200	4.3	31.3	4.1	10.1
White, Loaf, Sliced, Finest, Tesco*	1 Slice/50g	118	0.6	236	8.6	45.5	1.3	4.1
White, Med Sliced, Average	***1 Slice/39g***	***93***	***0.6***	***238***	***7.5***	***48.5***	***1.6***	***1.8***
White, Mega Thick, Roberts Bakery*	1 Slice/66g	154	1.2	233	8.3	46.2	1.8	2.2
White, Mighty, GF, Mini Loaf, Warburton's*	1 Slice/27g	67	1.8	249	6.7	37.9	6.5	5.8
White, Milk Roll, Warburton's*	1 Slice/18g	46	0.5	248	9.4	45	2.8	2.4
White, Multi Seeded, Farmhouse, Batch, Waitrose*	1 Slice/50g	139	3.8	278	10.6	39.1	7.7	4.9
White, Multiseed, Med Sliced, Batch, Tesco*	1 Slice/33g	88	2	267	9.9	40.3	6.1	5.5
White, Old English, Warburton's*	1 Slice/40g	99	1.2	248	9.8	44.3	2.9	2.8
White, Plain, Scottish, Sunblest*	1 Slice/57g	133	1.5	233	10.1	42.3	2.6	2.8
White, Sandwich, Bakery, Sainsbury's*	1 Slice/50g	121	0.4	242	9.1	48.1	0.9	2.7
White, Sandwich, Irish Pride*	1 Slice/38g	89	0.5	233	9.4	44.6	1.4	2.8
White, Scottish Plain, Medium, Mother's Pride*	1 Slice/50g	114	0.8	227	8.7	44.6	1.5	3
White, Seeds, Oats, & Honey, TTD, Sainsbury's*	1 Slice/50g	154	5.4	308	12.1	36.7	10.9	7.1
White, Sliced, Brennans*	1 Slice/40g	88	0.6	219	8.7	43	1.4	2.8
White, Sliced, Free From, Asda*	1 Slice/38g	98	2.8	256	1.9	41	7.2	9.6
White, Sliced, GF, Free From, Tesco*	1 Slice/42g	80	1.7	190	5.2	29.7	4	7.3
White, Sliced, Jacksons*	1 Slice/45g	125	3.9	278	10.9	34.5	8.7	9.4
White, Sliced, Roberts Bakery*	1 Slice/35g	87	0.7	249	10	48	2.1	2.5
White, Sm Loaf, Classic, Hovis*	1 Slice/33g	75	0.8	228	11.4	40.3	2.3	6.5
White, Soft, Batch Loaf, Sliced, Tesco*	1 Slice/50g	116	1	233	7.5	46.1	2.1	2.1
White, Soft, M&S*	1 Slice/47g	105	0.8	225	7.3	46.1	1.7	2.4
White, Soft, Med Sliced, 800g Loaf, Hovis*	1 Slice/40g	93	0.7	233	8.7	44.6	1.7	2.4
White, Soft, Med Sliced, Sainsbury's*	1 Slice/40g	95	0.9	239	8.1	45.6	2.2	2.3
White, Soft, No Crusts, Kingsmill*	1 Slice/22g	49	0.4	223	7.8	42.7	1.9	2.1
White, Soft, Sliced, Hovis*	1 Slice/25g	58	0.6	234	8.7	44.6	2.3	2.4
White, Soft, Thick Sliced, Kingsmill*	1 Slice/44g	105	0.9	238	8	45.6	2	2.7
White, Soft, Thick, Hovis*	1 Slice/50g	116	0.8	233	8.7	44.6	1.7	2.4
White, Soft, Toastie, Thick Sliced, Asda*	1 Slice/50g	120	1.1	239	8.1	46	2.2	2.3
White, Sourdough, Finest, Tesco*	1 Slice/50g	118	0.6	236	8.6	48.5	1.3	4.1
White, Sourdough, M&S*	1 Slice/50g	119	0.8	238	9.3	44.5	1.7	3.6
White, Sourdough, Specially Selected, Aldi*	1 Slice/58g	136	0.5	234	8.4	47	0.8	2.1
White, Sourdough, Waitrose*	1 Slice/50g	119	0.6	237	9	45.9	1.2	3.3
White, Square, Extra Thick Sliced, Hovis*	1 Slice/67g	155	1.3	231	8.5	44.7	2	2.6
White, Square, Med Sliced, Hovis*	1 Slice/40g	92	0.8	231	8.5	44.7	2	2.6
White, Square, Thick Sliced, Hovis*	1 Slice/50g	116	1	231	8.5	44.7	2	2.6
White, Thick Sliced, Brace's*	1 Slice/47g	117	0.6	248	7.6	50.4	1.3	2.1
White, Thick Sliced, M&S*	1 Slice/42g	96	0.5	228	7.3	46.7	1.3	2.8

	Measure INFO/WEIGHT	per Measure KCAL	FAT	Nutrition Values per 100g / 100ml KCAL	PROT	CARB	FAT	FIBRE

BREAD

White, Thick Sliced, Mighty White*	1 Slice/42g	96	0.8	229	7.4	43.3	1.9	4.6
White, Thick Sliced, Organic, Tesco*	1 Slice/44g	108	0.9	245	8.5	46.8	2.1	3.1
White, Thick Sliced, Sainsbury's*	1 Slice/44g	95	0.8	216	8.7	41.1	1.9	7.1
White, Thick Sliced, Sunblest*	1 Slice/40g	91	0.6	228	8	45.7	1.5	2.8
White, Thick Sliced, Super Toastie, Morrisons*	1 Slice/50g	128	1.5	257	8.7	48.9	3	2.1
White, Thick Sliced, Tesco*	1 Slice/44g	106	0.7	240	8.2	47.8	1.5	3
White, Thick, Super Soft, M&S*	1 Slice/48g	120	1.3	249	9	45.3	2.7	3.6
White, Thin Sliced, Sainsbury's*	1 Slice/29g	66	0.4	228	7.1	46.4	1.5	2.8
White, Tiger, Bloomer, Black Sheep*	1 Slice/57g	168	4	295	8.1	48.2	7	3.2
White, Toasted, Average	*1 Slice/33g*	*87*	*0.5*	*265*	*9.3*	*57.1*	*1.6*	*1.8*
White, Toastie, 400g Loaf, Warburton's*	1 Slice/29g	70	0.5	244	10.3	45.1	1.9	2.4
White, Toastie, GF, Genius*	1 Slice/33g	90	2	272	2.4	47	6.1	9.3
White, Toastie, Loved by Us, Co-Op*	1 Slice/50g	120	1.2	240	7.9	45.4	2.4	2.6
White, Toastie, Warburton's*	1 Slice/47g	116	0.9	244	9.1	46.4	2	2.3
White, Trio of Olive, Bloomer, Bakery, Tesco*	1 Slice/82g	199	4	243	6.8	41.3	4.9	3
Whole Seed, Cob, Crusty, Bakery, Tesco*	1 Slice/50g	179	6.1	359	13.7	45.7	12.3	5.2
Whole Seed, Loaf, Sliced, Tesco*	1 Slice/40g	109	2.9	272	10.9	38.4	7.2	5.3
Wholegrain, & Chia Seed, Staffords*	1 Slice/50g	150	3	301	12	46	6.1	7.8
Wholegrain, & Oats, Warburton's*	1 Slice/40g	98	1.4	245	11.7	38.8	3.5	5.9
Wholegrain, Average	*1 Slice/44g*	*117*	*1.9*	*265*	*13.4*	*43.3*	*4.2*	*7.4*
Wholegrain, Toasted, Average	*1 Slice/40g*	*117*	*1.9*	*288*	*14.5*	*47.1*	*4.6*	*8.1*
Wholemeal Loaf, British Farmers, Hovis*	1 Slice/47g	108	1.3	229	10	37.9	2.8	6.8
Wholemeal, Average	*1 Slice/40g*	*88*	*1*	*215*	*9.2*	*41.6*	*2.5*	*5.8*
Wholemeal, Batch, The Champion, Allison's *	1 Slice/46g	108	1.3	234	11	37.8	2.9	6.1
Wholemeal, Bloomer, Heroic, Sliced, Roberts*	1 Slice/37g	87	0.6	236	10.7	41	1.7	6.7
Wholemeal, Brown, Med Sliced, 400g, Hovis*	1 Slice/29g	64	0.5	221	10	37.8	1.8	6.8
Wholemeal, Crustless, Kingsmill*	1 Slice/22g	45	0.5	205	10.4	33.1	2.2	5.6
Wholemeal, Crusty, Finest, Tesco*	1 Slice/50g	103	0.8	206	10.8	37	1.7	6.9
Wholemeal, Danish, BFY, Morrisons*	1 Slice/17g	39	0.3	228	11.2	47.9	1.8	6.2
Wholemeal, Farmhouse, Bakery in Store, M&S*	1 Slice/35g	80	1	229	11.4	35.3	3	7.9
Wholemeal, Farmhouse, Loaf, Co-Op*	1 Slice/37g	84	0.8	230	11	38	2.1	6.3
Wholemeal, Farmhouse, Med Sliced, Waitrose*	1 Slice/36g	84	0.7	232	10.8	39.1	1.9	7.5
Wholemeal, Farmhouse, Sliced, Hovis*	1 Slice/44g	101	1.2	229	10	37.8	2.7	6.8
Wholemeal, Farmhouse, Thick Sliced, 400g, Waitrose*	1 Slice/33g	77	0.6	232	10.8	39.1	1.9	7.5
Wholemeal, Farmhouse, Thick Sliced, Tesco*	1 Slice/37g	82	0.7	222	9.4	38.7	1.9	6.1
Wholemeal, Farmhouse, Thick Sliced, Waitrose*	1 Slice/44g	103	0.8	232	10.8	39.1	1.9	7.5
Wholemeal, Granary, Med Sliced, Hovis*	1 Slice/47g	111	1.1	236	10.6	39.8	2.4	6.8
Wholemeal, High Protein, High Fibre, Warburton's*	1 Slice/29g	66	1	227	13.5	32	3.3	7.8
Wholemeal, Little Brown Loaf, Unsliced, Hovis*	1 Slice/40g	86	1.1	216	10	37.8	2.7	6.8
Wholemeal, Live Good, Hovis*	1 Slice/26g	67	0.4	258	10	46.9	1.5	6.9
Wholemeal, Loaf, Sliced, Thick, 800g, Hovis*	1 Slice/47g	104	0.8	221	10	37.8	1.8	6.8
Wholemeal, Lower Carb, Hovis*	1 Slice/36g	84	1.3	234	16	27	3.7	14.4
Wholemeal, Med Sliced, 800g Loaf, Hovis*	1 Slice/40g	88	0.7	221	10	37.8	1.8	6.8
Wholemeal, Med Sliced, Essential, Waitrose*	1 Slice/36g	78	0.6	217	10.7	36.2	1.7	7
Wholemeal, Med Sliced, H.W. Nevill's, Tesco*	1 Slice/33g	83	0.8	253	9.7	43.8	2.5	8.3
Wholemeal, Med Sliced, Loaf, 800g, Village Bakery, Aldi*	1 Slice/40g	90	0.9	225	11	37	2.3	6.2
Wholemeal, Med Sliced, M&S*	1 Slice/40g	80	1.2	200	10.5	32.7	3.1	6.7
Wholemeal, Med Sliced, Morrisons*	1 Slice/33g	72	0.5	216	9.6	38	1.4	6.5
Wholemeal, Med Sliced, Sainsbury's*	1 Slice/40g	93	1.2	234	11.9	36.7	2.9	6.6
Wholemeal, Med Sliced, Sunblest*	1 Slice/40g	94	1.2	235	11.5	36.9	3	7.1
Wholemeal, Med Sliced, Waitrose*	1 Slice/36g	76	0.9	213	10.1	37.6	2.4	7
Wholemeal, Medium, 400g Loaf, Warburton's*	1 Slice/24g	55	0.7	231	10.6	37.8	2.8	6.4
Wholemeal, Medium, 800g Loaf, Warburton's*	1 Slice/45g	103	1.3	231	10.6	37.8	2.8	6.4

BREAD

INFO/WEIGHT	Measure	per Measure		Nutrition Values per 100g / 100ml				
		KCAL	FAT	KCAL	PROT	CARB	FAT	FIBRE
Wholemeal, Medium, Sliced, Everyday Essentials, Aldi*	1 Slice/40g	85	0.7	213	10	36	1.7	6.3
Wholemeal, Multigrain, Sliced, Extra Special, Asda*	1 Slice/44g	108	2.2	246	11	35	5	7.7
Wholemeal, Multigrain, Soft Batch, Sainsbury's*	1 Slice/44g	106	2.9	242	11.3	34.5	6.5	5.6
Wholemeal, Multiseed, Batch, So Organic, Sainsbury's*	1 Slice/36g	104	3.1	289	12.1	35	8.7	10.9
Wholemeal, Multiseed, Farmhouse, Soft, TTD, Sainsbury's*	1 Slice/50g	140	4.4	280	12.6	33.8	8.8	8.2
Wholemeal, Nimble, Hovis*	1 Slice/22g	50	0.5	226	11.8	37	2.2	6.6
Wholemeal, No Added Sugar, Hovis*	1 Slice/45g	104	1.3	231	10.6	37.8	2.8	6.4
Wholemeal, No Added Sugar, Warburton's*	1 Slice/45g	103	1.2	231	10.6	37.8	2.8	6.4
Wholemeal, No Crusts, Kingsmill *	1 Slice/22g	45	0.5	205	10.4	33.1	2.2	5.6
Wholemeal, Our Ultimate Fibre, Roberts Bakery*	1 Slice/45g	95	0.7	212	9.2	35.7	1.5	8.7
Wholemeal, Premium, Thick Slice, M&S*	1 Slice/50g	95	1.5	190	9.8	30.8	3	6.4
Wholemeal, Scandalous Seeds, Allison*	1 Slice/46g	123	4.1	268	13.4	29.3	9	8.2
Wholemeal, Seeded Batch, Truly Irresistible, Co-Op*	1 Slice/47g	115	1.9	245	11.5	36.2	4	6.6
Wholemeal, Seeded, Farmhouse, Rowan Hill Bakery, Lidl*	1 Slice/33g	84	2.1	256	12.4	32.7	6.3	9.4
Wholemeal, Seeded, Farmhouse, M&S*	1 Slice/44g	116	2.9	263	11.4	35	6.7	8.4
Wholemeal, Seeds & Grains, 400g Loaf, Finest, Tesco*	1 Slice/33g	84	1.6	254	11.7	37.4	5	6.4
Wholemeal, Sliced, Loaf, Average	**1 Slice/40g**	**90**	**0.9**	**224**	**9.9**	**38.8**	**2.4**	**6.9**
Wholemeal, Soft, Sliced, Village Bakery, Aldi*	1 Slice/44g	103	1.1	235	12	38	2.6	6.5
Wholemeal, Soft, Thick Sliced, Rowan Hill Bakery, Lidl*	1 Slice/44g	97	0.8	221	10	37.8	1.8	6.8
Wholemeal, Sourdough, Half Bloomer, TTD, Sainsbury's*	1 Slice/40g	103	1.6	258	10.9	42.4	4	4.6
Wholemeal, Stoneground, Organic, Waitrose*	1 Slice/25g	57	0.9	228	10.8	38.2	3.6	7.1
Wholemeal, Supersoft, Eat Well, M&S*	1 Slice/33g	81	1.1	245	10.9	40	3.3	6.7
Wholemeal, Tasty, Medium, Kingsmill*	1 Slice/40g	93	1.1	233	10.2	38.6	2.8	6.3
Wholemeal, Tasty, Thick, Kingsmill*	1 Slice/44g	105	1.7	239	10.5	37.7	3.8	6.2
Wholemeal, The Champion, Batch, Allinson*	1 Slice/46g	108	1.3	234	11	37.8	2.9	6.1
Wholemeal, Thick Sliced, Great Everyday, Kingsmill*	1 Slice/44g	100	1.7	227	10.5	37.7	3.8	6.2
Wholemeal, Thick Sliced, Sainsbury's*	1 Slice/44g	103	1.3	234	11.9	36.7	2.9	6.6
Wholemeal, Thick Sliced, Toastie, Tesco*	1 Slice/50g	112	1.2	224	10.6	36.8	2.4	6.8
Wholemeal, Thick, Weight Watchers, Warburton's*	1 Slice/28g	64	0.6	225	10	38.4	2.2	6
Wholemeal, Toasted, Average	**1 Slice/26g**	**58**	**0.6**	**224**	**8.6**	**42.3**	**2.2**	**5.8**
Wholemeal. Medium, Brace's*	1 Slice/42g	95	0.9	226	10.2	44.3	2.2	6
Wholesome, Five Seeded, GF, Genius*	2 Slices/77g	229	9.3	297	5.1	37	12	12
Wholewheat, Nature's Own*	1 Slice/28g	66	1	236	14.3	39.3	3.6	10.7
Wrap, Indian Style, COU, M&S*	1 Pack/225g	331	5.6	147	5.9	23.4	2.5	3.5
Wrap, Mediterranean Herb, Soft, Village Bakery, Aldi*	1 Wrap/64g	188	2.6	294	8	54.7	4.1	2
Wrap, Original, Super Soft, Village Bakery, Aldi*	1 Wrap/62g	182	3.2	293	8.3	51	5.2	3.7
Wrap, Skinni, Tortilla, Plain, Deli Kitchen*	1 Wrap/31g	94	1.1	302	9	57	3.5	3
Wrap, Soft Taco, Gran Luchito*	1 Wrap/30g	92	2	307	8.5	52.5	6.5	0
Wrap, Tortilla, 8 Pack, Asda*	1 Wrap/50g	143	3	286	8	50	6	1.9
Wrap, Tortilla, Ancient Grain, Co-Op*	1 Wrap/40g	123	3	308	9.2	49	7.6	3.4
Wrap, Tortilla, Beetroot, Fibre Fest, Genius*	1 Wrap/40g	83	1.4	208	5.3	32	3.6	13
Wrap, Tortilla, Both in One, Mini, Village Bakery, Aldi*	1 Wrap/31g	97	2.1	313	7.9	53	6.8	5
Wrap, Tortilla, Both in One, Sunnyhills, Aldi*	1 Wrap/64g	184	2.9	287	8.1	52	4.5	3
Wrap, Tortilla, Carb Lite, Deli Kitchen*	1 Wrap/50g	127	3.2	254	13.8	29.3	6.5	12
Wrap, Tortilla, Chargrilled, Mission*	1 Wrap/60g	196	4.3	327	8	53.3	7.2	2
Wrap, Tortilla, Corn, & Wheat, Santa Maria*	1 Wrap/40g	118	2.2	294	7.7	50	5.6	0
Wrap, Tortilla, Large, Essential, Waitrose*	1 Wrap/64g	190	3.7	297	7.2	52.5	5.8	3.1
Wrap, Tortilla, Mediterranean Herb, Rowan Hill, Lidl*	1 Wrap/64g	178	2.2	278	7.3	53	3.5	2.5
Wrap, Tortilla, Mediterranean Style, Morrisons*	1 Wrap/64g	177	2.4	277	7.7	51.8	3.7	3
Wrap, Tortilla, Plain , Ocado*	1 Wrap/53g	154	4.4	291	6.7	45.7	8.4	3.1
Wrap, Tortilla, Plain, HL, Tesco*	1 Wrap/64g	182	3.2	284	8.2	49.7	5	3.7
Wrap, Tortilla, Plain, Rowan Hill Bakery, Lidl*	1 Wrap/64g	204	4.4	319	8.4	55.3	6.8	1.6
Wrap, Tortilla, Plain, Tesco*	1 Wrap/64g	182	3.2	284	8.1	49.7	5	3.8

BREAD

INFO/WEIGHT	Measure	per Measure		Nutrition Values per 100g / 100ml				
		KCAL	FAT	KCAL	PROT	CARB	FAT	FIBRE
Wrap, Tortilla, Plain, Village Bakery, Aldi*	1 Wrap/65g	194	4.9	298	7.8	49.6	7.6	2.7
Wrap, Tortilla, Seeded, Love Life, Waitrose*	1 Wrap/64g	185	3.6	290	8.8	46.6	5.7	4.3
Wrap, Tortilla, Seeded, Mission Deli*	1 Wrap/61g	185	3.8	304	8.6	50.1	6.2	6.2
Wrap, Tortilla, Seeded, Village Bakery, Aldi*	1 Wrap/62g	176	3	284	8.6	49	4.8	6.3
Wrap, Tortilla, Soft Flour, Sainsbury's*	1 Wrap/40g	123	2.6	307	8.5	52.5	6.5	2.3
Wrap, Tortilla, Soft Taco, M&S*	2 Tacos/68g	209	5.4	308	9	49.5	7.9	1.5
Wrap, Tortilla, Soft, M&S*	1 Wrap/64g	186	3.8	290	8	49.7	6	2.5
Wrap, Tortilla, Sweet Potato, GF, BFree*	1 Wrap/42g	91	0.8	217	5.4	33	1.9	15.2
Wrap, Tortilla, Wheat & Corn, Sainsbury's*	1 Tortilla/40g	126	1.9	314	9.4	58	4.8	0.5
Wrap, Tortilla, Wheat & White, Mini, Mission Deli*	1 Wrap/31g	93	2.1	299	7.5	50	6.9	3.6
Wrap, Tortilla, Wheat, Mountain Bread*	1 Wrap/25g	68	0.3	272	10.2	52.9	1.2	2.6
Wrap, Tortilla, White, Bakers Selection, Asda*	1 Wrap/62g	181	2.9	290	7.9	53	4.6	2.5
Wrap, Tortilla, White, GF, Free From, Tesco*	1 Wrap/40g	84	1.8	211	4.3	31	4.4	15.3
Wrap, Tortilla, White, GF, Warburton's*	1 Wrap/45g	138	2.6	306	3.9	57	5.8	5.3
Wrap, Tortilla, White, Mini, Asda*	1 Wrap/31g	90	1.2	289	8	54	4	2.6
Wrap, Tortilla, White, Mini, Tesco*	1 Wrap/31g	88	1.6	284	8.2	49.7	5	3.7
Wrap, Tortilla, White, Weight Watchers*	1 Wrap/48g	119	0.8	247	6.9	46.3	1.6	9.6
Wrap, Tortilla, Whole & White, HL, Tesco*	1 Wrap/64g	182	1.7	284	8.5	54.1	2.7	4.5
Wrap, Tortilla, Wholemeal , M&S*	1 Wrap/64g	160	2.4	250	11.2	42.5	3.8	6.5
Wrap, Tortilla, Wholemeal, Asda*	1 Wrap/61g	170	3.2	279	9	46	5.2	6.9
Wrap, Tortilla, Wholemeal, Discovery*	1 Wrap/40g	109	3.3	273	9.2	40.4	8.3	6.4
Wrap, Tortilla, Wholemeal, Mini, Tesco *	1 Wrap/31g	86	1.6	279	9	45.7	5.2	6.9
Wrap, Tortilla, Wholemeal, Mission Deli*	1 Wrap/60g	175	5	292	8.4	41.6	8.3	8.8
Wrap, Tortilla, Wholemeal, Weight Watchers*	1 Wrap/50g	118	0.8	236	8.1	52.8	1.5	11
Wrap. Tortilla, Plain, GF, Genius*	1 Wrap/40g	84	1.8	211	4.3	31	4.4	15.3
Wraps, Tortilla, Original, Mini, Soft, Village Bakery, Aldi*	1 Wrap/31g	91	1.6	293	8.3	51	5.2	3.7
Wraps, Tortilla, Sweet Potato, Free From, Sainsbury's*	1 Wrap/40g	73	1.3	182	4.4	26.2	3.2	15.3

BREAD & BUTTER PUDDING

Average	**1 Serving/250g**	**400**	**19.5**	**160**	**6.2**	**17.5**	**7.8**	**0.3**

BREAD MIX

Cheddar Cheese, & Onion, Made Up, Wrights*	1 Slice/45g	116	1.1	258	11.6	45.6	2.4	3.5
Focaccia, Garlic & Herb, Asda*	1 Serving/125g	385	10	308	11	48	8	3.3
Kornbrot, Saftiges, Made Up, Aurora*	1 Slice/50g	119	0.9	238	8	45	1.8	0
Multiseed, Baked, Sainsbury's*	1 Slice/44g	112	4.3	252	10.8	30.5	9.6	6.8
Multiseed, Crunchy Four Seed, Tesco*	1 Pack/500g	1370	37	274	11.3	38.1	7.4	4.9
Wholemeal, Hovis*	1 Serving/65g	148	3.1	227	10	35.8	4.8	6.8

BREADCRUMBS

Average	**1oz/28g**	**98**	**0.5**	**350**	**10.8**	**74.8**	**1.9**	**2.6**
Lemon & Pepper, Cooks' Ingredients, Waitrose*	1 Serving/25g	89	0.9	354	11.7	67.2	3.4	4.1
Panko, Blue Dragon*	1 Serving/30g	81	1.7	270	7.7	46.7	5.7	1.7
Southern Fried, Paxo*	1 Serving/24g	84	0.6	352	11.7	68.2	2.5	4.8

BREADFRUIT

Raw	**1oz/28g**	**19**	**0.1**	**67**	**0.9**	**16.4**	**0.2**	**0**

BREADSTICKS

Ciabatta, Garlic, Sainsbury's*	1 Breadstick/36g	147	7.2	412	10.5	45.8	20.1	3.3
Grissini, Italian, Sainsbury's*	1 Breadstick/5g	20	0.4	408	11.6	72.9	7.8	2.9
Grissini, Sesame, Buon Piemontesi*	1 Breadstick/10g	42	2	422	6.8	58.1	20.3	10.2
Grissini, Waitrose*	1 Breadstick/6g	25	0.4	397	12	72.5	6.2	3.1
Grissini, with Olive Oil, Cypressa*	1 Breadstick/8g	35	1	439	11	68	12.8	3.8
Italian Original, Tesco*	1 Breadstick/5.5g	23	0.4	414	11.2	73.1	7.9	2.8
Mini, Sainsbury's*	1 Breadstick/1g	4	0.1	416	10.4	71.9	8.8	3.8
Mini, Tesco*	1 Breadstick/2g	7	0.1	412	11.1	73.2	7.7	2.9
Sesame Seed Grissini, Sainsbury's*	1 Breadstick/6g	27	0.7	424	13.5	66.2	11	3.1

B

BREADSTICKS

	Measure INFO/WEIGHT	per Measure KCAL	FAT	Nutrition Values per 100g / 100ml KCAL	PROT	CARB	FAT	FIBRE
Sesame, Savour Bakes, Aldi*	1 Breadstick/8g	36	1.4	456	13.5	59.4	16.9	6.2
Traditional, Grissin Bon*	1 Breadstick/5g	21	0.4	415	13	71	8	4.3

BREAKFAST

All Day, Canned, Hunger Breaks, Princes*	1 Serving/393g	468	17.3	119	6.3	11.9	4.4	3.1

BREAKFAST CEREAL

	Measure INFO/WEIGHT	per Measure KCAL	FAT	Nutrition Values per 100g / 100ml KCAL	PROT	CARB	FAT	FIBRE
Porridge Oats, Protein, Original, Made Up, Quaker*	1 Sachet/38g	235	6.3	623	39.8	76.9	16.7	7.2
All Bran, Bran Flakes, & Fruit, Kellogg's*	1 Serving/40g	143	2.4	358	8	68	6	9
All Bran, Fibre Crunch, Kellogg's*	1 Serving/45g	184	5	409	7.6	63	11	13
All Bran, Golden Crunch, Kellogg's*	1 Serving/45g	182	5	405	8	62	11	13
All Bran, Oaty Clusters, Prebiotic, Kellogg's*	1 Serving/45g	163	5	388	14	45	12	22
All Bran, Original, High Fibre, Kellogg's*	1 Serving/40g	134	1.4	334	14	48	3.5	27
Alpen*, Crunchy Bran*	1 Serving/40g	120	1.9	299	11.8	52.3	4.7	24.8
Apple Jacks, Kellogg's*	1 Serving/40g	154	1.5	385	5.1	87.2	3.8	5.1
Apple, & Cinnamon, Flakes, M&S*	1 Serving/30g	113	0.4	377	11.3	78.7	1.3	3
Apricot Wheats, Harvest Morn, Aldi*	1 Serving/30g	101	0.4	337	7.6	72.3	1.4	8
Apricot Wheats, Whole Grain, Tesco*	1 Serving/40g	130	0.6	326	7.6	70.6	1.4	8
Balance, Oats & Honey, Sainsbury's*	1 Serving/30g	114	0.5	379	7.3	81.4	1.7	4.4
Balance, Sainsbury's*	1 Serving/30g	111	0.4	370	11.4	77.7	1.5	3.2
Benefit Flakes, Original, Harvest Morn, Aldi*	1 Serving/40g	154	0.5	384	12	80	1.3	2.2
Berries, Clusters, & Seeds, Protein, Special K, Kellogg's*	1 Serving/40g	148	1.3	371	12	69	3.2	8.9
Bircher Muesli, Love Life, Waitrose*	1 Serving/45g	153	3.5	341	8.8	57.7	7.7	6.8
Blueberry Wheaties, Asda*	1 Serving/45g	150	0.6	333	7.9	71	1.4	8.2
Blueberry Wheats, Harvest Morn, Aldi*	1 Serving/45g	150	0.6	333	7.9	71	1.4	8.2
Blueberry Wheats, Tesco*	1 Serving/50g	168	0.8	336	7.5	71.6	1.5	8.5
Bran Flakes, Asda*	1 Serving/30g	108	0.8	360	12	64	2.7	16
Bran Flakes, Kellogg's*	1 Serving/30g	108	1	359	12	63	3.2	15
Bran Flakes, Sultana Bran, Kellogg's*	1 Serving/40g	138	0.8	344	8	67	2	13
Bran Flakes, Tesco*	1 Serving/30g	107	0.7	356	10.8	64.3	2.4	16.8
Bran Flakes, Wholegrain, Essential, Waitrose*	1 Serving/30g	107	0.7	356	10.8	64.7	2.4	16
Bran Flakes, Wholegrain, Sainsbury's*	1 Serving/30g	109	0.9	363	10.1	67.1	3	13.6
Bran, High Fibre, Morrisons*	1 Serving/30g	102	1	341	13.3	51.6	3.3	25.9
Bran, High Fibre, Tesco*	1 Serving/40g	140	1.6	350	13.7	54	3.9	22.1
Cheerios, Honey, Nestle*	1 Serving/50g	184	1.4	369	6.6	79.2	2.8	5.8
Cheerios, Multigrain, Nestle*	1 Serving/30g	114	1.3	380	9.4	72	4.2	8.9
Cheerios, Nestle*	1 Serving/30g	114	1.1	381	8.6	74.5	3.8	7.1
Chocolate Chip, Crispy Minis, Weetabix*	1 Serving/40g	154	2	386	10	70	5.1	10
Chocolate Hoops, Average	**1 Serving/30g**	**116**	**1.3**	**386**	**7.2**	**79.3**	**4.4**	**3.4**
Chocolate Rice, Puffed, Average	**1 Serving/30g**	**117**	**1.2**	**389**	**5.7**	**81**	**4.1**	**3.2**
Cinnamon Chips, Harvest Morn, Aldi*	1 Serving/40g	166	4.4	416	6.8	70	11	0
Cinnamon Grahams, Nestle*	1 Serving/40g	164	3.9	411	4.7	76.1	9.8	4.2
Cinnamon Squares, Crownfield, Lidl*	1 Serving/40g	149	0.6	372	9.5	75.5	1.6	8.9
Coco Pops, Kellogg's*	1 Serving/30g	115	0.6	382	6.3	84	1.9	3
Coco Pops, Strawberry, & White Chocolate, Kellogg's*	1 Serving/30g	129	0.5	429	6	88	1.7	4.9
Coco Snaps, Value, Tesco*	1 Serving/30g	117	0.7	390	7	84.1	2.4	2.4
Corn Flakes, Honey Nut, Average	**1 Serving/30g**	**118**	**1.3**	**393**	**7**	**81.4**	**4.3**	**2.4**
Corn Flakes, Kellogg's*	1 Serving/30g	113	0.3	378	7	84	0.9	3
Cornflakes, GF, Nestle*	1 Serving/30g	115	0.3	384	7.4	84.6	1.1	3.1
Country Crisp with Real Strawberries, Jordans*	1 Serving/50g	214	7.8	428	7.5	64.1	15.7	7.1
Craze, Aldi*	1 Serving/40g	172	4.8	430	7.6	70.7	12	4.2
Crunchy Bran, Weetabix*	1 Serving/40g	140	1.4	350	11.9	57.6	3.6	20
Crunchy Nut, Clusters, Honey & Nut, Kellogg's*	1 Serving/40g	161	2	402	6	82	5	2.5
Crunchy Nut, Clusters, Milk Chocolate Curls, Kellogg's*	1 Serving/40g	183	7.2	458	8	66	18	4
Crunchy Nut, Corn Flakes, Kellogg's*	1 Serving/30g	118	1.2	392	6	83	4	2.5

BREAKFAST CEREAL

	Measure INFO/WEIGHT	per Measure KCAL	FAT	Nutrition Values per 100g / 100ml KCAL	PROT	CARB	FAT	FIBRE
Crunchy Nut, Oat Granola, with Chocolate, Kellogg's*	1 Serving/45g	224	11.2	497	8	57	25	6
Curiously Cinnamon Churros, Nestle*	1 Serving/30g	118	1.7	395	7.3	75.8	5.8	4.8
Curiously Cinnamon, Nestle*	1 Serving/30g	124	3	412	4.9	75.9	9.9	4.1
Fitness, Chocolate, Nestle*	1 Serving/30g	118	1.9	394	8.5	72.7	6.3	6.2
Frosted Flakes, Tesco*	1 Serving/30g	112	0.1	374	4.9	87.8	0.4	2.4
Frosted Wheats, Kellogg's*	1 Serving/30g	104	0.6	346	10	72	2	9
Frosties, Kellogg's*	1 Serving/30g	112	0.2	375	4.5	87	0.6	2
Fruit & Fibre, Morrisons*	1 Serving/30g	110	2.2	366	8.8	66.5	7.2	8.5
Fruit & Nut Crisp, Minis, Weetabix*	1 Serving/40g	148	1.6	371	9.9	69	4.1	9.3
Fruit & Fibre, Asda*	1 Serving/40g	155	2.6	387	8.8	69	6.5	8.8
Fruit & Fibre, Essential, Waitrose*	1 Serving/40g	153	2.6	383	7.8	68.5	6.6	9.3
Fruit & Fibre, Harvest Morn, Aldi*	1 Serving/30g	114	1.8	380	8.4	69	6.1	8
Fruit 'n' Fibre, Kellogg's*	1 Serving/40g	152	2.4	380	8	69	6	9
Fruit Wheats, Raisin, Harvest Morn*	1 Serving/45g	153	0.7	340	8.4	71	1.5	8.4
Golden Grahams, Nestle*	1 Serving/30g	112	0.9	375	6	81	3	3.4
Granola	**1 Serving/45g**	**194**	**8.7**	**430**	**17.5**	**48.8**	**19.4**	**16.8**
Granola, Apple, & Blueberry, Harvest Morn, Aldi*	1 Serving/45g	202	7.2	449	14	57	16	8.3
Granola, Apricot, & Cranberry, The Foodie Market, Aldi*	1 Serving/45g	198	7.2	441	27	44	16	6
Granola, Belgian Chocolate Praline, TTD, Sainsbury's*	1 Serving/45g	203	7.4	451	10.5	61.7	16.4	7.5
Granola, Berry & Orange, Wholegrain, M&S*	1 Serving/45g	178	4.3	396	8.5	65.5	9.6	6.7
Granola, Berry, Low Sugar, Sainsbury's*	1 Serving/45g	198	6.5	439	12.3	60.9	14.4	8.3
Granola, Berry, Morrisons*	1 Serving/45g	200	6.9	445	9.9	63.7	15.3	6.8
Granola, Buckwheat, Deliciously Ella*	1 Serving/45g	180	6.5	400	11.3	53.8	14.4	5.3
Granola, Cherries & Berries, Sainsbury's*	1 Serving/40g	176	5.4	439	10.4	65.1	13.6	7.3
Granola, Cherry Bakewell, Oat Pantry*	1 Serving/40g	157	6	393	9.5	52	15	7.3
Granola, Crunchy Nut Glorious Oat, Kellogg's*	1 Serving/45g	212	9.4	470	7	61	21	4.5
Granola, Crunchy Oat, Raisin, Almond, Harvest Morn, Aldi*	1 Serving/40g	166	4.6	416	8.2	66.9	11.4	6.4
Granola, Fruit & Nut, GF, Free From, Tesco*	1 Serving/30g	128	3.9	427	9.2	64.9	13	6.9
Granola, Fruit & Nut, Morrisons*	1 Serving/40g	190	11.8	476	17.1	32.9	29.6	4.7
Granola, Grain Free, Luxury, No Added Sugar, M&S*	1 Serving/45g	268	21.7	595	18.1	15.7	48.3	12.3
Granola, Grains & Seeds, Tesco*	1 Serving/50g	223	8	446	12.9	59	15.9	7.5
Granola, Gut-Loving, Super Seedy & Nutty, Bio & Me*	1 Serving/60g	278	12.5	463	13.3	48.3	20.9	14
Granola, Hazelnuts, & Pecans, Super Goodness, Quaker*	1 Serving/45g	187	5	416	9.6	67	11	8
Granola, High Protein, Lizi's*	1 Serving/40g	180	6.8	450	27	44	17	6.7
Granola, Honey & Seed, High Protein, Crownfield, Lidl*	1 Serving/45g	202	7.2	448	27.9	45.1	16.1	5.6
Granola, Honey, Dorset Cereals*	1 Serving/40g	204	12	511	13	44	30	7.4
Granola, Low Sugar, Eat Natural*	1 Serving/50g	248	15.7	495	13.7	33	31.4	12.8
Granola, Low Sugar, Harvest Morn, Aldi*	1 Serving/40g	186	7.2	465	13	58	18	7.9
Granola, Low Sugar, Make it Your Own, M&S*	1 Serving/45g	197	7	437	13.8	56	15.5	9.1
Granola, Mango, & Coconut, Wholegrain, M&S*	1 Serving/45g	196	6.7	435	10.5	61.3	14.8	7.4
Granola, Muesli, Fruit & Nut, The Best, Morrisons*	1 Serving/45g	174	4.4	387	8.5	63.2	9.8	6
Granola, Multigrain Nutty, G&B, Asda*	1 Serving/40g	178	7.6	444	12	52	19	7.6
Granola, Nut & Fruit, Lucury, M&S*	1 Serving/45g	205	8.9	455	10.5	55.1	19.8	7
Granola, Nuts, Pumpkin Seeds, & Fruit, Aldi*	1 Serving/45g	210	8.6	466	27	45	19	5
Granola, Nutty Fruit, 45g, Result Plan*	1 Serving/45g	194	6	431	9.8	62.2	13.3	6.9
Granola, Nutty, Dorset Cereals*	1 Serving/45g	223	11.9	496	11.6	49.3	26.4	7.4
Granola, Nutty, with Cinnamon, Troo*	1 Serving/45g	209	10	464	15.1	48.7	22.2	20.7
Granola, Oat, Golden Crunch, 30% Less Fat, Quaker*	1 Serving/45g	193	4.6	429	8.7	71.5	10.3	7.2
Granola, Oat, Simply Oat, Dorset Cereals*	1 Serving/40g	177	6.8	443	8.8	60	17	7.4
Granola, Original, Low Sugar, Crownfield, Lidl*	1 Serving/20g	100	5.1	499	14.2	49.7	25.6	6.5
Granola, Peanut, High Protein, Luxury, M&S*	1 Serving/45g	204	8.1	453	23.1	47.5	18	4.1
Granola, Protein, Eat Natural*	1 Serving/50g	256	16	512	18.4	34.3	32.1	6.5
Granola, Raisin, & Almond, Crownfield, Lidl*	1 Serving/50g	209	5.7	418	9.5	66.9	11.4	5.1

BREAKFAST CEREAL

	Measure INFO/WEIGHT	per Measure KCAL	FAT	Nutrition Values per 100g / 100ml KCAL	PROT	CARB	FAT	FIBRE
Granola, Raisin, Almond, & Honey, Waitrose*	1 Serving/40g	164	4.4	411	10.6	63.1	11.1	8.3
Granola, Really Nutty, Specially Selected, Aldi*	1 Serving/45g	203	7.4	451	12	60	16.4	7.3
Granola, Salted Toffee, & Pecan, Co-Op*	1 Serving/80g	358	12	447	13	62	15	6.5
Granola, Simply, Morrisons*	1 Serving/45g	168	2.5	374	11	66	5.6	7.7
Granola, Strawberry, Apple, & Raspberry, Asda*	1 Serving/50g	220	7.5	439	9.4	64	15	7.6
Granola, Super Berry, Deluxe, Lidl*	1 Serving/45g	201	7	447	10.3	64	15.6	6.8
Granola, Super Berry, Jordans*	1 Serving/45g	191	5.7	423	0.8	62.9	12.6	7.4
Granola, Super Berry, Tesco*	1 Serving/45g	195	6	434	9.2	66	13.3	6.5
Granola, Super Nutty, Deluxe, Lidl*	1 Serving/45g	211	8.9	469	10.7	58.4	19.8	6.4
Granola, Super Nutty, Finest, Tesco*	1 Serving/50g	229	8.7	457	12.2	59.3	17.4	7
Granola, Tropical, Sainsbury's*	1 Serving/45g	194	5.7	431	8.5	68	12.6	62
Granola, Very Berry, Aldi*	1 Serving/45g	191	5.4	424	11	64	12	8.1
Granola, with Nuts, & Seeds, Holie*	1 Serving/30g	121	4.5	404	12.6	49.1	14.9	13.3
Grape Nuts, Kraft*	1 Serving/45g	158	0.9	350	10.9	81.9	2	11.9
Grapenuts, Post Foods*	1 Serving/45g	162	0.9	359	11	68	2.1	12
High Bran, CBY, Asda*	1 Serving/40g	136	1.5	341	13.6	49.5	3.8	27.1
High Fibre Bran, Sainsbury's*	1 Serving/40g	140	1.6	350	13.7	54	3.9	22.1
Honey & Nut Crisp, Mini, Weetabix*	1 Serving/40g	150	0.8	375	9.4	75.1	2	9.3
Honey Hoops, Harvest Morn, Aldi*	1 Serving/30g	117	1	389	6.5	81	3.4	4
Honey Nut Crunch , Asda*	1 Serving/40g	176	5.2	441	10	68	13	5.3
Hoops, Multigrain, Asda*	1 Serving/30g	113	1.2	376	6.5	78.4	4	4.6
Hoops, Multigrain, Tesco*	1 Serving/30g	112	1.1	375	6.5	78.6	3.8	4.6
Hoops, Mutigrain, Harvest Morn, Aldi*	1 Serving/30g	114	1.4	381	10.2	69.6	4.5	10.8
Instant Oats, Dry Weight	**1 Sachet/36g**	**129**	**3.1**	**359**	**11.5**	**59.1**	**8.5**	**8.3**
Just Right, Kellogg's*	1 Serving/40g	148	0.8	371	7	79	2	4.5
Krave, Milk Chocolate, Kellogg's*	1 Serving/30g	132	3.9	440	7.1	72	13	3.5
Malted Wheats, Waitrose*	1 Serving/30g	110	0.6	365	10	72.7	1.9	8.5
Malties, Sainsbury's*	1 Serving/40g	146	0.8	366	10.1	71.8	1.9	10.8
Maple & Pecan Crisp, Tesco*	1 Serving/50g	215	7.6	430	10.5	62.5	15.2	10.2
Muesli Base, Wholesome, Waitrose*	1 Portion/50g	125	4.2	250	11.5	31.8	8.4	5
Muesli, Berry, & Cherry, Luscious, Dorset Cereals*	1 Serving/45g	163	2.5	363	9.6	64.1	5.5	9.2
Muesli, Five Grain, with Fruit, Kellogg's*	1 Sachet/45g	166	2.3	369	9.3	67	5.1	9.1
Muesli, Fruit & Nut, Luxury, Lidl*	1 Serving/57g	205	5.6	360	8	60	9.8	7.5
Muesli, Fruit & Nut, Luxury, Waitrose*	1 Serving/40g	145	3.8	363	9	60.3	9.5	6.5
Muesli, Fruit & Nut, M&S*	1 Serving/40g	128	1.1	320	7.4	74.5	2.8	7.4
Muesli, Fruit & Nut, Tesco*	1 Serving/50g	190	5.6	380	8.4	60.3	11.3	5.3
Muesli, Fruit & Nut, Essential, Waitrose*	1 Serving/45g	173	6.1	384	8.6	51.5	13.5	11
Muesli, Fruit & Nut, Jordans*	1 Serving/50g	180	4.7	361	8	61.2	9.4	7.5
Muesli, Fruit & Nut, Luxury, Sainsbury's*	1 Serving/50g	178	4.6	355	10.3	57.9	9.1	11.3
Muesli, Fruit & Nut, Sainsbury's*	1 Serving/30g	114	3.1	379	9.5	58.7	10.3	6.9
Muesli, Fruit & Nut, Wholegrain, M&S*	1 Serving/30g	105	1.6	349	9.5	60	5.5	10.8
Muesli, Fruit, M&S*	1 Serving/40g	145	2.6	362	7.3	64.2	6.4	9.3
Muesli, Fruit, Nut, & Seeds, Classic, Dorset Cereals*	1 Serving/45g	170	3.7	378	10.2	62	8.3	7
Muesli, Fruity, Free From, Sainsbury's*	1 Serving/50g	181	4.2	361	10.6	56.9	8.4	7.8
Muesli, Fruity, Sainsbury's*	1 Serving/20g	69	0.5	344	5.9	71.6	2.5	5.7
Muesli, Kavanagh's, Aldi*	1 Serving/45g	155	2.4	345	9.2	59.6	5.3	10.7
Muesli, Low Sugar, Rude Health*	1 Serving/40g	149	3.5	372	12.1	57	8.7	7.2
Muesli, Luxury Fruit, Harvest Morn, Aldi*	1 Serving/50g	179	2.3	358	7.2	69	4.6	5.6
Muesli, Natural, No Added Sugar or Salt, Jordans*	1 Serving/45g	165	1.8	366	10	68	3.9	9.2
Muesli, No Added Sugar, Crownfield, Lidl*	1 Serving/45g	168	2.7	373	12.4	63.1	6	8.4
Muesli, Orchard Fruit, & Berry, Waitrose*	1 Serving/45g	155	1.5	345	8.4	66.8	3.3	7.3
Muesli, Simply Delicious, Dorset Cereals*	1 Serving/45g	166	3.3	368	9.6	61.5	7.3	9
Muesli, Simply Fruity, As Sold, Dorset Cereals*	1 Serving/45g	157	1.3	349	8.6	68.4	2.9	7.3

| Measure | | per Measure | | Nutrition Values per 100g / 100ml | | | | |
INFO/WEIGHT		KCAL	FAT	KCAL	PROT	CARB	FAT	FIBRE

BREAKFAST CEREAL

	Measure INFO/WEIGHT	KCAL	FAT	KCAL	PROT	CARB	FAT	FIBRE
Muesli, Simply Sumptuous, Luxury Fruit, Lidl*	1 Serving/45g	154	1.5	343	6.5	68.7	3.3	6.2
Muesli, Simply, Sainsbury's*	1 Serving/45g	160	2.3	355	11.2	61.5	5.1	9.2
Muesli, Super, Glow, Lizis*	1 Serving/50g	214	8.1	429	13.4	52.1	16.2	10.8
Muesli, Swiss Style, Chocolate, Alpen*	1 Serving/45g	174	3.7	387	11	63	8.3	7.9
Muesli, Swiss Style, No Added Sugar, CBY, Asda*	1 Serving/45g	166	2.5	369	11	65	5.6	7.6
Muesli, Swiss Style, No Added Sugar, Lidl*	1 Serving/30g	111	1.8	371	10.9	64.5	6	7.8
Muesli, Swiss Style, No Added Sugar, Tesco*	1 Serving/50g	183	3	367	11.2	62.4	6.1	8.7
Muesli, Swiss Style, Tesco*	1 Serving/50g	189	3.1	378	10.4	67	6.2	6.4
Muesli, Swiss, No Added Sugar or Salt, Tesco*	1 Serving/40g	147	2.4	367	11.2	62.4	6.1	8.6
Muesli, The Ultimate, Organic, Rude Health*	1 Serving/50g	163	4.5	326	10.8	50.5	9	12.3
Muesli, Very Berry, Aldi*	1 Serving/45g	160	2.3	355	8	65	5.2	7.7
Muesli, with Berries, Swiss, Dry, Love Life, Waitrose*	1 Serving/45g	172	4.3	383	13.5	55.7	9.6	9.8
Multigrain Hoops, Free From, Tesco*	1 Serving/30g	113	1	376	7.4	77.3	3.2	4.2
Multigrain, Hoops, Average	*1 Serving/30g*	*112*	*1.1*	*374*	*6.6*	*77.4*	*3.6*	*6.1*
Nuts, Clusters, & Seeds, Protein, Special K, Kellogg's*	1 Serving/40g	157	2.8	392	13	65	7	8.3
Oat Granola, Raisin, Quaker*	1 Serving/45g	188	4.1	418	8	70.9	9.1	6.9
Oatbran 100%, Pure & Simple, Mornflake*	1 Serving/40g	146	3.8	364	13.4	47.3	9.4	18.2
Oatbran Sprinkles, Mornflake*	1 Serving/40g	146	3.8	364	13.4	47.3	9.4	18.2
Oatbran, Original Pure, Mornflake*	1 Serving/30g	104	2.9	345	14.8	49.7	9.7	15.2
Oatibix Flakes, Red Berries, Oatibix*	1 Serving/30g	121	2.5	403	11	67	8.3	8.1
Oatibix, Flakes, Weetabix*	1 Serving/50g	190	2.8	381	9.5	73.2	5.6	3.5
Oatibix, Weetabix*	2 Biscuits/48g	189	3.8	394	12.5	64.3	8	7.3
Oatmeal, Raw	*1oz/28g*	*112*	*2.4*	*401*	*12.4*	*72.8*	*8.7*	*6.8*
Oats, Easy, Original, Sachet, As Prepared, Sainsbury's*	1 Sachet/27g	190	5.4	704	35.2	90	20	10.7
Oats, Golden Syrup Flavour, Instant, Hot, Waitrose*	1 Serving/39g	153	2.3	393	7.8	77.4	5.8	6
Oats, Rolled, Jumbo, M&S*	1 Serving/40g	144	2.2	361	11.8	61.9	5.4	8.8
Oats, Vibrant, Forest Fruits, As Sold, Quaker*	1 Sachet/39g	148	2.5	375	9.7	66	6.3	7
Organic, Weetabix*	2 Biscuits/38g	134	0.7	358	11.5	68.6	2	10
Passion Fruit, & Pistachio, Lizi's Granola*	1 Serving/50g	238	11.9	476	9.5	52.1	23.8	7.5
Porage Oats, Old Fashioned, Dry Weight, Scott's*	1 Serving/30g	112	2.4	374	11	60	8	9
Porage Oats, Old Fashioned, Dry, Scotts*	1 Serving/40g	142	3.2	355	11	60	8	9
Porage Oats, Original, Dry, Scotts*	1 Serving/40g	142	3.2	355	11	60	8	9
Porage Oats, Syrup Swirl, So-Easy, Dry, Scotts*	1 Sachet/37g	135	2.2	366	8	70	6	6.5
Porridge Oats, As Sold, Shake That Weight*	1 Sachet/41g	149	4	368	36	36	9.9	6
Porridge Oats, Banana, Oat So Simple, Quaker*	1 Sachet/35g	134	2.3	385	9.1	67.6	6.5	7.4
Porridge Oats, Co-Op*	1 Serving/40g	144	3.2	360	12	61	8	9
Porridge Oats, Dry Weight, Value, Tesco*	1 Serving/50g	180	4	359	11	60.4	8.1	8.5
Porridge Oats, Everyday Essentials, Aldi*	1 Serving/40g	162	2.6	405	12	70	6.4	8.9
Porridge Oats, Golden Syrup, Asda*	1 Sachet/36g	137	2.1	381	9.3	70	5.7	6.8
Porridge Oats, Mornflake*	1 Serving/40g	147	3.4	367	12.1	56.1	8.4	9.1
Porridge Oats, Organic, Kavanagh's, Aldi*	1 Serving/40g	148	2.1	370	12	64	5.3	8.6
Porridge Oats, Organic, Tesco*	1 Serving/50g	184	4.2	368	12.1	56.1	8.4	10
Porridge Oats, Original, Asda*	1 Sachet/27g	101	2	375	12	61	7.4	8.4
Porridge Oats, Original, Big Pot, As Sold, Quaker*	1 Pot/67g	251	3.9	374	15	62.4	5.8	6.4
Porridge Oats, Raspberry, Chia, & Pumpkin, Moma Foods*	1 Pack/35g	132	3.9	378	13	51.8	11.1	9.9
Porridge Oats, Rolled, Tesco*	1 Serving/50g	180	4	359	11	60.4	8.1	8.5
Porridge Oats, Scottish, Hamlyns*	1 Serving/40g	154	3.1	384	11.2	63.2	7.7	8.7
Porridge Oats, Scottish, Organic, Sainsbury's*	1 Serving/45g	172	2.2	383	10	74.4	5	7.9
Porridge Oats, Scottish, Tesco*	1 Serving/50g	180	4	359	11	60.4	8.1	8.5
Porridge, Apple & Blueberry, Dry, Oat So Simple, Quaker*	1 Sachet/36g	136	2.2	378	8.6	68	6.2	7.2
Porridge, Apple, & Blueberry, Made Up, Quaker*	1 Sachet/36g	221	4.9	614	26.7	91.7	13.6	7.2
Porridge, Chocolate, Diet Chef Ltd*	1 Pack/37g	152	3.6	411	9.5	67.6	9.7	8.1
Porridge, Cinnamon, Protein, Dry, Oat So Simple, Quaker*	1 Sachet/46g	177	2.9	384	20	59	6.2	5.8

BREAKFAST CEREAL

INFO/WEIGHT	Measure	per Measure KCAL	FAT	Nutrition Values per 100g / 100ml KCAL	PROT	CARB	FAT	FIBRE
Porridge, Cranberry & Raisin, Dry, Moma Foods*	1 Serving/70g	248	2.7	355	13.9	63.6	3.9	6.2
Porridge, Fresh, Double Cream, & Demerara Sugar, M&S*	1 Pot/200g	244	13.6	122	3.9	10.8	6.8	1.2
Porridge, GF, Oat So Simple, Quaker*	1 Sachet/35g	130	2.5	370	13.2	58.5	7.2	9.2
Porridge, Golden Syrup, Dry, Oat So Simple, Quaker*	1 Sachet/36g	143	2.7	398	8.7	71	7.4	5.9
Porridge, Golden Syrup, High Protein, Pot, Fuel 10K*	1 Pot/70g	258	4.1	369	18.6	57.6	5.9	6.3
Porridge, Golden Syrup, Instant, As Consumed, Slim Fast*	1 Sachet/29g	99	1.3	340	17.4	53.2	4.6	7.9
Porridge, Golden Syrup, Made Up, Quaker*	1 Sachet/36g	228	5.8	633	26.7	94.4	16.1	5.8
Porridge, Golden Syrup, Pot, As Sold, Quaker*	1 Pot/57g	213	2.9	373	14	66	5.1	5.5
Porridge, Golden Syrup, Prepared, Oatilicious, Lidl*	1 Sachet/39g	140	1.5	358	8.8	69	3.9	6
Porridge, Instant, Keto, Apple & Cinnamon, Brave Ape*	1 Serving/30g	127	8.4	423	17	22	28	21
Porridge, Made with Semi Skimmed Milk, Waitrose*	1 Serving/50g	277	7.5	554	24.6	80.4	15	8.6
Porridge, Multi Grain, As Sold, Perfect Blends, Quaker*	1 Sachet/32g	120	2.5	376	12	60	7.8	9.4
Porridge, Multi-Grain, Apple, Raisin, Dry, Quaker*	1 Sachet/35g	131	2.5	374	11	62	7.1	9.3
Porridge, Oatbran, Fibreful, Mornflake*	1 Serving/40g	139	3.3	347	13	42.5	8.2	25.6
Porridge, Oats, Apple & Blueberry, Instant, Pot, Tesco*	1 Pot/205g	210	2.9	102	3.6	18.1	1.4	1.5
Porridge, Oats, Berry & Cherry, Instant, Pot, Tesco*	1 Pot/225g	207	2.9	92	3.2	16.2	1.3	1.4
Porridge, Oats, Dry, Smart Price, Asda*	1 Serving/50g	186	4	372	11	60	8	8
Porridge, Oats, Golden Syrup, Instant, Pot, Tesco*	1 Pot/55g	210	2.7	380	11.4	70	4.9	5.5
Porridge, Oats, Golden Syrup, Sainsbury's*	1 Sachet/39g	143	2.1	367	6.3	73.6	5.3	6.7
Porridge, Oats, Instant, Dry Weight, Essential, Waitrose*	1 Sachet/27g	99	1.6	365	11.9	61.6	5.9	8.9
Porridge, Oats, Irish, Multi Seed, Flahavans*	1 Serving/40g	166	5.3	415	14	55.4	13.3	9
Porridge, Oats, Jumbo, 100% Whole Grain, Dry, Quaker*	1 Serving/40g	150	3.2	374	11	60	8	9
Porridge, Oats, No Added Sugar, Love Life, Waitrose*	1 Pot/60g	224	3.8	373	17.5	57.8	6.4	7.2
Porridge, Oats, Original, Big Bowl, Dry, Quaker*	1 Sachet/39g	142	3	370	11	58	7.7	9
Porridge, Oats, Original, Big Bowl, Made Up Quaker*	1 Sachet/39g	254	7.1	660	31.2	88.3	18.4	9.1
Porridge, Oats, Original, Instant, Pot, Tesco*	1 Pot/256g	208	3.3	81	3.1	13.5	1.3	1.6
Porridge, Oats, Rolled, 100% Whole Grain, Dry, Quaker*	1 Serving/40g	150	3.2	374	11	60	8	9
Porridge, Oats, Twice the Fibre, M&S*	1 Portion/60g	230	3.5	384	10.4	62.6	5.9	19.5
Porridge, Oats, Whole, Chunky, Traditional, Jordans*	1 Serving/40g	143	2.7	358	6.7	63.6	6.8	7.9
Porridge, Original, Diet Chef Ltd*	1 Sachet/40g	157	2.5	392	12	67	6.3	9.8
Porridge, Original, Dry, Oat So Simple, Quaker*	1 Sachet/27g	100	2.1	370	11	59	7.7	9
Porridge, Original, Instant, Pot, Made Up, Aldi*	1 Pot/220g	187	2.9	85	4	14	1.3	1.3
Porridge, Original, Made Up, Oat So Simple, Quaker*	1 Sachet/27g	180	5	667	33	88.9	18.5	10.4
Porridge, Original, Pot, As Sold, Oat So Simple, Quaker*	1 Pot/45g	164	2.6	365	17	57	5.8	7
Porridge, Original, Pot, Made Up, Morrisons*	1 Pot/225g	205	2.7	91	3.5	16	1.2	1.1
Porridge, Original, Ready Brek, Weetabix*	1 Serving/40g	149	3.5	373	11.7	57.9	8.7	7.9
Porridge, Plain, Dry, Moma Foods*	1 Serving/65g	232	2.9	357	18.3	58.3	4.5	6.8
Porridge, Protein 360, The Protein Works*	1 Serving/50g	190	3.8	380	27	54	7.5	6.5
Porridge, Raspberry, Apple, & Acai, Dry, Quaker*	1 Sachet/36g	131	2.3	367	9.1	64	6.4	8.8
Porridge, Salted Caramel, Protein, Pot, Fuel 10K*	1 Pot/70g	258	4.3	369	18.6	56.6	6.1	6
Porridge, Strawberry, Raspberry & Cranberry, Dry, Quaker*	1 Sachet/33g	127	2.2	379	8.9	67.4	6.6	7.3
Porridge, Sultana, Raisin, Cranberry, & Apple, Dry, Quaker*	1 Sachet/39g	143	2.2	371	8.4	68.2	5.7	6.9
Porridge, Sweet Cinnamon, Dry, Oat So Simple, Quaker*	1 Sachet/33g	125	2.2	379	9	67.2	6.6	7.4
Porridge, Traditional, Scottish, Pot, As Sold, Stoats*	1 Pot/60g	216	3.6	361	17.6	59	6	6.6
Protein Crunch, Chocolate, Weetabix*	1 Serving/30g	114	1	379	20	64	3.2	7
Protein Crunch, Weetabix*	1 Serving/30g	114	0.8	379	20	66	2.5	6.1
Pure Oats, Free From, Tesco*	1 Serving/50g	179	2.3	357	11.5	63.6	4.6	8
Raisin & Almond, Crunchy, Jordans*	1 Serving/45g	186	5.7	412	9.9	61.6	12.6	6.6
Raisin Wheats, Kellogg's*	1 Serving/45g	104	0.6	345	9	69	2	9
Raisin, Bran Flakes, Asda*	1 Serving/50g	166	1.5	331	7	69	3	10
Red Berries, Special K, Kellogg's*	1 Serving/30g	113	0.4	376	8.9	79	1.5	5.3
Rice Krispies, Kellogg's*	1 Serving/30g	116	0.4	387	7	86	1.2	2
Rice Krispies, Multi-Grain, Shapes, Kellogg's*	1 Serving/30g	111	0.8	370	8	77	2.5	8

	Measure INFO/WEIGHT	per Measure KCAL	FAT	Nutrition Values per 100g / 100ml KCAL	PROT	CARB	FAT	FIBRE
BREAKFAST CEREAL								
Rice Pops, GF, Nestle*	1 Serving/30g	116	0.4	385	7.5	85	1.2	1.5
Shredded Wheat, Average	**2 Biscuits/45g**	**157**	**0.8**	**348**	**9**	**77**	**1.8**	**10**
Shredded Wheat, Bitesize, Nestle*	1 Serving/40g	148	0.9	369	11.8	69.6	2.2	11.8
Shredded Wheat, Honey Nut, Nestle*	1 Serving/40g	151	2.6	378	11.2	68.8	6.5	9.4
Shreddies, Cocoa, Nestle*	1 Serving/40g	148	0.8	371	9.2	75	1.9	9.3
Shreddies, Frosted, Nestle*	1 Serving/45g	166	0.7	370	9.2	76	1.5	9
Shreddies, Malt Wheats, Tesco*	1 Serving/45g	169	0.9	375	10.3	73.8	2	8.2
Shreddies, Nestle*	1 Serving/40g	146	0.8	365	13	68.9	2	11.8
Special Flakes, Gluten, Wheat, & Milk, Free From, Tesco*	1 Serving/30g	115	0.6	382	6.5	83	2	3
Special Flakes, Honey, Oats, & Almonds, Tesco*	1 Serving/30g	116	0.7	385	7.2	82.5	2.2	3.1
Special Flakes, Peach & Apricot, Morrisons*	1 Serving/30g	112	0.3	373	7	82.3	1.1	3.1
Special Flakes, Red Fruits, Asda*	1 Serving/30g	115	0.4	382	7.1	84	1.3	2.7
Special Flakes, Tesco*	1 Serving/20g	74	0.3	371	11	78.4	1.5	4.3
Special Flakes, with Red Berries, Crownfield, Lidl*	1 Serving/30g	113	0.5	377	6.5	81	1.6	6.4
Special K, Kellogg's*	1 Serving/30g	114	0.4	379	14	76	1.5	2.5
Special K, Oats & Honey, Kellogg's*	1 Serving/30g	114	0.9	381	9	77	3	5
Sultana Bran, HL, Tesco*	1 Serving/30g	98	0.6	325	8.2	68	1.9	12
Weetabix, Banana, Weetabix*	2 Bix/44g	159	0.8	361	11	70	1.9	10
Weetabix, Chocolate, Weetabix*	2 Biscuits/45g	166	1.8	368	10.1	67.9	4	10
Weetaflakes, Weetabix*	1 Serving/30g	102	0.4	340	8.9	72.9	1.4	11
Weetos, Chocolate, Weetabix*	1 Serving/30g	113	1.5	378	8.4	75.1	4.9	5.8
Wheat Biscuits, Average	**2 Biscuits/38g**	**130**	**0.8**	**347**	**11.7**	**68.4**	**2.2**	**9.9**
Wheat Puffs, Honey Monster*	1 Serving/30g	107	0.5	357	7.1	74	1.8	8.4
Wholegrain, Apricot, Wheats, Sainsbury's*	1 Serving/45g	151	0.6	335	8	71.3	1.4	8.3
Wholegrain, Fruit & Fibre, Sainsbury's*	1 Serving/40g	149	2.3	372	9.3	66.1	5.7	9.4
Wholegrain, Mini Wheats, Sainsbury's*	1 Serving/40g	144	0.7	359	11.8	68.2	1.8	11.2
Wholegrain, Minis, Weetabix*	1 Serving/40g	149	0.8	372	10.2	73.2	2	10
Yoghurt & Raspberry, Crisp, Sainsbury's*	1 Serving/45g	191	6.7	424	7.5	65.2	14.8	6.4
BRESAOLA								
Average	**1 Serving/28g**	**51**	**1**	**181**	**33.6**	**0.4**	**3.7**	**0.2**
BROCCOLI								
Green, Boiled, Average	**1 Serving/80g**	**19**	**0.6**	**24**	**3.1**	**1.1**	**0.8**	**2.3**
Green, Raw, Average	**1 Serving/80g**	**24**	**0.7**	**30**	**3.7**	**1.6**	**0.8**	**2.5**
Purple Sprouting, Boiled, Average	**1 Serving/80g**	**15**	**0.5**	**19**	**2.1**	**1.3**	**0.6**	**2.3**
Purple Sprouting, Raw	**1oz/28g**	**10**	**0.3**	**35**	**3.9**	**2.6**	**1.1**	**3.5**
Steamed, Average	**1 Serving/100g**	**24**	**0.8**	**24**	**3.1**	**1.1**	**0.8**	**2.3**
Tenderstem, Average	**1 Serving/80g**	**28**	**0.4**	**35**	**4.1**	**2.9**	**0.6**	**2.3**
BROWNIES								
Average	**1 Brownie/60g**	**243**	**10.1**	**405**	**4.6**	**0**	**16.8**	**0**
Billionaire, Fingers, Thorntons*	1 Finger/21g	87	4.1	423	5.8	54.5	19.7	0
Chocolate Chip, Cadbury*	1 Brownie/25g	116	7.2	465	4.8	46	29	3
Chocolate Chip, Free From, Morrisons*	1 Slice/30g	143	8	478	6	52.5	26.5	2.9
Chocolate, Average	**1 Serving/100g**	**446**	**22.3**	**446**	**5.9**	**55.6**	**22.3**	**2.2**
Chocolate, Chunky, Belgian, M&S*	1 Brownie/55g	242	11.2	440	6.2	57.7	20.3	2.5
Chocolate, Double, Bites, Amaze, Cadbury*	1 Bite/14g	65	3.3	470	5.3	56.7	24.1	3.1
Chocolate, Double, Mini Bites, Sainsbury's*	1 Bite/13g	61	3.3	469	5.4	54	25.4	1.3
Chocolate, Double, Weight Watchers*	1 Dessert/86g	174	3.5	202	4.5	35.9	4.1	1.9
Chocolate, Fudge, Fibre Yum, Crownfield, Lidl*	1 Square/24g	89	2.6	370	5.5	50	11	24.5
Chocolate, Fudge, Mini, Thorntons*	1 Bite/14g	61	2.8	435	5.6	57.4	20	0
Chocolate, Mini Bites, Asda*	1 Brownie/15g	62	3	420	5	55	20	1.4
Chocolate, Seriously Low-Carb Food*	1 Brownie/41g	142	12.7	346	6.5	9	31	0
Mini, The Skinny Bakery*	1 Brownie/17g	38	1.4	230	6.4	34.6	8.5	5.2

	Measure INFO/WEIGHT	per Measure KCAL	FAT	Nutrition Values per 100g / 100ml KCAL	PROT	CARB	FAT	FIBRE
BRUSCHETTA								
Cheese & Tomato, Asda*	1 Bruschetta/38g	68	1.7	180	8.6	26	4.6	2.9
Garlic, & Parsley, Valentina*	1 Bruschetta/10g	55	3.1	538	8.4	56.9	30.4	0
Olive Oil, Artisan Bread Company*	1 Piece/3g	12	0.4	398	10.3	59.1	12.2	0
Toasted, Olive Oil & Sea Salt, Tesco*	1 Serving/30g	126	4.6	420	11.5	58.7	15.5	4.5
Tomato, & Oregano, Valentina*	1 Piece/10g	47	2.2	473	9.8	58	21.5	0
Tomato, Tesco*	¼ Jar/48g	31	1.4	65	1.7	6.5	3	2.5
BRUSSELS SPROUTS								
& Sweet Chestnuts, Asda*	1 Serving/100g	73	1.7	73	3.1	11	1.7	4.2
& Bacon, Oven Baked, Iceland*	¼ Pack/83g	85	3.5	103	4.2	10	4.3	3.8
Boiled, Average	***1 Serving/80g***	***27***	***1***	***33***	***3***	***3***	***1.2***	***3.3***
Button, Raw, Average	***1 Serving/80g***	***28***	***1***	***36***	***3.3***	***2.8***	***1.3***	***3***
Canned, Drained	***1oz/28g***	***5***	***0.2***	***17***	***1.6***	***1.5***	***0.6***	***1.6***
Raw, Average	***1 Serving/80g***	***28***	***0.8***	***35***	***3.3***	***3.1***	***1***	***2.9***
Steamed, Average	***1 Serving/100g***	***35***	***1.3***	***35***	***3.1***	***3.2***	***1.3***	***3.5***
BUBBLE & SQUEAK								
Fried in Vegetable Oil	***1oz/28g***	***35***	***2.5***	***124***	***1.4***	***9.8***	***9.1***	***1.5***
BUCKWHEAT								
Average	***1oz/28g***	***102***	***0.4***	***364***	***8.1***	***84.9***	***1.5***	***2.1***
Puffed, GF, Holland & Barrett*	1 Serving/30g	112	1.2	375	9.7	78	3.9	5.1
BULGUR WHEAT								
Dry Weight, Average	***1oz/28g***	***99***	***0.5***	***353***	***9.7***	***76.3***	***1.7***	***8***
Vegetable, Mediterranean, Sainsbury's*	1 Sachet/135g	122	4.3	90	3.1	10.9	3.2	5.3
BUNS								
Belgian, Asda*	1 Bun/133g	464	19.9	350	4.8	49	15	2.2
Belgian, Iced, Essential, Waitrose*	1 Bun/89g	292	7.6	328	5.7	56	8.5	2.2
Brioche, Boosted, Gut Lovin' Greatness, Genius*	1 Bun/70g	165	4.3	236	4.4	35	6.2	11
Butterfly, GF, Free From, Asda*	1 Bun/37g	159	7.7	434	3.2	58	21	0.5
Chelsea	***1 Bun/78g***	***285***	***10.8***	***366***	***7.8***	***56.1***	***13.8***	***1.7***
Choux, Chocolate, Tesco*	1 Bun/74g	259	18.1	350	7.3	24.4	24.5	1.2
Cinnamon, Waitrose*	1 Bun/97g	379	19.1	389	6.3	46	19.6	1.7
Currant	***1 Bun/60g***	***178***	***4.5***	***296***	***7.6***	***52.7***	***7.5***	***0***
Finger, Iced, Essential, Waitrose*	1 Bun/40g	139	3.5	347	6.7	59.2	8.7	2.6
Fruit, Waitrose*	1 Bun/54g	155	2.3	287	8.1	54	4.3	1.6
Fruited, Iced & Spiced, M&S*	1 Bun/85g	270	4.6	318	4.9	61.3	5.4	2.2
Hot Cross	***1 Bun/50g***	***156***	***3.5***	***312***	***7.4***	***58.5***	***7***	***1.7***
Hot Cross, BGTY, Sainsbury's*	1 Bun/70g	186	2	266	7.1	51.7	2.8	2.7
Hot Cross, Bramley Apple, & Cinnamon, Finest, Tesco*	1 Bun/70g	191	3.7	273	7.5	47.4	5.3	3
Hot Cross, Extra Fruity, Finest, Tesco*	1 Bun/80g	205	2.2	256	7.2	48.9	2.7	3.7
Hot Cross, Free From, Tesco*	1 Bun/70g	161	2.6	231	4.2	41.2	3.7	7.8
Hot Cross, Fruited, Luxury, Specially Selected, Aldi*	1 Bun/85g	229	3.1	269	6.4	50	3.7	5.1
Hot Cross, Fruity, Free From, Sainsbury's*	1 Bun/70g	195	6.2	279	3.3	41.4	8.8	10.2
Hot Cross, Luxury, Rowan Hill Bakery, Lidl*	1 Bun/75g	204	3.5	272	8.3	47	4.7	4
Hot Cross, Marmite, M&S*	1 Bun/65g	187	5.1	288	14.6	38.5	7.9	2.3
Hot Cross, Wholemeal, Asda*	1 Bun/70g	182	4.2	262	9	43	6	6
Hot Cross, Wholemeal, Waitrose*	1 Bun/66g	176	3.2	267	9.6	43.2	4.9	5.7
Iced Finger, Average	***1 Bun/40g***	***130***	***3.1***	***325***	***7.2***	***57***	***7.7***	***2.3***
Vanilla Iced, Soft, M&S*	1 Bun/39g	125	3.1	320	7.6	54.9	8	2.9
BURGERS								
Aubergine, & Feta, Aromatic & Minty, Waitrose*	1 Burger/101g	238	12.9	235	5.2	22.3	12.7	5.3
Bean, BBQ, Monterey Jack, Oven Baked, Tesco*	1 Burger/131g	312	16.4	238	6.1	22.4	12.5	5.6
Bean, Mexican Style, Meat Free, Tesco*	1 Burger/106g	214	9.6	202	4.8	22	9.1	6.4
Bean, Nacho, Spicy, Iceland*	1 Burger/140g	326	16.5	233	6.9	20.1	11.8	4.4
Bean, Spicy Veg, with Chipotle Chilli, Good Life*	1 Burger/108g	227	10.5	210	5.8	20	9.7	8.9

BURGERS

INFO/WEIGHT	Measure	per Measure KCAL	FAT	Nutrition Values per 100g / 100ml KCAL	PROT	CARB	FAT	FIBRE
Bean, Spicy, BGTY, Sainsbury's*	1 Burger/113g	223	11.2	197	4.5	19.6	9.9	5.7
Bean, Spicy, in Herby Nacho Crumb, Morrisons*	1 Burger/102g	185	8.1	181	5.2	19.5	7.9	5.5
Bean, Spicy, Quarter Pounder, Mae's Kitchen, Aldi*	1 Burger/105g	287	13.6	274	5.4	30	13	9.7
Bean, Spicy, Vegetarian, Tesco*	1 Burger/106g	214	9.6	202	4.8	22	9.1	6.4
Beef, 100%, Average	*1 Burger/52g*	*148*	*11.6*	*286*	*20.5*	*0.6*	*22.3*	*0.1*
Beef, 3%, M&S*	1 Burger/100g	122	2.8	122	18.8	5.5	2.8	0.5
Beef, Applewood Smoke, Grilled, Waitrose*	1 Burger/80g	215	13.9	269	23.7	4	17.4	0.6
Beef, Best, Cheese, Gherkin, Tomato, & Mustard, M&S*	1 Burger/167g	414	32.2	248	15.4	3.2	19.3	0.1
Beef, British, Quarter Pounder, Grilled, Finest, Tesco*	1 Burger/99g	206	11.6	208	21.5	3.9	11.7	0.5
Beef, British, Quarter Pounders, 5% Fat, Morrisons*	1 Burger/114g	157	5.4	138	20.4	3.3	4.7	0.5
Beef, British, Quarter Pounders, Grilled, Fire Pit, Tesco*	1 Burger/92g	212	13.3	231	19.9	4.4	14.5	1.6
Beef, British, Waitrose*	1 Burger/113g	279	21	247	18.6	1.2	18.6	0
Beef, Caramelised Onion, Grilled, Finest, Tesco*	1 Burger/88g	196	11.4	223	19.1	7.4	12.9	0.5
Beef, Frozen, Tesco*	1 Burger/44g	117	8.4	266	18.9	4.6	19.1	0
Beef, Grilled, Supermarket, Gourmet Burger Kitchen*	1 Burger/130g	341	23.4	262	26	0.1	18	0.5
Beef, Half Pounder, Aberdeen Angus, Pan Fried, Iceland*	1 Burger/165g	390	25.7	237	23.3	0.4	15.6	1.1
Beef, Irish, Grilled, Fire Pit, Tesco*	1 Burger/76g	175	11	231	19.9	4.4	14.5	1.6
Beef, Original, with Onion, Grilled, Birds Eye*	1 Burger/38g	110	9.5	287	13.4	2.6	24.8	0.3
Beef, Our Best Ever, M&S*	1 Burger/170g	450	36.4	265	16.5	1.7	21.4	0
Beef, Quarter Pounder, Reduced Fat, Grilled, Asda*	1 Burger/94g	178	8	189	20	6.9	8.5	1.6
Beef, Quarter Pounders, Aberdeen Angus, Finest, Tesco*	1 Burger/88g	239	18	272	22.1	0.1	20.4	0.1
Beef, Quarter Pounders, Grilled, Morrisons*	1 Burger/94g	253	18.2	269	20.1	3.1	19.4	0.5
Beef, Quarter Pounders, Original, Birds Eye*	1 Burger/85g	251	21.2	296	15	2.7	25	0.5
Beef, Quarter Pounders, Reduced Fat, Grilled, Tesco*	1 Burger/98g	179	7.3	183	22.1	6.5	7.4	0.8
Beef, Quarter Pounders, Scotch, The Best, Morrisons*	1 Burger/97g	223	13.9	230	21	4	14.3	0.5
Beef, Rump, British, Grilled, Waitrose*	1 Burger/110g	262	15.1	238	24.2	4.1	13.7	0.6
Beef, Scotch, Ultimate, TTD, Sainsbury's*	1 Burger/119g	265	15.8	223	25.3	0.5	13.3	1
Beef, Seasoned, Grilled, Butchers Selection, Asda*	1 Burger/69g	159	10.4	230	20	5.1	15	0.5
Beef, Steak, 5oz, Inspirations, Birds Eye*	1 Burger/87g	293	25.4	335	17	1.4	29	0.5
Beef, Steak, Aberdeen Angus, As Sold, Deluxe, Lidl*	1 Burger/131g	285	19.8	217	18.7	1.1	15.1	0.5
Beef, Steak, Aberdeen Angus, Extra Special, Asda*	1 Burger/170g	362	20.4	213	23	3.2	12	0.5
Beef, Steak, British, Cooked, TTD, Sainsbury's*	1 Burger/110g	276	19.2	250	21.6	1.8	17.4	0.5
Beef, Steak, Mini, Waitrose*	1 Burger/45g	107	6.2	238	24.2	4.1	13.7	0.6
Beef, Steak, We Hae Meat*	1 Burger/114g	190	9.1	167	16.8	6.9	8	0
Beef, Wild Garlic, Pan Cooked, Slimming World*	1 Burger/170g	265	7.8	156	25.2	3.2	4.6	0.5
Beetroot, & Bean, Vegan, As Sold, Strong Roots*	1 Burger/75g	148	6.3	198	4.7	22	8.4	8
Cheese, Halloumi, Asda*	1 Burger/63g	202	15.8	320	22	2.3	25	0
Cheeseburger	*1 Burger/275g*	*706*	*29*	*257*	*13.7*	*25.6*	*10.6*	*1.8*
Cheeseburger, Bacon with Bun, Chargrilled, Tesco*	1 Burger/265g	726	42.1	274	13	19.6	15.9	1
Cheeseburger, Quarter Pounder, Rustlers*	1 Burger/190g	505	25.1	266	13.6	22.4	13.2	0
Chicken, 100% Breast, Golden Wholegrain, Birds Eye*	1 Burger/49g	119	5.9	243	13	20	12	1.4
Chicken, Average	*1 Burger/46g*	*111*	*5.6*	*242*	*14.9*	*18.7*	*12.1*	*1*
Chicken, Breast, Southern Fried, Asda*	1 Burger/95g	224	10.4	236	17	17	11	1.3
Chicken, Cajun Spiced, Tesco*	1 Burger/90g	207	8.9	230	19.5	15.7	9.9	0
Chicken, Cajun, Fillets, Birds Eye*	1 Pack/180g	275	8.8	153	21.5	5.8	4.9	0.3
Chicken, Cheese, & Bacon, Tesco*	½ Pack/129g	308	19.5	239	19.5	6.4	15.1	0.1
Chicken, Fillet, Southern Fried, Asda*	1 Burger/91g	192	7	210	20	14	7.7	1.6
Chicken, Italia, Grilled, Heck*	1 Burger/98g	126	3.8	129	22	1.6	3.9	0
Chicken, Southern Fried, M&S*	1 Burger/141g	240	10.3	170	18.1	7.2	7.3	1.5
Chicken, Southern Fried, Rustlers*	1 Burger/142g	410	18.3	289	10	32.3	12.9	0
Chicken, Style, Vegetarian, Quorn*	1 Burger/60g	122	5.1	205	12.1	16.5	8.6	6.6
Chicken, Thigh, Buttermilk, Gastro Roosters, Aldi *	1 Burger/153g	353	16.8	231	17	14	11	0.9
Chicken, Truffle, Grilled, Luxury, Iceland*	1 Burger/125g	258	14.8	207	16.7	7.9	11.9	0.5

BURGERS

INFO/WEIGHT	Measure	per Measure		Nutrition Values per 100g / 100ml				
		KCAL	FAT	KCAL	PROT	CARB	FAT	FIBRE
Cod, Fish Fillet, Breaded, Birds Eye*	1 Burger/118g	241	8.6	204	13	21	7.3	1
Dogs, Beef, British, Oven Baked, Iceland*	1 Burger Dog/100g	229	14.5	230	17.7	6.2	14.6	1.4
Fish, Fillet, Ultimate, Birds Eye *	1 Burger/117g	266	15.2	227	14	13	13	0.9
Halloumi, Specially Selected, Aldi*	1 Burger /70g	209	15.4	298	18	7.2	22	1.1
Hog Roast, & Apple, Irresistible, Co-Op*	1 Burger/142g	339	21.3	239	15	8	15	0.7
Hot & Spicy, Vegan, Quorn*	1 Burger/66g	139	5.7	211	11.1	20.3	8.7	3.4
Impossible Burger*	1 Burger/113g	240	14	212	16.8	8	12.4	2.6
Kale, & Quinoa, Vegetarian, Strong Roots*	1 Burger/80g	165	8.4	206	4.5	21.9	10.5	2.7
Lamb, Firecracker, Grilled, Shazans*	1 Burger/102g	191	9.5	187	17.4	8.2	9.3	0.6
Lamb, Minted, Average	**1 Burger/56g**	**125**	**7.4**	**223**	**20.6**	**5.5**	**13.2**	**0.2**
Lamb, Waitrose*	1 Burger/67g	99	4.7	148	15.7	5.4	7	0.9
Meat Free, Average	**1 Burger/113g**	**195**	**8.8**	**172**	**17.5**	**7.9**	**7.8**	**3**
Mushroom, & Chestnut, Oven Cooked, Waitrose*	1 Burger/113g	166	5	147	4.8	19.3	4.4	5.8
No Beef, Vegetarian, Plant Kitchen, M&S*	1 Burger/160g	339	22.7	212	11.2	73	14.2	5.3
No Chicken, Vegan, Plant Pioneers, Sainsbury's*	1 Burger/104g	310	17.2	298	8.5	27	16.5	3.7
Nut, with Carrot, & Parsnip, Oven Baked, Goodlife*	1 Burger/80g	197	11.8	246	5.3	22.1	14.8	2.2
Plant Based, Beyond Burger, Vegan, Beyond Meat*	1 Patty/114g	318	21.1	280	21.5	6.6	18.6	0.5
Plant Based, The Big Fry, Vegan, Fry's*	1 Burger/112g	161	4.5	144	17.7	8	4	3.1
Plant, Ultimate, Plant Pioneers, Sainsbury's*	1 Burger/86g	184	10	213	16.2	7.8	11.6	6.3
Pork, & Apple, Quarter Pounder, Grilled, Asda*	1 Burger/80g	147	6.4	184	23.9	4.1	8	0.5
Pork, Pulled, Quarter Pounder, Grilled, Linda McCartney*	1 Burger/97g	150	4.5	154	16.1	11.1	4.6	2
Pumpkin, & Spinach, Vegetarian, Strong Roots*	1 Burger/80g	162	7.5	202	3.9	24.6	9.3	2.3
Quarter Pounder, Cheddar, Vintage , Deluxe, Lidl*	1 Burger/78g	206	12.7	264	26.4	2.6	16.3	0
Quarter Pounder, Loved by Us, Co-Op*	1 Burger/114g	301	23.9	265	19	0.5	21	0
Quarter Pounder, Mozzarella, Vegetarian, Linda McCartney*	1 Burger/105g	265	15.4	252	19.8	7.9	14.7	5
Quarter Pounder, Quorn*	1 Burger/114g	170	6.8	150	14.4	7.7	6	4
Quinoa, Sweet Potato, & Lentil, Vegetarian, Sainsbury's*	1 Burger/88g	168	8.2	192	4.7	19.3	9.4	5.8
Red Lentil, & Sunflower Seed, Vegan, Biona Organic*	1 Burger/80g	207	8.8	259	7.8	29	11	6.8
Salmon, Thai, Grilled, Waitrose*	1 Burger/83g	161	8.4	194	18.6	6.7	10.1	1
Sausage, Plant Based, Moving Mountains*	1 Burger/114g	285	16	250	11	6.6	14	6.1
Soya, Quarter Pounders, Meat Free Butcher, Aldi*	1 Burger/108g	297	18.4	275	13	16	17	3.6
Spicy Bean, Vegan, Vemondo, Lidl*	1 Burger/106g	213	8.5	201	5.4	23.1	8	7.7
Steak, Peppered, M&S*	1 Burger/114g	310	24.4	272	18.8	0.8	21.4	0.7
Sweet Potato, & Edamame, Meat Free, Morrisons*	1 Burger/88g	144	8	164	6.4	10.6	9.1	7.2
Sweet Potato, & Chickpea, Veg, Plant Kitchen, M&S*	1 Burger/120g	221	8.9	184	7.5	18.3	7.4	7.1
Sweet Potato, Buckwheat, Vegan, Biona Organic*	1 Burger/80g	198	9.6	248	5.2	27	12	3.5
Sweet Potato, Chickpea, Carrot, Red Pepper, Aldi*	1 Burger/115g	172	2.6	150	4.2	25	2.3	6.1
Turkey, British, Grilled, Sainsbury's*	1 Burger/97g	171	6.5	176	24.6	4.1	6.7	0.5
Turkey, Sea Salt & Pepper, Butchers Selection, Asda*	1 Burger/96g	141	4.4	147	23	3.2	4.6	0.5
Turkey, Supervalu*	1 Burger/100g	105	1.4	105	19	3.5	1.4	1.4
Vegan, Quarter Pounder, Gro, Co-Op*	1 Burger/113g	189	11.3	167	10	3.7	10	9
Vegan, Vivera*	1 Burger/100g	169	7.3	169	18.5	4.8	7.3	5
Vegetable, Average	**1 Burger/56g**	**100**	**4.5**	**179**	**4.4**	**22.4**	**8**	**2.3**
Vegetable, Quarter Pounders, Meat Free, Vegan, Tesco*	1 Burger/106g	229	10.6	216	3.7	25.8	10	3.9
Vegetable, Quarter Pounders, Sainsbury's*	1 Burger/102g	226	10.1	221	4.8	26	9.9	4.4
Vegetarian, Average	**1 Burger/60g**	**112**	**5.3**	**187**	**17.2**	**2.9**	**8.8**	**3.3**
Vegetarian, Quarter Pounders, Grilled, Linda McCartney*	1 Burger/105g	232	12.5	220	17.3	9.8	11.9	2.4
Veggie, Frozen, Birds Eye*	1 Burger/125g	222	5.5	181	4.2	23	4.5	2.1
Veggie, Green Cuisine, Birds Eye*	1 Burger/127g	224	9.5	177	4.4	22	7.5	2
Veggie, Katsu Curry, Goodlife*	1 Burger/99g	154	7.3	156	7	13.4	7.4	4.3
Venison, Finnebrougue Estate*	1 Burger/142g	170	7	120	19.9	4.2	4.9	0.5

BURRITO

INFO/WEIGHT	Measure	per Measure		Nutrition Values per 100g / 100ml				
Bean, & Rice, Mexican, GF, Amy's Kitchen*	1 Burrito/158g	234	6	148	4.5	24	3.8	3.2

	Measure	per Measure		Nutrition Values per 100g / 100ml				
	INFO/WEIGHT	KCAL	FAT	KCAL	PROT	CARB	FAT	FIBRE
BURRITO								
Beef	**1 Serving/225g**	**536**	**20.2**	**238**	**12**	**27**	**9**	**2.2**
Beef, Chilli, Inspired Cuisine, Aldi*	1 Pack/400g	748	26.4	187	6.8	24	6.6	2.6
Beef, Spicy, Tex Mex, Tesco*	1 Burrito/192g	326	8.4	170	6.5	24.8	4.4	2.6
Tofu, Smoky, Oven Baked, Plant Based, Asda*	1 Pack/386g	618	19.7	160	5.3	21	5.1	3.6
BUTTER								
Brandy, Average	**1 Serving/10g**	**56**	**3.8**	**556**	**0.2**	**46.2**	**38.4**	**0.1**
Creamery, Average	**1 Serving/10g**	**74**	**8.1**	**736**	**0.5**	**0.4**	**81.4**	**0**
French, with Sea Salt Crystals, Waitrose*	1 Thin Spread/7g	51	5.6	727	0.7	1	80	0
Fresh, Average	**1 Thin Spread/7g**	**51**	**5.7**	**735**	**0.6**	**0.4**	**81.3**	**0**
Garlic, Crushed, Lurpak*	1 Serving/10g	69	7.5	692	1.3	3.7	75	0
Goat's, St Helen's Farm*	1 Thin Spread/7g	56	6.2	794	0.5	0	88	0
Guernsey Dairy*	1 Thin Spread/7g	53	5.8	755	0.6	0.6	83.4	0
Reduced Fat, Fresh, Average	**1 Thin Spread/7g**	**26**	**2.8**	**368**	**2.3**	**1.2**	**39.4**	**0.2**
Salted, Average	**1 Thin Spread/7g**	**51**	**5.7**	**729**	**0.4**	**0.3**	**81.1**	**0**
Spreadable, Fresh, Average	**1 Thin Spread/7g**	**51**	**5.7**	**730**	**0.4**	**0.3**	**80.8**	**0**
Spreadable, Reduced Fat, Average	**1 Thin Spread/7g**	**38**	**4.2**	**540**	**0.5**	**0.5**	**60**	**0**
Unsalted, Sainsbury's*	1 Spread/12g	89	9.9	745	0.6	0.6	82.2	0.5
with Olive Oil, Lighter, Spreadable, Lurpak*	1 Thin Spread/7g	38	4.2	543	0.3	0.4	60	0
BUTTERMILK								
Average	**1 Mug/400ml**	**177**	**1.3**	**44**	**4.2**	**5.9**	**0.3**	**0**
BUTTERNUT SQUASH								
Indian Spiced, Centrepieces, BOL Foods*	1 Serving/125g	170	11.2	136	1.7	10.8	9	0.6
Winter, Boiled, Flesh Only	**1 Serving/80g**	**27**	**0.1**	**34**	**0.7**	**8.8**	**0.1**	**2.6**
Winter, Butternut, Baked, Average	**1 Serving/100g**	**32**	**0.1**	**32**	**0.9**	**7.4**	**0.1**	**1.4**
Winter, Butternut, Raw, Prepared, Average	**1 Serving/80g**	**29**	**0.1**	**36**	**1.1**	**8.3**	**0.1**	**1.6**
Winter, Butternut, Raw, Unprepared, Average	**1 Serving/80g**	**24**	**0.1**	**30**	**0.9**	**6.8**	**0.1**	**1.3**
BUTTONS								
Milk Chocolate, Giant, Dairy Milk, Cadbury*	1 Button/2g	11	0.6	530	7.6	56.5	30.5	0.7
Milk Chocolate, M&S*	1 Pack/75g	375	19	500	8.6	59.8	25.3	1.9
Milk Chocolate, Tesco*	1 Bag/70g	359	19.3	513	7.1	59.1	27.6	2.1
White Chocolate, Co-Op*	½ Pack/35g	186	9.8	530	7	64	28	0
White Chocolate, Milkybar, Nestle*	1 Bag/30g	164	9.5	546	7.5	58.1	31.6	0
White Chocolate, Tesco*	1 Bag/70g	388	23.4	554	5.1	58	33.5	0

	Measure INFO/WEIGHT	per Measure KCAL	FAT	Nutrition Values per 100g / 100ml KCAL	PROT	CARB	FAT	FIBRE
CABBAGE								
& Leek, Ready Sliced, Sainsbury's*	1 Pack/240g	53	1.2	22	1.1	2.2	0.5	2.1
& Leek, Sliced, Tesco*	1/3 Pack/100g	32	0.6	32	2.1	3.4	0.6	2.6
Boiled, Average	**1 Serving/90g**	**14**	**0.3**	**15**	**1**	**2.2**	**0.3**	**1.7**
Raw, Average	**1 Serving/100g**	**21**	**0.4**	**21**	**1.3**	**3.2**	**0.4**	**1.8**
Red, Average	**1 Serving/90g**	**19**	**0.2**	**21**	**1**	**3.7**	**0.3**	**2.2**
Red, Braised with Red Wine, M&S*	½ Pack/150g	180	7.2	120	1.4	17.1	4.8	1
Red, Braised, with Bramley Apples, M&S*	½ Pack/150g	126	3	84	1	14	2	2.8
Red, Pickled, Average	**1 Serving/50g**	**13**	**0.1**	**26**	**0.9**	**4.6**	**0.2**	**1.6**
Red, with Apple, Finest, Tesco*	½ Pack/150g	177	8.8	118	1.6	14.7	5.9	4.6
Red, with Apple, Red Wine & Cranberries, Waitrose*	1/3 Pack/97g	116	5.7	120	1.4	14.2	5.9	2.6
Savoy, Boiled in Salted Water, Average	**1 Serving/90g**	**15**	**0.4**	**17**	**1.1**	**2.2**	**0.5**	**2**
Savoy, Raw, Average	**1 Serving/90g**	**24**	**0.4**	**27**	**2.1**	**3.9**	**0.5**	**3.1**
Spring Greens, Boiled, Average	**1 Serving/80g**	**16**	**0.6**	**20**	**1.9**	**1.6**	**0.7**	**2.6**
Spring Greens, Raw, Average	**1 Serving/80g**	**22**	**0.7**	**28**	**2.5**	**2.6**	**0.8**	**2.9**
Steamed, Average	**1 Serving/100g**	**15**	**0.3**	**15**	**1**	**2.2**	**0.3**	**1.7**
Sweetheart, Raw	**1 Serving/100g**	**26**	**0.6**	**26**	**2.1**	**3.2**	**0.6**	**2.8**
White, Raw, Average	**1oz/28g**	**8**	**0.1**	**27**	**1.4**	**5**	**0.2**	**2.1**
CACAO								
Nibs, Organic, Naturya*	1 Tbsp/15g	95	8.4	633	13	15	56	10
Powder, Organic, Naturya*	1 Serving/50g	184	6	367	27.2	22	12	29
CAKE								
After Dinner Mint Fancies, Mr Kipling*	1 Cake/28g	106	3.1	376	3	65.7	10.9	1.5
Almond, Bakewell, Mini, M&S*	1 Cake/52g	223	9.1	428	4.8	62.6	17.5	0.5
Almond, Slices, Mr Kipling*	1 Slice/35g	144	6.5	411	6	54.2	18.5	1.8
Almond, Slices, Sainsbury's*	1 Serving/27g	120	7.1	444	5.9	45.9	26.3	1.5
Angel Slices, 30% Less Sugar, Mr Kipling*	1 Slice/24g	98	4.8	410	3.5	53	19.9	2.5
Angel, Average	**1 Slice/44g**	**175**	**7.9**	**397**	**4.2**	**54.9**	**17.9**	**0.8**
Apple, Home Style, M&S*	1 Cake/54g	189	7.9	350	5.3	49.4	14.7	1.5
Apple, Slices, Delightful, Mr Kipling*	1 Slice/29g	92	1.1	317	4.4	66.2	3.9	1.3
Apple, Sticky Toffee, Finest, Tesco*	1 Slice/51g	247	9.2	487	3	52.7	18.1	0.6
Bakewell, Cherry, Co-Op*	1 Cake/47g	205	8	435	3.7	67.2	16.9	1.8
Bakewell, Cherry, Delightful, Mr Kipling*	1 Cake/45g	176	5.8	390	3.9	66.4	12.9	1.2
Bakewell, Cherry, M&S*	1 Cake/44g	185	7.8	420	4.5	61.7	17.7	1
Bakewell, Cherry, Mini, Sainsbury's*	1 Cake/27g	101	3.3	370	3.4	62.2	12	0.4
Bakewell, Cherry, Slices, GFY, Asda*	1 Slice/29g	98	0.7	337	3.4	75.4	2.4	0.7
Bakewell, Cherry, Waitrose*	1 Cake/44g	184	8.5	419	3.8	57.4	19.3	2.1
Bakewell, Lemon, Average	**1 Cake/42g**	**173**	**6.4**	**411**	**3.7**	**64.6**	**15.2**	**1.3**
Bakewell, Slices, Mr Kipling*	1 Slice/35g	146	6.2	414	4.1	59.2	17.6	1
Bakewell, Slices, Weight Watchers*	1 Slice/26g	84	0.6	324	3.7	71	2.4	2
Banana, Bread, Brilliant, Graze*	1 Cake/23g	72	3.6	312	5.2	40.4	15.6	3
Banana, J. Donald*	1 Slice/25g	38	4	152	2	0	16	0
Banana, Loaf, Tesco*	1 Slice/40g	152	6.9	380	5.3	50.3	17.2	1.6
Banana, Loaf, Waitrose*	1 Slice/70g	236	7.5	337	5	55.2	10.7	1.7
Battenberg, Mr Kipling*	1 Serving/38g	161	4.6	421	5	73.3	12	1.6
Birthday, M&S*	1 Serving/60g	240	7.1	400	2.3	70.9	11.9	0.8
Birthday, Piece of Cake, M&S*	1 Serving/85g	395	24.4	465	4.3	39.7	28.7	0.9
Birthday, Present, Tesco*	1 Serving/79g	347	13.9	439	3.5	66.6	17.6	0.4
Blueberry, Fitbakes*	1 Cake/17g	36	1	206	11	47	6	0
Butterfly, Mr Kipling*	1 Cake/29g	114	6.4	392	4.4	43.4	22.2	0.6
Butterfly, Vanilla, Bakery, Waitrose*	1 Cake/38g	163	7.3	430	3.5	60.6	19.2	0.5
Caramel, Salted, The Best, Morrisons*	1/6 Cake/63g	262	12.2	416	3.9	56.2	19.4	0.5
Carrot, & Orange, Finest, Tesco*	1/8 Cake/50g	205	10.2	410	4.6	51.2	20.5	2.1
Carrot, & Orange, Waitrose*	1/6 Cake/47g	164	7.4	350	5.3	46.8	15.7	1.8

CAKE

INFO/WEIGHT	Measure	per Measure KCAL	per Measure FAT	Nutrition Values per 100g / 100ml KCAL	PROT	CARB	FAT	FIBRE
Carrot, & Walnut, Aldi*	¼ Cake/100g	409	23	409	5.1	44	23	2.2
Carrot, & Walnut, Layered, Asda*	1 Serving/42g	172	8	409	4.6	55	19	1
Carrot, & Walnut, Mini Classics, Mr Kipling*	1 Cake/39g	172	9.8	440	4.5	48.6	25.2	1
Carrot, Average	*1 Slice/56g*	*211*	*10.4*	*377*	*4.6*	*47.6*	*18.6*	*1.4*
Carrot, Free From, Finest, Tesco*	1 Slice/67g	288	17.7	429	3	43.3	26.3	3.5
Carrot, Iced, Tesco*	1 Serving/61g	246	12	404	3.1	53.7	19.6	1.6
Carrot, TTD, Sainsbury's*	1 Slice/72g	287	13.7	398	4.5	51.1	19	2.5
Carrot, with Walnuts, M&S*	1 Pack/75g	290	13.5	387	4.5	50.6	18	2.4
Celebration Rose, Mary Berry*	1 Slice/100g	410	14.5	410	2.9	66.6	14.5	0
Cherry & Almond Slices, GF, Free From, Sainsbury's*	1 Slice/33g	144	7.9	442	6.5	48.7	24.3	1
Cherry Bakewell, Asda*	1 Cake/46g	189	6.9	411	3.8	63	15	2.1
Cherry Bakewell, Mr Kipling*	1 Bakewell/46g	200	8	435	3.4	65.5	17.4	1.4
Cherry Bakewell, Pearls, The Skinny Bakery*	1 Pearl/16g	41	1.2	255	6.1	42.9	7.8	3.7
Chocolate	*1oz/28g*	*128*	*7.4*	*456*	*7.4*	*50.4*	*26.4*	*1.7*
Chocolate & Caramel, Millionaire, M&S*	1 Serving/74g	329	18.6	444	3.8	50	25.1	1.6
Chocolate Chip, Co-Op*	1/6 Cake/63g	275	16.9	440	5	44	27	0.5
Chocolate Chip, Slices, Mr Kipling*	1 Slice/25g	109	5.1	442	6.2	57.4	20.5	1.6
Chocolate Slices, Mr Kipling*	1 Slice/32g	132	6	411	3.4	56.3	18.7	1.7
Chocolate, & Blood Orange, Bars, Lunchbox, Soreen*	1 Bar/30g	105	2.5	349	8.9	57.5	8.2	5.2
Chocolate, & Madeira, Marble Loaf, M&S*	1/6 Cake/88g	380	20.4	430	5	50	23.1	1
Chocolate, & Orange, Rolls, M&S*	1 Cake/60g	228	17	380	3.6	27	28.4	1.3
Chocolate, & Salted Caramel, Delice, TTD, Sainsbury's*	1 Serving/65g	207	12.3	319	3.6	32.5	19	1.9
Chocolate, Birthday Cubes, Sainsbury's*	1 Cube/49g	212	9.4	432	4.3	58.3	19.2	0
Chocolate, Celebration, Vegan, OGGS*	1 Serving/60g	259	14.7	431	5.3	45.5	24.5	3.6
Chocolate, Crispy Clusters, Mini, Tesco*	1 Cluster/8g	37	1.5	470	7	67.8	18.7	2.5
Chocolate, Free From, Finest, Tesco*	1 Slice/64g	279	16.1	438	4.1	46.9	25.3	3.2
Chocolate, Fudge	*1 Serving/110g*	*415*	*19.1*	*377*	*4.4*	*50.4*	*17.4*	*1.4*
Chocolate, Fudge, Oggs*	1 Cake/46g	185	10.3	402	5.5	40	22.3	2
Chocolate, Hand Finished, Co-Op*	1 Slice/65g	271	15	417	5.1	46.2	23.1	1.8
Chocolate, Indulgent, Ripple, Galaxy, Mars*	1 Slice/50g	216	11.5	433	4.7	50	23	0
Chocolate, Mousse, Galaxy, Mars*	1 Serving/71g	250	15.5	354	5.3	33	22	0
Chocolate, Mug, Foodpack, Lighter Life*	1 Pack/42g	153	4.5	364	30	29.8	10.7	11.5
Chocolate, Orange, Sponge, Asda*	1 Serving/70g	298	18.2	425	4.9	42.9	26	3
Chocolate, Rice Crispy, Knightsbridge, Lidl*	1 Cake/24g	88	4.2	368	3.9	48.7	17.5	0.1
Chocolate, Roll, Triple, Cadbury*	1 Serving/40g	165	6.7	410	4.3	60.1	16.6	1.5
Chocolate, Sponge, Tesco*	1 Serving/37g	129	3.6	358	5.1	60.8	10.1	1.7
Chocolate, Sponge, Victoria, Co-Op*	1 Slice/61g	201	9.8	330	5	42	16	1
Chocolate, Truffle, Mini, Finest, Tesco*	1 Cake/28g	125	6.6	448	5.9	52.9	23.7	0.3
Chocolate, Vegan, Just Love Food*	1 Slice/61g	249	13.4	409	3.4	48.4	22	0
Chocolate, White, Party, Asda*	1 Slice/100g	424	22	424	3.1	52	22	1.4
Chocolate, Wiggles The Caterpillar, Mini, Sainsbury's*	1 Cake/30g	139	6.7	462	4.8	59.9	22.2	1.8
Chocolate, with Butter Icing, Average	*1oz/28g*	*135*	*8.3*	*481*	*5.7*	*50.9*	*29.7*	*0*
Chocoramo, Ramo*	1 Cake/65g	290	15	446	6.2	52.3	23.1	3.1
Christmas, Connoisseur, M&S*	1 Slice/60g	216	5.5	360	4.1	64.7	9.2	3.3
Christmas, Rich Fruit, Organic, Tesco*	1 Serving/76g	282	7.6	374	3.9	67.1	10	2
Christmas, Rich Fruit, Tesco*	1 Serving/75g	261	7.2	348	3.8	60.6	9.6	2.1
Christmas, Slices, Mr Kipling*	1 Slice/43g	159	3.8	368	3	68.4	8.8	1.4
Cinnamon Roll, Nutrisystem*	1 Roll/58g	180	4.5	310	12.1	50	7.8	8.6
Cinnamon Scroll, Super, Wicked Kitchen, Tesco*	1 Scroll/98g	288	6.6	294	7.1	49.2	6.7	4.3
Coconut	*1 Slice/70g*	*304*	*16.7*	*434*	*6.7*	*51.2*	*23.8*	*2.5*
Coconut, & Raspberry, M&S*	1 Serving/52g	231	13.9	445	5	45.5	26.8	2.3
Coconut, & Raspberry, Loaf, Tesco*	1/6 Cake/46g	178	7.4	388	5.2	54.5	16.1	1.9
Coconut, Snowball, Tunnock's*	1 Cake/30g	134	6.2	446	4.2	56.7	20.8	3.6

C

CAKE

	Measure INFO/WEIGHT	per Measure KCAL	FAT	Nutrition Values per 100g / 100ml KCAL	PROT	CARB	FAT	FIBRE
Coconut, Sponge, Mini Classics, Mr Kipling*	1 Cake/38g	155	8.7	409	3.7	47	22.9	0.9
Coffee & Walnut, Hand Finished, Irresistible, Co-Op*	1 Slice/64g	271	13.4	424	3.4	56	21	0.9
Coffee, & Walnut Slices, HE, Tesco*	1 Slice/23g	69	0.5	301	4.4	65.7	2.3	2.8
Colin the Caterpillar, M&S*	1 Slice/60g	234	12.8	390	5.3	57.2	21.3	1.3
Cookies & Cream, Fitbakes*	1 Cake/78g	173	7	221	12	40	9	0
Cornflake Cluster, Chocolate, Sainsbury's*	1 Cluster/10g	46	1.7	463	7.3	69.7	16.8	0
Cornflake, Average	*1 Cake/18g*	*83*	*3.7*	*464*	*5.2*	*64.6*	*20.4*	*2*
Cornflake, Chocolate Clusters, Asda*	1 Cake/14g	64	2.6	460	8.2	65.2	18.5	2.7
Cornflake, Chocolate, Mini Bites, Tesco*	1 Bite/14g	62	2.5	446	7.1	64.1	17.9	5.9
Cream Sponge, Morrisons*	1 Serving/46g	138	6.4	302	3.8	39.8	13.9	1.2
Cream, Oysters, M&S*	1 Cake/72g	227	15.3	315	3.6	27.5	21.2	3
Cream, Slices, M&S*	1 Slice/80g	310	18.3	387	2.3	45.7	22.9	0.6
Date, & Walnut Loaf, Sainsbury's*	1/10 Slice/40g	148	8.2	371	6.7	40.1	20.4	1
Eccles, All Butter, M&S*	1 Cake/86g	345	14.8	400	4.5	57.4	17.2	3.2
Eccles, Fresh Baked	*1 Cake/45g*	*171*	*7.6*	*381*	*4.3*	*56.3*	*17*	*1.5*
Eccles, Giant, Bramble Foods*	1 Cake/125g	458	19	366	4.1	54.8	15.2	0
Fairy, Average	*1 Cake/23g*	*96*	*4.6*	*416*	*5.1*	*53*	*20.2*	*1.5*
Fairy, Chocolate, Ms Mollys*	1 Cake/23g	95	4.9	413	4.2	49.7	21.4	2.5
Fairy, Iced, Average	*1 Cake/23g*	*91*	*3.4*	*394*	*4.2*	*60.8*	*14.8*	*0.9*
Fairy, Lemon Iced, Average	*1 Cake/23g*	*90*	*3.1*	*393*	*4.4*	*63.2*	*13.6*	*1.1*
Fairy, Plain, Average	*1 Cake/23g*	*95*	*4.6*	*413*	*5.5*	*51.1*	*20.2*	*1.5*
Fairy, Strawberry Iced, Tesco*	1 Cake/24g	94	3.2	392	4.9	62.9	13.4	1.4
Fairy, Vanilla Iced, Average, Tesco*	1 Cake/23g	89	2.8	388	4.4	65.1	12.2	1.2
Fondant, Dark Chocolate, Graze*	1 Pack/40g	157	5.8	393	3.5	66.2	14.5	0
French Fancies, Average	*1 Cake/27g*	*100*	*2.5*	*371*	*2.7*	*69.6*	*9.1*	*0.8*
French Fancies, Lemon, Average	*1 Cake/28g*	*106*	*2.7*	*378*	*2.5*	*69.9*	*9.8*	*0.5*
Fruit, & Cherry, Loaf, Cakebasket*	1 Slice/30g	118	5.5	395	4.3	55.4	18.2	0
Fruit, Petit Cakes Aux Fruits, Bonne Maman*	1 Cake/25g	102	5.2	407	5.4	48	21	0
Fruit, Plain, Average	*1 Slice/90g*	*319*	*11.6*	*354*	*5.1*	*57.9*	*12.9*	*0*
Fruit, Rich, Average	*1 Slice/70g*	*225*	*8.8*	*322*	*4.9*	*50.7*	*12.5*	*1.7*
Fruit, Rich, Iced	*1 Slice/70g*	*249*	*8*	*356*	*4.1*	*62.7*	*11.4*	*1.7*
Fruit, Rich, Slices, Free From, Sainsbury's*	1 Slice/40g	144	5	361	4.5	57.4	12.6	3.7
Fruit, Slice, Lazy Day Foods*	1 Slice/50g	134	2.8	269	3	51.8	5.6	3
Genoa, Tesco*	1 Serving/44g	150	3.9	340	3.7	59.1	8.8	3.1
Genoa, Vegetarian, Co-Op*	1/8 Cake/40g	137	3	343	2.9	63	7.5	2.9
Ginger, & Syrup, Tesco*	1 Serving/32g	134	7	420	4.5	51.4	21.8	0.7
Ginger, Drizzle, Iced, Co-Op*	1/6 Cake/64g	226	7.7	350	3	58	12	1
Ginger, Jamaica, McVitie's*	1/9 Cake/26g	92	2.6	362	3.7	63.1	10.4	1.6
Ginger, Loaf , Stem, Waitrose*	1 Slice/35g	134	4.8	384	3.7	60.1	13.7	2.6
Granola, Square, All Butter, Finest, Tesco*	1 Square/72g	322	16.1	447	7.8	50.7	22.4	5.9
Granola, Square, M&S*	1 Square/72g	330	18.1	464	7.9	49.3	25.5	5
Hazelnut Choc, Fitbakes*	1 Cake/14g	40	1.5	284	14	43	11	0
Honey, & Apricot, Nevis*	1 Slice/45g	189	9.7	421	4.8	52	21.5	1
Hot Cross, Slices, Mr Kipling*	1 Slice/29g	118	4.7	410	4	61.3	16.2	1.5
Jaffa Chocolate, Fitbakes*	1 Cake/65g	169	5.2	259	13	43	8	0
Jam, & Cream, Split, Specially Selected, Aldi*	1 Slice/35g	141	6.6	402	4.5	53	19	0.9
Lattebit, Delicato*	1 Cake/30g	150	9.3	500	4.5	51	31	0
Lebkuchen, Chocolate, Dark, Mini, M&S*	1 Cake/9g	34	1.1	378	5.6	62.2	12.2	2.2
Lemon Curd, Bake, M&S*	1 Cake/45g	196	9.4	436	4.1	57.6	20.9	0.6
Lemon Drizzle, Deluxe, Lidl*	1 Slice/66g	269	11.5	407	3.8	58.5	17.4	0.7
Lemon Drizzle, Fitbakes*	1 Cake/77g	154	4.6	199	10	48	6	0
Lemon Slice, 30% Reduced Sugar, Mr Kipling*	1 Slice/24g	100	4.5	415	3.5	57.8	18.7	0.9
Lemon Slices, Mr Kipling*	1 Slice/33g	137	5.2	409	2.7	64.2	15.5	0.7

CAKE

	Measure INFO/WEIGHT	per Measure KCAL	FAT	Nutrition Values per 100g / 100ml KCAL	PROT	CARB	FAT	FIBRE
Lemon Zest, Nutrisystem*	1 Cake/62g	140	4	226	8.1	43.6	6.4	6.4
Lemon, & Orange, Finest, Tesco*	1 Serving/53g	216	10.7	410	4.5	52.4	20.3	1.1
Lemon, & Lime, Drizzle, No.1, Waitrose*	1/12 Cake/52g	209	9.2	402	3.1	57.5	17.6	0.8
Lemon, & Poppy Seed, Slices, Weight Watcher*	1 Slice/19g	69	2.1	364	3.7	60.9	11.3	1.9
Lemon, Average	**1 Slice/81g**	**320**	**14.5**	**396**	**4.1**	**54.8**	**18**	**0.6**
Lemon, Drizzle Cake, Asda*	1 Serving/50g	150	6	299	2.8	45	12	0.4
Lemon, Drizzle, Classic, M&S*	1 Serving/100g	333	13.6	333	4	47.5	13.6	2.2
Lemon, Drizzle, Finest, Tesco*	1 Slice/68g	266	11.2	391	3.6	56.3	16.5	1.6
Lemon, filled with Lemon Curd, TTD, Sainsbury's*	1 Slice/73g	299	13.5	407	3.9	56.1	18.4	0.7
Lemon, Hand Finished, Irresistible, Co-Op*	1/16 Cake/64g	241	9.6	377	3.9	57	15	0.6
Lemon, Iced, Asda*	1/8 Cake/36g	142	5.4	393	4.1	60	15	0.9
Lemon, Layer, Chocolate Coated, Cottage Bakery*	1 Box/150g	386	13.1	257	2.9	42.3	8.7	0.9
Lemon, Loaf, M&S*	1 Slice/47g	190	8.8	400	2.1	55.8	18.6	0.6
Lemon, Slice, GF, Free From, Sainsbury's*	1 Slice/35g	169	10.1	477	6.5	47.6	28.6	1.8
Lemon, Slices, Asda*	1 Slice/27g	113	5.3	424	3.8	56	20	1.8
Lemon, Slices, Free From, Tesco*	1 Slice/38g	156	6.6	410	3	59.5	17.5	1
Lemon, Slices, Iced, Tesco*	1 Slice/29g	114	4.9	394	3	56.1	17.1	2
Lemon, Slices, Low Fat, Weight Watchers*	1 Slice/22g	84	3.7	384	4.7	41.7	16.8	23
Lemon, Slices, Sainsbury's*	1 Slice/30g	130	6.3	432	4.1	56	20.9	1.7
Lemon, Zesty, Large, Vegan, OGGS*	1 Serving/64g	282	14.8	438	5	50.3	23	0.9
Lemon, Zesty, Vegan, OGGS*	1 Cake/46g	199	10.3	433	5.1	49.1	22.5	0.9
Leo the Lion, Birthday, Asda*	1 Slice/81g	325	12.9	402	2.6	62	16	0.5
Madeira	**1 Slice/40g**	**157**	**6.8**	**393**	**5.4**	**58.4**	**16.9**	**0.9**
Madeira, Cherry, Sainsbury's*	1 Slice/34g	117	2.6	349	4	64.8	7.9	1.3
Madeira, Cherry, Tesco*	1 Serving/38g	135	4.2	357	4.6	58.9	11	1.8
Madeira, Iced, Asda*	1/8 Cake/36g	141	5.1	388	3.9	61	14	1
Madeira, Iced, Tesco*	1 Slice/40g	157	5.8	393	3.8	60.7	14.6	1.7
Madeira, Lemon Iced, Co-Op*	1 Cake/290g	1131	52.2	390	4	53	18	0.6
Madeira, Lemon Iced, Tesco*	1 Slice/40g	169	7.4	418	4.9	58.1	18.2	1.1
Madeleine, Bonne Maman*	1 Madeleine/25g	114	6.8	456	6.3	46	27	2.1
Madeleine, with Lemon, Bonne Maman*	1 Madeleine/25g	100	5.5	402	5.6	45	22	0
Madeleines, Classic, French, GF, Mrs Crimbles*	1 Cake/30g	136	7.8	453	4.7	49	26	0
Madeleines, Tesco*	1 Cake/25g	122	7.3	486	4.8	50.5	29.1	1.5
Manor House, Mr Kipling*	1 Serving/69g	277	13.8	400	5.3	49.7	20	1.4
Marble, Half Moon, Bobby's*	1 Pack/350g	1572	73.5	449	5.1	60	21	0
Marble, Tesco*	1/8 Cake/45g	184	8.4	410	4.4	55.9	18.7	1.5
Marmalade, & Elderflower, Daylesford*	1 Cake/300g	1035	38.1	345	5.7	50.2	12.7	0
Mini Rolls, Cadbury*	1 Roll/26g	117	6.1	450	4.8	56.3	23.5	2.3
Mini Rolls, Chocolate, Average	**1 Cake/27g**	**122**	**6.2**	**453**	**4.8**	**56.9**	**22.9**	**0.9**
Mini Rolls, Jaffa, Average	**1 Cake/29g**	**111**	**3.3**	**382**	**3.5**	**67.2**	**11.2**	**1.4**
Mini Rolls, Jam, Average	**1 Cake/29g**	**115**	**4.5**	**395**	**3.8**	**59.8**	**15.6**	**1.8**
Pandoro, Italian	**1/8 Cake/87g**	**357**	**18.2**	**408**	**7.1**	**47.2**	**20.8**	**1.6**
Panettone, Average	**1 Portion/90g**	**345**	**15.3**	**383**	**8**	**52**	**17**	**0**
Panettone, Free From, Tesco*	1 Pack/100g	299	10.8	299	3.8	42.9	10.8	7.6
Patch the Panda, Tesco*	1 Serving/63g	261	9.3	414	2.2	67.6	14.8	1.1
Percy Pig, Cake Jar, M&S*	1 Jar/179g	736	24.3	411	1.9	69.9	13.6	0.7
Pineapple, Alba bakeries*	1 Serving/63g	258	9.4	410	1.5	66	15	2.6
Plum, & Ginger, Crumble, Graze*	1 Punnet/33g	119	9.1	361	6.2	35.1	27.6	3.3
Popdots, White, with Caramel, Popdots*	1 Popdot/21g	98	6.3	468	5.5	44	30	0
Pumpkin, Patch, Cadbury*	1 Cake/31g	149	7.1	480	5.3	61.7	22.9	2.4
Punchrulle Punsch Roll, Delicato*	1 Roll/40g	173	8	433	5	59	20	0
Raisin, Fruit Slab, Basics, Sainsbury's*	1 Slice/50g	183	6.2	367	5.3	57.3	12.5	1.9
Rasoberry, Almond, Crumb, Guilty*	1 Cake/104g	408	24.9	392	4.3	39.9	23.9	0.7

CAKE

	Measure INFO/WEIGHT	per Measure KCAL	FAT	Nutrition Values per 100g / 100ml KCAL	PROT	CARB	FAT	FIBRE
Raspberry Chocolate, Lava, Allplants*	1 Pot/93g	329	14.9	354	5.5	44	16	3.4
Raspberry, & Passion Fruit, Irresistible, Co-Op*	1/6 Cake/61g	242	10.4	396	3.2	56	17	1
Raspberry, Rockin' Raspberry, Slices, Mr Kipling*	1 Slice/21g	85	4.2	397	4.3	50.6	19.5	1
Raspberry, Slice, Dairy Milk, Cadbury*	1 Slice/29g	122	5.7	420	4.6	55	19.6	1.8
Raspberry, Sponge, Value, Tesco*	1 Slice/39g	130	4.6	334	3.4	53.4	11.9	0.7
Red Velvet, The Best, Morrisons*	1/6 Cake/63g	277	13.2	440	3.7	58.8	20.9	0.8
Red Velvet, TTD, Sainsbury's*	1 Slice/71g	302	16	428	2.8	52.8	22.7	0.8
Rock	**1 Sm Cake/40g**	**158**	**6.6**	**396**	**5.4**	**60.5**	**16.4**	**1.5**
Rose, Iced, Waitrose*	1 Serving/74g	303	10.4	409	2.2	68.3	14	0.5
Salted Caramel, Layered, Finest, Tesco*	1 Slice/75g	341	17	455	2.6	57.2	22.7	0.5
Shrek Birthday, Tesco*	1/16 Cake/72g	248	8.8	344	3.3	64	12.2	0.5
Slices, Dairy Milk, Cadbury*	1 Slice/29g	123	5.9	425	4.8	54.6	20.4	1.9
Snowballs, Sainsbury's*	1 Snowball/18g	80	4.1	445	2.5	55.6	23	3.6
Snowballs, Tesco*	1 Snowball/18g	79	4	432	2.5	55.8	22.1	5.4
Spelt, Ancient Grain, Morrisons*	1 Cake/8g	31	0.2	382	18.4	66.5	2.9	7.8
Sponge	**1 Slice/53g**	**243**	**13.9**	**459**	**6.4**	**52.4**	**26.3**	**0.9**
Sponge, Fatless	**1 Slice/53g**	**156**	**3.2**	**294**	**10.1**	**53**	**6.1**	**0.9**
Sponge, Jam Filled	**1 Slice/65g**	**196**	**3.2**	**302**	**4.2**	**64.2**	**4.9**	**1.8**
Sponge, with Butter Icing	**1 Slice/65g**	**318**	**19.9**	**490**	**4.5**	**52.4**	**30.6**	**0.6**
Sticky Toffee, Ginger Loaf, Bakedin*	1 Slice/65g	229	0.6	352	4.4	80	1	0
Sticky Toffee, Loaf, Mini, M&S*	1 Slice/74g	338	17.5	457	3.8	57.1	23.6	0.5
Stollen, Bites, Finest, Tesco*	1 Bite/17g	68	3.2	398	5	50.9	18.8	4.4
Stollen, Bites, Waitrose*	1 Bite/18g	71	3.1	395	4.6	54.5	17.1	2.2
Stollen, Chocolate & Rum, Finest, Tesco*	1/8 Cake/68g	262	9.5	381	5.3	57	13.8	3.9
Stollen, Christmas Range, Tesco*	1/8 Cake/62g	202	4.2	328	4.9	60.7	6.8	2.4
Stollen, Marzipan Butter, Mini, Favorina, Lidl*	1 Stollen/18g	81	4.2	452	9.5	49.2	23.3	0
Stollen, Slices, Average	**1 Slice/42g**	**160**	**6.3**	**381**	**5.5**	**55.8**	**15**	**3.1**
Strawberry, & Clotted Cream, Cornish, M&S*	1/6 Slice/68g	277	12.9	410	3.9	55.5	19.1	0.5
Strawberry, Sponge Roll, M&S*	1/6 Cake/49g	160	4.6	330	2.8	58	9.5	0.8
Sultana, & Cherry, M&S*	1 Slice/50g	180	5.8	360	0	59.5	11.5	2
Sultana, Fair Trade, Co-Op*	1/8 Cake/45g	155	4	345	5	60	9	1
Swiss Roll, Apricot, Co-Op*	1 Serving/44g	158	3.7	357	2.9	67	8.3	1
Swiss Roll, Average	**1oz/28g**	**77**	**1.2**	**276**	**7.2**	**55.5**	**4.4**	**0.8**
Swiss Roll, Cappuccino, Asda*	1 Slice/31g	112	3.8	356	3.7	58	12	1.3
Swiss Roll, Chocolate, Individual	**1 Roll/26g**	**88**	**2.9**	**337**	**4.3**	**58.1**	**11.3**	**0**
Swiss Roll, Lemon, Tesco*	1 Slice/32g	118	3	371	3.7	67.4	9.4	1
Swiss Roll, Raspberry, Average	**1 Slice/35g**	**107**	**1.2**	**305**	**3.8**	**64.8**	**3.5**	**0.6**
Swiss Roll, Sicilian Lemon, Deluxe, Lidl*	1 Slice/34g	124	3.3	365	2.6	66.5	9.7	1.5
Swiss Roll, Strawberry & Cream, Tesco*	1 Slice/32g	113	2.5	353	3.5	66.6	7.8	1.4
Tea Loaf, Rowan Hill Bakery, Lidl*	1 Slice/50g	135	0.4	270	3.8	63.3	0.9	3.4
Tiffin, Chocolate, Sainsbury's*	1 Cake/61g	184	11.6	301	2.7	29.8	19	1.3
Toffee, & Pecan Slices, M&S*	1 Slice/36g	160	8.5	445	4.7	54	23.7	1.3
Toffee, Apple, McVitie's*	1 Slice/26g	95	2.9	363	3.8	61.5	11	1.6
Toffee, Iced, Tesco*	1 Serving/35g	132	5.2	376	3.3	57.2	14.9	1.6
Toffee, Terror Whirls, Mr Kipling*	1 Whirl/28g	141	7.9	509	3.9	58.3	28.7	1.2
Vanilla, Mini, Vegan, OGGS*	1 Cake/20g	78	4	391	4.8	42.7	20.2	1
Vanilla, Slices, M&S*	1 Slice/103g	275	11.5	267	2.8	38.3	11.2	0.8
Vanilla, Sponge, Fresh Cream, Sainsbury's*	1 Slice/50g	152	5.1	304	7.5	45.6	10.2	0.4
Victoria Sandwich, Average	**1 Slice/68g**	**267**	**12.9**	**392**	**4.4**	**50.9**	**19**	**1**
Victoria Sponge, Free From, Finest, Tesco*	1 Slice/61g	238	11.8	393	2.9	51.3	19.4	0.8
Victoria Sponge, Lemon, Co-Op*	1 Slice/42g	151	8	360	4	44	19	0.7
Victoria Sponge, Mini, Bobby's*	1 Cake/35g	164	9.6	469	4	51.3	27.5	0.2
Victoria Sponge, Mini, Mr Kipling*	1 Cake/36g	152	6.9	420	3.9	58.5	19	0.8

	Measure INFO/WEIGHT	per Measure KCAL	FAT	Nutrition Values per 100g / 100ml KCAL	PROT	CARB	FAT	FIBRE
CAKE								
Victoria Sponge, Mini, Weight Watchers*	1 Cake/30g	103	2.5	343	5.7	57.2	8.3	8.4
Victoria Sponge, Vegan, OGGS*	1 Cake/46g	174	8	378	4	46.8	17.5	1
Viennese, Whirl, Average	*1 Cake/28g*	*131*	*6.9*	*467*	*4.1*	*56.7*	*24.8*	*1.1*
Viennese, Whirl, Chocolate, Mr Kipling*	1 Whirl/28g	134	7.8	484	4.6	53.1	28	2.1
Viennese, Whirl, Lemon, Mr Kipling*	1 Cake/28g	115	4.5	409	4.2	62.2	15.9	0.7
Walnut, Holly Lane, Aldi*	1/8 Cake/38g	154	6.8	404	6.2	54	18	1.4
Walnut, Lidl*	1 Serving/38g	150	6	395	6.3	56.4	15.7	1.3
Walnut, Sainsbury's*	1 Slice/40g	154	6	382	6	55.6	14.8	1.4
Walnut, Sandwich, Sainsbury's*	1/8 Cake/48g	182	8.3	379	5.4	53.8	17.3	1.3
Welsh, Average	*1oz/28g*	*121*	*5.5*	*431*	*5.6*	*61.8*	*19.6*	*1.5*
Winter Whirl, Mr Kipling*	1 Whirl/28g	145	8.1	515	3.6	59.4	28.7	2.4
Yorkshire Parkin, Bakers Delight*	1oz/28g	111	4.1	395	5.1	60.3	14.8	1.5
CAKE BAR								
Caramel, Tesco*	1 Cake/26g	103	4.9	395	5.1	50.8	19	8.2
Carrot, Tesco*	1 Bar/68g	239	12.6	351	4.7	41.4	18.5	2.4
Chocolate & Orange, Go Ahead, McVitie's*	1 Cake/33g	109	2	330	4.3	64.9	6	1
Chocolate Chip, Average	*1 Cake/28g*	*120*	*6*	*428*	*6.3*	*51.9*	*21.6*	*1.6*
Chocolate Dream, Go Ahead, McVitie's*	1 Bar/36g	141	4.8	391	4.6	63.2	13.4	0.9
Chocolate, Average	*1 Cake/28g*	*125*	*6.2*	*446*	*5.6*	*56.3*	*22.1*	*1.9*
Double Chocolate, Free From, Sainsbury's*	1 Cake/50g	196	7.9	391	4.2	58.2	15.7	1
Double Chocolate, Free From, Tesco*	1 Serving/45g	190	9.1	425	4.2	55.6	20.3	4.1
Flake, Cadbury*	1 Cake/25g	120	6.2	470	4.8	56.5	24.4	1.9
Galaxy, Salted Caramel, Festive, Galaxy, Mars*	1 Bar/26g	113	5.3	438	5.6	58.7	20.4	0
Golden Syrup, McVitie's*	1 Cake/33g	127	4.8	385	3.6	60.2	14.4	1.2
Jaffa Cakes, Spooky, McVitie's*	1 Bar/25g	96	3.5	390	3.2	62.1	14.2	2.7
Jaffa, McVitie's*	1 Bar/25g	96	3.5	395	3.1	62.9	14.5	2.5
Jamaica Ginger, McVitie's*	1 Cake/33g	128	4.9	388	3.5	60.2	14.7	1.2
Lemon, Fibre, WW*	1 Bar/18g	65	2.1	362	4	53	11.5	22.5
Milk Chocolate, Cadbury*	1 Bar/25g	110	5.6	445	4.9	53.8	22.8	2.9
Milky Way, McVitie's*	1 Cake/26g	124	6.2	476	5.1	58.5	23.6	1.2
Peanut, High Fibre, Squares, Tesco*	1 Square/24g	92	3.1	383	6	49	13	23
Vanilla, & Raspberry, Mini Rolls, Ms Mollys*	1 Roll/20g	74	2.2	368	4.7	62	11	1.2
CALLALOO								
Leaves, Raw, Unprepared	*1 Cup/28g*	*6*	*0.1*	*23*	*2.5*	*4*	*0.3*	*0*
CANNELLONI								
Beef, As Prepared, Waitrose*	1 Pack/360g	501	26.7	139	6.2	11.5	7.4	1
Beef, Meal for One, M&S*	1 Pack/400g	572	30.8	143	6.7	10.7	7.7	2.1
Bolognese, Pingo Doce*	1/4 Pack/250g	405	21.2	162	7.9	13	8.5	1.1
Mushroom, Italian, Sainsbury's*	1 Pack/450g	598	31	133	5.2	12.5	6.9	0.5
Ragu, Gino D'Acampo*	1 Pack/450g	680	40.5	151	6.4	11	9	1
Spinach, & Ricotta, Fresh, Ready Meal, Average	*1 Serving/300g*	*393*	*22*	*131*	*5*	*10.8*	*7.4*	*1.2*
Spinach, & Ricotta, Low Fat, COU, M&S*	1 Pack/400g	340	7.6	85	4.8	11.4	1.9	1.7
Spinach, & Ricotta, Ready Meal, Average	*1 Serving/300g*	*426*	*22*	*142*	*5.6*	*13.3*	*7.3*	*1.4*
Tubes, Dry, Average	*1oz/28g*	*101*	*1*	*361*	*12.5*	*69.1*	*3.6*	*1.2*
Vegetarian, Tesco*	1 Pack/400g	552	34.4	138	5.3	9.8	8.6	1.5
CAPERS								
in Vinegar, Average	*1 Tsp/5g*	*2*	*0*	*34*	*1.7*	*3*	*0.6*	*0*
CAPRI SUN								
Blackcurrant, No Added Sugar, Capri-Sun*	1 Pouch/200ml	10	0	5	0	0.9	0	0
Orange	*1 Pouch/200ml*	*90*	*0*	*45*	*0*	*11*	*0*	*0*
Orange, 100%, Juice	*1 Pouch/200ml*	*75*	*0*	*38*	*0.5*	*9.2*	*0*	*0.1*
CARAMAC								
Nestle*	1 Bar/31g	173	10.4	559	6.2	57.9	33.7	0

C

	Measure INFO/WEIGHT	per Measure KCAL	FAT	Nutrition Values per 100g / 100ml KCAL	PROT	CARB	FAT	FIBRE
CARBONARA								
Chicken, & Bacon, BFY, M&S*	1 Pack/375g	476	11.2	127	10.1	14.4	3	0.8
Chicken, & Bacon, Calorie Counted, Asda*	1 Pack/324g	311	4.9	96	7.5	12	1.5	1.5
Chicken, Mushroom, & Ham, Spaghetti, Asda*	1 Pack/700g	686	14	98	10	10	2	1.5
Chicken, Slimming World, Iceland*	1 Bowl/550g	556	3.8	101	10.2	12.5	0.7	2.2
Creamy, As Prepared, Pot Pasta*	1 Pot/260g	275	11.5	105	2.9	13	4.4	0.5
Mushroom, Vegan, Love Your Veg!, Sainsbury's*	1 Pack/400g	420	15.6	105	3.3	13.2	3.9	1.9
Mushroom, Vegan, Waitrose*	1 Pack/380g	437	19.4	115	2.3	14	5.1	2
Pasta, Snack Pot, Knorr*	1 Pot/71g	82	3.6	116	3.1	15	5	0
Pasta, Taste of Italy, Oven Baked, Iceland*	¼ Pack/281g	346	12.1	123	5.4	15.1	4.3	1.2
Penne, Taste of Italy, Tesco*	½ Pack/400g	604	18.5	151	7.9	19	4.6	0.9
Rigatoni, Allplants*	1 Serving/390g	534	23	137	6	14	5.9	2.3
Spaghetti, BGTY, Sainsbury's*	1 Pack/400g	392	7.6	98	5.9	14	1.9	0.7
Spaghetti, COU, M&S*	1 Pack/330g	346	7.2	105	6.1	15.7	2.2	0.8
Spaghetti, Extra Special, Asda*	1 Pack/350g	578	25.9	165	7.9	16	7.4	0.8
Spaghetti, Finest, Tesco*	1 Pack/370g	585	28.9	158	7.2	14.3	7.8	0.9
Spaghetti, Ready Meal, Average	**1 Pack/400g**	**524**	**21.5**	**131**	**5.9**	**14.4**	**5.4**	**1.1**
Tagliatelle, Ready Meal, Average	**1 Serving/400g**	**460**	**13.4**	**115**	**5.5**	**15.8**	**3.3**	**1**
CARDAMOM								
Black, Ground, Average	**1 Tsp/2g**	**6**	**0.1**	**311**	**10.8**	**68.5**	**6.7**	**28**
CAROB POWDER								
Average	**1 Tsp/2g**	**3**	**0**	**159**	**4.9**	**37**	**0.1**	**0**
CARP								
Fillet, Raw, Average	**1 Fillet/218g**	**244**	**10.2**	**112**	**17.5**	**0**	**4.7**	**0**
CARROT & SWEDE								
Diced, for Mashing, Average	**½ Pack/250g**	**58**	**0.7**	**23**	**0.6**	**4.7**	**0.3**	**1.9**
Mash, From Supermarket, Average	**1 Serving/150g**	**138**	**7.5**	**92**	**1.3**	**10.4**	**5**	**1.3**
Mash, Healthy Range, Average	**1 Serving/150g**	**98**	**4.2**	**66**	**1.3**	**8.6**	**2.8**	**2.1**
Mash, with Potato, British, Sainsbury's*	½ Pack/199g	143	3	72	1.3	12.2	1.5	2.1
CARROTS								
& Peas, Sainsbury's*	1 Serving/200g	100	1	50	3.3	8.3	0.5	3.8
& Houmous, On the Go, Sainsbury's*	1 Pack/100g	92	5.6	92	2.6	6.3	5.6	3
Baby, Canned, Average	**1 Can/195g**	**40**	**0.5**	**21**	**0.5**	**4.2**	**0.3**	**2.1**
Baby, Fresh, Average	**1 Serving/80g**	**28**	**0.1**	**35**	**0.6**	**8.2**	**0.1**	**2.9**
Batons, Fresh, Average	**½ Pack/150g**	**41**	**0.4**	**28**	**0.6**	**5.7**	**0.3**	**2.6**
Boiled, Average	**1oz/28g**	**6**	**0.1**	**22**	**0.6**	**4.4**	**0.4**	**2.3**
Canned, Average	**1oz/28g**	**6**	**0.1**	**20**	**0.5**	**4**	**0.2**	**1.9**
Chantenay, Wood Farm, Raw, Aldi*	1 Serving/80g	34	0.4	42	0.6	7.9	0.5	2.4
Raw, Average	**1 Med/61g**	**25**	**0.1**	**41**	**0.9**	**9.6**	**0.2**	**2.8**
Raw, Scrubbed, Average	**1 Serving/80g**	**24**	**0.4**	**30**	**0.7**	**6**	**0.5**	**2.4**
Sliced, Canned, Average	**1 Serving/180g**	**36**	**0.2**	**20**	**0.7**	**4.1**	**0.1**	**1.5**
Sliced, Fresh, Average	**1 Serving/60g**	**17**	**0.2**	**28**	**0.7**	**5.7**	**0.3**	**2**
Sticks, & Houmous, Reduced Fat, M&S*	1 Pack/130g	157	9.9	121	3.3	7.8	7.6	3.9
Whole, Raw, Peeled, Average	**1 Carrot/75g**	**21**	**0.2**	**29**	**0.6**	**6.4**	**0.3**	**2.2**
CASHEW NUTS								
& Jumbo Raisins, Iceland*	1 Serving/30g	123	5.4	411	8.5	52.2	18.1	2.5
BBQ, Co-Op*	1 Pack/40g	252	22	629	24	5.8	55	8.8
Cheese Flavour, Graze*	1 Pack/26g	140	10.8	540	15.3	35.7	41.5	0
Cracking Black Pepper, Graze*	1 Punnet/36g	216	16.6	600	19	26	46	4
Marmite, Graze*	1 Punnet/32g	185	14.1	577	21	21	44	4.2
Plain, Average	**½ Pack/25g**	**146**	**12.2**	**584**	**15.7**	**18.8**	**48.9**	**3.4**
Roasted & Salted, Average	**1 Serving/50g**	**306**	**25.6**	**612**	**18.8**	**19.6**	**51.1**	**3.1**
Wasabi, Roasted, Vitasia, Lidl*	1 Serving/30g	185	14.6	616	17.5	25.6	48.6	0

	Measure INFO/WEIGHT	per Measure KCAL	FAT	Nutrition Values per 100g / 100ml KCAL	PROT	CARB	FAT	FIBRE
CASSAVA								
Baked, Average	**1oz/28g**	**43**	**0.1**	**155**	**0.7**	**40.1**	**0.2**	**1.7**
Boiled in Unsalted Water, Average	**1oz/28g**	**36**	**0.1**	**130**	**0.5**	**33.5**	**0.2**	**1.4**
Gari, Average	**1oz/28g**	**100**	**0.1**	**358**	**1.3**	**92.9**	**0.5**	**0**
CASSEROLE								
Beef	**1 Serving/336g**	**490**	**23**	**146**	**16.3**	**4.6**	**6.8**	**0.6**
Beef, & Ale, Average	**1 Serving/300g**	**251**	**6.8**	**84**	**9.4**	**6.5**	**2.2**	**1.3**
Beef, & Red Wine, Average	**1 Serving/350g**	**290**	**7.3**	**83**	**7.2**	**8.2**	**2.1**	**1.5**
Beef, with Dumplings, Ready Meal, Average	**1 Serving/350g**	**464**	**21.1**	**132**	**9.5**	**10.1**	**6**	**1.5**
Beef, with Herb Potatoes, Ready Meal, Average	**1 Serving/475g**	**504**	**17.1**	**106**	**6.8**	**11.5**	**3.6**	**1.6**
Chicken, & Asparagus, HL, Tesco*	1 Serving/450g	342	10.3	76	6.3	8.3	2.3	0.5
Chicken, & Dumplings, Sainsbury's*	1 Serving/450g	612	24.8	136	9.1	12	5.5	1.2
Chicken, & Vegetable, Ready Meal, Healthy Range	**1 Serving/330g**	**265**	**11.9**	**80**	**4.7**	**7.6**	**3.6**	**1.1**
Chicken, & Bacon, Shake That Weight*	1 Pack/275g	256	12.4	93	11.2	2.4	4.5	1
Chicken, & Chorizo, Spanish Style, Oven Baked, Asda*	1 Pack/678g	1200	67.8	177	18	2.2	10	0.9
Chicken, & Dumpling, M&S*	1 Pack/450g	612	28.4	136	10.2	9	6.3	1.3
Chicken, & Dumplings, Lidl*	1 Pack/441g	538	22.5	122	8.3	10	5.1	1.1
Chicken, & Dumplings, Parsley Box*	1 Pack/270g	254	4.6	94	8.3	11	1.7	1
Chicken, & Mushroom, Slim Cook, Tesco*	1 Pack/467g	238	2.8	51	6.7	4.1	0.6	1.4
Chicken, Canned, M&S*	½ Can/200g	144	1.8	72	8.6	7	0.9	0.5
Chicken, Classic Kitchen, Canned, Tesco*	½ Can/198g	123	1.4	62	8.5	4.9	0.7	0.8
Chicken, Leek & Mushroom, Tesco*	1 Pack/350g	382	22	109	4.5	8.6	6.3	1
Pork, Apple, & Cider, Asda*	1 Pack/360g	443	15.5	123	14	6.3	4.3	1.1
Pork, Normandy Style, Finest, Tesco*	1 Pack/450g	405	21.6	90	7.6	4.1	4.8	2.3
Rabbit, Average	**1oz/28g**	**29**	**1.4**	**102**	**11.6**	**2.6**	**5.1**	**0.4**
Red Lentil, & Mixed Bean, Cook*	1 Serving/290g	218	4.4	75	4.5	14.2	1.5	6.6
Sausage, & Potato, M&S*	1 Serving/200g	190	11.8	95	3.3	7.5	5.9	0.9
Sausage, & Bean, Steam Fresh, Farmfoods*	1 Pack/350g	336	11.2	96	5	9.7	3.2	0
Sausage, CBY, Asda*	1 Pot/400g	240	15.2	60	3.6	1.9	3.8	2.1
Sausage, Lincolnshire, Easy to Cook, Waitrose*	1/3 Pack/240g	410	26.6	171	10.5	6.5	11.1	1.5
Sausage, Mini, 853, Oakhouse Foods*	1 Pack/270g	246	11.3	91	3.5	9.9	4.2	1.2
Steak, & Ale, Average	**1 Serving/275g**	**324**	**14.4**	**118**	**9**	**8.8**	**5.2**	**1**
Steak, & Dumplings, TTD, Sainsbury's*	1 Pack/382g	577	27.5	151	8.1	13.1	7.2	0.8
Steak, & Mushroom, Average	**1 Serving/275g**	**274**	**15.5**	**100**	**6.2**	**6**	**5.6**	**1**
Vegetable, Root, & Kale, Waitrose*	1 Pack/357g	343	15	96	1.9	11.6	4.2	2.1
Vegetables, Mix, Frozen, Boiled, Iceland*	1 Serving/80g	20	0.2	25	0.7	4.1	0.3	1.7
Veggie, Meal for One, M&S*	1 Pack/450g	436	16.6	97	2.2	12.5	3.7	2.3
CASSEROLE MIX								
Beef & Ale, Colman's*	1 Pack/45g	144	0.9	320	9.2	66.3	2	2.3
Beef, Recipe, Colman's*	1 Pack/42g	142	0.5	338	9.1	13.1	1.1	4
Beef, Recipe, Schwartz*	1 Pack/43g	123	0.9	287	7	56.6	2.1	6.6
Chicken Chasseur, Asda*	1 Pack/80g	273	0.8	341	9	74	1	1.4
Lamb, Authentic, Schwartz*	1 Pack/35g	116	1.2	332	7.7	68	3.3	1.3
Peppered Beef, Schwartz*	1 Pack/40g	129	2	323	7	62.9	4.9	7.3
Sausage, As Sold, Colman's*	1 Pack/39g	136	1	350	10	70	2.5	6
Sausage, Classic, Schwartz*	1 Pack/35g	96	0.9	275	12.4	50.1	2.7	14.9
CATFISH								
Cooked, Steamed, Weighed with Bone, Average	**1 Serving/100g**	**101**	**3.1**	**101**	**18.2**	**0**	**3.1**	**0.7**
CAULIFLOWER								
Bang Bang, Love Your Veg!, Sainsbury's*	½ Pack/62g	129	6	208	2.5	26.3	9.7	2.7
Bang Bang, Waitrose *	½ Pack/88g	214	14.9	243	2.2	19.4	16.9	2.4
Bites, Buffalo, Tesco*	½ Pack/115g	163	7.5	142	2.6	16.5	6.5	3.7
Boiled, Average	**1 Serving/80g**	**22**	**0.7**	**28**	**2.9**	**2.1**	**0.9**	**1.6**
Florets, Turmeric, Marinated, M&S*	½ Pack/85g	54	2.7	63	0.9	6.8	3.2	1.8

INFO/WEIGHT	Measure	per Measure		Nutrition Values per 100g / 100ml				
		KCAL	FAT	KCAL	PROT	CARB	FAT	FIBRE

CAULIFLOWER

Grills, Tesco*	1 Grill/96g	236	13.7	246	5.6	22	14.3	3.2
Popcorn, with Spicy Buffalo Dip, Plant Kitchen, M&S*	½ Pack/113g	213	12.7	189	2.3	18.7	11.3	1.6
Raw, Average	**1 Serving/80g**	**25**	**0.7**	**31**	**3.2**	**2.7**	**0.8**	**1.6**
Spiced, Roasted, Tesco*	½ Pack/70g	59	4.4	84	2.2	3.9	6.2	1.8
Spiced, Roasting, Sainsbury's*	1 Serving/107g	62	3	58	2.3	4.8	2.8	2.2
Steamed, Average	**1 Serving/100g**	**28**	**0.9**	**28**	**2.9**	**2.1**	**0.9**	**1.6**
Tikka Spiced, Twisted, & Bhaji, Wicked Kitchen, Tesco*	1 Pot/409g	429	13.9	105	6	9.5	3.4	6

CAULIFLOWER CHEESE

& Broccoli, Average	**1 Serving/200g**	**127**	**6.4**	**64**	**3.8**	**4.6**	**3.2**	**2**
A Bit on the Side, Oven Baked, Asda*	½ Pack/184g	167	10.9	91	4.6	4.3	5.9	1
Average	**1 Meal/400g**	**362**	**23.3**	**90**	**4.5**	**4.6**	**5.8**	**1.3**
Made with Semi-Skimmed Milk	**1oz/28g**	**28**	**1.8**	**100**	**6**	**5.2**	**6.4**	**1.3**
Made with Skimmed Milk	**1oz/28g**	**27**	**1.7**	**97**	**6**	**5.2**	**6**	**1.3**
Made with Whole Milk	**1oz/28g**	**29**	**1.9**	**105**	**6**	**5.2**	**6.9**	**1.3**
Truffled, M&S*	½ Pack/225g	245	17.1	109	5.8	3.7	7.6	1.4
with Wexford Mature Cheddar, M&S*	½ Pack/225g	263	17.6	117	6.7	4.3	7.8	1.3

CAVIAR

Average	**1oz/28g**	**25**	**1.3**	**89**	**11.6**	**0.5**	**4.6**	**0**

CELERIAC

Boiled in Salted Water, Average	**1oz/28g**	**5**	**0.1**	**18**	**0.9**	**1.9**	**0.4**	**3.2**
Raw, Average	**1 Serving/80g**	**17**	**0.3**	**21**	**1**	**1.9**	**0.4**	**3.2**
Remoulade, Waitrose *	1 Serving/110g	335	32.6	304	1.2	7.3	29.6	1.6

CELERY

Boiled in Salted Water	**1 Serving/50g**	**4**	**0.2**	**8**	**0.5**	**0.8**	**0.3**	**1.2**
Raw, Trimmed, Average	**1 Stalk/40g**	**3**	**0.1**	**7**	**0.5**	**0.9**	**0.2**	**1.1**

CHAMPAGNE

Average	**1 Glass/125ml**	**95**	**0**	**76**	**0.3**	**1.4**	**0**	**0**

CHANNA MASALA

Waitrose*	1 Pack/300g	300	18.3	100	3.7	7.4	6.1	7.9

CHAPATIS

Made with Fat	**1 Chapati/60g**	**197**	**7.7**	**328**	**8.1**	**48.3**	**12.8**	**0**
Made without Fat	**1 Chapati/55g**	**111**	**0.6**	**202**	**7.3**	**43.7**	**1**	**0**
Wholemeal, Patak's*	1 Chapati/42g	130	4	310	11.2	44.9	9.5	9

CHARD

Average	**1 Serving/80g**	**15**	**0.2**	**19**	**1.4**	**3.3**	**0.2**	**0.8**
Silverbeet, Fresh, Steamed	**1 Serving/100g**	**15**	**0**	**15**	**1.9**	**1.3**	**0**	**3.3**
Swiss, Boiled in Unsalted Water	**1oz/28g**	**6**	**0**	**20**	**1.9**	**4.1**	**0.1**	**2.1**
Swiss, Raw	**1oz/28g**	**5**	**0.1**	**17**	**1.7**	**3.4**	**0.2**	**1.5**

CHEDDARS

Baked, Mini, Blue Cheese, Jacob's*	1 Pack/25g	132	7.9	530	8.8	50.3	31.8	2.5
Baked, Mini, Red Leicester, Jacobs*	1 Pack/25g	132	7.9	528	8.8	50.4	31.6	2.4
Cheese, Baked, Mini, Original, Jacobs*	1 Bag/25g	129	7.2	516	9.2	53.2	28.8	2.8
Mini, Average	**1 Bag/26g**	**134**	**7.8**	**516**	**11.2**	**50.8**	**29.9**	**2.4**
Mini, BBQ, Jacob's*	1 Pack/25g	131	7.6	525	9.3	51.6	30.3	2.6
Mini, Lime & Chilli, Jacobs*	1 Bag/25g	129	7.2	516	9.1	53.3	28.7	2.8
Mini, Ploughmans Cheshire Cheese, Jacob's*	1 Pack/25g	129	7.2	516	9.1	53.2	28.7	2.8
Wee, Strathon Blue Cheese, Jacob's*	1 Pack/25g	129	7.2	516	9.1	53.3	28.7	2.7

CHEESE

Babybel, Cheddar Variety, Mini, Fromageries Bel*	1 Babybel/20g	75	6.2	375	24	0	31	0
Babybel, Cheddar, Light, Mini, Fromageries Bel*	1 Babybel/20g	59	4.4	296	24	0.5	22	0
Babybel, Emmental, Fromageries Bel*	1 Babybel/20g	63	4.9	316	23	1	24.5	0
Babybel, Light, Mini, Fromageries Bel*	1 Babybel/20g	42	2.4	208	25	0	12	0
Babybel, Original, Mini, Fromageries Bel*	1 Babybel/20g	61	4.8	304	22	0.1	24	0

CHEESE

INFO/WEIGHT	Measure	per Measure		Nutrition Values per 100g / 100ml				
		KCAL	FAT	KCAL	PROT	CARB	FAT	FIBRE
Beechwood, Smoked, Slices, Tesco*	1 Slice/25g	75	6	299	20.7	0	24	0
Blue, Castello, Soft, Castello*	¼ Pack/37g	162	15.6	432	14	0.5	41.5	0
Blue, Rich & Creamy, St Agur*	1 Serving/30g	108	9.9	361	16	0.5	33	0
Blue, Shropshire, The Delicatessen, Tesco*	1 Serving/30g	123	10.5	410	23.7	0.1	35	0
Brie, Average	*1 Serving/25g*	*74*	*6*	*296*	*19.7*	*0.3*	*24*	*0*
Brie, Breaded, Bites, Frozen, Tesco*	1 Bite/17g	54	3.4	319	8.6	24.2	20.2	2.8
Brie, Reduced Fat, Average	*1 Serving/50g*	*99*	*5.7*	*198*	*23*	*0.8*	*11.4*	*0*
Burrata, 1, Waitrose*	1 Serving/30g	67	5.6	222	13.4	0.2	18.6	0
Burrata, M&S*	1 Serving/30g	79	7.3	262	10	1.1	24.2	0.1
Caerphilly, Average	*1 Serving/50g*	*187*	*15.6*	*374*	*23*	*0.1*	*31.3*	*0*
Cambazola, Tesco*	1 Serving/30g	128	12.3	425	13.5	0.5	41	0
Camembert, Average	*1 Serving/50g*	*141*	*11.1*	*283*	*20.5*	*0.1*	*22.2*	*0*
Camembert, Breaded, Average	*1 Serving/90g*	*307*	*20.9*	*342*	*16.6*	*14.2*	*23.2*	*0.4*
Cantal, French, Sainsbury's*	1 Serving/30g	106	8.7	353	23	0.1	29	0
Cheddar, & Mozzarella, Grated, M&S*	1 Serving/30g	101	8.3	337	22	0.1	27.6	0.1
Cheddar, & Mozzarella, Grated, Morrisons*	1 Serving/30g	108	8.4	360	25.4	2.8	28	0
Cheddar, Average	*1 Serving/30g*	*123*	*10.3*	*410*	*25*	*0.1*	*34.4*	*0*
Cheddar, Canadian, Average	*1 Serving/30g*	*123*	*10.3*	*409*	*25*	*0.1*	*34.3*	*0*
Cheddar, Davidstow, Mature, Average	*1 Serving/28g*	*115*	*9.6*	*410*	*25*	*0.1*	*34.4*	*0*
Cheddar, Extra Mature, Average	*1 Serving/30g*	*123*	*10.3*	*410*	*25.1*	*0.1*	*34.4*	*0*
Cheddar, Grated, Average	*1 Serving/50g*	*206*	*17.2*	*413*	*24.4*	*1.5*	*34.3*	*0*
Cheddar, Mature, Average	*1 Serving/30g*	*123*	*10.3*	*410*	*25*	*0.1*	*34.4*	*0*
Cheddar, Mature, Grated, Average	*1 Serving/28g*	*113*	*9.3*	*404*	*24.7*	*1.6*	*33.2*	*0*
Cheddar, Mature, Lactose Free, Cathedral City*	1 Serving/30g	125	10.5	416	25.4	0.1	34.9	0
Cheddar, Mature, Lighter, Sandwich Slices, Cathedral City*	1 Slice/25g	83	6	331	28.6	0.1	24	0
Cheddar, Mature, Reduced Fat, Average	*1 Serving/25g*	*68*	*4.2*	*271*	*30*	*0.1*	*16.7*	*0*
Cheddar, Medium, Average	*1 Serving/30g*	*123*	*10.4*	*411*	*24.9*	*0.2*	*34.5*	*0*
Cheddar, Mild, Average	*1 Serving/30g*	*123*	*10.3*	*409*	*25*	*0.1*	*34.3*	*0*
Cheddar, Reduced Fat, Average	*1 Serving/30g*	*76*	*4.2*	*255*	*32.2*	*0.1*	*14*	*0*
Cheddar, Smoked, Average	*1 Serving/30g*	*123*	*10.3*	*411*	*25.2*	*0.1*	*34.4*	*0*
Cheddar, with Mixed Peppers, Sliced, Mexicana *	1 Slice/20g	79	6.3	396	23.7	4.7	31.3	0
Cheshire	*1oz/28g*	*106*	*8.8*	*379*	*24*	*0.1*	*31.4*	*0*
Cottage, Low Fat, 2% Fat, Natural, Average	*1 Serving/75g*	*68*	*1.4*	*90*	*13.7*	*3.6*	*1.9*	*0*
Cottage, Onion & Chive, Fat Free, Sainsbury's*	1 Serving/30g	22	0.2	75	11.8	6.4	0.5	0.5
Cottage, Organic, M&S*	1 Serving/30g	34	1.8	112	9.6	4.7	6.1	0.5
Cottage, Pineapple, Fat Free, Emporium, Aldi*	1 Serving/30g	25	0.2	82	12	7.6	0.5	0.5
Cottage, Pineapple, Low Fat, Morrisons*	1 Serving/30g	27	0.5	91	8	10.5	1.7	0.9
Cottage, Plain, Average	*1 Tbsp/20g*	*19*	*0.7*	*93*	*12*	*3.3*	*3.5*	*0.1*
Cottage, Plain, Reduced Fat, Average	*100g*	*85*	*1.9*	*85*	*12.3*	*4.4*	*1.9*	*0.1*
Cottage, Virtually Fat Free, Average	*1 Tbsp/20g*	*16*	*0.2*	*79*	*13*	*4.5*	*1*	*0*
Cottage, Whole Milk, Natural, Average	*1 Serving/75g*	*77*	*3.4*	*103*	*12.5*	*2.7*	*4.5*	*0*
Cottage, with Onion & Chive, GFY, Asda*	¼ Tub/75g	50	1	66	9.3	3.8	1.4	0.5
Cottage, with Onion, & Chive, Fat Free, Asda*	1 Serving/30g	17	0.2	58	9.3	4.6	0.5	0.5
Cottage, with Onion, & Chives, Low Fat, Co-Op*	1 Serving/30g	22	0.4	74	10	4.4	1.5	0.5
Cottage, with Pineapple, Fat Free, Tesco*	1 Serving/30g	22	0.1	73	8.8	8.6	0.4	0
Cream, Average	*1 Portion/30g*	*132*	*14.2*	*439*	*3.1*	*0*	*47.4*	*0*
Cream, Garlic & Herbs, Boursin*	1 Serving/30g	119	11.7	396	8.5	3	39	0
Cream, Marmite, M&S*	1 Spread/15g	42	3.4	283	8.1	10.9	22.8	0.7
Cream, Reduced Fat, Average	*1 Serving/20g*	*23*	*1.1*	*117*	*13*	*4*	*5.3*	*0.1*
Cream, Soft, Whipped, M&S*	1 Serving/30g	79	6.8	263	4.4	4.6	22.5	0.1
Dairylea, Light, Slices, Kraft*	1 Slice/25g	44	1.9	177	16	8.2	7.6	1.6
Danish Blue, Average	*1 Serving/30g*	*106*	*8.7*	*352*	*20.8*	*0*	*29.1*	*0*
Double Gloucester, Average	*1 Serving/30g*	*121*	*10.2*	*404*	*24.5*	*0.1*	*34*	*0*

	Measure INFO/WEIGHT	per Measure KCAL	FAT	Nutrition Values per 100g / 100ml KCAL	PROT	CARB	FAT	FIBRE
CHEESE								
Doux De Montagne, Average	**1 Serving/25g**	**88**	**7.1**	**352**	**22.9**	**1.5**	**28.3**	**0**
Edam, Average	**1 Serving/10g**	**33**	**2.5**	**326**	**25.3**	**0**	**24.9**	**0**
Edam, Slices, Average	**1 Slice/30g**	**96**	**7.2**	**320**	**25**	**0.4**	**24.1**	**0**
Emmental, Average	**1 Serving/10g**	**37**	**2.8**	**368**	**28.4**	**0**	**28.4**	**0**
Feta, Average	**1 Serving/30g**	**79**	**6.4**	**262**	**16.3**	**1**	**21.5**	**0**
Feta, Lactose Free, Greco*	1 Serving/30g	81	6.8	270	16.4	0.4	22.5	0
Fontina, Average	**1 Serving/28g**	**109**	**9**	**389**	**25**	**0**	**32.1**	**0**
for Pizza, Grated	**1 Serving/50g**	**163**	**12.2**	**326**	**25**	**1.6**	**24.4**	**0**
Four, Mix, Grated, Sainsbury's*	1 Serving/30g	112	8.8	373	22.2	5.3	29.2	0.5
Goats, Average	**1 Tsp/10g**	**26**	**2.1**	**262**	**13.8**	**3.8**	**21.2**	**0**
Goats, Blue, Beacon, Finest, Tesco*	1 Serving/30g	100	8.6	333	19	0.1	28.5	0
Goats, French, Mild, Average	**1 Serving/30g**	**49**	**3.5**	**163**	**11.2**	**3**	**11.8**	**0**
Goats, Premium, Average	**1 Serving/30g**	**98**	**7.8**	**327**	**20.5**	**0.6**	**26.1**	**0**
Goats, Soft, Average	**1 Serving/30g**	**79**	**6.3**	**262**	**16.7**	**1.8**	**20.8**	**0.5**
Gorgonzola, Average	**1 Serving/30g**	**100**	**8.1**	**334**	**20**	**0**	**27**	**0**
Gouda, Average	**1 Serving/30g**	**113**	**9.4**	**376**	**24**	**0**	**31.5**	**0**
Gouda, Light, Slices, Milbona, Lidl*	1 Slice/17g	42	2.7	250	23	3.5	16	0.5
Gouda, Popped, Crunchy, Cheesies*	1 Serving/20g	119	9.4	593	40	0	47	0
Grana Padano, Italian Cheese, Waitrose*	1 Serving/14g	54	4	388	33	0	28.4	0
Grana Padano, Reserva, Deluxe, Lidl*	1 Serving/10g	39	2.8	388	33	0	28.4	0
Greek Style, Salad, Light, Essential, Waitrose*	1 Serving/30g	57	3.6	190	20	0.6	12	0
Gruyere	**1oz/28g**	**115**	**9.3**	**409**	**27.2**	**0**	**33.3**	**0**
Halloumi, Average	**1 Serving/80g**	**253**	**19.7**	**316**	**20.8**	**1.6**	**24.7**	**0**
Halloumi, Light Average	**1 Serving/100g**	**245**	**15.3**	**245**	**24.7**	**1.7**	**15.3**	**0**
Halloumi, Pesto, The Grill, M&S*	½ Pack/113g	318	23.6	283	19.8	3.2	21	1.1
Healthy Range, Average	**1 Slice/20g**	**39**	**2.1**	**197**	**20.6**	**5.2**	**10.4**	**0**
Healthy Range, Slices, Average	**1 Slice/25g**	**45**	**2.2**	**180**	**19.5**	**5.4**	**9**	**0**
Iberico, & Serrano Ham, Rollitos, Tesco*	2 Rollitos/25g	72	4.9	289	26.3	1.9	19.5	0.9
Iberico, TTD, Sainsbury's*	1 Serving/30g	117	9.6	390	23.8	1	32.1	1
Italian Style, Grated, Morrisons*	1 Tsp/5g	24	1.6	479	47	2.9	31.1	0
Jarlsberg, Slices, Average	**1 Slice/15g**	**54**	**4**	**360**	**27**	**0**	**27**	**0**
Kvarg, Coconut, Lindahls, Nestle*	1 Serving/30g	18	0.1	60	11	3.4	0.2	0
Kvarg, Raspberry, Lindahls, Nestle*	1 Pot/150g	82	0.3	55	10	3.4	0.2	0
Kvarg, Stracciatella, Lindahls, Nestle*	1 Pot/150g	94	0.9	63	11	3.4	0.6	0
Kvarg, Stracciatella, Lindahls, Nestle*	1 Pot/150g	88	0.9	59	10	3.4	0.6	0
Kvarg, White Chocolate, Lindahls, Nestle*	1 Serving/50g	32	0.1	63	11	3.4	0.2	0
Kvarg, White Chocolate, Nestle*	1 Pot/151g	95	0.3	63	11	3.4	0.2	0
Lactose Free, Arla*	1 Serving/30g	103	8.1	344	25.3	1	27	0
Lancashire	**1oz/28g**	**104**	**8.7**	**373**	**23.3**	**0.1**	**31**	**0**
Leerdammer, Lighter, Sliced, M&S*	1 Slice/23g	62	3.9	271	29.5	0.1	17	0
Leerdammer, Original, Sliced, Leerdammer*	1 Slice/20g	71	5.5	356	27	0.1	27.5	0
Light, with Apple, & Grapes, Babybel*	1 Pack/75g	73	2.6	97	7.1	9.9	3.5	0.9
Manchego	**1 Serving/70g**	**340**	**30.8**	**485**	**22.2**	**0.1**	**44**	**0**
Mascarpone, Average	**1 Serving/30g**	**131**	**13.1**	**437**	**5.6**	**4.1**	**43.6**	**0**
Mature, Half Fat, Average	**1 Serving/25g**	**66**	**3.9**	**265**	**29.9**	**0.4**	**15.6**	**0.1**
Mild, Reduced Fat, Grated, Average	**1 Serving/30g**	**70**	**3.3**	**235**	**31.5**	**2.2**	**11.1**	**0**
Mimolette, Carrefour *	1 Slice/30g	118	8.6	393	35.7	0	28.7	0
Mozzarella & Cheese, Mix, Tesco*	1 Serving/30g	99	7.6	331	23.8	2.3	25.2	0
Mozzarella, Average	**½ Ball/63g**	**172**	**12.9**	**275**	**21.2**	**1.2**	**20.6**	**0**
Mozzarella, Reduced Fat, Average	**½ Ball/63g**	**115**	**6.4**	**184**	**21.2**	**1**	**10.2**	**0**
Mozzarella, Sticks, Breaded, Moreish, M&S*	1 Stick/20g	61	3.6	306	14.1	21.6	18	0.8
Mozzarella, Sticks, Free From, Tesco*	2 Sticks/25g	75	4.5	301	15.3	18.6	18	1.7
Mozzarella, Sticks, Melting, Crispy Golden Crumb, M&S*	½ Pack/75g	269	18.1	359	18.2	16.4	24.1	1.8

	Measure INFO/WEIGHT	per Measure KCAL	FAT	Nutrition Values per 100g / 100ml KCAL	PROT	CARB	FAT	FIBRE
CHEESE								
Norvegia, Sliced Light, Tine*	1 Slice/10g	27	1.6	272	32	0	16	0
Ossau-Iraty, Average	*1 Serving/30g*	*120*	*10.2*	*400*	*22.3*	*0.2*	*34*	*0*
Parmesan, Average	*1 Tbsp/10g*	*42*	*2.8*	*422*	*40*	*2*	*28.5*	*0*
Parmigiano Reggiano, Grated, Castelli*	1 Serving/10g	40	3	402	32	0	30	0
Pecorino, Romano, D.O.P., Sainsbury's*	1 Pack/10g	40	3.3	401	26	0	33	0
Protein, Eatlean*	1 Serving/30g	51	0.9	169	37	0.5	3	0.5
Provolone, Salami & Cheese Selection, The Deli, Aldi*	2 Slices/5g	16	1.2	318	22	2.2	24	0.9
Provolone, Ultra Thin, Slices, Sargento*	3 Slices/32g	110	9	344	25	3.1	28.1	0
Quark, Average	*1 Serving/20g*	*13*	*0*	*66*	*11.9*	*4*	*0.2*	*0*
Reblochon	*1 Serving/30g*	*95*	*8*	*318*	*19.7*	*0*	*26.6*	*0*
Red Leicester, Average	*1 Serving/30g*	*120*	*10.1*	*400*	*23.8*	*0.1*	*33.7*	*0*
Red Leicester, Reduced Fat, Average	*1 Serving/30g*	*78*	*4.6*	*261*	*30.2*	*0.1*	*15.4*	*0*
Ricotta, Average	*1 Serving/50g*	*67*	*4.8*	*134*	*9.3*	*2.9*	*9.5*	*0*
Roquefort, Average	*1oz/28g*	*105*	*9.2*	*375*	*19.7*	*0*	*32.9*	*0*
Roule, French, Sainsbury's*	1 Serving/30g	96	9.2	321	8.5	3	30.5	0
Sage Derby	*1oz/28g*	*113*	*9.5*	*402*	*24.2*	*0.1*	*33.9*	*0*
Salad, Greek Style, Simply, Lidl*	1 Serving/30g	78	6	259	18.2	0.5	20	0
Scamorza, M&S*	1 Serving/30g	93	7.3	310	22	0.5	24.4	0
Shropshire, Blue, Average	*1 Serving/50g*	*196*	*17.1*	*391*	*21*	*0*	*34.2*	*0*
Slices, Average	*1 Slice/23g*	*82*	*6.6*	*358*	*24*	*0.8*	*28.6*	*0*
Soft, Extra Light, Average	*1 Serving/20g*	*25*	*1.2*	*125*	*14.3*	*3.6*	*5.9*	*0.1*
Soft, Full Fat, Average	*1 Serving/50g*	*156*	*15.2*	*312*	*8.2*	*1.7*	*30.3*	*0*
Soft, Garlic, & Herb, Lighter, Sainsbury's*	1 Serving/30g	49	3.3	163	9.6	6.4	11	0
Soft, Garlic, & Herbs, Philadelphia*	1 Serving/30g	43	3	142	7.2	5.3	10	0.4
Soft, Herbs, Lightest, Philadelphia*	1 Serving/30g	26	0.8	87	11	4.9	2.5	0.4
Soft, Light & Herbs, with Breadsticks, Philadelphia*	1 Pack/41g	86	3.7	212	8.8	23	9	2.3
Soft, Light, Average	*1 Tbsp/30g*	*54*	*3.9*	*179*	*12.1*	*3.2*	*13.1*	*0*
Soft, Light, with Breadsticks, Philadelphia*	1 Serving/43g	103	4.7	242	7.9	26	11	1.2
Soft, Med Fat, Average	*1 Serving/30g*	*62*	*5.4*	*207*	*8.4*	*3*	*17.9*	*0*
Soft, Med Fat, with Chives, Philadelphia*	1 Serving/30g	44	3	146	7.4	5.1	10	0.6
Soft, Mediterranean Herbs, Full Fat, Philadelphia*	1 Serving/30g	64	5.7	213	5	4.1	19	0.3
Soft, Salmon & Dill, Light, Med Fat, Philadelphia*	1 Serving/20g	28	2	142	7.3	5.1	10	0.5
Soft, Sweet Chilli, Light, Med Fat, Philadelphia*	1 Serving/20g	30	2	148	6.8	7.3	10	0.5
Soft, White, Lactofree, Arla*	1 Serving/30g	59	5	197	8.6	3	16.5	0
Soft, with Chocolate, Milka, Philadelphia*	1 Serving/30g	86	3.9	285	6.3	34	13	1.7
Soft, with Garlic & Herbs, Full Fat, Deli, Boursin*	1 Serving/28g	84	8.3	299	3.5	5	29.5	0
Soft, with Garlic & Herb, Whipped, Milbona, Lidl*	1 Serving/30g	73	6.9	244	6	3	23	0
St Felicien, Du Dauphine, Finest, Tesco*	1 Serving/30g	80	7.2	266	12	0.5	24	0
Stilton, Average	*1 Serving/30g*	*123*	*10.6*	*410*	*22.4*	*0.1*	*35.5*	*0*
Stilton, Blue, Average	*1 Serving/30g*	*124*	*10.7*	*412*	*22.8*	*0.1*	*35.7*	*0*
Stilton, White, Average	*1oz/28g*	*101*	*8.8*	*362*	*19.9*	*0.1*	*31.3*	*0*
Taleggio D.o.p., Finest, Tesco*	1 Serving/30g	89	7.5	297	18	0	25	0
Twisted, Cheestrings*	1 String/20g	61	4.5	305	23	2.5	22.5	0
Wensleydale, Average	*1 Serving/25g*	*92*	*7.8*	*369*	*22.4*	*0.1*	*31*	*0*
Wensleydale, with Cranberries, Sainsbury's*	1 Serving/50g	180	13.9	359	20.7	6.4	27.8	0
CHEESE ALTERNATIVE								
Block, Original, Vegan, Waitrose*	1 Serving/30g	89	7	297	0.5	18.4	23.4	5.2
Blue Cheese, Free From, Asda*	1 Serving/30g	98	8.1	327	0.5	19	27	4.7
Camembert Style, Mouse's Favourite*	1 Serving/30g	130	10.4	432	14.7	15.2	34.7	0
Cheddar Style, Coconut Based, Sainsbury's*	1 Serving/30g	91	6.9	304	0.7	21.7	22.9	4
Cheddar, Coconut Base, Free From, Morrisons*	1 Serving/30g	97	7	323	1.7	26	23.2	1.5
Cheddar, Dairy Free, Koko*	1 Serving/30g	95	7.9	318	0.7	22.5	26.3	1.5
Cheddar, Mature, Free From, Asda*	1 Serving/30g	86	6.3	285	0.5	21	21	5.1

	Measure INFO/WEIGHT	per Measure KCAL	FAT	Nutrition Values per 100g / 100ml KCAL	PROT	CARB	FAT	FIBRE
CHEESE ALTERNATIVE								
Cheddar, Mature, Sliced, Free From, Asda*	1 Slice/20g	57	4.2	285	0.5	21	21	5.1
Cheddar, Slices, V Taste, Morrisons*	1 Slice/20g	59	4.8	297	0.3	19.8	24	0.1
Cheddar, V Taste, Morrisons*	1 Serving/30g	97	7	323	1.7	26	23.2	1.5
Coconut Oil, Jalapeno, & Chilli, Free From, Tesco*	1 Serving/30g	88	6.2	294	0.5	23.3	20.8	5.7
Edam, Slices, V Taste, Morrisons*	1 Slice/22g	67	5.2	305	1.1	21.4	23.8	0.5
Epic, Mature Cheddar Flavour, Violife*	1 Serving/30g	91	7.2	303	1.3	20	24	0
Greek Style, Cubes, in Mediterranean Herbs, Cauldron*	1 Serving/30g	44	3.3	147	10	1.7	11	1.9
Greek Style, V Taste, Morrisons*	1 Serving/30g	90	7.2	301	0.1	20.1	24.1	1.6
Greek, White, Block, Violife*	1 Serving/30g	92	8.7	305	0	11	29	0
Halloumi, Free From, Tesco*	1 Serving/30g	86	5.4	285	0.4	27.9	18.1	4.5
Hard, Italian Style, Free From, Tesco*	1 Serving/30g	92	5.9	306	1.2	29.5	19.6	3.6
Mature Style, Cheddar, Slices, Plant Kitchen, M&S*	4 Slices/50g	145	11.1	290	0.4	19.7	22.2	5
Mozzarella, Grated, Free From, Asda*	1 Serving/30g	94	7.8	313	0.5	18	26	3.2
Mozzarella, Grated, Free From, Tesco*	1 Serving/30g	94	7.8	313	0	18.3	26	3.2
Mozzarella, Slices, Dairy Free	**1 Slice/19g**	**80**	**6**	**420**	**10.5**	**10.5**	**31.5**	**0**
Natural, Almond, Spread, Nush Foods*	1 Serving/30g	64	5.4	215	7	5.9	18	0
Sheese, Spread, Sweet Chilli, Bute Island Foods Ltd*	1 Serving/30g	84	7.6	280	6.4	5.7	25.2	2.1
Smoked, Gouda Style, Slices, Follow Your Heart*	1 Slice/20g	57	4.6	285	0	20	23	0
Smoky, Vegan, Applewood*	1 Serving/30g	92	7.4	305	1.5	19.4	24.6	0.5
Soft, Coconut Based, Garlic & Herb, Sainsbury's*	1 Serving/30g	83	7.9	277	6.6	2.2	26.3	2.5
Soft, Cream Cheese, Koko*	1 Serving/30g	60	5.6	199	0.4	7.6	18.7	0.9
Soft, Garlic, & Herb, Free From, Tesco*	1 Serving/30g	75	7.5	250	0.3	5.4	25	1.2
Soft, V Taste, Morrisons*	1 Serving/30g	73	7.3	244	0.2	5.8	24.3	0.7
Treenut, Organic, Nutcrafter Creamery*	1 Serving/30g	163	16.3	543	27.7	7.4	54.3	6.7
Vegetarian, Average	**1 Serving/30g**	**110**	**8.4**	**368**	**28.2**	**0**	**28.1**	**0**
CHEESE PUFFS								
Average	**1 Bag/25g**	**129**	**7.4**	**517**	**7.8**	**54.8**	**29.5**	**1.5**
CHEESE SPREAD								
Average	**1 Serving/30g**	**76**	**6.4**	**254**	**9.4**	**5.9**	**21.4**	**0.1**
Cheese & Ham, Primula*	1 Serving/20g	43	2.9	214	12.8	7.8	14.6	0
Chickpea, & Herb, The Laughing Cow, Fromageries Bel*	1 Triangle/17g	36	2.6	216	11.5	7	15.5	0
with Chives, Primula*	1 Serving/30g	65	4.5	217	12.5	8.2	15	4.5
with Prawn, Primula*	1 Squeeze/25g	48	3.6	190	12.5	3.3	14.4	3.6
CHEESE STRAWS								
Homemade or Bakery, Average	**1 Straw/41g**	**173**	**12.6**	**422**	**12**	**24.2**	**30.7**	**0.7**
CHEESE TRIANGLES								
Average	**1 Triangle/14g**	**33**	**2.2**	**238**	**10.3**	**14.2**	**15.6**	**0.2**
Dairylea, Light, Kraft*	1 Triangle/16g	26	1.4	167	15	6.3	9	0.4
Light, Extra, The Laughing Cow, Fromageries Bel*	1 Triangle/18g	19	0.4	108	17	5.5	2	0
Light, with Blue Cheese, The Laughing Cow*	1 Triangle/16g	24	1.4	151	13	5.5	8.5	0
Lighter, Valley Spire, Lidl*	1 Triangle/17g	24	1.3	141	12	6	7.5	0.5
Reduced Fat, Average	**1 Triangle/18g**	**27**	**1.2**	**154**	**15.4**	**7**	**7**	**0**
CHEESE TWISTS								
Parmesan & Garlic, Sainsbury's*	1 Twist/8g	38	2	493	13.8	51	25.3	2.8
Parmesan, All Butter, TTD, Sainsbury's*	1 Serving/8g	38	2	487	13.8	51	25.3	2.8
Parmigiano Reggiano, & Garlic, The Best, Morrisons*	1 Twist/8g	40	2.1	505	14.3	60.6	26.6	3.1
Pre Packed, Average	**1 Twist/8g**	**41**	**2.2**	**515**	**13.7**	**47.9**	**27.7**	**2.3**
with Gruyere Cheese, M&S*	1 Twist/9g	46	2.6	515	12.1	50.5	28.7	3.3
CHEESECAKE								
Average	**1 Slice/115g**	**490**	**40.8**	**426**	**3.7**	**24.6**	**35.5**	**0.4**
Berry, Autumn, Waitrose*	1 Slice/92g	316	20.3	343	4.4	31.5	22.1	2
Berry, Red, Waitrose*	1 Slice/101g	350	22.5	346	4.6	31.3	22.2	1.4
Blackcurrant, Average	**1 Serving/90g**	**237**	**11.9**	**263**	**3.6**	**32.3**	**13.2**	**2.4**

CHEESECAKE

INFO/WEIGHT	Measure	per Measure		Nutrition Values per 100g / 100ml				
		KCAL	FAT	KCAL	PROT	CARB	FAT	FIBRE
Blackcurrant, Healthy Range, Average	**1 Serving/90g**	**182**	**4.7**	**203**	**4.7**	**33.6**	**5.3**	**2.1**
Blueberry, & Vanilla, TTD, Sainsbury's*	1 Serving/95g	353	24.8	372	5.4	28.9	26.1	2.1
Caramel, Salted, Frozen, Tesco*	1 Serving/75g	241	10.6	321	6.5	41.5	14.1	0.9
Caramel, Salted, Mini, Iceland*	1 Cake/22g	85	4.7	380	3.2	44.5	20.9	0.6
Caramel, Swirl, Cadbury*	1 Slice/91g	373	23.5	410	6	40.1	25.8	0
Caramel, Thorntons*	1 Pack/90g	481	27.9	534	6.7	56	31	0
Cherry, Healthy Range, Average	**1 Serving/90g**	**172**	**3**	**191**	**3.7**	**36.4**	**3.3**	**1.1**
Chocolate, & Honeycomb, Slice, Sainsbury's*	1 Slice/98g	333	20.3	340	3.7	33.7	20.7	2.4
Chocolate, & Irish Cream Liqueur, Tesco*	1 Serving/93g	385	28	414	5	30.7	30.1	0.8
Chocolate, & Vanilla, Reduced Fat, M&S*	1 Serving/114g	319	13.7	280	7	37.9	12	1.5
Chocolate, & Vanilla, Tesco*	1 Serving/90g	330	19.4	365	5.2	37.1	21.5	1.6
Chocolate, & Vanilla, Free From, Gu*	1 Pot/82g	320	21.3	390	2.9	36.4	26	1.5
Chocolate, Average	**1 Serving/75g**	**265**	**15.7**	**353**	**5.7**	**35.6**	**20.9**	**1.9**
Chocolate, Triple, Slices, M&S*	1 Slice/92g	377	21.5	410	4.3	44.2	23.4	1.7
Citrus, Good Choice, Mini, Iceland*	1 Cake/111g	198	4.7	178	3.5	31.6	4.2	0.4
Cookies & Cream, The Best, Morrisons*	1 Slice/90g	368	24.7	409	5	35.1	27.4	1
Fruit, Average	**1 Serving/75g**	**207**	**10.9**	**276**	**5.3**	**32.3**	**14.5**	**1.6**
Irish Cream, McVitie's*	¼ Slice/190g	616	36.9	324	4.4	33	19.4	0.4
Key Lime, Slices, Finest, Tesco*	1 Slice/90g	314	17.1	349	4.1	39.6	19	1.4
Lemon, & Blueberry, Light, Gu*	1 Pud/77g	150	8.5	195	2.6	21	11	0.5
Lemon, Average	**1 Serving/90g**	**307**	**19.5**	**341**	**4.1**	**33**	**21.6**	**1.8**
Lemon, Free From, Gu*	1 Ramekin/92g	327	19.3	355	1.8	40	21	0.6
Lemon, Meringue, Tesco*	1 Slice/94g	352	25	375	3.8	30.1	26.6	0.3
Lemon, Mousse, M&S*	1 Pot/125g	390	20.6	312	2.6	37.3	16.5	1.7
Madagascan Vanilla, Slices, Finest, Tesco*	1 Slice/90g	367	23.4	408	5.4	37.9	26	0.3
Mandarin, Morrisons*	1 Serving/135g	335	16.9	248	3.8	32.2	12.5	0.8
Millionaires, Pot, Tesco*	1 Pot/100g	274	14	274	3.8	32.9	14	0.6
New York, Baked, Waitrose*	1/12 Cake/83g	317	22.6	380	5.1	28.3	27.1	1.2
New York, Mini, Iceland*	1 Cake/22g	86	5.1	385	3.6	40.7	23	0.5
Oreo, Mondelez*	1 Serving/80g	283	13.6	354	4.5	45	17	1.2
Raspberry, & Vanilla, Slices, M&S*	1 Slice/100g	300	17.5	300	4.4	30.4	17.5	1.7
Raspberry, & Blackcurrant, Light, Gu*	1 Pud/77g	151	7.7	196	2.6	23	10	0.8
Raspberry, Rapture, Slices, Tesco*	1 Slice/110g	341	20.4	310	4.2	30.8	18.5	1.8
Raspberry, Ripple, Sainsbury's*	1 Portion/95g	355	21.8	373	4.5	37	22.9	0.9
Salted Caramel, Free From, Gu*	1 Ramekin/83g	287	16.6	346	1.6	39	20	0.5
Salted Caramel, Gu*	1 Pot/92g	333	21.3	362	3.7	34.5	23.1	0.7
Salted Caramel, Vegan, Gu*	1 Ramekin/83g	287	16.6	346	1.6	39	20	0.5
Strawberry, & Cream, Finest, Tesco*	1 Serving/104g	325	22.4	312	4.3	25.3	21.5	0.5
Strawberry, & Rhubarb, Slice, M&S*	1 Pack/100g	377	23.8	377	4.3	35.7	23.8	1.3
Strawberry, & Vanilla, Light, Gu*	1 Pud/77g	153	9.2	199	4.3	19	12	0.5
Strawberry, Devonshire, McVitie's*	1/6 Cake/66g	192	10.7	291	4.4	31.8	16.2	3.6
Strawberry, Finest, Tesco*	1 Slice/113g	383	25.1	339	4.8	30.1	22.2	0.9
Strawberry, Free From, Tesco*	1 Serving/77g	228	12.1	296	1.6	36.4	15.7	1.3
Strawberry, Frozen, Sainsbury's*	1/6 Cake/84g	277	14.2	332	4.3	40.4	17	2.3
Strawberry, Individual, Tesco*	1 Pot/100g	231	7.7	231	2.5	37.4	7.7	1
Strawberry, Slice, Asda*	1 Slice/95g	326	19.9	344	4.2	34	21	0.9
Strawberry, Wedges, Plant Kitchen, M&S*	1 Wedge/90g	273	14.6	303	1.6	37.1	16.2	1.2
Tiramisu, Allplants*	1 Serving/95g	338	24.7	356	9	20	26	3.9
Toffee, & Pecan, Wedge, Sainsbury's*	1 Serving/75g	296	21.8	395	5.4	28.1	29	3.1
Vanilla	**1 Serving/100g**	**395**	**26.2**	**395**	**5.3**	**42.8**	**26.2**	**1.1**
Vanilla Berry, Allplants*	1 Serving/95g	299	20	315	7.5	22	21	3.5
Vanilla, Creamy, New York, Slices, Tesco*	1 Slice/90g	314	21.4	349	5.1	28.3	23.7	0.8
Vanilla, New York, Slices, M&S*	1 Slice/105g	361	23.6	344	4.5	30.1	22.5	1.5

	Measure INFO/WEIGHT	per Measure KCAL	FAT	Nutrition Values per 100g / 100ml KCAL	PROT	CARB	FAT	FIBRE
CHEESECAKE								
White Chocolate, & Mixed Berry, Finest, Tesco*	1 Serving/70g	246	13.7	353	4.5	38.9	19.6	1.3
Zillionaires, Gu*	1 Pot/92g	362	22	396	3.6	42	24	1.3
CHERRIES								
Black in Syrup, Average	**1 Serving/242g**	**160**	**0**	**66**	**0.6**	**16**	**0**	**0.7**
Black, Fresh, Average	**1 Serving/80g**	**41**	**0.1**	**51**	**0.9**	**11.5**	**0.1**	**1.6**
Dark, Sweet, Morrisons*	1 Serving/80g	42	0.1	52	0.9	11.5	0.1	0.9
Glace, Average	**1oz/28g**	**79**	**0**	**280**	**0.4**	**71.2**	**0.2**	**1.1**
Picota, Average	**1 Serving/80g**	**42**	**0.1**	**52**	**0.9**	**11.4**	**0.1**	**1.2**
Raw, Average	**1oz/28g**	**14**	**0**	**49**	**0.9**	**11.2**	**0.1**	**1.4**
Stewed without Sugar, Average	**1oz/28g**	**12**	**0**	**42**	**0.8**	**10.1**	**0.1**	**0.8**
with Stone, Sweet & Juicy, Keelings*	1 Cherry/11g	7	0	63	1	16	0	2
CHESTNUTS								
Average	**1 Serving/100g**	**174**	**2.3**	**174**	**2.9**	**31**	**2.3**	**8.9**
Roasted, Peeled, Average	**1 Nut/10g**	**17**	**0.3**	**170**	**2**	**36.6**	**2.7**	**4.1**
CHEWING GUM								
Airwaves, Sugar Free, Wrigleys*	1 Pack/15g	23	0	155	0	62	0	0
Doublemint, Wrigleys*	1 Stick/3g	10	0	370	0	74.1	0	0
Extra, Cool Breeze, Wrigleys*	1 Piece/2g	3	0	153	0	64	0	0
Extra, Peppermint, Sugar Free, Wrigleys*	1 Piece/2g	3	0	155	0	39	0	0
Peppermint, Sugar Free, Active, Aldi*	2 Pieces/3g	4	0	146	0	61	0	0
Spearmint, Extra, Wrigleys*	1 Piece/1g	1	0	143	0	64.3	0	0
Spearmint, Wrigleys*	1 Piece/3g	9	0	295	0	73	0	0
CHICK PEAS								
Canned, Drained, Average	**1 Can/240g**	**276**	**6**	**115**	**7.4**	**15.2**	**2.5**	**4.6**
Charming, Annabel*	½ Pack/100g	134	1.5	134	8.3	19.9	1.5	4
Curried, Canned, East End*	½ Can/200g	258	11	129	5.7	11.9	5.5	4.4
Curried, Incredible, Jamie Oliver*	½ Pack/125g	169	5.4	135	6.1	15.6	4.3	4.5
Curried, Worldwide Foods, Aldi*	½ Pack/125g	172	4.8	138	7.3	15	3.8	6.5
Dried, Average	**1 Serving/100g**	**319**	**5.4**	**319**	**21.7**	**47.4**	**5.4**	**8**
Dried, Boiled, Average	**1 Serving/75g**	**85**	**1.7**	**114**	**7.3**	**16.4**	**2.2**	**2.6**
in Salted Water, Canned, Average	**1 Can/179g**	**204**	**5.2**	**114**	**7.2**	**14.9**	**2.9**	**4.1**
in Water, Canned, Average	**1 Can/250g**	**282**	**6.6**	**113**	**7.2**	**15.3**	**2.6**	**4.8**
Roasted, Curry, Cheeky P's*	1 Pack/50g	215	5	430	22	63	10	15
Roasted, Dark Choc, Brave*	1 Serving/30g	129	5.4	430	14	47	18	13
CHICKEN								
& Stuffing, Slices, Iceland*	1 Pack/70g	88	2.7	125	20.7	1.4	3.9	0.9
BBQ, Calorie Counted, Asda*	1 Pack/350g	287	3.5	82	6.1	11	1	2.7
Bites, Slow Roasted, Mini, Fridge Raiders, Mattessons*	1 Mini Bag/23g	43	2.2	190	21	3.2	10	0
Bites, Southern Style, Mini, Fridge Raiders, Mattessons*	1 Pack/23g	37	2.1	166	17	4.2	9.2	0
Bites, Tikka, Average	**1 Serving/50g**	**96**	**5.3**	**193**	**20.7**	**3.8**	**10.5**	**1.9**
Breast, Baked, Hoisin, Sticky, Hello Fresh*	1 Serving/456g	634	9.1	139	12	18	2	0
Breast, BBQ, Chunky, Pieces, Moy Park*	1 Pack/200g	254	3.6	127	20.2	7	1.8	0.2
Breast, BBQ, Sweet & Smokey, Slices, Sainsbury's*	1 Serving/89g	116	1.5	130	22.6	4.9	1.7	0.5
Breast, Butter Roast, Sliced, Extra Special, Asda*	2 Slices/79g	90	0.9	114	26	0.5	1.1	1.5
Breast, Chargrilled, Premium, Average	**1 Piece/10g**	**13**	**0.3**	**134**	**25.9**	**0.6**	**2.6**	**0.3**
Breast, Chargrilled, Sliced, Average	**1 Slice/19g**	**24**	**0.5**	**124**	**24.4**	**0.5**	**2.7**	**0.4**
Breast, Chunks, Tikka Marinated, Waitrose*	½ Pack/150g	226	7.2	151	23.1	3.7	4.8	0.5
Breast, Coronation, Slices, Sainsbury's*	½ Pack/80g	107	1.6	134	20.7	8	2	0.5
Breast, Diced, Average	**1 Serving/188g**	**242**	**4.4**	**129**	**26.9**	**0.1**	**2.4**	**0.1**
Breast, Fillet, Mini, Southern Fried, British, Waitrose*	½ Pack/131g	278	10.1	212	18	17.1	7.7	1
Breast, Fillets, Bacon, & Brie, Morrisons*	1 Fillet/183g	306	14.1	167	21.7	2.2	7.7	1.1
Breast, Fillets, Breaded, Average	**1 Fillet/112g**	**246**	**11.6**	**220**	**17.6**	**14**	**10.4**	**1.3**
Breast, Fillets, Cajun, Average	**1 Fillet/93g**	**124**	**2.6**	**134**	**23.6**	**3.5**	**2.8**	**0.3**

	Measure INFO/WEIGHT	per Measure KCAL	FAT	Nutrition Values per 100g / 100ml KCAL	PROT	CARB	FAT	FIBRE

CHICKEN

	Measure INFO/WEIGHT	KCAL	FAT	KCAL	PROT	CARB	FAT	FIBRE
Breast, Fillets, Chargrilled, Average	**1 Serving/100g**	**120**	**1.1**	**120**	**27.3**	**0.3**	**1.1**	**0.3**
Breast, Fillets, Coronation, Oven Baked, Asda*	½ Pack/141g	194	4.8	138	22	4.2	3.4	0.9
Breast, Fillets, Fajita Cooked, Mini, Tesco*	½ Pack/85g	100	0.8	118	19.5	7.5	1	0.4
Breast, Fillets, Garlic & Herb, Mini, Tesco*	½ Pack/86g	96	0.9	112	22.8	3.2	1	0
Breast, Fillets, Ginger, Coriander, & Lime, Waitrose*	½ Pack/103g	163	5.3	158	27.7	0.5	5.1	0.5
Breast, Fillets, Hunters, Morrisons*	½ Pack/172g	274	8.6	159	22.7	5.6	5	0.5
Breast, Fillets, Korma Style, Average	**1 Serving/100g**	**132**	**2.8**	**132**	**27.4**	**0.8**	**2.8**	**0.6**
Breast, Fillets, Mini, Raw, Average	**1oz/28g**	**34**	**0.4**	**121**	**26.9**	**0.2**	**1.5**	**0.1**
Breast, Fillets, Organic, Average	**1 Serving/150g**	**153**	**1.1**	**102**	**24**	**0**	**0.8**	**0**
Breast, Fillets, Skinless & Boneless, Raw, Average	**1 Breast/100g**	**129**	**2**	**129**	**27.7**	**0**	**2**	**0**
Breast, Grilled, Average	**1 Breast/130g**	**174**	**2.8**	**134**	**29**	**0.1**	**2.2**	**0**
Breast, Joint, Rotisserie, with Sticky Marinade, M&S*	½ Pack/233g	319	13	137	20.5	1	5.6	0.1
Breast, Meat & Skin, Raw, Average	**1 Serving/145g**	**249**	**13.4**	**172**	**20.8**	**0**	**9.2**	**0**
Breast, Meat & Skin, Weighed with Bone, Raw, Average	**1oz/28g**	**39**	**2.1**	**138**	**16.7**	**0**	**7.4**	**0**
Breast, Meat Only, Fried	**1 Serving/50g**	**68**	**1.7**	**137**	**24.4**	**0.4**	**3.4**	**0**
Breast, Pieces, Tikka, Average	**1 Serving/100g**	**154**	**3.4**	**154**	**28.2**	**2.8**	**3.4**	**0.4**
Breast, Piri Piri, Fillets, Cooked as per Instructions, Tesco*	1 Breast/141g	251	9.4	178	28.8	0.5	6.7	0.1
Breast, Piri Piri, Pieces, Cooked, Ready to Eat, Tesco*	1 Serving/90g	117	2.2	130	24	2.8	2.4	0.6
Breast, Roast, Sliced, From Supermarket, Average	**1 Slice/13g**	**17**	**0.4**	**139**	**25**	**1.8**	**3.5**	**0.2**
Breast, Roast, without Skin, Average	**1oz/28g**	**41**	**1.3**	**146**	**24.8**	**1**	**4.6**	**0.2**
Breast, Skewers, Mini, Asda*	1 Skewer/12g	17	0.3	140	24	5.5	2.5	0
Breast, Smoked, Sliced, Average	**1 Slice/20g**	**22**	**0.5**	**110**	**20.7**	**0.9**	**2.6**	**0.1**
Breast, Steaks, Cajun Style, Oven Cooked, Morrisons*	1 Steak/90g	138	2.7	153	28.1	2.8	3	0.9
Breast, Steaks, Garlic, & Herb, Tesco*	1 Steak/142g	201	4	142	26.6	2.7	2.8	0
Breast, Strips, Raw, Average	**1 Serving/280g**	**358**	**5.7**	**128**	**27.1**	**0.4**	**2**	**0.3**
Breast, Stuffed, M&S*	½ Pack/53g	78	2.5	147	23.5	2.3	4.7	0.5
Breast, Tandoori Style, Average	**1 Serving/180g**	**237**	**6.8**	**132**	**22.3**	**2.3**	**3.8**	**1**
Breast, Tikka, Sliced, Average	**1oz/28g**	**34**	**0.5**	**120**	**24.9**	**2**	**1.7**	**0.6**
Chargrills, BBQ, Asda*	1 Chargrill/85g	146	7.2	172	20	3.4	8.5	0.7
Chargrills, BBQ, Sweet & Sticky, Birds Eye*	1 Chargrill/87g	153	8	175	16	7.1	9.2	0.5
Chunks, No Chic'n, Plant Kitchen, M&S*	½ Pack/90g	86	0.6	95	18.9	1	0.7	6.4
Coconut, Bowl, COU, M&S*	1 Pack/300g	333	11.4	111	8.2	10.4	3.8	1.2
Coronation, Morrisons*	1 Serving/100g	176	9.3	176	11.9	11.1	9.3	0.5
Coronation, Sliced, M&S*	1 Serving/60g	96	2	160	26.7	4.9	3.3	1.7
Crown, Lemon, Salt & Pepper, Roast in the Bag, Tesco*	¼ Pack/131g	212	6.5	162	27.5	1.4	5	0.5
Diet Cola, Microwaved, Slimming World, Iceland*	1 Pack/550g	358	3.8	65	9.8	4.4	0.7	0.9
Dippers, Chicken Free, Vegan, Green Cuisine, Birds Eye*	5 Dippers/90g	257	15.3	286	8.8	23	17	3.1
Dippers, Crispy, Average	**5 Dippers/93g**	**231**	**14.3**	**249**	**13.2**	**14.4**	**15.4**	**0.6**
Drumsticks, BBQ Flavour, Average	**1 Serving/200g**	**348**	**16**	**174**	**22.6**	**3.1**	**8**	**0.4**
Drumsticks, Breaded, Fried, Average	**1oz/28g**	**66**	**3.9**	**237**	**18.7**	**9.4**	**13.9**	**0.6**
Drumsticks, Chinese Style, Average	**1 Serving/100g**	**178**	**8.1**	**178**	**22.6**	**3.6**	**8.1**	**0.7**
Drumsticks, Meat & Skin, Weighed with Bone, Raw	**1 Serving/133g**	**188**	**11**	**141**	**15.7**	**0.1**	**8.3**	**0**
Drumsticks, Meat Only, no Skin, Boneless, Raw	**1 Serving/100g**	**106**	**3.3**	**106**	**19.2**	**0**	**3.3**	**0**
Drumsticks, Meat Only, Weighed with Bone, Raw	**1 Serving/122g**	**159**	**9.3**	**130**	**14.4**	**0.1**	**7.6**	**0**
Drumsticks, Meat Only, Weighed with Bone, Roast	**1 Serving/100g**	**116**	**5.5**	**116**	**16**	**0.3**	**5.5**	**0.1**
Drumsticks, with Skin, Average	**1 Piece/125g**	**268**	**16.6**	**215**	**22.1**	**1.8**	**13.3**	**0.3**
Escalope, Breaded, Average	**1 Escalope/128g**	**361**	**21.6**	**282**	**13.4**	**19.1**	**16.9**	**0.7**
Escalope, Plain, Breast, Average	**1 Serving/100g**	**110**	**2.2**	**110**	**22.3**	**0.7**	**2.2**	**0.5**
Fillet, Chunks, Salt & Pepper, Oven Baked, Iceland*	5 Chunks/100g	224	7.8	224	17	20.6	7.8	1.4
Fillets, Battered, Average	**1 Fillet/90g**	**199**	**10.4**	**221**	**16.1**	**13.3**	**11.5**	**0.5**
Fillets, Breaded, Average	**1 Piece/98g**	**214**	**10.5**	**219**	**14.2**	**15.9**	**10.7**	**1.9**
Fillets, Breaded, Salt & Pepper, Mini, Waitrose*	½ Pack/144g	317	13	220	17	17.4	9	0.9
Fillets, Cajun, Ashfield Farm, Aldi*	1 Fillet/122g	161	3.3	132	26	0.7	2.7	0.5

CHICKEN

INFO/WEIGHT	Measure	per Measure KCAL	FAT	Nutrition Values per 100g / 100ml KCAL	PROT	CARB	FAT	FIBRE
Fillets, Cajun, Mini, Waitrose*	1 Serving/88g	126	3.3	143	25.8	1.4	3.8	0.5
Fillets, Chinese Style, Average	*1oz/28g*	*37*	*0.5*	*132*	*24.4*	*4.6*	*1.8*	*0.5*
Fillets, Honey & Mustard, Average	*1 Serving/100g*	*138*	*3.7*	*138*	*18.4*	*7.5*	*3.7*	*0.8*
Fillets, Hot & Spicy, Average	*1oz/28g*	*58*	*3.1*	*206*	*16.4*	*10.5*	*11*	*1.1*
Fillets, in Tempura Batter, Crispy, Birds Eye*	1 Fillet/89g	229	12.5	257	13	19	14	1.4
Fillets, Red Thai, Mini, Average	*1oz/28g*	*36*	*0.6*	*128*	*21.7*	*5.4*	*2*	*0.6*
Fillets, Southern Fried, Meat Only, Average	*1 Piece/100g*	*222*	*12*	*222*	*16.4*	*12.2*	*12*	*1.1*
Fillets, Tandoori Style, Mini, Average	*1 Serving/100g*	*128*	*2*	*128*	*24.7*	*2.6*	*2*	*0.4*
Fillets, Tikka, Average	*1 Serving/100g*	*141*	*5*	*141*	*22.4*	*1.7*	*5*	*1.1*
Fillets, Tikka, Mini, Average	*1oz/28g*	*35*	*0.6*	*124*	*25.1*	*1.3*	*2.2*	*1.2*
Fingers, Average	*1 Serving/75g*	*188*	*9.9*	*250*	*13.7*	*18.8*	*13.2*	*1.2*
Flatties, Coronation, M&S*	½ Pack/183g	322	15.6	176	19	5.4	8.5	1
Goujons, Breaded, Average	*1 Serving/114g*	*293*	*17.1*	*258*	*15.8*	*15.2*	*15*	*1*
Goujons, Breast, Fresh, Average	*1oz/28g*	*36*	*0.5*	*127*	*28*	*0*	*1.6*	*0*
Goujons, British, GF, Made Without Wheat, M&S*	¼ Pack/105g	236	13.4	225	11.2	15.6	12.8	1.5
Goujons, Southern Fried, Co-Op*	1 Pack/245g	657	44.1	268	13	13	18	2
Grill, BBQ, with Mango & Coconut, Ocado*	2 Pieces/159g	240	5.1	151	29	2.1	3.2	0.5
Joint, Butter Basted, with Salt & Pepper, M&S*	1 Serving/100g	156	5.5	156	20.4	6.2	5.5	0.1
Katsu, Crispy, Pieces, Finest, Tesco*	1 Serving/144g	323	15	224	15.9	16.1	10.4	1.2
Leg or Thigh, Hot & Spicy, Average	*1oz/28g*	*50*	*3*	*179*	*19.4*	*1*	*10.8*	*0.4*
Leg Portion, Roast, weighed with Bone, without Skin	*1 Portion/114g*	*175*	*11*	*153*	*30.9*	*0*	*9.6*	*0*
Leg Portion, Roasted Dry, with Skin, without Bone	*1 Portion/120g*	*188*	*11.8*	*156*	*16.7*	*0.2*	*9.8*	*0.2*
Leg, Meat Only, Cooked, Stewed, Average	*1 Serving/60g*	*111*	*4.8*	*185*	*26*	*0*	*8*	*0*
Leg, Meat Only, Raw, Average	*1oz/28g*	*34*	*1.1*	*120*	*20.1*	*0*	*3.8*	*0*
Leg, Meat Only, Raw, Weighed with Skin & Bone	*1oz/28g*	*21*	*0.7*	*76*	*12.8*	*0*	*2.4*	*0*
Leg, Meat Only, Stewed with Bone & Skin, Average	*1oz/28g*	*31*	*1.4*	*111*	*15.8*	*0*	*4.8*	*0*
Leg, with Skin, Raw, Average	*1 Serving/250g*	*430*	*26*	*172*	*19.1*	*0*	*10.4*	*0*
Leg, with Skin, Roasted, Weighed with Bone, Average	*1oz/28g*	*47*	*3.3*	*166*	*15.3*	*0.1*	*11.6*	*0*
Light Meat, Roasted	*1oz/28g*	*43*	*1*	*153*	*30.2*	*0*	*3.6*	*0*
Meat & Skin Portions, Deep Fried, Average	*1oz/28g*	*73*	*4.7*	*259*	*26.9*	*0*	*16.8*	*0*
Meat & Skin, Roasted, Average	*1oz/28g*	*60*	*3.9*	*216*	*22.6*	*0*	*14*	*0*
Meat Free, Nuggets, Tex-Mex, Oven Cooked, Quorn*	4 Nuggets/80g	191	8.8	239	11	21	11	6.5
Meat Free, Southern Fried, Green Cuisine, Birds Eye*	3 Strips/83g	227	14.1	274	9.6	19	17	3.1
Meat Free, Southern Fried, Grills, Green Cuisine, Birds Eye*	1 Grill/90g	286	15.3	318	12	26	17	6.3
Meat Free, Style Pieces, Plant Pioneers, Sainsbury's*	5 Pieces/48g	122	8	254	17.1	5.8	16.6	6.6
Meat Free, with Patatas Bravas, & Aioli, Gousto*	1 Serving/554g	554	25.5	100	4.4	10.7	4.6	2.9
Meat, Roasted, Average	*1oz/28g*	*47*	*1.9*	*167*	*25*	*0*	*6.6*	*0*
Mexican Chilli, Sliced, Eat Well, M&S*	1 Pack/130g	169	3.4	130	25.9	0.8	2.6	0.5
Mexican, Tray Bake, Tesco*	½ Pack/179g	315	14	176	16.7	9.1	7.8	1.2
Mince, Average	*1oz/28g*	*39*	*1.7*	*140*	*20.9*	*0.1*	*6*	*0.2*
Nuggets, Battered, Average	*1 Nugget/20g*	*50*	*2.9*	*251*	*13.5*	*16.9*	*14.4*	*0.9*
Nuggets, Breaded, Average	*1 Nugget/14g*	*37*	*2*	*263*	*14.8*	*19.8*	*13.8*	*1.9*
Nuggets, Frozen, M&S*	1 Serving/150g	346	17.7	231	14.4	16.3	11.8	1.2
Nuggets, Popcorn, Sklavenitis*	½ Pack/200g	472	20	236	16.8	19.7	10	0
Pieces, Boneless, Breaded, Fried, From Restaurant	*1 Piece/17g*	*51*	*3.3*	*301*	*17*	*14.4*	*19.4*	*0*
Pieces, Roast, Lemon & Herb, M&S*	½ Pack/64g	90	1.9	140	24.3	3.8	2.9	0.5
Plant-Based, This Isn't, This*	½ Pack/85g	142	4.1	167	23	3.3	4.8	7.5
Poppers, Ready to Eat, Tesco*	1 Popper/10g	27	1.6	273	11.5	19.9	16.2	0.7
Pulled, Chargrilled, Ready to Eat, Morrisons*	½ Pack/91g	107	1	118	26.2	0.7	1.1	0.3
Rashers, Oak Park*	1 Rasher/25g	25	0.6	100	19.6	0.5	2.2	0.5
Roll, Breast, Average	*1 Slice/10g*	*17*	*1*	*167*	*16.1*	*3.2*	*10*	*0.2*
Schnitzel, As Prepared, Easy to Cook, Waitrose*	½ Pack/99g	168	5.4	170	27	2.4	5.5	1.3
Shawarma, King Kebab, Waitrose*	1/6 Pack/113g	248	13.8	220	24.1	2.7	12.2	1.3

CHICKEN

Measure INFO/WEIGHT		per Measure		Nutrition Values per 100g / 100ml				
		KCAL	FAT	KCAL	PROT	CARB	FAT	FIBRE
Shawarma, Slow Cooked, Oven Cooked, Asda*	½ Pack/208g	356	18.3	171	21	1	8.8	1.7
Shredded, Crispy, Breaded, Oven Baked, Iceland*	¼ Pack/109g	291	15	267	16.4	18.8	13.8	0.9
Skewers, BBQ, Iceland*	1 Serving/76g	105	1.5	138	27.7	1.9	2	0.7
Skewers, BBQ, Morrisons*	1 Skewer/10g	21	0.9	209	20	10.7	9.2	1.9
Skewers, Salt & Chilli, Iceland*	2 Skewers/140g	183	2.7	131	26.1	1.8	1.9	1
Skewers, Satay, Tesco*	1 Skewer/15g	27	1.3	177	19.5	5	8.6	0.8
Skin, Dry, Roasted or Grilled, Average	**1 Serving/100g**	**501**	**46.1**	**501**	**21.5**	**0**	**46.1**	**0**
Skin, Moist, Roasted or Grilled, Average	**1 Serving/100g**	**452**	**42.6**	**452**	**17**	**0**	**42.6**	**0**
Sliced, Cooked, Average	**1 Slice/15g**	**18**	**0.4**	**118**	**22.4**	**1.6**	**2.4**	**0.1**
Slices, Hot & Spicy, Ready to Eat, Morrisons*	½ Pack/90g	118	1.8	131	24.7	3	2	1.4
Slices, Lemon, Garlic, & Herb, Morrisons*	¼ Pack/50g	66	0.6	132	25.1	4.4	1.3	1
Steaks, Average	**1 Serving/100g**	**205**	**9.4**	**205**	**21.1**	**9**	**9.4**	**0.7**
Steaks, Breaded, Birchwood, Lidl*	1 Steak/100g	252	18	252	16.9	17.5	18	1.6
Steaks, Breaded, Frozen, Morrisons*	1 Steak/95g	220	11.5	232	15.6	14.5	12.1	1.1
Strips, Mexican, Sliced, M&S*	½ Pack/70g	77	0.4	110	24.3	2.3	0.6	0.5
Style Pieces, What The Cluck , The Vegetarian Butcher*	1 Serving/80g	101	3.4	126	16	5.2	4.2	2.5
Style, Pieces, Frozen, Oven Cooked, Linda McCartney*	5 Pieces/55g	124	8	227	14.3	5.8	14.7	6.9
Style, Pieces, Vegan, V Taste, Morrisons*	¼ Pack/75g	189	12.5	252	17.1	5.8	16.6	0
Tandoori, Pieces, Tesco*	½ Pack/90g	153	6.8	170	19.9	5.4	7.5	0.5
Tenders, Crispy, Buttermilk, M&S*	½ Pack/150g	309	15.6	206	18.6	8.9	10.4	1
Thigh, Fillet, Buttermilk, Morrisons*	1 Thigh/114g	245	13.1	215	16.4	11.4	11.5	0
Thigh, Fillet, Jerk Spiced, Waitrose*	1 Thigh/70g	136	6.3	194	24.1	4	9	0.5
Thigh, Fillets, Tandoori, Ready to Eat, Morrisons*	½ Pack/75g	119	4.6	159	22.4	2.7	6.2	1.4
Thigh, Meat & Skin, Casseroled, Average	**1oz/28g**	**65**	**4.6**	**233**	**21.5**	**0**	**16.3**	**0**
Thigh, Meat & Skin, Raw, Average	**1 Serving/100g**	**218**	**14.7**	**218**	**21.4**	**0**	**14.7**	**0**
Thigh, Meat & Skin, Weighed with Bone, Raw, Average	**1 Serving/100g**	**186**	**14.1**	**186**	**13.8**	**0.2**	**14.1**	**0**
Thigh, Meat Only, Diced, Casseroled	**1oz/28g**	**50**	**2.4**	**180**	**25.6**	**0**	**8.6**	**0**
Thigh, Meat Only, Raw, Average	**1 Thigh/90g**	**144**	**9**	**160**	**18.5**	**0**	**10**	**0**
Thigh, Roast, Average	**1 Serving/100g**	**238**	**15.6**	**238**	**23.8**	**0.4**	**15.6**	**0**
Thighs, Southern Fried, Boneless, Oven Baked, Iceland*	2 Pieces/84g	176	8.5	210	17.1	12.2	10.1	0.9
Thighs, Stuffed, Pork & Apple, Waitrose*	1 Thigh/85g	198	12.2	233	23.9	1.9	14.3	0.3
Trimmings, Cooked, Iceland*	1 Serving/100g	103	2.5	103	16	2	2.5	0
Vegan, Fillets, Southern Fried, Plant Chef, Tesco*	1 Fillet/123g	268	12.8	218	17.4	11.7	10.4	4.1
Vegan, Goujons, Breaded, Plant Chef, Tesco*	3 Goujons/89g	213	7.7	239	13.7	24.9	8.6	3.5
Vegan, Slices, Deli Style, Quorn*	½ Pack/50g	47	1.2	94	11	4.1	2.3	6.2
Vegetarian, Bucket, Linda McCartney*	½ Pack/172g	449	25.8	261	14.6	14.8	15	4.6
Vegetarian, Fillets, Crispy, Quorn*	1 Fillet/100g	192	8.5	192	12.5	14.2	8.5	4
Vegetarian, Pieces, Chicken Style, Chilled, Quorn*	½ Pack/175g	173	4.6	99	13.8	1.7	2.6	7.1
Vegetarian, Pieces, Chicken Style, Frozen/Chilled, Quorn*	1 Serving/100g	113	2.8	113	15.3	3.9	2.8	5.3
Vegetarian, Roast Style, Quorn*	1/5 Roast/91g	96	1.8	106	15	4.5	2	4.9
Vegetarian, Roast, Family, Frozen, Cooked, Quorn*	1 Serving/80g	91	2.2	114	16.7	3	2.7	5
Wafer Thin, Average	**1 Slice/10g**	**12**	**0.4**	**120**	**19**	**2.8**	**3.6**	**0.2**
Whole, Roast, Average	**½ Chicken/685g**	**910**	**57.7**	**133**	**13.4**	**0.9**	**8.4**	**0.1**
Wing Quarter, Meat Only, Casseroled	**1oz/28g**	**46**	**1.8**	**164**	**26.9**	**0**	**6.3**	**0**
Wing, Breaded, Fried, Average	**1oz/28g**	**77**	**4.8**	**273**	**17.1**	**13**	**17.2**	**0.4**
Wing, Meat & Skin, Cooked, Average	**1 Wing/85g**	**216**	**14.3**	**254**	**23.8**	**0**	**16.9**	**0**
Wing, Meat Only, Cooked, Average	**1 Wing/21g**	**43**	**1.7**	**203**	**30.5**	**0**	**8.1**	**0**
Wing, Meat Only, Raw, Average	**1 Wing/29g**	**37**	**1**	**126**	**22**	**0**	**3.5**	**0**
Wings, BBQ Flavour, Average	**3 Wings/150g**	**330**	**18.7**	**220**	**20.3**	**6.6**	**12.4**	**0.6**
Wings, Chinese Style, Average	**1oz/28g**	**72**	**4.3**	**256**	**24.2**	**5.1**	**15.5**	**0.6**
Wings, Hot & Spicy, Average	**1oz/28g**	**65**	**3.8**	**231**	**21.8**	**5.2**	**13.6**	**0.8**
Wings, Meat & Skin, Raw, Average	**1 Wing/150g**	**286**	**19.3**	**191**	**17.5**	**0**	**12.8**	**0**
Wings, Salt, & Chilli, Oven Cooked, Tesco*	1 Pack/167g	389	22.4	233	24.7	2.4	13.4	1.8

CHICKEN &

	Measure INFO/WEIGHT	per Measure KCAL	per Measure FAT	KCAL	PROT	CARB	FAT	FIBRE
Black Bean Sauce, with Egg Fried Rice, Ready Meal	**1 Serving/400g**	**390**	**6.1**	**97**	**6.5**	**14.5**	**1.5**	**0.8**
Cashew Nuts, Chinese, Ready Meal, Average	**1 Serving/400g**	**497**	**24**	**124**	**9.2**	**7.5**	**6**	**1.2**
Chorizo Paella, Go Cook, Asda*	½ Pack/475g	591	10.5	124	10.2	15.9	2.2	2.6
Fries, Southern Fried Style, Tesco*	1 Pack/500g	930	40	186	11.5	16	8	1.4
King Prawn Special Fried Rice, Finest, Tesco*	1 Pack/450g	734	32	163	7.7	17	7.1	0.7
Mushroom with Rice, Egg Fried, Average	**1 Serving/400g**	**421**	**10.1**	**105**	**6.3**	**14.4**	**2.5**	**0.8**
Pineapple, Chilled, Tesco*	1 Pack/350g	364	8.4	104	9.6	11.1	2.4	5.5
Roasted Potatoes, Spanish, Charlie Bigham's*	½ Pack/387g	479	25.9	124	7.2	9.8	6.7	0

CHICKEN ARRABIATA

Arrabbiata, COU, M&S*	1 Pack/360g	396	6.7	110	8.5	14.5	1.9	1.3
COU, M&S*	1 Meal/360g	396	6.5	110	8.4	14.5	1.8	1.3
Italian Kitchen, Tesco*	1 Pack/414g	492	11.6	119	8.3	14.2	2.8	1.8
M&S*	1 Pack/396g	436	6.7	110	8.5	14.5	1.7	1.3
Meal for One, M&S*	1 Pack/400g	528	20.8	132	7.9	12.5	5.2	1.9
Morrisons*	1 Pack/400g	488	8.8	122	8.2	16.6	2.2	1.5

CHICKEN CHASSEUR

Average	**1 Serving/400g**	**363**	**9.2**	**91**	**12.2**	**4.9**	**2.3**	**0.9**
Mini, 336, Oakhouse Foods*	1 Pack/240g	161	2.6	67	8.4	5.4	1.1	0.9

CHICKEN CHILLI

Sweet, Pieces, Morrisons*	1 Pack/200g	282	5	141	25.5	4.1	2.5	0.5
Sweet, With Noodles, Ready Meal, Average	**1 Serving/400g**	**404**	**5.8**	**101**	**6.5**	**15.5**	**1.4**	**1.4**

CHICKEN CHINESE

Balls, M&S*	1 Ball/16g	45	2.2	280	10.8	29.2	13.6	2.1
Stir Fry, Morrisons*	1 Serving/319g	341	5.4	107	5.7	17	1.7	1.5
with Ginger & Spring Onion, Tesco*	1 Serving/350g	299	10.1	85	7.6	7.3	2.9	0.6

CHICKEN DINNER

Cooked, Eat Smart, Morrisons*	1 Pack/355g	245	4.3	69	8.2	4.4	1.2	4.1
Microwaved, Counted, Morrisons*	1 Pack/358g	283	2.9	79	9.2	8	0.8	1.7
Morrisons*	1 Pack/379g	375	6.1	99	7.4	12.7	1.6	1.9
Oven Cooked, Sainsbury's*	1 Pack/337g	330	7.7	98	9.3	9.3	2.3	1.5
Roast, 1301, Oakhouse Foods Ltd*	1 Serving/400g	408	14.8	102	7.5	8.6	3.7	2
Roast, Calorie Controlled, Tesco*	1 Pack/381g	274	3	72	8.1	7.2	0.8	1.8
Roast, Champ, Mixed Vegetables, Go Pig Or Go Home *	1 Pack/400g	350	5	88	8	10.8	1.2	0
Roast, Frozen, Inspired Cuisine, Aldi*	1 Pack/400g	404	11.6	101	8.3	9.3	2.9	1.9
Roast, Luxury, 1308, Oakhouse*	1 Pack/500g	550	21	110	7.8	9	4.2	1.7
Roast, Mini Meals, Tesco*	1 Pack/218g	234	7	108	6.9	12	3.2	1.7
Roast, Mini, 1001, Oakhouse Foods Ltd*	1 Serving/240g	259	5.3	108	7.9	8.5	2.2	2.3
Roast, Morrisons*	1 Pack/379g	375	6.1	99	7.4	12.7	1.6	1.9
Roast, Oven Baked, Asda*	1 Pack/384g	449	11.5	117	11	11	3	1.2
Roast, Taste The World, Aldi*	1 Pack/500g	500	15.5	100	6.8	10	3.1	1.6
Roast, What's Cooking, Lidl*	1 Pack/400g	360	7.2	90	7.7	10.4	1.8	0.6

CHICKEN IN

Barbeque Sauce, Breasts, COU, M&S*	1 Pack/350g	420	6.7	120	8.5	20.6	1.9	0.6
BBQ Sauce, Breast, Sainsbury's*	1 Serving/170g	199	1.2	117	14.5	13.1	0.7	1.3
BBQ, Smoky, SlimWell, Aldi*	1 Pack/500g	331	4.3	70	10	3.2	0.9	3.4
Black Bean Sauce, Sainsbury's*	1 Pack/465g	484	7.9	104	5	17.3	1.7	0.3
Dijon, with Rice, TTD, Sainsbury's*	1 Pack/368g	552	11.4	150	8	21.9	3.1	0.9
Gravy, Breast, Sainsbury's*	1 Box/200g	124	1	62	11.8	2.9	0.5	0.4
Hunter's BBQ Sauce, Asda*	½ Pack /190g	348	14.1	183	19.1	10.3	7.4	0
Mushroom, Sauce, Tesco*	1 Pack/370g	289	8	78	7.8	6.2	2.2	1.3
Oyster Sauce & Mushrooms, Tesco*	1 Pack/350g	252	5.6	72	8	6.3	1.6	0.7
Peppercorn Sauce, Counted, Morrisons*	1 Pack/353g	364	7.8	103	8.2	11.8	2.2	1.8
Prosecco Sauce, Finest, Tesco*	½ Pack/181g	245	10.9	135	17.7	2.3	6	0.6

	Measure INFO/WEIGHT	per Measure KCAL	FAT	Nutrition Values per 100g / 100ml KCAL	PROT	CARB	FAT	FIBRE
CHICKEN IN								
Red Wine, Gastropub, M&S*	½ Pack/233g	296	11.9	127	17	3	5.1	0.5
Sweet Chilli Sauce, Breast, Fresh Tastes, Asda*	½ Pack/180g	288	9	160	18.4	10.3	5	0.5
Teriyaki Sauce, with Noodles, Wat Kitchen*	1 Box/250g	352	7.2	141	3.7	24.6	2.9	1.4
Tomato & Basil Sauce, Breast Fillets, Morrisons*	½ Pack/171g	231	7.5	135	21.3	2.5	4.4	1.4
Tomato & Basil Sauce, Breast, GFY, Asda*	1 Pack/392g	447	13.3	114	12	9	3.4	1.5
White Sauce, Canned, 200g, Sainsbury's*	1 Can/200g	280	16	140	13.2	3.4	8	0.6
White Sauce, Canned, Princes*	½ Can/82g	109	6.6	133	10.4	4.5	8.1	0.5
CHICKEN TANDOORI								
& Basmati Rice, Aromatic, Asda*	1 Pack/380g	399	8	105	7.5	12	2.1	3.7
Breast, Fillets, with Creamy Sauce, Morrisons*	1 Fillet/144g	220	7.8	153	21.3	4.4	5.4	0.8
Fresh Tastes, Asda*	1 Pack/400g	356	5.6	89	6.4	12.7	1.4	2.1
Oven Baked, Asda*	½ Pack/141g	186	5.9	132	20	3.6	4.2	0.6
Sizzler, Sainsbury's*	1 Pack/400g	536	29.2	134	12.8	4.3	7.3	1.7
Sizzler, Tesco*	1 Serving/175g	243	11.6	139	10	10	6.6	1
with Rice, City Kitchen, Tesco*	1 Pack/385g	597	21.2	155	6.7	19.6	5.5	1.8
CHICKEN TERIYAKI								
& Noodles, Asda*	½ Pack/340g	445	8.8	131	9	18	2.6	0.9
Noodles, HL, Tesco*	1 Pack/367g	282	1.8	77	6.4	10.5	0.5	2.3
Teriyaki, Japanese, Sainsbury's*	1 Pack/380g	486	11.4	128	7.4	16.8	3	2.1
Teriyaki, Japanese, Street Kitchen*	1 Pack/255g	398	4.1	156	1.6	31	1.6	0
CHICKEN TIKKA								
& Lemon Rice, Deli Meal, M&S*	1 Pack/360g	342	7.2	95	9.8	10.2	2	0.7
& Cauliflower Rice, Spiced, BFY, M&S*	1 Pack/400g	276	8	69	8.4	3.3	2	1.9
& Rice, Lunch Bowl, Microwaved, Slimming World*	1 Pack/400g	316	5.2	79	5.8	10	1.3	2.3
& Roasted Sweet Potato, My Goodness, Sainsbury's*	1 Pack/350g	388	11.6	111	7.1	11.8	3.3	2.9
in Mayo, Aldi*	1 Serving/105g	288	21	274	17	5.2	20	0.8
Masala, & Pilau Rice, Charlie Bigham's*	½ Pack/403g	737	43.9	183	6.9	15.3	10.9	0
Masala, with Rice, Weight Watchers, Heinz*	1 Pack/310g	333	7.4	108	5.4	15.8	2.4	0.7
No Chicken, Plant Menu, Aldi*	½ Pack/90g	166	7.2	184	16.2	8.2	8	7.8
Takeaway	**1 Serving/350g**	**421**	**15**	**120**	**20.3**	**0**	**4.3**	**0.3**
The Gym Kitchen*	1 Pack/392g	384	6.7	98	8.5	10	1.7	3.5
CHICORY								
Fresh, Raw, Average	**1 Head/150g**	**30**	**0.9**	**20**	**0.6**	**2.8**	**0.6**	**0.9**
CHILLI								
& Rice, Bowl, BFY, M&S*	1 Pot/354g	418	7.8	118	8.2	15.3	2.2	2.2
& Rice, Calorie Controlled, Tesco*	1 Pack/365g	388	5.1	106	5.4	16.1	1.4	4.1
3 Bean, Chipotle, Hi Five*	1 Pack/467g	355	8.4	76	3.2	12.8	1.8	2.7
Bean, & Pepper, Easy Bean*	1 Pot/320g	195	6.1	61	2.7	7.5	1.9	3.2
Bean, & Rice, Little Kids, Microwaved, Asda*	1 Pack/150g	114	0.8	76	3	13	0.5	3.4
Bean, 3, Inspired Cuisine, Aldi*	1 Pack/380g	312	2.3	82	2.5	16	0.6	2.4
Bean, Bowl, Microwaved, Quorn*	1 Bowl/297g	300	1.2	101	5.1	17	0.4	4.4
Bean, Three, Mexican, Cook*	1 Serving/330g	300	5.9	91	4.1	17.4	1.8	5.4
Bean, Three, Slim Choice, Sainsbury's*	1 Pack/465g	437	2.8	94	3.7	16.1	0.6	4.9
Bean, Triple, Plant Chef, Tesco*	1 Pack/390g	417	6.6	107	3.2	17.9	1.7	3.4
Beef with Rice, GFY, Asda*	1 Serving/402g	354	6	88	4.7	14	1.5	0.9
Beef, & 3 Bean, with Wild Rice, Inspired Cuisine, Aldi*	1 Pack/377g	369	6.4	98	5.7	14	1.7	2
Beef, & Rice, HL, Tesco*	1 Pack/370g	370	5.9	100	5	13.7	1.6	5.5
Beef, & Rice, Tex Mex, Tesco*	1 Pack/450g	604	13	134	5.4	20.4	2.9	2.5
Beef, Asda*	½ Pack/200g	190	7.8	95	7	8	3.9	1.2
Beef, Chunky, Slimming World*	1 Pack/550g	418	6.6	76	8.8	5.9	1.2	3.1
Beef, Chunky, Slow Cooked, M&S*	½ Pack/268g	289	8.3	108	15.3	3.6	3.1	2.1
Beef, with Beans, Shake That Weight*	1 Pack/275g	280	11.8	102	7.2	6.3	4.3	4.5
Black Bean, Mexican, Power Pot, BOL Foods*	1 Pot/450g	351	5.4	78	4.7	9.9	1.2	6.3

CHILLI

INFO/WEIGHT	Measure	per Measure		Nutrition Values per 100g / 100ml				
		KCAL	FAT	KCAL	PROT	CARB	FAT	FIBRE
Con Carne with Rice, GFY, Asda*	1 Serving/400g	456	6.4	114	6	19	1.6	0.9
Con Carne with Rice, Healthy Choice, Asda*	1 Pack/400g	412	8.4	103	6	15	2.1	0.9
Con Carne with Rice, Morrisons*	1 Pack/400g	328	5.2	82	5.3	12.2	1.3	1.4
Con Carne, & Mexican Rice, Charlie Bigham's*	½ Pack/421g	589	25.2	140	7.2	14.1	6	0
Con Carne, & Rice, Fiesta, Aldi*	1 Pack/450g	648	24.3	144	6.7	16	5.4	2.3
Con Carne, Asda*	1 Can/392g	376	13.7	96	7	9	3.5	0
Con Carne, Beef, Slim Cook, Tesco*	1 Pack/476g	376	7.1	79	5.4	9.6	1.5	3.1
Con Carne, Canned, Morrisons*	1 Can/392g	368	11.8	94	8.8	8	3	2.4
Con Carne, Canned, Sainsbury's*	½ Can/200g	162	4.2	81	6.6	8.9	2.1	2.5
Con Carne, Classic, Canned, Stagg*	½ Can/200g	260	10	130	7	13	5	4.5
Con Carne, Donald Russell*	1 Pack/300g	396	19.5	132	9.1	9.3	6.5	2.2
Con Carne, From Restaurant, Average	**1 Serving/253g**	**256**	**8.3**	**101**	**9.7**	**8.7**	**3.3**	**0**
Con Carne, Frozen, Co-Op*	1 Pack/340g	306	3.4	90	6	15	1	1
Con Carne, Hunger Breaks*	½ Can/206g	196	8.2	95	6.7	6.8	4	2.3
Con Carne, M&S*	1 Pack/285g	285	10.5	100	8.7	7.4	3.7	2
Con Carne, Medium, Canned, Bramwells, Aldi*	1 Can/400g	408	17.6	102	8.8	4.7	4.4	4
Con Carne, Microwaved, Asda*	1 Pack/400g	532	15.2	133	5.9	18	3.8	1.5
Con Carne, Mild, Canned, Princes*	1 Can/392g	576	34.9	147	6.5	9.1	8.9	2
Con Carne, Recipe Mix, Colman's*	1 Pack/27g	84	2.1	312	12.3	37.8	7.7	22.9
Con Carne, with Long Grain Rice, COU, M&S*	1 Pack/390g	394	6.6	101	5.4	15	1.7	2.2
Con Carne, with Rice, BGTY, Sainsbury's*	1 Pack/374g	385	8.6	103	6.3	13.4	2.3	2.1
Con Carne, with Rice, Classic, Co-Op*	1 Pack/400g	464	13.6	116	5.9	14	3.4	2.7
Con Carne, with Rice, Counted, Morrisons*	½ Pack/158g	150	2.4	95	5.9	13.5	1.5	1.6
Con Carne, with Rice, Iceland*	1 Meal/375g	431	17.2	115	5.7	12.2	4.6	1.1
Con Carne, with Rice, Meal for One, M&S*	1 Pack/450g	536	12.2	119	5.5	18	2.7	0.5
Con Carne, with Rice, PB, Waitrose*	1 Pack/400g	404	7.2	101	5.8	15.3	1.8	1.7
Con Carne, with Rice, Tesco*	1 Pack/400g	468	8.4	117	6.1	17.6	2.1	2
Con Carne, with White Rice, Sainsbury's*	1 Pack/400g	469	13.6	117	5.1	16	3.4	1.2
Crushed, Cooks' Ingredients, Waitrose*	1 Tsp/5g	4	0.2	80	4.2	3.3	3.5	9.2
Four Bean, & Rice, Slimming World*	1 Pack/400g	356	2.8	89	3.1	15.3	0.7	4.4
Jackfruit, Microwaved, Slimming World*	1 Pack/550g	346	2.2	63	3.1	9.1	0.4	5.3
Mixed Vegetable, Tesco*	1 Pack/400g	352	11.6	88	3.9	11	2.9	3.2
Non Carne, Plant Pioneers, Sainsbury's*	1 Pack/360g	490	11.5	136	5.6	19.9	3.2	2.8
Non Carne, Vegan, The Gym Kitchen*	1 Pack/394g	343	5.5	87	5.6	12	1.4	2.7
Organic, Medium, Amy's Kitchen*	1 Can/416g	500	16	120	6.2	15.1	3.8	3.1
Quorn, Full of Beans, Microwaved, Quorn*	1 Pack/385g	366	4.2	95	4.7	15.2	1.1	2.6
Smoky, Soul, Allplants*	1 Serving/430g	555	17.2	129	5.1	16	4	3.9
Super Charged, Verde, Plant Pot, Foodologie*	1 Pot/400g	156	1.5	39	1.9	6	0.4	2.4
Vegan, Two Bean, Waitrose*	1 Pack/368g	254	5.9	69	3.1	9.4	1.6	2.4
Vegetable	**1oz/28g**	**16**	**0.2**	**57**	**3**	**10.8**	**0.6**	**2.6**
Vegetable & Rice, BGTY, Sainsbury's*	1 Pack/450g	410	5	91	3.5	16.7	1.1	3.5
Vegetable, Retail	**1oz/28g**	**20**	**0.6**	**70**	**4**	**9.4**	**2.1**	**0**
Vegetarian with Rice, Tesco*	1 Pack/500g	575	13	115	4	19	2.6	1.8
Vegetarian, Mexican, Chef's Selection, Quorn*	½ Pack/170g	143	4.3	84	6.6	6.5	2.5	4.5
Vegetarian, Soya Mince, & Rice, Waitrose*	1 Pack/402g	442	8.4	110	5.4	14.9	2.1	5.4
Vegetarian, with Rice, Ready Meal, Average	**1 Serving/400g**	**434**	**6**	**108**	**3.8**	**20**	**1.5**	**1.3**
Veggie, Packed, with Brown Rice, Hello Fresh*	1 Serving/739g	525	14.8	71	3	10	2	0
Veggie, Smoky, Jamie Oliver*	1 Serving/125g	111	2.6	89	4.6	10	2.1	5.1

CHILLI POWDER

INFO/WEIGHT	Measure	per Measure		Nutrition Values per 100g / 100ml				
		KCAL	FAT	KCAL	PROT	CARB	FAT	FIBRE
Average	**1 Tsp/4g**	**16**	**0.7**	**405**	**12.3**	**54.7**	**16.8**	**34.2**

CHIPS

	INFO/WEIGHT	KCAL	FAT	KCAL	PROT	CARB	FAT	FIBRE
& Curry Sauce, Microwaved, Iceland*	1 Serving/441g	454	11.9	103	1.9	16.4	2.7	2.7
& Gravy, Microwaved, Iceland*	1 Serving/440g	418	11	95	1.9	14.6	2.5	3.2
American Style, Oven, Co-Op*	1 Serving/150g	255	9	170	2	26	6	3
American Style, Thin, Oven, Tesco*	1 Serving/125g	210	8.1	168	2.7	24.6	6.5	2.1
Chip Shop, Fishnchickn*	1 Portion/311g	734	38.6	236	3.2	27.9	12.4	0
Chunky Oven, Harry Ramsden's*	1 Serving/150g	184	5.4	123	2.8	19.9	3.6	1.6
Chunky, Chilled, Waitrose*	1/3 Pack/150g	237	5.6	158	2.8	26.5	3.7	3.8
Chunky, COU, M&S*	1 Serving/150g	158	2.4	105	2.1	20.5	1.6	2.3
Chunky, Gastropub, M&S*	1 Pack/400g	520	12.4	130	2.6	22.4	3.1	2.3
Chunky, in Light Crisp Batter, M&S*	1 Serving/100g	119	2.9	119	2.1	19.6	2.9	3.2
Chunky, M&S*	½ Pack/200g	292	7.6	146	2	24.7	3.8	2.6
Chunky, Maris Piper, Oven Cooked, The Best, Morrisons*	½ Pack/176g	267	6.1	152	2.3	26.5	3.5	2.7
Chunky, Oven Cooked, Finest, Tesco*	1 Pack/387g	546	14.7	141	2.8	22.6	3.8	2.7
Chunky, Ready to Bake, M&S*	1 Serving/200g	310	8.4	155	2.2	26.8	4.2	2
Chunky, Skin On, Oven Baked, Tesco*	¼ Pack/125g	104	0.3	83	2.9	16.4	0.2	2.1
Crinkle Cut, Frozen, Fried in Corn Oil	*1 Serving/125*	*362*	*20.9*	*290*	*3.6*	*33.4*	*16.7*	*2.2*
Crinkle Cut, Oven Baked, Morrisons*	1/10 Pack/81g	131	3.3	161	3.2	26.3	4.1	3
Fine Cut, Frozen, Fried in Blended Oil	*1oz/28g*	*102*	*6*	*364*	*4.5*	*41.2*	*21.3*	*2.4*
French Fries, Crispy, Oven Baked, McCain*	1 Serving/100g	231	7.7	231	3.1	35.5	7.7	3.3
Fried, Average	*1 Serving/130g*	*266*	*10.9*	*204*	*3.2*	*29.6*	*8.4*	*1.2*
Fried, Chip Shop, Average	*1 Sm/100g*	*239*	*12.4*	*239*	*3.2*	*30.5*	*12.4*	*2.2*
Frites, M&S*	1 Sm Pack/100g	161	4.5	161	3.2	25.8	4.5	2.3
Frites, Oven Cooked, Waitrose*	½ Pack/150g	322	14	215	2.6	29.1	9.3	2.6
Fry or Oven, Oven Cooked, Smart Price, Asda*	1 Serving/125g	192	4.3	153	2.1	26.9	3.4	3.3
Home Chips, Crinkle Cut, Oven Baked, McCain*	1 Serving/100g	197	7.7	197	2.4	28	7.7	2.8
Home Chips, Straight Cut, Baked, McCain*	1 Serving/150g	312	10.8	208	3.3	31	7.2	2.9
Home, Straight Cut, Lighter, Reduced Fat, Baked, McCain*	1 Serving/100g	181	3.4	181	3.2	33	3.4	3.3
Homemade, Fried in Blended Oil, Average	*1oz/28g*	*53*	*1.9*	*189*	*3.9*	*30.1*	*6.7*	*2.2*
Homemade, Fried in Corn Oil, Average	*1oz/28g*	*53*	*1.9*	*189*	*3.9*	*30.1*	*6.7*	*2.2*
Homemade, Fried in Dripping, Average	*1oz/28g*	*53*	*1.9*	*189*	*3.9*	*30.1*	*6.7*	*2.2*
Homestyle Oven, Sainsbury's*	1 Serving/125g	206	5.4	165	2.4	29.2	4.3	2.1
Homestyle, BFY, Morrisons*	1 Serving/88g	175	5.2	199	2.8	32.1	5.9	3.6
Homestyle, Crispy & Fluffy, Oven Cooked, Aunt Bessie's*	1 Serving/100g	157	5.1	157	2.8	23	5.1	3.4
Homestyle, Crispy, Ovenbaked, Asda*	1 Serving/125g	249	7.4	199	2.8	32	5.9	3.6
Homestyle, Frozen, Aunt Bessie's*	1 Serving /125g	155	4.4	124	2.4	20	3.5	1.9
Homestyle, Harvest Basket, Lidl*	1 Serving/150g	202	5.8	135	2.4	21.5	3.9	2.3
Homestyle, Oven, Four Seasons, Aldi*	1 Serving/200g	350	9.4	175	3.3	28	4.7	3.4
Homestyle, Oven, Straight Cut , Tesco*	1 Serving/125g	218	5.1	174	2.1	30.9	4.1	2.5
Maris Piper, Oven, Chunky, Extra Special, Asda*	1 Serving/125g	211	4.4	169	2	31	3.5	2.7
Microwave, Cooked	*1oz/28g*	*62*	*2.7*	*221*	*3.6*	*32.1*	*9.6*	*2.9*
Oven, Chunky, Maris Piper, Oven Baked, Iceland*	1 Serving/100g	194	4.7	194	3.4	33.2	4.7	2.6
Oven, Cooked, SlimWell, Aldi*	1 Serving/100g	124	0.5	124	2.7	19	0.5	4.3
Oven, Crinkle Cut, As Sold, Aunt Bessie's*	1 Serving/200g	244	8.2	122	2	18	4.1	2.4
Oven, Crinkle Cut, Oven Baked, Tesco*	1 Serving/100g	162	4.3	162	2.8	26.7	4.3	2.8
Oven, Frozen, Baked	*1 Serving/125g*	*202*	*5.2*	*162*	*3.2*	*29.8*	*4.2*	*2*
Oven, Low Fat, Oven Baked, Savers, Morrisons*	1 Serving/100g	133	2.8	133	3	25	2.8	3.5
Oven, Steak Cut, Asda*	1 Serving/100g	153	4.1	153	2	27	4.1	2.5
Oven, Steak Cut, Sainsbury's*	1 Serving/165g	266	7.8	161	2.6	27.1	4.7	2.8
Oven, Steak Cut, Waitrose*	1 Serving/165g	218	5.6	132	2.7	22.7	3.4	1.7
Oven, Straight Cut, 5% Fat, Sainsbury's*	1 Serving/165g	280	8.1	170	3.4	28	4.9	2.5
Oven, Straight Cut, Asda*	1 Serving/100g	199	5	199	3.5	35	5	3
Oven, Straight Cut, BFY, Morrisons*	1 Serving/165g	249	5.8	151	2.8	27.1	3.5	2.1
Oven, Straight Cut, Naked, Oven Baked, McCain*	1 Serving/100g	162	3.9	162	2.3	28	3.9	2.1

	Measure INFO/WEIGHT	per Measure KCAL	FAT	Nutrition Values per 100g / 100ml KCAL	PROT	CARB	FAT	FIBRE
CHIPS								
Oven, Straight Cut, Oven Cooked, Essential, Waitrose*	1 Serving/125g	150	4.1	120	2.3	19.3	3.3	2.2
Oven, Straight Cut, Reduced Fat, Tesco*	1 Serving/100g	127	3	127	2.3	22.7	3	2.1
Oven, Straight Cut, Waitrose*	1 Serving/165g	219	6.1	133	2	23	3.7	1.7
Oven, Sweet Potato, Cooked, Tesco*	¼ Pack/87g	153	4.8	175	3	26.2	5.5	4.5
Oven, Thick Cut, Frozen, Baked	**1 Serving/125g**	**196**	**5.5**	**157**	**3.2**	**27.9**	**4.4**	**1.8**
Oven, Thin Cut, American Style, Asda*	1 Serving/100g	240	10	240	3.4	34	10	3
Oven, Thin Fries, Morrisons*	1 Serving/100g	161	6.1	161	2.9	23.6	6.1	1.2
Potato, Lights, Reduced Fat, Lay's*	1 Serving/25g	118	5.5	470	7.5	60	22	5
Proper, Frozen, Strong Roots*	1 Serving /125g	150	3.8	120	1.9	20	3	2.7
Salt & Pepper, Crinkle, Tesco*	1 Serving/112g	179	5.7	160	2.3	24.6	5.1	3.4
Salt & Pepper, Iceland*	1 Serving/100g	231	7.6	231	4.1	34.1	7.6	4.6
Steak Cut, Frying, Asda*	1 Serving/97g	181	6.8	187	2.9	28	7	2.8
Steak Cut, Harvest Basket, Lidl*	1 Serving/100g	155	4	155	2.7	26.6	4	1.2
Steak Cut, Iceland*	1 Serving/100g	156	4.1	156	3.3	24.6	4.1	3.6
Steak Cut, Morrisons*	1 Serving/125g	171	3.9	137	2.1	23.7	3.1	3.1
Steak Cut, Oven, Cooked, Tesco*	1/7 Pack/138g	247	6.3	179	3.7	29.3	4.6	3.2
Steak, Cut, Oven, Frozen, Essential, Waitrose*	1 Serving/180g	241	6.5	134	2.4	22.1	3.6	1.7
Steakhouse, Fry, Tesco*	1 Serving/125g	278	15.1	222	3.1	25.2	12.1	2
Straight Cut, Frozen, Fried in Blended Oil	**1 Serving/125g**	**341**	**16.9**	**273**	**4.1**	**36**	**13.5**	**2.4**
Straight Cut, Frozen, Fried in Corn Oil	**1 Serving/125g**	**341**	**16.9**	**273**	**4.1**	**36**	**13.5**	**2.4**
Thick Cut, Frozen, Fried in Corn Oil, Average	**1 Serving/125g**	**292**	**12.7**	**234**	**3.6**	**34**	**10.2**	**2.4**
Triple Cook, Oven Baked, Extra Special, Asda*	½ Pack/167g	411	20	246	3.4	29	12	3.3
Triple Cooked, Beef Dripping, Harvest Basket, Lidl*	1 Serving/150g	344	19.8	229	2.7	23	13.2	3.5
Triple Cooked, Finest, Tesco*	½ Pack/178g	262	6.8	147	2.6	24.1	3.8	3
Triple Cooked, Gastro, Frozen, McCain*	1 Serving/187g	379	22.2	203	1.9	21	11.9	2.2
Triple Cooked, Gastro, Oven Baked, McCain*	1 Serving/135g	379	20.5	281	2.9	31.6	15.2	3
Triple Cooked, Oven Cooked, TTD, Sainsbury's*	½ Pack/180g	264	8.6	147	2.7	22.1	4.8	2.3
Vegetable, Fries, Aldi*	1 Serving/100g	192	11	192	2.5	18	11	6.7
CHIVES								
Fresh, Average	**1 Tsp/2g**	**0**	**0**	**23**	**2.8**	**1.7**	**0.6**	**1.9**
CHOC ICES								
Chocolate, Real Milk, Sainsbury's*	1 Choc Ice/41g	126	8	311	3	29.9	19.8	0.6
Dark, Morrisons*	1 Choc Ice/70g	150	10.2	214	1.7	18.7	14.6	0.7
Dark, Sainsbury's*	1 Choc Ice/41g	115	7.2	283	2.7	27.2	17.8	1.5
Dark, Sainsbury's*	1 Choc Ice/41g	115	7.2	283	2.7	27.2	17.8	1.5
Dark, Tesco*	1 Choc Ice/43g	132	8.7	305	3.5	28	20	0.1
Essential, Waitrose*	1 Choc Ice/70g	124	8.4	177	1.7	15.4	12	0.7
Everyday, Value, Tesco*	1 Choc Ice/31g	95	6.3	300	2.3	26.7	19.9	1
Milk, Co-Op*	1 Choc Ice/42g	132	9.2	314	0	35.7	21.9	0
Plain, Co-Op*	1 Choc Ice/42g	123	8	293	3.1	26	19	0
CHOCOLATE								
100% Cocoa, M&S*	1 Square/10g	62	5.4	620	12.5	13.2	54	15.6
55% Milk, Organic, Rare, Original Beans*	1 Bar/70g	410	30.1	586	8	38	43	6
70% Ganache, Pots & Co*	1 Pot/50g	189	15	378	2	24	30	0
Acorns, Salted Caramel, M&S*	1 Chocolate/22g	112	6.1	508	4.6	59.2	27.7	1.6
Advent Calendar, Dairy Milk, Cadbury*	1 Chocolate/4g	22	1.3	525	7.5	56.6	30.1	0.7
Advent Calendar, Maltesers, Mars*	1 Chocolate/4g	21	1.2	537	6.8	57.9	30.9	0
Almond Butter, Cup, Dark, Pip & Nut*	1 Cup/17g	102	7.9	599	11.2	30.3	46.6	0
Alpine Milk , Milka*	1 Serving/25g	132	7.4	530	6.6	58.5	29.5	1.8
Balls, Protein, Exante Diet*	1 Pack/158g	713	27.8	451	42.9	28.9	17.6	2.9
Bar, Animal, Nestle*	1 Bar/19g	97	5	513	5.8	63.6	26.1	0
Bar, Bliss Truffle, Cadbury*	1 Bar/40g	226	14.9	565	6.6	48.8	37.3	2.8
Bar, Bubbly, Milk, Tesco*	1 Bar/25g	138	8.2	554	6.1	57.7	32.8	1.9

CHOCOLATE

	Measure INFO/WEIGHT	per Measure KCAL	FAT	Nutrition Values per 100g / 100ml KCAL	PROT	CARB	FAT	FIBRE
Bar, Cappuccino, Thorntons*	1 Bar/38g	201	13.2	529	5.2	49.7	34.7	0.5
Bar, Chocolate Cream, Fry's*	1 Piece/10g	42	1.3	415	2.8	70.8	13.2	1.2
Bar, Chopped Nuts, Dairy Milk, Cadbury*	6 Chunks/24g	130	7.8	547	7.9	52	33	2.5
Bar, Cookies & Cream, Hello, Lindt*	1 Square/10g	56	3.7	565	7	52	37	0
Bar, Dark, Thorntons*	1 Sm Bar/48g	250	17.7	521	7.3	39.9	36.9	10.9
Bar, Deliciously, Free From, Sainsbury's*	1 Bar/35g	190	12.2	543	2.5	48.2	35	12.4
Bar, Duplo, Ferrero*	1 Bar18g	101	6.1	555	6.1	56	33.5	5
Bar, Filled with Peanut Butter, Reeses*	1 Bar/120g	624	36.1	520	8.3	59.1	30.1	0
Bar, Free From, Asda*	1 Bar/35g	194	12.1	563	2.5	58	35	2.8
Bar, Fruit & Nut, Free From, Sainsbury's*	2 Squares/21g	120	7.7	573	4	54.3	36.8	4.1
Bar, Hazel Nut & Cashew, Dairy Milk, Cadbury*	3 Chunks/18g	96	6	540	8.8	50.6	33.5	1.8
Bar, Mandolin, Cadbury*	1 Bar/28g	139	4.6	495	3.5	66.5	16.5	0.6
Bar, Milk, Thorntons*	1 Sm Bar/50g	269	16	538	7.5	54.8	32	1
Bar, Orange Mousse, Moser Roth, Aldi*	1 Bar/38g	200	14	526	7.9	39.5	36.8	9
Bar, Orange Smarties, Nestle*	1 Row/15g	78	0.7	521	1	10	4.7	0.3
Bar, Salted Caramel, Aldi*	1 Bar/26g	138	7.8	532	5.1	57	30	5.4
Bar, Soft & Whippy, Sainsbury's*	1 Bar/22g	100	3.5	455	3.6	73.6	15.9	0
Bar, Truffle, M&S*	1 Bar/35g	168	11.4	480	5.9	41.7	32.5	8.3
Bar, White, Thorntons*	1 Bar/50g	274	15.6	547	6.5	59.5	31.3	0
Bars, Chocolate, Strawberry, Lindt*	1 Bar/100g	470	22.8	470	4.5	61.6	22.8	0
Bars, Milk Chocolate, Galaxy, Mars*	1 Bar/42g	229	13.6	546	6.7	56	32.4	1.5
Bars, Milk Chocolate, Gold, Lindt*	1 Bar/300g	1605	92.9	535	6.6	58.7	31	0
Bars, Milk Chocolate, Hazelnut, Lindt*	1 Bar/100g	570	38.8	570	8.5	47	38.8	0
Bars, Milk Chocolate, Lindt*	1 Bar/100g	622	47	622	4.6	44	47	0
Bars, Milk Chocolate, Raisin & Hazelnut, Lindt*	1 Bar/100g	530	31.6	530	3.1	54.7	31.6	0
Bars, Milk, Bubblies, Treat Size, Asda*	1 Bar/10g	53	3	528	7.1	57	30	0.6
Batons, Dark, 85%, Hotel Chocolat*	1 Baton/9g	56	4.6	625	9.4	22	51	19
Batons, Nutmilk, Hotel Chocolat*	1 Baton/8g	38	2.8	474	2.6	36.3	35.3	3.7
Batons, Supermilk, 65%, Hotel Chocolat*	3 Batons/24g	136	10.7	568	10.3	28.6	44.5	9.7
Beans, Coffee, Dark, Solid, M&S*	1 Serving/10g	53	3.8	532	4.7	42.4	37.6	11.6
Bear, Lindt*	1 Bear/11g	60	3.6	572	7.5	57.7	34.6	0
Belgian Milk, TTD, Sainsbury's*	1 Piece/10g	55	3.5	549	9.6	48.3	35.3	2
Belgian, Celeste, M&S*	2 Squares/34g	184	11.9	541	6	48.4	34.9	34.9
Belgian, Collection, M&S*	1 Chocolate/13g	71	4.6	549	6	50.9	35	3
Belgian, Dark, Lily O'briens*	1 Bag/110g	649	49.5	590	8	33	45	0
Belgian, Milk, Mini Eggs, M&S*	1 Egg/8g	43	2.5	535	7	55.8	31.7	2.7
Bittermints, Bendicks*	1 Mint/18g	77	3	428	3.5	62.8	16.8	0
Bloc, Hazelnut, Green & Black's*	1 Bloc/20g	116	8	578	6.8	43	40	7.4
Block, Orange Crisp, Thorntons*	1 Serving/100g	530	30	530	6.6	57	30	0
Blond, Swiss, M&S*	1/5th Bar/20g	119	8.3	597	6.3	49.1	41.7	0
Blueberry Intense, Excellence, Lindt*	1 Serving/40g	200	12.4	500	6	50	31	0
Bubbly Santa, M&S*	1 Santa/23g	124	7.3	540	7	55.8	31.7	2.7
Bubbly, Dairy Milk, Cadbury*	1 Bar/35g	185	10.5	525	7.7	56.9	29.7	0.7
Bunny, Kit Kat, Nestle*	1 Bunny/29g	156	9.1	537	6.2	55.6	31.4	2.9
Bunny, Lidl*	1 Rabbit/125g	676	38.9	541	7.2	57.1	31.1	1.9
Bunny, Lindt*	1 Bunny/11g	60	3.6	572	7.5	57.5	34.6	0
Bunny, with Vanilla Mousse, Dairy Milk, Cadbury*	1 Bunny/30g	168	10.4	560	6.4	54.5	34.5	1.2
Buttons, Bournville, Cadbury*	1 Serving/25g	128	6.8	510	3.9	60	27	6.2
Buttons, Caramel Crunch, Galaxy, Mars*	1 Serving/31g	161	8.4	519	6.5	62	27	0
Buttons, Caramel Filled, M&S*	6 Buttons/25g	127	7	509	5.7	57.6	28.1	1.3
Buttons, Dairy Milk, Cadbury*	1 Bag/30g	160	9	535	7.3	57	30	2.1
Buttons, Free From, Tesco*	1 Bag/25g	136	8.8	544	2.5	48.4	35	12.5
Buttons, Giant, Bourneville, Cadbury*	1 Pack/110g	563	29.5	512	0	60	26.8	6.4

CHOCOLATE

	Measure INFO/WEIGHT	per Measure KCAL	FAT	Nutrition Values per 100g / 100ml KCAL	PROT	CARB	FAT	FIBRE
Buttons, Giant, Dairy Milk, Cadbury*	1 Button/2g	11	0.6	535	7.3	57	30	2.1
Buttons, Giant, Orange, Dairy Milk, Cadbury*	1 Serving/25g	133	7.5	533	7.4	57	30	2.1
Buttons, Gigantic, M&S*	1/5 Pack/125g	704	40.8	563	7.7	58.8	32.6	1.6
Buttons, Maltesers, Mars*	1 Bag/32g	166	8.6	518	7.4	60	27	0
Buttons, Moo Free*	1 Pack/28g	150	8.7	536	3	57	31	0
Buttons, Orange, Dairy Milk, Cadbury*	10 Buttons/25g	133	7.5	533	7.4	57	30	2.1
Buttons, Orange, Smarties, Nestle*	6 Buttons/15g	78	4.1	518	6	61	27.3	2
Buttons, Smarties, Nestle*	1 Pack/90g	462	23.1	513	5.8	63.7	25.7	1.5
Buttons, White, Free From, Tesco*	1 Pack/25g	132	8.1	528	0.4	51.7	32.5	13.3
Buttons, White, Giant, Cadbury*	1 Serving/25g	134	7.2	535	4.8	63	29	0
Caramel & Sea Salt, Pure, Moser Roth, Aldi*	1 Tablet/25g	133	7.5	533	4.7	58	30	5.7
Caramel Crunch, Dairyfine, Aldi*	1 Bar/38g	196	10.6	515	5.5	59	28	1.3
Caramel, & Sea Salt, Vegan, Galaxy*	½ Bar/50g	290	19.4	581	3	53.4	38.9	0
Caramel, Bar, Dairy Milk, Cadbury*	1 Serving/37g	179	8.9	485	5.1	61	24	0.4
Caramel, Choceur, Aldi*	4 Squares/33g	158	7.6	479	5.1	62	23	2.7
Caramel, Chunk, Dairy Milk, Cadbury*	1 Chunk/33g	158	7.6	480	5	63	23	0
Caramelised Hazelnut, Vegan, Galaxy *	4 Squares/29g	173	12	596	3.4	50.8	41.5	0
Caramelles, Mister Choc, Lidl*	1/5 Pack/25g	120	5.1	482	4.2	69	20.5	2.2
Caramilk, Cadbury*	6 Chunks/30g	163	9.1	543	4.3	63.3	30.3	0
Chips, Dark, Tesco*	1 Serving/25g	134	8	536	6.7	51.3	32.2	7.3
Chips, Dark, The Pantry, Aldi*	1 Serving/25g	126	6.5	505	3.8	60	26	6.1
Chips, Milk, Tesco*	¼ Pack/25g	141	8.8	563	5.9	55.1	35	1.9
Chips, White, Tesco*	1 Serving/25g	146	9.2	582	4.6	58.1	36.8	0.1
Chocolat Noir, Lindt*	1/6 Bar/17g	87	5.4	510	6	50	32	0
Chocolate Favourites, Tesco*	½ Box/227g	1015	43.6	447	4.2	64.3	19.2	0.3
Chocolate Fingers, Bournville, Cadbury*	4 Fingers/21g	106	5.2	506	5.7	63	25	4.3
Chocowafer, Milka*	1 Biscuit/30g	159	8.8	530	7.2	57.7	29.5	0
Chomp, Cadbury*	1 Bar/24g	112	4.8	465	3.3	67.9	20	0.2
Chomp, Treat Size, Cadbury*	1 Bar/12g	56	2.4	466	2.8	68	20	0.7
Christmas Tree Decoration, Average	**1 Chocolate/12g**	**63**	**3.6**	**522**	**7.6**	**56.4**	**29.9**	**0.4**
Chunk Bar, Dairy Milk, Cadbury*	1 Chunk/7g	35	2.	525	7.5	57	29.8	0.1
Cocoa Fudge, Hotel Chocolat*	1 Bar/45g	170	6.3	378	1.8	62.1	13.9	2.1
Coconut, White, Excellence, Lindt*	1 Square/10g	61	4.4	610	6	48	44	0
Coins, Marzipan, & Cherry , Favorina, Lidl*	1 Serving/30g	132	5.7	439	5.3	58	19	3.3
Cranberry, Almond, & Hazelnut, Dark, Excellence, Lindt*	1 Pack/100g	518	29	518	5.1	55	29	0
Crisp Wafer, Milk, Sainsbury's*	1 Bar/19g	98	4.8	509	6.2	64.4	25	0.8
Crispies, Chunk, Dairy Milk, Cadbury*	1 Chunk/31g	158	8.5	510	7.6	58.6	27.4	0
Crispies, Dairy Milk, Cadbury*	1 Bar/49g	250	13.4	510	7.6	58.6	27.4	0
Crispy, Sainsbury's*	4 Squares/19g	99	5.4	521	9.1	56.9	28.5	2.1
Dairy Milk with Oreo, Dairy Milk, Cadbury*	3 Chunks/15g	85	5.4	560	6.1	53.5	35.5	0.7
Dairy Milk, 30% Less Sugar, Dairy Milk, Cadbury*	1 Sm Bar/35g	176	10.8	503	5.8	42	31	18
Dairy Milk, Cadbury*	1 Bar/45g	242	13.6	534	7.3	57	30	2.1
Dairy Milk, Oreo, Mint, Dairy Milk, Cadbury*	3 Chunks/15g	84	5.2	557	5.9	54	35	1.5
Dark & Milk, Aero, Nestle*	6 Pieces/29g	155	10.2	536	7.3	43.9	35.3	6.9
Dark Alternative, 30g, Pure Heavenly*	1 Bar/30g	132	15.3	443	5.4	23.6	51.2	11.5
Dark Alternative, Raspberry, 30g, Pure Heavenly*	1 Bar/30g	131	15.2	437	5.3	24.3	50.7	12.3
Dark Alternative, with Sea Salt, 30g, Pure Heavenly*	1 Bar/30g	128	11.1	427	1.6	43.1	37.1	13.9
Dark, Finest, 85% Cocoa, Moser Roth, Aldi*	1 Bar/25g	152	12.8	608	11	18	51	15
Dark, 56%, with Coffee, J D Gross, Lidl*	1 Square/10g	55	3.8	550	5	42.2	37.6	0
Dark, 60%, Amazonas, Lidl*	1 Square/13g	75	5.2	574	5.7	44	40	7.5
Dark, 64%, Almonds, Popped Quinoa, Moser Roth, Aldi*	1 Square /10g	57	4.1	573	8.7	39	41	8.4
Dark, 70% Cocoa Solids, Extra Fine, Lindt*	1 Square/10g	54	4.1	537	8	33	41	12.2
Dark, 70% Cocoa Solids, Organic, Green & Black's*	1 Serving/18g	104	7.5	580	9.1	36	42	10

CHOCOLATE

	Measure INFO/WEIGHT	per Measure KCAL	FAT	Nutrition Values per 100g / 100ml KCAL	PROT	CARB	FAT	FIBRE
Dark, 70%, with Raspberries, Divine Chocolate*	1 Square/5g	29	2.2	584	6.7	32.2	45	11.3
Dark, 70%, Irresistible, Co-Op*	2 Squares/20g	115	8.4	575	8.5	36	42	10
Dark, 70%, No Added Sugar, Live Cultures, Ohso*	1 Bar/14g	63	4.9	466	5.1	27.1	35.9	26.1
Dark, 70%, Peruvian, Moser Roth, Aldi*	1 Square/10g	58	4.3	584	9.1	35	43	9.3
Dark, 70%, Velvet, Green & Black's*	1 Bar/90g	557	44.1	619	6.1	33	49	9.7
Dark, 70%, with Salted Caramel Pieces, J D Gross, Lidl*	1 Square/13g	68	4.6	543	7.1	41.7	36.5	9.6
Dark, 72% Cranberry, Simpkins*	2 Squares/19g	94	7.9	509	7.5	24	42.5	20
Dark, 72%, Pure, Godiva*	1 Square/10g	57	4.2	567	9.1	32	42	0
Dark, 72%, Swiss, Aldi*	4 Squares/17g	98	7.4	591	6.9	35.8	44.3	0
Dark, 75%, Madagascan, Single Origin, No.1, Waitrose*	1 Square/10g	58	4.3	585	9.3	33.4	43.8	10.5
Dark, 80%, Single Origin, Peru, Waitrose*	1 Bar/30g	182	14.6	605	9.5	26.5	48.5	12.2
Dark, 85% Cocoa, Excellence, Lindt*	1 Serving/40g	234	18.4	584	12.5	19	46	16.3
Dark, 85% Cocoa, J D Gross, Lidl*	1 Square/12g	69	5.6	579	10.8	21.4	46.8	14.5
Dark, 85% Cocoa, Swiss, The Best, Morrisons*	1/5 Bar/20g	120	9.7	600	12.4	21	48.7	14.3
Dark, 85% Cocoa, TTD, Sainsbury's*	1 Serving/25g	149	12.8	596	9.6	16.8	51.4	14.1
Dark, 85%, J D Gross, Lidl*	1 Square/13g	75	6.1	579	10.8	21.4	46.8	14.5
Dark, 90% Cocoa, Godiva*	1 Serving/30g	193	16.8	643	9.5	22	56	0
Dark, 90% Cocoa, Lindt*	1 Square/10g	59	5.5	592	10	14	55	0
Dark, 90%, Ugandan, TTD, Sainsbury's*	1 Square/10g	65	5.6	648	9.1	20.7	56.3	10.7
Dark, 95% Cocoa, Arriba, J D Gross, Lidl*	1 Square/13g	75	6.5	594	12.5	12.7	51.1	16.7
Dark, Almond, & Sea Salt, Tony's Chocolonely*	1 Bar/180g	970	63	539	7.4	44	35	0
Dark, Basics, Sainsbury's*	3 Pieces/20g	103	5.8	516	4.4	56.1	29	6.3
Dark, Baton, 100%, Hotel Chocolat*	1 Baton/8g	47	4.2	586	11.9	0	52.9	29.3
Dark, Belgian, Rich, Intense, Waitrose*	1 Square/18g	98	7	547	10.6	30	39.1	16.1
Dark, Belgian, with Raisins, & Almonds, Waitrose*	1 Square/18g	92	5.5	510	7.7	45.9	30.8	9.3
Dark, Bournville, Classic, Cadbury*	1 Bar/45g	238	13.5	530	3.8	59.5	29.9	5.5
Dark, Buttons, Giant, Bourneville, Cadbury*	1 Serving/25g	128	6.8	510	3.9	60	27	6.2
Dark, Centres, Pistachio, Ombar*	1/6 Pack/12g	74	5.8	613	7.9	40.3	48.1	0
Dark, Chilli, Excellence, Lindt*	1 Serving/40g	202	12.8	506	5.4	49	32	7
Dark, Choco-Low, Dairyfine, Aldi*	2 Squares/20g	103	7.8	514	8.3	40	39	9.6
Dark, Classic, 74% Cocoa, Tesco*	1 Square/10g	56	4.1	561	9.7	32	41	12.7
Dark, Classic, Bourneville, Cadbury*	4 Squares/25g	125	6.8	505	4.7	58.8	27.3	2
Dark, Co-Op*	1 Bar/50g	252	14.5	505	4	57	29	6
Dark, Coconut, & Rum, Extra Special, Asda*	1/5 Bar/20g	113	7.6	563	5.9	45	38	8.6
Dark, Discs, Extra Fine, M&S*	1 Disc/5g	29	2.2	572	8	31.8	43.4	11.3
Dark, Everyday Essentials, Aldi*	½ Pack/50g	258	15	517	7.2	50	30	7.3
Dark, Fair Trade, Co-Op*	1 Bar/45g	214	13	475	4	49	29	6
Dark, Finest, 74% Cocoa, Fin Carre, Lidl*	1 Square/10g	57	4.2	571	9.9	32	42	12.6
Dark, Free'ist*	1 Bar/75g	340	24	453	6	48	32	0
Dark, Fudge, Salty, Johnny Doodle*	1 Block/13g	63	3.5	504	5	56	28	0
Dark, Ganache, Belgian, Godiva*	1 Piece/8g	48	3.1	582	6.7	53	37	0
Dark, Ginger, & Turmeric, 75% Cocoa, No.1, Waitrose*	1 Square/10g	57	4	568	8.3	38.5	40.3	9.2
Dark, Ginger, & Mandarin, Peruvian, Moser Roth, Aldi*	2 Squares//20g	108	6.8	539	7	48	34	7.2
Dark, Hazelnut Crisp, Mini Bar, Mister Choc, Lidl*	1 Mini Bar/18g	102	6.8	566	7.7	46.2	37.9	4.4
Dark, Hazelnut, Fin Carre, Lidl*	2 Squares/12g	71	4.9	569	7	42.4	39.6	7.6
Dark, Hazelnut, Tortina*	1 Serving/21g	116	7.8	554	8.3	45	37	0
Dark, Honeycomb, Excellence, Lindt*	1 Serving/20g	106	6	529	5.4	56	30	0
Dark, Intense, 85% Cocoa, Tesco*	1 Square/10g	58	4.7	585	11.2	22	47	14.7
Dark, Lovetts*	3 Pieces/20g	101	5.9	507	1.2	56.5	29.3	6.3
Dark, Madagascan, 70%, J D Gross, Lidl*	1 Square/10g	56	4.1	562	8.5	33.5	41.2	11.5
Dark, Madagascan, 80%, TTD, Sainsbury's*	2 Pieces/20g	118	9.1	592	9.4	30.6	45.5	10.8
Dark, Mint, Intense, Lindt*	1 Square/10g	53	3.2	529	5	51	32	0
Dark, Mint, Refreshing, Tesco*	2 Squares/20g	111	7	557	6.7	50.2	35.2	6.7

CHOCOLATE

	Measure INFO/WEIGHT	per Measure KCAL	FAT	Nutrition Values per 100g / 100ml KCAL	PROT	CARB	FAT	FIBRE
Dark, No Added Sugar, Majani*	¼ Bar/25g	127	7.8	507	4.4	57	31	0
Dark, No Added Sugar, Red*	1 Bar/26g	74	6.2	286	4.7	33	24	0
Dark, Orange & Almond, Moser Roth, Aldi*	1 Serving/25g	133	8	532	5.9	51	32	7.9
Dark, Orange, Vivani*	4 Squares/14g	82	6.3	585	7	32.5	44.9	0
Dark, Orange, Zesty, Tesco*	2 Squares/20g	111	7.1	554	5.7	50	35.3	6.9
Dark, Peruvian, 85%, Organic, Moser Roth, Aldi*	2 Squares/20g	119	9.6	597	11	24	48	13
Dark, Plain, Average	**1oz/28g**	**143**	**7.8**	**510**	**5**	**63.5**	**28**	**2.5**
Dark, Pure, Artisan, Raw, Raw Halo Ltd*	1 Bar/33g	201	16.9	610	7.7	30.1	51.1	0
Dark, Raspberry, Velvet Fruit, Green & Black's*	8 Pieces/26g	129	7.4	490	4.3	51	28	8.1
Dark, Rich, Tesco*	1 Serving/20g	98	6.1	491	5.8	60	30.4	11.5
Dark, Roasted Hazelnut, Excellence, Lindt*	1 Square/10g	55	3.5	546	6	47	35	0
Dark, Rum & Raisin, Old Jamaica, Bourneville, Cadbury*	4 Chunks/23g	105	5.3	465	4.2	59.6	23.4	2
Dark, Salted Caramel, Bars, Moser Roth, Aldi*	1 Bar/25g	133	7.5	532	5.1	57	30	5.4
Dark, Salted Caramel, Nespresso*	1 Piece/5g	27	1.7	543	7.9	48.4	33.7	7.3
Dark, Seriously Rich, 65%, Waitrose*	1 Sm Bar/30g	169	11.6	562	8.2	40.3	38.6	10.4
Dark, Simply, Lidl*	3 Squares/20g	98	5.6	491	4.6	51	28	8.1
Dark, Smooth, Bar, Galaxy, Mars*	1 Bar/125g	651	42	521	6.2	48	33.6	9.3
Dark, Smooth, No Added Sugar, Sainsbury's*	1 Piece/10g	53	4.2	529	8.2	34.3	42.2	11
Dark, Spiced Orange, Single Origin, No.1, Waitrose*	1 Square/10g	54	3.5	540	6.1	45.4	35.3	8.2
Dark, Sugar Free, Amul*	1 Serving/11g	52	3.7	475	6	57.3	33.7	0
Dark, Super Coconut, Plant Kitchen, M&S*	1 Bar/27g	149	11.4	552	4.7	34.7	42.1	7.5
Dark, Tiddly Pot, Hotel Chocolat*	1 Serving/58g	311	22.4	537	13.9	30.5	38.7	8.7
Dark, Whole Nut, Tesco*	1 Serving/13g	67	4.5	539	6.1	48.3	35.7	6.5
Dark, with Almonds, Green & Black's*	1 Lrg Bar/90g	560	45	622	9.2	29	50	9.4
Dark, with Blood Orange, Godiva*	2 Pieces/15g	76	4.4	509	5.4	60	29	0
Dark, with Coconut, Chateau, Aldi*	1 Piece/20g	104	6.6	518	5.5	48.1	33.2	0
Dark, with Hazelnut, Les Grandes, Lindt*	1 Square/15g	88	6.3	587	8	41	42	0
Dark, with Lime, & Ginger, Delicata *	1 Thin Bar/10g	52	3	520	4.5	54	30	7
Dark, with Mint, Velvet, Green & Black's*	1 Square/9g	56	4.4	619	6.1	33	49	9.7
Dark, with Orange, Co-Op*	2 Squares/20g	108	6.8	540	6.6	47	34	7.3
Dark, with Salted Caramel, Velvet, Green & Black's*	1 Lrg Bar/90g	540	40.5	600	5.2	39	45	8.2
Dark, with Sea Salt, Velvet, Green & Black's*	1 Lrg Bar/90g	554	44.1	616	6.1	33	49	9.7
Darker Milk, Galaxy, Mars*	1 Serving/22g	119	7	542	6.1	55	32	0
Darkmilk, Cadbury*	1 Bar/35g	197	13	562	5.8	49	37	4.8
Darkmilk, Salted Caramel, Cadbury*	3 Chunks/14g	77	4.9	551	5.2	52	35	4.3
Darkmilk, with Roasted Almonds, Cadbury*	3 Chunks/14g	79	5.3	567	7.2	45	38	5.3
Dessert, Milka*	3 Square/20g	112	7.4	562	6.6	48	37	4.3
Desserts, Collection, Lily O'briens*	1 Chocolate/12g	61	3.8	505	5.3	57.9	31.6	2.6
Discovery Collection, Box, Lir Chocolates Ltd*	1 Chocolate/10g	52	3.2	517	5.7	50.2	31.6	4.6
Domes, Raspberry Crunch, Godiva*	1 Dome/10g	51	3	511	6.9	50	30	0
Double, Caramel, Cups, Deliciously Ella*	1 Pack/36g	162	8.4	450	7.3	50.2	23.4	5.1
Drops, 40% Milk, Hotel Chocolat*	1 Pot/57g	329	22.6	577	7.3	45.8	39.6	3.1
Egg, Milk, Peanut Butter, Reese's, Hershey*	1 Egg/34g	170	10	500	11.8	52.9	29.4	2.9
Eggs, M&M*	1 Serving/22g	117	6.2	528	6.2	61	28	0
Eggs, Mini, Mister Choc, Lidl*	1 Egg/3g	15	0.7	500	5	68.4	22.8	0.8
Ferrero Rocher, Ferrero*	1 Chocolate/13g	75	5.3	603	8.2	44.4	42.7	0
Ferrero Rocher, Heart, Ferrero*	1 Chocolate/13g	75	5.3	603	8.2	44.4	42.7	0
Fingers, Milk, Mister Choc, Lidl*	1 Finger/18g	104	6.9	579	6.2	51.7	38.4	0.9
Freddo, Caramel, Dairy Milk, Cadbury*	1 Freddo/19g	93	4.7	490	5.5	60.5	24.8	0.5
Freddo, Dairy Milk, Cadbury*	1 Freddo/18g	95	5.4	530	7.5	57	29.8	0.7
Freddo, Rice Crisps, Dairy Milk, Cadbury*	3 Squares/25g	131	7.1	523	7.4	58.6	28.3	0
Frog, M&S*	1 Pack/23g	126	7.5	547	7.3	55.4	32.4	2.3
Fruit & Nut, Dark, Tesco*	4 Squares/25g	124	7	494	5.8	54.8	27.9	6.5

CHOCOLATE

	Measure INFO/WEIGHT	per Measure KCAL	FAT	Nutrition Values per 100g / 100ml KCAL	PROT	CARB	FAT	FIBRE
Fruit & Nut, Dairyfine, Aldi*	4 Squares/25g	131	8	525	8.1	50	32	4.2
Galaxy, Crispy, Galaxy, Mars*	1 Portion/20g	111	6.6	546	6.4	56.7	32.2	0
Golden Biscuit Crunch, Dairy Milk, Cadbury*	4 Chunks /25g	135	8.2	545	6.2	55.5	33	0.8
Golf Balls, Milk Chocolate, Lindt*	1 Pack/110g	619	39.5	563	6.5	53.6	35.9	0
Hazelnut Crunch, Choceur, Aldi*	1 Serving/40g	226	14.4	564	9.2	49.7	36	2.4
Hearts, Raspberry, Vegan, Extra Special, Asda*	1 Heart/81g	267	18.6	330	3.8	27	23	2.6
Honeycomb, & Nuts, Dairy Milk, Cadbury*	1 Serving/11g	58	3.3	525	7.3	59.1	29.5	0
Honeycomb, Asda*	1 Serving/35g	173	7.7	495	4.3	69	22	2.1
Honeycomb, Cone, M&S*	1 Cone/73g	210	11.2	287	3.9	32.9	15.4	0.5
Jazzies, Mini, Asda*	1 Jazzie/1g	4	0.1	449	3.4	81	12	0.6
Kinder Bueno, Bar, Ferrero*	1 Bar/21g	122	8	572	8.6	49.5	37.3	0
Kinder Maxi, Ferrero*	1 Bar/21g	116	7.1	550	10	51	34	0
Kinder Surprise, Ferrero*	1 Egg/20g	110	6.8	552	8.1	52.3	34.2	0
Kinder, Bar, Small, Ferrero*	1 Bar/13g	71	4.4	566	8.7	53.5	35	0
Kinder, Bueno, Bar, White, Ferrero*	1 Piece/20g	111	7	572	8.8	53	35.9	0
Kinder, Riegel, Ferrero*	1 Bar/21g	117	7.1	558	10	53	34	0
Kirsch, Lindt & Sprungli*	1 Bar/21g	98	4.8	467	4.5	57	23	0
Lime, & Sea Salt, Sea Dog, Montezuma's*	1 Bar/90g	519	37.8	577	9	36	42	9
Little Bars, Dairy Milk, Cadbury*	1 Bar/18g	96	5.4	534	7.3	57	30	2.1
Mars, Bites, Mars*	4 Bites/20g	90	3.3	449	4.1	70.2	16.6	0
Matchmakers, Mint, Cool, Quality Street, Nestle*	4 Sticks/17g	84	3.6	495	3.7	70.6	21.3	2.4
Matchmakers, Mint, Nestle*	1 Stick/4g	20	0.8	477	4.3	69.7	20.1	0.9
Matchmakers, Orange, Nestle*	4 Sticks/17g	84	3.6	492	3.7	70	21.3	2.4
Matchmakers, Yummy Honeycomb, Nestle*	4 Sticks/15g	72	3.1	495	3.7	70.6	21.3	2.4
Medley, Dark, Biscuit & Fudge, Dairy Milk, Cadbury*	1 Piece/9g	52	3.2	555	5.9	54.5	34	2
Mikado, Daim, Mikado *	11 Biscuits/25g	119	4.5	474	6.5	70	18	3.1
Milk Alternative, Banana, 30g, Pure Heavenly*	1 Bar/30g	128	11.1	427	1.7	43	37	14
Milk Alternative, Coconut, 30g, Pure Heavenly*	1 Bar/30g	128	11.1	427	1.7	43	37	14
Milk Alternative, Dark Cherry, 30g, Pure Heavenly*	1 Bar/30g	131	15.2	437	5.3	24.3	50.7	12.3
Milk Alternative, Mint, 30g, Pure Heavenly*	1 Bar/30g	128	11.1	427	1.7	43	37	14
Mllk Alternative, Orange Flavour, Pure Heavenly*	1 Bar/30g	128	11.1	427	1.6	43.1	37.1	13.1
Milk Alternative, Salted Caramel, 30g, Pure Heavenly*	1 Bar/30g	128	11.1	427	1.7	43	37	14
Milk Alternative, Silk, 30g, Pure Heavenly*	1 Bar/30g	128	11.1	427	1.7	43	37	14
Milk Alternative, Strawberry, 30g, Pure Heavenly*	1 Bar/30g	128	11.1	427	1.7	43	37	14
Milk for Baking, Value, Tesco*	½ Bar/50g	265	14.5	530	6.7	60	29	2.2
Milk with Honey & Almond Nougat, Swiss, Toblerone*	1 Piece/8g	42	2.4	525	5.4	59	29.5	2.2
Milk with Whole Almonds, Organic, Green & Black's*	1 Lrg Bar/90g	520	38	578	11.8	37.7	42.2	5.2
Milk, 65%, Cocoa Excellence, Lindt*	1 Square/8g	51	4.3	635	8.9	24	54	0
Milk, Almond Honey Nougat, Fairtrade, Tony's Chocolonely*	¼ Bar/45g	242	14.2	537	7.8	53.7	31.5	0
Milk, Almond, Choceur, Aldi*	1 Square/29g	171	12.2	589	13	38	42	3.5
Milk, Almond, Fin Carre, Lidl*	2 Squares/13g	78	5.4	603	11.8	42.8	41.7	5
Milk, Average	*1oz/28g*	*146*	*8.6*	*520*	*7.7*	*56.9*	*30.7*	*0.8*
Milk, Bars, M&S*	1 Bar/40g	214	12.8	535	7.8	54	32	1.9
Milk, Belgian, No Added Sugar, Chocologic*	4 Squares/13g	64	4.8	484	7.9	33.7	36.2	17
Milk, Biscuit Sticks, Mikado, Kraft*	1 Stick/2.3g	11	0.5	475	7.8	67	19.8	3.1
Milk, Bubbly, Mister Choc, Lidl*	4 Squares/17g	89	5.3	538	7.9	53.5	32	2.4
Milk, Bubbly, Swiss, M&S*	1 Serving/40g	218	13.7	545	8	52	34.3	2.5
Milk, Caramel Sea Salt, Tony's Chocolonely*	1 Piece/30g	161	9.5	537	7	54.3	31.7	0
Milk, Caramel, & Sea Salt, Peruvian, Moser Roth, Aldi*	2 Squares/20g	111	6.8	553	8.3	53	34	1.4
Milk, Creamy, Organic, Green & Black's*	1 Bar/90g	504	32	560	9.1	50.3	35.5	1.6
Milk, Easter Bunnies, Aldi*	1 Bunny/13g	67	3.8	538	6.4	58.3	30.5	2.5
Milk, Everyday Essentials, Aldi*	1 Serving/25g	130	6.5	519	6	64	26	1.9
Milk, Extra Au Lait, Milch Extra, Lindt*	½ Bar/50g	268	15.5	535	6.5	57	31	0

C

CHOCOLATE

	Measure INFO/WEIGHT	per Measure KCAL	FAT	KCAL	PROT	CARB	FAT	FIBRE
Milk, Extra Creamy, Excellence, Lindt*	1 Bar/100g	560	37.1	560	6	51.1	37.1	0
Milk, Extra Fine, Swiss, M&S*	1 Serving/25g	141	9.2	565	7.2	50.9	36.7	2.3
Milk, Fair Trade, Tesco*	1 Serving/45g	236	13.3	524	7.6	56.7	29.6	2
Milk, Figures, Hollow, Dairyfine, Aldi*	1 Serving/11g	58	3.2	523	5.5	59.9	29	3.1
Milk, Fin Carre, Lidl*	1 Serving/17g	88	5	528	6.8	57.2	29.7	2.1
Milk, Fin Carre, Lidl*	1 Pack/40g	227	14.6	568	6.2	52.8	36.5	1.8
Milk, Fruit & Nut, Fin Carre, Lidl*	4 Pieces/17g	83	4.5	499	6.4	56.7	26.7	3.4
Milk, Fruit & Nut, Tesco*	2 Sqaures/18g	95	5.9	528	9.9	47.4	32.6	2.5
Milk, Giant Buttons, M&S*	1 Button/8g	44	2.7	550	7.1	52.3	34.2	0.4
Milk, Latte Macchiato, Mini Bar, Mister Choc, Lidl*	1 Mini Bar/18g	106	7.4	588	7.7	46.2	41.2	2.8
Milk, Linden Lady Chocolates*	6 Squares/25g	141	9	563	7	51	36.2	0
Milk, Lindor, Lindt*	1 Square/11g	68	5.2	615	4.7	43	47	0
Milk, Mint, Truffle Balls, Mini, Lindt*	3 Balls/15g	92	6.8	612	5.4	45	45	0
Milk, No Added Sugar, Red*	1 Bar/26g	97	6.8	372	7.6	42	26	0
Milk, Orange, Bubbly, Mister Choc, Lidl*	1 Serving/17g	92	5.4	541	6.6	56.1	31.9	1.3
Milk, Organic, Tesco*	1 Serving/25g	140	9.1	558	6.3	51.4	36.3	2.3
Milk, Plus*	1 Piece/6g	33	2	549	7.3	52	34	2.7
Milk, Rich Coffee, Bar, Tesco*	2 Squares/20g	109	6.4	547	6.6	56.6	32.3	1.7
Milk, Sainsbury's*	4 Squares/25g	133	7.7	533	9.2	54.6	30.8	2.2
Milk, Salted Butterscotch, Extra Special, Asda*	1/5 Bar/20g	110	7	552	6.9	52	35	2.7
Milk, Salted Caramel, Godiva*	1 Square/10g	53	3	524	7.1	57	30	0
Milk, Santa, Lolly, Dairyfine, Aldi*	1 Lolly/15g	81	4.5	541	6.3	60	30	2.2
Milk, Santas, Tesco*	1 Bag/90g	433	21.8	481	4.5	61.4	24.2	1.4
Milk, Strawberry Yogurt, Mini Bar, Mister Choc, Lidl*	1 Mini Bar/18g	102	6.5	566	6	52.8	36.3	2.8
Milk, Swiss, Cooking, Menier*	1 Serving/17g	89	5	538	7.3	57.4	30.4	2.8
Milk, Swiss, Diabetic with Fruit & Nuts, Boots*	½ Bar/21g	97	6.7	462	7	55	32	2.7
Milk, Swiss, Finest, Tesco*	2 Squares/20g	112	7	558	8.5	50.6	35.2	2.3
Milk, Tesco*	1 Serving/25g	133	7.7	533	9.5	54.7	30.7	2.2
Milk, Thins, Earl Grey, Prestat*	1 Thin/7g	40	2.7	575	7.9	48.1	38.6	2
Milk, Tony's Chocolonely*	1 Sm Bar/50g	272	16.6	545	7.7	51.9	33.2	0
Milk, Value, Tesco*	1/6 Bar/16g	83	4.5	520	6.8	60	28	2.3
Milk, Whole Nut, Tesco*	1 Serving/25g	129	8.4	517	8.7	53.4	33.8	9
Milk, Wholenut, with Hazelnuts, Dairyfine, Aldi*	4 Squares/25g	144	9.5	574	8.3	47	38	4.2
Milk, Winnie the Pooh, Solid Shapes, M&S*	1 Chocolate/6g	32	1.9	540	8.1	54.1	32.4	1.3
Milk, with Crunchy Honeycomb, Thorntons*	1 Pack/90g	477	27	530	6.3	57	30	0
Milk, with Orange, Divine Chocolate*	1 Sm Bar/35g	189	11	541	6.2	57.3	31.4	1.7
Milk, with Salted Pistachio, Thorntons*	1 Pack/80g	434	25.6	543	7.9	55	32	0
Milky Bar, Giant Buttons, Mars*	1 Sweet/2g	11	0.6	546	7.5	57.7	31.6	0
Mini Eggs, Aero, Nestle*	8 Eggs/24g	129	7.3	537	6.8	57.3	30.4	2.1
Mini Eggs, Belgian, Doubly Divine, Moser Roth, Aldi*	1 Egg/11g	57	3.2	516	6.2	55	29	4.5
Mini Eggs, Cadbury*	1 Egg/3g	16	0.7	495	4.6	69.5	21.5	1.3
Mini Eggs, Caramel, Cadbury*	1 Mini Egg/11g	55	2.9	485	5.7	59	25.7	0.4
Mini Eggs, Daim, Cadbury*	1 Egg/11g	60	3.4	535	6.9	56.5	30.5	1.8
Mini Eggs, Kit Kat, Nestle*	1 Mini Egg/9g	49	2.9	542	6.1	54.8	32.2	3
Mini Eggs, Lindor, Lindt*	3 Eggs/15g	92	6.8	611	5.4	45	45	0
Mini Eggs, Oreo, Cadbury*	1 Egg/10g	58	3.7	565	5.9	53.5	36	1.3
Mini, Toblerone*	1 Serving/6g	32	1.8	525	5.6	57.5	30	3.5
Mint Chips, Dairy Milk, Cadbury*	1 Bar/49g	247	12.8	505	6.6	61.6	26.1	0.6
Mint Creme, Sainsbury's*	1 Serving/20g	93	4.9	467	2.8	62.7	24.5	2.1
Mint Crisps, M&S*	1 Mint/8g	40	2.4	494	5.4	54.8	29.6	3.1
Mint, Bar, Lindor, Lindt*	1 Bar/38g	232	17.1	611	5.3	45	45	0
Mint, Bubbly, Dairyfine, Aldi*	6 Squares/25g	137	7.8	547	5.7	60	31	0.5
Mint, Thins, Mister Choc, Lidl*	7 Thins/25g	133	7.8	533	7.6	51.5	31.3	7.6

CHOCOLATE

	Measure INFO/WEIGHT	per Measure KCAL	per Measure FAT	Nutrition Values per 100g / 100ml KCAL	PROT	CARB	FAT	FIBRE
Mint, Waves, Choceur, Aldi*	7 Waves/25g	129	7	516	6.4	56	28	6
Mints, Christmas, Cadbury*	1 Mint/13g	72	5	552	6.7	45	38.7	0
Mistletoe Kisses, Mars*	1 Pack /42g	209	11.5	498	5.3	57	27.3	0
Mix Mps, Milkybar, Nestle*	1 Pack/33g	175	10.2	538	10	53.2	31.3	1.2
Mojito & Mint, After Eight, Nestle*	1 Chocolate/8g	35	1.1	424	2.1	73.4	12.9	2.8
Mountain Bar, Dark, M&S*	1 Bar/100g	572	41.9	572	7.4	36.2	41.9	10.3
Mountain Bar, Fruit & Nut, M&S*	1 Bar/100g	551	34.3	551	7	52.4	34.3	2.5
Mountain Bar, Milk, M&S*	1 Bar/100g	552	33.9	552	6.9	53.8	33.9	2.1
Mountain Bar, White, M&S*	1 Bar/100g	574	36.9	574	6.3	54.1	36.9	0.2
Natural Orange, Excellence, Lindt*	1 Bar/100g	560	37	560	7	50	37	0
Natural Vanilla, Excellence, Lindt*	1 Bar/100g	590	40	590	6	51	40	0
Nuts About Caramel, Cadbury*	1 Bar/55g	272	15.1	495	5.8	56.6	27.4	0
Nutty Nougat, Bite Sized, Sainsbury's*	1 Bar/23g	111	5.5	481	7.6	59	23.8	0.6
Operetta, M&S*	1 Chocolate/12g	71	5	589	9	40	42	0
Orange Cream, Fry's*	1 Bar/50g	210	6.8	420	2.8	72.3	13.7	0
Orange, Dark, Terry's*	1 Segment/9g	45	2.6	511	4.3	57	29.3	6.2
Orange, Milk, Mini Segments, Minis, Terry's*	1 Segment/4g	21	1.1	520	5.8	59.5	28	2.4
Orange, Milk, Terry's*	1 Orange/157g	816	44	520	5.8	59.5	28	2.4
Orange, Mini Eggs, Terry's*	6 Eggs/23g	118	6	514	6.6	64	26	1
Orange, Plain, Terry's*	1 Orange/157g	801	43.2	510	5.2	55.5	27.5	7.6
Orange, Segsations, Terry's*	1 Segsation/7g	36	2	520	6.9	58.5	28.5	2.8
Orange, Tangs, Hotel Chocolat*	1 Piece/5g	19	0.6	381	2.4	62	12	4.5
Orange, Tuile, Lindt*	1 Tuile/3g	18	1	513	5	54	29	9.6
Oreo, Bar, Dairy Milk, Cadbury*	1 Bar/41g	226	13.7	550	6	55	33.5	1.6
Oreo, Bites, Dairy Milk, Cadbury*	1 Serving/25g	138	8.2	551	5	57	33	1.5
Oreo, Original, Milka*	1 Bar/37g	203	12.2	549	5.3	57	33	1.5
Oreo, Peanut Butter, Dairy Milk, Cadbury*	1 Chunk/5g	28	1.8	558	5.9	54	35	1.5
Overload, Reeses, Hershey*	1 Pack/42g	209	10.5	498	7.4	62.8	25.1	0
Panna Cotta & Raspberry, M&S*	1 Bar/36g	190	12.1	528	4.7	51.4	33.6	0.3
Peanut Butter Cup, Big Cup, Reese's, Hershey*	1 Cup/39g	210	12	538	10.3	53.8	30.8	2.6
Peanut Butter Cup, Mini, Reeses, Hershey*	2 Mini Cups/7g	38	2.1	542	8.8	58.3	30.5	0
Peanut Butter Cup, Miniature, Reese's, Hershey*	1 Cup/9g	44	2.6	500	9.1	59.1	29.6	2.3
Peanut Butter Cup, Reese's, Hershey*	1 Cup/21g	105	6.5	500	11.9	57.1	31	5.9
Peanut Butter Cups, Dark, Hershey*	1 Pack/39g	202	12.7	519	10.6	50.7	32.5	0
Peanut Butter Cups, Sugar Free, Reese's, Hershey*	1 Cup/11g	45	3.3	409	6.8	61.4	29.6	13.6
Peanut Butter Cups, Super Nature*	1 Cup/20g	119	9.4	597	8	31	47	0
Peanut Butter Cups. Dark, Reese's*	1 Bar/39g	207	12.7	532	10.6	50.8	32.5	0
Peanut Butter, Buttercup, LoveRaw*	1 Cup/17g	100	7.3	590	15	32	43	0
Peanut Butter, Crunchy, Superfoodio*	1 Serving/16g	91	6.5	570	19.3	32.3	40.7	7.5
Peanut Caramel Crisp, Big Taste, Dairy Milk, Cadbury*	1 Chunk/12g	63	3.9	547	9.8	49	34	2.5
Pen Pals, Hotel Chocolat*	1 Animal/40g	235	16.4	588	7.5	46.2	40.9	1.5
Peppermint Cream, Fry's*	1 Bar/51g	217	7.9	425	2.6	68.8	15.4	0
Peppermint, Ritter Sport*	1 Bar/100g	483	26	483	3	60	26	0
Pingui, Kinder, Ferrero*	1 Serving/30g	135	8.9	450	7	37.8	29.7	0
Plain with Hazelnuts, Tesco*	4 Squares/25g	135	8.9	539	6.1	48.3	35.7	6.5
Plain, 72% Cocoa Solids, Finest, Tesco*	1 Square/10g	60	4.4	603	7.7	44	44	3.7
Plain, Belgian, Organic, Waitrose*	1 Bar/100g	505	37.6	505	9.6	32	37.6	5.6
Plain, Couverture, Belbake, Lidl*	1 Serving/25g	133	8	531	6.9	49	32	0
Plain, Dark, Fruit & Nut, Rich, Sainsbury's*	4 Squares/25g	122	7	489	5.2	53.9	27.9	5.7
Plain, Ms Molly*	2 Squares/17g	88	5.3	520	5.7	51	31	7
Plain, Ms Mollys*	1 Bar/100g	520	31	520	5.7	51	31	7
Plain, Whole Nut, Belgian, Waitrose*	4 Squares/25g	135	9.5	540	6.3	45.4	38	7.8
Plain, with Mint, Tesco*	2 Squares/20g	111	7	557	6.7	50.2	35.2	6.7

C

CHOCOLATE

INFO/WEIGHT	Measure	per Measure		Nutrition Values per 100g / 100ml				
		KCAL	FAT	KCAL	PROT	CARB	FAT	FIBRE
Pocket Coffee, Ferrero*	1 Pocket/13g	55	2.6	440	3.5	58.8	20.5	0
Praline, Dizzy, Hotel Chocolat*	1 Chocolate/13g	74	5.4	589	8.3	42.2	43.2	3.9
Praline, M&S*	1 Bar/34g	185	12	545	7.3	49.6	35.2	3.1
Pretzel, Salted, Choceur, Aldi*	1 Rectangle/29g	151	8.1	520	8.4	58	28	2.5
Probiotic, Bar, Ohso*	1 Bar/14g	72	5	514	5	47	36	15.5
Rafaello, Roche, Ferrero*	1 Sweet/10g	60	4.7	600	9.7	35.4	46.6	0
Raspberry Intense, Lindt*	2 Squares/20g	102	6.2	510	5	51	31	0
Raspberry, Intense, Excellence, Lindt*	1 Square/10g	52	3.1	522	5.2	51	31	0
Reindeer, Baileys*	1 Reindeer/80g	440	27.2	550	7.7	52.2	34	2.2
Reindeer, Lindt*	1 Reindeer/107g	588	35.3	550	7.2	55	33	0
Rocky Road, Clusters, Tesco*	1 Bite/11g	52	2.2	470	5.6	65.2	20.3	2.1
Salted Butterscotch, Milk, The Best, Morrisons*	2 Squares/20g	112	7.1	558	6.2	53.1	35.3	1.6
Salted Caramel, Crunchy, Choceur, Aldi*	5 Squares/33g	181	10.6	548	6.6	57	32	1.3
Salted Caramel, Lindor, Lindt*	1 Bar/100g	624	47	624	4.8	44	47	0
Sesame Grille, Lindt*	1 Square/10g	52	3.2	525	7.1	50	32	0
Sharing Block, Smarties, Nestle*	3 Pieces/17g	88	4.8	529	6.6	59.6	28.9	1.8
Smooth Mint, Vegan, Galaxy*	1 Serving/25g	165	11	660	7.2	60	44	0
Smooth Orange , Galaxy, Mars*	1 Serving/22g	120	7	545	7.2	56	32	0
Smooth Praline, Choceur, Aldi*	1 Square/5g	27	1.6	544	7.8	52	33	3.9
Snack Bar, Kinder*	1 Bar/21g	116	7.1	554	10	52	34	0
Snack Size, Dairy Milk, Cadbury*	1 Bar/30g	159	9	530	7.8	57.1	29.9	0
Snickers, More Nuts, Snickers*	1 Bar/58g	299	17.3	515	10.1	52.8	29.8	0
Snowman, Mousse, Dairy Milk, Cadbury*	1 Snowman/29g	162	10.2	560	6.7	54.5	35	0.4
Tasters, Dairy Milk, Cadbury*	1 Bag/45g	238	13.7	530	7.6	56.4	30.5	0
Tasting Selection, Green & Black's*	1 Piece/15g	85	5.8	567	9	41	39	6.7
Tiffin, Honeycomb, Hare-Brained, McVitie's*	1 Slice/41g	197	9.3	480	4.2	64	22.6	2
Tiffin, Limited Edition, Dairy Milk, Cadbury*	6 Chunks/24g	120	6	502	6.7	60	25	2.1
Toffifee, Storck*	1 Sweet/8g	43	2.4	516	5.9	58.5	28.7	0
Treatsize, Dairy Milk, Cadbury*	1 Bar/14g	73	4.2	525	7.5	57	29.8	0.7
Truffle, Bomb, Giunduja, Hotel Chocolat*	1 Truffle/10g	60	4.9	595	9.6	26.1	48.8	11.7
Turkish Delight, Dairyfine, Aldi*	3 Squares/25g	119	6	475	3.4	62	24	0.5
Turkish Delight, Lge Bar, Dairy Milk, Cadbury*	1 Square/8g	35	1.6	470	5.6	63.2	21.4	0.5
Twirl, Bites, Cadbury*	1 Bite/2g	11	0.6	530	7.7	56.5	30.3	0.8
Vanilla, & Chocolate, Swirl, Milka*	1 Bar/71g	248	16.3	350	3.4	33	23	8
Vanilla, Madagascan, Moser Roth, Aldi*	1 Bar/25g	148	10.2	590	8.3	48	41	0.5
Wafer, Bar, Time Out, Cadbury*	1 Bar/21g	111	6.1	527	6.7	60	29	2.1
Whip, Nestle*	1 Whip/28g	142	7.5	507	6	61	26.9	1.4
Whips, Double Chocolate, M&S*	1 Whip/29g	140	7.3	485	6.6	57.8	25.3	1
White with Honey & Almond Nougat, Toblerone*	1 Serving/25g	132	7.2	530	6.2	60.5	29	0.2
White with Strawberries, Divine*	1 Piece/3g	16	0.9	534	7.6	59.9	29.3	0.1
White, 0% Sugar, Blanco, Torras*	1 Piece/13g	60	4.2	464	5	57	32	4
White, Average	**1oz/28g**	**148**	**8.7**	**529**	**8**	**58.3**	**30.9**	**0**
White, Bar, Sainsbury's*	1 Strip/25g	144	9.5	578	7.1	51.4	38.2	0.5
White, Bubbly, Milka*	1 Serving/24g	127	7	531	5.4	61	29	1
White, Buttons, Smarties, Nestle*	6 Buttons/15g	77	3.9	515	7.9	61.8	26.1	0.5
White, Creamy Vanilla, Green & Black's*	1 Lge Bar/90g	516	32.9	573	7.4	53.5	36.6	0.1
White, Mice, Morrisons*	¼ Pack/18g	95	5	529	4.8	63.9	28	1
White, Mousse Au Chocolate, Moser Roth, Aldi*	1 Bar/38g	233	17.6	621	7.1	43	47	0.5
White, Tiny, Toblerone*	1 Tiny/8g	43	2.4	535	6.1	62	29.5	0.2
White, Toblerone*	1 Triangle/33g	177	9.6	537	6.1	62	29	0.2
White, with Oreo, Cadbury*	3 Chunks/15g	83	5	560	4.4	59	34	0.5
Whole Nut, Dairy Milk, Cadbury*	1 Bar/49g	270	17.4	550	8.9	49.5	35.4	1.7
Whole Nut, Sainsbury's*	4 Chunks/25g	142	9.4	566	8.5	48.5	37.6	2.6

CHOCOLATE

	INFO/WEIGHT	KCAL	FAT	KCAL	PROT	CARB	FAT	FIBRE
Wildlife Bar, Cadbury*	1 Bar/21g	109	6.2	520	7.8	56.8	29.3	0
Winter Gingerbread, Dairy Milk, Cadbury*	3 Pieces/15g	82	5	549	6.1	56	33	1.8
Wispa, Bitsa Wispa, Cadbury*	¼ Bag/43g	238	14.7	550	7.3	53	34	0.9
with Crunchie Bits, Dairy Milk, Cadbury*	1 Bar/200g	1000	48.8	500	6.2	63.3	24.4	0
with Hazelnuts, Whole, Milka*	2 Squares/15g	83	5.3	554	8.1	50	35.5	2
with Shortcake Biscuit, Dairy Milk, Cadbury*	1 Square/6g	31	1.7	520	7.5	59	28	0

CHOCOLATE SPREAD

	INFO/WEIGHT	KCAL	FAT	KCAL	PROT	CARB	FAT	FIBRE
& Caramel, Gu*	1 Serving/25g	153	11.5	613	4.2	45	46	2
& Hazelnut, Smooth, Nutsy*	1 Serving/25g	136	7.6	542	1.6	66	30.2	0
Average	*1 Tsp/12g*	*68*	*4.5*	*569*	*4.1*	*57.1*	*37.6*	*0*
Caramel, Morrisons*	1 Tsp/5g	27	1.5	535	6.1	58.9	30.4	0.8
Chocaholic, The Skinny Food Co.*	1 Tsp/5g	25	1.9	494	5	53	38	2.8
Cocospread, Violife*	1 Spread/10g	24	1.6	235	1.5	21	16	0
Crunchie, Cadbury*	1 Tsp/5g	28	1.7	554	3.4	58	34	1.5
Crunchy, Hazelnut, Vego*	1 Tbsp/15g	84	5.4	563	6.1	51	36	5.5
Hazelnut, Jim Jams*	1 Tbsp/15g	74	5.5	494	6.4	49.4	36.6	0
Hazelnut, No Added Sugar, Tesco*	1 Tbsp/15g	75	5.6	502	6.3	49.5	37.5	2.8
Hazelnut, Nutella, Ferrero*	1 Tbsp/15g	80	4.6	533	6.6	56.4	31	3.5
Hazelnut, Nutoka, Aldi*	1 Tsp/5g	27	1.7	549	5.9	54	34	3.2
Hazelnut, Sainsbury's*	1 Serving/12g	67	4.2	555	6	53.5	34.5	3
Hazelnut, Smooth, Plant Kitchen, M&S*	1 Tbsp/15g	85	5.6	569	4.2	51.6	37.1	6
Hazelnut, Weight Watchers*	1 Serving/15g	50	1.8	333	4.7	45.3	12	12
La Crema, Vegan, Valsoia*	1 Serving/15g	77	4.2	514	5.2	57	28	6.8
White, Myprotein*	1 Tbsp/15g	81	6	540	22	33	40	0.1
with Nuts	*1 Tsp/12g*	*66*	*4*	*549*	*6.2*	*60.5*	*33*	*0.8*

CHOCOLATES

	INFO/WEIGHT	KCAL	FAT	KCAL	PROT	CARB	FAT	FIBRE
All Gold, Dark, Terry's*	1 Serving/30g	152	8.7	505	4	57.5	29	4.3
All Gold, Milk, Terry's*	1 Serving/30g	158	9.2	525	4.8	58	30.5	1.5
Alpini, Thorntons*	1 Chocolate/13g	70	4.2	538	7	54.6	32.3	2.3
Balls, Malt, WW*	1 Pack/15g	56	3	374	7	66	20	2.8
Bites, Maltesers*	1 Bag/32g	166	8.6	518	7.4	60	27	0
Buttons, Free From, Co-Op*	1 Serving/25g	136	8.8	543	2.5	48	35	12
Buttons, Giant, Aldi*	1 Bag/120g	665	38.4	554	7.7	58	32	2.4
Buttons, Milk Chocolate, Giant, Mister Choc, Lidl*	1 Serving/20g	109	6.5	543	6.5	55.8	32.5	0.5
Buttons, Milk, Giant, Organic, Montezuma's*	1 Lge Bag/180g	1033	70.2	574	6	50	39	2
Buttons, Mint, Maltesers, Mars*	1 Serving/34g	176	9.2	517	7.42760		27	0
Buttons, Twisted, Dairy Milk, Cadbury*	1 Serving/25g	134	7.5	535	6.1	60	30	1.1
Buttons, White Chocolate, Dairyfine, Aldi*	1 Pack/70g	386	22.4	551	4.4	61	32	0.5
Caramels, Sainsbury's*	1 Sweet/12g	57	2.6	490	3.5	69	22.2	0.2
Celebrations, Mars*	1 Sweet/8g	40	2	497	5.6	61.7	25	1.7
Coconut, Lindor, Lindt*	1 Ball/13g	79	6	632	5.4	42	48	0
Coffee Cream, Average	*1 Chocolate/12g*	*54*	*2*	*446*	*3.3*	*70.4*	*17*	*2.4*
Continental, Belgian, Thorntons*	1 Chocolate/13g	67	3.9	514	5.8	53.5	30.3	2.9
Continental, Thorntons*	1 Chocolate/15g	76	4.4	506	5.6	54.5	29.3	2.7
Cookies n Creme, Drops, Hershey's*	½ Pack/40g	205	10.4	512	6	63.9	26.1	0
Country Caramel, Milk, Thorntons*	1 Chocolate/9g	45	2.4	500	4.6	62.2	26.7	0
Cow Spots, Milka*	1 Serving/20g	106	5.8	530	6	60	29	1.6
Creme, Wafer Curls, Galaxy, Mars*	1/3 Pack/30g	151	6.9	502	8.4	64	23	0
Crunchie Rocks, Cadburys *	4 Pieces/24g	115	4.6	478	4.7	71	19	2
Dairy Box, Milk, Nestle*	1 Piece/11g	50	2.1	456	4.4	65.9	19.4	0.7
Dark Milk, Buttons, Giant, Cadbury*	1 Serving/25g	140	9.2	562	5.8	49	37	4.8
Dark, Ginger, Real Good Food Co.*	1 Serving/20g	91	3.9	453	2.7	65.6	19.5	0
Dark, Keto Nuggets, InnoFoods*	1 Serving/20g	114	9.2	572	12	23	46	9

CHOCOLATES

INFO/WEIGHT	Measure	per Measure		Nutrition Values per 100g / 100ml				
		KCAL	FAT	KCAL	PROT	CARB	FAT	FIBRE
Dark, Rondnoir, Ferrero*	1 Ball/12g	67	4.2	555	6.2	51.4	35	0
Dark, Rose & Violet Creams	*1 Chocolate/13g*	*55*	*1.6*	*422*	*2.2*	*76.1*	*12.5*	*1.7*
Dark, Swiss Thins, Lindt*	1 Pack/125g	681	46.2	545	4.8	49.2	37	0
Delishios, GF, Schar*	1 Pack/37g	188	9.2	509	6.3	64	25	1.9
Egg Box, Luxury, Moser Roth, Aldi*	1 Egg/12g	68	4.7	567	5.8	46.7	39.2	4.2
Eggs, Mini, Dairyfine, Aldi*	1 Pack/80g	400	18.2	500	5	68.4	22.8	0.8
Filled, Average	*1 Chocolate/13g*	*58*	*2.8*	*447*	*4.9*	*62.9*	*21.3*	*1.3*
Gnawables, Super Salted Caramel, Creative Nature*	1 Bag/30g	143	6.5	478	20	47.1	21.6	0
Hazelnut & Ginger, Hotel Chocolat*	1 Chocolate/13g	72	5.3	555	8	34	40.7	9.7
Heroes, Cadbury*	1 Sweet/8g	38	1.8	480	4.8	65.1	22.4	0.4
Holdsworth*	1 Chocolate/12g	63	4.1	524	5	47	34	0
Liqueurs, Brandy, Asda*	1 Chocolate/8g	34	1.4	409	4	60	17	0.8
Liqueurs, Brandy, Favorina, Lidl*	1 Keg/12g	53	2.6	444	1.7	54.3	21.4	0
Liqueurs, Cherry, Mon Cheri, Ferrero*	1 Chocolate/11g	50	2.2	455	3	52.8	20.3	0
Liqueurs, Cognac Truffle, Thorntons*	1 Chocolate/14g	65	3.8	464	7.3	40	27.1	2.9
Liqueurs, Cointreau, Plain, Barrels	*1 Chocolate/10g*	*44*	*1.8*	*435*	*3.5*	*57*	*18*	*0*
Little Robins, Dairy Milk, Cadbury*	1 Robin/11g	58	3.4	534	7.1	57	31	0
Milk Tray, Cadbury*	1 Chocolate/9g	47	2.4	495	4.7	61.5	25.8	0.7
Milk, Mini Eggs, Green & Black's*	1 Mini Egg/8g	42	2.7	562	8.6	48.3	35.5	3.8
Milk, Swiss Thins, Lindt*	1 Pack/125g	688	43.3	550	5.8	53.6	34.6	0
Mini Eggs, Mix, Cadbury*	1 Pack/276g	1419	74.5	514	1.6	60	27	1.6
Mini Eggs, Orange, Smarties, Nestle*	4 Eggs/69g	335	13.2	486	4	73.9	19.1	1
Mini Eggs, with Soft White Truffle Centre, M&S*	1 Egg/6g	33	2	550	6.5	56.3	33.9	1.4
Mint Batons, After Dinner, M&S*	¼ Pack/31g	165	8.8	531	3.5	63.2	28.5	3.6
Mint Creams, Dark, Smooth & Fragrant, Waitrose*	1 Sweet/10g	42	0.9	410	3	77.9	9.1	2.4
Mint Crisp, Bendicks*	1 Mint/8g	38	2.3	494	5.2	55	29.9	0
Mint Crisp, Dark, Elizabeth Shaw*	1 Chocolate/6g	27	1.2	458	1.9	68	20.7	0
Mint, & Orange, Thins, After Eight, Nestle*	2 Mints/17g	71	2.1	427	2.2	73.9	12.9	2.7
Mint, Selection, Sainsbury's*	1 Chocolate/10g	48	2.3	484	3.4	64.9	23.1	1.5
Mint, Thins, After Eight, Nestle*	1 Chocolate/8g	35	1.1	428	2.3	74.1	12.9	2.7
Mints, After Eight, Dark, Nestle*	1 Sweet/7g	32	0.9	461	5	63	12.9	2
Mints, After Eight, Straws, Nestle*	4 Straws/18g	97	5.6	528	5.2	55.3	30.7	4.7
Misshapes, Assorted, Cadbury*	1 Chocolate/8g	41	2.3	515	5.2	57.5	29.1	0
Moments, Thorntons*	1 Chocolate/7g	37	2	511	5.4	59.9	27.8	1.9
Mousse au Chocolat, Hotel Chocolat*	1 Chocolate/15g	76	5.2	505	7.2	38	34.9	7.1
Mushrooms, Meiji*	1 Pack/12g	69	4.3	575	8.3	53.3	35.8	1.6
Orange Cream, Average	*1 Chocolate/12g*	*53*	*2*	*440*	*3.2*	*69.3*	*16.7*	*0*
Peppermint Bliss, Sharing Box, Aero, Nestle*	3 Chocolates/25g	136	8	546	7.4	56.4	31.8	1.7
Peppermint Cream, Average	*1 Chocolate/12g*	*50*	*1.4*	*418*	*1.9*	*76.4*	*11.4*	*1.6*
Peppermint Cream, Buchanan'*	1 Chocolate/12g	50	1.1	413	1.9	80.6	9.2	0
Pinecones, Salted Caramel, M&S*	1 Pinecone/21g	107	5.8	508	4.6	59.2	27.7	1.6
Praline, Coffee, Thorntons*	1 Chocolate/7g	37	2.4	529	7	47.1	34.3	2.9
Praline, Hazelnut, Thorntons*	1 Chocolate/5g	27	1.8	540	7	48	36	4
Praline, Marzipan, Thorntons*	1 Chocolate/14g	63	3	450	5.9	58.6	21.4	2.1
Praline, Roast Hazelnut, Thorntons*	1 Chocolate/13g	70	4.4	538	6	51.5	33.8	3.1
Pralines, Mini, Lindt*	1 Chocolate/5g	26	1.6	530	7.5	54	31	0
Quality Street, Nestle*	1 Sweet/9g	44	1.9	470	3.5	67.3	20.5	1.5
Rainbow Buttons, Morrisons*	1/3 Pack/23g	114	4.9	496	2.5	73.5	21.2	0.5
Rose & Violet Creams, Hotel Chocolat*	1 Chocolate/11g	45	1.4	412	2.3	70.6	12.4	0
Roses, Cadbury*	1 Chocolate/9g	41	1.9	480	3.3	66	22.5	1.3
Sea Shells, Belgian, Guylian*	1 Chocolate/14g	78	5	555	7.7	50	36	0
Seashells, Milk & White, Belgian, Waitrose*	1 Serving/15g	77	4.6	511	5	53.1	31	2.8
Stars, Mini Wishes, Truffle Centre, Cadbury*	1 Star/13g	70	4.1	540	6.9	55.6	31.8	1.3

	Measure INFO/WEIGHT	per Measure KCAL	FAT	Nutrition Values per 100g / 100ml KCAL	PROT	CARB	FAT	FIBRE
CHOCOLATES								
Strawberries & Cream, Thorntons*	1 Chocolate/12g	64	3.9	533	5.1	54.2	32.5	0.8
Truffle, & Caramel, Selection, Vegan, M&S*	1 Chocolate/10g	51	3.1	506	5.4	46.7	31.3	8.1
Truffle, Amaretto, Thorntons*	1 Chocolate/14g	66	3.6	471	5.5	55	25.7	2.9
Truffle, Balls, Swiss Milk Chocolate, Waitrose*	1 Chocolate/13g	78	5.8	621	4.1	47	46	1.4
Truffle, Belgian Milk, Waitrose*	1 Truffle/14g	74	4.8	525	5.8	52.9	34.1	1.2
Truffle, Caramel Milk Chocolate, Aldi*	1 Truffle/12g	76	5.8	633	5.8	42.5	48.3	4.2
Truffle, Champagne, Premier, Thorntons*	1 Chocolate/17g	88	5.6	518	6.9	45.3	32.9	2.4
Truffle, Dark, Balls, Lindor, Lindt*	1 Ball/12g	76	6.2	630	3.4	38.5	51.4	0
Truffle, Filled, Swiss, Balls, Finest, Tesco*	3 Balls/37g	240	19	640	5	40.7	50.8	1.5
Truffle, French Cocoa Dusted, Sainsbury's*	1 Truffle/10g	57	4.5	570	4	37	45	0
Truffle, Hazelnut, Balls, Lindor, Lindt*	1 Ball/12g	76	6.1	632	5	39.1	50.6	0
Truffle, Lemon, White, Thorntons*	1 Chocolate/14g	63	3.5	450	4.6	64.3	25	0.7
Truffle, Milk Chocolate, Balls, Lindor, Lindt*	1 Ball/12g	75	5.6	623	4.9	44	47	2.8
Truffle, Mini Milk Chocolate Balls, Lindor, Lindt*	3 Balls/15g	90	7	600	6.7	40	46.7	0
Truffle, Rum, Average	**1 Truffle/11g**	**57**	**3.7**	**521**	**6.1**	**49.7**	**33.7**	**1.9**
Truffle, Selection, Tesco*	1 Chocolate/14g	75	4.2	539	5.1	62	29.8	0.5
Truffle, Seville, Thorntons*	1 Chocolate/14g	76	4.7	543	7.1	53.6	33.6	1.4
Truffle, Thorntons*	1 Chocolate/7g	33	1.9	471	6	48.6	27.1	1.4
Truffle, Vanilla, Thorntons*	1 Chocolate/13g	64	3.5	492	4.8	57.7	26.9	1.5
Truffle, Viennese, Dark, Thorntons*	1 Chocolate/10g	53	3.6	530	5.9	47	36	3
Truffle, Viennese, Milk, Thorntons*	1 Chocolate/10g	56	3.6	560	4.9	54	36	0
Truffle, White Chocolate, Balls, Lindor, Lindt*	1 Ball/12g	76	5.9	636	3.7	45	49	0
Truffles, Banana, Protein, Pure*	1 Protein Ball/14g	81	5.9	580	19.7	28	42.1	0
Truffles, Dark, & Hazelnut, Baci, Perugina*	1 Truffle/13g	71	4.8	565	7.1	45	38	6.5
Truffles, Extra Dark, Lindor, Lindt*	1 Truffle/12g	76	6.2	637	5	34	52	0
Truffles, Irish Cream Liqueur, M&S*	1 Truffle/12g	67	4.4	553	4.9	51.3	36.7	1.9
Truffles, Milk, Simple, Hotel Chocolat*	1 Truffle/11g	58	4.2	526	6.4	39.3	38.5	2.8
Truffles, Orange , Galaxy, Mars*	1 Truffle/21g	116	7.2	552	5.3	53.4	34.5	0
Truffles, Orange, Terry's*	1 Truffle/10g	53	3	532	5.1	59	30	2.6
Truffles, Salted Caramel, Intrigue, Quality Street, Nestle*	2 Chocolates/20g	93	5.1	461	3.8	52.8	25.4	3.2
Truffles, Salted Caramel, Irresistible, Co-Op*	1 Chocolate/11g	57	3.3	519	4.7	57	30	1.5
Truffles, Salted Caramel, Lindor, Lindt*	1 Ball/12g	75	5.6	623	4.9	43	47	0
Truffles, Salted Caramel, Plant Kitchen, M&S*	1 Truffle/12.5g	61	3.8	489	6.9	43.7	30.6	5.8
Whisky Creme, Shells, Hotel Chocolat*	1 Piece/11g	54	3.7	488	6.5	39.3	33.2	3.2
CHOW MEIN								
Beef, Ready Meal, Average	**1 Serving/400g**	**422**	**12.2**	**106**	**6**	**13.4**	**3**	**1**
Chicken, & Vegetable, COU, M&S*	1 Pack/380g	262	3.8	69	6.6	7.4	1	1.9
Chicken, & Vegetable, Slim Cook, Tesco*	1 Pack/490g	304	2.5	62	5.9	7.6	0.5	1.9
Chicken, Ready Meal, Average	**1 Serving/400g**	**375**	**9.4**	**94**	**6.5**	**11.5**	**2.4**	**1.2**
Pork, PB, Waitrose*	½ Pack/310g	332	2.8	107	7.6	17.2	0.9	1.6
Prawn, Takeaway, Chinese	**1 Portion/550g**	**792**	**60**	**144**	**5.6**	**6.1**	**10.9**	**2.8**
Special, Ready Meal, Average	**1 Serving/400g**	**383**	**9.7**	**96**	**6.5**	**12.1**	**2.4**	**1**
Vegetable, Ready Meal, Average	**1 Serving/400g**	**337**	**6.7**	**84**	**4.2**	**12.8**	**1.7**	**2**
CHRISTMAS PUDDING								
Alcohol Free, 450g, Sainsbury's*	1 Serving/114g	330	3.5	290	2.7	61.3	3.1	3.2
Average	**1oz/28g**	**81**	**2.7**	**291**	**4.6**	**49.5**	**9.7**	**1.3**
Free From, Sainsbury's*	1 Pudding/100g	303	6.2	303	1.9	58.1	6.2	3.8
GF, Made Without Wheat, M&S*	1 Pack/100g	336	6.7	336	2.2	64.5	6.7	4.6
Gluten & Wheat Free, Finest, Tesco*	1 Pudding/100g	305	7.1	305	3.3	55.1	7.1	3.7
Hidden Clementine, Heston, Waitrose*	1 Serving/114g	352	7.7	310	2.9	57.8	6.8	3.1
Luxury	**1 Serving/114g**	**416**	**18.8**	**365**	**2.5**	**48.6**	**16.4**	**1**
Nut Free & Alcohol Free, Tesco*	1 Serving/114g	395	7.6	347	2.2	68.2	6.7	2.6
Plant Kitchen, M&S*	1 Pudding/100g	341	6.9	341	2.2	65.4	6.9	4.2

CHUTNEY	Measure INFO/WEIGHT	per Measure KCAL	FAT	Nutrition Values per 100g / 100ml KCAL	PROT	CARB	FAT	FIBRE
Albert's Victorian, Baxters*	1 Tbsp/15g	23	0	151	1	35.2	0.3	1.8
Apple, & Pear, Spiced, M&S*	1 Tbsp/15g	34	0	230	0.8	55.5	0.2	1.6
Apricot, Sharwood's*	1 Tbsp/15g	21	0	131	0.6	32	0.1	2.3
Beetroot, & Orange, Extra Special, Asda*	1 Tbsp/15g	20	0.1	136	0.5	32	0.5	1.6
Bengal Spice Mango, Sharwood's*	1 Tbsp/15g	35	0	236	0.5	58	0.2	1.2
Caramelised Onion, Sainsbury's*	1 Tbsp/15g	17	0.2	111	1.1	23.5	1.4	1.1
Caramelised Red Onion, Shaws*	1 Tbsp/15g	28	0	186	0.9	44.5	0.1	0
Fig, Plum, & Date, Specially Selected, Aldi*	1 Tbsp/15g	30	0.1	202	1.4	46	0.9	2.9
Gooseberry, Hot, Tiptree, Wilkin & Sons*	1 Tbsp/15g	39	0	263	0	63	0	0
Lime & Chilli, Geeta's*	1 Tbsp/15g	38	0.2	253	1.9	57.5	1.3	1.7
Mango, Hot & Spicy, Waitrose*	1 Tbsp/15g	46	0.1	230	0.6	51.6	0.3	1.8
Mango, Sainsbury's*	1 Tbsp/15g	38	0.1	255	0.5	61.9	0.5	1.5
Mango, Spicy, Sainsbury's*	1 Tbsp/15g	33	0.1	222	0.5	53.8	0.5	1.9
Mango, Sweet	*1 Tbsp/15g*	*28*	*0*	*189*	*0.7*	*48.3*	*0.1*	*0*
Mixed Fruit	*1 Tbsp/15g*	*23*	*0*	*155*	*0.6*	*39.7*	*0*	*0*
Onion, Asda*	1 Tbsp/15g	19	0.1	126	0.7	29	0.5	1.1
Onion, Vitasia, Lidl*	1 Tbsp/15g	40	0.1	266	0.9	63.1	0.9	0
Ploughman's, M&S*	1 Tbsp/15g	22	0	150	0.8	34.6	0.3	2.9
Ploughmans, Mrs Bridges*	1 Tbsp/15g	32	0.1	212	1.6	49.6	0.9	0
Plum, & Apple, Deluxe, Lidl*	1 Tbsp/15g	20	0.1	134	0.3	31.4	0.4	1.6
Plum, Ploughman's, Tesco*	1 Tbsp/15g	23	0.1	154	1	34.1	0.4	5.3
Red Onion, Tesco*	1 Tbsp/15g	21	0	140	0.5	33.3	0.2	1.3
Red Onion, Tiptree, Wilkin & Sons*	1 Tbsp/15g	45	0.2	301	2.3	63	1.5	0
Sweet Mango, Patak's*	1 Tbsp/15g	39	0	259	0.3	67.4	0.1	0.7
Tamarind, Premium, Medium, Geeta's*	1 Tbsp/15g	40	0.1	264	1.1	64	0.4	1.5
Tamarind, Premium, Medium, Geeta's*	1 Tbsp/15g	40	0.1	264	1.1	64	0.4	1.5
Tomato	*1 Tbsp/15g*	*19*	*0*	*128*	*1.2*	*31*	*0.2*	*1.3*
Tomato & Chilli, Specially Selected, Aldi*	1 Tbsp/15g	21	0.1	138	12	32	0.5	1.3
Tomato, & Red Pepper, Arran Fine Foods*	1 Tbsp/15g	18	0	117	1.7	26	0	0
Tomato, Mediterranean, Branston*	1 Tbsp/15g	23	0.1	155	1.5	34.6	0.6	1.8
Tomato, Sundried, & Garlic, Woolliss & Sons Ltd*	1 Tbsp/15g	17	0	113	1.4	25.2	0.2	1.3
CIDER								
4.5%, M&S*	1 Bottle/500ml	180	0	36	0	0	0	0
Apple, Low Alcohol, Sainsbury's*	1 Glass/250ml	75	0.4	30	0.5	5.4	0.2	0
Apple, Medium, Inch's*	1 Bottle/500ml	215	0	43	0	0	0	0
Basics, Sainsbury's*	1 Glass/250ml	200	0	80	0	0	0	0
Berries, & Cherries, 4%, Old Mout*	1 Bottle/500ml	270	0	54	0	7.8	0	0
Berry, Irish, Magner's*	1 Bottle/500ml	215	0	43	0	4.3	0	0
Black Fox, Organic, Dunkertons*	1 Bottle/500ml	317	0	63	0	0	0	0
Cornish, Cloudy, Rattler Original*	1 Bottle/500ml	185	0	37	0	0	0	0
Cyder, Organic, Aspall*	1 Serving/200ml	120	0.2	60	0.1	3.1	0.1	0
Cyder, Perronelle's Blush, Aspall*	1 Serving/200ml	122	0.2	61	0.1	5.4	0.1	0.5
Cyder, Premier Cru, Aspall*	1 Serving/200ml	120	0	60	0	3.1	0	0
Cyder, Suffolk, Medium, Aspall*	1 Serving/200ml	134	0	67	0.1	4.4	0	0
Dabinett, 7.2%, M&S*	1 Bottle/500ml	260	0	52	0	0	0	0
Dry, Average	*1 Pint/568ml*	*205*	*0*	*36*	*0*	*2.6*	*0*	*0*
Dry, Strongbow*	1 Bottle/375ml	161	0	43	0	3.4	0	0
Founder's Reserve, Symonds*	1 Serving/200ml	72	0	36	0	2.6	0	0
Gold, Cornish Orchards*	1 Bottle/500ml	235	0	47	0	0	0	0
Gold, Thatchers*	1 Bottle/500ml	230	0	46	0	4.5	0	0
Haze, Cloudy, Thatchers*	1 Bottle/500ml	245	0	49	0	2.4	0	0
Laid Back, 2.5%, M&S*	1 Can/330ml	125	0	38	0	0	0	0
Light, Bulmers*	1 Can/500ml	140	0	28	0	0.8	0	0

	Measure INFO/WEIGHT	per Measure KCAL	FAT	Nutrition Values per 100g / 100ml KCAL	PROT	CARB	FAT	FIBRE
CIDER								
Low Alcohol	**1 Pint/568ml**	**97**	**0**	**17**	**0**	**3.6**	**0**	**0**
Low Carb, Stowford*	1 Bottle/500ml	140	0	28	0	0.2	0	0
Magner's*	½ Pint/284ml	105	0	37	0	2	0	0
Nordic Berries, Alska*	1 Bottle/500ml	195	0	39	0	1.1	0	0
Organic, Westons*	1 Serving/200ml	96	0	48	0	3.1	0	0
Original, Bulmers*	1 Serving/250ml	105	0	42	0	4	0	0
Passionfruit, Rekorderlig*	1 Bottle/500ml	315	0	63	0	8.5	0	0
Pear, Bulmers*	1 Serving/200ml	86	0	43	0	3.6	0	0
Pear, Magner's*	1 Bottle/568ml	179	0	32	0	0	0	0
Riserva, Craft, Italian, 6.8%, Angioletti*	1 Bottle/500ml	294	0	59	0	1	0	0
Rose, Craft, Italian, 4%, Angioletti*	1 Bottle/500ml	183	0	37	0	0.5	0	0
Rose, Irish, Magner's*	1 Can/330ml	125	0	38	0	0	0	0
Rose, Strongbow*	1 Can/440ml	189	0	43	0	0	0	0
Scrumpy, Average	**1 Serving/200ml**	**93**	**0**	**46**	**0**	**2.3**	**0**	**0**
Secco, Craft, Italian, 5%, Angioletti*	1 Bottle/500ml	202	0	40	0	1	0	0
Somerset Vintage, 7.4%, M&S*	1 Bottle/500ml	265	0	53	0	0	0	0
Somerset, Traditional, 4.5%, M&S*	1 Bottle/500ml	160	0	32	0	0	0	0
Strawberry & Lime, Non Alcoholic, Kopparberg*	1 Bottle/500ml	205	2.5	41	0.5	10.1	0.5	0
Strawberry, & Pomegranate, 4%, Old Mout*	1 Bottle/500ml	265	0	53	0	7.4	0	0
Sweet, Average	**1 Pint/568ml**	**239**	**0**	**42**	**0**	**4.3**	**0**	**0**
Vintage	**1 Pint/568ml**	**574**	**0**	**101**	**0**	**7.3**	**0**	**0**
Zero, Bulmers*	1 Bottle/330ml	66	1.6	20	0.5	5.1	0.5	0
CINNAMON								
Ground, Average	**1 Tsp/3g**	**8**	**0.1**	**261**	**3.9**	**55.5**	**3.2**	**0**
Stick, Average	**1 Stick/1g**	**3**	**0**	**246**	**3.9**	**77**	**1.5**	**53.1**
CLAMS								
in Brine, Average	**1oz/28g**	**22**	**0.2**	**79**	**16**	**2.4**	**0.6**	**0**
Raw, Average	**20 Sm/180g**	**133**	**1.7**	**74**	**12.8**	**2.6**	**1**	**0**
CLEMENTINES								
Raw, Weighed with Peel, Average	**1 Med/61g**	**22**	**0.1**	**35**	**0.6**	**9**	**0.1**	**1.3**
Raw, Weighed without Peel, Average	**1 Med/46g**	**22**	**0.1**	**47**	**0.8**	**12**	**0.2**	**1.7**
COCKLES								
Boiled	**1 Cockle/4g**	**2**	**0**	**53**	**12**	**0**	**0.6**	**0**
Bottled in Vinegar, Drained	**1oz/28g**	**8**	**0.1**	**28**	**6.3**	**0**	**0.3**	**0**
COCKTAIL								
Alcoholic, Juice Based, Average	**1 Glass/200ml**	**464**	**29.2**	**232**	**6.4**	**18.7**	**14.6**	**1.4**
Bloody Mary, Average	**1 Glass/250ml**	**86**	**0**	**42**	**0**	**2.3**	**0**	**0.6**
Bucks Fizz, Premixed, M&S*	1 Glass/250ml	152	0	61	0	9	0	0
Bucks Fizz, Tesco*	1 Serving/200ml	100	0	50	0	0	0	0
Cherry, & Amaretto, Fizz, M&S*	1 Glass/125ml	75	0	60	0	0	0	0
Cosmo, Skinny Brands*	1 Can/250ml	90	0.2	36	0	1.3	0.1	0
Cosmopolitan, Canned, M&S*	1 Serving/200ml	456	0	228	0	22	0	0
Daiquiri, Strawberry, Frozen, Average	**1 Glass/250ml**	**132**	**0**	**53**	**0**	**14.1**	**0**	**0**
Gin & Lemonade, Strawberry & Lime, Kopparberg*	1 Can/250ml	72	1.2	29	0.5	0	0.5	0
Grenadine, Orange Juice, Pineapple Juice	**1 Serving/200ml**	**158**	**0.3**	**79**	**0.5**	**19.2**	**0.1**	**0.2**
Long Island Iced Tea, Average	**1 Glass/250ml**	**282**	**0**	**113**	**0**	**13.6**	**0**	**0**
Mai Tai, Average	**1 Serving/200ml**	**209**	**0.1**	**105**	**0.2**	**13.9**	**0.1**	**0.1**
Mix, Bloody Mary, Bloody Ben's*	1 Serving/25ml	17	0	67	1.3	14.2	0.1	0.8
Mixer, Espresso Martini, Tipplesworth*	1 Serving/50ml	61	0	122	0.3	29.1	0.1	0
Mojito, Canned, M&S*	1 Can/250ml	208	0	83	0	8.9	0	0
Pina Colada	**1 Glass/250ml**	**592**	**20**	**237**	**1**	**28**	**8**	**0**
Raspberry Mojito, Shake Baby Shake*	1 Can/250ml	145	0	58	0	8.3	0	0

	Measure INFO/WEIGHT	per Measure KCAL	FAT	Nutrition Values per 100g / 100ml KCAL	PROT	CARB	FAT	FIBRE
COCOA								
Nibs, Naturya*	1 Serving/10g	58	5	578	13	18.2	50.3	13.4
COCOA POWDER								
Dark, Fine, Dr Oetker*	3 Tbsp/25g	89	5.2	357	20	8.9	21	28
Dry, Unsweetened, Average	*1 Tbsp/5g*	*11*	*0.7*	*229*	*19.6*	*54.3*	*13.7*	*33.2*
Hazelnut, Hotel Chocolat*	1 Pack/35g	37	2	105	4.8	8.7	5.6	0.5
Organic, Green & Black's*	1 Tsp/4g	16	0.8	405	22	19	21	27
COCONUT								
Creamed, Average	*1oz/28g*	*186*	*19.2*	*666*	*6*	*6.7*	*68.4*	*7*
Desiccated, Average	*1oz/28g*	*169*	*17.4*	*604*	*5.6*	*6.4*	*62*	*13.7*
Flaked, Neal's Yard*	1 Serving/30g	181	18.6	604	5.3	44.4	62	13.7
Flakes, Unsweetened, Dr Goerg*	1 Serving/100g	686	67	686	7	6	67	15.6
Fresh, Flesh Only, Average	*1oz/28g*	*69*	*7.1*	*246*	*2.2*	*2.6*	*25.2*	*5.1*
Ice, Average	*1oz/28g*	*104*	*3.6*	*371*	*1.7*	*66.7*	*12.7*	*2.6*
Rolls, Kiddylicious*	1 Pack/7g	37	2	529	2.9	64.7	27.9	1.5
Toasted, Julian Graves*	1 Serving/5g	33	3.2	655	8	9	65	13
COD								
Baked, Average	*1oz/28g*	*27*	*0.3*	*96*	*21.4*	*0*	*1.2*	*0*
Beer Battered, TTD, Sainsbury's*	1 Fillet/180g	356	17.1	198	11.5	16.4	9.5	0.5
Breaded, Chunky, GF, Free From, Waitrose*	1 Fillet/162g	290	12	179	12.4	15.4	7.4	0.6
Dried, Salted, Average	*1oz/28g*	*82*	*0.7*	*290*	*62.8*	*0*	*2.4*	*0*
Fillet, Battered, Jumbo, Arctic Royal*	1 Fillet/250g	420	18.8	168	8	15.2	7.5	0
Fillet, Beer Battered, M&S*	1 Fillet /190g	334	17.1	176	13.9	9	9	0.9
Fillet, Bites, M&S*	1 Serving/95g	189	7.6	199	13.7	17.5	8	1.1
Fillet, Breaded, Youngs*	1 Fillet/108g	251	15	232	12.3	14	13.9	1.2
Fillets, Battered, Average	*1 Fillet/125g*	*219*	*10.2*	*176*	*12.6*	*13*	*8.2*	*1*
Fillets, Breaded, Average	*1 Fillet/125g*	*258*	*12.2*	*206*	*13*	*16.7*	*9.8*	*1*
Fillets, Breaded, Chunky, Average	*1 Piece/135g*	*204*	*8*	*151*	*13.7*	*10.9*	*5.9*	*1.4*
Fillets, Breaded, Light, Healthy Range, Average	*1 Fillet/135g*	*209*	*6.9*	*154*	*13.6*	*13.3*	*5.1*	*1.2*
Fillets, Chunky, Average	*1 Fillet/198g*	*267*	*7.3*	*135*	*17.1*	*8.2*	*3.7*	*0.8*
Fillets, Skinless & Boneless, Raw, Average	*1 Fillet/140g*	*137*	*2.4*	*98*	*17.8*	*0*	*1.8*	*0.4*
Fillets, Smoked, Average	*1 Serving/150g*	*152*	*2.4*	*101*	*21.6*	*0*	*1.6*	*0*
Fillets, Tempura, Battered, Crispy, Gastro, Youngs*	1 Fillet/131g	252	12.1	192	12.9	14.1	9.2	0.8
Fillets, Wild, Icelandic, Eat Well, M&S*	1 Fillet/107g	81	1.3	76	16.2	0.1	1.2	0.1
Fillets, Wild, in Tomato & Rosemary Sauce, Birds Eye*	1 Fillet/136g	184	10.9	135	15	0.8	8	0.5
Fillets, with Cheese, & Chive, M&S*	½ Pack/175g	184	7.4	105	13	3.5	4.2	0.5
Fillets, with Puttanesca Sauce, Co-Op*	½ Pack/190g	150	4.9	79	11.6	2.1	2.6	0.6
Filltes, Breaded, GF, Free From, Tesco*	1 Fillet/135g	263	10.4	195	12.7	18	7.7	1.5
Loins, Average	*1 Serving/145g*	*116*	*1.2*	*80*	*17.9*	*0.1*	*0.8*	*0.2*
Mornay, with Mash & Peas, HL, Tesco*	1 Pack/364g	335	9.1	92	7.7	8.6	2.5	2
Poached, Average	*1oz/28g*	*26*	*0.3*	*94*	*20.9*	*0*	*1.1*	*0*
Smoked, Raw, Average	*1oz/28g*	*22*	*0.2*	*78*	*18.1*	*0*	*0.6*	*0*
Steaks, Battered, Chip Shop Style, Average	*1 Serving/150g*	*321*	*18*	*214*	*12.5*	*14.3*	*12*	*1.1*
Steaks, in Butter Sauce, Youngs*	1 Serving/137g	111	3.2	81	9.8	5.1	2.3	0.2
Steamed, Average	*1oz/28g*	*23*	*0.3*	*83*	*18.6*	*0*	*0.9*	*0*
COFFEE								
3 in 1, Kenco*	1 Sachet/20g	83	2.1	415	2.5	80	10.5	0
Amaretto Almond, Decaf, Instant, Beanies*	1 Tsp/4g	3	0	82	15	4.5	0.5	0
Americano, Azera, Made up, Nescafe*	1 Cup/200ml	2	2	1	0.1	3	1	0.3
Americano, Decaf, Pod, Kenco*	1 Pod/17g	0	0	1	0.2	0.1	0	0
Azera, Barista Style Instant, Nescafe*	1 Serving/200ml	2	0	1	0.1	0	0	0
Black, Average	*1 Mug/270ml*	*5*	*0*	*2*	*0.2*	*0.3*	*0*	*0*
Cafe Hazelnut, Nescafe*	1 Sachet/17g	73	2.4	428	9.3	66	14.1	0
Cafe Irish Cream, Cafe Range, Nescafe*	1 Sachet/23g	98	3.2	425	8.2	65.2	14.1	1.2

COFFEE

INFO/WEIGHT	Measure	per Measure KCAL	FAT	Nutrition Values per 100g / 100ml KCAL	PROT	CARB	FAT	FIBRE
Cafe Latte, Vita Coco*	1 Carton/330g	132	3.3	40	1.7	6	1	0
Cafe Mocha, Cafe Range, Nescafe*	1 Sachet/22g	92	2.9	418	8.5	66.6	13.1	0
Cafe Vanilla, Latte, Cafe Range, Nescafe*	1 Sachet/19g	73	1.6	395	9.2	68.3	8.5	4.1
Caffe Latte, Hotel Chocolat*	1 Sachet/35g	196	15.4	561	7.3	34.6	43.9	2.5
Cappuccino, Cafe Mocha, Dry, Maxwell House*	1 Serving/23g	100	2.5	434	4.3	78.2	10.8	0
Cappuccino, Cafe Specials, Dry, M&S*	1 Serving/14g	55	1.6	395	14	59	11.5	0.7
Cappuccino, Cappio, Iced, Kenco*	1 Can/200ml	138	6	69	3	7	3	0
Cappuccino, Decaff, Instant, Made Up, Nescafe*	1 Mug/200ml	68	2.3	34	1	5	1.2	0
Cappuccino, Decaff, Nescafe*	1 Sachet/16g	68	2.3	428	11.6	62.6	14.6	0
Cappuccino, Decaff, Unsweetened, Nescafe*	1 Sachet/16g	70	3.1	437	14.5	51.2	19.4	4.3
Cappuccino, Dry, Maxwell House*	1 Mug/15g	52	1.4	350	12	64	9.6	0.4
Cappuccino, Dry, Waitrose*	1 Sachet/13g	58	2.3	439	15.1	56	17.2	4.4
Cappuccino, for Filter Systems, Kenco*	1 Sachet/6g	22	0.8	375	19	44	13.5	0
Cappuccino, Gold, Hazelnut Flavour, Mokate*	1 Sachet/13g	56	1.2	428	5.1	80	9.4	0
Cappuccino, Gold, Nescafe*	1 Sachet/100g	60	1.3	60	1.4	10.3	1.3	0.7
Cappuccino, Iced, Cowbelle, Aldi*	1 Serving/250ml	169	4.5	68	3.3	9.6	1.8	0.3
Cappuccino, Iced, Dolce Gusto, Nescafe*	1 Cup/235ml	113	2.8	48	1.8	7.3	1.2	0.2
Cappuccino, Instant, Aldi*	1 Sachet/13g	49	1.7	393	12.5	55.1	13.6	0
Cappuccino, Instant, Asda*	1 Sachet/15g	60	2.3	399	13	53	15.2	0.9
Cappuccino, M&S*	1 Serving/164g	66	2.6	40	1.5	4.4	1.6	0
Cappuccino, Made Up, Dolce Gusto, Nescafe*	1 Serving/240ml	84	3.7	35	1.6	4	1.5	0.3
Cappuccino, Original, Sachets, Nescafe*	1 Sachet/18g	80	3.1	444	11.7	60.3	17.4	0
Cappuccino, Semi Skimmed Milk, Average	**1 Serving/200ml**	**63**	**2.3**	**31**	**2.2**	**3.2**	**1.2**	**0**
Cappuccino, Skinny, Sachets, Gold, Nescafe*	1 Sachet/15g	54	0.8	371	22.9	55	5.7	5
Cappuccino, Unsweetened, Gold, Bellarom, Lidl*	1 Sachet/10g	45	1.6	446	15	59	16	0
Cappuccino, Unsweetened, Gold, Nescafe*	1 Sachet/14g	55	1.8	392	12.9	52.5	13	5.7
Cappuccino, Whole Milk, Average	**1 Serving/150ml**	**87**	**4.6**	**58**	**2.9**	**4.8**	**3.1**	**0**
Capuccino, Alcafe, Aldi*	1 Sachet/135ml	61	1.6	45	0.5	8.2	1.2	0.4
Chococino, Made up, Dolce Gusto, Nescafe*	1 Serving/210g	147	5.4	70	2.3	9.4	2.6	0.7
Coconut, Caffe, Alpro*	1 Carton/250ml	88	2.8	35	0.2	5.2	1.1	0.9
Columbian, Nescafe*	1 Serving/2g	2	0	111	16.7	11.1	0	5.6
Compliment*	1 Serving/14ml	20	1.8	143	1.4	6.4	12.9	0
Cortado, Capsule, Dolce Gusto, Nescafe*	1 Capsule/80ml	23	1.1	29	1.5	1.9	1.4	1
Flat White, Duo, Instant, Made Up, Kenko*	1 Serving/22g	92	3.8	417	18.5	46.3	17.1	0
Flat White, Pods, As Sold, Dolce Gusto, Nescafe*	1 Pod/12g	50	2.3	425	19.7	36.8	19.7	4.3
Flat White, Tassimo, Kenco*	1 Cup/235ml	73	4.7	31	0.3	2.5	2	0.1
Gold Blend, Nescafe*	1 Cup 200ml/5g	3	0	63	7	9	0.2	27
Ground, Lazy Sunday, Dry Weight, Taylor's of Harrogate*	1 Scoop/7g	2	0	29	0	0	0	0
Ground, Made Up with Water, Average	**1 Serving/200ml**	**2**	**0**	**1**	**0**	**0**	**0**	**0**
Hazlenut, Caffe, Alpro*	1 Serving/250ml	78	2.2	31	0.2	5.2	0.9	1
Iced, Salted Caramel, As Prepared, Alcafe, Aldi*	1 Sachet/180ml	83	0.9	46	1.1	9.2	0.5	0.5
Iced, Soya, M&S*	1 Can/330ml	135	4.3	41	1.9	5.2	1.3	0.5
Infusion, Avg with Semi-Skimmed Milk	**1 Cup/220ml**	**15**	**0.4**	**7**	**0.6**	**0.7**	**0.2**	**0**
Infusion, Avg with Single Cream	**1 Cup/220ml**	**31**	**2.6**	**14**	**0.4**	**0.3**	**1.2**	**0**
Instant, 3 in 1, Original, As Sold, Nescafe*	1 Sachet/17g	68	2	402	2	68.3	11.6	7.5
Instant, Alta Rica, Nescafe*	1 Tsp/2g	2	0	98	13.8	10	0.3	21
Instant, Decaffeinated, Nescafe*	1 Tsp/2g	2	0	101	14.9	10	0.2	8.4
Instant, Dry Weight, Nycoffee*	1 Serving/17g	77	2	453	2.9	82.4	11.8	0
Instant, Fine Blend, Nescafe*	1 Tsp/2g	1	0	63	7	9	0.2	27
Instant, Made with Skimmed Milk	**1 Serving/270ml**	**15**	**0**	**6**	**0.6**	**0.8**	**0**	**0**
Instant, Made with Water & Semi Skimmed Milk	**1 Serving/350ml**	**24**	**0.7**	**7**	**0.4**	**0.5**	**0.2**	**0**
Instant, Made with Water, & Whole Milk	**1 Cup/220ml**	**18**	**0.9**	**8**	**0.5**	**0.6**	**0.4**	**0**
Instant, Original, Nescafe*	1 Tsp/2g	2	0	118	7.8	3.1	0.2	34.1

INFO/WEIGHT	Measure	per Measure		Nutrition Values per 100g / 100ml				
		KCAL	FAT	KCAL	PROT	CARB	FAT	FIBRE

COFFEE

Instant, Smooth, Dry Weight, Kenco*	1 Tsp/2g	2	0	100	7.5	15	0	0
Instant, Smooth, Made Up, Kenco*	1 Serving/200ml	4	0	2	0.2	0.3	0	0
Instant, with Skimmed Milk, Costa Rican, Kenco*	1 Mug/300ml	17	0.1	6	0.6	0.8	0	0
Irish Latte, Gold, Nescafe*	1 Mug/22g	90	2.2	411	8.3	70.6	9.9	2.6
Latte Macchiato, Made Up, Dolce Gusto, Nescafe*	1 Serving/220g	89	4.2	40	2	4.1	1.9	0.3
Latte, Azera My Way, Instant, As Sold, Nescafe*	1 Serving/11.5g	35	0	307	7.9	63.1	0.3	9.3
Latte, Cafe, M&S*	1 Serving/190g	142	5.3	75	4.3	8.3	2.8	0
Latte, Caramel, As Prepared with Water, Gold, Nescafe*	1 Mug/227ml	68	1.6	30	0.7	5	0.7	0.2
Latte, Caramel, Instant, Sachets, Sainsbury's*	1 Sachet/17g	70	1.7	412	8.2	71.2	10	0
Latte, Chocolate, & Caramelised Hazelnut, Gold, Nescafe*	1 Sachet/224ml	76	2	34	0.7	5.6	0.9	0.3
Latte, Cinnamon Bun, Gold, Nescafe*	1 Serving/20g	83	2.1	413	8.8	69.2	10.4	2.3
Latte, Costa, Made Up, Tassimo*	1 Cup/325ml	72	4.4	22	0.2	1.8	1.4	0.1
Latte, Double Shot, L'or, Tassimo*	1 Cup/336ml	74	4.7	22	0.3	1.8	1.4	0.1
Latte, Duo, Instant, Kenco*	1 Sachet/23g	97	3.9	423	18	50	17	0
Latte, Duo, Kenko*	1 Serving/224ml	99	3.9	44	1.8	5.4	1.7	0
Latte, Gingerbread, Costa, As Prepared, Tassimo*	1 Serving/310ml	83	4	27	0.2	3.2	1.3	0.1
Latte, Honest, Honest Organic Coffee*	1 Bottle/250ml	112	4.5	45	0	4.9	1.8	0
Latte, Iced, Salted Caramel, Dry Weight, Kenco*	1 Sachet /21g	83	1.5	391	7	75	7	0.4
Latte, Iced, Vanilla, Lavazza*	1 Can/250ml	154	3.2	62	2.8	9.8	1.3	0
Latte, Light, Dry Weight, Alcafe, Aldi*	1 Sachet/19g	75	0.9	395	22.1	63.2	4.7	2.6
Latte, Praline, Gold, Nescafe*	1 Mug/200ml	75	1.9	38	0.8	6.4	1	0.2
Latte, Sachet, Gold, Nescafe*	1 Sachet/19g	78	2.2	403	14.2	58.8	11.4	3.4
Latte, Skinny, Nescafe*	1 Sachet/20g	72	1.1	359	24.1	54.3	5.3	1.1
Latte, Skinny, Sachets, Made Up, Tesco*	1 Serving/219g	72	1.3	33	1.7	5.2	0.6	0.2
Latte, Smooth & Silky, Sachet, Kenco*	1 Sachet/20g	79	2.2	397	7	68	11	0
Latte, Soya, Caramel, Chilled, Alpro*	1 Serving/200ml	84	24	42	2.1	5.2	12	1.3
Latte, Toffee Nut, As Sold, Gold, Nescafe*	1 Sachet/19g	79	2	409	8.8	68.8	10.2	2.1
Latte, Toffee Nut, Dolce Gusto, Nescafe*	1 Pack/200ml	76	3	38	1.5	4.3	1.5	0.2
Latte, Toffee Nut, Pod, Tassimo*	1 Pod/280ml	81	4.1	29	0.2	3.6	1.5	0.1
Latte, Vanilla, Costa, Tassimo*	1 Cup/310ml	79	3.9	25	0.2	3.2	1.3	0.1
Latte, White Choco, Coconut, As Prepared, Tassimo*	1 Serving/280ml	81	4.2	29	0.2	3.6	1.5	0.1
Macchaito, Light, Chilled, Milbona, Lidl*	1 Serving/250ml	110	2	44	2.9	6.1	0.8	0.5
Made with 1% Milk, Average	**1 Mug/250ml**	**15**	**0.2**	**6**	**0.5**	**0.8**	**0.1**	**0**
Mocha, Cold Brew, Minor Figures*	1 Can/250g	160	6.2	64	0.9	9.3	2.5	0
Mocha, Double Chocolate, Gold, Nescafe*	1 Sachet/23g	93	2.3	403	9.4	66.3	9.8	5.1
Mocha, Made Up, Dolce Gusto, Nescafe*	1 Serving/210g	117	5.1	56	2.4	6.1	2.4	0.6
Mocha, Sachet, Gold, Nescafe*	1 Sachet/22g	86	2	392	8.2	66.6	9.1	4.4

COFFEE WHITENER

Alcafe, Aldi*	1 Tsp/5g	39	2.4	553	2	57	35	0.5
Light, Tesco*	1 Tsp/3g	12	0.2	406	1	85.5	6.7	0
Original, Coffee Mate, Nestle*	1 Tsp/3g	19	1.2	547	2.4	56.7	34.4	0
Tesco*	1 Tsp/3g	16	0.9	533	1.2	61.3	31.4	0

COGNAC

40% Volume	**1 Pub Shot/35ml**	**78**	**0**	**222**	**0**	**0**	**0**	**0**

COLA

Average	**1 Can/330ml**	**135**	**0**	**41**	**0**	**10.9**	**0**	**0**
Coke, Cherry, Coca-Cola*	1 Bottle/500ml	225	0	45	0	11.2	0	0
Coke, Cherry, Zero, Coca-Cola*	1 Can/330ml	1	0	0	0	0	0	0
Coke, Diet with Cherry, Coca-Cola*	1 Bottle/500ml	5	0	1	0	0	0	0
Coke, Diet, Caffeine Free, Coca-Cola*	1 Can/330ml	1	0	0	0	0.1	0	0
Coke, Mango, Exotic, Diet, Coca-Cola*	1 Bottle/500ml	2	0	0	0	0	0	0
Coke, Strawberry, Diet, Twisted, Coca-Cola*	1 Bottle/500ml	2	0	0	0	0	0	0
Coke, Vanilla, Coca-Cola*	1 Bottle/500ml	215	0	43	0	10.6	0	0

	Measure	per Measure		Nutrition Values per 100g / 100ml				
	INFO/WEIGHT	KCAL	FAT	KCAL	PROT	CARB	FAT	FIBRE
COLA								
Coke, with Vanilla, Diet, Coca-Cola*	1 Glass/200ml	1	0	0	0	0.1	0	0
Diet, Average	**1 Serving/200ml**	**1**	**0**	**1**	**0**	**0**	**0**	**0**
Light, 0% Sugar, Harboe*	1 Serving/200ml	2	1	1	0.5	0.5	0.5	0
Pepsi Max, Ginger, Pepsi*	1 Can/250ml	1	0	0	0	0	0	0
Pepsi Max, Raspberry, Pepsi*	1 Serving/250ml	1	0	0	0.1	0.1	0	0
Zero, Caffeine Free, Coca-Cola*	1 Glass/200ml	0	0	0	0	0	0	0
Zero, Coca-Cola*	1 Can/330ml	1	0	0	0	0	0	0
COLESLAW								
& Potato Salad, Baby, Finest, Tesco*	1 Serving/50g	105	9.6	210	1.4	7.2	19.2	1.4
Apple, Raisin & Walnut, TTD, Sainsbury's*	1 Serving/75g	212	19.6	283	2.3	8	26.2	2.8
Asian, Slaw, Moorish*	1 Serving/25g	24	1.6	95	2.6	7.4	6.4	2.7
Basics, Sainsbury's*	1 Serving/25g	27	2.4	107	1	3.7	9.8	1.6
Cheese, Deli Style, Waitrose*	¼ Tub/75g	247	24.3	330	3.8	5.1	32.5	0.9
Cheese, M&S*	1 Serving/57g	185	19.1	325	4.2	2	33.5	1.7
Cheese, Sainsbury's*	1 Serving/75g	184	16.8	246	3.8	6.5	22.4	1.4
Coronation, Sainsbury's*	¼ Pot/75g	145	11.6	193	1	11.4	15.5	1.9
COU, M&S*	½ Pack/125g	75	3.4	60	1.3	7.4	2.7	1.7
Creamy, Aldi*	1 Serving/50g	96	9	191	1.1	5.6	18	1.3
Creamy, Asda*	1 Serving/25g	62	6	248	0.9	7	24	1.8
Creamy, Co-Op*	1 Tbsp/15g	34	3.3	228	0.9	5.7	22	1.3
Creamy, Farmfoods*	1 Serving/50g	84	7.4	167	1	6.8	14.8	0
Creamy, LC, Tesco*	1/3 Pot/100g	105	8.8	105	1.2	4.9	8.8	1.6
Creamy, Meadow Fresh, Lidl*	1 Serving/50g	91	8.5	182	0.9	5.5	17	1.8
Creamy, Morrisons*	1 Serving/50g	112	10.9	224	0.7	5.4	21.8	1.5
Creamy, Tesco*	1 Serving/75g	142	13.4	190	1	5.5	17.8	1.5
Creamy, The Deli, Aldi*	1 Serving/50g	78	7	157	0.8	6.7	14	1.1
Crunchy & Creamy, Tesco*	1 Serving/50g	78	7.1	155	0.9	5.2	14.2	1.4
Deli Salad, Tesco*	1 Serving/50g	91	8.5	183	0.9	5.5	17.1	1.6
Deli Style, M&S*	1 Serving/50g	103	9.6	206	1.6	5.5	19.1	2.7
Eastmans, Tesco*	1 Serving/50g	58	5	116	0.9	4.7	10	1.4
Essential, Waitrose*	1 Tbsp/20g	50	4.9	248	0.8	5.4	24.6	1.2
Extra Crunchy, The Best, Morrisons*	1 Serving/50g	137	13.6	274	1.1	5	27.1	2.6
Extra Special, Asda*	1 Serving/50g	106	10.5	213	1.1	3.5	21	3.9
From Restaurant, Average	**3/4 Cup/99g**	**147**	**11**	**148**	**1.5**	**12.9**	**11.1**	**0**
Fruit, Celery, & Nut, Sainsbury's*	1 Serving/75g	143	11.6	191	2.1	96	15.5	2.4
Fruity, Waitrose*	1 Serving/90g	217	20.9	241	0.9	6.6	23.2	1.4
Half Fat, Waitrose*	1 Serving/100g	38	2.7	38	0.6	2.9	2.7	1.2
Iceland*	1 Serving/50g	80	6.9	160	0.8	6.9	13.8	2.3
Jalapeno, Sainsbury's*	1 Serving/75g	142	13.4	190	0.9	5.6	17.9	1.6
Lite, Butlers*	1 Serving/50g	75	7	150	1.1	4.2	14	2.7
Luxury, Asda*	1 Serving/50g	108	10.5	217	0.9	6	21	0
Luxury, Lidl*	1 Serving/50g	102	9.7	203	0.9	5.9	19.4	0
Luxury, TTD, Sainsbury's*	1 Serving/30g	60	5.6	200	1	6.8	18.5	1.4
Pink, Pickled, Tangy, Sainsbury's*	½ Pot/100g	43	0.5	43	0.9	8.7	0.5	1.5
Plant Based, V Taste, Morrisons*	1 Serving/50g	100	9.2	200	1	6.6	18.4	2.2
Plant Menu, Aldi*	1/6 Pack/50g	100	9	199	0.9	7.2	18	1.2
Rainbow, Finest, Tesco*	¼ Pack/84g	192	18.7	229	1.3	4.9	22.3	1.7
Red Cabbage, & Veg, M&S*	½ Pot/90g	72	1.4	80	1.1	15.5	1.6	3.4
Red, Tesco*	½ Pack/70g	53	1	76	1	13.5	1.5	2.4
Reduced Fat, Average	**1 Tbsp/20g**	**23**	**1.9**	**113**	**1**	**6.4**	**9.3**	**2**
Reduced Fat, Co-Op*	1 Serving/20g	26	2.2	132	0.9	5.6	11	1.5
Slaw, Pickled, Sainsbury's*	½ Pot/100g	43	0.5	43	0.9	8.7	0.5	1.5
Traditional, Reduced Fat, M&S*	1 Serving/50g	82	7.2	164	1	6.5	14.5	1.7

	Measure INFO/WEIGHT	per Measure KCAL	FAT	Nutrition Values per 100g / 100ml KCAL	PROT	CARB	FAT	FIBRE
COLESLAW								
TTD, Sainsbury's*	¼ Med Pot/75g	185	17.7	246	1.8	5.9	23.6	1.5
Vegan, Deli Style, Sainsbury's*	1 Serving/50g	83	7.7	166	1	5	15.4	1.6
Vegan, Gro, Co-Op*	1 Serving/50g	100	9	199	1	7	18	1
Vegan, Plant Chef, Tesco*	1 Serving/50g	96	8.8	192	1.1	6	17.7	2.3
Vegan, Plant Kitchen, M&S*	½ Pack/112g	161	14.2	143	1	5.3	12.6	2.4
with Real Mayonnaise, Hellmann's*	1 Serving/50g	134	13.4	268	1.2	4.6	26.9	0
with Reduced Calorie Dressing, Retail	*1 Serving/40g*	*27*	*1.8*	*67*	*0.9*	*6.1*	*4.5*	*1.4*
Yoghurt Dressed, Reduced Fat, Waitrose*	1 Serving/30g	36	2.6	121	1.5	8.9	8.6	1.2
Yoghurt Dressed, The Best, Morrisons*	1 Serving/50g	66	5.4	132	1.4	6.4	10.8	1.7
Yogurt, Deluxe, Lidl*	1 Serving/50g	73	6.4	146	1.3	5.7	12.8	1
COLEY								
Portions, Raw, Average	*1 Serving/92g*	*65*	*0.6*	*71*	*15.9*	*0*	*0.6*	*0*
Steamed, Average	*1oz/28g*	*29*	*0.4*	*105*	*23.3*	*0*	*1.3*	*0*
CONCHIGLIE								
Cooked, Average	*1 Serving/185g*	*247*	*1.6*	*134*	*4.8*	*26.6*	*0.8*	*0.6*
Dry Weight, Average	*1 Serving/100g*	*352*	*1.7*	*352*	*12.5*	*71.6*	*1.7*	*2.6*
Shells, Dry, Average	*1 Serving/100g*	*346*	*1.5*	*346*	*12.3*	*70.4*	*1.5*	*3*
Whole Wheat, Dry Weight, Average	*1 Serving/75g*	*237*	*1.5*	*316*	*12.6*	*62*	*2*	*10.7*
CONSERVE								
Apricot, Average	*1 Tbsp/15g*	*37*	*0*	*244*	*0.5*	*59.3*	*0.2*	*1.5*
Blackberry, Bramble, & Gin, M&S*	1 Tbsp/15g	35	0.2	233	0.8	54.2	1.1	1.4
Blackcurrant, Average	*1 Tbsp/15g*	*37*	*0*	*245*	*0.6*	*60*	*0.1*	*1.9*
Blueberry, M&S*	1 Tbsp/15g	31	0	206	0.3	51.1	0.1	1.3
Cherry, Black, Bonne Maman*	1 Tbsp/15g	36	0	243	0.7	59	0.2	1.1
Fig, Bonne Maman*	1 Tbsp/15g	36	0	240	0.5	59	0	1
Fig, Crosta & Mollica*	1 Tbsp/15g	28	0	188	0.7	43	0.3	3
Ginger, Tiptree, Wilkin & Sons*	1 Tbsp/15g	40	0	270	0	66	0	0
Hedgerow, TTD, Sainsbury's*	1 Tbsp/15g	41	0	276	0.5	68.2	0.1	0.5
Morello Cherry, Waitrose*	1 Tbsp/15g	39	0	258	0.4	64.2	0	1.4
Peach, Bonne Maman*	1 Tbsp/15g	36	0	241	0.4	59	0.1	1.3
Plum, Damson, Bonne Maman*	1 Tbsp/15g	36	0	241	0.4	59	0.1	1.3
Plum, Mirabelle, Bonne Maman*	1 Tbsp/15g	36	0	241	0.4	59	0.1	1.4
Plum, TTD, Sainsbury's*	1 Tbsp/15g	36	0.1	243	0.5	59.6	0.5	0.9
Raspberry, Average	*1 Tbsp/15g*	*37*	*0.1*	*249*	*0.6*	*61*	*0.3*	*1.3*
Rhubarb & Ginger, M&S*	1 Tbsp/15g	29	0	194	0.3	47.9	0.1	1
Rhubarb, & Ginger, The Best, Morrisons*	1 Tbsp/15g	37	0	248	0.4	60.8	0.2	1.1
Rhubarb, & Strawberry, Bonne Maman*	1 Tbsp/15g	36	0	241	0.3	59	0.1	1.2
Strawberry, Average	*1 Tbsp/15g*	*37*	*0*	*250*	*0.4*	*61.6*	*0.1*	*0.5*
CONSOMME								
Average	*1oz/28g*	*3*	*0*	*12*	*2.9*	*0.1*	*0*	*0*
Beef, Campbell's*	½ Can/149g	20	0	13	2.7	0.7	0	0
Beef, Canned, Sainsbury's*	1 Can/415g	46	0	11	2	0.7	0	0
Beef, Luxury, with Sherry, Baxters*	1 Can/415g	62	0	15	2.7	1	0	0
COOKIE MIX								
Chocolate, Mug Mix, Bakedin*	1 Mug/100g	388	6	388	5.8	76	6	0
Dough, Milk Choc Chip, Asda*	1 Serving/125g	615	28.8	492	5.7	65	23	1.6
COOKIES								
All Butter, Almond, Italian Style, M&S*	1 Cookie/23g	120	6.4	515	6.7	59.4	27.6	3.6
All Butter, Ginger Bread, M&S*	1 Cookie/23g	102	5	445	4.3	57.5	21.8	2.4
Almond, Ose*	1 Cookie/10g	46	1.4	456	8.4	74	14	0
Bounty, Mars*	1 Cookie/46g	215	9.6	468	5.7	63.4	20.9	0
Brazil Nut, Prewett's*	1 Cookie/50g	122	7.4	244	2.6	25.2	14.8	1
Butter & Sultana, Sainsbury's*	1 Cookie/13g	61	2.6	473	4.5	68.4	20.1	1.6

COOKIES

INFO/WEIGHT	Measure		per Measure		Nutrition Values per 100g / 100ml			
		KCAL	FAT	KCAL	PROT	CARB	FAT	FIBRE
Butter, Danesita*	1 Cookie/9g	45	2	529	5.9	67.6	23.5	2.9
Caramel, Mini, Dairy Milk, Cadbury*	1 Cookie/13g	62	2.7	474	5	65.7	20.9	1.8
Carrot Cake, Soft Bake, Asda*	1 Cookie/20g	88	3.4	440	5.4	64	17	2.1
Cheesecake, New York, Desserts, Maryland*	1 Cookie/10g	51	2.3	485	5.9	64.9	22.2	1.6
Choc Chip & Coconut, Maryland*	1 Cookie/10g	55	2.5	512	5.1	62.9	23.7	0
Choc Chip & Hazelnut, Maryland*	1 Cookie/11g	55	2.7	513	6.3	65.3	25	0
Choc Chip, Big, Treats, Maryland*	1 Cookie/16g	85	4.6	531	5.1	61.2	29	3.2
Choc Chip, Mini, Belmont Biscuit Co, Aldi*	1 Bag/20g	99	4.6	498	5.2	66	23	12.8
Choc Chip, Mini, Good to Go, Waitrose*	1 Bag/25g	127	6.6	508	6	60.4	26.4	2.4
Choc Chunk, Finest, Tesco*	1 Cookie/80g	355	14.1	445	5.7	65.3	17.7	1.8
Chocolate & Orange, COU, M&S*	1 Cookie/26g	90	0.7	350	5.7	77.2	2.6	3.2
Chocolate Chip & Hazelnut, Extra Special, Asda*	1 Cookie/25g	130	8.1	516	6	51	32	2.5
Chocolate Chip, Average	**1 Cookie/10g**	**49**	**2.5**	**489**	**5.5**	**64.1**	**24.7**	**2.9**
Chocolate Chip, Double, Vegan, Plant Menu, Aldi*	1 Cookie/25g	125	6.4	500	6.8	59.6	25.6	33.2
Chocolate Chip, Free From, Tesco*	1 Cookie/12g	59	2.6	488	5.2	65.6	22	3.4
Chocolate Chip, GF, Organic, Dove's Farm*	1 Cookie/17g	77	3.1	451	4.3	66.9	18.5	0
Chocolate Chip, Sugar Free, Siro *	1 Cookie/15g	66	3.3	440	5.9	60	22	6.5
Chocolate Chunk & Hazelnut, Tesco*	1 Cookie/22g	118	6.7	538	6.2	60.2	30.3	1.9
Chocolate Chunk & Hazelnut, TTD, Sainsbury's*	1 Cookie/25g	131	7.5	522	6.7	54.9	30	2.9
Chocolate Chunk, Cadbury*	1 Cookie/22g	119	6.9	540	6.5	58	31.2	0
Chocolate Chunk, Double, Belgian, M&S*	1 Cookie/25g	125	6.1	500	5.6	62.8	24.4	2.4
Chocolate Chunk, Triple, All Butter, Irresistible, Co-Op*	1 Cookie/25g	122	6	487	6.3	58	24	5.7
Chocolate Orange, Half Coated, Finest, Tesco*	1 Cookie/22g	107	5.6	488	4.9	59.6	25.5	1.2
Chocolate, Belgian, Extra Special, Asda*	1 Cookie/26g	138	8	535	6	58	31	2
Chocolate, Belgian, Specially Selected, Aldi*	1 Cookie/80g	393	17.6	491	5.6	67	22	1.7
Chocolate, Dark, & Ginger, Free From, Finest, Tesco*	1 Cookie/19g	92	4.2	485	4.6	66	22	2.1
Chocolate, Double, Sainsbury's*	1 Cookie/45g	202	8.5	450	5.8	63.1	18.9	2
Chocolate, Double, Tesco*	1 Cookie/42g	187	8.1	447	5.8	60.8	19.4	3.2
Chocolate, Milk, & Dark, Big & Chunky, Maryland*	1 Cookie/18g	91	4.7	507	5.2	61.1	26.3	0
Chocolate, Milk, Belgian, & Orange, Finest, Tesco*	1 Cookie/25g	132	7.6	529	6.1	57	30.3	1.9
Chocolate, Milk, Belgian, Puddle, Finest, Tesco*	1 Cookie/35g	171	8.5	488	6.3	60.2	24.2	1.9
Chocolate, Milk, Free From, Tesco*	1 Cookie/20g	100	6.1	500	5.6	50.4	30.7	4.1
Chocolate, Quadruple, Finest, Tesco*	1 Cookie/25g	128	6.9	512	6.3	58.3	27.5	3
Chocolate, Triple, Chunkie, Fox's*	1 Cookie/23g	115	5.8	500	4.9	63	25	3.4
Chocolate, Triple, Half Coated, Finest, Tesco*	1 Cookie/25g	131	7.3	525	5.7	58.7	29.3	2.3
Chocolate, Triple, Irresistible, Co-Op*	1 Cookie/19g	97	5.1	511	6.8	57.9	26.8	4.2
Chocolate, Triple, Wheat, & GF, Finest, Tesco*	1 Cookie/19g	97	5	508	5.8	60.4	26.2	3.5
Christmas, Selection, Waitrose*	1 Cookie/25g	124	6.3	496	6	60.3	25.1	2.5
Chunkie Extremely Chocolatey, Fox's*	1 Cookie/26g	130	6.8	506	6.2	61	26.3	2.6
Cocoa, Sandwich, No Added Sugar, Gullon*	1 Cookie/11g	43	1.8	408	5	65	17	9
Coconut & Raspberry, GF, Sainsbury's*	1 Cookie/20g	102	5.9	511	5.9	56	29.3	6.7
Coconut, Gluten-Free, Sainsbury's*	1 Cookie/20g	103	6.1	516	5.6	54.4	30.7	4.1
Coconut, Sugar Free, Free'ist*	1 Cookie/17g	78	5.6	461	4.8	35.2	32.7	0
Cranberry & Orange, Finest, Tesco*	1 Cookie/26g	125	5.8	490	4.1	67.4	22.6	3.2
Cranberry, & White Chocolate, Lean, Myprotein*	1 Cookie/50g	194	3	387	50	32	6	2
Danish Butter, Tesco*	1 Cookie/26g	133	6.6	516	4.7	66.7	25.6	1.3
Double Choc Chip, Mini, M&S*	1 Cookie/22g	108	5.2	490	5.3	63.6	23.7	1.8
Double Choc Chip, Tesco*	1 Cookie/11g	55	2.7	500	4.2	65.3	24.7	3
Double Choc, Maryland*	1 Cookie/10g	51	2.6	510	5.2	64.4	25.7	0
Double Choc, Minis, Maryland*	1 Mini Bag/20g	100	5	503	5.7	62.3	24.9	3.6
Double Chocolate & Walnut, Soft, Tesco*	1 Cookie/25g	116	6.4	463	5.8	52.1	25.7	4.7
Double Chocolate Chip, Co-Op*	1 Cookie/17g	87	4.6	510	5	63	27	2
Double Chocolate Chip, Organic, Waitrose*	1 Cookie/18g	96	5.6	535	5.1	58.6	31	1.9

	Measure INFO/WEIGHT	per Measure KCAL	FAT	Nutrition Values per 100g / 100ml KCAL	PROT	CARB	FAT	FIBRE
COOKIES								
Eton Mess, Finest, Tesco*	1 Cookie/66g	281	9.7	426	5.1	67.6	14.7	1.4
Flapjack, Fruity, Truly Irresistible, Co-Op*	1 Cookie/25g	116	5.1	464	5.2	64	20.4	2.4
Flapjack, Fruity, Vegan, Aldi*	1 Cookie/25g	107	4.7	428	4.4	60	18.8	3.4
Fortune, Average	*1 Cookie/8g*	*30*	*0.2*	*378*	*4.2*	*84*	*2.7*	*1.6*
Frui & Nut, Half Coated, Belmont Biscuit Co, Aldi*	1 Cookie/25g	122	6	488	6	61	24	2.5
Fruit & Nut, Half Coated, Belmont Biscuit Co, Aldi*	1 Cookie/25g	122	6	481	6.2	57.7	23.5	2.7
Fruit, & Oat, All Butter, The Best, Morrisons*	1 Cookie/25g	110	4.4	441	5.7	63	17.6	3.9
Fudge Brownie American Cream, Sainsbury's*	1 Cookie/12g	60	2.8	499	4.8	67.9	23.2	2.2
Galaxy, Galaxy, Mars*	1 Cookie/46g	207	8	451	5.6	67.3	17.4	0
Ginger & Choc Chip, BGTY, Sainsbury's*	1 Cookie/17g	69	3.2	415	5.8	55.3	19	12.1
Ginger, GF, Just Free, Lidl*	1 Cookie/19g	90	3.5	474	3.9	71.8	18.5	2.3
Half Coated, Milk Chocolate, Fabulous, Fox's*	1 Cookie/25g	125	6.2	500	5.6	62.7	24.8	1.9
Hazelnut, Heart, Sondey, Lidl*	1 Cookie/25g	129	6.8	515	5.7	60.1	27.3	3.2
Maple Syrup, & Pecan, Finest, Tesco*	1 Cookie/25g	127	6.6	507	6.7	59.9	26.4	1.7
Milk Chocolate Chunk, Average	*1 Cookie/25g*	*129*	*6.9*	*515*	*6.6*	*60*	*27.6*	*1.6*
Milk Chocolate, Hazelnut, Waitrose*	1 Cookie/21g	112	6.6	533	6.6	54.9	31.4	2.1
Mince Pie, Finest, Tesco*	1 Cookie/23g	104	4	453	4.1	68.7	17.5	2.1
Oat & Treacle, TTD, Sainsbury's*	1 Cookie/25g	121	5.9	482	5.7	61.8	23.6	3.7
Oat & Sultana, Free From, Sainsbury's*	1 Cookie/19g	87	3.7	462	6.2	62.6	19.8	4.2
Oat, & Raisin, Free From, Finest, Tesco*	1 Cookie/19g	80	2.8	422	6.2	63	15	5.1
Oat, with Honey, Violanta*	1 Cookie/18g	89	5.2	489	5.2	50.2	28.5	5.4
Oatflake & Raisin, Waitrose*	1 Cookie/17g	80	3.8	469	5.8	61.7	22.1	4.7
Oreo, Mini, Oreo*	1 Pack/25g	120	4.8	480	4.8	70	19.2	2.4
Oreo, Nabisco*	1 Cookie/11g	52	2.1	474	5.4	68	19	2.7
Pecan, & Caramel, Co-Op*	1 Cookie/25g	123	5.5	493	6	67	22	1.5
Pineapple, Coconut & White Chocolate, M&S*	1 Cookie/23g	119	5.7	518	5.1	56.7	24.9	2.9
Pistachio & Almond, All Butter, M&S*	1 Cookie/25g	132	8	528	10.7	46.9	32.1	4.5
Red Velvet, Filled, Bakery, Tesco*	1 Cookie/42g	170	5.5	405	4.6	66.6	13.1	1.3
Salted Caramel, M&S*	1 Cookie/25g	124	5.8	496	5.2	65.6	23.2	1.6
Stem Ginger, & Dark Chocolate, GF, The Best, Morrisons*	1 Cookie/19g	94	4.1	493	3.4	70.4	21.7	1
Stem Ginger, Aldi*	1 Cookie/13g	58	2.4	463	3.6	68.5	19.4	0
Stem Ginger, All Butter, Deluxe, Lidl*	1 Cookie/17g	80	3.6	468	5.1	62	21	5.4
Stem Ginger, All Butter, Waitrose*	1 Cookie/25g	115	4.3	459	4.7	70.7	17.1	1.8
Stem Ginger, Co-Op*	1 Cookie/25g	118	4.8	473	5	69	19	1.2
Stem Ginger, Deluxe, Lidl*	1 Cookie/17g	80	3.6	468	5.1	62	21	5.4
Stem Ginger, Reduced Fat, Waitrose*	1 Cookie/17g	75	2.7	448	4.5	71	16.2	1.6
Stem Ginger, Tesco*	1 Cookie/20g	98	4.8	489	4.2	64	24	2
Stem Ginger, The Best, Morrisons*	1 Cookie/25g	110	3.8	441	5.4	69	15.4	2.5
Stem Ginger, TTD, Sainsbury's*	1 Cookie/25g	124	6.2	496	4.9	62.3	24.7	2.2
Sticky Toffee, Finest, Tesco*	1 Cookie/63g	258	9.4	410	3.4	63.5	15	1.5
Sugar Free, Maryland*	1 Cookie/11g	47	2.4	434	6.1	60.6	22.3	3.6
Sultana, & Oat, Tesco*	1 Cookie/20g	91	3.9	454	5.5	61.6	19.7	4.4
Sultana, All Butter, Reduced Fat, M&S*	1 Cookie/17g	70	2.4	420	4.9	68.6	14.2	2.6
Sultana, Deluxe, Lidl*	1 Cookie/17g	77	3.2	453	5.3	64.7	18.8	2.9
Sultana, Soft & Chewy, Sainsbury's*	1 Cookie/25g	104	3.5	414	4.4	67.8	13.9	2.5
Triple Chocolate, Belgian, Bakery, Finest, Tesco*	1 Cookie/65g	310	14.9	478	6.1	60.1	23	2.9
Triple Chocolate, TTD, Sainsbury's*	1 Cookie/19g	95	4.9	508	5.9	61.1	26.1	2.7
White Chocolate & Raspberry, Finest, Tesco*	1 Cookie/76g	304	9.6	400	5.2	66.3	12.6	2.4
White Chocolate, Chunk, Average	*1 Cookie/25g*	*124*	*6.2*	*498*	*5.5*	*62.8*	*24.8*	*1*
COQ AU VIN								
Chicken, Parsley Box*	1 Pack/270g	221	6.8	82	14	0.9	2.5	0.4
Diet Chef Ltd*	1 Pack/300g	285	13.2	95	7.7	6.1	4.4	2.2
Donald Russell*	1 Pack/250g	230	7.2	92	10.7	3.5	2.9	0.4

	Measure INFO/WEIGHT	per Measure KCAL	FAT	Nutrition Values per 100g / 100ml KCAL	PROT	CARB	FAT	FIBRE
COQ AU VIN								
with Potato Gratin, TTD, Sainsbury's*	1 Pack/324g	385	15.5	119	6.8	11.5	4.8	1.1
CORDIAL								
Apple & Mango, Hi Juice, As Prepared, Morrisons*	1 Serving/250ml	69	0	28	0	6.7	0	0.1
Apple, & Blackcurrant, Diluted, Diet Rite*	1 Serving/250ml	7	0	3	0	0.7	0	0
Blackcurrant, & Liquorice, Undiluted, Mr Fitzpatricks*	1 Serving/17ml	11	0.1	64	0	76.8	0.6	0
Blackcurrant, New Zealand Honey Co*	1 Serving/30ml	109	0.3	363	1	88	1	0
Cherry, Sour, Super Concentrated, Optima*	1 Serving/30ml	78	0.1	260	1.5	63	0.2	0
Elderflower, Undiluted, Waitrose*	1 Serving/20ml	22	0	110	0	27.5	0	0
Lemon & Lime, High Juice, M&S*	1 Glass/250ml	75	0	30	0	7	0	0
Lime Juice, Concentrated	*1 Serving/20ml*	*22*	*0*	*112*	*0.1*	*29.8*	*0*	*0*
Lime Juice, Diluted	*1 Glass/250ml*	*55*	*0*	*22*	*0*	*6*	*0*	*0*
Lime, Crushed, & Mint, Diluted, Robinson's*	1 Serving/200ml	34	0	17	0	4.1	0	0
Pear, & Elderflower, Pressed, Diluted, Robinsons*	1 Serving/200ml	36	0	18	0	4.2	0	0
Pear, & Ginger, Undiluted, Urban Cordial*	1 Serving/10ml	10	0	100	0	24	0	0
Raspberry Ripple, Diluted, Waitrose*	1 Serving/250ml	48	0	19	0	4.9	0	0
Summer Fruits, Sun Quench, Aldi*	1 Serving/25ml	4	0.1	15	0.5	2	0.5	0.5
CORIANDER								
Ground, Sainsbury's*	1 Tsp/5g	13	0.9	262	12.4	13.1	17.8	0
Leaves, Dried, Average	*1oz/28g*	*78*	*1.3*	*279*	*21.8*	*41.7*	*4.8*	*0*
Leaves, Fresh, Average	*1 Bunch/20g*	*5*	*0.1*	*23*	*2.1*	*3.7*	*0.5*	*2.8*
CORN								
Baby, Average	*1 Serving/80g*	*21*	*0.3*	*26*	*2.5*	*3.1*	*0.4*	*1.7*
Baby, Canned, Drained, Average	*1 Serving/80g*	*18*	*0.3*	*23*	*2.9*	*2*	*0.4*	*1.5*
Cobs, Boiled, Weighed with Cob, Average	*1 Ear/200g*	*78*	*1.7*	*39*	*1.5*	*6.8*	*0.8*	*0.8*
Cobs, with Butter, From Restaurant, Average	*1 Ear/146g*	*155*	*3.4*	*106*	*3.1*	*21.9*	*2.4*	*0*
Creamed Style, Green Giant*	1 Can/418g	238	2.1	57	1.2	11.9	0.5	3
Crunchy, Smoked BBQ, Love Corn*	1 Pack/45g	190	5.8	423	7.3	63.3	12.9	7
Marmite, Graze*	1 Punnet/24g	107	4.1	445	8.4	61	17	8.9
Roasted, & Salted, Sunburst Snacks*	1 Serving/20g	90	2.2	449	7.8	79.3	11.2	0
Snack, Salt & Vinegar, Love Corn*	1 Pack/45g	194	5.7	430	7.1	68.3	12.7	7
Snack, Unsalted, Bodrun*	1 Serving/25g	108	3	430	8	70	12	6.5
CORN CAKES								
Apple, & Cinnamon, Kallo*	1 Corn Cake/10g	37	0.2	380	7.2	82	2.3	0
Harvest Morn, Aldi*	1 Corn Cake/7g	26	0	375	8.6	84	0.5	2.3
Milk Chocolate, Harvest Morn, Aldi*	1 Corn Cake/17g	82	3.4	482	6.5	70.6	20	2.9
Organic, Kallo*	1 Corn Cake/7g	26	0.1	383	7.6	83.6	1.1	7.2
The Best, Morrisons*	1 Corn Cake/7g	29	0.2	390	7.7	80.1	3.3	4.4
Unsalted, M&S*	1 Corn Cake/8g	30	0	381	6.5	87	0.3	1.9
with Chai Seeds, Kallo*	1 Corn Cake/7g	27	0.2	389	8	81	2.4	0
CORNED BEEF								
Average	*1 Slice/35g*	*75*	*4.3*	*214*	*25.9*	*0.7*	*12.2*	*0*
Lean, Healthy Range, Average	*1 Slice/30g*	*57*	*2.6*	*191*	*27*	*1*	*8.7*	*0*
Reduced Salt, Canned, Princes*	1 Can/340g	741	44.2	218	24.8	0.5	13	0
Sliced, Premium, Average	*1 Slice/31g*	*69*	*3.9*	*222*	*26.6*	*0.5*	*12.6*	*0*
CORNFLOUR								
Average	*1 Tsp/5g*	*18*	*0.1*	*355*	*0.6*	*86.9*	*1.2*	*0.1*
COURGETTE								
Baby, Raw, Average	*1 Courgette/29g*	*6*	*0.1*	*22*	*2*	*2*	*0.5*	*1.2*
Fried, Average	*1oz/28g*	*18*	*1.3*	*63*	*2.6*	*2.6*	*4.8*	*1.2*
Raw, Average	*1 Whole/224g*	*40*	*0.9*	*18*	*1.8*	*1.8*	*0.4*	*0.9*
Spaghetti, Waitrose*	½ Pack/80g	16	0.3	20	1.8	1.8	0.4	1.2
COUS COUS								
Caribbean, Ainsley Harriott*	1 Pack/260g	369	6.5	142	4.8	25	2.5	1.7

	Measure INFO/WEIGHT	per Measure KCAL	FAT	Nutrition Values per 100g / 100ml KCAL	PROT	CARB	FAT	FIBRE
COUS COUS								
Cooked, Average	**1 Tbsp/15g**	**24**	**0.3**	**158**	**4.3**	**31.4**	**1.9**	**1.3**
Cooked, From Restaurant, Average	**1 Cup/157g**	**176**	**0.3**	**112**	**3.8**	**23.2**	**0.2**	**1.4**
Coriander & Lemon, As Consumed, Sainsbury's*	½ Pack/140g	195	1	139	4.8	27.5	0.7	1.9
Dry, Average	**1 Serving/50g**	**178**	**0.7**	**356**	**13.7**	**72.8**	**1.5**	**2.6**
Fruity	**1 Pack/250g**	**450**	**10.8**	**180**	**3.7**	**30.7**	**4.3**	**2**
Giant, Cooked, Sainsbury's*	1 Serving/130g	126	2.1	97	3.6	16.2	1.6	1.7
Giant, Dry, Sainsbury's*	1 Serving/38g	126	2.1	332	12.4	55.5	5.5	5.8
Lemon, & Coriander, As Prepared, Morrisons*	½ Pack/139g	212	1.4	152	5.8	29.4	1	0.9
Lemon, & Coriander, As Prepared, Tesco*	½ Pack/140g	207	1.7	148	5.6	27.5	1.2	2.3
Mediterranean Inspired, As Prepared, Tesco*	½ Pack/141g	204	1.7	145	5.8	26.7	1.2	2.3
Mediterranean, Morrisons*	½ Pack/140g	204	1.5	146	5.6	27.7	1.1	1.4
Moroccan Inspired, Finest, Tesco*	½ Pack/115g	197	5.3	171	4.2	27	4.6	2.4
Moroccan Spiced, Fruity, Waitrose*	1 Serving/78g	146	3.7	187	4.5	29.2	4.8	4.4
Moroccan, Medley, Ainsley Harriott*	½ Sachet/130g	178	2	137	5.4	25.4	1.5	2.2
Moroccan, Style, Fruity, M&S*	1 Pack/200g	364	4.4	182	4.2	34.5	2.2	3.7
Moroccan, Style, TTD, Sainsbury's*	¼ Pot/100g	203	4.7	203	5.1	33.1	4.7	3.7
Moroccan, Twist'd Flavour Co.*	½ Pack/130g	177	2	136	4.9	24.9	1.5	1.8
Organic, Instant, GF, Dry Weight, Clearspring*	1 Serving/65g	231	1.5	355	6.9	75	2.3	2.7
Pilaf, The Levantine Table, Waitrose*	½ Pack/150g	240	3.8	160	4.4	29	2.5	2.1
Roasted Vegetable, As Prepared, Sainsbury's*	½ Pack/140g	211	2	151	4.5	29.2	1.4	1.5
Roasted Vegetable, Newgate, Lidl*	1 Serving/135g	186	2	138	4.6	26.2	1.5	2.2
Roasted Vegetable, Worldwide Foods, Aldi*	1 Serving/130g	182	1.5	140	5.1	26.2	1.2	1.9
Sun Dried Tomato, & Garlic, Morrisons*	½ Pack/140g	202	1.5	144	5.6	27.2	1.1	1.8
Tomato, Mediterranean, GFY, Asda*	½ Pack/141g	192	1.3	136	5	27	0.9	1.7
Tomato, Sun Dried, CBY, Asda*	1 Pack/310g	515	12.1	166	4.6	26.2	3.9	4
Turkish, & Grains, Ainsley Harriott*	1 Serving/125g	204	3.6	163	5	28.4	2.9	1.6
Vegetable, Chargrilled, Smoky, Finest, Tesco*	½ Pack/125g	194	5.6	156	4.3	23.2	4.5	2.6
Vegetable, Roasted, Dry, Ainsley Harriott*	½ Sachet/50g	180	2	360	14.6	66.4	4	6.8
Vegetable, Roasted, Fresh, Meadow Fresh, Lidl*	½ Pack/140g	211	7.3	151	4.6	20	5.2	0
Vegetable, Roasted, Made Up, Ainsley Harriott*	½ Pack/130g	177	1.6	136	4.8	25.5	1.2	1.9
Vegetable, Roasted, Snack Salad Pot, HL, Tesco*	1 Pack/60g	213	2.4	355	15.1	64.6	4	4.2
Vegetable, Roasted, Waitrose*	1 Serving/200g	328	13.2	164	3.9	22	6.6	0.9
Vegetable, Spicy, GFY, Asda*	½ Pack/55g	71	0.6	129	4.7	25	1.1	2
Vegetable, Spicy, Morrisons*	1 Pack/110g	187	5.5	170	5.1	26.2	5	2.9
Wholewheat, Cooked Weight, Tesco*	1 Serving/80g	131	0.8	164	6.5	30	1	4.5
CRAB								
Boiled, Meat Only, Average	**1 Tbsp/40g**	**51**	**2.2**	**128**	**19.5**	**0**	**5.5**	**0**
Chilli, British, M&S*	1 Pack/105g	371	35.3	353	9.4	2.8	33.6	0.3
Dressed, Average	**1 Can/43g**	**66**	**3.4**	**154**	**16.8**	**4.1**	**7.9**	**0.2**
Meat in Brine, Average	**½ Can/60g**	**41**	**0.2**	**69**	**15.6**	**0.8**	**0.4**	**0.1**
Meat, Raw, Average	**1oz/28g**	**28**	**0.2**	**100**	**20.8**	**2.8**	**0.6**	**0**
CRAB CAKES								
Goan, M&S*	1 Pack/190g	228	7.6	120	8	12.9	4	1.8
Iceland*	1 Serving/18g	52	3.2	288	7.2	25.6	18	1.3
Tesco*	1 Serving/130g	281	16	216	11	15.4	12.3	1.1
Thai Style, TTD, Sainsbury's*	1 Cake/141g	297	14.1	210	8.7	20.5	10	1.8
CRAB STICKS								
Average	**1 Stick/15g**	**14**	**0**	**94**	**9.1**	**13.9**	**0.3**	**0**
CRACKERBREAD								
Original, Ryvita*	1 Cracker/5g	20	0.2	390	10.5	77.5	3.7	2.5
Quinoa, Red, & Sesame, Protein, Ryvita*	1 Slice/10g	37	0.5	368	20.7	53.2	4.9	14.1
Wholegrain, Ryvita*	1 Cracker/5g	19	0.2	379	11.3	70.9	3.9	7.3

CRACKERS

	Measure INFO/WEIGHT	per Measure KCAL	FAT	Nutrition Values per 100g / 100ml KCAL	PROT	CARB	FAT	FIBRE
Ale, Miller's Elements*	1 Cracker/5g	20	0.5	406	10.7	66.3	10.4	0
Bath Oliver, Jacob's*	1 Cracker/12g	52	1.6	432	9.6	67.6	13.7	2.6
Beetroot, & Seed, Finest, Tesco*	2 Crackers/15g	75	3.7	497	12.2	53.1	24.8	6.4
Beetroot, Apple, & Chilli, Specially Selected, Aldi*	1 Cracker/4g	17	0.4	423	8.7	70	11	4.3
Black Olive, M&S*	1 Cracker/4g	20	1	485	8.3	59.4	23.5	4.3
Black Olive, Melts, Carr's*	1 Cracker/4g	22	1.1	504	7.7	60.4	25.3	2.2
Black Pepper for Cheese, Ryvita*	1 Cracker/7g	27	0.2	384	13.2	72.9	2.9	6.8
Black Pepper, Savoury, Gourmet, Specially Selected, Aldi*	1 Cracker/5g	24	1.1	490	8.6	62	22	3.2
Bran, Jacob's*	1 Cracker/7g	32	1.3	454	9.7	62.8	18.2	3.2
Breaks, Original, Ritz*	1 Cracker/6g	29	1.1	463	8.4	65	18	3.5
Buckwheat & Chia, Rude Health*	1 Cracker/7g	29	0.7	388	14	56	8.8	15
Butter Puff, Sainsbury's*	1 Cracker/10g	54	2.7	523	10.4	60.7	26.5	2.5
Butter Puffs, Jacob's*	1 Cracker/11g	55	2.7	502	9.3	59	24.8	3.1
Buttermilk, Wafer, Miller's Damsel*	1 Cracker/5g	24	0.8	484	13.4	70.6	15.8	0
Caramelised Onion, Ciabatta, Jacob's*	1 Cracker/10g	43	1	426	12.5	68.6	10.3	4.3
Cheese & onion, Triangles, Eat Well, M&S*	1 Bag/30g	128	3.3	425	9.8	69.4	11	4.7
Cheese Thins, Asda*	1 Cracker/4g	21	1.3	532	12	49	32	0
Cheese Thins, Co-Op*	1 Cracker/4g	21	1.3	530	12	49	32	3
Cheese Thins, Oven Baked, Rivercote, Lidl*	1 Cracker/4g	21	1.3	534	10.9	45.8	33.6	2.3
Cheese Thins, Savour Bakes, Aldi*	1 Thin/4g	19	0.8	475	15	62.5	20	0
Cheese Thins, Tesco*	1 Biscuit/4g	20	1.2	543	11.3	47.5	33.7	2.5
Cheese Thins, Waitrose*	1 Cracker/4g	21	1.2	545	11.9	52.6	31.9	2.5
Cheese, Cheddar, Crispies, TTD, Sainsbury's*	1 Thin/4g	21	1.5	576	14.2	39	40.4	2.2
Cheese, GF, Made Without Wheat, M&S*	1 Cracker/6g	26	0.8	425	5	72.5	12.5	5
Cheese, Oat Bakes, Nairn's*	1 Bag/30g	130	4.7	432	15	57.4	15.8	1.3
Cheese, Ritz*	1 Cracker/4g	17	0.9	486	10.1	55.9	24.7	2.2
Chive, & Extra Virgin Olive Oil, Fine Cheese Co*	1 Cracker/5g	20	0.6	402	12.5	65.4	12	0
Christmas, Festive, Extra Special, Asda*	¼ Pack/79g	144	8.7	182	11.9	7.9	11	1.8
Ciabatta, Sundried Tomato & Basil, Jacobs*	1 Cracker/10g	42	1	424	12.4	68.5	10.2	4.3
Corn Thins, 97% Fat Free, Real Foods*	1 Cracker/6g	23	0.2	378	10.2	81.7	3	8.6
Corn, Chilli, & Lime, Cofresh*	1/3 Pack/20g	104	6	522	6.3	56	30	3.7
Cracked Pepper, & Chia Seed, Raw, Cru8*	1 Cracker/16g	106	7.4	660	13.2	39	46	33
Cream Cheese & Onion Flavour, Bakefuls, Ritz*	1 Bag/23g	109	4.8	474	7	63	21	2.7
Cream, Average	*1 Cracker/7g*	*31*	*1.1*	*440*	*9.5*	*68.3*	*16.3*	*2.2*
Cream, Light, Jacob's*	1 Cracker/8g	31	0.5	388	10.6	72.2	6.3	4.1
Crispy Cheese, M&S*	1 Cracker/4g	20	1	470	9.4	58.1	22.1	3
Crispy Chickpea, M&S*	¼ Pack/25g	99	1.4	396	17.6	67.8	5.5	2.5
Digestive, Savour Bakes, Aldi*	1 Cracker/11g	51	2.1	467	8.1	62	19	6.1
Emmental, Netto*	1 Serving/25g	130	7	520	13	53	28	3.1
Extra Wheatgerm, Hovis*	1 Serving/6g	27	1.1	447	10.2	60	18.5	4.4
Flatbread, Multigrain, Carr's*	1 Cracker/10g	42	0.7	411	11	73.8	6.8	5.3
Flatbread, Multigrain, Jacob's*	1 Cracker/10g	42	0.7	411	11	73.8	6.8	5.3
Galletas Habaneras, Gamesa*	1 Cracker/8g	31	0.7	393	10	69.1	8.5	7.5
Garlic & Herb, Jacob's*	1 Cracker/10g	45	1.7	450	10	68.3	16.7	3.3
Garlic, CBY, Asda*	2 Biscuits/12g	58	2.6	483	7	63.3	21.5	4.2
Garlic, Rivercote, Lidl*	1 Cracker/6g	27	1.2	488	8	63.4	21.5	4.4
Grain Free, Chilli, Life Bake*	2 Crackers/15g	35	1.6	231	19.3	2.5	10.5	25.9
Harvest Grain, Sainsbury's*	1 Cracker/6g	27	1.1	458	8.5	64.5	18.4	4.1
Herb, & Onion, Free From, Morrisons*	1 Cracker/7g	31	0.9	448	1.7	78.6	12.8	5.7
Herbs & Spice Selection, Jacob's*	1 Cracker/6g	27	0.9	451	9.5	68	15.7	2.7
Integrali, MOLINO BIANCO*	1 Serving/25g	99	2	396	14	60.4	8	13.2
Lightly Salted, Italian, Jacob's*	1 Cracker/6g	26	0.8	429	10.3	67.6	13	2.9
Lightly Salted, Savoury Bakes, Aldi*	7 Crackers/25g	128	6.2	511	7.7	62	25	2.1

CRACKERS

Measure INFO/WEIGHT	per Measure KCAL	FAT	Nutrition Values per 100g / 100ml KCAL	PROT	CARB	FAT	FIBRE
Luxury, Selection, Lidl*	1 Cracker/5g	22	0.7	437	9.8	67.5	13.2	4.3
Matzos, Flame Baked, Rakusen's*	1 Cracker/21g	75	0.2	357	10	79	1	4.3
Matzos, Tea, Flamed Baked, Round, Rakusen's*	1 Cracker/5g	19	0	382	9.9	85.7	0.8	3.7
Mini, Savoury, Huntley & Palmers*	1 Serving/25g	127	6.5	508	6	62	26	0
Mixed Seed, Lunch Bakes, Jacobs*	1 Cracker/9g	45	1.6	497	10.6	71.1	18	4.3
Mixed Seed, Multi Grain, Asda*	1 Cracker/6g	28	1.1	445	11	62	17	4.4
Multi Seed, Thins, Ryvita*	1 Thin/9g	39	1.3	434	16.4	56.2	14.1	8.1
Multi-grain, Aldi, Savour Bakes, Aldi*	1 Cracker/5g	20	0.8	404	8.3	55	16.8	5.1
Multigrain Pops, Original, Slims*	1 Cracker/5g	18	0.1	367	11.4	75.5	1.4	3.4
Multigrain, Choice Grain, Jacobs*	1 Cracker/8g	34	1.1	429	8.8	63.9	14.2	5.5
Multigrain, Morrisons*	10 Crackers/20g	76	2.2	379	8.8	61.3	11	5.1
Multigrain, Savour Bakes, Aldi*	1 Cracker/5g	23	1.1	491	9.9	58	23	5.5
Multigrain, Tesco*	1 Cracker/5g	24	1	477	8.8	60.8	20.8	5.7
Naan, Multiseed, Tesco*	1 Cracker/3g	14	0.6	477	11.4	61.2	20	3.2
Naan, Tandoori, Tesco*	1 Cracker/2g	11	0.4	451	10.9	65.8	15.4	2.9
Oat & Wheat, Weight Watchers*	4 Crackers/20g	74	0.5	370	10.5	75	2.5	4
Olive Oil & Oregano, Mediterraneo, Jacob's*	1 Cracker/6g	25	0.7	412	12.4	65.5	11.2	6
Olive Oil, & Sea Salt, The Fine Cheese Co*	1 Cracker/5g	20	0.6	390	11.8	63.4	11.6	0
Olive Oil, Sea Salt & Black Pepper, Deliciously Ella*	1 Serving/30g	128	3	427	6.7	76.7	10	6.7
Oriental, Asda*	1 Serving/30g	115	6	383	1.7	49	20	4.3
Original, Ritz*	5 Crackers/16g	80	4.5	500	6.2	62.5	28.1	0
Paprika, & Nigella Seed, The Best, Morrisons*	1 Cracker/7g	31	1.2	448	10	61.4	16.9	4.9
Pizza Flavour, Mini, Sainsbury's*	1 Serving/25g	113	4	454	7.6	68.7	15.9	2.7
Plain, Free From, Morrisons*	1 Cracker/6g	27	0.8	443	1.5	77.9	12.7	5.4
Poppy & Sesame Seed, Sainsbury's*	1 Cracker/4g	20	1	482	9.5	57	23	4.2
Poppy Oat, Cracker Selection, TTD, Sainsbury's*	1 Cracker/4g	19	0.7	467	9.8	65	17.7	4.1
Poppy Seed, Savour Bakes, Aldi*	1 Cracker/4g	19	0.7	463	13	61	18	2
Poppy, & Sesame Seed, Thins, M&S*	1 Thin/4g	19	0.9	487	10.5	57.9	22.8	4
Pops, Multigrain, Onion Flavour, Slim's*	1 Cracker/5g	15	0	300	20	60	0	0
Pumpkin Seed, & Cheese, Bettabuy, Morrisons*	1 Cracker/23g	97	3	421	20.8	51.7	13	6.9
Quelitas, Rustic, Quely*	1 Cracker/3g	13	0.5	467	9.2	66	18	3.1
Rosemary, Co-Op*	1 Cracker/6g	29	1.4	499	7.6	61	24	2.6
Rosemary, Free From, Morrisons*	1 Cracker/6g	27	0.8	455	1.3	80.7	12.7	6.4
Rosemary, Rivercote, Lidl*	1 Cracker/6g	30	1.4	493	8.1	61.2	23.3	2.9
Rosemary, Sainsbury's*	1 Cracker/6g	30	1.4	502	7.8	65.1	22.7	3.1
Rye Cakes, Lightly Salted, Ryvita*	1 Cake/6g	23	0.1	363	8.9	69.9	2	13.7
Rye Cakes, Multigrain, Ryvita*	1 Rye Cake/7g	23	0.2	352	9.4	66.3	2.5	13.3
Rye, Sourdough,, The Best, Morrisons*	1 Cracker/4g	15	0.2	380	10.2	67.1	5.5	10.6
Salt & Black Pepper, Jacob's*	1 Cracker/6g	27	1	457	9.5	67.5	16.5	2.7
Salt & Black Pepper, Eat Well, M&S*	1 Pack/25g	106	3.7	422	9.6	62.9	14.7	5.1
Salt & Pepper, Sainsbury's*	1 Cracker/6g	29	1.3	504	8.1	65.8	22.5	3.2
Salt & Pepper, Tesco*	1 Cracker/6g	30	1.4	499	8.2	62.5	23.4	2.7
Salt & Pepper, WW*	1 Serving/30g	108	0.2	360	11.8	74.1	0.8	4.7
Salt, & Pepper, Asda*	1 Cracker/6g	30	1.4	497	8.2	63	23	2.7
Saltine, Wholewheat, Savour Bakes, Aldi*	1 Cracker/4g	19	0.9	478	10	58	22	5.6
Sea Salt & Vinegar Flavour, Bakefuls, Ritz*	1 Bag/23g	108	4.8	471	7	61	21	2.8
Sea Salt, & Black Pepper, Free From, Co-Op*	1 Cracker/6g	25	0.4	424	2.6	84	6.5	10
Sea Salt, Asda*	1 Serving/24g	123	5.8	508	8.1	65	24	2.8
Sea Salt, Gourmet, Savour Bakes, Aldi*	1 Cracker/3g	15	0.6	454	11	60	18	6.1
Sea Salt, Gourmet, Specially Selected, Aldi*	4 Crackers/20g	94	4	471	8.7	63	20	4.1
Sea Salt, Tesco*	5 Crackers/30g	149	7	496	8.1	61.8	23.5	2.8
Seeded, Gail's*	1 Cracker/10g	40	2.2	396	12	33.2	22.2	7.6
Selection, Finest, Tesco*	1 Serving/30g	136	4.3	452	9.6	71	14.4	0

	Measure	per Measure		Nutrition Values per 100g / 100ml				
	INFO/WEIGHT	KCAL	FAT	KCAL	PROT	CARB	FAT	FIBRE

CRACKERS

Sesame & Poppy Thins, Tesco*	1 Cracker/4g	20	1	485	9.9	57.6	23.5	4.4
Sesame, Am-mak Bakeries*	5 crackers/28g	110	2	393	17.9	67.9	7.1	10.7
Sesame, Osem*	1 Cracker/6g	29	1.1	469	11	68	17	0
Smokehouse BBQ Crunch, Graze*	1 Box/31g	137	4.7	441	10	62	15	5.4
Snackers, Tesco *	1 Cracker/3g	14	0.6	471	8.1	65.8	18.9	2.9
Sourdough, Rosemary, No.1, Waitrose*	1 Cracker/4g	15	0.2	379	10.4	69.5	4.5	9.2
Sourdough, Sesame, & Tomato, Market St, Morrisons*	1 Cracker/6g	26	0.9	435	15.4	54.1	15.7	7.9
Spicy Indonesian Vegetable, Waitrose*	1 Pack/60g	295	16.3	492	1.2	60.6	27.2	2.2
Spicy, Asda*	¼ Pack/25g	126	6.5	504	0.9	65	26	2
Super Seed, Sunflower, Sesame, & Linseed, M&S*	2 Crackers/14g	73	5.5	509	23.3	3	38.5	29.3
Sweet Chilli, Dipping, Tesco*	1 Cracker/3g	12	0.5	470	9.3	63.2	19.6	2
Sweet Chilli, Oat Bakes, Nairn's*	1 Bag/30g	128	4	426	8.1	68.4	13.3	7.2
Sweet Chilli, Thins, Ryvita*	1 Thin/8g	31	0.1	382	12	77.5	1.5	5.2
Sweet Potato, M&S*	1 Serving/25g	117	4.9	467	7.3	61.9	19.7	6.6
Tapas, Mediterranean, Feta & Oregano, Jacobs*	1 Cracker/6g	31	1.5	509	9.1	58.2	25.4	1.8
Tapas, Quely*	1 Cracker/6g	25	0.9	451	9.1	66	16	3.2
Tapas, Tomato & Basil, Mediterraneo, Jacob's*	1 Cracker/6g	28	1.3	500	9	61	24	1.4
Tarallini with Fennel Seeds, Crosta & Mollica*	1 Cracker/4g	21	0.9	529	8.2	67.5	22	4.2
Thai Spicy Vegetable, Sainsbury's*	1 Pack/50g	231	10.4	462	7.2	61.5	20.8	2.6
The British Barbecue, Graze*	1 Punnet/25g	127	8	508	17.4	36.8	32.2	7.4
Thins, Thai Sweet Chilli, Crisps, Jacob's*	1 Pack/25g	119	4.8	476	8.2	65.6	19.3	3.1
Tuc, Cheese Sandwich, Jacob's*	1 Cracker/14g	72	4.3	531	8.4	53.8	31.4	0
Tuc, Cheese, Mini, Jacobs*	¼ Pack/50g	242	11.5	485	9.2	59	23	2.4
Tuc, Jacob's*	1 Cracker/5g	25	1.4	518	6.9	54.2	29.9	2.6
Tuc, Mini with Sesame Seeds, Jacob's*	1 Biscuit/2g	10	0.5	523	9.7	63.1	25.8	3.9
Tuc, Original, Jacob's*	1 Cracker/4g	17	0.7	478	8.3	67	19	2.4
Veggie, Chickpea, & Paprika, Deliciously Ella*	1 Pack/30g	129	2.4	430	6.5	81	8	4.3
Water Biscuits, High Bake, M&S*	1 Cracker/5g	22	0.4	409	9.8	75.1	6.8	3.9
Wheat, Tesco*	6 Crackers/30g	139	5.6	464	11.2	60.2	18.8	4.6
Wheaten, M&S*	1 Cracker/4g	20	0.9	450	10.2	57	20.2	5

CRANBERRIES

& White Chocolate, Shot, Asda*	1 Pack/25g	94	2	375	2.8	71	8.1	3
Dried, Sweetened, Average	**1 Serving/10g**	**34**	**0.1**	**335**	**0.3**	**81.1**	**0.8**	**4.4**
Fresh, Raw, Average	**1oz/28g**	**4**	**0**	**15**	**0.4**	**3.4**	**0.1**	**3**
Yoghurt Coated, Wilko*	1 Serving/25g	117	4.8	469	1.5	71.4	19	3

CRAYFISH

Raw	**1oz/28g**	**19**	**0.2**	**67**	**14.9**	**0**	**0.8**	**0**
Tails, Cooked & Peeled, Waitrose*	1 Pack/100g	77	0.5	77	17.6	0.5	0.5	0.5
Tails, Sainsbury's*	1 Pack/80g	58	0.4	73	17.5	0.5	0.5	0.5

CREAM

Aerosol, Average	**1oz/28g**	**87**	**8.7**	**309**	**1.8**	**6.2**	**30.9**	**0**
Aerosol, Reduced Fat, Average	**1 Serving/55ml**	**33**	**3**	**60**	**0.6**	**2**	**5.4**	**0**
Brandy, Extra Thick, TTD, Sainsbury's*	1 Serving/30ml	131	12.3	436	1.4	10.4	40.8	0.5
Brandy, Really Thick, Finest, Tesco*	½ Pot/125ml	579	49.5	463	1.3	19.7	39.6	0
Chantilly, TTD, Sainsbury's*	2 Tbsp/30g	136	14	455	1.4	6.9	46.8	0
Clotted, Fresh, Average	**1 Serving/28g**	**162**	**17.5**	**579**	**1.6**	**2.3**	**62.7**	**0**
Double, Average	**1 Tbsp/15ml**	**68**	**7.3**	**452**	**1.6**	**2.4**	**48.4**	**0**
Double, Reduced Fat, Average	**1 Serving/30g**	**73**	**7**	**243**	**2.7**	**5.6**	**23.3**	**0.1**
Real Dairy, Lighter, Spray, Tesco*	1 Spray/13g	29	2.4	221	2.5	11	18.6	0
Real Dairy, Spray, Tesco*	1 Portion/13g	44	4.4	338	2.2	5.9	34	0
Single, Average	**1 Tbsp/15ml**	**28**	**2.7**	**188**	**2.6**	**3.9**	**18**	**0.1**
Single, Extra Thick, Average	**1 Serving/38ml**	**72**	**6.9**	**192**	**2.7**	**4.1**	**18.4**	**0**
Single, Soya, Fresh, Plant Based, Cuisine, Alpro*	1 Tbsp/15ml	18	1.5	122	2	4.5	10.2	0.4

C

CREAM

INFO/WEIGHT	Measure	per Measure KCAL	FAT	Nutrition Values per 100g / 100ml KCAL	PROT	CARB	FAT	FIBRE
Single, Soya, UHT, Plant Based, Cuisine, Alpro*	1 Tbsp/15g	23	2.2	151	2	1.2	15	0.3
Soured, Fresh, Average	*1 Tsp/5ml*	*10*	*0.9*	*191*	*2.7*	*3.9*	*18.4*	*0*
Soured, Reduced Fat, Average	*1 Tsp/5ml*	*6*	*0.4*	*119*	*5.2*	*6.7*	*8.6*	*0.4*
Soured, Squeezy, Old El Paso*	1 Tbsp/15g	20	1.7	130	0.7	6.8	11	0.5
Whipping, Average	*1 Tbsp/15ml*	*52*	*5.5*	*348*	*2.1*	*3.2*	*36.4*	*0*

CREAM ALTERNATIVE

Creamy Oat, Single, Oatly*	½ Carton/125ml	188	16.2	150	0.9	5.8	13	0.8
Double, Light, Elmlea*	1 Serving/30g	73	7.2	243	2.7	4.1	24	0
Double, Vegan, Plant, Elmlea*	1 Serving/25ml	72	7.8	289	0.6	2	31	0
Oat, Single, Free From, Asda*	1 Serving/110g	128	10.9	116	0.5	6.3	9.9	0.5
Single, Oatly*	½ Carton/125ml	188	16.2	150	1	6	13	0.7
Single, Vegan, Plant, Elmlea*	1 Serving/25ml	38	3.8	153	1.5	2.4	15.4	0
Whipped, Vegan, Heavenly, Food Heaven*	1 Squirt/10ml	20	1.6	203	0	15	16	0

CREAM SODA

American with Vanilla, Tesco*	1 Glass/313ml	75	0	24	0	5.9	0	0
Barr's*	1 Can/330ml	33	0	10	0.5	2.2	0	0
Diet, Sainsbury's*	1 Serving/250ml	2	0	1	0	0	0	0
Shapers, Boots*	1 Bottle/300ml	3	0	1	0	0	0	0
Traditional Style, Tesco*	1 Can/330ml	139	0	42	0	10.4	0	0

CREME BRULEE

Average	*1 Serving/100g*	*313*	*26*	*313*	*3.8*	*15.7*	*26*	*0.2*
Reduced Fat, M&S*	1 Serving/89g	186	13.1	210	4.9	14.2	14.8	0.5
Vanilla, Pots & Co*	1 Pot/90g	376	33.1	418	4	17.8	36.8	0

CREME CARAMEL

Average	*1 Serving/128g*	*140*	*2.8*	*109*	*3*	*20.6*	*2.2*	*0*

CREME EGG

Cadbury*	1 Egg/40g	177	6	440	3.2	73	15	0.4
Minis, Cadbury*	1 Egg/12g	50	1.9	435	4.2	67	16.5	0.5

CREME FRAICHE

Average	*1 Pot/295g*	*1067*	*112.2*	*362*	*2.2*	*2.6*	*38*	*0*
Half Fat, Average	*1 Tbsp/15g*	*27*	*2.4*	*181*	*3.1*	*5.5*	*16.2*	*0*
Low Fat, Average	*1 Tbsp/30ml*	*43*	*3.6*	*143*	*3.3*	*5.6*	*12.1*	*0.1*
Oat, Creamy, Oatly*	1 Tbsp/15ml	27	2.2	177	1	9.1	15	1

CREPES

Chocolate Filled, Saint Albert *	1 Crepe/30g	143	6.6	478	6.1	60	22	0
Chocolate Filled, Tesco*	1 Crepe/32g	137	5.2	429	5.9	63.5	16.2	3
Chocolate Filled, Whaoo*	1 Crepe/32g	150	7.4	468	6.7	57	23	3
Duc De Coeur, Lidl*	1 Crepe/50g	78	3.5	156	5.6	17	7	0
Galette, Buckwheat, Average	*1 Serving/100g*	*161*	*1.7*	*161*	*5.8*	*30.2*	*1.7*	*1*
Mushroom, M&S*	1 Pack/186g	195	4.5	105	5.7	17.1	2.4	2.5
Praline, At Home, Cote*	½ Pack/125g	533	26.8	427	7.8	49.6	21.5	1.4

CRISPBAKES

Cheddar & Onion, Cooked, Free From, Tesco*	1 Bake/125g	291	15.1	232	7.1	22.8	12.1	2
Cheese & Onion, Tesco*	1 Bake/116g	233	12.6	201	5.4	18.6	10.9	3.3
Cheese & Onion, Meat Free, Morrisons*	1 Bake/136g	282	13.8	207	1.5	23.5	10.1	4.9
Cheese & Onion, Ovenbaked, Iceland*	1 Bake/76g	131	5.7	173	5.1	20.6	7.5	1.4
Cheese & Onion, Sainsbury's*	1 Bake/114g	201	8.7	177	4.9	21.1	7.7	2
Cheese, & Onion, British Classic, Sainsbury's*	1 Bake/110g	272	17.5	247	7	18.2	15.9	1.4
Cheese, & Bacon, Crestwood, Aldi*	1 Bake/114g	316	19.3	278	6.9	23	17	2
Cheese, & Onion, Asda*	1 Bake/130g	315	14.3	242	7.6	28	11	1.6
Cheese, Spring Onion & Chive, Sainsbury's*	1 Bake/107g	232	10.2	216	6.4	25.1	9.5	2.2
Dutch, Asda*	1 Bake/8g	31	0.3	388	14.7	74.9	3.3	4.2
Dutch, Co-Op*	1 Bake/10g	38	0.4	375	16	69.6	3.5	6.5

	Measure INFO/WEIGHT	KCAL	FAT	Nutrition Values per 100g / 100ml				
				KCAL	PROT	CARB	FAT	FIBRE
CRISPBAKES								
Dutch, HL, Tesco*	1 Bake/8g	30	0.2	385	14.7	74.9	2.7	4.2
Dutch, Original, Van Der Meulen*	1 Bake/8g	30	0.2	386	14.4	73.4	3.1	3.4
Dutch, Sainsbury's*	1 Bake/10g	38	0.5	392	14.5	72.3	5	5.8
Dutch, Tesco*	1 Bake/10g	40	0.5	397	13.6	71.7	5.3	4.2
Garlic & Mushroom, Eatwell*	1 Bake/113g	213	10.4	188	5.3	19.9	9.2	2.4
Minced Beef, M&S*	1 Bake/113g	226	12.3	200	10	15.6	10.9	1.5
Minced Beef, M&S*	1 Bake/114g	218	10.2	192	9.2	17.6	9	1.9
Roast Vegetable & Basil, Cauldron Foods*	1 Bake/115g	242	11	210	3.5	26	9.6	2.9
Vegetable, Crunchy, Vegetarian, Waitrose*	1 Bake/113g	234	10.4	207	4.5	27.5	9.2	3.5
Vegetable, M&S*	1 Bake/114g	200	10.3	175	2.5	19.2	9	2.6
CRISPBREAD								
3 Grain 3 Seed, Foodie Market, Aldi*	1 Crispbread/25g	109	4.2	436	15	52	17	8.8
3 Seed, Classic, Gourmet, Dr Karg*	1 Crispbread/25g	108	4.9	430	16.5	46.6	19.7	10.9
Apple & Cinnamon, Ryvita*	1 Crispbread/15g	54	0.2	356	7.2	72.5	1.6	11.8
Cheese & Pumpkin Seed, Oven Baked, M&S*	1 Crispbread/25g	120	5.4	480	17.1	50.9	21.7	6.4
Chestnut, Organic, Amisa*	1 Crispbread/6g	21	0.1	343	6.9	77	1.2	4.3
Chia Seed, & Buckwheat, Protein, Ryvita*	1 Crispbread/10g	38	0.4	371	21.5	56.9	3.7	12
Cracked Black Pepper, Thins, Ryvita*	1 Crispbread/10g	35	0.2	344	8.8	66.6	1.6	14.5
Currant, Seed, & Oat, Fruit Crunch, Ryvita*	1 Crispbread/15g	54	0.8	358	8.3	61.8	5.4	14.9
Dark Rye, Ryvita*	1 Crispbread/10g	34	0.1	342	8.5	66.5	1.2	15.2
Dill, Ikea*	1 Crispbread/25g	100	1.9	399	14	69	7.5	0
Fibre Plus, Wholegrain with Sesame, Wasa*	1 Crispbread/10g	35	0.7	350	13	47	7	24
Fruit Crunch, Ryvita*	1 Crispbread/12g	45	0.7	358	8.3	61.8	5.4	14.9
GF, Average	**1 Crispbread/8g**	**25**	**0.1**	**331**	**6.4**	**72.9**	**1.5**	**0**
Krispies, Toasted Rolls, Wholegrain, Papadopoulou *	1 Crispbread/11g	41	0.7	386	15	59	7.1	12
Mixed Grain, Jacobs*	1 Crispbread/10g	41	1.3	436	9.1	66.7	13.9	4.2
Multigrain, Rye, Crunchy, Ryvita*	1 Crispbread/10g	37	0.5	354	12.8	55.7	5.1	17.2
Multigrain, Ryvita*	1 Crispbread/11g	41	0.8	370	11.2	56	7.2	18.3
Original Rye, Thin, Finn Crisp*	1 Crispbread/6g	22	0.2	339	10	59	2.6	20
Original, Rye, Rivercote, Lidl*	1 Crispbread/10g	36	0.1	357	9.8	71.2	0.9	12.6
Original, Ryvita*	1 Crispbread/10g	35	0.2	350	8.5	66.9	1.7	16.5
Protein Punch, GF, Genius*	1 Crispbread/24g	120	7.7	501	17	27	32	21
Pumpkin Seeds & Oats, Ryvita*	1 Crispbread/13g	46	0.8	366	13.5	54.7	6.6	16.8
Rye, Morrisons*	1 Crispbread/3g	10	0.1	326	10.3	54.7	3.1	18.8
Rye, Original, Tesco*	1 Crispbread/9g	32	0.3	357	11.6	62.4	2.8	18
Rye, Vegan, Melvit*	1 Crispbread/15g	66	3.2	441	13	58	21	0
Scan Bran, Slimming World*	1 Crispbread/10g	31	0.5	310	14.9	29	5.3	42.1
Sesame & Rye, Tesco*	1 Crispbread/9g	34	0.8	385	12.5	55.6	8.7	17.2
Sesame, Ryvita*	1 Crispbread/10g	37	0.7	373	10.5	58.3	7	17.5
Sesame, Savour Bakes, Aldi*	1 Crispbread/9g	31	0.5	344	10	57.8	5.6	15.6
Sesame, Simply, Ryvita*	1 Crispbread/10g	40	0.7	383	13.4	57.5	6.9	18.5
Sourdough, Original, Peter's Yard*	1 Crispbread/3g	11	0.1	381	12.9	68.3	4.1	9.5
Sweet Onion, Ryvita*	1 Crispbread/12g	43	0.2	356	9	70.6	1.4	12.6
Wheat, Morrisons*	1 Crispbread/8g	28	0.3	377	11.5	73.1	3.4	4.2
Wholegrain, Rye, with Sesame Seeds, Rivercote, Lidl*	1 Crispbrea/10g	38	0.7	383	11.4	62.1	7	13.1
with Chives, Lunch Bakes, Jacob's*	1 Crispbread/10g	49	1.5	487	9.6	75.2	15.3	4.7
CRISPS								
Apple, Eat Smart, Morrisons*	1 Pack/20g	68	0.1	338	1.9	75.3	0.7	11.4
Apple, Thyme & Sage, M&S*	1 Bag/55g	253	13.4	460	5.5	55.3	24.3	6.1
Bacon Bites, Asda*	1 Bag/25g	126	6.2	502	6.6	62	25	2
Bacon Rashers, Happy Shopper*	1 Serving/23g	113	5.7	493	5.9	60	25	1.8
Bacon Rashers, M&S*	1 Pack/18g	72	1.4	398	8.4	72.1	7.8	3.1
Bacon, Brown Bag*	1 Pack/40g	199	10.7	498	5.6	58.7	26.7	2.5

C

CRISPS

	Measure INFO/WEIGHT	per Measure KCAL	FAT	Nutrition Values per 100g / 100ml KCAL	PROT	CARB	FAT	FIBRE
Bacon, Crispies, Sainsbury's*	1 Bag/25g	117	5.7	468	19.9	45.8	22.8	4.8
Bacon, Rashers, BGTY, Sainsbury's*	1 Pack/10g	34	0.2	340	10.8	70.3	1.6	3.5
Bacon, Rashers, COU, M&S*	1 Pack/20g	72	0.6	360	9.4	77.5	2.9	3.5
Bacon, Rashers, Iceland*	1 Bag/75g	330	13.2	440	8.3	61.9	17.6	2.9
Bacon, Rashers, Snackrite, Aldi*	1 Bag/18g	89	4.3	496	5.6	63	24	1.7
Bacon, Rice Bites, Asda*	1 Bag/30g	136	4.8	452	7	70	16	0.4
Bacon, Shapers, Boots*	1 Bag/23g	99	3.4	431	8	66	15	3
Bacon, Sizzler, Ridge Cut, McCoys*	1 Bag/32g	165	9.7	516	7.1	53.6	30.3	3.9
Bacon, Sizzler, Ridged, Snackrite, Aldi*	1 Pack/30g	160	9.3	532	7.2	55	31	3.9
Bacon, Smith's, Walkers*	1 Bag/23g	113	5.3	488	7.5	62	23	1.3
Bacon, Smoky, BGTY, Sainsbury's*	1 Bag/25g	118	5.9	472	6.5	58.5	23.6	5.7
Bacon, Smoky, Select, Tesco*	1 Bag/25g	134	8.7	536	6.4	49	34.9	4.3
Bacon, Smoky, Snackrite, Aldi*	1 Bag/25g	130	7.2	522	6	57	29	3.3
Bacon, Smoky, Sunseed Oil, Walkers*	1 Bag/35g	183	11.4	530	6.5	51	33	4
Bacon, Smoky, Tayto*	1 Bag/35g	184	11.9	526	7.6	47.3	34	4.5
Baked, Average	**1 Bag/25g**	**93**	**1.5**	**374**	**6.5**	**73.5**	**5.9**	**5.8**
Barbecue Beef, Ridge Cut, Kettle Chips*	1 Pack/40g	202	11.2	505	7.3	53.6	27.9	5
Barbecue, Corn Chips, Popchips*	1 Bag/17g	73	2.9	430	6	65	17	1.6
Barbecue, Pirato*	1 Pack/29g	156	8.4	539	6.5	56	29	0
Barbecue, Pop Outs, Passions, Aldi*	1 Pack/100g	422	13	422	5.8	69	13	3
Barbecue, Potato Crisps, Popchips*	1 Pack/23g	97	3.4	420	5.7	62	15	3.9
BBQ Rib, Double Crunch, Max, Walkers*	1 Serving/30g	145	7.4	483	7.7	55.3	24.7	5.7
BBQ, Double, Max, Walkers*	1 Serving30g	146	7.4	485	7.7	55.3	24.6	5.8
BBQ, Popped Chips, Asda*	1 Serving/21g	91	3.2	432	6.2	67	15	4.5
BBQ, Southern Style, Bugles, Walkers*	1 Pack/20g	105	6	525	6.5	56	30	3.5
BBQ, Spicy, Popped Chips, Co-Op*	1 Pack/23g	92	1.4	399	6.7	77	6.3	3.5
BBQ, Stackers, Snackrite, Aldi*	1 Serving/25g	134	8.5	538	3.1	53	34	4
Beasty Bites, Pickled Onion, Asda*	1 Bag/22g	111	5.5	505	6.2	64	25	0.5
Beef Wellington, M&S*	1 Pack/40g	203	11.4	507	7.3	51.6	28.5	7.4
Beef, & Onion Flavour, Average	**1 Bag/25g**	**131**	**8.3**	**524**	**6.5**	**50**	**33.1**	**4.3**
Beef, & Red Wine, Specially Selected, Aldi*	1 Serving/25g	130	7.3	519	5.1	59	29	2.5
Beef, Barbecue, Select, Tesco*	1 Pack/25g	134	8.7	536	6.4	49.2	34.8	4.4
Beef, Chinese Sizzling, McCoys*	1 Bag/35g	177	10.6	506	6.9	51.8	30.2	4
Beef, Maize & Potato, Happy Shopper*	1/3 Pack/23g	120	6.7	520	7.3	58	29	1.6
Beef, Roast, Monster Claws, Snackrite, Aldi*	1 Pack/17g	87	4.4	511	6.3	62	26	1.2
Beef, Space Raiders, KP Snacks*	1 Pack/13g	64	2.9	495	6.5	65.3	22.8	1
Beefy, Smiths, Walkers*	1 Bag/25g	133	9.2	531	4.3	45.2	37	0
Beetroot, Eat Smart, Morrisons*	1 Pack/20g	63	0.1	313	15.1	52	0.4	20.5
Beetroot, with Sweet Chilli Jam, Baked with Veg, Walkers*	1 Pack/23g	100	3.2	434	7.2	67	14	3.4
Black Truffle, & Olive Oil, M&S*	1 Serving/30g	148	8.1	493	4.3	54.7	27	8.3
Burger Bites, Happy Shopper*	1 Serving/23g	120	6.7	520	7.3	58	29	1.6
Cheddar, & Chive, Mature, Tyrrells*	1 Serving/30g	134	6.9	447	6.9	53.7	23.1	2.4
Cheddar, & Onion, Crinkles, Walkers*	1 Pack/28g	150	9.3	538	6	51.5	33.3	3.5
Cheddar, & Red Onion Chutney, Sensations, Walkers*	1 Bag/40g	198	11.2	495	6.5	54	28	4.5
Cheddar, & Red Onion, Mature, Finest, Tesco*	1 Bag/40g	208	8.3	519	5.1	58.6	20.8	2.5
Cheddar, & Jalapeno, Popchips*	1 Pack/85g	351	12.8	413	6.4	64	15	4.2
Cheddar, & Onion, Double Crunch, Max, Walkers*	1 Serving/30g	146	7.5	486	7.7	55	24.9	5.8
Cheddar, & Onion, McCoys*	1 Pack/25g	132	7.5	530	7.4	54	30	4.3
Cheddar, & Red Onion, Specially Selected, Aldi*	1 Pack/25g	126	7	504	9	50	28	6.6
Cheddar, Mature, & Onion, Hand Cooked, Spar*	1 Serving/22g	109	5.4	495	8	58.4	24.7	3.6
Cheddar, Mature, & Red Onion, Hand Cooked, M&S*	1 Pack/40g	206	11.7	515	7.8	52.5	29.2	5.6
Cheddars, Mini, Sticks, Jacobs*	1 Pack/25g	116	4.7	464	10.8	62.4	18.8	2
Cheese & Onion, 30% Less Fat, Sainsbury's*	1 Pack/25g	115	5.4	459	7.5	58.1	21.8	5.4

CRISPS

INFO/WEIGHT	Measure	per Measure KCAL	per Measure FAT	Nutrition Values per 100g / 100ml KCAL	PROT	CARB	FAT	FIBRE
Cheese & Onion, Crinkle Cut, Low Fat, Waitrose*	1 Bag/25g	122	5.8	490	7.7	62.6	23.2	4.7
Cheese & Onion, GFY, Asda*	1 Pack/26g	122	5.7	470	7	61	22	4.2
Cheese & Onion, M&S*	1 Bag/25g	134	8.9	535	5.5	48.8	35.5	5
Cheese & Onion, Max, Walkers*	1 Pack/50g	266	16.4	533	6.8	51	32.9	2.9
Cheese & Onion, Organic, Tesco*	1 Bag/25g	128	8.2	514	5.2	49.9	32.6	7
Cheese & Onion, Sainsbury's*	1 Bag/25g	132	8.7	527	4.6	48.8	34.8	3.9
Cheese & Onion, Squares, Walkers*	1 Bag/25g	108	4.5	430	6.5	61	18	5.5
Cheese & Onion, Value, Tesco*	1 Bag/20g	108	7.2	541	6	48.3	36	4.8
Cheese & Onion, Walkers*	1 Pack/22g	95	3.5	430	5	66	16	5
Cheese & Onion Flavour, Asda*	1 Bag/25g	130	7.8	519	5.6	53.6	31.4	3.7
Cheese & Onion, Baked, Walkers*	1 Bag/32g	164	5.1	436	6.7	68.6	13.6	6.2
Cheese & Onion, Crinkle, Seabrook*	1 Pack/32g	170	10.5	536	5.9	51.1	33.1	5.2
Cheese & Onion, Discos, KP Snacks*	1 Pack/28g	146	8.2	520	5.1	59.1	29.3	2.5
Cheese & Onion, Golden Wonder*	1 Bag/25g	132	8	530	6.1	53	31.9	3
Cheese & Onion, Oven Baked, Asda*	1 Bag/25g	95	2	380	5.1	72	8	3.3
Cheese & Onion, Oven Baked, Tesco*	1 Bag/25g	102	1.6	410	5.3	74.7	6.6	7.7
Cheese & Onion, Pom Bear, KP Snacks*	1 Bag/13g	68	3.6	521	3.9	63	28	2.4
Cheese & Onion, Pop, Protein, Corners*	1 Pack/85g	343	7.7	403	27.4	47.7	9.1	10.5
Cheese & Onion, Shake That Weight*	1 Pack/25g	90	2.5	360	44.8	14.4	10	16
Cheese & Onion, Smiths*	1 Pack/25g	130	10.1	518	6.2	52.9	40.4	4.2
Cheese & Onion, Snackrite, Aldi*	1 Pack/25g	137	8.2	548	7.2	55	33	1.5
Cheese & Onion, Sunseed Oil, Walkers*	1 Bag/33g	171	10.7	525	7	50	33	4
Cheese & Onion, Tesco*	1 Pack/25g	135	8	535	5.4	54.8	31.8	3.2
Cheese & Onion, Walkers*	1 Multi Bag/25g	124	6.7	495	5.6	55.9	26.7	4.4
Cheese Balls, Free From, Tesco*	1/6 Pack/25g	123	5.8	492	5.6	65.1	23.1	0.4
Cheese Curls, Morrisons*	1 Bag/17g	95	6.1	557	3.1	54.8	35.6	2.6
Cheese Curls, Sainsbury's*	1 Pack/16g	87	5.5	546	3.3	55.6	34.1	1.9
Cheese Curls, Snaktastic, Lidl*	1 Pack/12g	65	4.2	545	3.4	54.1	34.6	1.8
Cheese Curls, Tesco*	1 Bag/14g	75	4.5	520	4.5	54.4	31.1	1.9
Cheese Puffs, Happy Shopper*	1 Serving/23g	120	6.4	522	7.1	59	28	1.1
Cheese Puffs, Happy Shopper*	1 Serving/23g	120	6.4	522	7.1	59	28	1.1
Cheese Puffs, Tesco*	1 Bag/17g	99	6.7	580	4.6	52.1	39	0.9
Cheese Tasters, M&S*	1 Pack/30g	156	8.7	521	8.2	56.2	29	1
Cheese Tasters, Reduced Fat, M&S*	1 Pack/80g	380	15.9	475	8	65.5	19.9	0.9
Cheese, & Chives, Walkers*	1 Bag/33g	172	10.7	530	6.5	50	33	4.1
Cheese, & Onion, Reduced Fat, Tesco*	1 Pack/25g	116	5.1	463	8.7	57.3	20.4	7.6
Cheeseburger, Classic, Walkers*	1 Multipack/25g	124	6.8	497	5.7	55	27	4.6
Cheesy Wiggles, Asda*	1 Pack/16g	85	4.6	529	7.1	59	29	1.2
Chicken & Thyme, Oven Baked, Walkers*	1 Pack/25g	109	3.4	436	7.1	68	13.6	6.1
Chicken Katsu Curry, Ridge Cut, M&S*	1 Pack/40g	202	11.6	506	7.5	51	28.9	5.7
Chicken Wings, Hot, Strong, Max, Walkers*	1 Bag/30g	160	9.9	532	6.3	51	33	3
Chicken, & Thyme, Oven Roasted, Tesco*	1 Pack/150g	728	40.5	485	6.5	54	27	4.5
Chicken, & Chorizo, Double, Max, Walkers*	1 Pack/140g	683	35	488	7.8	54.9	25	6
Chicken, Chargrilled, Ridged, Snackrite, Aldi*	1 Pack/30g	157	9	524	6.5	54	30	4
Chicken, Roast, Select, Tesco*	1 Bag/25g	134	8.8	536	6.6	48.6	35	4.4
Chicken, Roast, Snack Rite*	1 Bag/25g	132	8.3	526	5.3	51.3	33.3	0
Chickpea Chips, Cheese & Onion, Sainsbury's*	1 Pack/20g	79	1.9	395	11	62.5	9.5	7.5
Chickpea Snack, Bean & Rosemary, WW*	1 Pack/21g	87	2.4	412	15.1	60.4	11.3	4.3
Chilli, & Lime, Strong, Max, Walkers*	1 Pack/30g	160	9.9	532	6.6	50.9	32.9	3.1
Chip Sticks, Salted, Lidl*	1 Serving/25g	137	8.8	548	5.5	51	35	0
Chip Sticks, Salted, Morrisons*	1/6 Bag/25g	127	7	508	5.2	57	28.2	2.8
Chiplets, Salt & Vinegar, Reduced Fat, M&S*	1 Pack/30g	122	3.8	407	6.7	65	12.7	4.3
Chipsters, Potato Snacks, Belin*	1 Serving/30g	142	6	472	4.3	66	20	4

CRISPS

INFO/WEIGHT	Measure	per Measure KCAL	FAT	Nutrition Values per 100g / 100ml KCAL	PROT	CARB	FAT	FIBRE
Chunky, Egg & Chips, Slabs*	1 Pack/80g	372	15	465	5.6	67.5	18.8	1.7
Combo Mix, Ready Salted, M&S*	1 Serving/30g	139	6	463	5	63.7	20.1	3.7
Combo Mix, Sour Cream, & Onion, Tesco*	1 Serving/25g	116	4.7	466	4.4	67.9	18.8	3.6
Corn Chips, Popped Not Fried, M&S*	1 Serving/23g	95	2.1	415	6.1	72.3	9.2	6.1
Corn Sticks, Rymut*	1 Pack/60g	215	1	359	7.9	75	1.7	3
Crinkle Cut, Lower Fat, No Added Salt, Waitrose*	1 Bag/40g	193	10	483	6.5	58	25	3.9
Crinkle Cut, Ready Salted, Snackrite, Aldi*	1 Bag/25g	122	6	488	7.2	59	24	3.9
Crinkle Cut, Salt & Vinegar, Coles*	1 Serving/25g	126	7.7	502	0	48.6	30.7	3.6
Crinklys, Baked, Cheese & Onion, Jacob's*	1 Pack/25g	122	5.4	489	8.5	63.4	21.6	2.9
Crinklys, Baked, Chilli Beef, Jacob's*	1 Pack/25g	123	5.6	492	8.3	63.2	22.2	2.6
Crunchy Fries, Snaktastic, Lidl*	1 Bag/15g	69	3.2	461	4.4	61.3	21.2	3.9
Crunchy Sticks, Ready Salted, M&S*	1 Pack/75g	398	24.8	530	5.6	52.2	33	3.8
Crunchy Sticks, Ready Salted, Tesco*	1 Serving/25g	119	5.9	475	5.6	60.3	23.5	3
Crunchy Sticks, Salt & Vinegar, Sainsbury's*	1 Bag/25g	118	6.1	474	5.9	58	24.3	2.4
Crunchy Sticks, Salt & Vinegar, Value, Tesco*	1 Bag/22g	112	5.7	509	5	64	25.8	0.8
Duck & Hoisin, Crispy, Walkers*	1 Bag/25g	131	8.2	523	5.8	51.5	32.6	4
Fiery Peri Peri, Max Strong, Walkers*	1 Pack/27g	139	8.4	515	7	51.8	31.1	4.4
Firecracker Ribs, Ridge Cut, TTD, Sainsbury's*	1 Serving/30g	160	10	532	7.4	47.7	33.5	4.8
Flamin' Hot, Fiercely, Max, Walkers*	1 Pack/50g	265	16.4	530	6.5	50.8	32.8	3
Flatbread Chips, Indian Spiced, TTD, Sainsbury's*	1 Serving/30g	135	4.7	449	11.2	61.8	15.5	8.7
Footballs, Cheese Flavour, Cheetos*	1 Serving/30g	156	8.3	520	5.4	61.4	27.8	1.4
French Fries, Worcester Sauce, Walkers*	1 Pack/18g	79	3	441	5.9	64.1	16.8	4.8
Fries, Loaded, Salt & Vinegar, Seabrook*	1 Bag/19g	89	4.5	467	5	59	23.5	1.3
Fruit, Apple, Air Dried, 100% Fruit, Spare Snacks*	1 Pack/22g	76	0.1	346	2.3	76.8	0.6	12.2
Fruit, Apple, Air Dried, M&S*	1 Bag/16g	54	0.1	339	1.8	75.9	0.8	10.3
Fruit, Pineapple, Air Dried, M&S*	1 Pack/16g	55	0	341	3.1	76.6	0.1	10.4
Funyuns, Smiths*	1 Serving/30g	158	8.7	525	6.2	59	29	1.7
Garden Greens, Emily Crisps Ltd*	1 Pack/23g	97	3.4	420	8.5	56.9	14.6	13.7
Ham, Honey Roast, Hand Cooked, Finest, Tesco*	1 Serving/25g	130	7.3	515	5.1	58.6	28.8	2.5
Ham, Honey Roast, Reduced Fat, M&S*	1 Serving/30g	140	6	467	7.9	61.4	20.1	4.5
Handcooked, Lightly Salted, Fairfields Farm Crisps*	1 Pack/40g	200	11.3	499	6.1	56.2	28.3	2.5
High Fives, Tayto*	1 Pack/20g	97	4.6	485	6.5	62.5	23	2
Hint of Salt, Natural Sea Salt, Walkers*	1 Pack/25g	126	7	506	6	54.3	28.3	4.7
Honey & Mustard, Mackie's*	1 Pack/30g	150	7.8	499	5.8	60	26	2.7
Hoops, Ready Salted, Snackrite, Aldi*	1 Bag/25g	124	6	494	3.3	65	24	2.6
Hummus Bites, The Foodie Market, Aldi*	1 Bag/20g	94	4.2	468	7.9	59	21	6.1
Hummus, Tomato & Basil, Eat Real*	1 Serving/45g	216	10.8	481	6.4	57.5	24	5.4
Jagabee BBQ, Calbee*	1 Pack/14g	80	5.6	569	5.1	50.5	40	2.7
Jalapeno, & Cheese, Strong, Max, Multipack, Walkers*	1 Multipack/27g	139	8.4	515	7.3	49.5	31	4.3
Jalapeno, & Cheese, Strong, Max, Walkers*	1 Pack/30g	159	9.9	531	6.5	51	33	3.1
Katsu Curry, Yo!, Walkers*	1 Pack/25g	124	6.8	496	6	56	27.2	4.8
Kentucky Fried Chicken, Max, Walkers*	½ Bag/70g	354	20.3	505	7	51.9	29	4.3
Lamb & Mint, Slow Roasted, Sensations, Walkers*	1 Bag/35g	170	9.4	485	6.5	54	27	4.5
Lamb, & Mint, Seabrook*	1 Pack/25g	126	7.2	505	6.3	53.3	28.7	0
Lentil Bites, Sea Salt, Snaktastic, Lidl*	1 Serving/23g	110	4.8	478	8	62.1	21	4.5
Lentil Chips, Sea Salt, Proper Crisps*	1 Serving/20g	96	4.2	482	9.7	63.6	20.8	0.7
Lentil Chips, Sour Cream, & Chive, Proper Chips*	1 Pack/20g	93	3.9	466	9.8	63	19.3	1
Lentil Curls, Chilli & Lime, Nudie Snacks*	1 Pack/35g	153	6.7	422	9.5	54	18.6	5.3
Lentil Curls, Sour Cream & Chive, Sainsbury's*	1 Pack/20g	95	4.1	476	10.5	61.3	20.3	3.1
Lentil Curls, Sour Cream & Onion, Asda*	1 Pack/20g	98	4.6	490	11	59	23	3.4
Lentil Curls, Sour Cream, & Chive, Tesco*	1 Pack/20g	90	3.1	448	11.3	64.1	15.6	3.3
Lentil Curls, Thai Sweet Chilli, Passions Deli*	1 Pack/20g	91	3.4	456	11	63	17	4.1
Lentil Curls, Thai Sweet Chilli, Snaktastic, Lidl*	1 Pack/20g	92	3.6	460	11	61.5	18	3.5

CRISPS

INFO/WEIGHT	Measure	per Measure		Nutrition Values per 100g / 100ml				
		KCAL	FAT	KCAL	PROT	CARB	FAT	FIBRE
Lentil Curls, Tomato & Garlic, Snaktastic, Lidl*	1 Pack/20g	92	3.6	460	10.7	62	18.1	3.3
Lentil Waves, Salt & Vinegar, Burts*	1 Pack/20g	92	3.7	462	10.2	62.3	18.3	3.7
Lightly Salted, Crinkle Cut, Finest, Tesco*	1/6 Pack/25g	124	6.8	495	6.8	53.7	27.4	3.4
Maize, Cheese, Tayto*	1 Multipack/17g	79	4	463	6.9	55.1	23.4	0
Marmite, Sunseed, Walkers*	1 Bag/33g	168	9.9	517	7.3	51.1	30.5	4.3
Mature Cheddar, & Onion, Happy Shopper*	1 Serving/50g	254	14.5	509	6.8	54	29	0
Mature Cheddar, & Onion, The Best, Morrisons*	1 Serving/25g	131	7.5	525	6.3	55.9	29.9	3.4
Monster Claws, Flamin' Hot, Snackrite, Aldi*	1 Pack/18g	91	4.7	503	5.9	60	26	1.4
Monster Claws, Flamin' Hot, Snaktastic, Lidl*	1 Pack/18g	92	5	511	6.1	58.3	27.8	0.6
Monster Claws, Pickled Onion, Snackrite, Aldi*	1 Pack/18g	92	4.9	511	6.1	61.1	27.2	2.8
Multi Grain Waves, Sweet Chilli, The Foodie Market, Aldi*	1 Pack/25g	117	5.1	468	8	60	20.4	4.8
Multigrain Bites, Snaktastic, Lidl*	1 Pack/25g	115	4.4	460	7.2	66	17.6	5.2
Multigrain Waves, Sour Cream & Black Pepper, Tesco*	1 Bag/20g	97	4.6	483	6.4	60.4	23.1	3.9
Multigrain Waves, Sweet Chilli, Tesco *	1 Pack/20g	96	4.6	480	6.5	59.5	23	4
Nacho Cheese, Muchos, Mccoys*	1 Serving/30g	160	9.6	535	6.2	55	32	2.7
Nacho Cheese, Tortitos*	1 Pack/30g	123	4.8	410	40	17.3	16	15
Naked, Tyrrells*	1 Serving/30g	152	8.6	507	7.1	52	28.7	5.2
Oat, Snackers, Smoked Paprika, GF, Nairn's*	1 Bag/23g	101	4	440	9.7	56.6	17.4	9.3
Onion Rings, Corn Snacks, Average	**1 Bag/25g**	**122**	**6.1**	**486**	**5.8**	**60.9**	**24.2**	**2.7**
Onion, Pickled, Golden Wonder*	1 Bag/25g	131	8.5	524	5.6	49	34	2
Onion, Pickled, Space Raiders, KP Snacks*	1 Bag/13g	64	2.9	495	6.5	65.3	22.8	1
Onion, Pickled, Sunseed, Walkers*	1 Bag/33g	171	10.7	525	6.5	50	33	4
Pancetta, Italian Style, M&S*	1 Pack/25g	155	13.1	620	36.6	0.9	52.3	1.3
Paprika Mix, Warm & Smoky, Waitrose*	1 Serving/25g	127	7.1	509	4	57.5	28.3	3.9
Paprika, Corn Snacks, Shapers, Boots*	1 Pack/13g	64	3.5	494	8.7	54	27	2.2
Paprika, Double Crunch, Max, Walkers*	½ Bag/75g	398	24.4	530	6.5	51.2	32.6	3.1
Paprika, Hand Cooked, M&S*	1 Pack/40g	210	12.5	524	5.9	52.3	31.3	4.5
Paprika, Max, Walkers*	1 Bag/50g	265	16.3	530	6.5	51.2	32.6	3.1
Parmesan, & Prosciutto, M&S*	1 Pack/40g	206	11.9	516	8.5	50.6	29.8	5.9
Parsnip, Honey Roast, M&S*	1 Serving/50g	275	21.3	550	4.1	30.5	42.6	14.3
Pastrami & Cheese, Crinkle, M&S*	1 Bag/25g	120	5.9	485	6.5	61	24	3.5
Pea Snacks, Paw Patrol, Seabrook*	1 Pack/15g	64	2.2	429	19.6	48.9	14.8	11
Pea Snacks, Snackrite, Aldi*	1 Pack/21g	87	2.7	415	20	49	13	13
Pea Snacks, Sour Cream, & Chive, Passions, Aldi*	1 Bag/21g	89	3	424	18.6	47.6	14.3	13.3
Pea Snacks, Soy, & Balsamic Vinegar, Snaktastic, Lidl*	1 Bag/21g	87	2.9	416	18.6	47.9	13.7	13.5
Peri Peri Chicken, Nandos, Walkers*	1 Pack/25g	124	6.7	496	5.6	56	26.8	4.8
Pickled Onion, Mackie's*	1 Serving/30g	150	7.8	500	6.7	59	26	3.8
Pickled Onion, Walkers*	1 Std Bag/22g	108	5.5	490	6	60	25	1.7
Pigs in Blankets, Hand Cooked, Christmas, Waitrose*	1 Serving/30g	148	7.8	495	7.3	55.9	26	4
Pigs in Blankets, Irresistible, Co-Op*	¼ Bag/38g	193	11	509	7.6	51	29	5.2
Pigs in Blankets, Walkers*	1 Bag/25g	126	6.7	504	6	56.8	26.8	4.4
Pitta Chips, Red Pepper, M&S*	1 Serving/25g	116	4.1	464	11.1	65.2	16.4	4.1
Plain, Crinkle Cut, Weight Watchers*	1 Pack/16g	79	3.6	492	8	61.6	22.5	5.5
Pom Bear, Original, KP Snacks*	1 Pack/13g	65	3.4	503	3	63	26	3.9
Popchips, Sea Salt & Vinegar	1 Serving/23g	95	3.2	411	5.1	63	14	4
Poppables, BBQ Rib, Walkers*	1 Serving/30g	153	7.8	510	5	63	26	3.7
Popped Chips, BBQ, Lite Bites*	1 Pack/23g	97	3	422	21	51.3	13.1	8.3
Popped Chips, Salt & Vinegar, Light Bites*	1 Pack/23g	92	3	402	20	47.5	13	8.2
Popped, Barbecue, Sainsbury's*	1 Pack/88g	350	7.7	398	6.3	70.9	8.8	5
Popped, Houmous & Lime, Eat Well, M&S*	1 Serving/23g	94	2.2	410	6.1	73.2	9.4	3.9
Popped, Popworks*	1 Pack/30g	140	4.5	465	6.8	74.8	15.1	1.3
Popped, Sea Salt, & Apple Cider Vinegar, COU, M&S*	1 Pack/20g	83	2.1	414	6	72.4	10.4	3.5
Popped, Sea Salted, Sainsbury's*	1 Serving/22g	87	1.7	395	6.9	73.2	7.6	3.3

CRISPS

Measure INFO/WEIGHT	KCAL	FAT	KCAL	PROT	CARB	FAT	FIBRE
			Nutrition Values per 100g / 100ml				

CRISPS

	Measure INFO/WEIGHT	KCAL	FAT	KCAL	PROT	CARB	FAT	FIBRE
Popped, Smoky BBQ, M&S*	1 Pack/20g	84	2.1	419	6.4	72.6	10.5	4.1
Popped, Sour Cream, & Onion, Protein, Popworks *	1 Serving/30g	119	3.1	397	26.1	44.1	10.2	12.3
Popped, Sweet BBQ, Protein, Popworks*	1 Serving/30g	119	2.9	397	24.5	47.8	9.7	11.7
Potato	*1oz/28g*	*148*	*9.6*	*530*	*5.7*	*53.3*	*34.2*	*5.3*
Potato Chips, Cooked, GF, Jumbo Country Chips*	1 Serving/30g	156	9.6	521	6	50.2	32	4.3
Potato Chips, Hand Cooked, Burts*	1 Pack/40g	208	11.5	519	5.1	58.6	28.8	2.5
Potato Loops, Asda*	1 Pack/24g	110	4	458	4.6	70.8	16.7	1.7
Potato Snacks, Original, Snaktastic, Lidl*	1 Serving/50g	266	15	533	4	60	30	3.4
Potato Squares, Ready Salted, Sainsbury's*	1 Bag/50g	192	8	384	6.5	53.8	15.9	7.8
Potato Sticks, Salt & Vinegar, Snaktastic, Lidl*	1 Serving/30g	163	10.2	543	5.6	52	34	3.4
Potato Twirls, Sainsbury's*	1 Serving/50g	218	7.3	435	3	72.8	14.6	3.1
Potato Twists, Salt & Vinegar, Asda*	1/6 Bag/20g	93	3.6	464	4	71	18	2.5
Potato, Low Fat	*1oz/28g*	*128*	*6*	*458*	*6.6*	*63.5*	*21.5*	*5.9*
Potato, Sea Salted, Specially Selected, Aldi*	1 Pack/25g	126	7	504	7.9	53	28	5.2
Prawn Cocktail, Oven Baked, Walkers*	1 Pack/25g	110	3.2	440	6.8	71.3	13	5.1
Prawn Cocktail, Posh, Tyrells*	1 Serving/30g	152	8.4	505	5.6	55.9	28	3.3
Prawn Cocktail, Snaktastic, Lidl*	1 Pack/25g	134	8	535	5.9	54	32	3.5
Prawn Cocktail, Spirals, Shapers, Boots*	1 Bag/15g	73	3.8	489	3.3	61	25	3
Prawn Cocktail, Sunseed Oil, Walkers*	1 Bag/33g	171	10.7	525	6.5	50	33	4
Prawn Cocktail, Tayto*	1 Bag/35g	185	12.3	526	7.5	46.6	35	4.5
Prawn Crackers, Tesco*	1 Pack/40g	220	13.3	550	2.2	60.4	33.2	0.6
Prawn Marie Rose, Finest, Tesco*	1 Serving/25g	129	7.7	517	7.4	50.3	30.7	4.7
Prawn Shells, Co-Op*	¼ Bag/20g	108	6.2	540	7.2	57	31	1.1
Prawn, Spirals, Shapers, Boots*	1 Pack/100g	468	22	468	3.1	64	22	2.8
Puffs, Chickpea, & Carrot, Tesco*	1 Pack/20g	87	2.5	435	14.3	63.8	12.6	4.4
Puffs, Chickpeas, Salt & Vinegar, Snackrite, Aldi*	1 Serving/30g	132	6	440	11	48	20	15
Puffs, Sweet Chilli, Apetina*	1 Pack/25g	120	5.4	482	7.4	63	21.7	2.9
Ready Salted, Crinkle Cut, Lite, Snackrite, Aldi*	1 Bag /25g	122	5.8	486	7	61	23	3.7
Ready Salted, Crinkle Cut, Reduced Fat, Tesco*	1 Pack/25g	118	5.4	474	5.6	61.3	21.8	4.9
Ready Salted, Crinkle Cut, Weight Watchers*	1 Bag/16g	77	3.6	481	5.2	62	22.3	5.6
Ready Salted, Sainsbury's*	1 Pack/25g	137	9	550	6.2	48.6	36	3.5
Ready Salted, Stockwell & Co., Tesco*	1 Bag/25g	133	8.2	533	5	52.8	32.7	3.8
Ready Salted, Tesco*	1 Pack/25g	136	8.3	544	5.2	55.6	33.2	2
Ready Salted, Walkers*	1 Bag/21g	91	3.4	434	5	65	16	5
Reggae Reggae, Grove Cut, Levi Roots*	1 Pack/40g	200	11.5	500	5.1	58.6	28.8	2.5
Ridge Cut, Snaktastic, Lidl*	1 Pack/30g	156	9.3	521	7.6	50.2	31.2	4.6
Ridged, Flame Grilled Steak, Sainsbury's*	1 Pack/27g	141	8.2	521	6.4	53.4	30.5	3.9
Ringos, Sour Cream, & Onion, Golden Wonder*	1 Bag/13g	60	3	483	4.2	61.7	23.9	2.1
Roast Beef, & Horseradish, Crinkle Cut, Finest, Tesco*	1 Serving/25g	130	7.4	518	7.3	53.3	29.6	4.5
Roast Beef, Walkers*	1 Bag/40g	196	10	490	7	59	25	1.7
Roast Chicken, Walkers*	1 Pack/33g	162	8.8	499	5.7	56	27	4.4
Salt & Pepper, Black, Cracked, Hand Cooked, M&S*	1 Bag/40g	206	11.8	516	7.5	52.2	29.5	6
Salt & Vinegar, Balsamic, Cracker, Jacob's*	1 Serving/25g	118	4.8	470	5.2	67	19.3	2.4
Salt & Vinegar, Balsamic, Delux, Lidl*	1 Pack/25g	121	6.3	484	6	56.8	25.2	4.4
Salt & Vinegar, Balsamic, Handcooked, M&S*	1 Bag/40g	208	12.1	521	6.7	52.8	30.4	4.6
Salt & Vinegar, Balsamic, Kettle Chips*	1 Bag/40g	204	11.2	509	5.7	55.8	28.1	4.9
Salt & Vinegar, Chiplets, M&S*	1 Bag/30g	132	5.7	440	5.7	61.3	18.9	4.7
Salt & Vinegar, Cider Vinegar & Sea Salt, Tyrrells*	1 Pack/40g	192	9.8	481	7.2	60.1	24.6	2.4
Salt & Vinegar, Cider Vinegar, Crinkle Cut, Finest, Tesco*	¼ Pack/38g	186	10	495	6.7	54.6	26.7	4.5
Salt & Black Pepper, Mix, Waitrose*	1 Serving/25g	122	6.1	488	4.4	61.2	24.4	3.2
Salt & Shake, Walkers*	1 Pack/24g	128	7.8	533	6.2	52.2	32.3	4.4
Salt & Vinegar, Average	*1 Bag/25g*	*130*	*8.2*	*519*	*5.5*	*50.3*	*32.9*	*3.4*
Salt & Vinegar, Crinkle Cut, Seabrook*	1 Pack/25g	126	7.2	502	5.9	52.9	28.7	3.9

CRISPS

INFO/WEIGHT	Measure	per Measure		Nutrition Values per 100g / 100ml				
		KCAL	FAT	KCAL	PROT	CARB	FAT	FIBRE
Salt & Vinegar, Kettle Cooked, Lays*	1 Serving/28g	150	8	536	7.1	60.7	28.6	3.6
Salt & Vinegar, Reduced Fat, Crinkle, M&S*	1 Pack/40g	183	7.7	457	6.8	61.9	19.2	4.5
Salt & Vinegar, Squares, Walkers*	1 Bag/28g	122	5	443	6.5	61	18	5.5
Salt & Vinegar, Sunseed Oil, Walkers*	1 Bag/33g	171	10.7	525	6.5	50	33	4
Salt & Vinegar, Thick Ridged, Snackrite, Aldi*	1 Bag/30g	159	9.3	529	5.8	55	31	3.4
Salt Your Own, Excluding Salt, Aldi*	1 Pack/24g	130	8.1	536	6	52.6	33.5	4.5
Salt Your Own, Sainsbury's*	1 Pack/24g	127	7.9	520	5	52.2	32.3	3.7
Salt Your Own, Snackrite, Aldi*	1 Pack/24g	130	8.1	536	6	52.6	33.5	4.5
Salted, Average	**1 Bag/25g**	**127**	**7.4**	**508**	**6.1**	**53.4**	**29.7**	**4**
Salted, Crinkle Cut, Lights, Snackrite, Aldi*	1 Bag/25g	122	5.8	486	7	61	23	3.7
Salted, Reduced Fat, Crinkle, M&S*	1 Pack/40g	188	8.2	471	6.3	62.8	20.6	4.6
Salted, Reduced Fat, Tesco*	1 Pack/25g	114	6.2	456	6.3	52	24.7	5.9
Salted, Sea, Anglesey Sea Salt, Red Sky*	1 Serving/40g	185	8.7	463	6.8	59.8	21.8	5
Salted, Sea, Crinkle Cut, Seabrook *	1 Bag/32g	165	10	517	5.7	53.7	31.1	0
Salted, Sea, Hand Cooked, Specially Selected, Aldi*	¼ Lge Bag/38g	182	9	486	6.2	59	24	4.5
Salted, Sea, Houmous Chips, Eat Real*	1 Serving/28g	126	4.8	449	6.5	68.4	17	4.5
Salted, Sea, Lentil Chips, Eat Real*	1 Serving/28g	133	5.9	478	8	62.1	21	4.5
Salted, Sea, Lightly, Hand Cooked, English, Tyrrells*	1 Pack/25g	125	6.4	501	5.9	49	25.4	5.3
Salted, Sea, Lightly, Potato Chips, Tyrrells*	1 Pack/150g	740	38.1	493	7.7	58.9	25.4	2.6
Salted, Sea, Popchips*	1 Bag/23g	94	3.2	410	5.5	62	14	4.3
Salted, Sea, Potato, Mackies*	1 Pack/40g	200	10.8	499	7.4	55	27	4.5
Salted, Squares, Walkers*	1 Pack/25g	109	4.8	435	6.5	60	19	6
Salted, Sunseed Oil, Walkers*	1 Bag/33g	175	11.1	537	5.9	49.7	34.1	4.2
Sausage, & Tomato, Golden Wonder*	1 Pack/25g	132	7.9	530	6.2	53.8	31.5	3.1
Sausage, & Onion, Mackie's*	1 Serving/30g	148	7.8	492	7.6	55	26	5
Scampi, Smiths, Walkers*	1 Bag/27g	134	7	496	13	52.5	26	0
Sea Salt & Balsamic Vinegar, Hand Cooked, Waitrose*	1 Serving/30g	151	8.3	503	5.8	55.4	27.7	4.6
Sea Salt & Cider Vinegar, Finest, Tesco*	1 Serving/25g	123	6.4	491	6.8	56.3	25.4	5.2
Sea Salt & Malt Vinegar, Baked, M&S*	1 Serving/30g	149	7.9	497	5.4	57.1	26.5	4.2
Sea Salt, & Aspall Cyder Vinegar, Fairfields Farm Crisps*	1 Pack/40g	201	11.3	502	7.1	57	28.3	4.7
Sea Salt, Anglesey, Pipers Crisps*	1 Bag/40g	213	12.3	532	5.1	57.2	30.7	3.5
Sea Salt, Original, Terra*	1 Pack/28g	150	9	536	3.6	57.1	32.1	10.7
Sea Salted, Furrows, Tyrrells*	1 Pack/50g	262	15.4	524	6.7	52.8	30.9	0
Sea Salted, Morrisons*	1 Serving/50g	257	14.2	514	5.1	57.8	28.3	3.8
Sea Salted. Lightly, Hand Cooked, M&S*	1 Pack/150g	776	44.1	517	5.8	55.2	29.4	4.2
Sheese, & Red Onion, Vegan, Kettle Chips*	1 Serving/30g	154	8.8	514	8	51.7	29.4	5.4
Shells, Prawn Cocktail, Asda*	1 Bag/18g	90	5.3	501	4.6	54.9	29.2	6.2
Skips, Prawn Cocktail, Tayto*	1 Bag/17g	91	5.6	534	3.3	55	33.1	0
Smoked Chipotle Chilli, Kent Crisps*	1 Pack/40g	208	11.5	519	5.1	58.6	28.8	2.5
Smoked Paprika, San Nicasio *	½ Pack/75g	428	30	571	6.8	45	40	0
Smoky Bacon Flavour, Average	**1 Bag/25g**	**132**	**8.4**	**527**	**6.2**	**49.7**	**33.7**	**3.2**
Smoky Chilli Chicken, Muchos, McCoys*	1 Serving/30g	152	7.8	507	6.1	60	26	2.9
Snax, Original, Asda*	1 Serving/25g	126	6.5	504	4.5	61	26	4.2
Sour Cream & Onion, Potato Chips, Popchips*	1 Pack/23g	95	3.5	413	28.3	69.6	15.2	4.3
Sour Cream, & Chilli Lentil Curls, M&S*	1 Pack/60g	243	5.2	405	13.6	65.3	8.7	4.3
Sour Cream, & Chive Flavour, Average	**1 Bag/25g**	**127**	**7.7**	**508**	**6.8**	**50.7**	**30.9**	**4.6**
Sour Cream, & Chive, Crinkle, Reduced Fat, M&S*	1 Bag/40g	187	8.1	468	6.7	62.2	20.3	4.6
Sour Cream, & Chives, Quinoa Chips, Eat Real*	1 Pack/30g	165	8.6	550	8	66.4	28.8	2.5
Sour Cream, & Onion, Corn Chips, Popchips*	1 Multipack/17g	72	2.9	422	6.5	65	17	1.9
Sour Cream, & Chive, Hummus Chips, Eat Real*	1 Pack/45g	213	10.4	474	6.7	58	23	5.8
Sour Cream, & Jalapeno, Party Mix, Golden Cross*	1 Serving/25g	116	4.9	464	4.4	68.4	19.6	1.8
Sour Cream, & Mexican Lime, Deluxe, Lidl*	1 Serving/25g	124	5.8	496	6	63.2	23.3	4.5
Sour Cream, & Onion, Stackers, Snackrite, Aldi*	1 Serving/25g	139	9.2	557	3.1	52	37	2.8

	Measure INFO/WEIGHT	per Measure KCAL	FAT	Nutrition Values per 100g / 100ml KCAL	PROT	CARB	FAT	FIBRE
CRISPS								
Spirals, Salt & Vinegar, Bobby's*	1 Serving/21g	100	6.7	477	4	65	32	0
Stackers, Salt & Vinegar, Snackrite, Aldi*	½ Pack/83g	401	19.9	483	4.4	62	24	3.5
Steak, & Peppercorn Sauce, Crinkle Cut, Co-Op*	¼ Bag/38g	198	11.8	522	6.6	53	31	3.8
Steak, Flame Grilled, Ridge Cut, McCoys*	1 Bag/47g	250	14.7	526	6.9	53	31	3.9
Steak, Flamed Grilled, Max, Walkers*	1 Pack/50g	266	16.4	533	6.5	51.6	32.8	2.8
Steak, T Bone, Bubble Chips, Roysters*	1 Pack/28g	151	8.9	540	5.5	55	32	2.6
Sticks, Salt & Vinegar, Asda*	1 Serving/25g	126	6.2	504	5.2	63	25	2
Sun Bites, Lightly Sea Salted, Grain Waves, Walkers*	1 Pack/25g	120	5.4	480	7.5	80.7	21.6	6.6
Sunbites, Cheddar & Caramelised Onion, Walkers*	1 Bag/25g	120	5.4	480	7.6	60.8	21.6	6.4
Sunbites, Onion, & Turmeric, Wholegrain, Walkers*	1 Bag/25g	119	5.2	475	7.5	61.2	20.6	7.7
Sundried Tomato, & Garlic, Quinoa Chips, Eat Real*	1 Bag/22g	121	6.4	551	8	66.4	28.9	2.7
Sweet & Salty, Katy's Kettle Corn, Popchips*	1 Serving/28g	128	4	455	6.9	65.9	14.1	5.4
Sweet & Smokin', Hippeas*	1 Pack/22g	90	3.8	411	13.2	51.1	17.4	7.3
Sweet Chilli, & Red Pepper, Potato Chips, Tyrrells*	¼ Pack/37g	180	9.2	481	7.9	59.7	24.5	2.4
Sweet Chilli, & Irish Red Pepper, Keoghs*	1 Bag/50g	263	13.2	526	7.2	49	26.5	5
Sweet Chilli, Average	***1 Bag/25g***	***115***	***5.6***	***461***	***5.1***	***59.9***	***22.6***	***4.6***
Sweet Chilli, Hand Cooked, Fairfields Farm Crisps*	1 Pack/70g	361	20.8	516	6	58.4	29.7	4.3
Sweet Chilli, Lentil, Curls, Bites, Kettle Chips*	1 Pack/22g	94	2.6	428	13.2	65	11.9	4
Sweet Chilli, Multigrain, Waves, Sainsbury's*	1 Pack/20g	104	5.6	520	6.3	58.6	28	4
Sweet Chilli, Thai, Lentil Waves, Burts*	1 Pack/20g	91	3.3	453	11.7	62.6	16.3	4.9
Sweet Chilli, Thai, Sensations, Walkers*	1 Bag/40g	198	9.9	494	6.9	59	24.7	3.7
Sweet Chilli, Thai, Velvet Crunch, King*	1 Pack/20g	81	1.9	404	1.6	77.5	9.7	2
Sweet Potato Sticks, Sea Salt, Emily Crisps Ltd*	1 Pack/35g	176	9.2	503	3.4	58.6	26.3	9.1
Sweet Potato, Paprika, Oven Baked, with Veg, Walkers*	1 Bag/23g	101	3.4	437	7	66	15	3.9
Sweet Potato, Thai Sweet Chilli, Kettle Chips*	1 Serving/30g	151	7.9	502	7.1	56.5	26.4	4.9
Take it Cheesy, Chickpea Puffs, Organic, Hippeas*	1 Pack/15g	61	2.5	406	14.6	48.8	16.8	8.2
Tangy Toms, Golden Wonder*	1 Pack/81g	411	21	507	5.4	63	25.9	0.5
Tapas Fries, Made For Drink*	1 Pack/35g	180	10.8	514	14.4	44.3	31	0
Thai Bites, Mild, Jacob's*	1 Bag/25g	93	0.8	373	6.9	79	3.3	1
Tomato & Basil, Houmous Chips, Eat Real*	1 Serving/28g	126	4.8	449	6.5	68.4	17	4.5
Tomato & Herbs, Baked Fusions, Snacks, Walkers*	1 Pack/25g	109	3.4	434	6.7	68.3	13.5	6.4
Tomato Ketchup, Golden Wonder*	1 Bag/25g	135	8	521	5.1	54	30.8	3.6
Turkey, & Stuffing, Walkers*	1 Bag/25g	126	6.8	504	6.4	56.4	27.2	4.4
Twirls, Salt & Vinegar, Tesco*	1 Bag/80g	349	14	436	3.9	65.8	17.5	2.4
Twists, Salt & Vinegar, Zack's Snacks*	1 Serving/18g	86	3.8	479	3.4	67	21	2.6
Unsalted, Seabrook*	1 Bag/30g	163	10.7	544	5.7	47.9	35.8	4.1
Veg Thins, Sea Salt, Emily Crisps Ltd*	1 Serving/20g	80	1.8	398	14.9	59.2	9	10.4
Vegetable, Average	***1 Bag/25g***	***118***	***7.4***	***470***	***4.1***	***46.5***	***29.6***	***12.1***
Vegetable, Paprika, Punchy, Great Shape, Asda*	1 Pack/23g	99	3	432	3.9	73	13	3.7
Veggie & Kale, Straws, Eat Real*	1 Bag/22g	109	5.6	497	3.1	65.1	25.5	2.8
Veggie Puffs, Pickled Onion, The Foodie Market, Aldi*	1 Pack/21g	87	2.7	415	20	48	13	11
Veggie Puffs, Roast Beef, The Foodie Market, Aldi*	1 Pack/21g	87	2.8	414	21.9	45.7	13.3	11.9
Veggie Straws, Cheesy Flavour, Kiddylicious*	1 Pack/12g	65	3.7	542	2.5	60.8	30.8	2.5
Veggie Straws, The Foodie Market, Aldi*	1 Bag/22g	122	7.7	553	3.2	54	35	3.3
Veggie Straws, WW*	1 Bag/15g	78	4.4	520	3.3	59.3	29.3	3.3
Veggie Straws, WW*	1 Pack/15g	78	4.4	519	3.1	59.3	29.3	3.1
Veggie, Lightly Sea Salted, M&S*	¼ Pack/25g	103	4.9	411	7.4	49	19.5	5.1
Veggie, Popped, Aldi*	1 Pack/23g	90	1.5	393	7.4	74	6.6	4.7
Wasabi, Strong, Max, Walkers*	1 Pack/30g	160	9.9	534	6.3	51.7	32.9	2.9
Wheat Crunchies, Cheese & Onion, KP Snacks*	1 Pack/20g	100	5	498	9.4	57	25	3.6
Wheat Crunchies, Golden Wonder*	1 Pack/35g	172	8.7	491	11.1	55.9	24.8	0
Wheelies, Bacon, Tayto*	1 Pack/20g	98	4.6	492	6.7	63.3	23.1	0

	Measure INFO/WEIGHT	KCAL	FAT	Nutrition Values per 100g / 100ml KCAL	PROT	CARB	FAT	FIBRE
CRISPY PANCAKE								
Beef Bolognese, Findus*	1 Pancake/65g	104	2.6	160	6.5	25	4	1
Chicken, Bacon & Sweetcorn, Findus*	1 Pancake/63g	101	2.5	160	5.5	26	4	1.1
Minced Beef, As Consumed, Findus*	1 Pancake/115g	178	2.9	155	6.2	26	2.5	1.9
CROISSANT								
All Butter, Bakers Selection, Asda*	1 Croissant/40g	164	8.4	412	6.9	48	21	1.9
All Butter, Finest, Tesco*	1 Croissant/62g	258	14.3	415	7.9	42.9	23.1	1.9
All Butter, Frozen, Sainsbury's*	1 Croissant /44g	169	9	384	8.8	40.1	20.4	2.5
All Butter, Irresistible, Co-Op*	1 Croissant/62g	272	16.1	438	8.6	41	26	2.5
All Butter, Light & Flaky, Specially Selected, Aldi*	1 Croissant/40g	174	10	436	9.2	42	25	1.4
All Butter, M&S*	1 Croissant/40g	179	10.8	447	10.1	40.1	27	1.6
All Butter, Ready to Bake, M&S*	1 Croissant/48g	194	11.2	404	9	38.5	23.3	2.3
All Butter, Reduced Fat, M&S*	1 Croissant/40g	154	7.1	384	10.9	44.1	17.7	2.2
All Butter, Reduced Fat, Tesco*	1 Croissant/52g	164	5.5	315	7.5	47.4	10.6	1.8
All Butter, Sainsbury's*	1 Croissant/44g	170	8.1	385	8.5	44.9	18.3	3.5
All Butter, Tesco*	1 Croissant/44g	168	7.5	383	9	47.2	17	2.6
All Butter, The Best, Morrisons*	1 Croissant/64g	261	13.7	407	9.4	43.5	21.3	2
Almond, Bakery, Tesco*	1 Crossant/84g	342	17.7	407	9.3	43.8	21	2.4
Average	**1 Croissant/50g**	**180**	**10.2**	**360**	**8.3**	**38.3**	**20.3**	**1.6**
Butter, Bakery, Tesco*	1 Croissant/72g	285	13.7	396	9.3	46.1	19	1.6
Butter, Charentes, No.1, Waitrose*	1 Croissant/68g	309	19.3	454	8	40.5	28.4	2.1
Butter, Morrisons*	1 Croissant/44g	196	12.5	446	9.3	38.2	28.4	2
Cheese & Ham, Delice de France*	1 Croissant/91g	225	12.3	247	7	24.4	13.5	2.5
Chocolate Filled, All Butter, Finest, Tesco*	1 Croissant/75g	267	11.3	355	7.4	45.9	15.1	2.8
Chocolate, & Hazelnut, Bakery, Sainsbury's*	1 Croissant/81g	345	19	426	8.6	43.9	23.4	2.7
Cocoa Cream, Elka*	1 Croissant/50g	213	12.5	426	10.4	39.9	25	2.6
Cornetti, Italian, with Apricot Conserve, Crosta & Mollica*	1 Croissant/89g	323	17	363	7.4	40.4	19.1	2.5
Flaky Pastry with a Plain Chocolate Filling, Tesco*	1 Croissant/83g	369	20.8	445	8.6	45	25.1	2.6
GF, Free From, Tesco*	1 Croissant/70g	244	11.8	348	3.3	44.5	16.8	2.8
Multiseed, Bakery, Sainsbury's*	1 Croissant/69g	262	16	379	8.7	31.8	23.2	4.1
PresbyrÃƒÆ'Ã‚Â¥n*	1 Croissant/48g	185	10.5	385	7.9	38	21.8	0
Ready to Bake, Frozen, M&S*	1 Croissant/48g	194	11.2	405	9	38.6	23.3	2.3
Strawberry Jam, Elka*	1 Croissant/50g	186	8.7	373	6.9	47.1	17.4	2.5
with Cocoa Filling, Max, 7 Days*	1 Croissant/28g	128	7.8	456	6	44	28	0
CROQUETTES								
Cheese, Cheddar, Inspired Cuisine, Aldi*	1 Croquette/42g	129	7.1	306	7.2	24	17	2.5
Mac 'n' Cheese, Paramount*	1 Croquette/50g	133	6.6	266	8.9	27.4	13.2	1.1
Potato, Fried in Blended Oil, Average	**1 Croquette/80g**	**171**	**10.5**	**214**	**3.7**	**21.6**	**13.1**	**1.3**
Potato, Frozen, HFC, Tesco*	1 Serving/128g	266	11.7	208	3.3	26.5	9.1	3.2
CROUTONS								
Baked, Cooks' Ingredients, Waitrose*	½ Pack/50g	222	7.4	444	12	64	14.7	4.2
Black Pepper, & Sea Salt, Oven Baked, Asda*	½ Pack/20g	90	2.6	450	11	69	13	4.8
Cheese, & Shallot, Waitrose*	1 Serving/10g	45	1.4	449	13.1	64.4	14.5	3.4
d'Ail, Tipiak*	1 Serving/22g	89	3.2	406	8.2	58.9	14.7	2.5
Fresh, M&S*	1 Serving/10g	53	3.3	530	11.4	50	32.8	3.2
Garlic, Waitrose*	1 Serving/40g	209	12	522	10.8	52.1	30	2.7
Herb, Sainsbury's*	1 Serving/15g	64	1.7	429	13.4	68.2	11.4	2.8
Lightly Sea Salted, Asda*	1 Serving/20g	83	1.9	414	12.9	69.7	9.3	4.3
Mini, Osem*	1 Serving/20g	104	5	522	9.2	65	25	0
Prepacked, Average	**1 Serving/15g**	**74**	**3.6**	**495**	**10.8**	**58.7**	**24**	**2.6**
Sea Salt, & Black Pepper, Belbake, Lidl*	1 Serving/20g	92	3.2	461	11	66	16	4.4
Sea Salt, & Black Pepper, M&S*	½ Pack/43g	210	9.6	488	10.8	58.6	22.4	4.4
Sun Dried Tomato, Sainsbury's*	¼ Pack/15g	75	3.8	497	11.7	55.2	25.5	2.5

	Measure INFO/WEIGHT	per Measure KCAL	FAT	Nutrition Values per 100g / 100ml KCAL	PROT	CARB	FAT	FIBRE
CRUDITES								
Vegetable Sticks, Average	**1 Serving/100g**	**24**	**0.2**	**24**	**0.7**	**4.5**	**0.2**	**1.9**
with Cheese & Chive Dip, Tesco*	1 Pack/115g	132	10.5	115	1.6	5.9	9.1	1.5
with Soured Cream & Chive, Reduced Fat, Dip, Tesco*	1 Pack/53g	30	1.6	56	1.8	5	3	1.9
CRUMBLE								
Almond, & Apricot, Devondale*	1 Cake/80g	314	13.2	392	3.6	57	16.5	9.8
Apple, & Blackberry, M&S*	1 Serving/135g	398	15.1	295	3.5	44.9	11.2	1.6
Apple, & Blackberry, Sainsbury's*	1 Serving/110g	232	6.2	211	3	37.1	5.6	2.1
Apple, & Blackberry, Tesco*	1/6 Pie/90g	286	11.7	318	3	45.8	13	2.8
Apple, & Custard, Asda*	1 Serving/125g	250	8.8	200	2.3	32	7	0
Apple, & Blackberry, Waitrose*	¼ Crumble/125g	296	9.4	236	3.1	38	7.5	2.1
Apple, Average	**1 Serving/240g**	**497**	**12**	**207**	**0.9**	**40.5**	**5**	**1.1**
Apple, Flapjack, Finest, Tesco*	¼ Pack/125g	310	13.2	248	5.1	31.2	10.6	3.8
Apple, Golden, Allplants*	1 Serving/100g	242	15	242	3.5	22	15	3.1
Apple, Slices, Frozen, Tesco*	1 Slice/54g	173	8	321	4.9	40.6	14.9	2.8
Apple, with Custard, Green's*	1 Serving/79g	171	5.3	216	1.9	37	6.7	1.2
Apple, with Sultanas, Weight Watchers*	1 Dessert/110g	196	4.3	178	1.4	34.2	3.9	1.3
Berry, Winter, Aldi*	1/6 Crumble/99g	279	9.9	282	3.3	43	10	2.9
Blackberry, & Lemon, Parsley Box*	1 Pack/155g	324	9	209	2.4	37	5.8	0.5
Blackcurrant, & Apple, Devondale*	1 Cake/80g	314	13.2	393	3.6	57	16.5	9.8
Bramley Apple, Waitrose*	¼ Crumble/125g	296	9.6	237	3.1	37.8	7.7	1.9
Fruit	**1 Portion/170g**	**337**	**11.7**	**198**	**2**	**34**	**6.9**	**1.7**
Fruit, Wholemeal	**1oz/28g**	**54**	**2**	**193**	**2.6**	**31.7**	**7.1**	**2.7**
Fruit, with Custard	**1 Serving/270g**	**463**	**17.6**	**171**	**2.4**	**27**	**6.5**	**1.3**
Gooseberry, M&S*	1 Serving/133g	379	14.2	285	3.5	43.3	10.7	1.7
Lemon Meringue, Holly Lane*	1 Tart/50g	213	8.5	426	4.8	63	17	1.8
Rhubarb, Average	**1 Portion/150g**	**330**	**11.1**	**220**	**2.7**	**35.5**	**7.4**	**1.9**
Summer Fruit, Parsley Box*	1 Serving/155g	347	10.2	224	3	35	6.6	6.6
CRUMPETS								
Asda*	1 Crumpet/45g	85	0.4	188	6	39	0.9	2.1
Bakers Selection, Asda*	1 Crumpet/50g	106	0.6	211	6.7	42	1.2	2.7
Bunny, Morrisons*	1 Crumpet/57g	107	0.4	187	5.5	38.4	0.7	2.6
Buttermilk, TTD, Sainsbury's*	1 Crumpet/52g	102	0.6	195	6.5	38.5	1.1	2.6
Christmas Tree, Village Bakery, Aldi*	1 Crumpet48g	86	0.3	180	5.5	37	0.7	2.6
Co-Op*	1 Crumpet/40g	70	0.3	175	7	35	0.7	2
Creations, Co-Op*	1 Crumpet/60g	113	0.4	188	5.7	38	0.7	2.5
Essential, Waitrose*	1 Crumpet/52g	94	0.6	182	6.5	35.1	1.1	2.6
Fluffy, Village Bakery, Aldi*	1 Crumpet/57g	117	0.6	206	6.4	42	1	2.4
Golden Sun, Lidl*	1 Crumpet/43g	83	0.7	193	7.8	37.1	1.6	1.6
Ham, Pulled, & Rarebit, M&S*	1 Crumpet/24g	41	0.7	169	9.4	24.7	3	2.7
Jones Village Bakery*	1 Crumpet/55g	95	0.4	172	5.6	34.9	0.7	2
Mcgee's*	1 Crumpet/47g	96	1.1	204	4.8	42.5	2.4	0
Morrisons*	1 Crumpet/40g	90	0.2	225	7.8	47.2	0.5	3.2
Planet Deli*	1 Crumpet/48g	88	0.5	183	6.1	36.6	1	1
Premium, Sainsbury's*	1 Crumpet/50g	96	0.7	191	6.1	38.6	1.4	1.7
Rowan Hill Bakery, Lidl*	1 Crumpet/44g	78	0.5	178	5.5	34.5	1.2	0
Sourdough, Finest, Tesco*	1 Crumpet/55g	100	0.4	181	6	36.5	0.7	2.3
Sourdough, Irresistible, Co-Op*	1 Crumpet /54g	101	0.6	187	6.1	37	1.1	2.2
Sourdough, TTD, Sainsbury's*	1 Crumpet/55g	93	0.3	169	5.6	34.1	0.6	2.4
Sourdough, Waitrose*	1 Crumpet/55g	95	0.4	172	5.6	34.9	0.7	2
Square, Tesco*	1 Crumpet/60g	101	0.5	168	6.3	33.8	0.8	2.7
Tesco*	1 Crumpet/55g	100	0.4	181	6	36.2	0.8	2.3
Thick & Fluffy, Rowan Hill Bakery, Lidl*	1 Crumpet/55g	98	0.4	178	5.8	35.8	0.8	2.3
Toasted, Average	**1 Crumpet/40g**	**80**	**0.4**	**199**	**6.7**	**43.4**	**1**	**2**

	Measure INFO/WEIGHT	per Measure KCAL	FAT	Nutrition Values per 100g / 100ml KCAL	PROT	CARB	FAT	FIBRE
CRUMPETS								
Waitrose*	1 Crumpet/62g	116	0.7	188	6.3	37.9	1.2	2.1
Warburton's*	1 Crumpet/55g	97	0.4	176	6	35.3	0.8	1.9
Wholemeal, Bakers Selection, Asda*	1 Crumpet/50g	94	0.4	189	7.3	36	0.8	3.7
CRUNCHIE								
Blast, Cadbury*	1 Serving/42g	199	8.3	480	4.7	69.6	20.1	0.7
Cadbury*	1 Bar/40g	185	7.5	465	4	69.5	18.9	0.5
Nuggets, Cadbury*	1 Bag/125g	569	20.5	455	3.8	73.1	16.4	0
Treat Size, Cadbury*	1 Bar/17g	79	2.9	463	3	75	17	1.3
CUCUMBER								
& Miso Houmous, Taiko Foods*	1 Pack/130g	101	6	78	2.3	6.2	4.6	0
Average	*1 Serving/80g*	*8*	*0.1*	*10*	*0.7*	*1.5*	*0.1*	*0.6*
Baby, Pickled, Always Fresh*	1 Serving/30g	14	0.1	47	2	8	0.3	0
Baby, Raw, M&S*	1 Cucumber/40g	6	0.2	15	1	1.2	0.6	0.7
Baby, Raw, Tesco*	2 Cucumbers/80g	12	0.5	16	1	1.2	0.6	0.7
Mini, Love Me Tender*	1 Cucumber/33g	6	0.2	19	0.7	3.5	0.5	0.5
CUMIN								
Seeds, Whole, Average	*1 Tsp/2g*	*8*	*0.5*	*375*	*17.8*	*44.2*	*22.7*	*10.5*
CUPCAKES								
Assorted, Sainsbury's*	1 Cake/38g	130	2.3	341	2.2	69.3	6.1	0.4
Birthday, Hostess*	1 Cake/46g	190	8.5	413	1.1	58.7	18.5	0
Carrot, Average	*1 Cake/40g*	*157*	*8.6*	*392*	*3.6*	*45.4*	*21.6*	*0.6*
Celebration, Tesco*	1 Cake/61g	310	17.8	510	2.6	58.5	29.3	1
Chocolate Filled, Free From, Tesco*	1 Cake/52g	238	13.1	459	3.4	53.6	25.3	1.6
Chocolate Fudge, Party Pack, Tesco*	1 Cake/63g	300	17.5	476	4.2	50.7	27.8	3
Chocolate Fudge, Vegan, OGGS*	1 Cake/63g	270	16.1	428	4.9	40	25.6	2.1
Chocolate, Average	*1 Cake/40g*	*159*	*6.4*	*398*	*3.5*	*59.9*	*16*	*1.2*
Chocolate, Mini, GF, Free From, Morrisons*	1 Cake/18g	79	3.7	438	4.9	57.3	20.5	2.3
Lemon, Average	*1 Cake/40g*	*184*	*10.1*	*461*	*3*	*55.5*	*25.3*	*1.1*
Lemon, Healthy Option, Average	*1 Cake/40g*	*131*	*1.5*	*328*	*2.7*	*68.9*	*3.7*	*5.2*
Lemon, Mini Fruity Selection, M&S*	1 Cake/23g	105	5.6	458	3.6	55.4	24.6	0.5
Milkshake Flavour, Mini, Co-Op*	1 Cake/22g	23	1.3	106	0	9.5	5.8	0
Raspberry, Mini Fruity Selection, M&S*	1 Cake/23g	104	4.8	453	3.2	62.7	20.9	0.5
Red Velvet, Party Pack, Tesco*	1 Cake/62g	308	17.5	497	2.5	56.8	28.3	2.6
Red Velvet, Tesco*	1 Cake/63g	308	16.6	490	3.1	59.3	26.4	1.2
Sponge Top, Individual, Tesco*	1 Cake/50g	220	10.5	443	3	59.5	21.1	1.3
Strawberry & Cream, Party Pack, Tesco*	1 Cake/65g	316	17.8	486	2.5	56.8	27.3	1.8
Strawberry, Party Selection, Tesco*	1 Cake/46g	229	13.3	496	2	55.8	28.8	2.8
Sweetie, Fiona Cairns*	1 Cake/80g	350	16.9	437	3.1	58.3	21.1	0
Unicorn, Tesco*	1 Cake/63g	316	17.6	502	3.2	58.6	28	1.1
Vanilla, & Chocolate, Mini, Waitrose*	1 Cake/21g	93	4.8	441	4.1	53.7	22.9	2.2
Vanilla, Mini Fruity Selection, M&S*	1 Cake/23g	106	5.2	463	3.3	61.2	22.7	0.5
Vanilla, Mini, GF, Free From, Morrisons*	1 Cake/18g	29	4.1	162	3.5	60.3	22.8	0.8
Vanilla, Party Platter, Holly Lane, Aldi*	1 Cake/57g	282	16	494	2.6	56	28	2.1
Vanilla, Party Selection, Tesco*	1 Cake/46g	230	13.1	495	2.6	57.2	28.1	1.5
White Chocolate, & Vanilla, Tesco*	1 Cake/76g	390	22.5	513	1.7	59.7	29.6	0.8
CURACAO								
Average	*1 Pub Shot/35ml*	*109*	*0*	*311*	*0*	*28.3*	*0*	*0*
CURLY WURLY								
Cadbury*	1 Bar/26g	118	4.7	453	3.1	70	18	0.7
Squirlies, Cadbury*	1 Squirl/3g	13	0.5	442	3.5	69.2	17.3	0.8
CURRANTS								
Average	*1oz/28g*	*75*	*0.1*	*267*	*2.3*	*67.8*	*0.4*	*1.9*

C

	Measure INFO/WEIGHT	KCAL	FAT	Nutrition Values per 100g / 100ml KCAL	PROT	CARB	FAT	FIBRE
Aubergine	**1oz/28g**	**33**	**2.8**	**118**	**1.4**	**6.2**	**10.1**	**1.5**
Aubergine, Masala, TTD, Sainsbury's*	½ Pack/115g	135	11.4	117	2.9	4.1	9.9	5.8
Beef Massaman, Thai, Musclefood*	1 Serving/470g	498	17.4	106	8.5	9.8	3.7	1.1
Beef Rendang, COOK!, M&S*	½ Pack/269g	377	10.8	140	21.3	4.2	4	1.1
Beef, Canned, Tesco*	½ Can/200g	264	15.8	132	9.5	4.3	7.9	2.8
Beef, Sainsbury's*	1 Serving/400g	552	32.8	138	10.7	5.4	8.2	0.9
Beef, Thai, Finest, Tesco*	1 Serving/500g	770	29	154	9	16.5	5.8	1.2
Beef, with Rice, Iceland*,	1 Pack/500g	580	14.5	116	5	16.7	2.9	1.5
Blackeye Bean, Gujerati	**1oz/28g**	**36**	**1.2**	**127**	**7.2**	**16.1**	**4.4**	**2.8**
Butternut & Spinach, Allplants*	1 Serving/376g	425	22.6	113	3.4	9.9	6	2.7
Butternut Squash, & Chickpea, Plant Based, Asda*	1 Pack/388g	400	8.5	103	3.2	17	2.2	1.2
Butternut Squash, & Coconut, Cook*	1 Pack/285g	208	7.7	73	3	10	2.7	1.5
Cabbage	**1oz/28g**	**23**	**1.4**	**82**	**1.9**	**8.1**	**5**	**2.1**
Cambodian Amok, Mindful Chef*	1 Serving	642	28	642	49	52	28	0
Cauliflower & Potato	**1oz/28g**	**17**	**0.7**	**59**	**3.4**	**6.6**	**2.4**	**1.8**
Cauliflower, Chickpea, & Potato, Vegan, Waitrose*	½ Pack/205g	166	7.4	81	3.2	6.4	3.6	5.2
Chana Saag, Slimming World*	1 Pack/350g	256	4.9	73	4.4	7.3	1.4	6.8
Chettinad, Prawn, King, M&S*	1 Serving/200g	184	7.6	92	8.7	5.1	3.8	1.5
Chick Pea, Whole, Average	**1oz/28g**	**50**	**2.1**	**179**	**9.6**	**21.3**	**7.5**	**4.5**
Chick Pea, Whole, Basic, Average	**1oz/28g**	**30**	**1**	**108**	**6**	**14.2**	**3.6**	**3.3**
Chicken Panang, Taste Thailand, M&S*	½ Pack/115g	170	11.2	148	9.3	5.2	9.7	1.2
Chicken Tikka, Fake Away, The Skinny Food Co.*	1 Pouch/300g	189	3.6	63	5.2	7.2	1.2	0
Chicken, & Potato, Massaman, Hello Fresh*	1 Serving/607g	704	25.9	116	7.1	12.2	4.3	0
Chicken, & Prawn, Thai Green, Gousto*	1 Serving/452g	529	26.2	117	11.5	3.7	5.8	2.4
Chicken, & Rice, Calorie Controlled, Tesco*	1 Pack/315g	293	3.8	93	5.4	14.5	1.2	1.6
Chicken, & Rice, Calorie Counted, Asda*	1 Pack/350g	283	3.6	81	4.6	13.1	1	0.9
Chicken, & Rice, Calorie Counted, Asda*	1 Pack/350g	322	4.2	92	5	15	1.2	1
Chicken, & Rice, Dinner, Tesco*	1 Pack/500g	520	12	104	8.2	11.7	2.4	1.3
Chicken, & Rice, Microwaved, Asda*	1 Pack/400g	588	22.2	148	5.5	18	5.6	1.8
Chicken, & Rice, Microwaved, Calorie Counted, Asda*	1 Pack/308g	283	3.7	92	5	15	1.2	1
Chicken, Butter Masala, Asda*	½ Pack/189g	261	14.4	138	13	4.3	7.6	0.7
Chicken, Butter, & Rice, Taste of India, Tesco*	1 Pack/427g	624	29.9	146	6.4	12.8	7	3.1
Chicken, Butter, Takeaway, Tesco*	½ Pack/175g	224	13.3	128	7.9	6.4	7.6	1.2
Chicken, Canned, Grants'*	½ Can/196g	155	4.5	79	8.8	5.4	2.3	0.7
Chicken, Canned, Stockwell & Co., Tesco*	½ Can/196g	131	2.7	67	4.5	8	1.4	2.3
Chicken, Chinese Style, Slimming World*	1 Pack/500g	315	5	63	8.1	4.9	1	1.1
Chicken, Chinese Style, with Basmati Rice, Musclefood *	1 Pack/420g	382	8	91	7.5	11	1.9	1.1
Chicken, Chinese with Rice, Ready Meal, Average	**1 Serving/450g**	**490**	**11.5**	**109**	**7.2**	**14.1**	**2.6**	**1.3**
Chicken, Fiery Andhra, Waitrose*	½ Pack/175g	226	11.2	129	13.3	3.7	6.4	1.9
Chicken, Fruity, 1330, Oakhouse Foods Ltd*	1 Serving/401g	706	29.7	176	6.4	20.7	7.4	1
Chicken, Fruity, Meal for One, M&S*	1 Pack/400g	508	15.6	127	6.7	15.6	3.9	1.1
Chicken, Fruity, Mini Meal, M&S*	1 Pack/200g	262	7.4	131	8.2	15.7	3.7	1.1
Chicken, Fruity, Mini, 339, Oakhouse Foods Ltd*	1 Serving/240g	389	14.2	162	6.4	20.2	5.9	1.4
Chicken, Garlic, Cook*	1 Pack/320g	358	13.7	112	10.7	7.5	4.3	0.5
Chicken, Green Thai, Charlie Bigham's*	½ Pack/300g	342	21	114	8.7	4.8	7	0
Chicken, Green Thai, Cook*	1 Serving/270g	327	16.5	121	11.7	4.4	6.1	0
Chicken, Green Thai, with Water Chestnuts, & Rice, M&S*	1 Pack/380g	414	10.3	109	6.4	14.3	2.7	1.1
Chicken, Green, Thai Inspired, TTD, Sainsbury's*	1 Pack/384g	545	22.3	142	8	13.8	5.8	1.2
Chicken, Green, Thai, Jasmine Rice, Sainsbury's*	½ Pack/188g	184	4.7	98	7.9	10.5	2.5	1.3
Chicken, Hot, Can, Tesco*	1 Can/418g	514	26.3	123	9.7	6.9	6.3	0.9
Chicken, Hot, Canned, M&S*	½ Can/200g	246	10.8	123	12.8	4.9	5.4	1.9
Chicken, Kashmiri, Waitrose*	1 Serving/400g	640	36.4	160	14.5	5	9.1	0.6
Chicken, Malaysian, Finest, Tesco*	1 Pack/375g	375	8.3	100	7.4	12.2	2.2	0.8

CURRENT

CURRY

INFO/WEIGHT	Measure		per Measure		Nutrition Values per 100g / 100ml				
			KCAL	FAT	KCAL	PROT	CARB	FAT	FIBRE
Chicken, Microwave Pot, Fray Bentos*	1 Pot/250g		235	9.2	94	6.1	8.5	3.7	0.9
Chicken, Mild, Box Ingredients Only, Gousto*	1 Serving/415g		722	28.2	174	9.2	19.1	6.8	1.2
Chicken, Mild, Canned, Bilash, Aldi*	½ Can/200g		180	7.6	90	9.5	4.5	3.8	0.7
Chicken, Mild, with Fluffy Rice, M&S*	1 Pack/225g		238	5.8	106	6.9	13.3	2.6	0.9
Chicken, Piri Piri, & Cajun Rice, Asda*	1 Pack/380g		410	8.7	108	6.7	14	2.3	2.6
Chicken, Red Thai Style, M&S*	½ Pack/175g		254	17.2	145	8.5	5.1	9.8	1.1
Chicken, Red Thai, BFY, M&S*	1 Pack/380g		399	8.7	105	7.5	13.1	2.3	1
Chicken, Red Thai, Waitrose*	½ Pack/175g		287	19.4	164	9.4	5.8	11.1	2
Chicken, Sweet & Sour, Chinese, Tesco*	1 Pack/507g		684	21.8	135	6.6	16.7	4.3	1.6
Chicken, Thai Green, 1521, Oakhouse Foods Ltd*	1 Serving/400g		444	14.4	111	6	13.3	3.6	1.1
Chicken, Thai Green, Donald Russell*	1 Serving/250g		285	15.5	114	7.9	6	6.2	1.3
Chicken, Thai Green, Fake Away, The Skinny Food Co.*	1 Pouch/300g		264	4.5	88	8.2	9.5	1.5	0
Chicken, Thai Red, & Fragrant Rice, Charlie Bigham's*	½ Pack/416g		658	25	158	7.5	17.8	6	0
Chicken, Thai, Green, & Jasmine Rice, Ready Meal	*1 Serving/450g*		*520*	*17.2*	*116*	*7.7*	*12.6*	*3.8*	*1.1*
Chicken, Thai, Green, No Rice, Average	*1 Serving/200g*		*174*	*7*	*87*	*8.2*	*5*	*3.5*	*1.4*
Chicken, Thai, Red, & Jasmine Rice, Ready Meal	*1 Serving/450g*		*500*	*15.3*	*111*	*7.5*	*12.6*	*3.4*	*1*
Chicken, Thai, Red, & Rice, Ready Meal, Healthy	*1 Serving/400g*		*400*	*7.8*	*100*	*6.4*	*14*	*2*	*1*
Chicken, Thai, Red, & Sticky Rice, Ready Meal	*1 Serving/450g*		*527*	*15.7*	*117*	*6.7*	*14.2*	*3.5*	*1.7*
Chicken, Thai, Red, No Rice, Average	*1 Serving/200g*		*194*	*6.9*	*97*	*7.2*	*9*	*3.4*	*1.4*
Chicken, Tikka, Biryani, Tesco*	1 Pack/365g		599	13.9	164	10.2	20.7	3.8	3.5
Chicken, Weight Watchers*	1 Pack/350g		346	4.6	99	5.2	16.2	1.3	1.1
Chicken, with Brown Rice, Shake That Weight*	1 Pack/273g		199	3.8	73	9	7	1.4	2.2
Chicken, with Rice, 264, Wiltshire Farm Foods*	1 Serving/360g		407	7.2	113	5.5	18	2	0
Chicken, with Rice, Average	*1 Serving/400g*		*465*	*11*	*116*	*5.1*	*17.8*	*2.8*	*0.8*
Chicken, Yellow Thai Style, HL, Tesco*	1 Pack/450g		504	12.2	112	9.3	12.6	2.7	0.5
Chickpea, & Coconut, Tangy, Fiid*	½ Pack/200g		198	4	99	5.1	12.3	2	5.9
Chickpea, & Lentil, Bowl, Spiced, Quorn*	1 Bowl/300g		281	6.6	94	5.3	10.7	2.2	5
Chickpea, Green, Super Nature*	1 Pack/350g		298	11.2	85	3.5	10.4	3.2	3.8
Chickpea, South Indian Spiced, BOL Foods*	1 Serving/380g		391	10.6	103	2.5	14.9	2.8	2.7
Chinese, Chicken, with Rice, Meal for One, M&S*	1 Pack/400g		528	15.6	132	7.8	15.7	3.9	1.2
Coconutty, with Lentils, Annabel Food*	½ Pack/250g		150	2.2	60	3	8.2	0.9	3.1
Cod, Squid, & King Prawn, Keralan, Waitrose*	½ Pack/185g		211	9.6	114	13.5	3	5.2	0.6
Cod, Thai Inspired, Beautifully Balanced, Tesco*	1 Pack/357g		336	4.6	94	5.2	14.4	1.3	2
Cod, Yellow Thai, with Lime Rice, Hello Fresh*	1 Serving/569g		597	30.7	105	5.8	8.6	5.4	0.4
Coronation Chickpea, Plant Menu, Aldi*	1 Pack/380g		429	7.6	113	2.9	19.4	2	2.7
Courgette, & Potato	*1oz/28g*		*24*	*1.5*	*86*	*1.9*	*8.7*	*5.2*	*1.2*
Delhi Biryani, Meal Kit, The Spice Tailor*	1 Pack/360g		461	10.4	128	0	22	2.9	1.3
Dupiaza, Lamb, Cook*	1 Pack/300g		468	29.1	156	10.1	6	9.7	0
Fish, & Vegetable, Bangladeshi, Average	*1oz/28g*		*33*	*2.4*	*117*	*9.1*	*1.4*	*8.4*	*0.5*
Fish, Bangladeshi, Average	*1oz/28g*		*35*	*2.2*	*124*	*12.2*	*1.5*	*7.9*	*0.3*
Fish, Goan, with Rice, Fodmap, Field Doctor*	1 Serving/389g		486	26.4	125	5.5	9.1	6.8	1.9
Fish, Red Thai, Waitrose*	1 Pack/500g		275	11	55	5.2	3.7	2.2	1
Fish, Yellow Thai, Asian Fusion, Waitrose*	½ Pack/175g		222	15.8	127	6.8	3.9	9	1.4
Goan, Fiery, Meal Kit, The Spice Tailor*	1 Pack/300g		558	45	186	1.9	9	15	2.6
Goan, Meal Kit, Pataks*	½ Pack/157g		248	18.8	158	2.2	8.3	12	0
Gobi, Sri Lankan, Vegan, Hi Five*	1 Pack/487g		316	12.2	65	1.9	9.1	2.5	2.3
In a Naan, Chicken Tikka, Tuk In*	1 Pack/180g		396	13.3	220	7.4	27.1	7.4	1.9
Karagee, Chicken, Asian Fusion, Waitrose*	½ Pack/75g		205	10.6	273	16.3	19.3	14.1	2.1
Karahi, Prawn, Cook*	1 Pack/310g		223	10.2	72	5.3	4.3	3.3	0
Katsu, Chicken, & Rice, G&B, Asda*	1 Pack/370g		388	8.1	105	9.4	11	2.2	1.4
Katsu, Chicken, Naked, Nourish, Morrisons*	1 Pack/400g		436	10.4	109	10	10.5	2.6	1.5
Katsu, Chicken, with Sticky Rice, Asian Fusion, Waitrose*	1 Pack/350g		581	21.7	166	8.3	18.1	6.2	2.1
Katsu, Pumpkin, with Rice, Wasabi*	1 Pack/448g		694	29.6	155	2.1	20.8	6.6	0

CURRY

	Measure INFO/WEIGHT	per Measure KCAL	per Measure FAT	Nutrition Values per 100g / 100ml KCAL	PROT	CARB	FAT	FIBRE
Katsu, Sweet Potato, Leon*	1 Pack/380g	376	11.4	99	3	13.9	3	2.3
Katsu, Sweet Potato, Plant Kitchen, M&S*	1 Pack/400g	536	16.8	134	3.2	19.8	4.2	2
Kerala, Vegetable, By Ruby*	1 Pack/700g	525	33.1	75	2.2	7.7	4.7	1.2
Keralan, Butternut Squash, Waitrose*	1 Serving/351g	393	22.1	112	2.8	9.8	6.3	2.6
Keralan, Coconut, Veg Pot, BOL Foods*	1 Pot/345g	361	9.6	105	3.5	15.5	2.8	1.9
Lamb, Aromatic, BFY, M&S*	1 Pack/380g	483	7.6	127	9.9	16.3	2	2.3
Lentils, Indian Madras, Tasty Bite*	½ Pack/143g	136	6.1	95	4.2	8.2	4.3	3.6
Madras, Beef, Canned, Sainsbury's*	½ Can/200g	246	13.2	123	11.3	3.9	6.6	2.8
Massaman, Beef, Slow Cooked, Oven Baked, Asda*	½ Pack/188g	269	10	143	18	5	5.3	1.3
Mushroom, & Pea, Masala, Indian, Sainsbury's*	1 Pack/300g	264	14.7	88	3.3	5.2	4.9	5.1
Mutton, with Rice, Island Delight*	1 Pack/400g	548	18.4	137	9	15.6	4.6	0
Panang, Chicken, Cook*	1 Serving/250g	420	25.8	168	14.2	5.3	10.3	0
Panang, Coconut, Thai, BOL Foods*	1 Pack/405g	450	19.4	111	3.2	12.7	4.8	2.1
Paneer, Spinach, Daylesford*	½ Pack/225g	214	13	95	3.7	5.8	5.8	2.5
Peanut, Chickpea, Red Rice, Soulful Food Co*	1 Pot/380g	346	11	91	3.5	15	2.9	4
Pork, & Lentil, with Naan Bread, Hello Fresh*	1 Serving/611g	788	32.9	129	6.8	12.4	5.4	0
Potato & Pea	**1oz/28g**	**26**	**1.1**	**92**	**2.9**	**13**	**3.8**	**2.4**
Prawn, & Mushroom	**1oz/28g**	**47**	**4**	**168**	**7.3**	**2.5**	**14.4**	**1**
Prawn, & Mango, Keralan, Cook*	1 Pack/260g	260	13	100	7.5	5.8	5	0
Prawn, 977, Oakhouse Foods*	1 Pack/400g	476	14.8	119	6.4	15.9	3.7	0.4
Prawn, Coconut & Lime, King, Sainsbury's*	½ Pack/351g	207	8.8	59	3.7	5.4	2.5	1
Prawn, Goan, King, M&S*	1 Pack/400g	680	44.4	170	5.1	11.6	11.1	1.5
Prawn, King, Taste Sri Lanka, M&S*	1 Pack/350g	413	23.4	118	6.3	7.3	6.7	1.6
Prawn, Malay, King, Waitrose*	1 Pack/350g	364	19.2	104	6.6	7.1	5.5	0.9
Prawn, Red Thai, Hello Fresh*	1 Serving/467g	579	23.3	124	5	16	5	0
Prawn, Red Thai, Sainsbury's*	1 Pack/300g	546	39.6	182	6.3	9.4	13.2	1.7
Prawn, Takeaway, Average	**1 Serving/350g**	**410**	**29.8**	**117**	**8.2**	**2.2**	**8.5**	**2**
Prawn, Yellow Thai, Cook*	1 Serving/295g	215	8	73	6.4	5.7	2.7	0.4
Red Kidney Bean, Punjabi	**1oz/28g**	**30**	**1.6**	**106**	**4.7**	**10.1**	**5.6**	**3.8**
Red Thai, Vegetarian, Tesco*	1 Pack/429ml	588	21.9	137	5.4	17.3	5.1	1.6
Rendang, Naked, Finnebrogue*	1 Pack/305g	238	4.3	78	3.4	12.4	1.4	1.5
Rendang, Tempeh, Allplants*	1 Pack/360g	464	24.1	129	3.8	12	6.7	2.6
Roasted Cauliflower, & Paneer, Higgidy*	1 Meal/365g	456	28.8	125	4.4	7.4	7.9	3.7
Saag, Aloo Gobi, Chef Select, Lidl*	½ Pack/139g	125	7.2	90	2.3	6.8	5.2	3.4
Salmon, Green, Waitrose*	1 Pack/401g	581	40.5	145	9.1	4.5	10.1	2.7
Sambar, Cauli-Coconut, Sri Lankan, BOL Foods*	1 Pot/345g	304	9.7	88	4.6	7.9	2.8	6.2
Satay, Golden Peanut, Allplants*	1 Serving/377g	611	27.5	162	6.8	15	7.3	3.7
South Indian Style, Microwaved, Plant Based, Asda*	1 Pack/323g	371	9	115	3.2	17	2.8	3.8
Sweet Potato, & Aubergine, Sri Lankan, Cook*	1 Pack/280g	297	12	106	2.2	15.9	4.3	2.5
Sweet Potato, & Cashew, Plant Kitchen, M&S*	1 Pack/340g	411	10.9	121	4.4	16.7	3.2	3.8
Sweet Potato, & Coconut, Plant Based, Asda*	½ Can/196g	149	8	76	1	8.1	4.1	1.4
Sweet Potato, Katsu, with Rice, Sainsbury's*	1 Pack/377g	550	19.6	146	2.2	21.7	5.2	2
Sweet Potato, Slimfree, Aldi*	1 Pack/500g	250	3	50	2.3	6.5	0.6	4.8
Sweet Potato, What's Cooking, Lidl*	1 Serving/550g	335	7.3	61	2.6	7.9	1.3	3.3
Thai Chicken, Jane Plan*	1 Pack/300g	309	10.2	103	6.6	10.5	3.4	2
Thai Green, & Rice, Co-Op*	1 Pack/380g	429	14.1	113	6.3	13	3.7	0.6
Thai Green, Allplants*	1 Serving/405g	446	23.9	110	4.1	9.1	5.9	2
Thai Green, Creamy, Veg Pot, BOL Foods*	1 Pot/345g	259	8.3	75	2.2	10	2.4	2.3
Thai Green, Meal Kit, The Spice Tailor*	½ Pack/137g	200	16.4	146	1.9	7.5	12	1.3
Thai Green, with Chargrilled Chicken Breast, Tweakd*	1 Pack/620g	915	54	148	13.3	3.1	8.7	2.1
Thai Red, & Rice, GF, Co-Op*	1 Pack/373g	422	9	113	4.8	15	2.4	5.5
Thai Red, Kit, Asda*	½ Pack/122g	160	13.4	131	1.7	5.1	11	0.9
Thai, Chicken, & Rice, Pot, Musclefood*	1 Pack/311g	336	7.5	108	11	10	2.4	1.1

	Measure INFO/WEIGHT	per Measure		Nutrition Values per 100g / 100ml				
		KCAL	FAT	KCAL	PROT	CARB	FAT	FIBRE
CURRY								
Thai, Yellow, Plant Menu, Aldi*	1 Pack/400g	500	18.8	125	2.6	17	4.7	2.1
Tofu, Red Thai, 1, Waitrose*	½ Pack/175g	345	25.9	197	8.7	6.7	14.8	1.1
Vegetable, & Chickpea, Cook*	1 Serving/321g	218	6.1	68	3.2	7.9	1.9	3.3
Vegetable, Canned, Sainsbury's*	½ Can/200g	200	12.2	100	1.4	9.8	6.1	1.8
Vegetable, Canned, Tesco*	1 Can/400g	308	11.2	77	2	9.7	2.8	2.4
Vegetable, Classic, Jane Plan*	1 Pack/300g	261	7.8	87	2.3	12.8	2.6	1.7
Vegetable, Creamy, Meal for One, M&S*	1 Pack/400g	572	30	143	2.4	15.7	7.5	1.4
Vegetable, Creamy, Steam & Serve, Morrisons*	1 Pack/350g	399	22	114	3.1	9.5	6.3	3.4
Vegetable, Frozen, Mixed Vegetables, Average	**1oz/28g**	**25**	**1.7**	**88**	**2.5**	**6.9**	**6.1**	**0**
Vegetable, Goan, M&S*	½ Pack/200g	204	12.4	102	1.8	8.9	6.2	1.4
Vegetable, Green Thai, Cook*	1 Pack/270g	364	21.6	135	4.1	10.1	8	0
Vegetable, in Sweet Sauce, Average	**1 Serving/330g**	**162**	**6.9**	**49**	**1.4**	**6.7**	**2.1**	**1.3**
Vegetable, Indian Meal for One, Tesco*	1 Serving/200g	218	14.4	109	2	9	7.2	1.2
Vegetable, Indian, Sainsbury's*	½ Pack/200g	206	14.6	103	2.5	6.8	7.3	4.6
Vegetable, Indian, Tesco*	1 Serving/225g	257	17.8	114	2.1	8.6	7.9	1.6
Vegetable, Medium, Tesco*	1 Pack/350g	326	21.7	93	2.3	7.1	6.2	1.9
Vegetable, Pakistani, Average	**1oz/28g**	**17**	**0.7**	**60**	**2.2**	**8.7**	**2.6**	**2.2**
Vegetable, Red Thai, with Rice, Tesco*	1 Pack/385g	381	11.5	99	4.4	12.6	3	2.1
Vegetable, Sabzi Tarkari, Patak's*	1 Pack/400g	500	31.2	125	2.5	11.1	7.8	2.2
Vegetable, Takeaway, Average	**1 Serving/330g**	**346**	**24.4**	**105**	**2.5**	**7.6**	**7.4**	**0**
Vegetable, Thai Green, Waitrose*	1 Serving/175g	187	12.9	107	1.3	7.7	7.4	2.3
Vegetable, Tinned, Morrisons*	½ Can/196g	135	3.3	69	2.4	10.2	1.7	1.7
Vegetable, with Rice, Healthy Range, Average	**1 Serving/400g**	**351**	**4.6**	**88**	**2.3**	**16.8**	**1.1**	**1.9**
Vegetable, with Rice, Ready Meal, Average	**1 Serving/400g**	**408**	**12**	**102**	**3.3**	**16.4**	**3**	**0**
Vegetable, with Rice, Shake That Weight*	1 Pack/275g	242	7.7	88	8.3	5.2	2.8	4.7
Vegetable, with Yoghurt, Average	**1oz/28g**	**17**	**1.1**	**62**	**2.6**	**4.6**	**4.1**	**1.4**
Vegetable, Yellow Thai, Sainsbury's*	1 Pack/400g	624	48.8	156	2.2	9.4	12.2	1.1
Vegetable, Yellow, Cook*	1 Serving/270g	367	25.1	136	2.4	10	9.3	1.6
CURRY LEAVES								
Fresh	**1oz/28g**	**23**	**0.3**	**81**	**6.6**	**11**	**1.1**	**0**
CURRY PASTE								
Balti, Sainsbury's*	¼ Jar/50g	73	4.9	147	3.4	7.6	9.9	6.7
Curry, Katsu, Mild, M&S*	¼ Jar/48g	88	4.2	186	4.8	19.6	8.8	4.7
Green Thai, Average	**1 Tsp/5g**	**6**	**0.4**	**128**	**2.1**	**11.7**	**7.9**	**3.1**
Green, Thai Style, Sainsbury's*	¼ Jar/45g	38	2.5	84	1.1	6.5	5.5	2.2
Gulyaskrem Cispos, Le Gusto*	1 Serving/15g	18	1	118	2	9	7	0
Hot Madras, M&S*	¼ Jar/50g	90	5.4	179	2.2	16	10.8	4.4
Jalfrezi, Spice, Pataks*	1/8 Jar/35g	101	8.6	285	3.2	7.8	24.3	7.5
Katsu, M&S*	¼ Pot/48g	76	3.8	161	3	17.6	8.1	2.6
Korma, Asda*	1 Tube/100g	338	23.5	338	5.1	26.6	23.5	1.2
Korma, Asian Home Gourmet*	¼ Sachet/13g	35	2.9	271	3.4	11.1	22.4	0
Korma, Cooks' Ingredients, Waitrose*	1 Serving/50g	76	5	152	3.2	10.6	10	3.4
Madras, Cumin & Chilli, Hot, Patak's*	¼ Jar/70g	202	18.1	289	4.7	7.6	25.9	10.8
Madras, Pot, Patak's*	½ Pot/35g	98	8.1	279	4.4	7	23.1	0
Massaman, Thai, Pot, Blue Dragon*	½ Pot/25g	89	6.8	357	4.9	24	27	9.2
Panang, Sainsbury's*	1 Tbsp/15g	17	0.9	115	2.1	10.4	5.7	6.9
Red, Thai, Average	**1 Tsp/5g**	**7**	**0.5**	**132**	**2.3**	**9.5**	**9.1**	**3**
Rogan Josh, Cooks' Ingredients, Waitrose*	1 Serving/50g	50	3	100	2.6	6.8	6	4.1
Rogan Josh, Easy Paste, Sharwood's*	1 Serving/23g	102	8.9	443	5.2	12.5	38.8	11.5
Rogan Josh, Sainsbury's*	¼ Jar/50g	68	3.7	136	2.7	10.4	7.4	8.7
Rogan Josh, Tomato & Paprika, Patak's*	1 Serving/30g	119	11	397	4.1	12.7	36.7	5.9
Stir Fry, Katsu, Chop*	1 Pot/50g	118	7	235	3.2	24	14	3.4
Tandoori, Cooks' Ingredients, Waitrose*	1 Serving/45g	56	3.5	125	3.9	5.4	7.9	8.3

	Measure INFO/WEIGHT	per Measure KCAL	FAT	Nutrition Values per 100g / 100ml KCAL	PROT	CARB	FAT	FIBRE
CURRY PASTE								
Tikka Masala, Spice, Patak's*	1 Tbsp/15g	40	3.4	270	3	7.8	22.9	6.8
Tikka, Geeta's*	1 Pack/80g	210	15.3	262	1.8	20.7	19.1	2.3
Tikka, M&S*	¼ Jar/50g	110	7.8	219	2.8	13.8	15.5	6.4
Tikka, Sainsbury's*	¼ Jar/50g	40	1.4	80	2.5	8.6	2.7	5.9
Tom Yum, Thai Taste*	1 Tsp/13g	35	2	269	5.4	30.8	15.4	7.7
Yellow Thai, Tesco*	1 Tbsp/15g	15	0.6	100	1.9	13.6	4.1	4.9
Yellow, Thai, Barts*	1 Serving/30g	84	3.8	281	2.7	30.4	12.8	8.3
CURRY POWDER								
Average	**1 Tsp/2g**	**6**	**0.3**	**325**	**12.7**	**41.8**	**13.8**	**0**
CUSTARD								
Banana, Ambrosia*	1 Pot/55g	47	1.6	86	2.9	12.1	2.9	0
Banana, Pot, Ambrosia*	1 Pot/150g	134	4.4	89	2.8	12.8	2.9	0.5
Canned, Essential, Waitrose*	¼ Can/100g	101	3.2	101	2.7	15.3	3.2	0
Chocolate Flavour, Pot, Average	**1 Pot/125g**	**138**	**3.4**	**111**	**3.1**	**18.2**	**2.7**	**0.6**
Devon, Individual Pot, Ambrosia*	1 Pot/125g	120	3.6	96	2.8	14.8	2.9	0.5
Fresh, Tesco*	¼ Pot/125g	121	4.6	97	2.6	12.9	3.7	0.6
Low Fat, Average	**1/3 Pot/141g**	**116**	**1.6**	**82**	**2.9**	**15**	**1.2**	**0**
Powder	**1 Tsp/5g**	**18**	**0**	**354**	**0.6**	**92**	**0.7**	**0.1**
Ready to Serve, Average	**1 Serving/50g**	**59**	**2.3**	**118**	**3.3**	**16.1**	**4.6**	**0.2**
Salted Caramel Flavour, Morrisons*	½ Pot/150g	167	4.8	111	2.9	17.4	3.2	0.5
Soya, Vanilla, Dairy Free, Deliciously, Alpro*	1 Tbsp/15g	12	0.3	81	3	13.3	1.8	0.5
Strawberry, Canned, Ambrosia*	1/3 Can/130g	116	3.8	89	2.8	12.9	2.9	0.5
Strawberry, Pot, Ambrosia*	1 Pot/150g	134	4.4	89	2.8	12.9	2.9	0.5
Vanilla Flavour, Pot, Average	**1 Pot/125g**	**128**	**3.5**	**102**	**2.8**	**16.4**	**2.8**	**0**
CUSTARD APPLE								
Cherimoya, Weighed without Skin & Seeds, Average	**1 Serving/312g**	**234**	**2.1**	**75**	**1.6**	**17.7**	**0.7**	**3**

	Measure INFO/WEIGHT	per Measure KCAL	per Measure FAT	Nutrition Values per 100g / 100ml KCAL	PROT	CARB	FAT	FIBRE
DAB								
Raw	**1oz/28g**	**21**	**0.3**	**74**	**15.7**	**0**	**1.2**	**0**
DAIM								
Mondelez*	1 Bar/28g	148	8.7	530	2.9	59	31	1.2
DAMSONS								
Raw, Weighed with Stones, Average	**1oz/28g**	**9**	**0**	**31**	**0.4**	**7.7**	**0**	**1.4**
Raw, Weighed without Stones, Average	**1oz/28g**	**11**	**0**	**38**	**0.5**	**9.6**	**0**	**1.8**
DANISH PASTRY								
Apple & Sultana, Tesco*	1 Pastry/72g	293	16.4	407	5.4	45	22.8	1.4
Apple Danish, Bakery, Waitrose*	1 Pastry/123g	400	22.2	325	5.1	35.7	18	2.4
Apple, Fresh Cream, Sainsbury's*	1 Pastry/67g	248	14.6	368	3.1	40.2	21.6	0.4
Average	**1 Pastry/110g**	**411**	**19.4**	**374**	**5.8**	**51.3**	**17.6**	**1.6**
Fruit Bears Claw , Waitrose*	1 Pastry/97g	339	15.8	349	4.6	45	16.3	2
Fruit Filled, Average	**1 Pastry/94g**	**335**	**15.9**	**356**	**5.1**	**47.9**	**17**	**0**
Maple, & Pecan, Plait, Bakery, Sainsbury's*	1 Plait/82g	408	28.1	498	5.5	41.1	34.3	1.4
Maple, & Pecan, Plait, Frozen, Tesco*	1 Pastry/78g	348	22.8	447	5.6	39	29.3	2.7
Mini, Selection, Tesco*	1 Pastry/38g	154	8.4	404	5.7	44.3	22.2	2.2
DATES								
Dried, Average	**1 Date/20g**	**53**	**0.1**	**266**	**2.8**	**64.1**	**0.4**	**4.1**
Dried, Medjool, Average	**1 Date/20g**	**56**	**0.1**	**279**	**2.2**	**69.3**	**0.3**	**4.3**
Fresh, Raw, Yellow, Average	**1 Date/20g**	**21**	**0**	**107**	**1.3**	**27.1**	**0.1**	**1.5**
Medjool, Stuffed with Walnuts, Tesco*	2 Dates/40g	98	2.3	245	4.4	44	5.7	3.4
Milk Chocolate Covered, Holland & Barrett*	1 Date/17g	65	1.9	384	4.5	66	11.3	2.6
DELI FILLER								
Cheese & Onion, Essential, Waitrose*	1 Pot/170g	692	64.8	407	10.8	4.5	38.1	1.5
Chicken & Bacon, Co-Op*	1 Pack/200g	420	29.6	210	17.6	1	14.8	2.6
Chicken, Bacon, & Sweetcorn, M&S*	1 Serving/30g	65	5	216	10.5	5.7	16.7	0.5
King Prawn & Avocado, M&S*	1 Pack/170g	425	38.8	250	9.5	1.4	22.8	0.5
Prawn & Mayonnaise, M&S*	1 Serving/60g	150	13.8	250	11.3	1	23	0.5
Prawn Cocktail, Eat Well, M&S*	½ Pot/85g	119	7.3	140	9.1	6.4	8.6	0.6
Seafood, & Prawn Cocktail, M&S*	1 Serving/50g	100	7.8	199	5.8	9	15.5	0.5
Tuna, & Sweetcorn, Reduced Fat, M&S*	¼ Pot/55g	86	5.7	157	9.1	6.4	10.3	0
DESSERT								
Apple Crumble, Sainsbury's*	1 Pot/136g	291	10.5	214	3.2	33	7.7	2.7
Banana Split	**1 Serving/175g**	**368**	**25.5**	**210**	**2.2**	**18**	**14.6**	**0.2**
Banoffee, Layered, Sainsbury's*	1 Pot/115g	270	14.7	235	2.2	27.8	12.8	1
Banoffee, Pot, The Coconut Collaborative*	1 Pot/45g	104	9	232	0.7	13	20	1
Banoffee, Sainsbury's*	1 Pot/140g	360	19.1	257	2.7	30.9	13.6	1.3
Billionaire's, Pots, Gastropub, M&S*	1 Pot/80g	293	16.2	366	1.8	43.1	20.3	2
Black Forest, Bonne Maman*	1 Pot/100g	245	13	245	2.5	26	13	1.1
Buche, Aldi*	1 Buche/200g	484	34	242	3	20	17	0.8
Caramel, Pots Of Joy, Dairy Milk, Cadbury*	1 Pot/70g	150	7.3	215	2.5	27.1	10.5	0.1
Caramel, Soya, Creamy, Sweet, Alpro*	1 Pot/125g	106	2.2	85	3.2	13.7	1.8	0.5
Choc Delight, Brooklea, Aldi*	1 Pot/80g	74	1.2	92	4.5	15	1.5	0.6
Chocolate Fix, Belgian, with Mint, Mullerlight, Muller*	1 Pot/100g	97	2.9	97	3.5	14.7	2.9	0
Chocolate Surprise , Essential, Waitrose*	1 Pot/150g	254	13.2	169	3.5	18.8	8.8	0.5
Chocolate, & Cherry, Wicked Kitchen, Tesco*	1 Pot/90g	186	7.7	207	1.3	27	8.6	4
Chocolate, & Orange, Pot, Finest, Tesco*	1 Pot/80g	212	12.3	265	3.9	27	15.4	1.3
Chocolate, & Salted Caramel, Pot, Finest, Tesco*	1 Pot/80g	227	12.6	283	4	31	15.7	1
Chocolate, Brownie, Double, Weight Watchers*	1 Pot/86g	167	3.3	194	5.1	33.7	3.8	2.4
Chocolate, Buttons, Milk, Cadbury*	1 Pot/100g	280	14.9	280	6.2	30.8	14.9	0
Chocolate, Buttons, Twin Pot, Cadbury*	1 Pot/90g	220	11.7	245	4.4	27.5	13	0.6
Chocolate, Creme, King Frais, Lidl*	1 Pot/125g	131	3.6	105	2.6	17	2.9	0
Chocolate, Dark, Soya, Alpro*	1 Pot/125g	118	2.9	94	3	14.7	2.3	1.4

	Measure INFO/WEIGHT	per Measure KCAL	per Measure FAT	Nutrition Values per 100g / 100ml KCAL	PROT	CARB	FAT	FIBRE

DESSERT

	Measure INFO/WEIGHT	KCAL	FAT	KCAL	PROT	CARB	FAT	FIBRE
Chocolate, Everyday Value, Tesco*	1 Pot/100g	121	4	121	2.7	18.4	4	0.4
Chocolate, Fix, Mullerlight, Muller*	1 Pot/100g	94	1.9	94	3.2	15.2	1.9	0
Chocolate, Frappe, Skinny, COU, M&S*	1 Pot/100g	116	2.6	116	6.2	16.9	2.6	0.5
Chocolate, Little Choc Pots, The Coconut Collaborative*	1 Pot/45g	103	5.8	228	2.5	24.8	13	1.5
Chocolate, Mini Egg, Cadbury*	1 Pack/85g	230	11.3	271	4.4	33.7	13.3	0.9
Chocolate, Muffin, Skinny, Low Fat, COU, M&S*	1 Pot/110g	154	3.1	140	5.2	23.5	2.8	0.5
Chocolate, Pots Of Joy , Dairy Milk, Cadbury*	1 Pot /70g	158	8.2	225	4.2	25.6	11.7	0.1
Chocolate, Salted Caramel, Pot, M&S*	1 Pot/85g	341	25	401	5.2	30.3	29.4	0
Chocolate, Soya, Silky Smooth, Alpro*	1 Pot/125g	104	2.4	83	3	13	1.9	1.1
Chocolate, White Buttons, Pots of Joy, Cadbury*	1 Pot /70g	158	6.6	225	4.8	30.4	9.4	0
Coconut, & Berry, Chia Pot, Allplants*	1 Pot/295g	463	18	157	5	18	6.1	4.7
Coconut, Blueberry, Pot, Plant Kitchen, M&S*	1 Pot/120g	146	10.8	122	0.8	9.4	9	0.1
Coconut, Pot, Plant Kitchen, M&S*	1/3 Pot/117g	146	12.1	125	1.2	6.8	10.3	1
Coconut, Vanilla, Pot, Plant Kitchen, M&S*	1/3 Pot/117g	141	11.7	121	1.2	6.6	10	0.1
Coffee, 414, Wiltshire Farm Foods*	1 Serving/77g	129	4.2	167	4.1	23	5.4	0
Coffee, Italian Style, Free From, Tesco*	1 Pot/90g	210	8.2	233	1.3	36.2	9.1	0.6
Compote, Peaches, & Apricots, Bonne Maman*	1 Pot/130g	107	0.4	82	0.9	18	0.3	1.9
Creme Caramel, Sainsbury's*	1 Pot/100g	116	1.6	116	2.6	22.9	1.6	0
Creme, Caramel, Salted, Bonne Maman*	1 Pot/90g	220	13.5	245	1.6	25	15	0.5
Creme, Coffee, Bonne Maman*	1 Pot/90g	178	12.6	198	2.1	15	14	0.5
Creme, Vanilla, Bonne Maman*	1 Pot/90g	190	13.1	211	2.1	17.9	14.6	0
Darkmilk, Cadbury*	1 Pot/90g	213	12.1	237	4.3	25.2	13.4	1.1
Jaffa, COU, M&S*	1 Pot/107g	155	4.9	145	3.4	22.4	4.6	0.5
Jaffa, Skinny, M&S*	1 Pot/107g	167	4	156	2.7	27	3.7	1.7
Key Lime Pie	**1 Serving/125g**	**431**	**25**	**344**	**4.1**	**37.9**	**20**	**1.4**
Lemon, Layered, Free From, Sainsbury's*	1 Dessert/80g	237	11.9	296	2.3	37.8	14.8	0
Limone, Italiamo, Lidl*	1 Serving/75g	191	5	255	2.6	43.4	6.6	0
Mango, & Turmeric, Chia Pot, Allplants*	1 Serving/188g	299	11.3	159	4.8	19	6	3.9
Meringue Roulades, Toffee & Pecan, M&S*	1 Roll/93g	352	13.7	378	4	57.3	14.7	0.1
Milk, & Chocolate, with Hazelnut, Monte Maxi*	1 Pot/100g	195	13.3	195	2.8	15.9	13.3	0
Milky Bar, White Chocolate, Nestle*	1 Pot/70g	105	5.5	150	4.4	18.4	7.9	0
Millionaire's Shortbread, M&S*	1 Dessert/120g	440	27.8	365	3.2	35.5	23.1	1
Mississippi Mud Pie	**1 Serving/125g**	**480**	**32**	**384**	**5.3**	**33.1**	**25.6**	**1.8**
Mochi, Brown Rice, Sweet, Clearspring*	1 Mochi/42g	98	0.9	233	4.4	48	2.1	0
Mochi, Wao, Coconut, Aldi*	1 Pack/210g	525	13.2	250	2.2	45.8	6.3	0.4
Posset, Zesty Citrus, Pots & Co*	1 Pot/50g	169	13.5	338	1.9	22	27	0
Quark, Vanilla, with Strawberry Sauce, Fluffy, Danio*	1 Pot/125g	178	6.5	142	5	18.7	5.2	0
Raspberry, Royale, Essential, Waitrose*	1 Pot/150g	216	10.6	144	1.1	18.9	7.1	0.5
Rolo, Nestle*	1 Pot/70g	170	8.3	243	3.3	30.8	11.9	0.5
Strawberry, & Raspberry, Charlotte, COU, M&S*	1 Pot/110g	153	1.2	139	2.1	29.7	1.1	1.1
Tiramisu	**1 Serving/150g**	**420**	**20.8**	**280**	**4.4**	**34**	**13.9**	**0.8**
Trifle, Chocolate, Cadbury*	1 Pot /90g	234	13.8	260	4.8	22.5	15.3	0
Vanilla, Soya, Heavenly Velvet, Alpro*	1 Pot/125g	94	2.8	75	3.7	9.5	2.2	1
White Chocolate, & Raspberry, Pot, Finest, Tesco*	1 Pot/80g	206	15.4	258	3.2	17	19.2	1.5

DHAL

	Measure INFO/WEIGHT	KCAL	FAT	KCAL	PROT	CARB	FAT	FIBRE
Black Gram, Average	**1oz/28g**	**21**	**1**	**74**	**4.2**	**7**	**3.4**	**1.7**
Cauliflower, & Chickpea, Slimming World*	1 Pack/550g	286	3.8	52	2.9	6.7	0.7	4
Cauliflower, Coconut, & Lentil, Plant Kitchen, M&S*	1 Pot/300g	270	9.6	90	4.5	9.2	3.2	3.3
Chick Pea	**1oz/28g**	**42**	**1.7**	**149**	**7.4**	**17.7**	**6.1**	**3.8**
Lentil, & Spinach, Meal Pot, Tideford Organics*	1 Pot/300g	141	5.4	47	2	5.1	1.8	1.2
Lentil, Co-Op*	1 Pack/200g	336	22	168	4.9	10	11	4.9
Lentil, Red Masoor & Tomato with Butter, Average	**1oz/28g**	**26**	**1.4**	**94**	**4**	**9.7**	**4.9**	**0.9**
Lentil, Red Masoor & Vegetable, Average	**1oz/28g**	**31**	**1.1**	**110**	**5.8**	**14.7**	**3.8**	**1.8**

	Measure INFO/WEIGHT	per Measure KCAL	FAT	Nutrition Values per 100g / 100ml KCAL	PROT	CARB	FAT	FIBRE
DHAL								
Lentil, Red Masoor with Vegetable Oil, Average	*1oz/28g*	*48*	*2.2*	*172*	*7.6*	*19.2*	*7.9*	*1.8*
Lentil, Red Masoor, Punjabi, Average	*1oz/28g*	*39*	*1.3*	*139*	*7.2*	*19.2*	*4.6*	*2*
Lentil, Red Masoorl & Mung Bean, Average	*1oz/28g*	*32*	*1.9*	*114*	*4.8*	*9.9*	*6.7*	*1.6*
Lentil, Turmeric, Biona Organic*	1 Serving/175g	135	3.2	77	3.9	9.6	1.8	2.4
Mung Bean, Bengali	*1oz/28g*	*20*	*0.9*	*73*	*4.2*	*7.4*	*3.3*	*1.7*
Mung Beans, Dried, Boiled in Unsalted Water	*1oz/28g*	*26*	*0.1*	*92*	*7.8*	*15.3*	*0.4*	*0*
Split Peas, Yellow, Chana, Asda*	1 Serving/275g	300	19.2	109	2.6	9	7	1.8
Tarka, Asda*	½ Pack/150g	216	12	144	6	12	8	6
Tarka, Indian, Waitrose*	1 Pack/300g	432	21.9	144	6.5	7.2	7.3	11.6
Tarka, M&S*	1 Serving/250g	235	8.8	94	4.3	9.4	3.5	3.7
Vegetable, Microwaved, Slimming World*	1 Pack/350g	259	2.1	74	5.4	8.3	0.6	7
DHANSAK								
Butternut, Slim Cook, Tesco*	1 Pack/485g	364	3.9	75	3.8	10.5	0.8	5.1
Chicken with Bagara Rice, Waitrose*	1 Pack/450g	549	8.1	122	8.2	18.2	1.8	1.2
Vegetable, Curry, Microwaved, Slimzone, Asda*	1 Portion/459g	225	2.3	49	2.5	7.7	0.5	2.6
Vegetable, Sainsbury's*	1 Serving/200g	148	5.6	74	3.1	8.9	2.8	2.8
DILL								
Dried, Average	*1 Tsp/1g*	*3*	*0*	*253*	*19.9*	*42.2*	*4.4*	*13.6*
Fresh, Average	*1 Tbsp/3g*	*1*	*0*	*25*	*3.7*	*0.9*	*0.8*	*2.5*
DIP								
Aubergine, Eridanous, Lidl*	½ Pack/125g	275	25.5	220	1.2	7.8	20.4	0
Aubergine, Fresh, Waitrose*	1 Serving/85g	159	12.8	187	2.5	10.5	15	1.7
Baba Ganoush, Sabra*	1 Serving/75g	188	17.6	251	3.9	4.4	23.5	0
Babaganoush, Delphi*	1 Serving/30g	51	4.8	169	2.8	2.2	16	2.5
Bean, Mexican, Doritos, Walkers*	1 Tbsp/20g	18	0.7	89	2.7	12.1	3.3	2.4
Beetroot, & Mint, Meadow Fresh, Lidl*	¼ Pack/50g	58	3	116	3.1	10.6	6	3.6
Beetroot, & Mint, The Deli, Aldi*	¼ Pot/50g	66	3.8	131	3.5	10	7.6	4.2
Beetroot, Feta, & Seed, Sainsbury's*	½ Pack/80g	128	8.6	160	5.5	9.1	10.8	2.6
Caramel, Salted, for Mini Doughnuts, Tesco*	1 Dip/3g	11	0.3	386	2.9	68.7	11.1	0
Carrot, & Houmous, Co-Op*	1 Pack/105g	85	4.9	81	2.3	6.3	4.7	2.1
Cheese & Chive, 50% Less Fat, Asda*	1 Pot/125g	261	21.5	209	4.5	9	17.2	0
Cheese & Chive, Asda*	1 Serving/43g	190	19.6	447	4.9	3.4	46	0
Cheese & Chive, Tesco*	1 Serving/28g	76	7.2	273	3.7	6.6	25.7	0.1
Cheese & Chive, The Deli, Aldi*	1 Serving/31g	107	10.5	345	4.6	5.7	34	0.5
Cheese, & Chive, Sainsbury's*	¼ Pot/50g	146	14	292	4.1	5.4	28.1	0.5
Cheese, with Crackers, Dip-it, Emporium, Aldi*	1 Pot/45g	111	4.5	246	11	27	10	0.6
Chilli Cheese, Asda*	1 Serving/50g	131	11	262	8	8	22	1.1
Chilli, M&S*	1 Pot/35g	103	0.1	295	0.4	73.2	0.2	0.4
Cracked Corn, Hella Hot, Wicked Kitchen, Tesco*	1 Serving/30g	27	1.3	90	2	10.2	4.3	1.2
Edamame, & Ginger, Meadow Fresh, Lidl*	¼ Pot/50g	59	3	118	3.3	10.6	5.9	4.6
Endamame & Pea, Waitrose*	¼ Pot/51g	85	5.9	166	6.3	8	11.6	2
French Onion, Frito-Lay*	1 Tsp/5ml	10	0.8	200	4	14	16	0
Garlic & Herb	**1 Serving/100g**	**584**	**62.4**	**584**	**1.4**	**4.1**	**62.4**	**0.2**
Garlic, & Onion, 30% Less Fat, Asda*	1 Serving/30g	50	3.9	166	3.9	8.2	13	0.5
Garlic, Takeaway Pizza, Goodfella's*	1 Pot/18g	57	5.4	319	0.3	12	30	0
Guacamole, Tex-Mex Multipack Selection, Tesco*	½ Pot/53g	76	6.8	142	1.1	4	12.8	3
Nacho Cheese, Average	**1 Serving/50g**	**175**	**17.2**	**350**	**6.3**	**3.4**	**34.4**	**0.9**
Nacho Chilli Cheese, The Deli, Aldi*	¼ Pot/50g	94	6.3	188	4.4	13.8	12.6	1.2
Onion & Garlic, Average	**1 Tbsp/15g**	**62**	**6.4**	**410**	**1.7**	**4.8**	**42.7**	**0.4**
Onion & Garlic, Gro, Co-Op*	¼ Pack/45g	122	11.2	270	1.6	9	25	0.5
Onion, & Garlic, Meadow Fresh, Lidl*	1/8 Pack/33g	90	8.1	272	2	10.6	24.6	1
Onion, & Garlic, Reduced Fat, Tesco*	¼ Pot/50g	64	4.8	128	3.7	6.5	9.6	0.6
Onion, Three, Toasted, Wicked Kitchen, Tesco*	½ Pot/85g	269	26.3	317	2.2	7.6	30.9	0.3

DIP	Measure INFO/WEIGHT	per Measure KCAL	FAT	Nutrition Values per 100g / 100ml KCAL	PROT	CARB	FAT	FIBRE
Pea & Spinach, Tesco*	¼ Pot/46g	34	1	75	4	7.7	2.1	4.4
Pea, & Mint, The Deli, Aldi*	¼ Pack/50g	52	3	103	3.3	6.4	6.1	4.4
Pea, & Spinach, Tesco*	¼ Pot/46g	61	4	132	3.1	8.6	8.6	3.9
Pea, Yogurt & Mint, Sainsbury's*	¼ Pack/50g	119	10.8	238	3.4	7.5	21.6	2.1
Pea-Lentiful, Supermarket, Leon Restaurants*	1 Serving/30g	90	8.1	301	6.9	5.9	27	4.9
Peanut, Satay Selection, Occasions, Sainsbury's*	1 Serving/2g	4	0.2	186	7.1	13.8	11.4	1.1
Pecorino, Basil & Pine Nut, Fresh, Waitrose*	½ Pot/85g	338	33.7	398	5.1	5.1	39.7	0
Ponzu, for Gyoza, Plant Kitchen, M&S*	1 Pot/22g	12	0	55	2.7	10.4	0.2	0.5
Raita, Tesco*	1 Serving/40g	81	7.8	203	1.6	4.8	19.6	0.3
Red Pepper, Chilli, & Garlic, Morrisons*	¼ Pot/50g	88	7.3	177	2.2	8.8	14.6	0.8
Red Pepper, Meadow Fresh, Lidl*	¼ Pot/50g	59	3	118	3.3	10.6	5.9	4.6
Red Pepper, Sainsbury's*	1 Pot/100g	103	4	103	2.3	14.6	4	0
Red Pepper, Smoky, Love Your Veg!, Sainsbury's*	¼ Pot/40g	36	1.4	89	2.5	10.3	3.5	3
Red Pepper, The Deli, Aldi*	¼ Pot/50g	60	3	119	3.6	11	6	4
Salsa, Chunky Tomato, Tesco*	1 Pot/170g	68	2.2	40	1.1	5.9	1.3	1.1
Salsa, Chunky, Fresh, Sainsbury's*	1 Serving/100g	51	1.7	51	1.1	7.8	1.7	1.2
Salsa, Hot, Snaktastic, Lidl*	1 Serving/50g	17	0.1	34	1.3	6.1	0.2	1.5
Salsa, Mild, Asda*	1 Portion/100g	38	0.5	38	1.5	6.7	0.5	0.6
Salsa, Mild, Doritos, Walkers*	1 Tbsp/30g	9	0.1	30	0.8	6	0.3	1.5
Salsa, Mild, Snaktastic, Lidl*	1 Serving/50g	21	0.2	42	1.6	7.7	0.4	0.6
Sour Cream & Chive, Half Fat, Waitrose*	½ Pot/85g	133	9.9	157	5.5	7.6	11.6	0.1
Sour Cream & Chive, Reduced Fat, Tesco*	¼ Pot/50g	80	6.1	159	4.2	7.9	12.2	0.2
Sour Cream & Chive, Average	**1 Tbsp/15g**	**48**	**4.8**	**317**	**3.2**	**4**	**32**	**0.3**
Sour Cream, & Chive, 30% Less Fat, Asda*	¼ Pot/50g	60	4.2	119	3.9	6.9	8.3	0.7
Sour Cream, & Chive, Reduced Fat, M&S*	1 Pack/230g	389	32.7	169	4.7	4.9	14.2	1.5
Sour Cream, & Chive, Reduced Fat, Morrisons*	¼ Pot/50g	70	5.5	139	4	5.8	11	0.1
Soy, Gyoza Selection, Tesco*	1 Pot/30g	30	0.2	100	1.7	21.4	0.7	0.7
Sweetcorn, & Chilli, Tesco*	¼ Pot/46g	53	1.6	115	2.9	17.3	3.4	1.7
Taramasalata, Sainsbury's*	¼ Pot/57g	267	26.6	465	3.3	8.6	46.3	0.5
DOLMADES								
Stffed Vine Leaves, Delphi*	1 Dolmade/30g	36	0.8	119	2.2	21.9	2.5	1.1
Stuffed with Rice, M&S*	1 Leaf/38g	40	1.6	105	2.6	14.2	4.1	1.2
DOPIAZA								
Chicken, Indian, Waitrose*	½ Pack/175g	243	14.5	139	10.2	5	8.3	1.6
Chicken, M&S*	1 Pack/350g	402	21.4	115	11.5	3.7	6.1	2.5
Chicken, Slimming World*	1 Pack/500g	335	6	67	9.1	4.2	1.2	1.6
Mushroom, Retail	**1oz/28g**	**19**	**1.6**	**69**	**1.3**	**3.7**	**5.7**	**1.1**
DORITOS								
Chilli Heatwave, Walkers*	1 Bag/30g	148	7.6	495	6.3	57.3	25.3	6.7
Cool, Original, Walkers*	1 Bag/70g	349	17.8	498	5.9	58.1	25.5	5.6
Dippas, Hint of Lime, Walkers*	1 Bag/35g	173	8.8	495	7	60	25	3.5
Dippas, Lightly Salted, Dipping Chips, Walkers*	1 Serving/25g	128	6.8	510	6.5	60	27	3
Lighly Salted, Corn Chips, Doritos*	1 Bag/30g	149	7.1	497	6.9	62.9	23.6	3.3
Stax, Ultimate Cheese, Walkers*	1 Serving/30g	158	8.1	527	4.5	63	27	5.2
Sweet Chilli, Walkers*	1 Serving/28g	140	7	500	7.1	64.3	25	3.6
Tangy Cheese, Walkers*	1 Bag/40g	200	10.8	500	7	57	27	3
DOUBLE DECKER								
Cadbury*	1 Bar/54.5g	253	9.3	464	3.7	73	17	1.6
Dinky Deckers, Cadbury*	1 Piece/5g	22	0.8	456	4.2	71	17	1.5
Snack Size, Cadbury*	1 Bar/36g	165	7.4	465	4.8	64.5	20.9	0
DOUGH BALLS								
Garlic, Cooked, Morrisons*	¼ Pack/42g	146	5	349	9.4	50.2	11.9	1.9
Garlic, M&S*	4 Balls/60g	230	12.2	384	7.7	40.9	20.3	3.6

D

	Measure INFO/WEIGHT	per Measure KCAL	FAT	Nutrition Values per 100g / 100ml KCAL	PROT	CARB	FAT	FIBRE
DOUGH BALLS								
with Garlic & Herb Butter, Aldi*	1 Ball/12g	45	2.2	365	7.7	46.7	18.2	1.8
with Garlic Butter Dip, Supermarket, Pizza Express*	4 Balls/46g	130	1	280	10.6	53.1	2.2	2.7
DOUGHNUTS								
Caramel Cream, Baker's Soft, Tesco*	1 Doughnut/61g	200	10.6	328	6.2	35.2	17.4	2.7
Chocolate, Bakery, Tesco*	1 Doughnut/66g	250	12.8	379	6.6	43.5	19.4	2.2
Chocolate, Iced, Ring, Bakery, Sainsbury's*	1 Doughnut/55g	212	10.3	386	6.3	47.4	18.8	1
Custard Filled, Average	**1 Doughnut/75g**	**268**	**14.2**	**358**	**6.2**	**43.3**	**19**	**0**
Glazed, Bakery, Tesco*	1 Doughnut/52g	202	10.1	389	6.5	45.9	19.5	2
Glazed, Ring, Bakery, Sainsbury's*	1 Doughnut/62g	229	12	369	5.5	42.8	19.3	1.1
Iced, Raspberry Filled, Morrisons*	1 Doughnut/65g	245	10.7	378	5.5	51	16.5	1.5
Jam, & Cream, Asda*	1 Doughnut/41g	139	7.4	336	4.9	39	18	0.6
Jam, & Cream, Cream Cake Selection, Tesco*	1 Doughnut/71g	225	10.2	317	6	40.4	14.4	1
Jam, & Fresh Cream, Tesco*	1 Doughnut/71g	223	9.5	314	5.6	41.7	13.4	1.7
Jam, Filled, Average	**1 Doughnut/75g**	**252**	**10.9**	**336**	**5.7**	**48.8**	**14.5**	**0**
Jam, Jazzy, Wicked Kitchen, Tesco*	1 Doughnut/45g	139	4.6	309	5.7	47.5	10.3	1.8
Mini, Sainsbury's*	1 Doughnut/14g	53	2.7	379	5.2	47.9	18.9	2.1
Plain, Ring, Average	**1 Doughnut/60g**	**238**	**13**	**397**	**6.1**	**47.2**	**21.7**	**0**
Raspberry Jam, Sainsbury's*	1 Doughnut/58g	203	8.9	350	5.5	46.4	15.3	2.3
Ring, Iced, Average	**1 Doughnut/70g**	**268**	**12.2**	**383**	**4.8**	**55.1**	**17.5**	**0**
Ring, Mini, Bakers Selection, Asda*	1 Doughnut/13g	55	2.8	409	5.2	49	21	1.4
Selection, Bakers Selection, Asda*	1 Doughnut/75g	273	17.9	365	4.5	32	24	1.4
Strawberry, Iced, Ring, Bakery, Tesco*	1 Doughnut/58g	248	14.3	428	5.4	45.3	24.7	1.4
Strawberry, Iced, Ring, Mini, Bakery, Tesco*	1 Doughnut/15g	62	3.1	415	4.9	51.5	20.8	1.3
Sugar, Ring, Bakery, Sainsbury's*	1 Doughnut/51g	222	14	435	5.7	40.7	27.4	2.1
Vanilla, Bakery, Sainsbury's*	1 Doughnut/66g	248	12.9	376	6.1	42.7	19.6	2
White Iced, Ring, Bakery, Sainsbury's*	1 Doughnut/55g	211	10.2	383	7	46.4	18.6	1
Yum Yums, Glazed, Sweet, Waitrose*	1 Doughnut/45g	172	10	382	4	41.6	22.2	2
Yum Yums, M&S*	1 Doughnut/37g	155	8.9	420	4.9	45.7	23.9	1.6
Yum Yums, Sainsbury's*	1 Doughnut/50g	214	12.4	428	4.8	45.8	24.7	1.3
DOVER SOLE								
Fillet, Raw, Average	**1oz/28g**	**25**	**0.5**	**89**	**18.1**	**0**	**1.8**	**0**
DR PEPPER*								
Coca-Cola*	1 Can/330ml	66	0	20	0	4.9	0	0
Zero, Coca-Cola*	1 Can/330ml	2	0	0	0	0	0	0
DRAGON FRUIT								
Raw, Edible Portion, Average	**1 Serving/100g**	**41**	**0.5**	**41**	**0.7**	**9.6**	**0.5**	**3.6**
DRAMBUIE								
39% Volume	**1 Pub Shot/35ml**	**125**	**0**	**358**	**0**	**23**	**0**	**0**
DRESSING								
French, Style, BGTY, Sainsbury's*	1 Tbsp/15ml	11	0.4	76	0.7	12.6	2.5	0.5
Balsamic, & Olive Oil, Tesco*	1 Tbsp/15ml	45	4.2	297	1.1	10.6	27.8	0
Balsamic, BGTY, Sainsbury's*	1 Tbsp/15ml	11	0.1	74	0.5	17.3	0.5	1
Balsamic, Fig Glaze, Tesco*	1 Tbsp/15ml	31	0	208	1.4	47.9	0	0
Balsamic, Low Fat, Tesco*	1 Tbsp/15ml	10	0.2	65	0.2	13.3	1.1	0.9
Balsamic, Sainsbury's*	1 Tbsp/15ml	21	0.8	138	0.5	21.9	5.4	0.5
Beetroot, & Balsamic, Morrisons*	1 Tbsp/15ml	11	0	73	0.7	16.9	0.2	0.6
Beetroot, & Honey, Tigg's Perfect Match*	1 Tbsp/15ml	40	3.3	268	1.5	16.4	21.7	0
Blue Cheese, Hellmann's*	1 Tbsp/15ml	69	7.1	459	0.7	6.3	47.2	1.1
Blue Cheese, Waitrose*	1 Tbsp/15ml	90	9.2	598	1.4	9.6	61.2	1.7
Caesar, Asiago, Briannas*	1 Tbsp/15ml	70	7.5	467	3.3	3.3	50	0
Caesar, Classic, Sainsbury's*	1 Tbsp/15ml	66	6.9	442	2.7	4.6	45.9	0.5
Caesar, Creamy, Asda*	1 Tbsp/15ml	34	3.3	225	1.5	12	22	1
Caesar, Creamy, M&S*	1 Tbsp/15ml	66	6.5	437	2.6	9.1	43.1	1

D

DRESSING

INFO/WEIGHT	Measure	per Measure		Nutrition Values per 100g / 100ml				
		KCAL	FAT	KCAL	PROT	CARB	FAT	FIBRE
Caesar, Fat Free, Average	**1 Tbsp/15ml**	**13**	**0.6**	**84**	**4.6**	**11**	**4.1**	**0.2**
Caesar, Finest, Tesco*	1 Tbsp/15ml	72	7.6	477	1.9	2.8	50.9	0.2
Caesar, Low Fat, Average	**1 Tbsp/15ml**	**12**	**0.4**	**77**	**2.3**	**11.1**	**2.6**	**0.2**
Caesar, Original, Cardini's*	1 Tbsp/15ml	83	9	555	2.3	1.5	60	0.2
Caesar, Rich & Creamy, Waitrose*	1 Tbsp/15ml	78	8.3	518	2.2	2.4	55.4	0.8
Caesar, Tesco*	1 Tbsp/15ml	59	6.1	393	1	4.9	40.9	0.4
Caesar, The Best, Morrisons*	1 Tbsp/15ml	48	4.7	322	3.2	7.1	31.1	0.6
Caesar, Vegan, Plant Chef, Tesco*	1 Tbsp/15ml	51	5.2	343	1.2	4.1	35	3.5
Caesar, Vegan, Sacla*	1 Tbsp/15ml	65	6.9	432	0.3	4.1	46	0
Caesar, with Smoked Garlic, Hellmann's*	1 Tbsp/15ml	35	3.3	231	2	6.4	22	0
Chilli, & Herb, Morrisons*	1 Tbsp/15ml	21	1.1	140	1.1	17	7.3	0.9
Cucumber, & Mint, M&S*	1 Tbsp/15ml	46	3.9	305	0.7	16.7	26.1	0.1
Drizzle, with Balsamic Vinegar of Modena, Tesco*	1 Tbsp/15ml	27	0	183	0.7	44.4	0	1.1
French, BGTY, Sainsbury's*	1 Tbsp/15ml	11	0.3	73	0.5	13.5	1.7	0
French, Chilled, Tesco*	1 Tbsp/15ml	63	5.9	421	1.1	15.1	39.6	0
French, Classics, M&S*	1 Tbsp/15ml	77	8	516	0.6	8.2	53.1	0.2
French, Fresh, Organic, Sainsbury's*	1 Tbsp/15ml	45	4.6	301	0.4	5.5	31	0.4
French, Fresh, Sainsbury's*	1 Tbsp/15ml	64	6.7	429	0.6	6.6	44.6	0.6
French, LC, Tesco*	1 Tbsp/15ml	8	0.2	50	0.8	7.6	1.6	1.1
French, Light & Tangy, Lucy's*	1 Tbsp/15ml	47	4.8	313	2	2.5	32.2	0.5
French, Reduced Fat, M&S*	1 Tbsp/15ml	10	0.4	70	0.7	11.5	2.8	0.7
French, Reduced Fat, Tesco*	1 Tbsp/15ml	10	0.2	65	0.5	13	1.3	0
Garlic & Herb, Sainsbury's*	1 Tbsp/15ml	44	4.4	292	0.5	6.4	29.3	0.5
Glaze, with Balsamic Vinegar Of Modena, Asda*	1 Tbsp/15ml	31	0.1	204	1	49	0.5	1
Honey & Mustard, BGTY, Sainsbury's*	1 Tbsp/15ml	12	0.2	78	0.5	16.1	1.3	0.5
Honey & Mustard, Hellmann's*	1 Tbsp/15ml	27	0.2	182	0.7	13.7	1.6	0.3
Honey & Mustard, Light, Asda*	1 Tbsp/15ml	9	0.2	62	0.5	11	1.3	1.3
Honey & Mustard, M&S*	1 Tbsp/15ml	47	3.8	313	2.7	16.8	25.5	2.8
Honey & Mustard, Mellow Yellow*	1 Tbsp/15ml	88	8.8	588	2.6	11.7	58.8	0
Honey & Mustard, Tesco*	1 Tbsp/15ml	33	2.3	220	0.8	18.8	15.2	2.5
House, Classic, Salad, Hellmann's*	1 Tbsp/15ml	38	3.9	254	0.5	5.7	26	0
House, Light, Supermarket, Pizza Express*	1 Tbsp/15ml	45	4.5	300	0.7	4.3	30	0.3
House, Supermarket, Pizza Express*	1 Tbsp/15ml	62	6.6	415	0.7	3.3	44	0.3
Kalamata, Balsamic Glaze, Fig, Vrionis*	1 Tbsp/15ml	30	0	201	1.5	48	0	0
Lemon, & Black Pepper, Fat Free, Tesco*	1 Tbsp/15ml	11	0	74	0.1	17.8	0.1	0.9
Lemon, & Herb, Counted, Morrisons*	1 Tbsp/15ml	6	0.3	39	0.5	4.9	1.7	1.2
Light, Salad, Mary Berry*	1 Tbsp/15ml	34	2.8	230	0.8	14	19	0.6
Mango, & Chilli, Tesco*	1 Tbsp/15ml	33	2.9	223	0.2	11.3	19.3	1.5
Mary Berry*	1 Tbsp/15ml	77	6.6	513	0.8	28.5	44	0.1
Moroccan Style, TTD, Sainsbury's*	1 Tbsp/15ml	25	1.6	168	0	16.3	10.5	2.7
Mustard, & Maple, Specially Selected, Aldi*	1 Tbsp/15ml	45	3.7	301	0.6	17	25	2.3
Oil & Lemon	**1 Tbsp/15ml**	**97**	**10.6**	**647**	**0.3**	**2.8**	**70.6**	**0**
Peri Peri, M Kitchen, Morrisons*	1 Tbsp/15ml	38	3.4	253	1.6	10.1	22.8	0.5
Pesto, TTD, Sainsbury's*	1 Tbsp/15ml	22	1.8	144	2.1	5.8	12.1	1.3
Ranch, Light, Hidden Valley*	1 Tbsp/15ml	30	2.5	200	0	13.3	16.7	0
Salad, Balsamic Vinaigrette, Specially Selected, Aldi*	1 Tbsp/15ml	44	3.8	293	3.3	15.3	25.3	3.3
Salad, Balsamic, with Garlic, Spray, Heinz*	1 Spray/1ml	1	0.1	82	0.4	10.3	4.3	0
Salad, Caesar, Inspired Vegan*	1 Tbsp/15ml	51	4.8	340	4	7.7	32.3	0.5
Salad, Lemon, & Thyme, Specially Selected, Aldi*	1 Tbsp/15ml	23	1.2	157	0.5	21	7.9	1.2
Salad, Moroccan Style, Irresistible, Co-Op*	1 Tbsp/15ml	9	0.5	60	0.6	6.2	3.3	1.6
Salad, Raspberry Balsamic, Spray, Heinz*	20 Sprays/15ml	23	1.9	156	0.4	9.3	13.1	0
Salad, Specially Selected, Aldi*	1 Tbsp/15ml	45	3.7	300	3.3	17.3	24.7	3.3
Soy, Chilli, & Ginger, Counted, Morrisons*	1 Tbsp/15ml	8	0	51	0.2	11.8	0.3	0.3

	Measure INFO/WEIGHT	per Measure KCAL	FAT	Nutrition Values per 100g / 100ml KCAL	PROT	CARB	FAT	FIBRE
DRESSING								
Soy, Chilli, & Ginger, Specially Selected, Aldi*	1 Tbsp/15ml	19	1.2	124	0.5	11	8.3	1.2
Sweet Chilli, & Coriander, Sainsbury's*	1 Tbsp/15ml	38	2.4	255	1.1	26.5	16	0.5
Thousand Island	**1 Tbsp/15ml**	**48**	**4.5**	**323**	**1.1**	**12.5**	**30.2**	**0.4**
Thousand Island, Reduced Calorie	**1 Tbsp/15ml**	**29**	**2.3**	**195**	**0.7**	**14.7**	**15.2**	**0**
DRIED FRUIT								
Apricots, Soft, Alesto, Lidl*	1 Serving/30g	81	0.1	269	2	61.3	0.3	6.4
Berry, Mix, Diet Chef Ltd*	1 Pack/25g	84	0.2	337	1.4	77.6	0.8	4.8
Fruity Biscuit Shot, Whitworths*	1 Pack/25g	93	2.1	372	2.8	69.2	8.4	4.5
Mango, & Raspberries, Freeze-Dried, 5th Season*	1 Pack/14g	48	0.3	341	4.9	54.2	2.2	16.2
Mixed, Trio, Holland & Barrett*	1 Serving/30g	82	0.2	273	2.3	69.2	0.5	2
Raisin & Chocolate, Shot, Whitworths*	1 Pack/25g	91	2.3	364	4	63.2	9.2	5.6
Summer Berry Burst, Graze*	1 Punnet/26g	80	0.2	306	1.4	69	0.6	7.1
Trail Mix, Kick Start, Wholefoods, Asda*	1 Serving/50g	194	10.2	387	10.9	40	20.4	10.7
Tropical Mix, Alesto, Lidl*	1 Serving/25g	104	4.8	416	3.4	55.9	19	4
Vine, Mixed, Jumbo, BuyWholeFoodsOnline*	1 Serving/30g	83	0.2	278	2.5	71.1	0.5	2.4
DRIED FRUIT MIX								
Average	**1 Tbsp/25g**	**67**	**0.1**	**268**	**2.3**	**68.1**	**0.4**	**2.2**
Berry, Love Life, Waitrose*	1 Serving/30g	89	0.3	296	1.9	70	0.9	3
Continente Puro Prazer*	1 Serving/25g	150	11.2	601	15	32	45	7.8
Garden of England, Graze*	1 Punnet/25g	70	0.2	280	1	71.2	0.7	5.6
Partially Rehydrated, Whitworths*	1 Serving/25g	75	0.2	300	2.4	70	0.6	0.5
Sultanas Raisins & Cranberries, Dunnes*	1 Handful/15g	47	0.1	315	2	80.2	0.9	4.7
with Cranberry, & Apricots, Tesco*	1 Serving/30g	94	0.3	314	2.6	71.2	1	5.1
DRINK								
Almond, with Caramel Coffee, Free From, Asda*	1 Serving/200ml	72	2.8	36	1	4.5	1.4	0.5
Aloe, Original, Green Globe*	1 Serving/200ml	36	0	18	0	4.5	0	0.1
AloeMax, Herbalife*	1 Serving/15ml	2	0	13	0	2.9	0	0
Amalfi Spritz, Non Alcoholic, Lyre's*	1 Can/250ml	72	0	29	0	6.6	0	0
Aperitif, Bitter, Non Alcoholic, AEcorn *	1 Measure/50ml	24	0	47	0.4	8.6	0	0
Aperitif, Bittersweet, Non Alcoholic, Everleaf*	1 Measure/50ml	26	0	51	0	12.6	0	0
Aperitif, Non Alcoholic, Vibrante, Martini*	1 Serving/75ml	45	0	60	0	14	0	0
Apple Cider Vinegar, with Apple Juice, OSU*	1 Bottle/500ml	910	2.5	182	0.5	39.9	0.5	0.6
Citrus, & Ginger, Hot Shot, M&S*	1 Shot/100ml	32	0.1	32	0.7	6.9	0.1	0.4
Classico, Non-Alcoholic, Lyre's*	1 Can/250ml	44	0	18	0	3.8	0	0
Coconut, Milk Free, Sweetened, Sainsbury's*	1 Serving/100ml	15	0.8	15	0	1.9	0.8	0
G&T, Pre Mixed, Reduced Calorie, Tesco*	1 Can/250ml	70	0	28	0	0	0	0
Ginger Zinger, M&S*	1 Bottle/100ml	41	0.1	41	0.2	10.6	0.1	0.1
Ginger, Immune Support, M&S*	1 Bottle/100g	41	0.1	41	0.2	10.6	0.1	0.1
Limone e Menta, Sparkling, Vive, Aldi*	1 Serving/250ml	5	1.2	2	0.5	0.5	0.5	0.5
Malted, Instant, As Sold, Morrisons*	1 Serving/30g	130	2.7	433	8.3	79	9	1.3
Mango & Ginger, Nix And Kix*	1 Can/250ml	50	0.2	20	0.1	5	0.1	0
Oat, Provamel*	1 Serving/200ml	94	2.6	47	0.3	8.1	1.3	0.8
Protein, Mango, & Passion Fruit, Up Beat*	1 Serving/18g	55	0	316	71.5	6.2	0.1	1.9
Raspberry, Isotonic, Sports, Tesco*	1 Bottle/500ml	115	0	23	0	5.3	0	0
Soda, Mexican Lime, Fever Tree*	1 Bottle/300ml	48	0	16	0	4	0	0
Soda, Pink Guava, Hopt*	1 Bottle/330ml	66	0.3	20	0.1	4.9	0.1	0
Soda, Raspberry & Rose, Fever-Tree*	1 Bottle/500ml	100	0	20	0	4.9	0	0
Soda, Sparkling, Feijoa, Pear, & Elderflower, Mac's*	1 Bottler/330ml	107	0	32	0	8.6	0	0
Soya, Original, Essential, Waitrose*	1 Serving/200ml	82	3.8	41	3.4	2.6	1.9	0
Soya, Unsweetened, Essential, Waitrose*	1 Serving/200ml	70	3.8	35	3.4	0.8	1.9	0.6
Sparkling, Cherry, Dalston's*	1 Can/330ml	50	0	15	0	3.2	0	0
Turmeric, & Cayenne, Shot, Eat Well, M&S*	1 Bottle/100ml	42	0.1	42	0.3	10	0.1	0.6
Turmeric, Raw, Original, Shot, The Turmeric Co*	1 Shot/60ml	22	0.2	37	0.6	7.9	0.3	0

	Measure INFO/WEIGHT	per Measure KCAL	FAT	Nutrition Values per 100g / 100ml KCAL	PROT	CARB	FAT	FIBRE
DRINKING CHOCOLATE								
Cacao A La Taza, Dry Weight, El Canari*	1 Tbsp/15g	51	0.4	340	5.5	72.1	2.9	3.1
Ginger, & Orange, Christmas, Montezuma*	1 Disk/15g	85	6.4	566	8	31	43	11
Made Up with Semi-Skimmed Milk, Average	*1 Mug/227ml*	*129*	*4.3*	*57*	*3.5*	*7*	*1.9*	*0.2*
Made Up with Skimmed Milk, Average	*1 Mug/227ml*	*100*	*1.1*	*44*	*3.5*	*7*	*0.5*	*0*
Made Up with Whole Milk, Average	*1 Mug/227ml*	*173*	*9.5*	*76*	*3.4*	*6.8*	*4.2*	*0.2*
Mint, Organic, 54%, Montezuma*	1 Disk/15g	82	5.7	547	5	45	38	7
Mochachino, 54%, Montezuma*	1 Disk/15g	79	5.2	526	5	42	35	7
DRIPPING								
Beef	*1oz/28g*	*249*	*27.7*	*891*	*0*	*0*	*99*	*0*
DUCK								
Breast, Meat Only, Cooked, Average	*1oz/28g*	*48*	*2*	*172*	*25.3*	*1.8*	*7*	*0*
Breast, Meat Only, Raw, Average	*1 Serving/160g*	*206*	*6.8*	*128*	*22.6*	*0*	*4.2*	*0.2*
Confit, Bistro, Gressingham*	½ Pack/125g	272	16.2	218	23	1.1	13	0.5
Confit, from South West, Picard*	½ Pack/180g	549	43.2	305	22	0.2	24	0
Crackling, Wildings*	1 Pack/25g	168	14.1	672	34	6.4	56.4	0.8
Leg, Meat & Skin, Average	*1oz/28g*	*80*	*5.6*	*286*	*17.2*	*0.5*	*20*	*0.4*
Raw, Meat, Fat & Skin	*1oz/28g*	*109*	*10.4*	*388*	*13.1*	*0*	*37.3*	*0*
Roasted, Meat Only, Weighed with Fat, Skin & Bone	*1 Serving/100g*	*41*	*2.2*	*41*	*5.3*	*0*	*2.2*	*0*
Roasted, Meat, Fat & Skin	*1oz/28g*	*118*	*10.7*	*423*	*20*	*0*	*38.1*	*0*
Shredded, Peking, Hoisin Sauce, & Pancakes, Sainsbury's*	1 Pack/210g	487	9	232	17	31	4.3	0.9
Shredded, Portuguese Style, Porsi*	½ Pack/200g	328	24	164	12	2.1	12	0.5
Shredded, with Hoisin Sauce, Asda*	1 Pack/191g	387	11.2	203	9	27	5.9	2.3
Vegetarian, Shredded, Hoisin, Frozen, Linda McCartney*	1 Serving/75g	159	6.5	212	24.7	6.7	8.7	4.4
DUCK AROMATIC								
Crispy, Ā,¼, Hoisin Sauce & 6 Pancakes, Tesco*	1/6 Pack/40g	92	3.3	231	13.3	25.3	8.3	1
Crispy, Ā,¼, Hoisin Sauce, Pancakes, M&S*	½ Pack/155g	290	12.1	187	10.5	18.1	7.8	1
Crispy, Ā,½, Duck & Pancakes, M&S*	½ Pack/311g	590	26.7	190	13.9	14	8.6	2.1
Crispy, Ā,½, Hoisin Sauce, & 12 Pancakes, Tesco*	3 Pancakes/106g	263	9.5	248	17.9	23.4	8.9	1
DUMPLINGS								
Average	*1oz/28g*	*58*	*3.3*	*208*	*2.8*	*24.5*	*11.7*	*0.9*
Dim Sum, Assorted Stuffing, Steamed, Restaurant	*1 Serving/100g*	*230*	*8.2*	*230*	*7.9*	*32*	*8.2*	*3*
Dim Sum, Chicken, Steamed, Restaurant	*1 Serving/100g*	*230*	*5.9*	*230*	*7.5*	*37*	*5.9*	*2.1*
Dim Sum, Chinese, Deep Fried, Restaurant	*1 Serving/100g*	*430*	*23*	*430*	*4.9*	*50*	*23*	*1.8*
Dim Sum, From Restaurant, Average	*1 Piece/12g*	*50*	*2.4*	*433*	*28.9*	*31.3*	*20.4*	*0*
Dim Sum, Meat Dumpling, Deep Fried, Restaurant	*1 Serving/100g*	*340*	*16*	*340*	*4.9*	*43*	*16*	*1*
Dim Sum, Pork, Restaurant, Average	*1 Serving/100g*	*270*	*7.3*	*270*	*7.3*	*43*	*7.3*	*1.6*
Dim Sum, Prawn, Steamed, Eat Well, M&S*	1 Dim Sum/20g	28	0.2	138	6.7	25.1	1.1	0.6
Dim Sum, Steamed, Prawn, M&S*	6 Dim Sum/120g	222	3.2	185	1.1	39	2.7	1.5
Dim Sum, Vegetable & Meat, Steamed, Restaurant	*1 Serving/100g*	*240*	*7.9*	*240*	*5.9*	*37*	*7.9*	*2.5*
Dim Sum, Wonton, Deep Fried, Restaurant	*1 Serving/100g*	*430*	*29*	*430*	*9.7*	*32*	*29*	*1.2*
Gyoza, Beef, Korean, Supermarket, Itsu*	1 Gyoza/20g	38	1.6	191	11.3	18	7.8	2.8
Gyoza, Chicken & Vegetable Selection, Sainsbury's*	1 Pack/150g	300	11.1	200	7.2	24	7.4	1.7
Gyoza, Chicken, Sainsbury's*	1 Pack/150g	219	7	146	8.1	17.2	4.7	1
Gyoza, Chicken, Yutaka*	1 Gyoza/20g	29	0.6	147	7	22	3	3
Gyoza, Duck, Aromatic, Supermarket, Itsu*	1 Gyoza/20g	35	0.9	175	4.4	28	4.5	2.1
Gyoza, Legumes, Lidl*	¼ Pack/100g	133	0.9	133	4.9	26	0.9	1.2
Gyoza, Pork, Itsu*	5 Gyoza/100g	185	6.6	185	8.1	22	6.6	2.1
Gyoza, Prawn, Classic, Itsu*	½ Pack/110g	198	5.7	180	5.5	27	5.2	1.9
Gyoza, Prawn, King, Steamed	5 Gyoza/75g	135	3.9	180	5.5	27	5.2	1.9
Gyoza, Prawn, Thai Tapas*	1 Gyoza/28g	59	2.3	211	6.4	27.8	8.2	1.1
Gyoza, Vegetable, with Ponzu Dip, Ready to Eat, M&S*	1 Pack/68g	87	2.1	128	3.7	20.6	3.1	1.5
Gyoza, with Spicy Vegetables, & Tofu, Vitasia, Lidl*	1 Serving/100g	146	2.3	146	6.1	23.2	2.3	0
Gyozas, Chicken, Microwaved, Iceland*	1 Gyozas/18g	31	0.5	176	8.3	28	2.7	3.3

D

	Measure INFO/WEIGHT	per Measure KCAL	FAT	Nutrition Values per 100g / 100ml KCAL	PROT	CARB	FAT	FIBRE
DUMPLINGS								
Hearty, Frozen, As Sold, Aunt Bessies*	1 Dumpling/49g	161	7.3	330	4.7	43	15	1.7
Homestyle, Baked Weight, Frozen, Aunt Bessie's*	1 Dumpling/53g	177	7.9	337	5.4	47	15	3.5
Lamb, & Leek, Chinese, Hong's*	1 Dumpling/25g	50	2	199	12	20	8	1
Mix, Cooked as Directed, Aunt Bessie's*	2 Dumpling/53g	126	4.9	238	4.5	33	9.2	2.4
Pork & Garlic Chive, Waitrose*	1 Pack/115g	215	8.1	187	9.4	20.4	7	1.1
Pork, & Beef, Kuljanka*	1 Serving/250g	612	20.8	245	10.4	31.1	8.3	0
Pork, Beijing, Red Sun *	1 Dunmpling/25g	55	2	220	11.1	25.3	7.9	3.8
Pork, Sichuan Style, Spicy, Hong's*	1 Dumpling/25g	66	3.8	262	12	18	15	1
Potato, Half & Half, Kartoffel Knodel, Pfanni*	1 Serving/190g	220	1.3	117	2.2	24	0.7	2.1
Prawn Sui Mai, Selection, M&S*	6 Sui Mai/120g	143	0.8	119	9.4	13.3	0.7	1.5
Prawn, Siu Mai, Chinese, M&S*	1 Dumpling/20g	22	0.3	108	9.4	13.3	1.6	1.5

D

	Measure INFO/WEIGHT	per Measure KCAL	FAT	Nutrition Values per 100g / 100ml KCAL	PROT	CARB	FAT	FIBRE
EASTER EGG								
Aero, Medium, Egg Shell Only, Aero, Nestle*	1 Egg/131g	702	38.9	534	6.2	59.9	29.6	1.6
Buttons, Chocolate Egg Shell Only, Cadbury*	1 Egg/100g	537	31	537	7.3	56	31	2.1
Caramel, Chocolate Egg Shell Only, Cadbury*	1 Egg/343g	1801	102.9	525	7.5	56.8	30	0.7
Chocolate Egg Shell Only, Dairy Milk, Cadbury*	1 Egg/343g	1818	104.6	530	7.6	56.5	30.5	0.7
Chocolate Egg Shell Only, Small, Dairy Milk, Cadbury*	1 Egg/72g	386	22.3	537	7.3	56	31	2.1
Chocolate Orange, Terry's*	1 Egg/196g	1015	52.9	518	8.1	59	27	2.3
Chocolate, Free From, Sainsbury's*	1 Egg/100g	581	35.8	581	3	59.5	35.8	4.5
Creme Egg, Chocolate Egg Shell Only, Cadbury*	1 Egg/178g	956	55.2	537	7.3	56	31	2.1
Crunchie, Cadbury*	1 Egg/200g	1072	61.9	537	7.3	56	31	2.1
Dairy Milk, Caramel, Egg Shell Only, Cadbury*	1 Egg/176g	945	54.6	537	7.3	56	31	2.1
Dark Chocolate, & Mint, Deluxe, Lidl*	¼ Egg/50g	270	17.4	541	4.9	48.2	34.8	7.5
Ferrero Rocher, Egg Shell Only, Ferrero*	1 Egg/175g	1064	80.2	608	7.3	39.8	45.8	0
Flake, Chocolate Egg Shell Only, Cadbury*	1 Egg/200g	1074	62	537	7.3	56	31	2.1
Freddo Faces, Chocolate Egg Shell Only, Cadbury*	1 Egg/72g	382	22	530	7.6	56.5	30.5	0.7
Kit Kat, Chunky, Nestle*	1 Egg/107g	572	31.5	534	6.1	60.4	29.4	1.5
Malteser, Malteaster, Egg Shell Only, Mars*	1 Egg/149g	785	43.2	527	7	59	29	0
Maltesers, Bunny, Egg Shell Only, Mars*	1 Egg/175g	922	50.8	527	7	59	29	0
Maltesers, Truffles, Egg Shell Only, Mars*	1 Egg/175g	922	50.8	527	6.7	59	29	0
Milk Chocolate, Nestle*	½ Egg/42g	205	9.7	489	5	65.2	23.1	0.5
Milky Bar, Nestle*	¼ Egg/18g	97	5.7	543	10.6	53.1	31.7	0
Mini Eggs, Chocolate Egg Shell Only, Cadbury*	¼ Egg/25g	134	7.7	537	7.3	56	31	2.1
Minstrels, Egg Shell Only, Galaxy, Mars*	1 Egg/200g	1056	58	528	7.1	58.9	29	0
Oreo, Cadbury*	1 Egg/31g	175	11.2	563	5	55	36	1.4
Roses, Chocolate Egg Shell Only, Cadbury*	1 Egg/200g	1060	61	530	7.6	56.5	30.5	0.7
Smarties, Nestle*	¼ Egg/31g	160	8.4	524	6	62	27.7	1.4
Twirl, Chocolate Egg Shell Only, Cadbury*	1 Egg/325g	1745	100.8	537	7.3	56	31	2.1
White Chocolate, Thorntons*	1 Egg/360g	1958	109.1	544	5.5	62.2	30.3	2.1
ECLAIR								
Caramel, Asda*	1 Eclair/58g	215	15.1	371	5.6	29	26	0.7
Chocolate, 25% Less Fat, Sainsbury's*	1 Eclair/58g	171	9.3	295	6.8	31.1	16	1.2
Chocolate, Asda*	1 Eclair/33g	144	11	436	6.7	27.3	33.3	4.8
Chocolate, Belgian, & Cream, Essential, Waitrose*	1 Eclair/39g	148	9.5	379	6.2	33	24.4	1.6
Chocolate, Belgian, Fresh Cream, Tesco*	1 Eclair/61g	233	15.4	382	7.3	30.6	25.3	1
Chocolate, Belgian, Sainsbury's*	1 Eclair/34g	127	8.4	374	6.1	30.8	24.8	1.5
Chocolate, Fresh Cream, M&S*	1 Eclair/44g	170	12.2	390	6.3	28.4	27.9	2
Chocolate, Fresh Cream, Morrisons*	1 Eclair/39g	146	9.4	373	6.6	32.3	23.9	1.5
Chocolate, Fresh Cream, Sainsbury's*	1 Eclair/35g	130	8.3	372	6.5	32.2	23.8	1.5
Chocolate, Frozen, Free From, Tesco*	1 Eclair/25g	81	4.2	327	4.1	38.9	17	0.8
Chocolate, Frozen, Morrisons*	1 Eclair/31g	116	9.6	374	5	18.8	31	1.3
Chocolate, Our Best Ever, M&S*	1 Eclair/118g	479	34	406	5.2	30.6	28.8	1.2
EEL								
Cooked or Smoked, Dry Heat, Average	**1 Serving/100g**	**236**	**15**	**236**	**23.6**	**0**	**15**	**0**
Jellied, Average	**1oz/28g**	**26**	**1.9**	**93**	**8**	**0**	**6.7**	**0**
Raw, Average	**1oz/28g**	**32**	**2.1**	**113**	**11.1**	**0**	**7.6**	**0**
EGG SUBSTITUTE								
Easy Egg, Vegan, Dry , Orgran*	1 Serving/50g	175	1.6	350	14.9	46.8	3.2	16
Egg Replacer, Free From, Vegan, Free & Easy*	1 Tsp/3g	1	0	30	0.1	8.3	0.1	2.6
Vegan Egg, Follow Your Heart*	1 Serving/10g	40	1.7	401	5	0	17	40
EGGS								
Araucana, Bluebell, Free Range, Finest, Tesco*	1 Egg/50g	66	4.5	131	12.6	0.1	9	0
Blue, Old Cotswold Legbar, Clarence Court*	1 Egg/60g	79	5.4	131	12.4	0	9	0
Duck, Boiled & Salted, Weight with Shell	**1 Egg/75g**	**148**	**11.6**	**198**	**14.6**	**0**	**15.5**	**0**
Duck, Whole, Raw, Weight with Shell	**1 Egg/75g**	**122**	**8.8**	**163**	**14.3**	**0**	**11.8**	**0**

	Measure INFO/WEIGHT	per Measure KCAL	FAT	Nutrition Values per 100g / 100ml KCAL	PROT	CARB	FAT	FIBRE
EGGS								
Free Range, Large, Weight with Shell	1 Egg/68g	97	6.8	143	12.6	0.8	9.9	0
Fried in Veg Oil, Average	1 Med/60g	107	8.3	179	13.6	0.7	13.9	0
Golden Yolk, Specially Selected, Aldi*	1 Egg/52g	68	4.7	131	13	0	9	0
Goose, Whole, Fresh, Raw, Weight with Shell	1 Egg/144g	232	16.6	161	12.1	1.2	11.5	0
Large, Weight with Shell	1 Egg/68g	97	6.8	143	12.6	0.8	9.9	0
Medium, Boiled, Weight with Shell	1 Egg/60g	86	6	143	12.6	0.8	9.9	0
Medium, Weight with Shell	1 Egg/56g	80	5.6	143	12.6	0.8	9.9	0
Poached, Weight with Shell	1 Med/58g	83	5.8	143	12.6	0.8	9.9	0
Quail, Whole, Raw, Weight with Shell	1 Egg/13g	20	1.4	151	12.9	0.4	11.1	0
Scotch, Retail	1 Egg/120g	301	20.5	251	12	13.1	17.1	0
Scrambled, Average	1 Lge Egg/68g	97	6.8	143	12.6	0.8	9.9	0
Very Large, Average, Weight with Shell	1 Egg/78g	112	7.8	143	12.6	0.8	9.9	0
Whites Only, Raw, Average	1 Lg Egg/33g	17	0.1	52	10.9	0.7	0.2	0
Yolks, Raw	1 Yolk/17g	55	4.5	322	15.9	3.6	26.5	0
ELK								
Raw, Meat only	1 Serving/100g	111	1.4	111	23	0	1.4	0
Roasted, Meat only	1 Serving/100g	146	1.9	146	30.2	0	1.9	0
ENCHILADAS								
3 Bean, Ready Meal, Average	1 Pack/400g	505	16.6	126	4.4	16.9	4.2	3.2
Beans, & Rice, Big Bros, Wicked Kitchen, Tesco*	1 Pack/404g	565	15.3	140	4.2	20.5	3.8	3.4
Cheesy, Baked, Meal Kit, Old El Paso*	1 Enchilada/83g	152	2.4	183	5.6	32	2.9	3.2
Chicken, Average	1 Serving/295g	483	18.8	164	11.6	16	6.4	1.7
with Cheese & Beef, From Restaurant	1 Serving/295g	496	27.1	168	6.2	15.9	9.2	0
with Cheese, From Restaurant	1 Serving/163g	319	18.8	196	5.9	17.5	11.6	0
ENDIVE								
Raw	1oz/28g	2	0	8	1.1	0.6	0.1	1.3
ENERGY DRINK								
Average	1 Can/250ml	118	0	47	0	11.4	0	0
BPM Energy*	1 Bottle/500ml	345	0	69	0	14	0	0
Cherry, Lucozade*	1 Bottle/500ml	345	0	69	0	17.1	0	0
Espresso, Vanilla, Monster*	1 Can/250ml	150	5	60	2.2	8.3	2	0
KX, Sugar Free, Diet, Tesco*	1 Can/250ml	5	0	2	0	0	0	0
Mango Loco, Monster*	1 Can/500ml	245	0	49	0	12	0	0
Monster*	1 Can/500ml	240	0	48	0	12	0	0
Natural, Tenzing*	1 Can/250ml	48	0	19	0	4.5	0	0
Origin, Relentless*	1 Can/500ml	110	0	22	0	6.1	0	0
Pacific Punch, Monster*	1 Can/500ml	230	0	46	0	12	0	0
Pipeline Punch , Monster*	1 Can/500ml	180	0	36	0	9	0	0
Red Thunder, Diet, Low Calorie, Aldi*	1 Can/250ml	5	0	2	0.1	0	0	0
Relentless, Original, Relentless*	1 Can/500ml	230	0	46	0	10.4	0	0
Ultra, Zero Calorie, Monster*	1 Can/500ml	10	0	2	0	0.9	0	0
ESCALOPE								
Chicken Style, Vegan, Ocado*	1 Escalope/67g	143	4.5	213	17	19	6.7	4.5
Chicken, Garlic & Herb, with Sourdough, Finest, Tesco*	1 Escalope/153g	343	14.2	224	16.3	18.2	9.3	1.1
Escalope, Average	1 Escalope/138g	341	19.3	247	13.5	16.7	14	0.6
Escalope, Lemon & Pepper, Average	1 Escalope/143g	371	22.6	260	12.6	16.7	15.8	0.4
Plant, Vivera*	1 Escalope/100g	188	7.2	188	13	16	7.2	4.7
The Great, The Vegetarian Butcher*	1 Escalope/90g	238	11.7	264	15	20	13	3.7
Turkey, Picard*	1 Escalope/125g	254	10.5	203	16.8	14.4	8.4	1.2
Turkey, Viennese, Picard*	1 Escalope/125g	253	10	202	16.8	14.4	8	1.4
Vegetarian, Garlic & Mushroom, Creamy, Quorn*	1 Escalope/120g	259	12.3	216	10.4	18.8	10.3	3.7
Vegetarian, Gruyere Cheese, Quorn*	1 Escalope/110g	267	15.4	243	10	18	14	2.6
Vegetarian, Mozzarella & Pesto, Quorn*	1 Escalope/112g	228	6.3	203	11	25	5.6	4.8

	Measure INFO/WEIGHT	per Measure KCAL	FAT	Nutrition Values per 100g / 100ml KCAL	PROT	CARB	FAT	FIBRE
FAJITA								
Chicken, & Vegetable, Asda*	½ Pack/350g	289	11	83	1.5	7.4	3.1	2.8
Chicken, & Vegetable, with Rice, Stir Fried, G&B, Asda*	½ Pack/325g	289	10.7	89	5.3	8.1	3.3	3
Chicken, Average	**1 Serving/240g**	**357**	**12.8**	**149**	**10.2**	**15**	**5.4**	**2.3**
Kit, Crunchy Nacho, Inspired Cuisine, Aldi*	1 Fajita/63g	207	6	328	7.6	50	9.6	5.8
Kit, Medium, Tesco*	1 Serving/120g	286	6	238	6.4	40.6	5	2.5
Meal Kit, Extra Mild, Old El Paso*	1 Fajita/59g	152	3.6	256	7	42.1	6.1	2.1
Meal Kit, Mild, Tesco*	1 Wrap/59g	144	3.4	247	6.9	40.5	5.8	2.5
Meal Kit, Sainsbury's*	¼ Pack/118g	280	5.8	237	6.5	40.5	4.9	2.3
Meal Kit, Sizzling, Smoky BBQ, As Sold, Old El Paso*	1 Fajita/63g	141	2.3	224	6.8	40	3.7	1.8
Meal Mix, Asda *	½ Pack/200g	62	1	31	0.9	5.4	0.5	2.1
Medium, Dinner Kit, As Prepared, Inspired Cuisine, Aldi*	1 Fajita/62g	141	2.9	226	6.3	38	4.7	2.7
Mix, Fish, Tesco*	½ Pack/148g	142	3.3	96	13.9	3.9	2.2	2.5
Vegetable	**1 Serving/275g**	**472**	**14.9**	**172**	**4.9**	**25.6**	**5.4**	**1.9**
FALAFEL								
& Houmous, Gro, Co-Op*	1 Pack/105g	269	15.8	256	7.9	20	15	6.5
Balls, Meat Free, Meat Free, Tesco*	3 Balls/67g	135	5.3	205	7.1	21.7	8.1	6.3
Beetroot, & Feta, World Deli, Waitrose*	1 Falafel/21g	59	3.3	279	7.5	25.1	15.5	4.6
Beetroot, with Red Pepper, & Chilli, Gosh*	4 Falafel/88g	150	6	170	5.4	25.1	6.8	6.4
Chickpea, Cumin, & Coriander, Goodlife*	1 Falafel/19g	39	2	207	7.9	14.1	10.4	12.6
Classic, Vegan, Delphi*	1 Falafel/28g	56	1	200	11.5	31.6	3.7	5.8
Fresh Herb, M&S*	1 Falafel/18g	45	2.2	248	8.3	22.6	12	8.1
Fried in Vegetable Oil, Average	**1 Falafel/25g**	**45**	**2.8**	**179**	**6.4**	**15.6**	**11.2**	**3.4**
Mediterranean, Aldi*	1 Pack/200g	470	24	235	6.4	21	12	7.6
Mezze, Rainbow, Allplants*	1 Serving/360g	457	16.9	127	4.6	15	4.7	3.7
Mini, M&S*	1 Falafel/14g	43	2.5	310	7.9	28.1	18.4	2.6
Moroccan Spiced, Cauldron Foods*	1/3 Pack/60g	143	3.9	239	6	36	6.5	6
Red Pepper, & Chipotle, Love Your Veg!, Sainsbury's*	1 Falafel/20g	44	1.4	219	10.5	25.1	7.1	6.4
Sweet Chilli, & Pumpkin, The Deli, Aldi*	1 Pack/200g	456	22	228	6.5	22	11	6.7
Sweet Potato, Bites, Tesco*	¼ Pack/36g	75	2.9	209	6.7	23.4	8	8.7
FANTA								
Grape, Coca-Cola*	1 Can/355ml	170	0	48	0	12.4	0	0
Grape, Zero, Coca-Cola*	1 Can/325ml	13	0	4	0	0.7	0	0
Icy Lemon, Coca-Cola*	1 Can/330ml	112	0	34	0	8.3	0	0
Icy Lemon, Zero, Coca-Cola*	1 Can/330ml	7	0	2	0	0.2	0	0
Lemon, Coca-Cola*	1 Can/330ml	165	0	50	0	12	0	0
Orange, Coca-Cola*	1 Can/330ml	63	0	19	0	4.6	0	0
Orange, Zero, Coca-Cola*	1 Can/330ml	11	0	3	0	0.5	0	0
Pink Grapefruit, Zero Sugar, Coca-Cola*	1 Can/330ml	10	0	3	0	0.3	0	0
Strawberry, Coca-Cola*	1 Can/355ml	160	0	45	0	12.7	0	0
FARFALLE								
Bows, Dry, Average	**1 Serving/75g**	**265**	**1.4**	**353**	**11.4**	**72.6**	**1.9**	**1.9**
FENNEL								
Florence, Boiled in Salted Water	**1oz/28g**	**3**	**0.1**	**11**	**0.9**	**1.5**	**0.2**	**2.3**
Florence, Raw, Unprepared, Average	**1 Bulb/250g**	**24**	**0.4**	**10**	**0.7**	**1.4**	**0.2**	**1.9**
Florence, Steamed	**1 Serving/80g**	**9**	**0.2**	**11**	**9**	**1.5**	**0.2**	**2.3**
FENUGREEK								
Leaves, Raw, Fresh, Average	**10g**	**4**	**0**	**35**	**4.6**	**4.8**	**0.2**	**1.1**
FETTUCCINE								
Chicken, & Parmesan, Italian, Microwaved, Morrisons*	1 Pack/400g	556	15.6	139	9.3	16.2	3.9	1
Edamame & Mung Bean, Explore Asian*	¼ Pack/50g	168	2.1	335	47.2	16.8	4.2	20.6
Edamame, & Mung Bean, Dried Weight, Explore Cuisine*	¼ Pack/50g	162	3.4	325	42.3	11.3	6.9	24.4
Konjac, Clean Foods*	½ Pack/100g	6	0.2	6	0.1	0.1	0.2	3.6
Mushroom, Plant Chef, Tesco*	1 Pack/366g	436	9.5	119	3.5	18.8	2.6	3.3

F

	Measure INFO/WEIGHT	per Measure KCAL	FAT	Nutrition Values per 100g / 100ml KCAL	PROT	CARB	FAT	FIBRE
FETTUCCINE								
Slim Pasta, Eat Water*	½ Pack/100g	9	0	9	0.2	0	0	4
with Tomato & Mushroom, Easy Cook, Napolina*	1 Pack/120g	461	8.6	384	11.8	67.9	7.2	0
FIGS								
Dried, Average	**1 Fig/14g**	**32**	**0.1**	**232**	**3.6**	**53.2**	**1.1**	**8.6**
Dried, with Honey, Intermarche *	4 Figs/30g	80	0.4	268	3.2	57.1	1.2	8.4
Partially Rehydrated, Sainsbury's*	1 Serving/30g	75	0.4	250	3.3	48.6	1.5	14.3
Raw, Fresh, Average	**1 Fig/35g**	**16**	**0.1**	**45**	**1.3**	**9.8**	**0.2**	**1.5**
FINGERS								
Fishless, Aldi *	1 Finger/30g	76	3.6	253	11	25	12	2
Fishless, Powered by Plants, Green Cuisine, Birds Eye*	1 Finger/28g	72	3.6	257	7.9	26	13	2
Fishless, Squeaky Bean*	1 Finger/27g	68	3	250	13	24	11	3
Vegetarian, Fishless, Vegan, Quorn*	1 Finger/20g	37	1.4	187	4.4	24.1	7.1	4.7
FISH								
3 Fish, Roast, Aldi*	1 Serving/100g	171	10	171	15	5	10	0.7
Ball, Tvi*	4 Balls/60g	61	0.2	101	9.5	15	0.3	0.3
Balls, Fried, Small, Mr Freeds*	1 Ball/19g	35	1.2	188	16.1	16.1	6.6	0
Battered, Extra Large, Captain Birds Eye, Birds Eye*	1 Fillet/159g	345	19.1	217	11	16	12	0.5
Char, Arctic, Whole, Raw	**1 Serving/100g**	**137**	**6**	**137**	**20.8**	**0**	**6**	**0**
Chargrills, Sun Ripened Tomato, Basil, Birds Eye*	1 Chargrill/163g	127	2.5	75	14	1.4	1.5	0.5
Chargrills, with Tomato & Herb, Oven Baked, Birds Eye*	1 Serving/163g	122	2.4	75	14	1.4	1.5	0.5
Fillet, Battered Or Breaded, & Fried, From Restaurant	**1 Portion/256g**	**594**	**31.5**	**232**	**14.7**	**17**	**12.3**	**0.5**
Fillet, Breaded, Mini, Cooked, Whitby Seafoods*	1 Fillet/100g	224	9.8	224	11.2	22.2	9.8	1.3
Fillet, Breaded, Simply, Extra Large, Oven Baked, Youngs*	1 Fillet/143g	310	15.9	217	10.8	18	11.1	1
Fillet, Fishless, Battered, Totally Vegan, Quorn*	1 Fillet/97g	202	8.3	209	4.5	27	8.6	2.9
Fillet, Omega 3, in Bubbly Batter, Chip Shop, Youngs*	1 Fillet/91g	225	13.1	247	10.8	17.9	14.4	1.4
Fillet, White, in Breadcrumbs, Ocean Sea, Lidl*	1 Fillet/161g	201	1.3	125	13	16	0.8	0
Fillets, Beer Battered, Extra Large, Chip Shop, Youngs*	1 Fillet/138g	326	20.8	237	9.9	14.8	15.1	1.1
Fillets, Lemon & Pepper, Breaded, Gastro, Youngs*	1 Fillet/131g	280	13.5	214	12	17.7	10.3	1.2
Filllet, Strips, Salt & Vinegar, Oven Baked, Iceland*	1 Serving/200g	484	27	242	14.6	15	13.5	0.9
Fishless, Fillets, Breaded, Morrisons*	1 Fillet/88g	182	7.2	207	5.6	26	8.2	3.2
Goujons, Tempura, Fishmonger, Aldi*	½ Pack/100g	222	11	222	10	20	11	0.5
Goujons, Vegetarian, Vivera*	1 Goujon/35g	87	3.5	248	13	25	10	2.7
Grouper	**1 Serving/100g**	**92**	**1**	**92**	**19.4**	**0**	**1**	**0**
Kippers, Smoked, Co-Op*	1 Serving/100g	183	12	183	19	0.6	12	0
Steak, in Creamy Butter Sauce, Youngs*	1 Pouch/121g	104	2.9	86	10.8	5.2	2.4	0.3
Vegan, Fillets, Battered, Fish Free, Plant Chef, Tesco*	1 Fillet/123g	274	8.7	223	13.3	24.7	7.1	3.4
Vegan, Plant, Fillet, Vivera*	1 Fillet/85g	175	7.6	206	14	15	8.9	3.4
White, Breaded, Fillets, Iceland*	1 Fillet/92g	201	8.9	219	12.5	19.9	9.7	1
White, Smoked, Average	**1 Serving/100g**	**108**	**0.9**	**108**	**23.4**	**0**	**0.9**	**0**
FISH & CHIPS								
Cod, & Peas, Mini, 528, Oakhouse Foods Ltd*	1 Serving/240g	408	15.6	170	7.3	20.5	6.5	2.9
Meal for One, M&S*	1 Serving/310g	521	17.1	168	6.1	23	5.5	1.1
Oven Cook Only, 7503, Wiltshire Farm Foods*	1 Serving/300g	447	15.9	149	5.8	19	5.3	0
with Mushy Peas, Kershaws*	1 Pack/400g	556	20	139	4.4	18.3	5	1.7
FISH & CHIPS								
Cod, Chips, & Peas, Birds Eye*	1 Pack/396g	574	23	145	5	17	5.8	2.4
Feel Good, Gousto*	1 Serving/485g	509	23.3	105	5.3	11.1	4.8	1.5
Haddock, Breaded, Scottish, M&S*	1 Pack/300g	507	18.6	169	7.5	20.1	6.2	1.2
Mini Meal, 093, Wiltshire Farm Foods*	1 Serving/185g	255	8.3	138	6.9	17.7	4.5	2.8
Takeaway or Fast Food, Average	**1 Serving/470g**	**1000**	**70.5**	**213**	**12**	**12**	**15**	**2.6**
with Mushy Peas, Classic, Oven Baked, Iceland*	1 Serving/350g	480	14.4	137	4.3	19.1	4.1	3
FISH CAKES								
Breaded, Freshly, Fish Counter, Waitrose*	1 Fishcake/124g	188	5.7	152	10.7	16.3	4.6	0.9

F

FISH CAKES

	Measure INFO/WEIGHT	per Measure KCAL	FAT	Nutrition Values per 100g / 100ml KCAL	PROT	CARB	FAT	FIBRE
Breaded, Oven Baked, Youngs*	1 Fishcake/48g	92	4.4	192	8	18.9	9.1	1.2
Cod, & Parsley, Waitrose*	1 Fishcake/85g	147	6.5	173	9.2	16.9	7.6	1.1
Cod, & Chorizo, Aldi*	1 Fishcake/137g	266	11.5	194	11	18	8.4	1.3
Cod, & Chorizo, Deluxe, Lidl*	1 Fishcake/139g	296	14.6	213	10.2	18.8	10.5	1.2
Cod, & Chorizo, Finest, Tesco*	1 Fishcake/131g	222	9.4	170	11.6	13.8	7.2	1.6
Cod, & Parsley Sauce, The Best, Morrisons*	1 Fishcake/150g	278	13	185	10.2	16.1	8.7	0.7
Cod, & Parsley, Melt in the Middle, Co-Op*	1 Fishcake/135g	248	9.7	184	9.1	20	7.2	1.7
Cod, & Pea, Battered, Mini, M&S*	1 Fishcake/60g	102	4.6	170	7.8	16.6	7.6	2.1
Cod, & Prawn, Red Thai Style, Extra Special, Asda*	1 Fishcake/140g	227	8.5	162	10	16	6.1	1.4
Cod, Battered, & Crushed Pea, M&S*	1 Fishcake/145g	244	11.3	168	8.9	14.9	7.8	1.1
Cod, Battered, with Mushy Pea Center, Co-Op*	1 Fishcake/135g	247	12.4	183	7.8	16	9.2	1.9
Cod, Breaded, Frozen, Oven Baked, Iceland*	1 Fishcake/40g	95	4.8	238	8.7	23.1	12.1	1.4
Cod, Breaded, Oven Baked, Youngs*	1 Fishcake/48g	100	4.9	209	8	20.5	10.3	1.4
Cod, Chunky, Breaded, Chilled, Youngs*	1 Fishcake/90g	192	11.5	213	9.5	14.9	12.8	1.2
Cod, Fillet, Free From, Morrisons*	1 Fishcake/131g	252	10.8	193	8.8	20.1	8.3	1.5
Cod, Fillet, GF, Made Without Wheat, M&S*	1 Fishcake/85g	145	6.7	171	8.3	16	7.9	1.4
Cod, Fillet, in Farmhouse Crumb, M&S*	1 Fishcake/85g	142	5.8	167	7.7	18.2	6.8	1.1
Cod, Fillet, in Golden Farmhouse Crumb, M&S*	1 Fishcake/85g	142	5.8	167	7.7	18.2	6.8	1.1
Cod, HFC, Tesco*	1 Fishcake/48g	86	3.3	181	8.6	20.2	7	1.4
Cod, Homemade, Average	**1 Fishcake/50g**	**120**	**8.3**	**241**	**9.3**	**14.4**	**16.6**	**0.7**
Cod, Katsu, M&S*	1 Fishcake/145g	239	10.6	165	9.1	15.1	7.3	1
Cod, Katsu, Specially Selected, Aldi*	1 Fishcake/140g	260	12	186	8.7	17	8.6	2
Cod, Melt in the Middle, Specially Selected, Aldi*	1 Fishcake/141g	261	13.7	185	8.1	16	9.7	0.6
Cod, Mornay, Easy to Cook, Waitrose*	1 Fishcake/149g	248	9.4	166	10.6	16.2	6.3	1.4
Cod, Oven Baked, Asda*	1 Fishcake/115g	187	7.2	162	8.5	18	6.2	1.1
Cod, Oven Cooked, Sainsbury's*	1 Fishcake/124g	211	8.3	170	8	19.2	6.7	0.8
Cod, with Lemon & Herb, Tesco*	1 Fishcake/135g	201	5.8	149	10.2	16.5	4.3	1.6
Cod, with Parsley Centre, TTD, Sainsbury's*	1 Fishcake/136g	266	13.4	196	8	18.6	9.9	0.5
Crab, Thai Style, Oven Cooked, TTD, Sainsbury's*	1 Fishcake/141g	296	14.1	210	8.7	20.5	10	1.8
Fried in Blended Oil	**1 Fishcake/50g**	**109**	**6.7**	**218**	**8.6**	**16.8**	**13.4**	**1.2**
Frozen, Average	**1 Fishcake/85g**	**112**	**3.3**	**132**	**8.6**	**16.7**	**3.9**	**0**
Haddock, & Vintage Cheddar, Smoked, Saucy Fish Co*	1 Fishcake/135g	220	7.6	163	9.7	18	5.6	0.9
Haddock, Fillet, in Golden Farmhouse Crumb, M&S*	1 Fishcake/145g	245	9.9	169	7.7	18.6	6.8	1.2
Haddock, Fillet, Smoked, M&S*	1 Fishcake/145g	245	11.5	169	9.8	15.4	7.9	1
Haddock, Fillet, Smoked, Morrison's*	1 Fishcake/130g	238	9.1	183	11.7	17.7	7	1.6
Haddock, Fishmonger, Aldi*	1 Fishcake/131g	220	7.7	168	9.2	18.7	5.9	1.4
Haddock, GF, Free From, Sainsbury's*	1 Fishcake/129g	233	10.4	180	10.6	15.8	8	1
Haddock, Melting, Cheddar & Leek, TTD, Sainsbury's*	1 Fishcake/138g	276	13.5	200	9.7	17.8	9.8	0.9
Haddock, Sainsbury's*	1 Fishcake/135g	253	10	188	10.8	18.7	7.4	1.5
Haddock, Smoked, Cheddar, & Leek, TTD, Sainsbury's*	1 Fishcake/138g	276	13.5	200	9.7	17.8	9.8	0.9
Haddock, Smoked, Extra Special, Asda*	1 Fishcake/115g	218	10.9	190	12.8	13.2	9.5	1.3
Haddock, Smoked, Lighthouse Bay, Lidl*	1 Fishcake/127g	236	9.3	186	8.9	20.3	7.3	1.6
Haddock, Smoked, Tesco*	1 Fishcake/135g	208	6.2	154	9.9	17.9	4.6	0.7
Haddock, Smoked, with Cheddar Sauce, Asda*	1 Fishcake/142g	302	15.6	213	11	17	11	1.7
No Fish, Melt in the Middle, Plant Kitchen, M&S*	1 Fishcake/145g	209	9.1	144	2.1	18.9	6.3	1.5
Prawn, Cod, Sweet Potato, & Sweet Chilli, Co-Op*	1 Fishcake/135g	293	11.9	217	5.7	27	8.8	2.8
Prawn, Thai Style, Finest, Tesco*	1 Fishcake/135g	196	6.8	145	9.5	14.6	5	1.8
Salmon Fillet, Market St, Morrisons*	1 Fishcake/130g	289	13.5	222	11	20.1	10.4	1.7
Salmon, & Dill, Waitrose*	1 Fishcake/85g	206	11.9	242	11.5	17.5	14	1.8
Salmon, & Cheddar, Melt in the Middle, Morrisons*	1 Fishcake/132g	337	18.7	255	8.9	22	14.2	1.8
Salmon, & Watercress, Melt in the Middle, Waitrose*	1 Fishcake/137g	259	12.1	189	11.1	16	8.8	0.9
Salmon, Fillet, Lochmuir, M&S*	1 Fishcake/85g	180	10.1	212	9	16.5	11.9	1.3
Salmon, Fillet, with Hollandaise Sauce Center, M&S*	1 Fishcake/145g	348	22.2	240	10.7	14.3	15.3	1.1

F

	Measure INFO/WEIGHT	per Measure KCAL	FAT	Nutrition Values per 100g / 100ml KCAL	PROT	CARB	FAT	FIBRE
FISH CAKES								
Salmon, Frozen, Oven Baked, Asda*	1 Fishcake/115g	208	8.6	181	11	17	7.5	1.5
Salmon, Homemade, Average	**1 Fishcake/50g**	**136**	**9.8**	**273**	**10.4**	**14.4**	**19.7**	**0.7**
Salmon, Morrisons*	1 Fishcake/90g	241	11.8	268	10.1	27.6	13.1	1.5
Salmon, Rocket, & Watercress, Essential, Waitrose*	1 Fishcake /135g	289	13.9	214	10.5	19	10.3	1.4
Salmon, Scottish, Sainsbury's*	1 Fishcake/130g	240	11.3	184	9.5	16.8	8.7	0.6
Salmon, Scottish, with Hollandaise, TTD, Sainsbury's*	1 Fishcake/140g	301	16.8	215	10.1	16.2	12	0.9
Salmon, Spinach & Sicilian Lemon, Finest, Tesco*	1 Fishcake/133g	297	15	223	11.6	17.6	11.3	2.4
Salmon, Sweet Chilli, Aldi*	1 Fishcake/145g	299	12.8	206	8.3	23	8.8	0.9
Salmon, Sweet Chilli, Specially Selected, Aldi*	1 Fishcake/138g	284	12.1	206	8.3	23	8.8	0.9
Salmon, Thai Style, Chapmans*	1 Fishcake/115g	154	5.7	134	10.6	12.4	4.9	1.2
Salmon,Spinach, & Lemon, Finest, Tesco*	1 Fishcake/133g	297	15	223	11.6	17.6	11.3	2.4
Vegetarian, Linda McCartney*	1 Fishcake/100g	195	9	195	12.6	13.5	9	4.7
FISH FINGERS								
Breaded, Fishmonger, Aldi*	3 Fingers/86g	168	7.2	195	12	17	8.4	1
Breaded, Frozen, Grilled, Iceland*	4 Fingers/91g	192	8.8	210	13	17.4	9.6	1
Chunky, Birds Eye*	2 Fingers/117g	229	8.6	196	13	19	7.4	0.7
Chunky, Cooked, Tesco*	2 Fingers/98g	230	10	235	13.2	21.6	10.2	1.3
Chunky, Crispy Batter, Captain Birds Eye, Birds Eye*	1 Finger/60g	132	6.6	220	12	18	11	0.7
Chunky, Extra Large, Captain Birds Eye, Birds Eye*	2 Fingers/120g	247	9.6	206	13	20	8	0.8
Cod, Chunky, Aldi*	1 Finger/38g	82	3.8	217	11.5	18.4	10.1	0.6
Cod, Fried in Blended Oil, Average	**1 Finger/28g**	**67**	**3.9**	**238**	**13.2**	**15.5**	**14.1**	**0.6**
Cod, Frozen, Average	**1 Finger/28g**	**48**	**2.2**	**170**	**11.6**	**14.2**	**7.8**	**0.6**
Cod, Grilled, Average	**1 Finger/28g**	**56**	**2.5**	**200**	**14.3**	**16.6**	**8.9**	**0.7**
Cod, Oven Cooked, Ocean Sea, Lidl*	1 Finger/30g	74	3.3	243	16	19	11	2.1
Free From, Sainsbury's*	1 Finger/30g	56	2.3	188	11.4	18	7.8	0.7
Haddock, Fillet, Chunky, TTD, Sainsbury's*	2 Fingers/113g	244	10.3	216	13.8	19.3	9.1	0.6
Haddock, Fillets, Asda*	1 Finger/30g	62	2.7	205	14	17	9	0
No Fish, Vegan, Iceland*	2 Fingers/60g	102	2.5	170	13	18	4.1	3.5
Pollock, Omega 3, Birds Eye*	4 Fingers/100g	203	8.2	203	13	19	8.2	0.8
Pollock, Sainsbury's*	3 Fingers/85g	160	6.7	188	13	15.9	7.9	0.8
FIVE SPICE								
Powder, Sharwood's*	1 Tsp/2g	3	0.2	172	12.2	11.6	8.6	23.4
FLAKE								
Dipped, Cadbury*	1 Bar/41g	215	12.5	530	7.6	56.1	30.8	0.8
Luxury, Cadbury*	1 Bar/45g	240	13.6	533	7.3	57.8	30.2	0
Praline, Cadbury*	1 Bar/38g	201	12.9	535	7.7	49.5	34.3	0
FLAN								
Pastry with Fruit	**1oz/28g**	**33**	**1.2**	**118**	**1.4**	**19.3**	**4.4**	**0.7**
Sponge with Fruit	**1oz/28g**	**31**	**0.4**	**112**	**2.8**	**23.3**	**1.5**	**0.6**
FLAN CASE								
Sponge, Average	**1oz/28g**	**90**	**1.5**	**320**	**7**	**62.5**	**5.4**	**0.7**
FLAPJACK								
Lemon Curd, Graze*	1 Punnet/53g	248	12.7	468	6	60	24	6
Apricot & Raisin, Waitrose*	1 Flapjack/38g	143	4.2	376	4.7	64.3	11.1	5.8
Average	**1 Sm/50g**	**242**	**13.3**	**484**	**4.5**	**60.4**	**26.6**	**2.7**
Bites, Sainsbury's*	1 Bite/15g	67	2.9	448	5.9	61.6	19.2	2.9
Caramel Fudge, Brynmor*	1 Bar/80g	369	18.4	461	6.2	56.2	23	4
Cherry Bakewell, Fibre, Graze*	1 Punnet/53g	243	12.7	458	7.1	51	24	15
Chocolate Dipped, M&S*	1 Flapjack/96g	442	21.5	460	6.1	61.3	22.4	3
Chocolate, Belgian, M&S*	1 Bar/80g	372	19.8	465	5.5	52.9	24.7	4.6
Chunky Chocolate, M&S*	1 FlapJack/80g	348	15.1	435	5.8	59.9	18.9	2.2
Cranberry, & Orange, Free From, Tesco*	1 Flapjack/30g	131	5.5	440	5.9	60.4	18.5	4.3
Cranberry, Apple & Raisin, LC, Tesco*	1 Flapjack/30g	98	1.7	325	5.7	63.1	5.6	5.7

	Measure INFO/WEIGHT	per Measure KCAL	FAT	Nutrition Values per 100g / 100ml KCAL	PROT	CARB	FAT	FIBRE
FLAPJACK								
Free From, Morrisons*	1 Bar/55g	232	7.9	422	4.2	66.9	14.3	4.3
Fruity, M&S*	1 Flapjack/68g	287	11.7	422	5.5	59.3	17.2	4.1
Golden Oaty Fingers, Tesco*	1 Flapjack/34g	142	5.7	420	5.7	59.7	16.8	3.7
Honey, & Seed, Protein, Graze*	1 Pack/52g	246	14	473	15.8	42.3	26.9	13.8
Lemon Drizzle, Graze*	1 Punnet/53g	248	12.7	468	5.9	54	24	5.8
Lemon, Smooth, Protein, Trek*	1 Flapjack/50g	234	10.8	467	18.4	48.8	21.7	2.5
Lively Lemon, Fibre, Graze*	1 Pack/53g	247	13.2	466	6.6	52	25	16
Maple, Protein, Graze*	1 Pack/53g	244	12.7	461	19	43	24	14
Mini, Sainsbury's*	1 Slice/15g	65	2.9	431	5.6	59.3	19	2.7
Oat, Morrisons*	1 Flapjack/50g	228	11	455	5.6	56.3	22.1	3.9
Oats, & Protein, Oatein*	1 Flapjack/40g	161	4.1	402	25	50.6	10.2	3.3
Peanut Butter, Chocolate, Oat Boosts, Graze*	1 Serving/30g	141	8.7	470	15	31	29	15
Peanut Butter, Chocolate, Protein, Graze*	1 Punnet/50g	237	14	473	18	32	28	12
Protein, Cocoa, Vanilla, Graze*	1 Punnet/53g	243	12.7	459	15	44	24	15
Slices, Free From, Morrisons*	1 Slice/38g	164	6.6	431	4.5	61.7	17.5	4.1
Slices, Free From, Tesco*	1 Flapjack/30g	132	5.8	442	6.2	59	19.3	4
Slices, Sainsbury's*	1 Slice/38g	168	7.2	448	5.9	61.6	19.2	2.9
Toffee, Finest, Tesco*	1 Flapjack/35g	156	6.7	446	4.9	63.6	19.1	1.3
FLATBREAD								
7 Spiced Chicken, Wrap, The Levantine Table, Waitrose*	1 Pack/232g	395	5.8	170	9.8	26.3	2.5	1.7
Brioche, Folded, Deli Kitchen*	1 Flatbread/35g	122	3.4	349	8.3	55.4	9.7	3.1
Cheese, & Tomato, Tesco*	¼ Pack/54g	152	3.8	282	10.3	43.4	7	1.9
Cheese, Three, Thins, Ryvita*	1 Flatbread/7g	29	0.7	420	19.1	60	10.5	4.4
Chicken, Chargrilled, COU, M&S*	1 Pack/163g	245	3.1	150	10.8	23	1.9	5.2
Chicken, Harissa, & Roasted Vegetable, M&S*	1 Pack/186g	342	4.8	184	10.7	19.7	2.6	0
Chicken, Mexican, Stonebaked, Finest, Tesco*	1 Pack/155g	280	5.1	180	11.7	25.1	3.3	1.6
Chicken, Moroccan, Shapers, Boots*	1 Pack/164g	289	2.1	176	9.8	30	1.3	2.2
Chicken, Tikka, BGTY, Sainsbury's*	1 Flatbread/186g	292	4.5	157	11.6	20.5	2.4	3.5
Chicken, Tikka, Shapers, Boots*	1 Flatbread/175g	270	4.9	154	11	21	2.8	1.7
Chickpea, & Sesame, Thomas Fudge*	1 Flatbread/11g	48	1.6	439	15	57	15	7
Coronation Chicken, Waitrose*	1 Serving/25g	111	3.6	444	11.2	65.8	14.3	3.5
Crispy, Marmite*	2 Flatbreads/18g	79	2.7	441	20.1	57.4	15.1	0
Extra Virgin Olive Oil, & Roasted Garlic, Waitrose*	¼ Pack/40g	149	6.2	374	9.9	46.9	15.6	2.9
Feta, COU, M&S*	1 Pack/180g	225	4	125	6.3	20.6	2.2	1.9
Garlic, & Cheese, Co-Op*	1 Serving/66g	194	4.4	294	9.5	39	6.7	1.9
Garlic, & Herb, Morrisons*	¼ Flatbread/66g	200	5.7	303	8.7	46.4	8.7	2.2
Garlic, & Herb, Oven Baked, Asda*	¼ Pack/61g	185	5.1	302	9.2	46	8.4	2.5
Garlic, Deep Filled, Tesco*	¼ Flatbread/61g	170	4	278	9	44.1	6.5	3.6
Garlic, Mini, Sainsbury's*	½ Flatbread/56g	169	5.1	302	9.3	44.3	9.1	2.5
Garlic, Roasted, & Olive Oil, TTD, Sainsbury's*	¼ Flatbread/53g	168	5.7	319	9.6	44.1	10.8	3.2
Mozzarella, & Basil, Stonebaked, Carlos, Aldi*	½ Flatbread/175g	506	28	289	9.9	26	16	3.1
Multiseed, Thins, Savour Bakes, Aldi*	1 Flatbread/10g	41	1.2	413	17	56	12	7.7
Olive Oil, Extra Virgin, & Garlic, M&S*	1 Flatbread/41g	135	5.8	330	8.7	40.9	14.2	1.7
Olive Oil, Extra Virgin, & Garlic, Waitrose*	¼ Flatbread/41g	146	5.8	357	9	46.9	14.2	2.5
Olive, M&S*	1 Flatbread/25g	113	4.4	453	9.3	61.6	17.4	6.5
Plain, Thins, Deli Kitchen*	1 Flatbread/35g	103	1.9	295	8.5	51.4	5.3	4.1
Prawn, Tikka, King, Waitrose*	1 Pack/165g	257	3.3	156	9.4	25.1	2	1.5
Roasted Garlic, Waitrose*	¼ Flatbread/61g	181	5.2	297	8.9	44.8	8.6	2.1
Roasted Red Pepper Pesto, & Chicken, Nutrisystem*	1 Pack/124g	230	7	185	8.9	25	5.6	2.4
Rosemary, & Sea Salt, GF, Nairn's*	1 Flatbread/13g	54	1.8	430	9	63	14.2	7.2
Rosemary, & Sea Salt, Thins, Ryvita*	1 Slice/7g	28	0.4	401	14.8	70.8	5.4	5.2
Salami, Calabrese, Carlos, Aldi*	½ Pizza/181g	490	21.7	271	10	30	12	1.7
Sea Salt, Peters Yard*	1 Flatbread/8g	32	0.8	399	11	72.3	9.4	9.5

	Measure INFO/WEIGHT	per Measure KCAL	FAT	Nutrition Values per 100g / 100ml KCAL	PROT	CARB	FAT	FIBRE
FLATBREAD								
Seeded, Folded, M&S*	1 Flatbread/35g	113	3.1	324	9.3	49.6	8.8	4.5
Seeded, Olinas*	1 Biscuit/17g	83	5.7	488	22.9	12.9	33.5	26.5
Thins, Multi-Seed, Rivercote, Lidl*	1 Thin/10g	44	1.4	437	15.2	56.3	14.5	10
Tomato, & Garlic, Asda*	½ Pack/133g	360	7.4	272	8.7	46	5.6	2.1
White, Folded, Subwich, Deli Kitchen*	1 Flatbread/55g	142	0.6	258	11.2	49.5	1	3
FLAXSEED								
& Goji Berries, Linwoods*	1 Serving/30g	151	11.7	503	20	7.9	39	22
Cold Milled, Organic, Virginia Health Food*	1 Serving/30g	160	12.6	534	18.3	1.6	42.2	27.3
Golden, Ground, P H Foods*	1 Serving/10g	51	4.2	514	18.3	1.6	42.2	27.3
Golden, Tesco*	1 Serving/25g	124	9	495	23.1	9.2	36	21.1
Milled, 100% Natural, The Foodie Market, Aldi*	1 Serving/25g	122	9.5	490	21	1.3	38	29
Milled, Organic, Linwoods*	1 Serving/5g	25	2	508	22.1	3	40	23.7
FLOUR								
Arrowroot, Average	*1oz/28g*	*100*	*0*	*357*	*0.3*	*88.2*	*0.1*	*3.4*
Bread, White, Strong, Average	*1oz/28g*	*94*	*0.4*	*336*	*11.8*	*68.4*	*1.5*	*3.4*
Brown, Chapati, Average	*1 Tbsp/20g*	*67*	*0.2*	*333*	*11.5*	*73.7*	*1.2*	*0*
Brown, Wheat	*1oz/28g*	*90*	*0.5*	*323*	*12.6*	*68.5*	*1.8*	*6.4*
Chick Pea	*1oz/28g*	*88*	*1.5*	*313*	*19.7*	*49.6*	*5.4*	*10.7*
Coconut, Average	*1 Serving/100g*	*344*	*13.6*	*344*	*18.2*	*15.4*	*13.6*	*43.8*
Corn, Harina de Maiz, Hacendado*	1 Tbsp/15g	52	0	350	0.3	87	0.1	0
Hemp, Organic, Forest Whole Foods*	1 Tsp/5g	11	0.5	229	27	54.1	9.5	46
Konjac, Gum, Powder, Special Ingredients*	1 Pinch/2g	4	0	179	0.9	4.1	0	83.5
Plain, Average	*1oz/28g*	*98*	*0.4*	*349*	*10.3*	*73.8*	*1.5*	*2.2*
Rice	*1 Tsp/5g*	*18*	*0*	*366*	*6.4*	*80.1*	*0.8*	*2*
Soya, Low Fat, Average	*1oz/28g*	*99*	*2*	*352*	*45.3*	*28.2*	*7.2*	*13.5*
Spelt, Average	*1 Serving/57g*	*216*	*1.7*	*381*	*14.3*	*74.5*	*3*	*6.4*
Vital Wheat Gluten, Good Stuff*	1 Serving/100g	403	5	403	81	9	5	1
White, Average	*1oz/28g*	*89*	*0.3*	*319*	*9.8*	*66.8*	*1*	*2.9*
White, Chapati, Average	*1 Tbsp/20g*	*67*	*0.1*	*335*	*9.8*	*77.6*	*0.5*	*0*
White, Self Raising, Average	*1oz/28g*	*94*	*0.4*	*336*	*9.9*	*71.8*	*1.3*	*2.9*
Wholemeal, Average	*1oz/28g*	*87*	*0.6*	*312*	*12.6*	*61.9*	*2.2*	*9*
FOOL								
Apricot, Fruit, Tesco*	1 Pot/113g	200	12.7	177	2.6	16.4	11.2	0.3
Apricot, Spanish, The Best, Morrisons*	1 Pot/114g	198	11.6	174	2.7	17.5	10.2	0.5
Fruit, Average	*1 Pot/120g*	*196*	*11.2*	*163*	*1*	*20.2*	*9.3*	*1.2*
Gooseberry, Fruit, Co-Op*	1 Pot/114g	211	11.4	185	3	22	10	1
Gooseberry, Tesco*	1 Pot/112g	225	14.1	200	3	17.8	12.5	0.7
Lemon, Fruit, BGTY, Sainsbury's*	1 Pot/113g	94	3.8	83	3.4	9.7	3.4	0.3
Lemon, Signature, Morrisons*	1 Pot/114g	213	11.8	187	3	20	10.4	0.5
Lemon, Tesco*	1 Pot/114g	213	12	187	2.7	20.3	10.5	0.3
Lemon, Whipped, Sainsbury's*	1 Pot/114g	218	13.9	191	2.9	17.3	12.2	0.5
Raspberry, Fruit, Tesco*	1 Pot/113g	234	12.8	207	2.6	23.6	11.3	0.3
Rhubarb, Fruit, Waitrose*	1 Pot/114g	182	12.9	160	2.7	11.9	11.3	0.3
Strawberry, Fruit, BGTY, Sainsbury's*	1 Pot/120g	100	3.1	83	3.7	11.1	2.6	0.8
Strawberry, Fruit, Co-Op*	1 Pot/114g	188	10.3	165	2	18	9	0.8
FRANKFURTERS								
Average	*1 Sausage/42g*	*123*	*11.2*	*292*	*12*	*1.3*	*26.6*	*0*
Vegetarian, Quorn*	1 Sausage/45g	92	6.3	205	13.5	4.5	14	3.5
Vegetarian, Tivall*	1 Sausage/30g	73	4.8	244	18	7	16	3
FREEKEH								
Dry Weight, Suma*	1 Serving/50g	165	1.4	330	12.6	55.5	2.7	16.5
Smoky, Dry Weight, Zaytoun*	1 Serving/50g	178	2.4	355	13	71.1	4.7	11.9

F

FRIES	Measure INFO/WEIGHT	per Measure KCAL	FAT	Nutrition Values per 100g / 100ml KCAL	PROT	CARB	FAT	FIBRE
As Sold, Aunt Bessie's*	1 Serving/100g	150	3.7	150	2.4	26	3.7	1.9
Carrot, & Parsnip, Mash Direct*	½ Pack/150g	231	14	154	1.9	12.8	9.3	5.5
Chips, From Restaurant, Average	*1 Serving/105g*	*294*	*16.3*	*280*	*3.3*	*34*	*15.5*	*2.1*
Crinkle, Home, Cooked, McCain*	1 Serving/100g	197	7.7	197	2.4	28	7.7	2.8
Crispy, Frozen, McCain*	1 Serving/100g	184	7	184	2.3	26.9	7	2.3
Criss Cross, Oven Baked, Iceland*	1 Serving/125g	324	14.1	259	3.5	33.7	11.3	4.4
Curly, Cajun, Weighed Frozen, McCain*	1 Portion/100g	156	8.7	156	1.6	17.7	8.7	1.8
Curly, Lightly Seasoned, McCain*	1 Serving/125g	239	10.8	191	2.3	25.1	8.6	2.4
Curly, Ovenbaked, Iceland*	1 Serving/150g	370	11.1	247	3.5	39.5	7.4	4.4
Curly, Southern Style, Tesco*	1 Serving/50g	95	2.8	189	2.6	29.6	5.6	4.9
Dirty, Carlos, Aldi*	½ Pack/230g	444	20.5	193	5.7	21	8.9	3.3
Dirty, Cheesy, M&S*	½ Pack/250g	518	30	207	7	16.7	12	2
Dirty, Oven Baked, Plant Based, Asda*	½ Pack/183g	201	5.7	110	2.1	18	3.1	1.6
Dirty, Plant Kitchen, M&S*	1 Pack/400g	564	22.8	141	3	18.4	5.7	1.9
Halloumi, Brew city*	1 Pack/150g	513	36	342	15	15	24	2.2
Halloumi, Iceland*	8 Fries/85g	277	21.7	326	22.5	1.8	25.5	0
Halloumi, Oven Cooked, Deluxe, Lidl*	1 Stick/17g	57	3.8	333	16.7	16.2	22.1	1
Loaded, Tasty, Oven Baked, Aldi*	½ Pack/232g	429	20.6	185	5.5	19	8.9	2.6
Seasoned, Frozen, Ovenbaked, Asda*	1/6 Pack/125g	286	10.9	229	3.1	33	8.7	3
Skin On, Bacon Flavour, Oven Baked, Asda*	¼ Pack/77g	144	5.7	186	2.1	26	7.4	2.8
Skin On, Crispy, Deep Fried, McCain*	1 Serving/100g	253	10	253	3.4	36	10	2.9
Skin On, Crispy, Four Seasons, Aldi*	1 Serving/100g	198	6.3	198	2.7	31	6.3	2.2
Skin On, Crispy, McCain*	1 Serving/100g	139	3.6	139	2.3	23	3.6	2.5
Sweet Potato, Co-Op*	¼ Bag/125g	172	6.9	138	1.6	19	5.5	2.9
Sweet Potato, Crispy, McCain*	1 Serving/125g	170	5.7	136	1.6	20.4	4.6	3.5
Sweet Potato, Crispy, Tesco*	½ Pack/150g	320	18.2	213	2.6	21.6	12.1	3.8
Sweet Potato, Lightly Coated, Sainsbury's*	¼ Pack/125g	236	7.5	189	1.3	30.1	6	4.6
Sweet Potato, Oven Baked, Asda*	½ Pack/150g	302	16.5	201	2.6	19	11	4.7
Sweet Potato, Oven Cooked, Savers, Morrisons*	¼ Pack/88g	212	6.7	241	3.3	37.1	7.6	5.7
Sweet Potato, Ready to Roast, Cooked, Sainsbury's*	½ Pack/116g	201	8.3	174	2.1	23.7	7.2	3.2
Sweet Potato, Seasoned, Oven Baked, Morrisons*	¼ Pack/88g	136	3.4	154	1.2	26.4	3.9	4.1
Takeaway, Carlos, Aldi*	1 Pack/186g	420	15.2	226	2.9	33	8.2	3.9
Waffle, Frozen, Leon*	1 Serving/125g	335	10.2	268	4.3	41.5	8.2	5.7
Waffle, Potato, Frozen, McCain*	1 Serving/90g	163	6.4	181	2.6	25	7.1	2.5
FRITTATA								
Cheddar, & Bacon, Summer Edition, Sainsbury's*	1 Frittata/25g	45	2.4	178	13.7	9.2	9.3	1.4
Goats Cheese, & Butternut Squash, Chef Select, Lidl*	1 Pack/130g	189	10.1	145	8.9	9.1	7.8	1.4
Mediterranean Style, Morrisons*	¼ Frittata/85g	122	7.1	143	9.4	7	8.3	1.4
Mushroom, Bacon, & Spinach, Morrisons*	1 Frittata/130g	186	10.3	143	10.8	6.9	7.9	0.6
Spinach & Courgette, Meat Free, Tesco*	1 Frittata/120g	199	12.8	166	5.8	10.2	10.7	2.9
Tomato, Pepper & Mozzarella, Morrisons*	1 Frittata/130g	170	7.9	131	9.9	8.7	6.1	0.6
Vegetable, Mediterranean Inspired, Crestwood, Aldi*	1 Pack/130g	193	10.3	148	7.8	11	7.9	1.2
FRITTERS								
Black Pudding, Oven Baked, Tony's Chippy*	1 Fritter/85g	234	12.6	275	5.5	28.8	14.8	0
Corn, Plant Chef, Tesco*	2 Fritters/126g	218	10.3	173	3	19.5	8.2	4.7
Courgette, Pea, & Mint, Waitrose*	½ Pack/70g	155	9.7	221	4.9	17.7	13.9	3.4
Courgette, Summer Edition, Sainsbury's*	1 Fritter/27g	45	2.4	168	4.8	15.4	9	2.8
Supergreen, with Pea, & Mint Dip, Morrisons*	1 Pack/104g	156	5.7	150	5.9	16.3	5.5	5.8
Sweetcorn, Tesco*	1 Fritter/25g	53	2.9	212	5.2	19.9	11.5	4.1
FROMAGE FRAIS								
0% Fat, Isigny Ste Mere*	2 Tbsp/30g	16	0.2	54	8.5	4.7	0.5	0
Apricot, Family Pack, Simply, Lidl*	1 Pot/50g	43	1.2	86	5.3	10.5	2.4	0.5
Fat Free, Average	*1 Pot/60g*	*35*	*0.1*	*58*	*7.7*	*6.8*	*0.2*	*0*

F

	Measure INFO/WEIGHT	per Measure KCAL	per Measure FAT	Nutrition Values per 100g / 100ml KCAL	PROT	CARB	FAT	FIBRE
FROMAGE FRAIS								
Fruit Tubes, Kids, Milbona, Lidl*	1 Tube/37g	31	0.7	84	5.4	11.1	1.9	1.4
High Protein, Tesco*	1 Serving/30g	16	0	54	8.8	4.6	0	0
Kids, Yeo Valley*	1 Serving/90g	111	4.8	123	6.6	12.6	5.3	0
Munch Bunch, Nestle*	1 Pot/42g	44	1.3	105	6.7	12.6	3	0
Plain, Average	**1oz/28g**	**32**	**2**	**113**	**6.8**	**5.7**	**7.1**	**0**
Raspberry, Creamfields*	1 Pot/50g	40	0.4	80	6.9	11.2	0.8	0.2
Raspberry, Savers, Morrisons*	1 Pot/55g	43	1	78	5.5	9.4	1.8	0.4
Strawberry, Family Pack, Simply, Lidl*	1 Pot/50g	43	1.2	86	5.3	10.6	2.4	0.5
Strawberry, Petits Filous, Yoplait*	1 Pot/50g	52	1.4	104	6.7	12.6	2.9	0.2
with Fruit, Average	**1 Avg Pot/90g**	**74**	**2.2**	**83**	**6.1**	**9**	**2.5**	**0.8**
with Fruit, Healthy Range, Average	**1 Avg Pot/90g**	**40**	**0.1**	**45**	**5.8**	**5.1**	**0.2**	**0.3**
FROZEN YOGHURT								
Black Cherry, M&S*	1 Pot/125g	164	1.4	131	3.1	27.1	1.1	0.5
Cherry Garcia, Low Fat, Ben & Jerry's*	1 Serving/100g	143	2.4	143	3	26	2.4	1
Chocolate, Average	**1 Portion/100g**	**120**	**1.9**	**120**	**4.3**	**22**	**1.9**	**2.1**
Coconut, Pinkberry*	1 Sm Pot/140g	196	0	140	4	30	0	0
Green Tea, Pinkberry*	1 Sm Pot/100g	110	0	110	4	25	0	0
Mango, Pinkberry*	1 Sm Cup/140g	140	0	100	3	23	0	0
Nakedmoo, Yoomoo*	1 Serving/125g	168	2	134	3.3	24.5	1.6	4.1
Natural, Average	**1 Portion/100g**	**101**	**0.8**	**101**	**3.8**	**19.9**	**0.8**	**0.9**
Original, Pinkberry*	1 Sm Pot/140g	140	0	100	3	21	0	0
Strawberry, Average	**1 Portion/100g**	**114**	**2.2**	**114**	**2.6**	**21.2**	**2.2**	**0.5**
Strawberry, Lolly, Yoomoo *	1 Lolly/57g	73	0.8	128	2.8	25.5	1.4	0.5
Tropical, Lolly, Yoomoo *	1 Lolly/57g	74	0.8	130	2.9	26.1	1.4	0.6
Vanilla, Greek Style, 3% Fat, M&S*	1/5 Pot/69g	97	1.9	141	6.1	22.8	2.8	0.5
FRUIT & NUT MIX								
Alesto, Lidl*	1 Serving/30g	146	8.5	485	13.7	40.5	28.4	6.1
Billionaires Shortbread, Graze*	1 Serving/43g	197	10.7	459	8.6	56	25	6.5
Chocolate, & Hazelnut, Shots, Whitworths*	1 Pack/25g	99	3.5	397	5.7	59.9	14	4.2
Chocolate, The Best, Morrisons*	1 Serving/40g	187	10.3	467	7.7	47.7	25.6	7.5
Christmas, Waitrose*	1 Serving/30g	132	6.8	439	9.9	45.9	22.6	6.3
Cranberry, The Best, Morrisons*	1 Serving/40g	192	12.7	481	11.1	34.3	31.8	6.7
Island Mix, Growers Harvest, Tesco*	1 Serving/30g	105	0.3	349	2.2	79.9	1.1	5.1
Pina Colada, Graze*	1 Punnet/32g	141	7.4	441	8.1	54	23	6.2
Selection, Asda*	1 Serving/35g	164	9.8	470	12	42	28	3.7
Trail Mix, Average	**1oz/28g**	**121**	**8**	**432**	**9.1**	**37.2**	**28.5**	**4.3**
Unsalted, Stockwell & Co, Tesco*	1 Serving/25g	120	7.1	478	19.4	33.5	28.3	5.7
with Milk Chocolate Raisins, Market St, Morrisons*	1 Pack/60g	284	14.7	473	12.6	48.1	24.5	4.7
FRUIT COCKTAIL								
Canned, in Grape Juice, Freshona, Lidl*	1 Can/410g	221	2	54	0.4	12.2	0.5	1.3
Canned, in Light Syrup, Prince's*	1 Can/410g	258	0.4	63	0.3	15	0.1	1.1
Fresh & Ready, Sainsbury's*	1 Pack/300g	117	0.3	39	0.6	9	0.1	1.2
in Apple Juice, Asda*	1/3 Can/80g	40	0.1	50	0.3	12	0.1	1.6
in Juice, Del Monte*	1 Can/415g	203	0.4	49	0.5	11.2	0.1	1
in Light Syrup, Del Monte*	1 Serving/70g	43	0	61	0.2	14	0	0.7
in Light Syrup, Sunnysouth*	1 Can/250g	155	0.2	62	0.3	14.5	0.1	0.3
in Syrup, Morrisons*	½ Can/205g	129	0.2	63	0.3	14.9	0.1	0
in Syrup, Smart Price, Asda*	1 Can/411g	173	0.4	42	0.3	10	0.1	1.6
Tropical, Canned, Asda*	½ Can/200g	120	0	60	0	15	0	1.6
FRUIT COMPOTE								
Apple, & Pear, No Added Sugar, Andros*	1 Tbsp/15g	7	0	46	0.2	9.6	0.3	2.1
Apricot & Prune, Yeo Valley*	1 Pot/225g	207	0.2	92	0.6	22.3	0.1	1.6
Apricot, Bonne Maman*	1 Serving/15g	16	0	108	0.8	25	0.2	1.4

F

	Measure INFO/WEIGHT	per Measure KCAL	FAT	Nutrition Values per 100g / 100ml KCAL	PROT	CARB	FAT	FIBRE
FRUIT COMPOTE								
Cherry, Bonne Maman*	1 Serving/15g	17	0	115	1.1	26	0.3	1.9
Mixed Berry, Organic, Yeo Valley*	1 Pot/220g	185	1.1	84	0.7	19.3	0.5	0
Peach, Bonne Maman*	1 Serving/15g	16	0	104	0.6	24	0.2	1.7
Rhubarb, Bonne Maman*	1 Serving/15g	15	0	103	0.5	24	0.1	2
Strawberry & Raspberry, M&S*	1 Serving/80g	72	0.1	90	0.7	23.5	0.1	2.3
Summer Berry, Opies*	1 Tbsp/15g	16	0.2	106	0.8	26	1.6	0
FRUIT MIX								
Berry Bowl, Morrisons*	1 Pack/350g	119	1.8	34	0.7	6.2	0.5	1.1
Berry Medley, Asda*	1 Pack/220g	121	1.1	55	0.7	12	0.5	1
Black Forest Fruit, Four Seasons, Aldi*	1 Serving/80g	40	0.4	50	0.8	11	0.5	2.1
Date, & Banana, Dried, Asda*	1 Serving/30g	117	4.2	389	2.9	61	14	5.5
Exotic, Frozen, Tesco*	1 Serving/80g	33	0	41	0.6	8.7	0	1.9
Frozen, Tesco*	1 Serving/80g	39	0.2	49	0.7	9	0.3	2.9
in Pineapple Juice, Dole*	1 Pot/100g	54	0	54	0.5	12	0	1
Melon, & Mango, Morrisons*	1 Pot/150g	52	0.2	35	0.6	7.3	0.1	1.2
Pear, Plum, Mandarin, & Grapes, Asda*	1 Pot/160g	86	0.8	54	0.6	11	0.5	2.1
Pieces, in Juice, Freshona, Lidl*	1 Pot/110g	53	0.1	48	0.3	11.2	0.1	1
Pineapple, Grape, & Apple, Asda*	1 Serving/80g	44	0.4	55	0.5	12	0.5	1.8
Pineapple, Melon, Mango, Tesco*	1 Pack/440g	242	0.9	55	1.1	11.4	0.2	1.3
Pineapple, Watermelon, & Grapes, Asda*	1 Serving/160g	75	0.8	47	0.5	10	0.5	0.9
Plum, & Berries, Eat Well, M&S*	1 Serving/100g	41	0.2	41	0.8	7.8	0.2	2.3
Red, Frozen, Crops*	3 Tbsp/80g	28	0.1	35	1	5.2	0.1	4.6
Sour Mango Tangtastic, Graze*	1 Pack/34g	110	0.2	323	1.3	79.8	0.6	2
Strawberry, & Grapes, Co-Op*	1 Pack/90g	54	0.4	60	0.6	13	0.5	0.7
Summer Fruits, British, Frozen, Waitrose*	1 Pack/300g	111	0.6	37	1.1	6.2	0.2	3.2
Summer Fruits, Frozen, Asda*	1 Serving/100g	28	0	28	0.9	6	0	2.5
Summer Fruits, Frozen, Del Monte*	1 Serving/80g	21	0	26	0.9	4.3	0	2.5
Summer Fruits, Frozen, Four Seasons, Aldi*	1 Serving/80g	26	0	33	1.1	5.2	0	3.2
Summer Fruits, Frozen, Sainsbury's*	1 Serving/80g	43	0.1	54	0.9	6.9	0.1	2
Tropical, Fruit Bowl, Dole*	1 Bowl/113g	61	0	54	0.5	12	0	1.1
Watermelon, & Mango, Fingers, Tesco*	½ Pack/136g	64	0.4	47	0.5	9.8	0.3	1.6
Watermelon, Mango, & Blueberries, Tesco*	1 Pack/220g	99	0.7	45	0.6	9.6	0.3	1.1
FRUIT SALAD								
Apple, Melon, & Berries, Nutritious, Boots*	1 Pack/257g	118	0.8	46	0.6	9.4	0.3	1.8
Apple, Orange, Pineapple & Grape, Morrisons*	1 Serving/64g	40	0.1	62	0.8	13.1	0.1	2.6
Autumn, Fresh, M&S*	½ Pack/160g	64	0.2	40	0.7	9.4	0.1	2.9
Berry, Seasonal, Asda*	1 Pack/300g	93	0.3	31	0.6	7	0.1	2.1
Canned, in Fruit Juice, Asda*	1/3 Can/136g	60	0.7	44	0.5	10	0.5	0.5
Citrus, Fresh, M&S*	½ Pack/225g	79	0.2	35	0.9	7.7	0.1	1.5
Classic, Fresh, Prepared, Sainsbury's*	1 Pack/320g	157	0.3	49	0.6	10.3	0.1	2
Classic, Waitrose*	1 Pack/330g	162	0.7	49	0.8	10.4	0.2	1.2
Dried, M&S*	½ Pack/125g	269	0.5	215	1.8	51.4	0.4	5.9
Exotic, Co-Op*	½ Pack/150g	70	0.8	47	0.6	9.6	0.5	1.5
Exotic, Waitrose*	1 Pack/300g	126	0.6	42	0.6	9.5	0.2	1.1
Fresh for You, Tesco*	1 Pack/160g	59	0.3	37	0.6	8.2	0.2	1.1
Fresh, Morrisons*	1 Tub/350g	150	0.4	43	0.7	9.9	0.1	0
Fresh, Tesco*	1 Pack/200g	84	0.4	42	0.7	9.3	0.2	1.5
Freshly Prepared, M&S*	1 Pack/350g	140	0.7	40	0.5	9.3	0.2	1
Frozen, Asda*	1 Serving/80g	37	0.4	46	0.6	9	0.5	2.4
Frozen, Tesco*	1 Serving/80g	26	0.4	32	0.5	6.1	0.5	1.7
Fruity Cocktail, M&S*	1 Serving/80g	33	0.1	41	0.6	8.5	0.1	1.7
Grapefruit & Orange, Fresh, M&S*	1 Serving/250g	88	0.2	35	0.9	7.4	0.1	1.6
Homemade, Unsweetened, Average	**1 Serving/140g**	**77**	**0.1**	**55**	**0.7**	**13.8**	**0.1**	**1.5**

F

	Measure INFO/WEIGHT	per Measure KCAL	FAT	Nutrition Values per 100g / 100ml KCAL	PROT	CARB	FAT	FIBRE
FRUIT SALAD								
in Juice, Freshona, Lidl*	1 Pot/114g	57	0.1	50	0.1	12	0.1	1
Juicy Melon, Pineapple & Grapes, Asda*	1 Pot/300g	111	0.3	37	0.5	8.4	0.1	0.9
Kiwi, Pineapple & Grape, Fresh Tastes, Asda*	1 Pack/200g	106	0.6	53	0.6	11	0.3	1.8
Mango, Pineapple & Passion Fruit, Waitrose*	1 Serving/80g	42	0	52	0.8	10.4	0	2.5
Melon & Red Grape, Freshly Prepared, M&S*	1 Pack/450g	158	0.4	35	0.5	8.4	0.1	0.7
Melon & Mango, Shapers, Boots*	1 Pack/80g	29	0.1	36	0.6	7.8	0.1	1.2
Melon, & Grape, Sainsbury's*	1 Pack/159g	59	0.8	37	0.6	7.8	0.5	1.2
Mixed, Average	**1 Bowl/100g**	**42**	**0.2**	**42**	**0.6**	**9.4**	**0.2**	**1.5**
Pineapple, Apple & Strawberries, Tesco*	1 Pack/190g	80	0.2	42	0.4	9.8	0.1	1.4
Pineapple, Melon & Grape, Eat Well, M&S*	1 Pot/130g	53	0.3	41	0.5	8.6	0.2	1.6
Pineapple, Melon, & Mango, Nutritious, Boots*	1 Pack/250g	111	0.5	44	0.6	9.2	0.2	1.6
Pineapple, Strawberry, Grape & Carrot, M&S*	1 Pack/240g	101	1	42	0.6	8.3	0.4	1.4
Plum, Blackberries, & Fig, Tesco*	1 Pot/260g	109	0.5	42	0.8	8.2	0.2	2.5
Rainbow Layers, Tesco*	1 Pack/270g	122	0.5	45	0.5	9.8	0.2	1.1
Rainbow, Fresh, Tesco*	1 Tub/270g	105	0.5	39	0.5	8.8	0.2	0.9
Rainbow, M&S*	1 Pack/300g	126	0.6	42	0.5	9.1	0.2	0.9
Rainbow, Waitrose*	1 Pack/285g	154	1.4	54	0.7	11.4	0.5	1.5
Seasonal, Fresh, Asda*	1 Pack/125g	55	0.1	44	0.5	10.4	0.1	1.2
Selection, M&S*	½ Pack/275g	140	0.8	51	0.6	10.3	0.3	2.1
Summer, Red, Fresh, M&S*	1 Pack/400g	160	0.8	40	0	10	0.2	1.2
Sunshine, Fresh, M&S*	1 Serving/200g	70	0.2	35	0	8.3	0.1	1.3
Super Fruity, M&S*	1 Pot/150g	88	0.4	59	1	11.6	0.3	3
SuperValu*	1 Serving/200g	110	1	55	0.6	11	0.5	2
Tropical Mix, Tesco*	½ Pack/140g	71	0.3	51	0.5	11	0.2	1.5
Tropical, Fresh, Asda*	1 Pack/400g	164	0.8	41	0.7	9	0.2	1.8
Tropical, in Juice, Natures Finest*	1 Pot/125g	61	0.6	49	0	13	0.5	1
Tropical, Tropical Harvest*	1 Serving/100g	52	0	52	0.3	12.8	0	1.4
Virgin Trains*	1 Serving/140g	56	0.1	40	0.4	10	0.1	0.8
FRUIT SPREAD								
Cherries & Berries, Organic, Meridian Foods*	1 Tbsp/15g	16	0	109	0.5	26	0.3	1.1
Cherry & Berry, Meridian Foods*	1 Serving/10g	14	0.1	138	0.7	33.7	0.6	3.2
Seville Orange, Weight Watchers*	1 Tsp/15g	17	0	111	0.2	27.5	0	0.3
FU YUNG								
Chicken, Chinese Takeaway, Tesco*	1 Pack/350g	315	3.5	90	5.6	14.5	1	0.8
Egg, Average	**1oz/28g**	**67**	**5.8**	**239**	**9.9**	**2.2**	**20.6**	**1.3**
FUDGE								
All Butter, Finest, Tesco*	1 Sweet/10g	43	1.4	429	1.3	73.4	14.5	0
Butter Tablet, Thorntons*	1oz/28g	116	3.1	414	0.9	77.6	11.1	0
Butter, Milk, Thorntons*	1 Sweet/13g	60	2.5	462	3.7	68.5	19.2	0
Cadbury*	1 Bar/25g	118	4	445	2.5	74.5	15	0.5
Caramel, & Sea Salt, Lidl*	2 Pieces/25g	114	4.7	456	1.5	69.8	18.9	0
Chocolate, Average	**1 Sweet/30g**	**132**	**4.1**	**441**	**3.3**	**81.1**	**13.7**	**0**
Chocolate, Belgian, Vegan, Mrs Tilly's*	1/3 Pack/50g	233	7	466	0.5	80	14	0
Chunks for Baking	**1 Serving/100g**	**428**	**12.2**	**428**	**1.7**	**77.2**	**12.2**	**0.6**
Clotted Cream, M&S*	½ Pack/68g	300	9.6	444	0.6	78.2	14.2	0.5
Clotted Cream, Sainsbury's*	1 Sweet/8g	35	0.9	430	1.9	81.5	10.7	0.5
Dairy, Co-Op*	1 Sweet/9g	39	1.2	430	2	76	13	0
Dairy, Morrisons*	3 Sweets/24g	107	3.6	447	1.8	76.1	14.9	0.5
Maple Salt, Specially Selected, Aldi*	3 Pieces/30g	134	4.2	445	0.5	78	14	0.5
Minis, Cadbury*	1 Piece/5g	23	0.9	455	2.6	73	17	0.7
Vanilla, Bar, M&S*	1 Bar/43g	205	10	476	3.7	63	23.3	0.4
Vanilla, Julian Graves*	1 Serving/10g	41	1	407	1	78.9	9.7	0
Vanilla, Thorntons*	1 Bag/100g	465	21.9	465	1.8	65.9	21.9	0

F

	Measure INFO/WEIGHT	per Measure KCAL	FAT	Nutrition Values per 100g / 100ml KCAL	PROT	CARB	FAT	FIBRE
FUSILLI								
Cooked, Average	**1 Serving/210g**	**248**	**1.4**	**118**	**4.2**	**23.8**	**0.6**	**1.2**
Dry Weight, Free From, Co-Op*	1/6 Pack/83g	300	1.5	360	8	77	1.8	2
Dry, Average	**1 Serving/90g**	**316**	**1.4**	**352**	**12.3**	**72**	**1.6**	**2.2**
Fresh, Cooked, Average	**1 Serving/200g**	**329**	**3.6**	**164**	**6.4**	**30.6**	**1.8**	**1.8**
Fresh, Dry, Average	**1 Serving/75g**	**208**	**2**	**277**	**10.9**	**53.4**	**2.7**	**2.1**
GF, Dry, Average	**1 Serving/60g**	**205**	**0.8**	**341**	**6.8**	**73.7**	**1.3**	**3**
Green Pea, Cooked, Sainsbury's*	1 Serving/170g	291	1.7	171	11	27.5	1	3.8
Red Lentil, Dry, Cook Italian*	1 Serving/80g	283	1.6	354	23	58	2	6
Red Lentil, GF, Dry, Tesco*	1 Serving/70g	296	1.1	423	27.9	70.4	1.6	7.2
Tricolore, Dry, Average	**1 Serving/75g**	**264**	**1.3**	**351**	**12.2**	**71.8**	**1.7**	**2.7**
Whole Wheat, Dry Weight, Average	**1 Serving/90g**	**290**	**2.1**	**322**	**13.1**	**62.3**	**2.3**	**9**
FYBOGEL								
Lemon, Reckitt Benckiser*	1 Serving/4g	4	0	95	2.4	11.3	1.1	64.8
Orange, Reckitt Benckiser*	1 Serving/4g	5	0	106	2.4	12.7	1.1	64.4

F

	Measure INFO/WEIGHT	per Measure KCAL	FAT	Nutrition Values per 100g / 100ml KCAL	PROT	CARB	FAT	FIBRE
GALANGAL								
Raw, Root, Average	**100g**	**71**	**0.6**	**71**	**1.2**	**15.3**	**0.6**	**2.4**
GALAXY								
Caramel & Sea Salt, Galaxy, Mars*	½ Bar/50g	276	17	552	3.1	57	34	0
Cookie Crumble, Mars*	1 Bar/114g	627	37.6	550	6.2	56	33	1.9
Hazelnut, Mars*	1 Piece/6g	37	2.5	582	7.8	49.4	39.2	0
Smooth Caramel, Galaxy, Mars*	1 Serving/25g	124	6.4	498	5.4	60.5	25.7	0
GAMMON								
Breaded, Average	**1oz/28g**	**34**	**0.9**	**120**	**22.5**	**1**	**3**	**0**
Hocks, with Honey & Mustard Sauce, TTD, Sainsbury's*	1 Pack/748g	1114	49.3	149	17.1	4.5	6.6	1.6
Honey & Mustard, Average	**½ Pack/190g**	**294**	**13.5**	**155**	**19.1**	**3.6**	**7.1**	**0.1**
in Somerset Cider Sauce, 4227, Wiltshire Farm Foods*	1 Serving/381g	339	13	89	6	7.4	3.4	0
Joint, Boiled, Average	**1 Serving/60g**	**122**	**7.4**	**204**	**23.3**	**0**	**12.3**	**0**
Joint, Honey Glaze, Just Cook, Sainsbury's*	1/3 Pack/123g	242	12.8	197	23.4	2.1	10.4	0
Joint, Oven Baked, Iceland*	1 Serving/100g	217	11.2	217	27.8	1.4	11.2	0
Joint, Raw, Average	**1 Serving/100g**	**138**	**7.5**	**138**	**17.5**	**0**	**7.5**	**0**
Joint, Smoked, Morrisons*	1 Serving/150g	152	3.3	101	19.9	0.3	2.2	0
Joint, with Honey Glaze, Tesco*	¼ Pack/124g	170	2.2	137	22.6	7.2	1.8	1
Shanks, with Caramelised Apple Sauce, M&S*	½ Pack/166g	226	6.5	136	14.7	10.5	3.9	0.3
Slow Cooked, British, Thick Sliced, Asda*	1 Slice/33g	40	0.8	121	24	1	2.4	0.7
Steak, Smoked, Tesco*	1 Steak/225g	333	19.6	148	17.4	0.1	8.7	0
Steak, with Cheese, & Pineapple, Ready to Cook, Tesco*	½ Pack/155g	203	5.7	131	21	3.3	3.7	0.4
Steak, with Maple, & Bourbon Sauce, Cooked, Tesco*	½ Pack/105g	197	4.5	188	26.8	10.1	4.3	0.7
Steaks, Honey Roast, Average	**1 Steak/100g**	**142**	**5.3**	**142**	**21.5**	**2.3**	**5.3**	**0**
Steaks, Smoked, Average	**1 Steak/110g**	**150**	**5.5**	**137**	**22.7**	**0.1**	**5**	**0.1**
Steaks, Unsmoked, Grilled, Morrisons*	1 Steak/104g	136	2.4	131	26.7	0.5	2.3	0.5
Steaks, with Cheese, & Pineapple, Iceland*	½ Pack/117g	170	4.6	145	21.5	5.7	3.9	0.6
Steaks, with Pineapple & Mango Salsa, Easy, Waitrose*	1 Steak/163g	239	11.6	146	14.1	6.5	7.1	0.5
with Honey & Mustard Glaze, Just Cook, Sainsbury's*	½ Pack/240g	351	6.7	146	23.8	6.1	2.8	0.8
GARAM MASALA								
Dry, Ground, Average	**1 Tbsp/15g**	**57**	**2.3**	**379**	**15.6**	**45.2**	**15.1**	**0**
GARLIC								
Black	**1 Clove/5g**	**13**	**0**	**264**	**13.3**	**53.3**	**0**	**20**
Powder, Average	**1 Tsp/3g**	**7**	**0**	**246**	**18.7**	**42.7**	**1.2**	**9.9**
Raw, Average	**1 Clove/3g**	**3**	**0**	**98**	**7.9**	**16.3**	**0.6**	**2.1**
Wild	**1 Leaf/1g**	**0**	**0**	**23**	**2.8**	**1.7**	**0.6**	**1.9**
GARLIC PUREE								
Average	**1 Tbsp/18g**	**68**	**6**	**380**	**3.5**	**16.9**	**33.6**	**0**
GATEAU								
Black Forest, 500g Size, Tesco*	1 Cake/500g	1125	55	225	4	27.1	11	1.8
Black Forest, M&S*	1/8 Cake/77g	207	10.9	269	3.1	31.6	14.1	1.5
Black Forest, Mini, Tesco*	1 Serving/55g	136	5.1	247	5.7	35.3	9.2	1
Caramel, Salted, Profiterole, Tesco*	1 Slice/88g	248	13.6	282	4.3	31	15.5	0.9
Chocolate Layer, M&S*	1 Serving/86g	278	15.7	323	4.2	35.9	18.3	0.9
Chocolate, & Vanilla, Ice Cream, Iceland*	1 Serving/130g	252	12.2	194	3.3	24.1	9.4	0.6
Chocolate, Double, Frozen, Tesco*	1/5 Gateau/70g	115	4.4	255	5.5	34.2	9.8	3.5
Chocolate, Iceland*	1/8 Gateau/75g	201	9.7	268	4.9	31.7	12.9	3
Chocolate, Rich, Tesco*	1 Slice/84g	210	8.6	251	5.1	32.9	10.2	3.4
Chocolate, Swirl, Tesco*	1 Serving/83g	230	13.3	277	3.8	29.3	16	0.2
Strawberry, Co-Op*	1 Serving/77g	222	12.9	288	5.1	29.2	16.7	1
GHEE								
Butter	**1oz/28g**	**251**	**27.9**	**898**	**0**	**0**	**99.8**	**0**
Vegetable	**1oz/28g**	**251**	**27.8**	**895**	**0**	**0**	**99.4**	**0**

G

	Measure INFO/WEIGHT	per Measure KCAL	FAT	Nutrition Values per 100g / 100ml KCAL	PROT	CARB	FAT	FIBRE
GHERKINS								
Pickled, Average	**1 Gherkin/36g**	**4**	**0**	**12**	**0.8**	**2.1**	**0.1**	**1**
GIN								
& Diet Tonic, Can, Greenalls*	1 Can/250ml	95	0	38	0	0	0	0
& Tonic, Canned, Ready to Drink, M&S*	1 Can/250ml	175	0.8	70	0.2	5.6	0.3	0.1
& Tonic, Premixed, Can, Gordons*	1 Can/250ml	208	0	83	0	0	0	0
37.5% Volume	**1 Pub Shot/35ml**	**72**	**0**	**207**	**0**	**0**	**0**	**0**
40% Volume	**1 Pub Shot/35ml**	**78**	**0**	**224**	**0**	**0**	**0**	**0**
41% Volume	**1 Pub Shot/35ml**	**83**	**0**	**237**	**0**	**0**	**0**	**0**
Alcohol free, 0%, Tanqueray*	1 Single/25ml	3	0	12	0	0	0	0
Average, 43%	**1 Serving/25ml**	**60**	**0**	**241**	**0**	**0**	**0**	**0**
Citrus, Grove 42, Non Alcoholic, Seedlip Ltd*	1 Shot/30ml	0	0	0	0	0	0	0
Clean G, Rhubarb, Low Alcohol, 0.5%, Clean Co.*	1 Serving/50ml	12	0	24	0	5	0	0
Clean G, Rhubarb, Low Alcohol, 1.2%, Clean Co.*	1 Serving/50ml	15	0	30	0	5.7	0	0
Clean, Raspberry, Low Alcohol, 1.2%, Clean Co.*	1 Serve/50ml	13	0	26	0	6.1	0	0
Flor De Sevilla, Tanqueray*	1 Single/25ml	64	0	254	0	0	0	0
Gordons & Schweppes Slimline Tonic, Canned, Diageo*	1 Can/250ml	75	0	30	0	0	0	0
Gordons & Schweppes Tonic, Canned, Diageo*	1 Can/250ml	152	0	61	0	6.2	0	0
London, Special Dry, 30%, Gordons*	1 Serve/25ml	52	0	208	0	0	0	0
Mango & Passionfruit, 37.5%, Haysmith's*	1 Serve/25ml	56	0	225	0	0	0	0
Peach, & Orange Blossom, 37.5%, Haysmith's*	1 Shot/25ml	57	0	227	0	0	0	0
Pink Grapefruit, Whitley Neill*	1 Shot/25ml	60	0	240	0	0.6	0	0
Pink, & Tonic, Mixed, Can, Gordons*	1 Can/250ml	168	0	67	0	8.7	0	0
Raspberry, Liqueur, Edinburgh Gin Distillery*	1 Serving/25ml	46	0	184	0	18.2	0	0
Rhubarb, & Ginger, Whitley Neill*	1 Shot/25ml	68	0	273	0	0	0	0
Sicilian Lemon, 37.5%, Gordons*	1 Serving/50ml	110	0	221	0	2	0	0
GINGER								
Chunks, Crystallised, Julian Graves*	1 Serving/10g	28	0	283	0.2	70.1	0.2	1.5
Ground, Average	**1 Tsp/2g**	**5**	**0.1**	**258**	**7.4**	**60**	**3.3**	**0**
Root, Raw, Pared, Average	**1 Tsp/2g**	**2**	**0**	**81**	**1.8**	**18**	**0.8**	**2**
Root, Raw, Unprepared, Average	**1 Tsp/2g**	**1**	**0**	**74**	**1.7**	**16.3**	**0.7**	**1.8**
Stem in Sugar Syrup, Sainsbury's*	1 Ball/10g	29	0	292	0.5	71.3	0.5	1.6
GINGER ALE								
Dry	**1 Glass/250ml**	**38**	**0**	**15**	**0**	**3.9**	**0**	**0**
Low Calorie, Schweppes*	1 Bottle/250ml	50	0	20	0	4.6	0	0
Orange, Light Spiced, Fever-Tree*	1 Serving/200ml	36	0	18	0	4.3	0	0
GINGER BEER								
Alcoholic, Crabbies*	1 Bottle/500ml	254	0	51	0	7.1	0	0
Bundaberg*	1 Bottle/375ml	79	0	21	0	5.2	0	0
Diet, Crabbies*	1 Bottle/700ml	7	0	1	0	0	0	0
Light, Belvoir Fruit Farms*	1 Serving/200ml	42	0	21	0	4.4	0	0
Light, Waitrose*	1 Glass/250ml	2	0.2	1	0	0	0.1	0.1
No Added Sugar, Canned, Tesco*	1 Can/330ml	3	0.3	1	0	0.1	0.1	0.1
Refreshingly Light, Fever-Tree*	1 Bottle/200ml	38	0	19	0	4.9	0	0
GINGERBREAD								
Average	**1oz/28g**	**106**	**3.5**	**379**	**5.7**	**64.7**	**12.6**	**1.2**
Man, Free From, Co-Op*	1 Biscuit/25g	115	3.7	461	4.2	77	15	1.3
Men, GF, Free From, Asda*	1 Biscuit/25g	113	3.5	451	4.3	76	14	1.8
GNOCCHI								
Cheesy Brocolli, Allplants*	1 Serving/480g	422	14.9	88	4.2	9.7	3.1	2.4
Chorizo, Spinach, & Courgette, Hello Fresh*	1 Portion/514g	714	28	139	5	17.3	5.4	0
Cooked, Tesco*	¼ Pack/132g	217	0.4	164	3.5	36.1	0.3	1.7
Four Cheese, Filled, Rana La Famiglia*	½ Pack/140g	332	7.3	237	6.8	38	5.2	5.5
Fresh, Cooked, Essential, Waitrose*	¼ Pack/134g	242	0.5	181	4.7	39	0.4	1

G

	Measure INFO/WEIGHT	per Measure KCAL	FAT	Nutrition Values per 100g / 100ml KCAL	PROT	CARB	FAT	FIBRE
GNOCCHI								
Fresh, Italian, Chilled, Sainsbury's*	½ Pack/250g	355	1.2	142	2.5	29.9	0.5	4
GF, Farabella*	¼ Pack/125g	231	0.6	185	3.8	41	0.5	1.8
Italian, Boiled, Asda*	1 Pack/498g	573	2.5	115	1.4	25	0.5	2.2
Italian, Cooked, Morrisons*	1 Serving/250g	385	2.5	154	3.1	32.2	1	1.8
Pan Fried, Rana La Famiglia*	1 Serving/150g	231	1.4	154	2.6	34	0.9	0
Potato, Cooked, Average	**1 Serving/150g**	**200**	**0**	**133**	**0**	**33.2**	**0**	**0**
Potato, Fresh , Dell Ugo *	1 Serving/225g	299	1.8	133	4.7	25	0.8	2.8
Potato, Fresh Pasta Co*	½ Pack/200g	328	0.4	164	3.1	36.5	0.2	1.5
Pumpkin, Fresh, Dell'ugo*	½ Pack/226g	325	2	144	4.5	28	0.9	3.3
Roasted Mushroom, Finest, Tesco*	½ Pack/297g	410	13.4	138	4.4	19.5	4.5	1
Spinach, GF, Difatti*	½ Pack/125g	204	0.6	163	3.5	36	0.5	0
Tomato, & Mozzarella, Aldi*	1 Serving/225g	336	4.7	149	3.4	28	2.1	2.6
Tomato, & Mozzarella, Italiamo, Lidl*	1 Serving/250g	365	4.8	146	3.5	28	1.9	2.3
Tricolore, Mini, De Marlino*	1 Serving/100g	162	0.5	162	3.6	36	0.5	1.7
Uncooked, As Sold, Essential, Waitrose*	1 Pack/500g	844	6	169	4.2	33.6	1.2	3.4
Vegetable, Chargrilled, Plant Based, Asda*	1 Pack/384g	338	3.1	88	2.7	17	0.8	1.5
Wholewheat, Cooked, Tesco*	¼ Pack/132g	185	1.1	140	4.7	26.5	0.8	4.3
Wholewheat, Uncooked, Tesco*	¼ Pack/125g	185	1	148	5	27.9	0.8	4.5
GOAT								
Meat, Uncooked	**1 Serving/100g**	**109**	**2.3**	**109**	**20.6**	**0**	**2.3**	**0**
GOJI BERRIES								
Average	**1 Serving/100g**	**287**	**0.7**	**287**	**6.6**	**65.1**	**0.7**	**6.8**
GOOSE								
Meat & Skin, Roasted	**½ Goose/774g**	**2361**	**169.5**	**305**	**25.2**	**0**	**21.9**	**0**
Meat, Raw	**1 Portion/185g**	**298**	**13**	**161**	**23**	**0**	**7**	**0**
Meat, Roasted	**1 Portion/143g**	**340**	**18.1**	**238**	**29**	**0**	**12.7**	**0**
GOOSEBERRIES								
Dessert, Raw, Tops & Tails Removed	**1oz/28g**	**11**	**0.1**	**40**	**0.7**	**9.2**	**0.3**	**2.4**
Stewed with Sugar	**25g**	**14**	**0.1**	**54**	**0.7**	**12.9**	**0.3**	**4.2**
Stewed without Sugar	**25g**	**4**	**0.1**	**16**	**0.9**	**2.5**	**0.3**	**4.4**
GOULASH								
Beef, Average	**1 Serving/300g**	**310**	**9.5**	**103**	**8.1**	**10.4**	**3.2**	**0.9**
Meatball, Beef, with Rice, Hello Fresh*	1 Serving/796g	621	20	78	5.5	8.8	2.5	0
GRAINS								
Five, Mix, M&S*	½ Pack/125g	196	2.2	157	5.6	25.4	1.8	8.2
Italian Infused, Pesto-ey, Merchant Gourmet*	1 Pack/250g	452	12.7	181	6.1	25.8	5.1	3.4
Korean Style, Zingy, Merchant Gourmet*	½ Pack/125g	199	3.5	159	6.4	24.8	2.8	4.2
Mediterranean Style, Microwave, Sainsbury's*	½ Pack/125g	222	3.8	178	5.3	29.8	3	5.3
Mexican, 3 Bean, Wonder Grains, Quorn*	1 Pot/200g	256	7	128	6.4	15	3.5	6.5
Middle Eastern Style, Golden Sun, Lidl*	½ Pack/125g	220	6.2	176	5.5	24.5	5	5.3
Mixed, Nutty & Versatile, Microwave, Tesco*	½ Pack/125g	204	2.9	163	5	28.7	2.3	3.6
Mixed, Sun Dried Tomato, Merchant Gourmet*	1 Serving/125g	220	3.4	176	6.2	29.5	2.7	4.6
Pesto Infused, Good Grains, Worldwide Foods, Aldi*	½ Pack/125g	206	4.4	165	5.7	25	3.5	5.5
Piri Piri, Spicy, Merchant Gourmet*	½ Pack/110g	194	4.3	176	4	28.3	3.9	6
Quinoa & Lentils, Persian Style, Merchant Gourmet*	½ Pack/125g	220	3.5	176	6.7	28.6	2.8	4.9
Spanish Style, Worldwide Foods, Aldi*	½ Pouch/125g	231	7.4	185	4.2	27	5.9	4.6
Super, Garlic, & Ginger, Tilda*	½ Pack/110g	165	5.8	150	4.5	19	5.3	4.2
Super, Sweet Potato, Chilli, & Coconut, Tilda*	½ Pouch/110g	161	5.1	146	3.1	22	4.6	2.3
Trahana, Sour, Andritsaina*	1 Serving/50g	188	2.2	377	14	71	4.4	4
Wheatberries, & Kale, Sainsbury's*	½ Pack/150g	195	6.8	130	6.6	12	4.5	7.6
Wonder, Mediterranean, Stir & Eat, Quorn*	1 Pot/200g	212	4	106	5.5	14	2	4.9
Wonder, Thai Style, Stir & Eat, Quorn*	1 Pot/200g	252	9.4	126	5.5	14	4.7	3.6

G

	Measure INFO/WEIGHT	per Measure KCAL	FAT	Nutrition Values per 100g / 100ml KCAL	PROT	CARB	FAT	FIBRE
GRAPEFRUIT								
in Juice, Canned, Average	**1/3 Can/179g**	**82**	**0.1**	**46**	**0.5**	**10.6**	**0**	**0.4**
in Syrup, Average	**1oz/28g**	**19**	**0**	**69**	**0.5**	**16.8**	**0.1**	**0.5**
Raw, Flesh Only, Average	**½ Fruit/160g**	**48**	**0.2**	**30**	**0.8**	**6.8**	**0.1**	**1.3**
Raw, Weighed with Skin & Seeds, Average	**1 Lge/340g**	**54**	**0.2**	**16**	**0.3**	**4**	**0**	**0.6**
Ruby Red in Juice, Average	**1 Serving/135g**	**54**	**0.1**	**40**	**0.6**	**9.4**	**0**	**0.5**
GRAPES								
Black, Seedless, Sable, TTD, Sainsbury's*	1 Serving/80g	56	0.4	70	0.5	15.4	0.5	0.7
Candy Floss, Seedless, Raw, Tesco*	1 Serving/80g	58	0.1	73	0.6	17	0.1	0.6
Candy Snaps, No.1, Waitrose*	1 Serving/80g	53	0.4	66	0.5	15.4	0.5	0.9
Cotton Candy, 1, Waitrose*	1 Serving/80g	53	0.1	66	0.4	15.4	0.1	0.9
Green, Average	**1 Grape/5g**	**3**	**0**	**62**	**0.4**	**15.2**	**0.1**	**0.7**
Red & Green Selection, Average	**1 Grape/5g**	**3**	**0**	**62**	**0.4**	**15.2**	**0.1**	**0.8**
Red, Average	**1 Grape/5g**	**3**	**0**	**65**	**0.4**	**15.8**	**0.1**	**0.6**
Sable, 1, Waitrose*	1 Pack/400g	264	0.4	66	0.4	15.4	0.1	0.9
Sable, Finest, Tesco*	1 Serving/80g	53	0.1	66	0.4	15.4	0.1	0.7
Seedless, Red, Average	**1 Grape**	**4**	**0**	**74**	**0.6**	**17**	**0.3**	**0.6**
GRAPPA								
Average	**1 Serving/30ml**	**85**	**0**	**283**	**0**	**6.7**	**0**	**0**
GRATIN								
Broccoli, & Cauliflower, Creamy, Iceland*	1 Gratin/112g	204	17.1	182	3.1	7	15.3	1.9
Cottage Garden, Cook*	1 Pack/370g	533	32.9	144	3.8	9.8	8.9	3.1
Dauphinois, Mini, Duc De Coeur, Lidl*	1 Gratin/120g	163	9.7	136	3.2	11.8	8.1	1.4
Garden Vegetable, 4253, Wiltshire Farm Foods*	1 Serving/374g	595	30.3	159	6.9	14	8.1	0
Haddock, Smoked, & Bacon, Cook*	1 Pack/390g	526	28.5	135	7.2	10.8	7.3	1.2
Mushroom, Portobello, Waitrose*	½ Pack/170g	178	10.5	105	4.7	6.5	6.2	2.2
Potato Au, Chilled, Aldi *	1 Serving/400g	504	15.2	126	2.5	19	3.8	3.3
Potato Dauphinoise, Gastropub, M&S*	½ Pack/225g	304	20.5	135	2.8	10.2	9.1	0.6
Potato, & Spinach, M&S*	1 Serving/225g	259	16	115	2.9	9.1	7.1	1.3
Potato, Chef Select, Lidl*	½ Pack/250g	380	22.2	152	2.8	14	8.9	2
Potato, Creamy, M&S*	½ Pack/225g	360	25	160	2.2	11.9	11.1	0.9
Potato, Dauphinois, Peka *	½ Pack/225g	328	21.6	146	2.1	12.1	9.6	1.4
Potato, Dauphinoise, Finest, Tesco*	1 Gratin/107g	210	14.1	196	3.3	15	13.1	2
Potato, Individual, Waitrose*	1 Gratin/120g	230	16.8	192	3.8	11.8	14	1.6
Potato, Oven Cooked, Sainsbury's*	1 Serving/100g	195	12.8	195	2.8	16	12.8	2.4
Potato, Tasty, Aldi*	1 Pack/400g	640	30.4	160	4.8	17	7.6	1.9
Potato, Tesco*	1 Pack/450g	504	26.1	112	2.3	12	5.8	0.8
Potato, Waitrose*	½ Pack/207g	275	16.7	133	4.7	9.9	8.1	1.1
Sweet Potato, & Vegetable, Sainsbury's*	1 Gratin/100g	180	14.1	180	2.9	9.1	14.1	2.3
Vegetable, Root, Finest, Tesco*	½ Pack/214g	365	23.9	171	2.4	14	11.2	2
GRAVY								
Beef, Aunt Bessie's*	1 Serving/100g	73	5.3	73	1	5.3	5.3	0.5
Beef, Favourite, Granules, Made Up, Bisto*	1 Serving/50ml	13	0.5	26	0	4.2	1	0
Beef, Fresh, Sainsbury's*	1 Serving/83g	47	2.7	56	2.4	4.5	3.2	0.6
Beef, Roast, Best in Glass Jar, Made Up, Bisto*	1 Serving/70ml	21	0.3	30	0.3	6.1	0.4	0
Beef, Roast, Traditional, Finest, Tesco*	¼ Pot/125g	68	3	54	2.4	5.5	2.4	0.3
Chicken, Granules, Dry, Average	**1 Tsp/4g**	**17**	**0.9**	**428**	**4.5**	**49.4**	**23.6**	**1.2**
Chicken, Granules, Made Up, Average	**1 Serving/50ml**	**15**	**0.8**	**30**	**0.4**	**3.6**	**1.5**	**0.1**
Granules, Chicken, As Sold, Best, Bisto*	1 Serving/4g	14	0.3	350	4.1	67.7	6.7	1.3
Granules, Instant, Made Up	**1oz/28g**	**10**	**0.7**	**34**	**0.3**	**3**	**2.4**	**0**
Granules, Low Salt, Organic, Made Up, Kallo*	1 Serving/70ml	227	8.5	32	0.3	5.1	1.2	0
Granules, Onion, As Prepared, Tesco*	1 Serving/75ml	24	1.5	32	0.2	3.3	2	0.1
Granules, Onion, Dry	1 Tbsp/15g	17	1.1	116	1.9	10.9	7.5	1.9
Granules, Southern Style, As Sold, Bisto*	1 Serving/7g	28	1	422	5.7	64.7	15.1	2

	Measure	per Measure		Nutrition Values per 100g / 100ml				
	INFO/WEIGHT	KCAL	FAT	KCAL	PROT	CARB	FAT	FIBRE
GRAVY								
Granules, Vegetable, Dry Weight, Morrisons*	1 Tsp/5g	23	1.5	460	2	48	30	2
Lamb, Granules, Dry, Average	**1 Tsp/4g**	**14**	**0.3**	**344**	**10.8**	**56.2**	**8.4**	**2.8**
Onion, Caramelised, Made Up, Bisto*	1 Serving/50ml	14	0.2	29	0.1	6.1	0.4	0.1
Onion, Fresh, Asda*	1/6 Pot/77g	30	1.6	39	1.7	3.3	2.1	0.4
Onion, Granules, Dry Weight, Bisto*	4 Tsp/20g	78	2.9	391	2.4	62.3	14.7	2.3
Onion, Granules, Made Up, Bisto*	1 Serving/50ml	14	0.3	28	0.2	5.6	0.6	0
Onion, Rich, M&S*	½ Pack/150g	60	1.8	40	2	5.9	1.2	0.3
Pork, & Sage, Roast, Classic, Dry, Schwartz*	1 Pack/25g	88	1.4	354	11.8	63.8	5.8	0
Pork, Best, Made Up, Bisto*	1 Serving/50ml	13	0.5	26	1	5.8	1	1
Reduced Salt, Granules, Chicken, As Prepared, Bisto*	1 Tsp/5g	1	0	28	1	4.4	1	1
Reduced Salt, Granules, Chicken, Dry Weight, Bisto*	1 Tsp/5g	21	0.8	415	2.3	65.5	15.6	1.7
Southern Style, Mayflower, Made Up, Iceland *	1 Serving/50ml	32	1.7	65	0.8	8	3.4	0.3
Turkey, Finest, Tesco*	¼ Pouch/88ml	49	1.4	56	3.9	6.4	1.6	0
Vegan, Plant Kitchen, M&S*	1 Serving/50g	20	0.4	39	1	6.4	0.9	0.4
Vegetable, GF, As Sold, Free From, Tesco*	1 Serving/20g	87	5.6	437	1.4	43.7	28.2	1.4
Vegetable, Granules, Dry Weight, Bisto*	1 Tsp/4g	15	0.5	380	2.1	63	13.3	4.5
Vegetable, Granules, Made Up, Bisto*	1 Serving/50ml	14	0.2	28	0.2	5.6	0.4	0.2
Vegetarian, Granules, Dry Weight, Bisto*	1 Serving/28g	100	3.7	356	2.7	56	13.3	4.5
Vegetarian, Granules, Made Up, Sainsbury's*	1 Serving/50ml	16	1.1	32	0.2	2.8	2.2	0.8
GROUSE								
Meat Only, Roasted	**1oz/28g**	**36**	**0.6**	**128**	**27.6**	**0**	**2**	**0**
GUACAMOLE								
Average	**1 Tbsp/17g**	**33**	**3.3**	**194**	**1.6**	**3.4**	**19.2**	**2.4**
Jalapeno, & Red Pepper, Holy Moly*	1 Serving/30g	38	3.6	126	1.2	1.5	12	4.7
GUAVA								
Canned in Syrup	**1oz/28g**	**17**	**0**	**60**	**0.4**	**15.7**	**0**	**3**
Raw, Flesh Only, Average	**1 Fruit/55g**	**37**	**0.6**	**68**	**3**	**14**	**1**	**5**

G

	Measure INFO/WEIGHT	per Measure KCAL	FAT	Nutrition Values per 100g / 100ml KCAL	PROT	CARB	FAT	FIBRE
HADDOCK								
Fillet, Lightly Dusted, Scottish, Waitrose*	1 Fillet/133g	189	5.5	142	17.3	8.2	4.1	1.4
Fillets, Battered, Average	*1oz/28g*	*64*	*3.4*	*228*	*13.4*	*16.3*	*12.2*	*1.1*
Fillets, in Breadcrumbs, Average	*1 Fillet/125g*	*253*	*12.4*	*203*	*13.5*	*14.9*	*9.9*	*1.2*
Fillets, in White Wine & Onion Sauce, Birds Eye*	1 Fillet/137g	169	7.8	123	16	1.8	5.7	0.5
Fillets, Raw, Average	*1 Fillet/140g*	*111*	*1.2*	*79*	*17.7*	*0.2*	*0.8*	*0*
Fillets, Smoked, Cooked, Average	*1 Pack/300g*	*337*	*7.7*	*112*	*21.9*	*0.4*	*2.6*	*0.1*
Fillets, Smoked, Raw, Average	*1 Pack/227g*	*190*	*1*	*84*	*19.9*	*0.1*	*0.4*	*0.2*
Fillets, Smoked, with Cheese Crumb, Sainsbury's*	1 Fillet/174g	325	23	187	13.6	3.4	13.2	0.5
Fingers, Battered, M&S*	½ Pack/115g	247	13.6	215	12	14.9	11.8	0.7
Flour, Fried in Blended Oil	*1oz/28g*	*39*	*1.1*	*138*	*21.1*	*4.5*	*4.1*	*0.2*
Goujons, Batter, Crispy, M&S*	1 Serving/100g	250	14.1	250	11.7	18.5	14.1	0.8
HAGGIS								
Bon Bons, Simon Howie*	1 Serving/120g	253	10	211	11.3	23	8.3	0
Sliced, Breakfast Pack, As Sold, Simon Howie*	1 Slice/50g	102	4.8	204	11.8	17.6	9.7	0
Slices, Uncooked, Malcolm Allan*	1 Slice/56g	178	11.8	318	10.4	21.6	21.1	0
Traditional, Average	*1 Serving/454g*	*1119*	*66.5*	*246*	*12.4*	*17.2*	*14.6*	*1*
Vegetarian, Macsween*	1/3 Pack/151g	412	24.6	273	6	22.9	16.3	6.7
HAKE								
Fillets, in Breadcrumbs, Average	*1oz/28g*	*66*	*3.7*	*234*	*12.9*	*16*	*13.4*	*1*
Goujons, Average	*1 Serving/150g*	*345*	*17.8*	*230*	*12.4*	*18.6*	*11.9*	*1.3*
Raw, Average	*1oz/28g*	*28*	*0.6*	*100*	*20.1*	*0*	*2.2*	*0*
HALIBUT								
Cooked, Dry Heat, Average	*1oz/28g*	*38*	*1.1*	*135*	*24.6*	*0.4*	*4*	*0*
Raw	*1oz/28g*	*28*	*0.5*	*101*	*21.1*	*0*	*1.9*	*0*
HALVA								
Average	*1oz/28g*	*107*	*3.7*	*381*	*1.8*	*68*	*13.2*	*0*
HAM								
Applewood Smoked, Average	*1 Slice/28g*	*31*	*0.8*	*112*	*21.2*	*0.6*	*2.8*	*0.2*
Baked, Average	*1 Slice/74g*	*98*	*3.7*	*133*	*21*	*1*	*5*	*0*
Bavarian, Smoked, Finely Sliced, Asda*	2 Slices/35g	36	0.6	102	21	0.5	1.6	0
Black Forest, Slices, Dulano, Lidl*	1 Slice/11g	26	1.6	240	25	1	15	0.5
Boiled, Average	*1 Pack/113g*	*154*	*6.5*	*136*	*20.6*	*0.6*	*5.8*	*0*
Breaded, Average	*1 Slice/37g*	*57*	*2.3*	*155*	*23.1*	*1.8*	*6.3*	*1.6*
Breaded, Dry Cured, Average	*1 Slice/33g*	*47*	*1.8*	*142*	*22.2*	*1.4*	*5.4*	*0*
Brunswick, Average	*1 Slice/20g*	*32*	*1.8*	*160*	*19.5*	*0.6*	*8.8*	*0*
Cooked, Sliced, Average	*1 Slice/17g*	*18*	*0.5*	*109*	*19*	*1*	*3.2*	*0.1*
Crumbed, Sliced, Average	*1 Slice/28g*	*33*	*0.9*	*117*	*21.5*	*0.9*	*3.1*	*0*
Danish, Average	*1 Slice/11g*	*14*	*0.6*	*125*	*18.4*	*1*	*5.4*	*0*
Dry Cured, Average	*1 Slice/18g*	*26*	*1*	*144*	*22.4*	*1*	*5.6*	*0.2*
Extra Lean, Average	*1 Slice/11g*	*10*	*0.2*	*90*	*18*	*1.4*	*1.4*	*0*
Gammon, Breaded, Average	*1 Serving/25g*	*31*	*0.8*	*122*	*22*	*1.5*	*3.1*	*0*
Gammon, Dry Cured, Sliced, Average	*1 Slice/33g*	*43*	*1.4*	*131*	*22.9*	*0.4*	*4.2*	*0*
Gammon, Honey Roast, Average	*1 Serving/60g*	*81*	*2.8*	*134*	*22.4*	*0.4*	*4.8*	*0*
Gammon, Smoked, Average	*1 Slice/43g*	*59*	*2.1*	*137*	*22.3*	*0.7*	*4.9*	*0.2*
Garlic & Herb, Tesco*	1 Slice/33g	36	0.7	109	21	1.2	2.1	0.5
German Black Forest, Average	*½ Pack/35g*	*93*	*6*	*267*	*27.2*	*1.3*	*17*	*0.5*
Hock, Cooked, Shredded, Sainsbury's*	½ Pack/55g	100	4.1	182	27.6	0.5	7.5	1
Hock, Mustard Sauce, with Mash, & Peas, Tesco*	1 Pack/450g	387	13	86	7.5	6.8	2.9	1.4
Hock, Pulled, M&S*	1 Pack/100g	165	6.5	165	26.5	0.1	6.5	0.1
Hock, Wiltshire, Pulled, M&S*	½ Pack/100g	158	4.3	158	28.4	0.9	4.3	0.9
Honey & Mustard, Average	*1oz/28g*	*39*	*1.2*	*140*	*20.8*	*4.6*	*4.3*	*0*
Honey Roast, Average	*1 Slice/20g*	*25*	*0.8*	*123*	*20.3*	*1.6*	*3.8*	*0.1*
Honey Roast, Dry Cured, Average	*1 Slice/33g*	*46*	*1.5*	*140*	*22.7*	*2.3*	*4.4*	*0.2*

H

	Measure INFO/WEIGHT	per Measure KCAL	FAT	Nutrition Values per 100g / 100ml KCAL	PROT	CARB	FAT	FIBRE
HAM								
Honey Roast, Lean, Average	1 Serving/25g	28	0.8	111	18.2	2.7	3.1	0
Honey Roast, Wafer Thin, Average	1 Slice/10g	11	0.3	113	17.4	3.7	3.2	0.3
Jambon de Bayonne, Natoora*	1 Pack/70g	155	6.5	221	33.9	0.1	9.3	0
Joint, Cured, Roasted, Average	1 Serving/100g	138	5.2	138	21.7	1	5.2	0.1
Lean, Average	1 Slice/18g	19	0.4	104	19.5	1.1	2.4	0.3
Lean, Prime Cuts, on the Bone, Tesco*	1 Slice/31g	36	0.9	115	21.4	0.9	2.8	0.5
Oak Smoked, Average	1 Slice/20g	26	0.9	130	21	1	4.7	0.3
Parma, Average	1 Slice/10g	21	1.1	213	29.3	0	10.6	0
Parma, Premium, Average	1 Slice/14g	36	2.3	258	27.9	0.3	16.1	0
Peppered, Average	1 Slice/12g	13	0.3	110	18.5	2	2.7	0
Prosciutto, Average	1 Slice/12g	27	1.5	226	28.7	0	12.4	0.4
Roast, Cooked On The Bone, Finest, Tesco*	1 Slice/25g	32	0.6	130	26.3	0.2	2.6	0.5
Roast, Thick Cut, M&S*	1 Slice/40g	56	1.9	140	23	1	4.8	1
Roast, Thick Sliced, Finest, Tesco*	1 Slice/63g	78	1.6	124	24.7	0.2	2.6	0.5
Roast, Thickly Carved, Extra Special, Asda*	1 Slice/40g	48	0.6	119	25	1	1.5	0.7
Roasted, Free Range, with Rosemary & Thyme, Waitrose*	½ Pack/50g	90	4.4	181	23.5	1.2	8.9	0.8
Serrano, Average	1 Slice/20g	46	2.4	230	30.5	0.4	11.8	0
Serrano, Spanish, Slices, Tesco*	1 Slice/16g	40	2.2	250	30.1	0.9	13.7	1
Smoked, Average	1 Slice/18g	21	0.7	117	19.7	0.9	3.7	0
Smoked, Dry Cured, Average	1 Slice/28g	38	1.2	137	23	1.4	4.4	0.2
Smoked, Wafer Thin, Average	1 Serving/40g	41	1.2	102	17.7	1.2	2.9	0.2
Thick Cut, Average	1 Slice/74g	94	2.9	127	22.4	0.6	3.9	0.1
Tinned, Average	½ Can/100g	136	8.8	136	12.2	2	8.8	0
Torchon, Aldi*	1 Slice/50g	58	1.4	116	22	1	2.8	0.5
Torchon, French, Sainsbury's*	1 Slice/50g	57	1.5	114	21	0.7	3	0
Torchon, French, Unearthed*	1 Slice/40g	46	1.2	114	21	0.8	3	0
Trimmings, Cooked, Blue Mountain*	1 Serving/180g	200	3.6	111	20	1	2	0
Vegan, Simply Vamm, Vdeli Slices, Vbites Foods *	3 Slices/33g	70	3.7	212	23.2	4.4	11.3	0.2
Vegetarian, Slices, Quorn*	¼ Pack/25g	30	0.5	122	16	6.5	2.2	5.8
Vegetarian, Slices, Quorn*	2 Slices/28g	34	0.8	123	17	5.2	2.7	5.4
Wafer Thin, Average	1 Slice/10g	10	0.3	101	17.9	1.4	2.6	0.1
Wiltshire, Average	1oz/28g	41	1.7	148	23.1	0	6	0
Wiltshire, Breaded, Average	1oz/28g	41	1.4	145	23.9	1	5	0
HARIBO*								
American Hard Gums, Haribo*	1 Pack/175g	630	3.3	360	0.3	85.5	1.9	0.2
Cola Bottles, Fizzy, Haribo*	1 Pack/175g	595	0.4	340	6.3	78.3	0.2	0.3
Cola Bottles, Haribo*	1 Pack/16g	56	0	348	7.7	78.9	0.2	0.3
Dolly Mixtures, Haribo*	1 Pack/175g	719	8.4	411	1.8	90.2	4.8	0.2
Fantasy Mix, Haribo*	1 Pack/100g	344	0.2	344	6.6	79	0.2	0.3
Gold Bears, Haribo*	1 Pack/100g	343	0.5	343	6.9	77	0.5	0
Happy Cherries, Haribo*	1 Serving/40g	139	0.1	348	7.7	78.9	0.2	0.3
Horror Mix, Haribo*	1 Pack/100g	344	0.2	344	6.6	79	0.2	0.3
Jelly Babies, Haribo*	1 Serving/25g	87	0	348	4.5	82.1	0.2	0.5
Kiddies Super Mix, Haribo*	1 Pack/100g	344	0.2	344	6.6	79	0.2	0.3
Liquorice Favourites, Haribo*	1 Serving/40g	143	1.2	357	2.8	78.8	3	2.3
Milky Mix, Haribo*	1 Pack/175g	607	0.4	347	7.1	79.6	0.2	0.4
Pontefract Cakes, Haribo*	1 Serving/40g	118	0.1	296	5.3	68.2	0.2	0.5
Snakes, Haribo*	1 Snake/8g	28	0	348	7.7	78.9	0.2	0.3
Starmix, Haribo*	1 Pack/100g	344	0.2	344	6.6	79	0.2	0.3
Tangfastics, Haribo*	1 Pack/100g	359	2.3	359	6.3	78.3	2.3	0.5
HARISSA PASTE								
Al'fez*	1 Tsp/5g	7	0.2	138	2.7	19.7	4.5	4.1
Average	1 Tsp/5g	6	0.3	123	2.9	12.9	6.7	2.8

H

	Measure INFO/WEIGHT	per Measure KCAL	FAT	Nutrition Values per 100g / 100ml KCAL	PROT	CARB	FAT	FIBRE
HARISSA PASTE								
Ruby Rose, Cooks' Ingredients, Waitrose*	1 Tsp/5g	4	0.2	88	1.5	11.3	3.2	4.2
HASH								
Beef, Steak, Specially Selected, Aldi*	1 Pack/383g	452	14.9	118	7.4	12	3.9	1.8
Chicken, & Stuffing, Dinner, M&S*	1 Pack/400g	480	18.4	120	8	10.9	4.6	1.3
Corned Beef, Homestyle, Hormel*	1 Can/400g	644	40.7	161	7.2	9.8	10.2	0.8
Corned Beef, Waitrose*	1 Pack/385g	516	20.4	134	6.8	13.9	5.3	1.7
Steak, Hash, Extra Special, Asda*	1 Pack/354g	450	11	127	7.5	16	3.1	2.4
Steak, with Ale Gravy, Oven Cooked, The Best, Morrisons*	1 Pack/400g	460	16	115	7.3	11.9	4	1.3
HASH BROWNS								
Cauliflower, Strong Roots*	1 Piece/40g	74	4.3	185	1.7	19.4	10.7	1.8
Fries, Oven Baked, Iceland*	1 Serving/150g	375	15	250	3.4	34.7	10	3.5
Iceland*	1 Piece/36g	69	3.2	193	2.2	24.4	9	2.8
Oven Baked, Tesco*	3 Pieces/141g	249	11.2	176	2.7	22.4	7.9	2.2
Oven Baked, Weighed Frozen, McCain*	1 Piece/40g	60	2.4	150	1.6	21.3	6	2.1
Potatoes, From Restaurant, Average	**1 Portion/150g**	**489**	**32.5**	**326**	**2.6**	**32.1**	**21.6**	**2.7**
Roasted Onion, & Rosemary, Sainsbury's*	1 Hashbrown/52g	96	4.5	185	3	22.3	8.6	3.1
Uncooked, Average	**1 Piece/45g**	**78**	**3.7**	**173**	**2**	**22.5**	**8.3**	**1.9**
HAZELNUTS								
Blanched, Average	**1 Serving/25g**	**164**	**15.9**	**656**	**15.4**	**5.8**	**63.5**	**6.5**
Chopped, Average	**1 Serving/10g**	**67**	**6.4**	**666**	**16.8**	**5.6**	**64**	**6.6**
Dark Chocolate, Picks*	1 Pack/90g	503	32.4	559	7.7	47	36	6.8
White Chocolate, & Coconut, Finest, Tesco*	1 Serving/30g	182	13.8	606	9	37	46	4.2
Whole, Average	**10 Whole/10g**	**66**	**6.4**	**655**	**15.4**	**5.8**	**63.5**	**6.5**
HEART								
Lambs, Average	**1 Heart/75g**	**92**	**4.5**	**122**	**16**	**1**	**6**	**0**
Ox, Raw	**1oz/28g**	**23**	**0.8**	**82**	**14.4**	**0**	**2.8**	**0**
Ox, Stewed	**1oz/28g**	**44**	**1.4**	**157**	**27.8**	**0**	**5.1**	**0**
HERRING								
Canned in Tomato Sauce, Average	**1oz/28g**	**57**	**4.3**	**204**	**11.9**	**4.1**	**15.5**	**0.1**
Dill Marinated, Silver Tide*	1 Pot/200g	370	16	185	9.1	19.1	8	0
Fillets, Marinated, in Cream Sauce, Lisner*	1 Serving/70g	201	18.8	287	5.4	5.9	26.8	0
Fillets, Raw, Average	**1 Herring/100g**	**139**	**9.4**	**139**	**13.8**	**0**	**9.4**	**0**
Grilled, Average	**1oz/28g**	**51**	**3.1**	**181**	**20.1**	**0**	**11.2**	**0**
Pickled, Average	**1oz/28g**	**42**	**2.9**	**149**	**8.1**	**5.5**	**10.3**	**0**
HONEY								
Acacia, Tiptree, Wilkin & Sons*	1 Tbsp/15g	43	0	288	0	76	0	0
Blossom, Everyday, Hilltop Honey*	1 Tbsp/15g	46	0	307	0	76	0	0
Clear, with a Hint of Cinnamon, Rowse*	1 Tbsp/15g	49	0.1	329	0.5	81.5	0.5	0.5
Greek, Waitrose*	1 Tsp/6g	18	0	307	0.4	76.4	0	0
Manuka, 40 Mgo, Manuka Doctor*	1 Tsp/5g	17	0	335	0.2	81.9	0.2	0
Manuka, Mgo 50+, Hiltop*	1 Tsp/5g	17	0	333	0.5	83	0.5	0.5
Manuka, Npa 5+, Deluxe, Lidl*	1 Tbsp/15g	52	0	350	0.1	86.9	0.1	0.5
Manuka, Rowse*	1 Tsp/5g	17	0	348	0	86.9	0.1	0
Pure, Clear, Average	**1 Tbsp/20g**	**63**	**0**	**315**	**0.5**	**78.5**	**0**	**0**
Pure, Set, Average	**1 Tbsp/20g**	**62**	**0**	**312**	**0.4**	**77.6**	**0**	**0**
Raw, & Unfiltered, 100%, Louisiana, Nature Nates*	1 Tbsp/15g	50	0	333	0	85.7	0	0
Raw, British Wildflower, Hilltop*	1 Tsp/5g	17	0	333	0.2	83.1	0.2	0
Spanish Lavender, Hilltop Honey*	1 Tbsp/15g	50	0.1	333	0.5	83	0.5	0.5
Spanish Orange Blossom, Sainsbury's*	1 Tbsp/15g	51	0	339	0.1	84.7	0	0.3
HONEYCOMB								
Chocolate Dipped, M&S*	1 Serving/40g	180	4.6	451	2.6	83.4	11.6	1.1
Natural, Epicure*	1 Serving/100g	290	4.6	290	0.4	74.4	4.6	0

H

	Measure INFO/WEIGHT	per Measure KCAL	FAT	Nutrition Values per 100g / 100ml KCAL	PROT	CARB	FAT	FIBRE
HORLICKS								
Malted Drink, Instant, Dry Weight, Horlicks*	2 Tbsp/30g	108	0.6	359	13.1	74.4	1.9	1.9
Malted Drink, Light, Dry Weight, Horlicks*	1 Serving/32g	116	1.2	364	14.8	72.2	3.8	1.9
Powder, Made Up with Semi-Skimmed Milk	**1 Mug/227ml**	**184**	**4.3**	**81**	**4.3**	**12.9**	**1.9**	**0**
Powder, Made Up with Whole Milk	**1 Mug/227ml**	**225**	**8.9**	**99**	**4.2**	**12.7**	**3.9**	**0**
HORSERADISH								
Cream, Strong, Tracklement's*	1 Tsp/5g	15	1.3	299	4.3	7.5	26.5	4.9
Creamed, Sainsbury's*	1 Tsp/10ml	25	1.4	253	2.8	26.9	14.3	2.3
Prepared, Average	**1 Tsp/5g**	**1**	**0**	**28**	**2**	**5**	**0.1**	**2.8**
HOT CHOCOLATE								
Belgian Choc, Options*	1 Sachet/11g	40	0.8	365	8.9	59	7.3	0
Belgian Chocolate, Options, Ovaltine*	1 Serving/11g	40	0.8	365	8.9	59	7.3	0
Caramel, Whittards of Chelsea*	1 Serving/20g	71	1.5	355	7.5	64.5	7.5	13
Choc Mint, Highlights, Made Up, Cadbury*	1 Serving/200ml	40	1.4	20	1	2.5	0.7	0.3
Chocolate Au Lait, Options, Ovaltine*	1 Sachet/10g	36	1	355	11.8	54.5	10	7.3
Classic, Hotel Chocolat*	1 Serving/35g	172	2.2	490	4.6	11.7	6.2	1.9
Cocoa, Lidl*	1 Serving/20g	77	1.2	386	6.1	74.1	6.2	0
Dairy Fudge, Highlights, Dry Weight, Cadbury*	1 Serving/11g	38	1.2	347	16	41	11	9.7
Dreamy Caramel, Options, Ovaltine*	1 Sachet/11g	39	0.9	354	12.3	48.5	7.8	0
Drink, Organic, Green & Black's*	1 Tsp/5g	20	0.4	396	8.6	67	7.5	12
Fairtrade, Whittards of Chelsea*	4 Tsp/20g	68	0.8	342	7.8	69	3.9	10.9
Frothy, Ultimate, Dry Mix, Galaxy*	1 Serving/25g	97	2	387	4.5	72	8.1	0
Galaxy, Mars*	1 Sachet/25g	97	1.9	386	4.8	71.9	7.7	4.7
Highlights, Instant, Made Up, Cadbury*	1 Cup/200ml	40	1.4	20	1	2.5	0.7	0.3
Instant Break, Cadbury*	1 Sachet/28g	119	3.9	425	10.9	64.2	14	0
Instant, As Prepared, Smart Price, Asda*	1 Serving/227g	109	1.1	48	0.8	10	0.5	0.5
Instant, Dry Weight, Morrisons*	1 Serving/28g	113	1.7	403	7.8	78.2	6.1	2.8
Instant, Fairtrade, Sainsbury's*	1 Serving/231g	111	1.8	48	0.5	8.6	0.8	1.4
Instant, Highlights, Cadbury*	1 Sachet/22g	80	2.8	364	17.3	44.6	12.7	0
Instant, Tesco*	1 Serving/30g	120	2.5	401	7.1	71.6	8.4	5.4
Instant, Vegan, Dry Weight, Galaxy, Mars*	1 Serving/25g	102	2.5	408	4.7	75	9.9	0
Low Calorie, Dry Weight, As Sold, Average	**1 Sachet/11g**	**41**	**1.2**	**374**	**14.6**	**50**	**10.7**	**11.1**
Milk, Swiss, Powder, Twinings*	1 Serving/20g	78	0.7	389	5	81.3	3.5	0
Milky, 50%, Sachet, Hotel Chocolat*	1 Sachet/35g	199	14.7	568	8.6	33.7	41.9	9.4
Mint Madness, Belgian, Options, Ovaltine*	1 Sachet/11g	38	0.8	348	12.3	49.2	6.9	20
Mint, Highlights, Cadbury*	1 Serving/200ml	40	1.4	20	1	2.5	0.7	0
Mint, Sachet, As Sold, Hotel Chocolat*	1 Sachet/35g	196	14.5	561	7.4	32.9	41.5	11.7
Original, Dry Weight, Cadbury*	1 Serving/18g	73	1	404	6.4	76	5.8	9.3
Outrageous Orange, Options, Ovaltine*	1 Serving/11g	38	0.8	348	12.3	49.3	6.9	20
Pods, Galaxy, Mars*	1 Pod/17g	69	1.8	406	5.3	70.6	10.6	0
Skinny, Powder, Nomu*	1 Tsp/6g	20	0.4	331	22	35	7.5	17.2
Wicked White, Options, Ovaltine*	1 Sachet/11g	44	1.1	398	10.5	64.6	10	3.7
Wispa, Hot Frothy, Cadbury*	1 Sachet/27g	107	1.4	395	11	74	5.3	2.9
HOT DOG								
Beef, Campofrio*	1 Hotdog/120g	257	20.4	214	11	3.8	17	0
Bunlimited*	1 Hot Dog/70g	208	18	297	15.7	0.9	25.7	0
Meat-Free, Plant Menu, Aldi*	1 Hotdog/58g	93	3.8	160	10.1	11.1	6.5	8.2
Plain, From Restaurant, Average	**1 Hot Dog/98g**	**242**	**14.5**	**247**	**10.6**	**18.4**	**14.8**	**0**
Plant Based, Moving Mountains*	1 Hot Dog/60g	77	5.4	128	7	3	9	3.2
Pork, Maple, & Bacon, Finest, Tesco*	1 Hot Dog/75g	203	14.3	271	14.5	9.4	19.1	1.5
Posh Dogs, The Grill, M&S*	1 Hot Dog/100g	264	20.9	264	13.1	5.6	20.9	0.7
Posh Dogs, Vegan, Plant Kitchen, M&S*	1 Hot Dog/80g	174	13.4	218	8.4	4.5	16.7	7.9
Sausage, American Style, Average	**1 Hot Dog/75g**	**180**	**14.3**	**241**	**11.6**	**6.2**	**19**	**0**
Sausage, Average	**1 Hot Dog/23g**	**40**	**3**	**175**	**10.8**	**4.3**	**12.8**	**0.3**

H

	Measure INFO/WEIGHT	per Measure KCAL	FAT	Nutrition Values per 100g / 100ml KCAL	PROT	CARB	FAT	FIBRE
HOT DOG								
Vegetarian, Meat Free, Sainsbury's*	1 Hot Dog/30g	72	5.1	240	17.4	3.8	16.8	2
Vegetarian, Tesco*	1 Hot Dog/30g	66	4.7	222	17.1	1.6	15.8	2.2
HOT POT								
Beef, Minced, 3% Fat, Calorie Counted, Asda*	1 Pack/310g	319	7.1	103	4.5	15	2.3	2.2
Beef, Minced, Bisto*	1 Pack/375g	363	13.5	97	4.1	11.3	3.6	1.4
Beef, Minced, Classic, Asda*	1 Pack/400g	424	18.4	106	6.8	8.7	4.6	1.1
Beef, Minced, Frozen, Tesco*	1 Pack/360g	377	10.1	105	5.2	11.7	2.8	1.6
Beef, Minced, HFC, Tesco*	1 Pack/362g	347	10	96	5.2	11.7	2.8	1.6
Beef, Minced, Iceland*	1 Pack/462g	448	17.1	97	2.7	12.2	3.7	1.6
Beef, Minced, Morrisons*	1 Pack/369g	487	17.3	132	6.7	14.2	4.7	2.9
Beef, Minced, Sainsbury's*	1 Pack/450g	464	22.1	103	5.3	9.5	4.9	2.2
Chicken, Classic Recipe, Tesco*	1 Pack/365g	314	10.6	86	4.4	10.3	2.9	0.8
Chicken, Counted, Morrisons*	1 Pack/350g	196	1.6	56	6.6	6	0.5	0.8
Chicken, Oven Baked, Asda*	1 Pack/368g	364	12.9	99	5.1	11	3.5	1.2
Chicken, Oven Baked, Iceland*	1 Pack/485g	500	18.9	103	4.4	12	3.9	1.4
Chicken, Oven Cooked, Morrisons*	1 Pack/285g	348	13.7	122	6.7	12	4.8	1.8
Chicken, Oven Cooked, Morrisons*	1 Pack/400g	488	19.2	122	6.7	12	4.8	1.8
Chicken, Sainsbury's*	1 Pack/400g	340	11	85	5.2	9.8	2.8	1.3
Chicken, Waitrose*	1 Pack/400g	353	13.5	88	4.9	8.9	3.4	1.3
Chicken, Weight Watchers*	1 Pack/320g	296	6.7	93	6.3	11.8	2.1	1.1
Lamb, Chef Select, Lidl*	1 Serving/450g	463	20.8	103	6.1	8.4	4.6	1.6
Lamb, Diet Chef Ltd*	1 Pack/270g	275	14	102	6.3	7.5	5.2	1.2
Lamb, Minced, & Vegetable, COU, M&S*	1 Pack/400g	340	10.8	85	5.7	12.5	2.7	1.8
Lamb, Minced, Classic Kitchen, Tesco*	1 Pack/427g	384	12.8	90	5.6	9.4	3	1.5
Lamb, Minced, Morrison*	1 Pack/400g	376	11.6	94	4.1	11.7	2.9	2.2
Lamb, Mini Meal, Meal for One, M&S*	1 Pack/200g	244	7.6	122	7.3	13.8	3.8	1.8
Lamb, Onion & Pearl Barley Gravy, BFY, M&S*	1 Pack/375g	304	3	81	7.1	10.7	0.8	1.5
Lamb, Shank, Extra Special, Asda*	1 Pack/450g	508	20.2	113	10.2	7.8	4.5	1.3
Lancashire, M&S*	1 Pack/450g	441	13.5	98	8.4	8.8	3	1.3
Lancashire, Tesco*	½ Pack/225g	205	7	91	6	9.7	3.1	0.5
Pork, & Apple Cider, Parsley Box*	1 Pack/270g	248	10	92	5	9.1	3.7	0.9
Sausage, & Vegetable, Vegetarian, Linda McCartney*	1 Pot/400g	516	20.4	129	6.4	15.7	5.1	2.3
Steak, Parsley Box*	1 Pack/270g	281	8.9	104	5.9	12	3.3	1.3
Vegetarian, Quorn*	1 Pack/400g	252	8	63	3.3	8	2	1.9
HOUMOUS								
30% Less Fat, BGTY, Sainsbury's*	¼ Pot/50g	82	4.4	164	6.9	12.2	8.7	4.8
Caramelised Onion, M&S*	¼ Pot/50g	134	10.4	268	5.8	12.8	20.7	3.8
Caramelised Onion, Meadow Fresh, Lidl*	1 Serving/50g	112	7	224	7.4	14.8	14.1	4.1
Caramelised Onion, Reduced Fat, Tesco*	1 Sm Pot/67g	123	6.9	184	5.8	14.8	10.3	4.4
Caramelised Onion, Sainsbury's*	1 Serving/30g	68	4.4	225	6.3	15.2	14.5	4.5
Caramelised Onion, Tesco*	¼ Pot/46g	105	7.7	229	5.3	12	16.8	4.1
Chickpea, Italian, Natoora *	¼ Pot/50g	157	13.6	315	5	10.5	27.1	3.6
Classic, Meadow Fresh, Lidl*	1 Serving/50g	176	15	351	6.6	12	30	3.1
Classic, Sabra*	1 Serving/30g	75	5.4	250	7.1	14.3	17.9	3.6
Classic, Sainsbury's*	1 Serving/50g	113	7.9	226	7.3	11.3	15.8	5
Classic, So Organic, Sainsbury's*	¼ Pot/50g	146	11.9	292	6.7	10.9	23.8	4
Classic, The Deli, Aldi*	1 Serving/50g	151	11.5	302	7.7	12	23	5.5
Coronation, Chunky, The Deli, Aldi*	¼ Pot/43g	75	3.2	177	6.3	17	7.5	8.3
Jalapeno, & Red Pepper, Tesco*	¼ Pot/46g	92	5.9	199	6.3	12.3	12.9	3.9
Jalapeno, Mexican, Morrisons*	¼ Pot/50g	162	13.6	325	7.5	9.8	27.3	5.1
Jalapeno, Pepper, Hot & Spicy, Tesco*	¼ Pot/46g	104	6.8	227	8.1	12.8	14.9	4.8
Lemon & Coriander, Tesco*	¼ Pot/46g	116	8.9	253	6.8	9.9	19.4	5.7
Lemon & Coriander, Waitrose*	¼ Pot/50g	129	9.7	258	6.3	11.8	19.4	5.4

H

	Measure INFO/WEIGHT	per Measure KCAL	FAT	Nutrition Values per 100g / 100ml KCAL	PROT	CARB	FAT	FIBRE
HOUMOUS								
Lentil, Original, Pulse*	1 Serving/30g	70	4.1	232	8.5	15.3	13.8	6.5
Marmite, Marmite*	1 Serving/50g	128	8	257	11	16	16	4.7
Marvellously Moreish, Organic, Abel & Cole*	1 Serving/50g	90	6	181	6.4	12.4	12.1	0
Moroccan, Inspired, Finest, Tesco*	¼ Pot/43g	130	10.7	305	5.3	12	25.1	4.7
Moroccan, Sainsbury's*	¼ Pot/50g	114	8.3	229	6	11.1	16.6	5.5
Onion, Caramelised, The Deli, Aldi*	½ Pack/42g	94	5.9	224	7.4	15	14	4.1
Organic, Duchy, Waitrose*	¼ Pot/50g	166	14.2	332	6.8	10.7	28.3	3.5
Organic, M&S*	1 Serving/25g	83	7.4	332	7.2	5.9	29.4	7.3
Red Pepper, & Chilli, 30% Less Fat, Asda*	¼ Pack/50g	77	4	154	5.5	13	7.9	5
Red Pepper, Deluxe, Lidl*	1 Serving/30g	90	7	300	6.9	13.3	23.4	4.5
Red Pepper, Reduced Fat, Tesco*	¼ Pot/46g	81	4.8	176	6.1	12.2	10.5	4.1
Red Pepper, Roasted, M&S*	1 Pack/200g	534	41.8	267	6.1	11.8	20.9	3.8
Red Pepper, Roasted, Reduced Fat, M&S*	¼ Pack/50g	91	5.5	182	5.8	12.7	11	4.5
Red Pepper, Tesco*	1 Serving/25g	56	4.1	223	5.9	11	16.3	4.5
Red Pepper, The Deli, Aldi*	1 Serving/50g	140	10.5	281	7.8	12	21	5.7
Reduced Fat, Average	**1 Tbsp/30g**	**72**	**5**	**241**	**9.2**	**13.3**	**16.8**	**3.6**
Roasted Beetroot, & Mint, Waitrose*	¼ Pot/50g	112	8.1	224	5.9	11.6	16.2	4.1
Smoked, Moorish*	1 Pack/150g	448	36.3	299	7.1	11.5	24.2	3.4
Smoked, Waitrose*	¼ Pot/50g	141	11.2	282	7.2	10.6	22.4	4.5
Sweet Chilli, Tesco*	¼ Pot/46g	106	6.8	231	7.1	15	14.7	5.2
Sweet Chilli, with Breadsticks, Tesco*	1 Pack/57g	186	8.5	326	8.4	36.9	14.9	5.3
HULA HOOPS								
BBQ Beef, KP Snacks*	1 Pack/24g	120	5.8	500	3.8	65	24	2.2
Beef Puft, KP Snacks*	1 Pack/15g	72	3	478	9	64	20	4
Beef, 55% Less Saturated Fat, KP Snacks*	1 Pack/34g	172	9	505	3.7	61.8	26.4	2.2
Beef, Big Hoops, KP Snacks*	1 Pack/50g	250	12	499	3.8	65	24	2.8
Cheese & Onion 55% Less Saturated Fat, KP Snacks*	1 Pack/34g	175	9.7	515	3.6	61	28.5	1.9
Cheese & Onion, KP Snacks*	1 Pack/24g	120	5.8	502	3.8	66	24	2.5
Original, KP Snacks*	1 Pack/24g	121	5.8	503	3.4	66	24	2.3
Ready Salted, Puft, KP Snacks*	1 Pack/15g	72	3.2	482	8.3	64	21	4
Salt & Vinegar, 50% Less Saturated Fat, KP Snacks*	1 Pack/25g	128	7	510	3.1	60.9	28.2	1.8
Salt & Vinegar, KP Snacks*	1 Pack/24g	122	5.8	507	3.4	66	24	2.2
Salt & Vinegar, Puft, KP Snacks*	1 Pack/15g	72	3	478	8.1	63	20	3.9
Sweet Chilli, Puft, KP Snacks*	1 Pack/15g	71	3	474	8.1	64	20	4

H

ICE CREAM

INFO/WEIGHT	Measure		per Measure		Nutrition Values per 100g / 100ml				
			KCAL	FAT	KCAL	PROT	CARB	FAT	FIBRE
Banana, Pot, Yeo Valley*	1 Pot/100g		171	5.6	171	3.6	26.1	5.6	0.2
Banoffee Fudge, Sainsbury's*	1/8 Pot/67g		119	4	178	2.8	28.7	5.9	0.2
Belgian Chocolate, Haagen-Dazs*	1 Sm Tub/78g		249	16.2	318	4.6	28.4	20.7	0
Belgian Milk Chocolate, Tesco*	1 Lolly/75g		241	15.4	321	3	31.2	20.5	0
Berry Neighbourly, Ben & Jerry's*	1 Scoop/44g		123	7	279	3.5	29	16	0
Birthday Cake, Asda*	1 Scoop/50g		65	1.3	131	6.5	18.9	2.7	7.1
Birthday Cake, Halo Top*	1 Scoop/50g		60	1.6	121	5.2	19	3.2	0
Blondie Brownie, Ben & Jerry's*	1 Scoop/43g		109	6	253	4.2	29	14	0
Blueberries & Cream, Minicup, Haagen-Dazs*	1 Minicup/87g		212	14	244	4.1	20.3	16.1	0.5
Blueberry Crumble, Halo Top*	½ Tub/68g		84	2.3	123	6.8	20	3.4	0
Bob Marleys One Love, Ben & Jerry's*	1 Scoop/45g		123	6.3	273	3.2	33	14	0
Candy Bar, Halo Top*	¼ Tub/118g		90	3.7	76	4.3	14	3.1	2.3
Cappuccino, Tesco*	1 Scoop/54g		121	4.5	224	2.3	34.8	8.3	0.2
Caramel Biscuit & Cream, Minicup, Haagen-Dazs*	1 Minicup/87g		249	16.1	286	4.6	25.5	18.4	0.1
Caramel Chocolate Crunch, Oppo*	1 Scoop/50g		74	3.8	147	4.3	17	7.5	5
Caramel Chocolate Pretzel, Plant Based, Halo Top*	1 Scoop/50g		70	2.5	141	0.5	21.7	5	0
Caramel Latte, Morrisons*	1 Scoop/50g		99	4.3	199	2.4	27.9	8.5	0.5
Caramel Popcorn, Asda*	1 Scoop/50g		66	1.4	133	6.3	19.3	2.7	8.6
Caramel Swirl, Gelato, Minicup, Haagen-Dazs*	1 Mini Tub/72g		139	5.3	193	5.1	23.2	7.4	6.4
Caramel, Chew Chew, Ben & Jerry's*	1 Scoop/45g		122	6.8	270	3.5	28	15	0
Caramel, Pecan, Praline, Vegan, Booja-Booja*	1 Scoop/50g		133	6.5	267	4.1	30	13.1	0
Caramella, Tesco*	1 Serving/51g		120	5.5	235	2.6	32	10.7	1.1
Cheesecake Brownie, Ben & Jerry's*	1 Serving 100g		260	16	260	4	26	16	0
Cheesecake, Strawberry, Haagen-Dazs*	2 Scoops/86g		226	12.3	262	3.8	29.4	14.3	0.4
Cherry Bakewell, Ripple, Kelly's Of Cornwall*	1 Scoop/50g		112	4.4	223	3.2	32.8	8.7	0.3
Choc Choc Chip, Minicup, Haagen-Dazs*	1 Minicup/87g		245	15.9	281	4.5	24.3	18.2	0.9
Chocolate Brownie, Vegan, Jude's*	1 Scoop/50g		105	3.3	210	1.4	35.5	6.6	0
Chocolate Chip Cookie Dough, Halo Top*	1 Scoop/50g		68	2	135	5.2	22	3.9	2.5
Chocolate Chip, Hacendado*	1 Scoop/50g		146	8.5	292	4.6	29	17	2.2
Chocolate Drizzle, Gelato, Mini Cup, Haagen-Dazs*	1 Minicup/72g		136	4.9	190	5.9	22.4	6.8	7.5
Chocolate Flavour, Average	**1 Serving/70g**		**149**	**7.9**	**212**	**4.1**	**23.7**	**11.3**	**0.6**
Chocolate Honeycomb, Co-Op*	¼ Pot/81g		186	10.5	230	4	26	13	0.3
Chocolate, Dark, Finest, Tesco*	1 Scoop/50g		128	8.2	257	4.8	22.5	16.3	1
Chocolate, Finest, Tesco*	1 Scoop/70g		254	17.7	363	4.4	28.9	25.3	1.1
Chocolate, Fudge, Brownie, Ben & Jerry's*	1 Scoop/42g		102	5.4	245	4.2	29	13	0
Chocolate, Fudge, Oatly*	1 Scoop/50g		118	5.5	235	1.2	32	11	1.4
Chocolate, Gelatelli, Lidl*	1 Portion/50g		126	6.8	251	3.8	27.3	13.6	2.1
Chocolate, Non Dairy, V Taste, Morrisons*	1 Scoop/50g		78	4.5	157	2.5	16	9	1
Chocolate, Plant Kitchen, M&S*	1/5 Tub/62g		119	6.6	192	1.8	19.9	10.6	5.1
Chocolate, Salted Caramel, Vegan, Booja-Booja*	1 Scoop/50g		125	4.8	249	5	28.4	9.6	0
Chocolate, Santo Domingo, 1, Waitrose*	1 Serving/66g		220	16.4	333	4.5	22.8	24.8	0.5
Chocolate, Triple, Giannis, Aldi*	1 Scoop/50g		103	4.4	206	2.5	29	8.7	0.7
Chocolate, Vegan, Jude's*	1 Scoop/50g		58	2.4	115	1.4	17.5	4.7	0
Chunky Monkey, Non-Dairy, Ben & Jerry's*	1 Scoop/42g		109	5.8	262	2.4	30	14	0
Cinnamon Roll, Tub, Halo Top*	1 Serving/118g		90	3	76	4	15	2.5	2.5
Clotted Cream, Cornish, Kelly's Of Cornwall*	1 Serving/125g		282	18.6	226	2.9	20.1	14.9	0.1
Coconut Milk, Chocolate, Gelatelli, Lidl*	1 Ice Cream/60g		122	8.3	204	1.4	17.5	13.8	0
Coffee, Arabica, Carte d'Or*	1 Scoop/50g		115	4.4	230	3.1	34	8.9	0
Coffee, Carrefour *	1 Scoop/50g		114	4.6	227	3.5	32	9.3	0
Coffee, Colombian, No.1, Waitrose*	1 Sm Pot/81g		197	10.7	243	3.8	27	13.2	0.5
Coffee, Finest, Tesco*	¼ Pot/93g		236	14.9	254	4.9	22.5	16	0
Cookie Dough, Ben & Jerry's*	1 Scoop/43g		115	6.4	270	4	30	15	0
Cookie Dough, High Protein, Giannis, Aldi*	1 Scoop/50g		77	2	154	10	17	4.1	3.1

ICE CREAM

	Measure INFO/WEIGHT	per Measure KCAL	FAT	Nutrition Values per 100g / 100ml KCAL	PROT	CARB	FAT	FIBRE
Cookie Dough, High Protein, Morrisons*	1 Scoop/50g	57	1.8	114	6.6	14.7	3.6	6.2
Cookie Dough, Tesco*	1 Serving/125g	301	14.2	241	3.3	31	11.4	0.6
Cookie Dough, Vegan, Wicked Kitchen, Tesco*	1 Scoop/50g	117	6.1	234	1.7	28.5	12.2	1.5
Cookies & Cream, Haagen-Dazs*	1 Sm Tub/100g	226	14.7	226	4	19.5	14.7	0
Cornish Clotted, Honeycomb, M&S*	1 Scoop/50g	129	7.8	258	2.5	26.8	15.6	0.2
Dairy, Flavoured	*1oz/28g*	*50*	*2.2*	*179*	*3.5*	*24.7*	*8*	*0*
Damson, & Sloe Gin, Snugburys*	1 Scoop/50g	98	5.5	196	4	20	11	0
Double Chocolate, Nestle*	1 Serving/78g	248	14.3	320	4.8	33.7	18.4	0
Dulce De Leche, Minicup, Haagen-Dazs*	1 Minicup/87g	231	13.6	265	4.4	26.7	15.6	0.1
Espresso Caramel, Gelatelli, Lidl*	1 Scoop/50g	38	1	77	4.6	8.6	2	3
Eton Mess, Gelateria, Carte d'Or*	2 Scoops/100g	181	5.8	181	2.2	30	5.8	0
Fig & Orange Blossom Honey, Waitrose*	1 Serving/100g	219	11.8	219	3.9	24.3	11.8	0.4
Gelato, Vanilla	*1 Serving/100g*	*162*	*7.2*	*162*	*2.4*	*22.6*	*7.2*	*0.3*
Gingerbread, Specially Selected, Aldi*	1 Scoop/64g	169	8.3	264	4	33	13	0.6
Gooey Brownie, Halo Top*	1 Scoop/50g	69	2.2	138	5.7	22	4.3	0
Half Baked, Ben & Jerry's*	1 Scoop/41g	107	5.3	262	4.1	32	13	0
Hazelnut Swirl, Vegan, Oatly*	1 Scoop/50g	123	7	246	1.4	28	14	1.1
Home Sweet Honeycomb, Ben & Jerry's*	1 Scoop/43g	114	6.4	266	3.8	30	15	0
Honeycomb, Scottish, Aberdoyle*	1 Scoop/50g	158	9.4	315	3.1	33.4	18.7	0.5
Lavazza, Carte d'Or*	1 Serving/55g	120	5.4	218	3.5	29	9.9	0
Lemon, & Ginger, Vitasia, Lidl*	1 Scoop/50g	96	3.4	191	3.1	28.8	6.8	0
Luscious Mint Choc Chip, Morrisons*	1 Serving/50g	99	5.2	198	2.9	23.1	10.5	0.7
Magnum, Classic, Tub, Wall's*	1 Scoop/50g	108	7	217	2.4	21	14	0
Magnum, White, Tub, Wall's*	1 Scoop/50g	109	6.5	218	2.5	23	13	0
Maltesers, Mars*	1 Scoop/50g	64	3	128	1.4	17	6	0
Mango & Raspberry, Minicup, Haagen-Dazs*	1 Minicup/87g	211	11.5	243	3.3	27.2	13.3	0.6
Mango, & Raspberry, Haagen-Dazs*	1 Scoop/50g	124	6.7	247	3.4	27.9	13.4	0.6
Mango, Swirl, Passionate, Alpro*	1 Scoop/50g	76	3	153	2.1	16.9	6	10.5
Mince Pie, Farmhouse Dairy, TTD, Sainsbury's*	¼ Pot/100g	272	14.9	272	4.5	29.3	14.9	1.3
Mint & Chocolate Flavour, Average	*1 Serving/70g*	*129*	*6.3*	*184*	*3*	*22.6*	*9*	*1.2*
Mint Chocolate Chip, High Protein, Gelatelli, Lidl*	1 Scoop/50g	40	1.4	81	4.4	7.7	2.9	3
Mint Chocolate Chip, Ice Dream, Wicked Kitchen, Tesco*	1 Scoop/50g	110	5.1	220	1.7	29.2	10.2	2.1
Mint, After Dinner, Co-Op*	1/6 Tub/82g	143	5	174	2.3	27	6.1	0.6
Mint, Majestic Luxury, Iceland*	1 Serving/80g	269	14.6	337	3.8	39.3	18.3	1.3
Mint, Specially Selected, Aldi*	1 Scoop/50g	112	6.5	224	6	22	13	0.6
Mint, Viennetta, Wall's*	1 Scoop/50g	125	8	250	2.5	25	16	0
Minter Wonderland, Ben & Jerry's*	1 Scoop/44g	117	7.5	266	4	24	17	0
Mochi, Coconut, Little Moons*	1 Ball/32g	81	3.5	253	2.8	34.4	10.9	0
Neapolitan, Average	*1 Serving/70g*	*111*	*4.6*	*158*	*3.1*	*21.9*	*6.5*	*0.6*
Netflix & Chill'd, Ben & Jerry's*	2 Scoops/100g	276	16	276	4.9	28	16	0
Non-Dairy, Reduced Calorie	*1oz/28g*	*33*	*1.7*	*119*	*3.4*	*13.7*	*6*	*0*
Peanut Butter Chocolate Overload, Plant Based, Halo Top*	1 Scoop/50g	72	2.8	145	0.9	21	5.6	0
Peanut Butter Crunch, Haagen-Dazs*	2 Scoops/100g	343	24.4	343	8.4	21.7	24.4	1.7
Peanut Butter Cup, Ben & Jerry's*	1 Scoop/43g	138	9	320	7	25	21	0
Peanut Butter Cup, Halo Top*	1 Scoop/50g	54	1.9	107	9	14.7	3.8	2.6
Peanut Butter, & Cookies, Non-Dairy, Ben & Jerry's*	1 Scoop/50g	144	8	288	4.2	30	16	0
Phish Food, Ben & Jerry's*	1 Scoop/43g	116	5.2	270	3.5	36	12	0
Pistachio, Joe Deluccis Gelato*	1 Scoop/70g	148	6.6	211	2.4	28	9.4	0
Pistachio, West Country, Luxury, M&S*	1 Scoop/50g	95	4.6	190	5.4	21.4	9.1	0.6
Poppin' Popcorn, Moophoria, Ben & Jerry's*	2 Scoops/100g	197	7.9	197	3.3	25	7.9	0
Pralines & Cream, Haagen-Dazs*	1 Sm Tub/78g	213	12.9	272	3.9	27.2	16.5	0
Raspberry Ripple, Average	*1 Serving/70g*	*93*	*3.3*	*134*	*1.9*	*20.8*	*4.7*	*0.1*
Raspberry Ripple, Plant Kitchen, M&S*	1 Scoop/50g	90	4.8	181	0.8	21.1	9.6	3.4

ICE CREAM

	Measure INFO/WEIGHT	per Measure KCAL	FAT	Nutrition Values per 100g / 100ml KCAL	PROT	CARB	FAT	FIBRE
Real, Dairy, Marshfield Farm*	1 Scoop/50g	132	8	263	3.7	27	16	0
Really Creamy Chocolate, Asda*	1 Serving/100g	227	11	227	4.1	28	11	0.4
Rhubarb, & Ginger, Ronaldos*	2 Scoops/100g	164	6	164	3	24	6	1
Rocky Road, Sainsbury's*	1/8 Pot/67g	137	4.9	205	3.8	30.9	7.3	1
Rum & Raisin, TTD, Sainsbury's*	¼ Pot/100g	220	10.4	220	3.8	27.7	10.4	1
Salted Caramel Brownie, Moophoria, Ben & Jerry's*	1 Scoop/50g	93	2.8	186	3.6	28	5.5	0
Salted Caramel Crunch, Dairy Free, Morrisons*	1 Scoop/50g	95	2.8	191	0.3	34.4	5.7	0.6
Salted Caramel Swirl, Double, Oppo*	1 Scoop/50g	59	2.6	118	3.9	14.8	5.2	5.8
Salted Caramel Swirl, Gro, Co-Op*	1 Scoop/50g	100	3.3	199	0.9	33	6.6	1.3
Salted Caramel, & Macadamia, Plant Based, Roar*	1 Scoop/50g	123	5.5	246	1.6	34	11	1.2
Salted Caramel, & Praline, Deluxe, Lidl*	1 Scoop/50g	77	4.6	154	2.5	15.2	9.1	0.5
Salted Caramel, Almond, Alpro*	1 Scoop/50g	91	4.4	182	0.8	18.3	8.7	12.9
Salted Caramel, Carte D'or*	1 Scoop/50g	100	4	200	3	29	8	0
Salted Caramel, Fair Trade, Co-Op*	1/5 Tub/54g	59	1.6	110	6.2	15	2.9	0.6
Salted Caramel, Finest, Tesco*	1 Scoop/50g	108	6.7	215	3.1	19.9	13.4	0.8
Salted Caramel, High Protein, Jude's*	1 Scoop/50g	58	2.4	115	3.9	16.7	4.9	0
Salted Caramel, High Protein, Morrisons*	1 Scoop/50g	48	1.1	96	6	12.5	2.2	6.9
Salted Caramel, Low Sugar, Gelatelli, Lidl*	1 Scoop/50g	64	1.6	128	7.1	22.6	3.3	0
Salted Caramel, Mini Cup, Specially Selected, Aldi*	1 Mini Cup/63g	147	7.6	233	3.1	28	12	0.5
Salted Caramel, Minicup, Haagen-Dazs*	1 Minicup/87g	246	15	282	4.1	27.8	17.2	0
Salted Caramel, Premium, Gelatelli, Lidl*	1 Scoop/50g	56	2.3	112	1.7	15.7	4.6	0.5
Salted Caramel, Salcombe Dairies *	1 Tub/120g	287	15.8	239	4.6	25.4	13.2	0
Salted Caramel, Vegan, Jude's*	1 Scoop/50g	110	4.2	219	1	34.2	8.4	0
Salted Caramel, Vegan, Oatly*	1 Scoop/50g	110	6	220	0.7	27	12	0.7
Salted Carmael, Good As Gold, Co-Op*	1 Scoop/50g	53	1.2	106	7.1	14	2.3	0.6
Save Our Swirled Now, Non Dairy, Ben & Jerry's*	1 Scoop/50g	136	7	273	1.6	34	14	0
Scottish Tablet, Deluxe, Lidl*	1 Scoop/50g	104	5.5	208	4.5	22.4	11	0.5
Sea Salt Caramel (SWE), Nicks*	1 Sm Tub/72g	43	1.6	60	3.5	9.6	2.2	4.2
Sea Salt Caramel, Dairy Free, Halo Top*	1 Scoop/50g	61	2.2	122	3.3	25.6	4.4	6.7
Semifreddo, Gin & Tonic, Individual, Cook*	1 Serving/50g	152	10	303	2.3	23.3	20.1	0
Sicilian Lemon, M&S*	1 Scoop/50g	118	7	237	3.5	24	14	0.3
Sofa So Good , Ben & Jerry's*	1 Scoop/43g	110	5.5	259	4	31	13	0
Soy, Vanilla, Swedish Glace, Wall's*	1 Scoop/50g	87	2.9	174	1	29	5.8	0
Speculoos? Specu-Love, Ben & Jerry's*	1 Scoop/42g	129	8.3	310	3.8	28	20	0
Sticky Toffee Pudding, Co-Op*	1 Scoop/50g	110	5	220	1.9	30	10	0.6
Strawberries & Cream, Minicup, Haagen-Dazs*	1 Minicup/87g	211	13.5	243	3.9	21.8	15.5	0.3
Strawberries & Cream, Haagen-Dazs*	1 Scoop/50g	122	7.8	244	3.9	22.2	15.5	0.3
Strawberries, & Cream, Luxury, Iceland*	1 Scoop/56g	113	3.9	202	2.4	32.3	7	0
Strawberry Cheesecake, Ben & Jerry's*	1 Serving 100g	240	14	240	3	27	14	0
Strawberry Cheesecake, Co-Op*	1/6 Pot/86g	163	6	190	3	29	7	0.2
Strawberry Cheesecake, Halo Top*	1 Scoop/50g	66	2	133	4.8	21	4	0
Strawberry, & Vanilla, Free From, Co-Op*	1 Cone/65g	188	7.8	289	3.5	41.5	12	0.8
Strawberry, Les Classiques, From Multipack, Carte d'Or*	1 Portion/50g	84	3	167	2.8	25	5.9	0
Strawberry, Soft Scoop, Tesco*	1 Serving/46g	78	3.4	170	2.8	23.1	7.4	0.1
Summer Berries & Cream, Minicup, Haagen-Dazs*	1 Minicup/88g	225	14.1	255	3	24.4	16	0.8
Toblerone*	1 Ice Cream/66g	234	13.9	355	3.8	37	21	1.6
Toffee Fudge, Soft Scoop, Asda*	1 Serving/50g	92	3.5	185	2.6	28	7	0
Toffee Vanilla, HE, Tesco*	1 Serving/73g	106	1.8	145	2.5	28.1	2.5	0.5
Toffee, & Vanilla, Giannis, Aldi*	1 Scoop/50g	108	5	216	1.7	29	10	0.6
Toffee, & Vanilla, Morrisons*	1 Scoop/50g	88	3.5	175	1.9	25.9	6.9	0.5
Triple Chocolate, Carte d'Or*	1 Serving/58g	122	5.7	210	3.7	27	9.8	0
Triple Chocolate, Italy, Iceland*	1 Scoop/50g	108	5.2	216	3.4	26.8	10.3	1.4
Tutti Frutti, Tesco*	1 Scoop/50g	78	2.4	157	2.3	25.7	4.7	0.6

	Measure INFO/WEIGHT	per Measure KCAL	FAT	Nutrition Values per 100g / 100ml KCAL	PROT	CARB	FAT	FIBRE
ICE CREAM								
Vanilla & Caramel, Tesco*	1 Scoop/53g	117	4.4	222	2.4	34.5	8.3	0.1
Vanilla Bean, High Protein, Jude's*	1 Scoop/50g	58	2.5	115	3.9	16.4	5	0
Vanilla Bean, Light, Deluxe, Lidl*	1 Serving/64g	110	2.5	172	4.7	26.6	3.9	0
Vanilla Caramel Brownie, Minicup, Haagen-Dazs*	1 Minicup/83g	228	13.7	275	4.4	26.9	16.5	0.4
Vanilla Chocolate Brownie, Haagen-Dazs*	1 Pot/78g	217	13.1	278	4.4	27	16.8	0
Vanilla Flavour, Soft Scoop, Sainsbury's*	1 Serving/71g	96	3.9	136	2.9	18.8	5.5	0.2
Vanilla Florentine, Specially Selected, Aldi*	1 Scoop/62g	148	7.4	238	4.4	28	12	0.7
Vanilla, & Chocolate, Viennetta, Wall's*	2 Scoops/100g	125	7	250	2.5	27	14	0
Vanilla, & Salted Caramel, Free From, Tesco*	1 Scoop/50g	96	5.2	193	1	22.9	10.3	2.1
Vanilla, Alpro*	1 Serving/100g	166	8	166	2.3	16.4	8	9.8
Vanilla, Dairy Milk, Cadbury*	1 Serving/120g	259	13.9	216	3.5	26	11.6	0.1
Vanilla, Dairy, Average	**1 Scoop/40g**	**80**	**4.4**	**201**	**3.5**	**23.6**	**11**	**0.7**
Vanilla, High Protein, Asda*	1 Scoop/50g	35	0.9	70	3.9	9.9	1.8	2.7
Vanilla, Les Classiques, From Multipack, Carte d'Or*	1 Portion/50g	86	3.3	172	2.1	26	6.6	0
Vanilla, Low Fat, Average	**1 Scoop/50g**	**59**	**1.7**	**118**	**2.3**	**19.4**	**3.4**	**0.6**
Vanilla, Madagascan, Carte D'or*	1 Scoop/50g	96	3.8	193	2.1	29	7.5	0
Vanilla, Madagascan, Finest, Tesco*	1 Scoop/50g	108	7.5	216	3.9	16	15	0.5
Vanilla, Madagascan, Light, 4.5% Fat, Carte d'Or*	1 Scoop/50g	71	2.2	142	2.3	21	4.4	0
Vanilla, Madagascan, Low Fat, COU, M&S*	1 Scoop/50g	52	0.2	104	3.9	20.1	0.5	1.5
Vanilla, Made with Madagascan Vanilla, Sainsbury's*	1 Serving/56g	101	4	181	3	25.6	7.2	0.6
Vanilla, Mini Cup, Specially Selected, Aldi*	1 Mini Cup/63g	138	8.2	219	3.2	23	13	0.5
Vanilla, Non-Dairy, Average	**1 Serving/60g**	**107**	**5.2**	**178**	**3.2**	**23.1**	**8.7**	**0**
Vanilla, Pecan, Praline, Oppo*	1 Scoop/50g	70	3.6	141	4.2	17	7.1	4.2
Vanilla, Vanilla Collection, Minicup, Haagen-Dazs*	1 Minicup/87g	217	14.7	249	4.3	19.9	16.9	0
Vanilla, Vegan, Free From, Sainsbury's*	1 Scoop/50g	89	5.9	178	1.4	16.3	11.8	0.5
Vanilla, Vegan, Oatly*	1 Scoop/50g	109	6.5	218	0.8	24	13	0.8
Vanilla, with Cherry Sauce, Tesco*	1 Scoop/56g	114	4.1	204	2.1	32.4	7.3	0.2
Viennese Munt, Mini, Aldi*	1 Ice Cream/35g	87	5	249	4.6	25.1	14.3	1.4
White Chocolate, & Raspberry, Giannis, Aldi*	1 Scoop/50g	84	3	169	8.8	18	6.1	3.1
with Honeycomb Pieces, Giannis, Aldi*	1 Scoop/50g	96	3.8	191	3.3	27	7.6	0
ICE CREAM BAR								
Caramel, Biscuits, Gateau, Tesco*	½ Pack/200g	614	33.4	307	5.7	33.3	16.7	0.6
Caramel, Soft Dipped, Haagen-Dazs*	1 Bar/79g	270	18	342	3.8	30.4	22.8	1.3
Chocolate Covered	**1 Bar/40g**	**128**	**9.3**	**320**	**5**	**24**	**23.3**	**0**
Chocolate, Dark, & Nordic Berry, Nuii*	1 Bar/66g	235	15.2	356	3.8	33	23	3.3
Cookies, & Mint, Idaho Valley, Nuii*	1 Bar/61g	232	13.4	381	4.3	41	22	0
Crunchie, Cadbury*	1 Bar/60g	165	9.7	275	3	29.5	16.2	0.5
Dairy Milk, Caramel, Cadbury*	1 Bar/60g	175	10.3	290	3.6	30.2	17.1	0
Maltesers, Mars*	1 Bar/45g	113	7	252	2.9	25	15.6	0.7
Milk Chocolate, Co-Op*	1 Bar/100g	296	19	296	4.3	27	19	0.8
Peanut Nutter, Carb Killa, Grenade*	1 Bar/43g	137	9	318	16	17	21	7
Salted Caramel, Vegan, Giannis, Aldi*	1 Bar/68g	222	14.3	327	2.2	32	21	1.2
Sea Salt Caramel, Halo Top*	1 Bar/57g	80	1.5	140	6.7	26	2.6	6.4
Snickers, Mars*	1 Bar/53g	179	10.4	337	6.5	33.2	19.6	0
Titan, Dairyfine, Aldi*	1 Bar/42g	152	9.2	362	4.1	36	22	0.7
Twix, Mars*	1 Bar/27g	123	6	451	4.3	56.8	22.1	0
ICE CREAM CONE								
Average	**1 Cone/75g**	**140**	**6.4**	**186**	**3.5**	**25.5**	**8.5**	**0**
Brownie, & Cream, Extreme, Nestle*	1 Cone/71g	207	9.9	292	3.5	38	14	1.5
Chocolate & Nut, Co-Op*	1 Cone/110g	307	17	279	3.9	31	15.5	0.6
Chocolate & Honeycomb, Swirl Top, Waffle, Co-Op*	1 Cone/140g	206	8.7	147	1.9	20.7	6.2	0.6
Chocolate & Orange, Cornetto, Wall's*	1 Cone/56g	188	10.6	335	3.8	35	19	0
Chocolate Fudge, Gooey, Extreme, Nestle*	1 Cone/73g	218	10.4	299	3.8	37.4	14.3	2.5

	Measure INFO/WEIGHT	per Measure KCAL	FAT	Nutrition Values per 100g / 100ml KCAL	PROT	CARB	FAT	FIBRE
ICE CREAM CONE								
Chocolate, Double, Waffle Cone, Co-Op*	1 Cone/135g	209	9	155	2.3	21	6.7	0.9
Chocolate, Mini, Cornetto, Wall's*	1 Cone/36g	110	5.9	300	3.5	34	16	2
Chocolate, Mini, Cornetto, Wall's*	1 Cone/19g	67	3.8	354	4.2	39	20	0
Chocolate, Vanilla & Hazelnut, Sainsbury's*	1 Cone/62g	190	10.5	306	4.5	33.9	16.9	0.6
Classic, Mini, Gelatelli, Lidl*	1 Cone/17g	54	2.7	319	3.6	40.1	15.7	0
Classico, Mini, Cornetto, Wall's*	1 Cone/19g	65	3.6	342	3.8	38	19	0
Cookies & Cream, Tesco*	1 Cone/71g	197	7.9	277	3.9	39.8	11.1	1.4
Cornetto, GFY, Asda*	1 Cone/67g	162	6	241	3	37	9	0.1
Cornetto, Soy & GF, Cornetto, Wall's*	1 Cone/60g	179	8.4	299	1.8	40	14	0
Cornetto, Wall's*	1 Cone/75g	195	9.7	260	3.7	34.5	12.9	0
Cup Cornet, Wafer Cone, Askeys*	1 Cone/4g	13	0.1	376	10.7	77.6	2.5	0
Extreme Raspberry, Cornetto, Nestle*	1 Cone/76g	177	6.2	233	2.4	36.4	8.2	1.5
Flake 99, Cadbury*	1 Cone/125g	245	12.7	196	2.5	23.4	10.2	0.3
Mint Choc, Morrisons*	1 Cone/74g	200	8	270	3.3	39.1	10.8	1.8
Mint, & Chocolate, Tesco*	1 Cone/74g	219	8.8	296	3.5	43.1	11.9	1.6
Mint, Cornetto, Wall's*	1 Cone/60g	169	8.4	282	3.4	37	14	0
Nutty Chocolate, Morrisons*	1 Cone/72g	204	8.8	283	3.8	38.9	12.2	1.4
Rainbow, Tesco*	1 Cone/70g	175	6.6	250	3.1	37.8	9.5	0.6
Rainbow, Uni Cone, Co-Op*	1 Cone/135g	198	8.6	147	2	20	6.4	0.7
Salted Butter Caramel, Gelatelli*	1 Cone/76g	216	8.1	284	3.6	43.4	10.6	0
Salted Caramel, Tesco*	1 Cone/65g	189	7	289	3.2	44.1	10.7	1.9
Salted Caramel, Wall's*	1 Cone/81g	211	9.7	261	2.9	35	12	0
Strawberry & Vanilla, Iceland*	1 Cone/62g	147	5.9	236	2.9	34.7	9.4	0.6
Strawberry & Vanilla, Tesco*	1 Cone/69g	181	7	262	3.3	39	10.1	0.8
Strawberry & Vanilla, Bon Gelati, Lidl*	1 Cone/75g	194	7.2	258	3.2	39.2	9.6	1.2
Strawberry Rose, Co-Op*	1 Cone/130g	204	9.3	157	1.8	21.5	7.2	0.4
Strawberry, Cornetto, Wall's*	1 Cone/75g	198	8.2	264	2.1	40	11	0
Strawberry, Swirl Top, Co-Op*	1 Cone/75g	200	8.2	267	3	40	11	0.6
Strawberry, Vegan, No Moo, Iceland*	1 Cone/65g	188	7.8	290	3.6	42	12	0.5
Toffee & Vanilla, Giannis, Aldi*	1 Cone/71g	195	7.1	275	4.5	42	10	0.6
Toffee, & Vanilla, Free From, Tesco*	1 Cone/65g	185	8.9	285	2.1	38	13.7	0.6
Toffee, & Vanilla, Sainsbury's*	1 Cone/72g	176	6.8	244	2.8	37.1	9.4	0.5
Vanilla, & Chocolate, Classico, Cornetto, Wall's*	1 Cone/60g	178	9.6	296	3.1	33	16	0
Vanilla, & Chocolate, Ms Molly*	1 Cone/61g	160	7.1	263	3.4	35.9	11.6	0.6
Vanilla, Premium, Bon Gelati, Lidl*	1 Cone/71g	211	10	297	3.9	37.8	14.1	1.4
Waffle Cone, Tesco *	1 Cone/12g	49	0.7	411	6.7	81.9	5.6	3.3
ICE CREAM SANDWICH								
'Wich, Ben & Jerry's*	1 Pack/117g	398	19.9	340	4	44	17	1
Choc Chip Cookie, Giannis, Aldi*	1 Sandwich/65g	248	12.4	382	5.1	48	19	2.2
Cookies, & Ice Cream, Giannis, Aldi*	1 Sandwich/36g	109	4	303	5.6	45	11	1.7
Freddo, Dairy Milk, Cadbury*	1 Sandwich/34g	98	4	289	4.2	40.8	11.7	2.1
Neapolitan, Gelatelli, Lidl*	1 Sandwich/90g	134	8	149	1.8	15.1	8.9	0.8
ICE CREAM STICK								
Birthday Cake, Halo Top*	1 Ice Cream/56g	90	3.5	160	6.6	15	6.2	6.4
Biscoff, Lotus*	1 Ice Cream/71g	312	20.6	440	3.4	41	29	0.7
Black Forest, Majestic, Iceland*	1 Ice Cream/63g	210	13.2	333	3.4	30.8	20.9	3.6
Blood Orange, & Milk Chocolate, M&S*	1 Ice Cream/65g	217	12.8	333	3.4	35.5	19.7	0.6
Bobble Mania, Giannis, Aldi*	1 Ice Cream/53g	155	8.5	293	2	35	16	0.4
Brunch, Wall's*	1 Ice Cream/90g	166	9.9	184	2.4	18	11	0
Caramel, Double, Gelatelli, Lidl*	1 Ice Cream/73g	238	14.7	326	3.2	32	20.2	0
Caramel, White Chocolate, & Texan Pecan, Nuii*	1 Ice Cream/43g	163	10.3	380	5.2	37	24	0.6
Choc Sticks, Free From, Tesco*	1 Ice Cream/70g	234	15.8	335	2.9	28.6	22.6	2.9

	Measure	per Measure		Nutrition Values per 100g / 100ml				
	INFO/WEIGHT	KCAL	FAT	KCAL	PROT	CARB	FAT	FIBRE

ICE CREAM STICK

	Measure	KCAL	FAT	KCAL	PROT	CARB	FAT	FIBRE
Chockas, Dark, Mini Selection, Morrisons*	1 Ice Cream/50g	123	8.2	245	2.5	21.7	16.3	1.1
Chockas, Milk, Mini Selection, Morrisons*	1 Ice Cream/50g	114	7.4	228	2.2	21.7	14.7	0.5
Chockas, White, Mini Selection, Morrisons*	1 Ice Cream/50g	116	7.4	232	3	21.7	14.7	0.6
Chocolate & Mint, Tesco*	1 Ice Cream/79g	250	15.6	316	3.2	31.3	19.7	0.7
Chocolate, & Almond, Tesco*	1 Ice Cream/77g	268	18	348	4.5	29.2	23.4	1.2
Chocolate, & Caramel, Tesco*	1 Ice Cream/78g	240	14.7	306	3.1	30.5	18.8	0.6
Chocolate, Belgian, Mini, M&S*	1 Ice Cream/35g	113	7	324	3.9	31.9	19.9	0.6
Chocolate, Feast, Wall's*	1 Ice Cream/70g	245	16.1	350	3.6	31	23	0
Chocolate, Milk, Mini, Tesco*	1 Ice Cream/35g	119	7.7	341	3.1	31.9	22.2	0.9
Chocolate, Milk, Sainsbury's*	1 Ice Cream/75g	240	14.8	320	2.9	32.4	19.7	0.7
Chocolate, Mini Milk, Wall's*	1 Ice Cream/23g	32	0.7	138	4.4	22	3.2	0
Chocolate, White, Tesco*	1 Ice Cream/75g	255	17.5	341	3.3	29.4	23.4	0
Coconut, & Mango, Indian, Nuii *	1 Ice Cream/71g	236	14.2	333	3.7	35	20	0.5
Cookies, & Cream, Tesco*	1 Ice Cream/73g	238	14.6	326	3.3	33	20	0.7
Crunchie Blast, with Popping Candy, Cadbury*	1 Ice Cream/100g	247	14.9	247	3	24.7	14.9	0.5
Exotic, Solero, Wall's*	1 Ice Cream/68g	98	2.1	144	1.7	27	3.1	0
Heavenly Moments, Chocolate Almond Crunch, Asda*	1 Ice Cream/50g	124	8	247	3.4	21	16	1.5
Heavenly Moments, Milk Chocolate Classic, Asda*	1 Ice Cream/50g	112	7	225	2	22	14	0.6
Heavenly Moments, White Chocolate Dream, Asda*	1 Ice Cream/50g	111	7	222	1.6	23	14	0.6
Kinder*	1 Ice Cream/27g	62	3	229	3.1	30	11	0
Maltesers, Mint, Mars*	1 Ice Cream/100g	235	14.4	235	2.2	24.2	14.4	0
Milk Chocolate, & Chopped Almonds, Minis, Lolly, Aldi*	1 Ice Cream/38g	144	9.5	380	4.5	34	25	1.1
Milk Chocolate, Majestic, Iceland*	1 Ice Cream/83g	267	15.5	320	4.4	33.3	18.6	0.6
Milk Chocolate, Minis, Lolly, Multipack, G, Aldi*	1 Ice Cream/34g	120	7.5	353	3.4	35	22	0.5
Mini Mix, Chocolate Coated, Gelatelli, Lidl*	1 Ice Cream/36g	123	7.8	342	3.9	32	21.8	1.2
Mint Choc, Giannis, Aldi*	1 Ice Cream/58g	87	2.3	150	6.3	21	3.9	5.1
Oreo, Coated, Sandwich, Cadbury*	1 Ice Cream/51g	185	10.2	362	4.8	40	20	1.6
Peace Pop, Cookie Dough, Ben & Jerry's*	1 Ice Cream/69g	243	15.2	352	4.6	33	22	0
Peanut Butter, Haagen-Dazs*	1 Ice Cream/70g	290	22.1	414	8.4	23.1	31.5	2.3
Peanut Butter, Swirl, Halo Top*	1 Ice Cream/58g	100	5	172	9.1	16	8.6	6.9
Raspberry, Low Calorie, Morrisons*	1 Ice Cream/60g	81	1.6	135	5.1	22.5	2.6	0.5
Raspberry, Luxury, M&S*	1 Ice Cream/67g	211	12.5	315	1.6	34.4	18.7	1.5
Salted Caramel, & Australian Macadamia, Mini, Nuii*	1 Ice Cream/55g	206	12.1	375	3.8	39	22	0.8
Salted Caramel, & Australian Macadamia, Nuii*	1 Ice Cream/68g	246	14.3	361	3.8	38	21	0.8
Salted Caramel, & Glazed Almond, Magnum*	1 Ice Cream/74g	236	15	319	3.4	29.7	20.3	0
Salted Caramel, Minis, Jude's*	1 Ice Cream/50g	94	5.7	189	2.7	18.2	11.4	0
Salted Caramel, No.1, Waitrose*	1 Ice Cream/78g	277	16.4	353	4.2	36.1	20.9	1.6
Salted Caramel, Specially Selected, Aldi*	1 Ice Cream/81g	285	17	353	2.9	37	21	1
Salted Caramel, Tesco*	1 Ice Cream/69g	209	11.6	301	3.2	34.1	16.7	0.6
Stem Ginger with Belgian Chocolate, Waitrose*	1 Ice Cream/110g	255	14.4	232	2.9	25.5	13.1	1.7
Strawberry Cheesecake, Halo Top*	1 Ice Cream/59g	100	4.3	170	6.3	15	7.3	6.1
Strawberry Split, Essential, Waitrose*	1 Ice Cream/73g	80	1.9	110	1.8	19.5	2.6	0.6
Vanilla, Chocolate Covered, Swedish Glace, Wall's*	1 Ice Cream/37g	105	6.6	285	1	30	18	0
Vanilla, Dark Coco Nutters, Coconut Collaborative*	1 Ice Cream/69g	134	9.7	194	1	11	14	0
Vanilla, Mini Milk, Wall's*	1 Ice Cream/23g	30	0.7	130	3.9	22	3.1	0
Vanilla, with White Chocolate, Mini, Jude's*	1 Ice Cream/50g	88	5.8	177	2.8	15.1	11.6	0
Vienna, Vanilla, Mini, Iceland *	1 Ice Cream/35g	75	4.1	214	3.2	23.8	11.7	0.1
White Chocolate, Giannis, Aldi*	1 Ice Cream/100g	237	14	237	2.4	24	14	0

ICE LOLLY

	Measure	KCAL	FAT	KCAL	PROT	CARB	FAT	FIBRE
Apple, Blackcurrant, & Raspberry, Sorbet, Oasis*	1 Lolly/40g	44	0.2	110	0.5	26.8	0.5	0.9
Assorted, Iceland*	1 Lolly/51g	33	0	65	0	16.2	0	0
Baby, Tesco*	1 Lolly/32g	26	0	80	0.1	20	0	0.1
Berry, Mixed, Gelatelli, Lidl*	1 Lolly/73g	104	1.8	143	1.7	27.5	2.5	0

ICE LOLLY

INFO/WEIGHT	Measure	per Measure		Nutrition Values per 100g / 100ml				
		KCAL	FAT	KCAL	PROT	CARB	FAT	FIBRE
Birthday Cake, Halo Top*	1 Lolly/58g	89	3.4	153	6.4	19	5.8	6.4
Blackcurrant Split, Iceland*	1 Lolly/75g	61	2.4	81	1.1	12	3.2	0.1
Blackcurrant, Sainsbury's*	1 Lolly/74g	62	0.4	84	0.5	19.9	0.5	0.6
Bubblegum Swirl, Iceland*	1 Lolly/55g	74	1.4	135	3.1	24.3	2.6	0.6
Bubblegum, Calippo, Wall's*	1 Lolly/106g	90	0.5	85	0.5	21	0.5	0
Bubblegum, Morrisons*	1 Lolly/51g	57	1.2	112	2.4	20.2	2.4	0.4
Bubblegum, Tesco*	1 Lolly/59g	60	1.1	102	1.8	19.2	1.9	0.6
Chai Latte, Waitrose*	1 Lolly/58g	63	1.8	108	0.9	18.8	3.1	0.6
Chocolate Wonderpops, Sainsbury's*	1 Lolly/43g	118	8.3	276	2.6	21.8	19.4	0.7
Chocolate, Plain, Mini, Tesco*	1 Lolly/31g	94	6.6	304	3.1	24.8	21.4	1.2
Cloudy Apple, Sainsbury's*	1 Lolly/73g	64	0.4	88	0.5	21.5	0.5	0
Coconut, Creamy, Finest, Tesco*	1 Lolly/77g	77	1.6	100	0.4	19.6	2.1	0.6
Coconut, Mango, & Passion Fruit, Sorbet, Oasis*	1 Lolly/40g	47	0.4	118	0.5	26	1.1	0.5
Coconut, Specially Selected, Aldi*	1 Lolly/73g	68	2	93	0.5	16	2.8	0.5
Cola, Morrisons*	1 Lolly/40g	24	0	59	0.1	14.6	0	0
Dip Dab, Barratt*	1 Lolly/67g	84	0.1	126	0.1	31	0.2	0.1
Drumstick Squashies, Swizzels*	1 Lolly/44g	82	4.1	187	2.7	22.6	9.4	0.5
Exotic Burst, Solo, Iceland*	1 Lolly/75g	100	2.8	134	2.3	22.5	3.7	0.6
Exotic Fruit, Ice Cream, Gelatelli, Lidl*	1 Lolly/110g	148	2.8	135	1.8	25.6	2.5	0
Exotic Fruit, Mini, HL, Tesco*	1 Lolly/31g	41	0.6	131	1	26.4	2	1
Fab, Nestle*	1 Lolly/58g	82	2.9	142	0.6	23.1	5.1	0.3
Flumps, Barratt*	1 Lolly/35g	55	2.4	158	2.9	20.9	6.9	0.1
Forest Fruit, Dairy Free, Giannis, Aldi*	1 Lolly/67g	216	14.1	322	2.5	29	21	2.1
Freeze Pops, Premium, R Whites*	1 Lolly/60g	17	0	29	0	7	0	0
Frozen Yoghurt, Mango, Greek Style, Claudi & Fin*	1 Lolly/26g	29	1.3	112	2.7	12.9	5.2	0.5
Frozen Yoghurt, Mixed Berry, Yoo Moo*	1 Lolly/57g	74	0.8	129	2.8	25.8	1.4	0.5
Frozen Yoghurt, Strawberry, Yoo Moo*	1 Lolly/57g	73	0.8	128	2.8	25.5	1.4	0.5
Frozen Yoghurt, Tropical, Yoo Moo*	1 Lolly/57g	74	0.8	130	2.9	26.1	1.4	0.6
Fruit Pastille, Rowntree's*	1 Lolly/65g	57	0.1	88	0.1	21.1	0.1	0.1
Fruit Salad, Barratt*	1 Lolly/65g	100	3.6	154	1.4	24.4	5.6	0
Fruit Spiral, Sainsbury's*	1 Lolly/70g	58	0.4	83	0	20.3	0.5	0
Fruit Split, Waitrose*	1 Lolly/73g	91	2.6	124	2.5	21.7	3.6	0.4
Fruit Splits, Farmfoods*	1 Lolly/49g	48	1.4	98	1.4	16.9	2.8	0
Fruit Splits, Pineapple, Gelatelli, Lidl*	1 Lolly/62g	69	1.6	112	1.5	20.3	2.6	0.6
Fruits of the Forest, Ice Cream, Gelatelli, Lidl*	1 Lolly/110g	145	2.8	132	1.9	24.5	2.5	0
Fruity Swirly Pops, Co-Op*	1 Lolly/70g	52	0.4	75	0.5	18	0.5	0.5
Ice Breakers, Lemon & Orange, Iceland*	1 Lolly/60g	51	0.2	85	0.4	20.4	0.3	0
Ice Breakers, Raspberry & Cherry, Iceland*	1 Lolly/61g	46	0.1	76	0	18.3	0.2	0.3
Ice Burst, Aldi*	1 Lolly/60g	67	1.1	112	0.5	24	1.8	0.5
Ice Cooler, Cola, Giannis, Aldi*	1 Lolly/80g	62	0.1	78	0	19	0.1	0
Lemon & Blackcurrant, Twister, Wall's*	1 Lolly/71g	68	0.4	96	0.7	21	0.6	0
Lemon & Lime, Mini, Calippo, Wall's*	1 Lolly/78g	70	0.4	90	0.5	21	0.5	0
Lemon & Lime, Mini, Lemon Core, Twister, Wall's*	1 Lolly/39g	42	0.5	107	0.6	22	1.2	0
Lemon & Lime, Mini, Strawberry Core, Twister, Wall's*	1 Lolly/39g	41	0.5	105	0.6	22	1.2	0
Lemon & Lime, Tornado, Iceland*	1 Lolly/69g	59	0.2	85	0.3	20.1	0.3	0.1
Lemon & Lime, Twister, Wall's*	1 Lolly/71g	76	0.9	107	0.5	22	1.2	0
Lemonade Flavour, R White*	1 Lolly/75g	71	0	95	0	22.7	0	0.2
Mango, & Fresh Mint, Ice Kitchen*	1 Lolly/75g	60	0	80	0.5	18.2	0	1.1
Mango, Max, Wall's*	1 Lolly/75g	74	0.5	98	0.6	21	0.7	0
Mango, Strawberry, Vanilla, 3Ster, Twister, Wall's*	1 Lolly/72g	70	0.5	98	0.6	21	0.7	0
Milk, Strawberry, Little, Jude's*	1 Lolly/28g	31	0.7	111	2.4	19.7	2.5	0
Mini Whirlz, Giannis, Aldi*	1 Lolly/40g	46	0.6	114	1	24	1.6	0.5
Mint Chocolate, Tesco*	1 Lolly/47g	160	10.9	342	2.7	30	23.2	1.1

	Measure INFO/WEIGHT	per Measure		Nutrition Values per 100g / 100ml				
		KCAL	FAT	KCAL	PROT	CARB	FAT	FIBRE
ICE LOLLY								
No Added Sugar, Tesco*	1 Lolly/32g	26	0	80	0.1	20	0	0.1
Nougat, Barratt*	1 Lolly/62g	123	6.5	199	4.6	21.1	10.5	0.6
Orange, Average	**1 Lolly/72g**	**66**	**0**	**92**	**0.4**	**22.4**	**0**	**0.1**
Parma Violet, Swizzels*	1 Lolly/70g	69	0.1	99	0.2	24	0.2	0.1
Pineapple & Coconut, Cooler, Co-Op*	1 Lolly/68g	105	3.3	154	1.2	26.5	4.8	0
Rainbow, Iceland*	1 Lolly/65g	54	0.1	83	0.1	20.2	0.2	0.1
Raspberry Smoothie, Del Monte*	1 Lolly/88g	85	0	97	0.3	23	0	1.3
Raspberry, Real Fruit Juice, Sainsbury's*	1 Lolly/72g	62	0.1	86	0.3	21	0.1	0.1
Refresher, Fruit Flavour, Bassett's*	1 Lolly/45g	56	0.7	125	1.6	26	1.6	0.3
Rocket, Asda*	1 Lolly/60g	44	0.3	73	0.5	17	0.5	0.6
Rocket, Co-Op*	1 Lolly/60g	42	0	70	0	17	0	0
Rocket, Sainsbury's*	1 Lolly/60g	50	0.3	83	0.5	19.9	0.5	0.5
Rocket, Sour, Tesco*	1 Lolly/59g	43	0.1	73	0.3	17.3	0.2	0.6
Rocket, Sourz, Iceland*	1 Lolly/58g	32	0.1	55	0.3	12.7	0.2	0.6
Rocket, Tesco*	1 Lolly/60g	39	0.1	66	0.4	15.2	0.2	0.6
Rollercoaster, Ice King*	1 Lolly/65g	102	4.2	157	0.5	25	6.4	0.5
Scottish Raspberry, The Best, Morrisons*	1 Lolly/73g	63	0.1	86	0.5	20.3	0.2	0.6
Solo Smoothies, Iceland*	1 Lolly/44g	53	0.2	121	0.1	29.1	0.5	0
Sorbet, Banana, Pineapple, & Coconut, Gelatelli, Lidl*	1 Lolly/63g	78	1.6	124	1.3	22.8	2.5	0
Sorbet, Fruit, Mini, Oasis*	1 Lolly/40g	45	0.2	112	5	27.7	0.5	0.5
Sorbetto, Alphonso Mango, Remeo*	1 Stick/70g	79	0.4	113	0.6	24.7	0.6	0
Sorbetto, Trentino Blackcurrant, Remeo*	1 Stick/70g	80	0.1	114	0.7	26.6	0.1	0
Sour Cherry, & Raspberry, Blasters, Co-Op*	1 Lolly/51g	39	0.3	77	0.5	19	0.5	0.5
Spiral, Aldi*	1 Lolly/70g	47	0.4	67	0.5	16	0.5	0.5
Spiral, Cherry Cola, Aldi*	1 Lolly/70g	37	0	53	0	12	0	0
Strawberries, & Cream, Ice Kitchen*	1 Lolly/75g	111	5.8	148	0.7	18.4	7.7	0
Strawberry & Lemonade, Helter Skelter, Tesco*	1 Lolly/71g	52	0.1	73	1	16.8	0.1	0.5
Strawberry Flavour, Real Fruit Split, Tesco*	1 Lolly/64g	70	1.5	109	1.2	20.5	2.3	0.6
Strawberry Split, Average	**1 Lolly/72g**	**78**	**2.3**	**108**	**1.5**	**18.5**	**3.2**	**0.2**
Strawberry Sprinkles, Asda*	1 Lolly/60g	65	0.4	109	0.5	25	0.7	0.5
Strawberry, Blackcurrant & Vanilla, Mini, Twister, Wall's*	1 Lolly/50g	38	0.3	77	0.7	16	0.7	0
Strawberry, Fruit Split, Iceland*	1 Lolly/54g	57	1.6	105	1.5	17.9	2.9	0.7
Strawberry, Orange & Pineapple, Rocket, Iceland*	1 Lolly/61g	51	0.2	84	0.3	20.2	0.3	0.1
Strawberry, Push Up, Rowntree's*	1 Lolly/80g	55	0.1	69	0.1	15.6	0.1	0.3
Tornados, Sour Cherry & Raspberry, Iceland*	1 Lolly/70g	54	0.1	77	0.1	18.8	0.1	0.1
Traffic Light, Co-Op*	1 Lolly/52g	55	0.4	105	0.4	25	0.8	0
Tropical, Giannis, Aldi*	1 Lolly/75g	112	3.2	150	1.8	26	4.3	0.6
Tropical, Mmmm, Tesco*	1 Lolly/73g	109	3.1	150	1.2	26.6	4.3	0.4
Tropical, Sorbet, Oasis*	1 Lolly/40g	45	0.2	113	0.5	28	0.5	0.5
Twistys, Morrisons*	1 Lolly/70g	51	0.1	73	0.2	17.5	0.2	0
Watermelon, Rowntree's*	1 Lolly/73g	61	0.3	83	0.1	19	0.4	0.3
IRN BRU								
Diet, Sugar Free, Barr's*	1 Can/330ml	2	0	1	0.5	0	0	0
Original, Barr's*	1 Bottle/500ml	100	0	20	0.5	4.8	0	0
Xtra, Barr's*	1 Can/330ml	3	0	1	0.5	0	0	0

	Measure INFO/WEIGHT	per Measure KCAL	FAT	Nutrition Values per 100g / 100ml KCAL	PROT	CARB	FAT	FIBRE
JACKFRUIT								
Bon Bons, BBQ, Plant Chef, Tesco*	1 Bonbon/17g	29	1	171	2.1	24.3	6	5.6
Canned, in Brine, Drained, Tropical Sun*	½ Can/125g	34	0	27	0.8	6.1	0	0.8
Caribbean, Allplants*	1 Serving/410g	549	12.3	134	4.4	20	3	4.6
in Chilli Sauce, Vegan, Waitrose*	1 Pot/350g	259	13	74	2.8	4.7	3.7	5.1
Mexican Style, Plant Pioneers, Sainsbury's*	1 Serving/150g	105	3.6	70	1.9	9.6	2.4	1.4
Raw, Average, Flesh Only	*1 Portion/165g*	*155*	*0.5*	*94*	*1.5*	*24.4*	*0.3*	*1.6*
Shredded, in Mexican Sauce, Vegan, Tesco*	1 Pouch/150g	117	4.6	78	2.3	8.9	3.1	2.4
Shredded, in Thai Green Sauce, Vegan, Tesco*	1 Pack/150g	120	8.8	80	1.4	4.6	5.9	1.6
Shredded, in Thai Red Curry Sauce, Morrisons*	1 Pack/150g	136	8.1	91	1.1	8.4	5.4	2
Thai Green, with Brown Rice, One Pot, Aldi*	1 Pot/383g	287	14.5	75	1.3	8.1	3.8	1.8
JALFREZI								
Chicken, & Pilau Rice, Co-Op*	1 Pack/425g	455	15.7	107	5.9	12	3.7	1.9
Chicken, & Rice, Rice Pot, Sharwood's*	1 Pot/270g	248	1.9	92	3	17.9	0.7	1.1
Chicken, 1138, Oakhouse Foods*	1 Pack/400g	448	13.6	112	6.2	13.6	3.4	1.1
Chicken, Asda*	½ Pack/191g	201	8	105	12	4.2	4.2	1.9
Chicken, Cook*	1 Pack/300g	249	7.8	83	9.8	5.9	2.6	0
Chicken, G&B, Asda*	1 Pack/400g	352	3.2	88	6	13.2	0.8	1.8
Chicken, Hot & Spicy, Sainsbury's*	½ Pack/200g	228	11.4	114	12.8	2.9	5.7	1
Chicken, Ready Set... Cook!, Aldi*	½ Pack/205g	293	13.9	143	17.2	2.5	6.8	1.6
Chicken, Takeaway for One, M&S*	1 Pack/210g	265	12.4	126	12.1	5.3	5.9	1.7
Chicken, with Pilau Rice, Morrisons*	1 Pack/359g	456	11.5	127	6.4	17.6	3.2	1.1
Chicken, with Rice, Ready Meal	*1 Serving/450g*	*557*	*18.9*	*124*	*6.9*	*14.5*	*4.2*	*1.5*
Chicken, with Rice, Ready Meal, Healthy Range	*1 Serving/400g*	*363*	*5.7*	*91*	*7.1*	*12.3*	*1.4*	*1.4*
Paneer, with Saffron Rice, Aromatic, TTD, Sainsbury's*	1 Pack/400g	624	32.4	156	6.1	13.9	8.1	1.5
Vegetable, Waitrose*	1 Pack/400g	256	16	64	2.2	4.7	4	3.7
JAM								
Apricot, Average	*1 Tbsp/15g*	*37*	*0*	*248*	*0.2*	*61.6*	*0*	*1.5*
Bacon, Eat 17*	1 Tbsp/15g	32	0.9	214	7.4	31	6.3	0
Black Cherry, Average	*1 Tbsp/15g*	*37*	*0*	*247*	*0.4*	*61.2*	*0.3*	*0.4*
Blackberry, Extra Special, Asda*	1 Tbsp/15g	29	0.1	190	0.9	45	0.7	0
Blackcurrant, Average	*1 Tbsp/15g*	*38*	*0*	*250*	*0.2*	*62.3*	*0*	*1*
Blackcurrant, Reduced Sugar, Average	*1 Tbsp/15g*	*27*	*0*	*178*	*0.4*	*44.4*	*0.2*	*1*
Blueberry, Best, Hartley's*	1 Tbsp/15g	37	0	244	0.3	60.6	0.1	0
Chilli, M&S*	1 Tbsp/15g	39	0	262	3	62.4	0.3	4.1
Chilli, Mackays*	1 Tbsp/15g	42	0.3	283	0.9	65.9	1.7	0
Chilli, Medium, Sweet, Supermarket, Nando's*	1 Tbsp/15g	21	0	138	0.6	32	0.1	0
Cloudberry, Wild, Scandi Kitchen*	1 Tbsp/15g	25	0.1	169	0.5	42	0.5	3.5
Damson, Extra Fruit, Best, Hartley's*	1 Tbsp/15g	37	0	244	0.2	60.8	0	0
Festive Fruit, Cottage Delight Ltd*	1 Tbsp/15g	40	0	269	0.5	63.9	0.1	0
Fig	*1 Tbsp/15g*	*36*	*0*	*242*	*0.5*	*60*	*0*	*0*
Jalapeno Chilli, Specially Selected, Aldi*	1 Tbsp/15g	41	0.1	271	0.5	67	0.5	0.6
Kiwi & Gooseberry, 66% Fruit, Asda*	1 Tbsp/15g	28	0.1	187	0.5	45	0.5	0
Lingonberry, Rarorda Lingon, Felix*	1 Tbsp15g	28	0	190	0.5	45	0	0
Mixed Fruit, Average	*1 Tbsp/15g*	*38*	*0*	*252*	*0.3*	*63.5*	*0*	*0.5*
Peach, & Ginger, Eswatini*	1 Tbsp/15g	38	0	252	0.5	66	0.1	0
Peach, Pure, Summerland Sweets*	1 Tbsp/15g	75	0	500	0	130	0	0
Plum, & Damson, Soft Set, British, M&S*	1 Tbsp/15g	40	0.1	264	0.4	63.7	0.5	1.3
Plum, Tesco*	1 Tbsp/15g	39	0	261	0.2	64.4	0	0.6
Raspberry, & Lychee, Seasonal, Bonne Maman*	1 Tbsp/15g	36	0	241	0.6	58	0.2	2.3
Raspberry, Average	*1 Tbsp/15g*	*36*	*0*	*239*	*0.6*	*58.6*	*0.1*	*0.9*
Raspberry, Reduced Sugar, Average	*1 Tbsp/15g*	*24*	*0*	*160*	*0.5*	*39.3*	*0.2*	*0.6*
Raspberry, Seedless, Average	*1 Tbsp/15g*	*39*	*0*	*257*	*0.4*	*63.6*	*0*	*0.3*
Rhubarb & Ginger, Baxters*	1 Tbsp/15g	40	0	264	0.4	65	0.1	0.8

J

	Measure INFO/WEIGHT	per Measure KCAL	FAT	Nutrition Values per 100g / 100ml KCAL	PROT	CARB	FAT	FIBRE
JAM								
Stem Ginger, Cottage Delight Ltd*	1 Tbsp/15g	49	0	327	0.1	84.7	0.1	0
Strawberry, & Champagne, Fortnum & Mason*	1 Tbsp/15g	40	0	267	0	61	0	0
Strawberry, Average	***1 Tbsp/15g***	***37***	***0***	***243***	***0.3***	***60.2***	***0.1***	***0.7***
Strawberry, Reduced Sugar, Average	***1 Tbsp/15g***	***28***	***0***	***187***	***0.4***	***45.8***	***0.3***	***0.2***
Wild Blackberry Jelly, Baxters*	1 Tbsp/15g	32	0	210	0	53	0	1.2
JAMBALAYA								
Cajun Chicken, Cooked, BGTY, Sainsbury's*	1 Pack/389g	389	7.4	100	6.2	12.7	1.9	3.3
Chicken & Prawn, World Cafe, Waitrose*	1 Pack/350g	413	12.2	118	5.3	15.3	3.5	2.3
Chicken, HL, Tesco*	1 Pack/385g	319	5.2	83	7.7	9	1.3	2.1
Chicken, Microwaved, G&B, Asda*	1 Pack/380g	353	5.7	93	6.6	12	1.5	2.1
Ready Meal, Average	***1 Pack/450g***	***569***	***18.2***	***126***	***6.4***	***15.7***	***4***	***1.3***
JELLY								
Apple, & Watermelon, 10 Cal, Hartley's*	1 Pot/175g	7	0.2	4	0.1	0.2	0.1	0
Apple, No Added Sugar, Hartley's*	1 Pot/115g	7	0.3	6	0	1.1	0.3	0
Black Forest Gateau, 10 Cal, Hartley's*	1 Pot/175g	9	0.2	5	0.1	0.2	0.1	0
Blackcurrant & Tahitian Vanilla, M&S*	¼ Pack/143g	77	0.4	54	0.3	12.1	0.3	0.6
Blackcurrant, Low Cal, Pot, Asda*	1 Pot/175g	4	0	2	0	0.5	0	0
Blackcurrant, Made Up, Rowntree's*	¼ Jelly/140ml	100	0.1	71	1.4	16.4	0.1	0
Blackcurrant, Made Up, Sainsbury's*	¼ Jelly/150g	98	0	65	1.2	15.1	0	0
Blackcurrant, Ready to Eat, Pot, Hartleys*	1 Pot/124g	51	0.1	41	0.1	9.5	0.1	0
Blueberry & Blackcurrant, 10 Cal, Hartley's*	1 Pot/175g	4	0.2	2	0.1	0.2	0.1	0.1
Cherry Flavoured, Waitrose*	1 Pot/175g	87	0.5	50	0.3	11.3	0.3	0.2
Cloudy Lemonade, Pot, Hartley's*	1 Pot/183g	11	0.9	6	0.5	0.9	0.5	0
Cranberry & Raspberry, Chivers*	1 Pot/150g	9	0	6	0	0.8	0	0
Cranberry, Tiptree, Wilkin & Sons*	1 Serving/15g	39	0	260	0	65	0	0
Crystals, Strawberry, Made Up, Tesco*	1 Serving/145g	9	0	6	1.3	0.3	0	0
Exotic Fruit, M&S*	1 Pot/175g	140	0.4	80	0.1	18.9	0.2	0.9
Fresh Fruit, M&S*	1 Pot/175g	131	0.2	75	0.2	18.4	0.1	0.3
Fruit Salad, Waitrose*	1 Pot/151g	77	0.8	51	0.5	12	0.5	0.5
Juicy, Naturelly*	1 Pot/120g	38	0.1	32	0.5	7.8	0.1	2.5
Juicy, Pouches, Orange, Hartley's*	1 Pouch/90g	27	0.4	30	0.5	7.1	0.5	0
Juicy, Pouches, Strawberry, Hartley's*	1 Pouch/90g	29	0.4	32	0.5	7.8	0.5	0
Juicy, Strawberry, Hartley's*	1 Pouch/90g	36	0.4	40	0.5	9.6	0.5	0
Lemon & Lime, Ready to Eat, Pot, Hartley's*	1 Pot/125g	51	0.1	41	0.1	9.7	0.1	0
Lemon Cheesecake, 10 Cal, Hartley's*	1Pot/175g	7	0.2	4	0.1	0.1	0.1	0
Lemon, Jell-0*	¼ Pack/8g	25	0	312	0	75	0	0
Lime Flavour, Cubes, Hartley's*	1 Cube/12g	36	0	296	5.1	68.9	0	0
Lime, Made Up, Rowntree's*	¼ Jelly/140ml	100	0.1	71	1.4	16.4	0.1	0
Made Up with Water, Average	***1oz/28g***	***17***	***0***	***61***	***1.2***	***15.1***	***0***	***0***
Mandarin & Pineapple, Sainsbury's*	1 Pot/125g	95	0.1	76	0.2	18.9	0.1	1.2
Mango, Low Cal, Asda*	1 Pot/175g	1	0	1	0	0.3	0	0
Orange, 10 Cal, Hartley's*	1 Pot/175g	4	0.2	2	0.1	0.3	0.1	0
Orange, Sugar Free, Made Up, Hartley's*	1 Serving/145g	9	0.8	6	1.3	0.5	0.5	0
Orange, Sugar Free, Rowntree's*	1 Serving/140ml	8	0	6	1.4	0.1	0	0
Orange, Unprepared, Rowntree's*	1 Square/11g	33	0	296	4.4	69.6	0	0
Orange, with Mandarin Pieces, Tesco*	1 Pot/120g	92	0.1	77	0.1	18.7	0.1	0.5
Passion Fruit, & Orange, M&S*	1 Pot/175g	96	0.5	55	0.5	12.2	0.3	0.7
Pink Lemonade, Waitrose*	1 Pot/150g	81	0.8	54	0.5	12.6	0.5	0.5
Raspberry, Aldi*	¼ Pack/34g	79	0.2	231	6.6	51	0.5	0
Raspberry, Individual Pot, Waitrose*	1 Pot/175g	94	0.9	54	0.5	12.5	0.5	0.5
Raspberry, M&S*	1 Pot/175g	100	0.5	57	0.4	12.7	0.3	0.7
Redcurrant, Average	***1oz/28g***	***70***	***0***	***250***	***0.2***	***64.4***	***0***	***0***
Strawberry & Raspberry, Sainsbury's*	½ Pot/280g	230	0	82	0.2	20.2	0	1.2

	Measure INFO/WEIGHT	per Measure KCAL	FAT	Nutrition Values per 100g / 100ml KCAL	PROT	CARB	FAT	FIBRE

JELLY

	Measure INFO/WEIGHT	KCAL	FAT	KCAL	PROT	CARB	FAT	FIBRE
Strawberry Flavour, Sugar Free, Made Up, Rowntree's*	1 Serving/140ml	10	0	7	1.5	0.1	0	0
Strawberry, Glitter, Made Up, Hartley's*	1 Serving/150g	94	0	63	0	15.4	0	0
Strawberry, Sugar Free, Made Up, Hartley's*	1 Serving/145ml	8	0	6	1.1	0.3	0	0
Strawberry, Unprepared, Co-Op*	1 Pack/135g	402	0.1	298	5.5	69.1	0	0
Sugar Free, Dry, Tesco*	1 Pack/13g	36	0	285	55.4	15.6	0	0.2

JELLY BABIES

Bassett's*	1 Sweet/6g	20	0	335	3.5	79.7	0	0
M&S*	1 Pack/125g	418	0	334	5.2	78	0	0
Mini, Rowntree's*	1 Sm Bag/35g	128	0	366	4.6	86.9	0	0

JELLY BEANS

Average	*1 Serving/100g*	*365*	*0.1*	*365*	*0.1*	*91.2*	*0.1*	*0.1*

JERKY

Bacon, Marinated Strips, Kings*	1 Bag/45g	213	14	473	20.2	28	31	0.5
Bacon, Specially Selected, Aldi*	1 Pack/45g	107	3.4	238	35.7	6.8	7.5	0
Beef, BBQ, British, Kings*	1 Pack/25g	68	1.2	273	32	24.9	5	1.1
Beef, British, Texan BBQ, Billy Franks*	1 Pack/30g	96	1.6	320	62	4.7	5.3	2.7
Beef, Honey & Chipotle, Tesco*	1 Pack/40g	123	2.2	307	29.1	34.7	5.4	1.8
Beef, Original, Jack Link's*	1 Pack/25g	65	0.9	260	42	15	3.5	0
Beef, Wagyu, Kings*	1 Pack/25g	94	4.9	374	27	22.5	19.5	0.6
Veggie, Black Bean , Kings*	1 Pack/47g	150	3.3	320	22.5	38.2	7.1	6.8

JUICE

12 Fruits, Multivitamins, Tropicana*	1 Glass/150ml	70	0	47	0.5	11	0	0.6
Activated Charcoal, Fuel Station*	1 Bottle/330ml	103	0.2	31	0.6	6.2	0.1	0
Apple & Cranberry, Average	*1 Glass/250ml*	*114*	*0*	*46*	*0.1*	*10.2*	*0*	*0*
Apple & Elderflower, Copella*	1 Glass/250ml	108	0.2	43	0.4	10.2	0.1	0
Apple & Mango, Average	*1 Glass/200ml*	*108*	*0.1*	*54*	*0.3*	*12.6*	*0*	*0.1*
Apple & Orange, Fresh Up*	1 Serving/150ml	63	0	42	0	10.3	0	0
Apple & Raspberry, Average	*1 Serving/150ml*	*67*	*0.1*	*44*	*0.4*	*10.2*	*0*	*0.2*
Apple & Cherry, Sainsbury's*	1 Serving/150ml	72	0	48	0.3	10.8	0	0.8
Apple & Rhubarb, Caxton Vale*	1 Glass/250ml	115	1	46	0.2	9.7	0.4	0
Apple, & Pear, Gut Health, Waitrose*	1 Serving/150ml	63	0.8	42	0.5	8.7	0.5	0.5
Apple, Cloudy, Pressed, Copella*	1 Glass/100ml	46	0	46	0.2	10.7	0	0.7
Apple, Juhayna*	1 Serving/200ml	96	0	48	0	12	0	0
Apple, Pineapple, & Grape, Dia*	1 Serving/150ml	75	0	50	0.6	11.8	0	0
Apple, Pure, Average	*1 Glass/250ml*	*116*	*0.1*	*47*	*0.1*	*11.2*	*0*	*0*
Apple, Raspberry, & Rhubarb, Waitrose*	1 Serving/150ml	63	0	42	0.2	10.2	0	0.4
Apricot, Nectar, Carrefour*	1 Serving/200ml	100	0.2	50	0.2	12.1	0.1	0.1
Apricot, Nectar, Granini*	1 Glass/200ml	94	1	47	0.5	10.7	0.5	0
Beet Me, Fuel Station*	1 Bottle/330ml	99	0.4	30	0.6	6	0.1	0
Beetroot, Apple, & Rhubarb, Morrisons*	1 Glass/150ml	68	0.2	45	0.7	9.9	0.1	0.7
Breakfast, Ruby, Tropicana*	1 Glass/200ml	90	0	45	0.8	9.7	0	0.7
Brilliant Beetroot, Cawston Press*	1 Glass/200ml	84	0.2	42	0.9	9.3	0.1	0
Carrot, & Ginger, Natures Choice*	1 Serving/330ml	80	1	24	0.5	3.6	0.3	0.2
Carrot, Average	*1 Glass/200ml*	*48*	*0.2*	*24*	*0.5*	*5.7*	*0.1*	*0*
Cherry, Concentrate, Montmorency, Holland & Barrett*	1 Serving/30ml	102	0	340	3.7	81.7	0	8.7
Citrus Shield, Super Juice, Innocent*	1 Serving/150ml	60	0	40	0	10	0	0
Clementine, 100% Pure Squeezed, Tesco*	1 Serving/150ml	71	0	48	0.4	10.7	0	0.2
Clementine, Morrisons*	1 Serving/100ml	48	0.1	48	0.5	10.9	0.1	0.1
Cranberry, Average	*1 Bottle/250ml*	*139*	*0.2*	*56*	*0.1*	*13.4*	*0.1*	*0.3*
Cranberry, No Added Sugar, Average	*1 Glass/200ml*	*11*	*0.1*	*6*	*0.1*	*0.8*	*0*	*0*
Elderberry, Pressed, Pure, Biona Organic*	1 Serving/200ml	76	0	38	2	7.4	0	0.2
Exotic, No Added Sugar, Morrisons*	1 Glass/150ml	24	0	16	0	3.6	0	0
Fruit, Tropical, Pure Premium, Tropicana*	1 Glass/200ml	98	0	49	0.5	11	0	0.8

	Measure INFO/WEIGHT	per Measure KCAL	FAT	Nutrition Values per 100g / 100ml KCAL	PROT	CARB	FAT	FIBRE
JUICE								
Ginger Fix, B Fresh*	1 Bottle/70ml	29	0.2	42	0.7	9.1	0.3	0
Grape, Red, Average	*1 Glass/250ml*	*155*	*0*	*62*	*0.2*	*15.2*	*0*	*0*
Grape, White, Average	*1 Can/160ml*	*95*	*0.1*	*60*	*0.2*	*14.3*	*0.1*	*0.1*
Grapefruit, Pink, Average	*1 Glass/200ml*	*81*	*0.1*	*40*	*0.6*	*9*	*0*	*0.2*
Grapefruit, Pure, Average	*1 Glass/200ml*	*77*	*0.2*	*38*	*0.5*	*8.5*	*0.1*	*0.1*
Green & Clean, Cold Pressed, M&S*	1 Bottle/250g	35	0	14	0.8	2.7	0	0.5
Lemon, Fresh, Average	*1 Lemon/36ml*	*2*	*0*	*7*	*0.3*	*1.6*	*0*	*0.1*
Lemon, from Concentrate, Solevita, Lidl*	1 Tbsp/15ml	4	0.1	28	0.4	2.2	0.5	0.5
Lemon, Jif*	1 Tbsp/15ml	5	0.1	31	0.5	6.9	0.5	0.5
Lime, Fresh, Average	*1 Tsp/5ml*	*0*	*0*	*9*	*0.4*	*1.6*	*0.1*	*0.1*
Multivitamin, Fruit, Vitafit, Lidl*	1 Carton/250ml	135	0.2	54	0.3	12.5	0.1	0.5
Orange & Pineapple, Average	*1 Glass/120ml*	*56*	*0.6*	*46*	*0.4*	*10.5*	*0.5*	*0.5*
Orange & Grapefruit, Average	*1 Carton/250ml*	*106*	*0.2*	*42*	*0.8*	*9.2*	*0.1*	*0.4*
Orange & Lime, Tropicana*	1 Serving/150ml	69	0	46	1.1	9.4	0	0.6
Orange & Mango, Average	*1 Bottle/375ml*	*176*	*0.4*	*47*	*0.5*	*10.7*	*0.1*	*0.2*
Orange & Passionfruit, Tropicana*	1 Serving/150ml	70	0	47	0.8	10	0	0.7
Orange & Raspberry, Tropicana*	1 Bottle/330ml	139	0	42	0.4	9	0	0.8
Orange, Apple & Mango, Calypso*	1 Carton/200ml	92	0.4	46	0	11	0.2	0.1
Orange, Freshly Squeezed, Average	*1 Serving/150ml*	*50*	*0*	*33*	*0.6*	*8.1*	*0*	*1*
Orange, from Concentrate, with Bits, Tesco*	1 Serving/150ml	70	0.2	47	0.5	10.5	0.1	0.1
Orange, Jaffa Gold*	1 Serving/200ml	40	1	20	0.5	4.5	0.5	0.5
Orange, Lemon, & Carrot, Solevita*	1 Pack/200ml	42	0	21	0	5	0	0
Orange, Pure with Bits, Average	*1 Glass/200ml*	*90*	*0.1*	*45*	*0.6*	*10.2*	*0.1*	*0.1*
Orange, Pure, Smooth, Average	*1 Glass/200ml*	*88*	*0.1*	*44*	*0.7*	*9.8*	*0*	*0.2*
Orange, Sparkling, 55, Britvic*	1 Bottle/275ml	135	0.3	49	0.3	11.3	0.1	0.1
Pear, Granini*	1 Serving/200ml	104	1	52	0.5	12.5	0.5	0
Pineapple, Average	*1 Glass/200ml*	*100*	*0.1*	*50*	*0.3*	*11.7*	*0.1*	*0.2*
Pineapple, Kiwi, & Lime, Morrisons*	1 Serving/151ml	77	0.8	51	0.5	11	0.5	0.5
Pomegranate, Pomegreat*	1 Serving/200ml	96	0	48	0.1	12	0	0
Prune, Average	*1 Serving/200ml*	*123*	*0.1*	*61*	*0.6*	*15.3*	*0.1*	*1.8*
Red Fruit, Hacendado*	1 Serving/200ml	64	0.2	32	0.2	5.5	0.1	0.4
Tomato, 100% Pressed, Sainsbury's*	1 Serving/150ml	30	0.8	20	0.6	3	0.5	0.7
Tomato, Average	*1 Glass/200ml*	*40*	*0.1*	*20*	*0.8*	*4*	*0*	*0.4*
Tropical, Farmfoods*	1 Serving/150ml	8	0	5	0	0.9	0	0
Tropical, Jaffa Gold*	1 Serving/200ml	10	1	5	0.5	1	0.5	0.5
Tropical, Pure, Sainsbury's*	1 Glass/200ml	104	0.2	52	0.5	12	0.1	0.1
Tropical, with Kale, M&S*	1 Glass/200ml	94	0.2	47	0.3	11.2	0.1	0.5
Vegetable, Original, V8*	1 Glass/150ml	26	0.2	17	0.9	2.8	0.1	0.9
Yuzu, Cooks' Ingredients, Waitrose*	1 Tbsp/15g	6	0	38	1	8.5	0	0
JUICE DRINK								
Aloe Vera, OKF*	1 Bottle/500ml	175	0	35	0	9	0	0
Aloe Vera, Strawberry, Light, Lidl*	1 Bottle/500ml	95	0	19	0	4.6	0	0
Apple & Raspberry, Sainsbury's*	1 Serving/150ml	84	0.2	56	0.1	13.8	0.1	0.1
Apple & Strawberry, Sainsbury's*	1 Serving/150ml	8	0.1	5	0	1	0	0
Apple & Raspberry, Tesco*	1 Serving/300ml	138	0	46	0.1	11.2	0	0
Apple, & Blackberry, Classic, Fentimans*	1 Glass/200ml	82	0	41	0	10.3	0	0
Apple, & Elderflower, Presse, Sparkling, Finest, Tesco*	1 Serving/150ml	32	0	21	0	5.1	0	0.5
Berries, Mixed, Sparkling, Pressed, Shloer*	1 Can/330ml	66	0	20	0.1	4.6	0	0
Blood Orange, Sparkling, Aranciata Rossa, San Pellegrino*	1 Can/330ml	73	0	22	0.1	4.9	0	0
Cherry, No Added Sugar, Sainsbury's*	1 Carton/250ml	25	0.1	10	0.2	1.9	0	0
Citrus Punch, Zero, Oasis*	1 Bottle/500ml	50	0	10	0	1.3	0	0
Clarity, Nutriseed*	1 Bottle/250ml	99	0.8	40	0	9.2	0.3	0.5
Cranberry & Raspberry, BGTY, Sainsbury's*	1 Glass/250ml	10	0.2	4	0.1	0.7	0.1	0.1

J

JUICE DRINK

	Measure INFO/WEIGHT	per Measure KCAL	FAT	Nutrition Values per 100g / 100ml KCAL	PROT	CARB	FAT	FIBRE
Cranberry Blend, Ocean Spray*	1 Serving/150ml	89	0	59	0.1	13.9	0	0
Cranberry, & Raspberry, Tesco*	1 Serving/150ml	28	0	19	0	4.4	0	0
Cranberry, Asda*	1 Serving/150ml	30	0	20	0	4.5	0	0
Cranberry, Classic, Ocean Spray*	1 Bottle/500ml	115	0	23	0	5.8	0	0
Cranberry, Light, Classic, Ocean Spray*	1 Glass/200ml	16	0	8	0	1.4	0	0
Cranberry, No Added Sugar, HL, Tesco*	1 Glass/200ml	8	0	4	0	1.1	0	0
Cranberry, Tesco*	1 Serving/150ml	30	0	20	0	4.4	0	0.1
Cranberry, Waitrose*	1 Serving/250ml	145	0	58	0.1	13.9	0	0.1
Elderflower, Presse, Sparkling, Bottle Green*	1 Serving/250ml	50	0	20	0	4.8	0	0
Grape, Apple & Raspberry, Asda*	1 Glass/200ml	82	1	41	0.5	9.8	0.5	0.5
Grape, Red, Sparkling, Light, Shloer*	1 Serving/250ml	48	0	19	0.1	4.4	0	0
Grape, Red, Sparkling, Shloer*	1 Serving/250ml	52	0	21	0	4.8	0	0
Grape, Rose, Sparkling, Shloer*	1 Serving/200ml	42	0	21	0.1	4.8	0	0
Grape, White, Sparkling, Shloer*	1 Serving/250ml	52	0	21	0.1	4.8	0	0
Grapefruit, Ruby Red, Ocean Spray*	1 Serving/200ml	83	0	42	0	11.7	0	0
J20, Apple & Raspberry, Britvic*	1 Bottle/275ml	88	0	32	0.1	7.3	0	0.3
J20, Apple, & Watermelon, Spritz, Britvic*	1 Bottle/275ml	55	0	20	0	4.8	0	0
J20, Orange & Passion Fruit, Britvic*	1 Bottle/275ml	63	0	23	0	4.8	0	0
J20, Pear & Guava, Summer Shine, Britvic*	1 Bottle/275ml	47	0	17	0	3.7	0	0
J2O, Apple & Watermelon, Sparkling, Spritz, Britvic*	1 Serving/250ml	58	0	23	0	5.4	0	0
Lemon, Lime, & Apple, Sparkling, Bubbles, Innocent*	1 Can/333ml	90	0	27	0	6.8	0	0
Lemonade, Asda*	1 Glass/200ml	88	0	44	0.1	11	0	0
Limonata, Organic, San Pellegrino*	1 Bottle/200ml	70	0	35	0	10	0	0
Mango, No Added Sugar, Morrisons*	1 Serving/150ml	21	0	14	0.1	2.8	0	0.5
Mango, Rubicon*	1 Serving/100ml	54	0.1	54	0.1	13.1	0.1	0
Mulled Lemonade, Sainsbury's*	1 Serving/150ml	67	0.8	44	0.5	10.8	0.5	0.5
Orange & Lime, Sparkling, Innocent*	1 Can/330ml	93	0	28	0.6	6.5	0	0
Orange & Mango, Spring Water, Sparkling, Rubicon*	1 Bottle/500ml	15	0	3	0	0.5	0	0
Orange, & Clementine, Lean, Tropicana*	1 Serving/150ml	40	0	27	0.4	6.3	0	0
Orange, Caprisun*	1 Pouch/200ml	89	0	45	0	10.8	0	0
Orange, Value, Tesco*	1 Glass/250ml	32	0	13	0	3.3	0	0
Orange, Zero, Vive, Aldi*	1 Serving/200ml	2	1	1	0.5	0.5	0.5	0.5
Passion Fruit, Exotic, Rubicon*	1 Serving/200ml	110	0	55	0.1	13.6	0	0
Peach, & Apricot, Fibre, Still, Get More Vits*	1 Serving/240ml	7	0	3	0	0	0	1.2
Pear, Partially Made with Concentrate, Tesco*	1 Glass/200ml	110	0	55	0	12.4	0	0.2
Pink Cranberry Lemonade, Diet, Sparkling, M&S*	1 Bottle/500ml	15	0.5	3	0.1	0.5	0.1	0.1
Pink, Bubbly, Shloer*	1 Serving/125ml	29	0	23	0.1	5.4	0	0
Pomegranate, Rubicon*	1 Can/330ml	108	0	54	0	13.5	0	0
Raspberry, & Apple, Still, Refresh'd, Robinson's*	1 Bottle/500ml	45	0	9	0	2	0	0
Rhubarb, & Apple, Sparkling, Pressed, Shloer*	1 Can/330ml	63	0	19	0.1	4.4	0	0
Shot, Vitamin D, Moju*	1 Shot/60ml	20	0	33	0.7	7.2	0	0
Sicilian Lemon & Garden Mint, Presse, Finest, Tesco*	1 Serving/250ml	50	0	20	0	5	0	0
Summer Fruits, Fresh, Tesco*	1 Glass/250ml	112	0.2	45	0.1	10.8	0.1	0.3
Summer Fruits, Oasis*	1 Bottle/500ml	90	0	18	0	4.2	0	0
Super, Juicemaster*	1 Bottle/420g	206	7.1	49	0.7	6.9	1.7	1.6
Tangerine & Strawberry, Essenza, San Pellegrino*	1 Can/330ml	3	0	1	0	0	0	0
Tropical Fruit, Tesco*	1 Glass/250ml	118	0	47	0	11.4	0	0
Tropical, Lightly Sparkling, Rio*	1 Bottle/248ml	109	0	44	0	10.6	0	0
Turbo Express, Juicemaster*	1 Bottle/420g	202	8.4	48	0.5	6.4	2	1.4
Vitamin, Energy, Waitrose*	1 Serving/150ml	66	0.2	44	0.3	10.3	0.1	0.4
White, Bubbly, Shloer*	1 Serving/125ml	29	0	23	0.1	5.3	0	0

J

	Measure INFO/WEIGHT	per Measure KCAL	FAT	Nutrition Values per 100g / 100ml KCAL	PROT	CARB	FAT	FIBRE
KALE								
Black, Cavolo Nero, Aldi*	1 Serving/80g	23	0.9	29	2.4	1	1.1	2.8
Curly, Boiled in Salted Water, Average	*1 Serving/60g*	*14*	*0.7*	*24*	*2.4*	*1*	*1.1*	*2.8*
Curly, Raw, Average	*1 Serving/90g*	*25*	*1.2*	*28*	*2.9*	*1.2*	*1.4*	*2.6*
KATSU								
Chicken, Heat to Eat, M&S*	1 Pack/390g	421	8.6	108	6.9	13.6	2.2	2.8
Chicken, Pot, Tesco*	1 Pack/132g	187	4.1	141	7.1	20.4	3.1	1.7
Chicken, Red Pepper, & Jasmine Rice, BFY, M&S*	1 Pack/380g	384	8.4	101	9.2	10.5	2.2	1.4
Yakisoba, Wasabi Co Ltd*	1 Pack/450g	891	32.8	198	8	24.6	7.3	0
KEBAB								
Beef ,& Pepper, Kofta, Waitrose*	1 Kebab/138g	223	13.9	162	14.8	2.9	10.1	0.6
Beef, BBQ, 5% Fat, Ashfield Farm, Aldi*	1 Kebab/80g	120	2.9	150	21	7.4	3.6	1.2
Beef, BBQ, Sweet & Smoky, Fire Pit, Tesco*	1 Kebab/84g	214	15.1	255	20.7	1.9	18	1.1
Beef, Kofta, Spicy, Oakhurst, Aldi*	1 Kebab/45g	112	6.8	248	20	6.5	15	2.8
Beef, Kofta, Uncooked, Tesco*	1 Kebab/73g	163	12.5	225	14	3.2	17.3	1.2
Cheese, & Vegetable, Firepit, Tesco*	1 Kebab/110g	126	8.3	115	7.1	4.1	7.6	0.5
Chicken, & Chorizo, Fire Pit, Tesco*	1 Kebab/59g	93	3	157	26.4	1.7	5	0.1
Chicken, Breast, Cajun, Ocado*	2 Skewers/150g	238	4.8	159	31	1.5	3.2	0.4
Chicken, Buttermilk, King, Waitrose*	1/6 Pack/106g	192	9.8	181	24.1	1.6	9.2	0
Chicken, Coronation, Co-Op*	½ Pack/65g	93	1.7	143	28	1.6	2.6	0
Chicken, Indian Spiced, Morrisons*	½ Pack/112g	159	2.7	142	26.7	3.1	2.4	0.5
Chicken, Mango & Coconut, Tesco*	½ Pack/175g	320	15.2	183	21.6	4	8.7	0.6
Chicken, Peri Peri, King, Oakhurst, Aldi*	¼ Pack/177g	301	11	170	24.3	4.3	6.2	1
Chicken, Shawarma, Ashfield Farm, Aldi*	½ Pack/95g	149	3.9	157	17	12	4.1	1.1
Chicken, Shawarma, Specially Selected, Aldi*	1 Pack/270g	300	8.1	111	5.8	15	3	1.3
Chicken, Shish in Pitta Bread with Salad	*1 Kebab/250g*	*388*	*10.2*	*155*	*13.5*	*17.2*	*4.1*	*1*
Chicken, Shish, Meat Only, Average	*1 Kebab/250g*	*312*	*5.2*	*125*	*25.7*	*0.9*	*2.1*	*0.1*
Chicken, Skewers, Chimichurri, Oakhurst, Aldi*	1 Skewer/83g	135	3.9	163	23	3.9	4.7	1
Chicken, Sweet Chilli, Birchwood Farm, Lidl*	1 Kebab/80g	110	1.8	138	28.1	1.1	2.2	0
Chicken, Sweet Chilli, Waitrose*	2 Kebabs/125g	219	3.8	175	30.2	6.6	3	0.5
Chicken, Teriyaki, Ashfield Farm, Aldi*	1 Skewer/62g	102	3.7	165	21	6.7	6	0.5
Chicken, Thigh, Sticky Barbecue, M&S*	1 Pack/100g	189	6.8	189	26.3	5.7	6.8	0.1
Chicken, Thigh, Yakitori, Skewers, M&S*	½ Pack/150g	248	14.2	165	17.3	2.2	9.5	0.7
Chicken, Tikka, Morrisons*	1 Pack/64g	125	5.8	195	18.2	9.3	9	1.8
Courgette, & Feta, Kofta, Vegetarian, Waitrose*	½ Pack/75g	166	7.8	222	5.8	24.2	10.4	4.1
Doner, in Pitta, with Salad, Average	*1 Serving/400g*	*1020*	*64.8*	*255*	*14.2*	*14*	*16.2*	*0.8*
Doner, Koftas, Oven Baked, Iceland*	1 Kofta/69g	196	15.3	285	16.7	4.3	22.2	0.7
Doner, Meat, & Chips, Heat Me Eat Me*	1 Pack/165g	307	14.9	186	5.4	20	9	2.6
Doner, Meat, Ready Cooked & Sliced, Babek*	1 Serving/100g	300	28	300	14.7	8.1	28	0
Handmade, Seekh, Mumtaz*	½ Pack/94g	201	14.6	214	15.8	2.9	15.5	0
Kofta, Tandoori, Vegan, Waitrose*	1 Kebab/64g	82	2.8	128	5.1	13	4.3	8.5
Lamb, & Chicken, Kofta, Tesco*	2 Koftas/38g	97	5.3	255	14.6	16.8	13.9	2
Lamb, Kofta, Citrus Tikka, Sainsbury's*	1 Kebab/84g	199	11.6	235	18.1	9.8	13.7	2.6
Lamb, Kofta, The Butcher's Hook*	1 Kebab/70g	171	13.3	244	13.3	3.5	19	3
Lamb, Mint, Birchwood Farm, Lidl*	1 Kebab/80g	189	10.5	236	23.3	5.8	13.1	1.2
Lamb, Minted, Ashfield Farm, Aldi*	1 Kebab/54g	137	9.2	254	18.5	5.7	17	0
Lamb, Minted, Grilled, Butchers Choice, Asda*	1 Kebab/49g	126	8.8	257	19	3.4	18	2.7
Lamb, Minted, Iceland*	1 Kebab/33g	92	6.2	277	21.7	4.2	18.7	2.8
Lamb, Minted, Shish, As prepared, Waitrose*	1 Kebab/57g	123	7.3	217	17.2	7.9	12.9	0.1
Lamb, Moroccan, Tesco*	1 Kebab/83g	185	10.4	223	19.3	7.3	12.5	2.5
Lamb, Shami with a Mint Raita Dip, M&S*	½ Pack/90g	189	12.1	210	12.8	9.7	13.4	3.5
Lamb, Shish, The Grill, M&S*	1 Kebab/74g	168	12.6	227	14.6	3.5	17	0.6
Lamb, with Mint, Tesco*	1 Serving/80g	192	13.4	240	16	5.5	16.7	0.4
Meat, Tasty, Heron*	¼ Pack/125g	364	28.6	291	16.5	4.4	22.9	0.3

K

	Measure INFO/WEIGHT	per Measure KCAL	FAT	Nutrition Values per 100g / 100ml KCAL	PROT	CARB	FAT	FIBRE
KEBAB								
Pork, BBQ, Ashfield Farm, Aldi*	1 Kebab/67g	165	9.4	246	23	6.6	14	0.5
Pork, BBQ, Sainsbury's*	1 Serving/90g	65	2.2	72	11	1.4	2.4	0.9
Pork, Greek Inspired, Fire Pit, Tesco*	1 Kebab/73g	161	9.4	221	24	1.8	12.9	0.7
Pork, Outdoor Bred, Co-Op*	1 Kebab/100g	174	9.5	174	17	4.5	9.5	0.7
Pork, Sticky Masala, Tesco*	1 Kebab/79g	182	9.4	231	23.4	7.2	11.9	0.6
Salmon, Chilli & Lime, Fire Pit, Tesco*	2 Kebabs/79g	182	9.4	231	21.8	8.4	11.9	1.2
Salmon, Teriyaki, Waitrose *	1 Kebab/50g	90	4.4	181	20.7	4.3	8.8	0.8
Shish, with Onions & Peppers	**1oz/28g**	**59**	**4.5**	**212**	**12.9**	**3.9**	**16.2**	**1.2**
Veggie, Greek Style, Vivera*	1 Pack/175g	273	15.8	156	15	1.5	9	4.6
KEDGEREE								
Average	**1oz/28g**	**48**	**2.4**	**171**	**15.9**	**7.8**	**8.7**	**0.1**
Haddock, Smoked, Big Dish, M&S*	1 Pack/450g	585	22.5	130	8.5	13	5	1.9
KETCHUP								
Barbeque, Asda*	1 Tbsp/15g	20	0	136	0.9	33	0	0
BBQ, Heinz*	1 Tbsp/15g	21	0	137	1.3	31.3	0.3	0.3
Chilli, Smoked, Gran Luchito*	1 Tbsp/15g	54	0.1	358	1.8	18.4	0.9	0
Curry, Scharf, Hela*	1 Tbsp/15g	21	0	137	0.8	30.8	0.3	0
Mayo, Heinz*	1 Tbsp/15g	65	6.1	432	0.9	14.7	40.8	0
Mustard, Sweet, Tracklements*	1 Tbsp/15g	51	2.6	337	8.3	35.3	17.4	4.5
Tomato, Average	**1 Tbsp/15g**	**18**	**0**	**120**	**1.5**	**28.1**	**0.2**	**0.8**
Tomato, GF, Chippa *	1 Tbsp/15g	14	0.1	90	0.9	21.2	0.5	0
Tomato, Reduced Sugar, Average	**1 Tbsp/15g**	**13**	**0.2**	**87**	**2**	**16.9**	**1.2**	**0.9**
KIDNEY								
Lamb, Fried, Average	**1oz/28g**	**53**	**2.9**	**188**	**23.7**	**0**	**10.3**	**0**
Lamb, Raw, Average	**1oz/28g**	**25**	**0.7**	**91**	**17**	**0**	**2.6**	**0**
Ox, Raw	**1oz/28g**	**22**	**0.5**	**77**	**15.1**	**0**	**1.8**	**0**
Pig, Fried	**1oz/28g**	**57**	**2.7**	**202**	**29.2**	**0**	**9.5**	**0**
Pig, Raw	**1oz/28g**	**22**	**0.7**	**77**	**14**	**0**	**2.4**	**0**
Pig, Stewed	**1oz/28g**	**43**	**1.7**	**153**	**24.4**	**0**	**6.1**	**0**
Veal, Raw, Average	**1 Serving/100g**	**99**	**3.1**	**99**	**15.8**	**0.8**	**3.1**	**0**
KIEV								
Chicken, & Garlic, M&S*	1 Kiev/143g	352	23	246	12.8	11.9	16.1	1
Chicken, Cheese & Ham, Morrisons*	1 Kiev/128g	282	16	221	14.3	12	12.5	1.8
Chicken, COU, M&S*	1 Kiev/150g	188	2.7	125	15.8	10.8	1.8	0.5
Chicken, Garlic & Parsley Butter, Breaded, Waitrose*	1 Kiev/156g	375	21.3	241	17.5	11.1	13.7	1.4
Chicken, Garlic & Herb Butter, Tesco*	1 Kiev/106g	318	22.3	300	13.6	14	21	0.7
Chicken, Garlic & Herb, Birchwood Farm, Lidl*	1 Kiev/120g	356	26	297	13.1	11.3	21.7	1.9
Chicken, Garlic & Herb, M&S*	1 Kiev/130g	359	27	276	14.3	7.3	20.8	1.2
Chicken, Garlic & Herb, Oven Baked, Asda*	1 Kiev/122g	321	20.7	263	13	14	17	1.9
Chicken, Garlic & Herb, Sainsbury's*	1 Kiev/113g	317	22.8	281	11.5	12.5	20.2	1.2
Chicken, Garlic & Herb, Whole Breast, Iceland *	1 Kiev/153g	358	20.2	234	16	11.5	13.2	2.2
Chicken, Garlic & Parsley, BGTY, Sainsbury's*	1 Kiev/125g	267	15.5	213	14.7	10.6	12.4	0.5
Chicken, Garlic, & Herb, Iceland*	1 Kiev/120g	343	24.7	286	13.1	12	20.6	0.2
Chicken, Garlic, Breaded, Tesco*	1 Kiev/128g	373	27.9	291	12.5	11	21.8	0.8
Chicken, Garlic, Oven Baked, Morrisons*	1 Kiev/113g	376	27.3	333	14.7	14	24.2	0.4
Chicken, Garlic, Ready to Cook, Co-Op*	1 Kiev/170g	289	13.9	170	18	6	8.2	0.8
Chicken, Garlic, Whole Breast Fillets, Sainsbury's*	1 Kiev/169g	403	23	238	19.8	8.6	13.6	1.2
Chicken, Garlic, Wild, & Cornish Butter, Gastropub, M&S*	1 Kiev/225g	493	32.2	219	17.3	5	14.3	0.6
Chicken, Ham, & Cheese, Tesco*	1 Kiev/143g	307	18.6	215	14.4	9.3	13	1.3
Chicken, Hunters, Fresh, Sainsbury's*	1 Kiev/113g	241	12.7	214	12.4	15	11.3	1.4
Chicken, Hunters, Tesco*	1 Kiev/122g	285	15.5	234	13.8	15.1	12.7	1.7
Chicken, Wild Garlic, & Jersey Butter, Aldi*	1 Kiev/175g	387	21	221	18.9	9.1	12	0.5
Chicken, with Garlic, & Herb, Inspirations, Birds Eye*	1 Kiev/150g	357	19.5	238	16	14	13	0.5

K

	Measure INFO/WEIGHT	per Measure KCAL	FAT	Nutrition Values per 100g / 100ml KCAL	PROT	CARB	FAT	FIBRE
KIEV								
Fish Fillet, Breaded, with Garlic & Herb, Iceland*	1 Kiev/131g	299	20.1	228	9.1	12.8	15.3	1.4
Garlic, Plant Based, The Vegan Factor*	1 Kiev/119g	315	18.8	265	14.3	16	15.8	0.5
Garlic, Vegan, Plant Chef, Tesco*	1 Kiev/124g	327	19.6	264	14.3	16	15.8	0.5
Haddock, M&S*	1 Kiev/163g	357	21.4	219	12.7	12	13.1	0.9
Mushroom, & Spinach, Oven Baked, Goodlife*	1 Kiev/119g	295	14.8	248	6.9	25.2	12.4	3.7
No Chicken, Garlic, & Herb, Plant Menu, Aldi*	1 Kiev/140g	326	19.6	233	12.3	12.8	14	3.4
No Chicken, Mini, Plant Kitchen, M&S*	1 Kiev/30g	79	4.9	264	13.7	13.9	16.4	2.8
No Chicken, Plant Kitchen, M&S*	1 Kiev/140g	340	21.1	243	12.1	13	15.1	3.3
No-Chick-In, Vegan, V Taste, Morrisons*	1 Kiev/128g	311	16.9	243	5.5	22.9	13.2	5.4
Vegetable, Veggie, M&S*	1 Kiev/155g	267	15.5	172	3.4	15.9	10	2.6
KIMCHI								
Ramyun, Nongshim*	1 Serving/30g	125	3.6	418	7.7	69	12	0
Raw, Vadasz*	1 Serving/50g	8	0.2	15	1.1	1	0.4	1.8
Sliced, Bibigo*	1 Serving/30g	10	0.1	32	1.9	5.4	0.3	0
Spicy, Biona Organic*	1 Serving/50g	12	0.1	24	1.1	3.7	0.2	1.8
Unpasteurised , Kim Kong*	1 Serving/15g	6	0.1	37	2.3	4.4	0.7	2.1
KIPPER								
Baked, Average	**1oz/28g**	**57**	**3.2**	**205**	**25.5**	**0**	**11.4**	**0**
Fillets, Raw, Average	**1 Serving/200g**	**384**	**29.1**	**192**	**14.5**	**0**	**14.6**	**0**
Grilled, Average	**1oz/28g**	**71**	**5.4**	**255**	**20.1**	**0**	**19.4**	**0**
Smoked, Average	**1 Serving/150g**	**322**	**23**	**214**	**18.9**	**0**	**15.4**	**0**
Whole, with Bone, Grilled, Average	**1 Serving/100g**	**161**	**12.2**	**161**	**12.7**	**0**	**12.2**	**0**
KIT KAT								
2 Finger, Dark, Nestle*	2 Fingers/21g	107	5.4	510	5.4	62.2	25.5	5.4
2 Finger, Nestle*	2 Fingers/21g	104	5.1	502	6.7	62.7	24.4	2.1
4 Finger, Dark, Nestle*	4 Fingers/42g	226	14.2	542	8	46.7	34	8.7
4 Finger, Nestle*	4 Fingers/42g	208	10.2	502	6.7	62.7	24.5	2.1
Chunky, Caramel, Nestle*	1 Bar/48g	259	15.3	539	5.2	58.6	31.8	0
Chunky, Double Caramel, Nestle*	½ Bar/21g	109	5.8	520	6.5	61	27.6	1
Chunky, Nestle*	1 Bar/40g	206	10.2	516	5.4	65.1	25.6	1.7
Chunky, Orange, Nestle*	1 Bar/48g	247	12.5	515	5.8	62	26.1	0
Chunky, Peanut, Nestle*	1 Bar/42g	226	13.2	537	8.4	54.9	31.5	0
Chunky, Salted Caramel, Fudge, Nestle*	1 Bar/42g	222	12.5	529	9.2	55.1	29.7	1.9
Chunky, Snack Size, Nestle*	1 Bar/26g	133	7.1	513	6.6	60.4	27.2	1.1
Cookies & Cream, 2 Finger, Nestle*	1 Bar/21g	106	5.3	507	7.6	60.9	25.4	1.4
Dark, & White, Zebra, 4 Finger, Nestle*	1 Pack/42g	216	11.5	521	5.7	60.3	27.6	4.2
Dark, Mint, 2 Finger, Nestle*	1 Bar/21g	105	5.3	502	5.4	60.6	25.3	5.3
Mini, Nestle*	1 Bar/15g	75	3.9	502	7.5	59.4	26	0
Orange, 2 Finger, Nestle*	2 Fingers/21g	107	5.6	507	5.5	61.7	26.5	0
Peanut Butter, Bites, Nestle*	4 Pieces/23g	121	6.5	525	10.8	55.3	28.3	2.1
Ruby, 4 Finger, Kit Kat*	1 Pack/42g	225	13	541	6.5	56.8	31.4	1.4
Senses, Millionaires Shortbread, Nestle*	1 Bar/23g	117	6.1	514	8.1	58.8	26.8	1.5
Senses, Nestle*	1 Bar/31g	165	9.5	531	7.5	56.3	30.7	0
White, Chunky, Nestle*	1 Bar/40g	206	10.6	516	8.1	60.8	26.4	0.5
KIWI FRUIT								
Fresh, Raw, Flesh & Seeds, Average	**1 Kiwi/60g**	**29**	**0.3**	**49**	**1.1**	**10.6**	**0.5**	**1.9**
Weighed with Skin, Average	**1 Kiwi/60g**	**25**	**0.3**	**42**	**0.9**	**9.1**	**0.4**	**1.6**
KOHLRABI								
Boiled in Salted Water	**1oz/28g**	**5**	**0.1**	**18**	**1.2**	**3.1**	**0.2**	**1.9**
Raw	**1oz/28g**	**5**	**0**	**16**	**1.1**	**2.6**	**0.1**	**1.5**
KOMBUCHA								
Captain Kombucha*	1 Bottle/333ml	60	0	18	0	4.4	0	0
Classic, Kinoko*	1 Can/330ml	86	0.3	26	0.5	4.6	0.1	0.1

K

KOMBUCHA

	Measure INFO/WEIGHT	per Measure KCAL	FAT	KCAL	PROT	CARB	FAT	FIBRE
Dry Dragon, Non Alcoholic, Real Kombucha*	1 Serving/250ml	40	0	16	0	3	0	0
Elderflower & Lemon, Naturally Sugar Free, Nexba*	1 Serving/250ml	5	0	2	0	0	0	0
Ginger & Lemon, Organic, Lo Bros Living Drinks*	1 Bottle/330ml	18	1.5	6	0.1	1.1	0.5	0.1
Ginger Beer, Lo Bros Living Drinks*	1 Bottle/330ml	46	1.6	14	0.5	3.4	0.5	0.1
Ginger, & Lemon, The Gutsy Captain*	1 Bottle/400ml	72	0	18	0	4.4	0	0
Ginger, & Turmeric, SynerChi*	1 Can/250ml	8	0	3	0.2	0.6	0	0
Ginger, Organic, Equinox*	1 Can/250ml	32	0.2	13	0.1	3.1	0.1	0.5
No Sugar, Remedy*	1 Can/250ml	25	0.2	10	0.1	2.2	0.1	0.5
Original, Lo Bros Living Drinks*	1 Bottle/330ml	26	0	8	0	2	0	0
Pomegranate, Zero, The Gutsy Captain*	1 Bottle/400ml	0	0	0	0	0	0	0
Raspberry Lemonade, No Sugar, Remedy*	1 Can/250ml	8	1.2	3	0.5	1.5	0.5	0.5
Raspberry, & Elderflower, Equinox*	1 Bottle/275g	38	0.3	14	0.1	3.5	0.1	0.5
Raspberry, & Lemon, Lo Bros Living Drinks*	1 Bottle/330ml	30	0	9	0	1.8	0	0
Raspberry, The Gutsy Captain*	1 Bottle/400ml	72	0	18	0	4.4	0	0
Royal Flush, Non Alcoholic, Real Kombucha*	1 Serving/250ml	40	0	16	0	3	0	0

KORMA

	Measure INFO/WEIGHT	per Measure KCAL	FAT	KCAL	PROT	CARB	FAT	FIBRE
Cashew, & Chickpea, with Black Rice, Mindful Chef*	1 Pack/450g	504	21.2	112	4	11.8	4.7	2.9
Cashew, & Basmati Rice, Passage To India*	1 Pack/280g	420	9	150	2.9	26.4	3.2	1.5
Chicken, & Rice, Free From, Tesco*	1 Pack/369g	565	18.8	153	8.3	17.8	5.1	1.5
Chicken, Donald Russell*	1 Pack/440g	664	45.3	151	9.3	5.5	10.3	1.2
Chicken, Kashmiri, Sainsbury's*	1 Pack/400g	582	26.6	146	7.6	13.3	6.6	1
Chicken, Meal for 2, Sainsbury's*	½ Pack/184g	235	11.6	128	12.5	4.2	6.3	2
Chicken, Rice Pot, As Prepared, Sharwoods*	1 Pot/270g	273	5.9	101	3	17.1	2.2	0.6
Chicken, with Peshwari Coriander Rice, Finest, Tesco*	1 Pack/550g	908	48.4	165	7.5	13.9	8.8	0.9
Chicken, with Pilau Rice, Inspired Cuisine, Aldi*	1 Meal/450g	673	28	150	6.7	16.2	6.2	1.4
Chicken, with Rice, Ready Meal	**1 Pack/400g**	**740**	**34.7**	**185**	**8.4**	**18.1**	**8.7**	**1.7**
Mushroom, & Chickpea, Allplants*	1 Serving/390g	499	26.1	128	3.8	12	6.7	3
Vegetable, Takeaway or Restaurant	**1 Serving/300g**	**336**	**13.5**	**112**	**3.4**	**15.4**	**4.5**	**2.6**
Veggie, The Happy Pear*	1 Pack/400g	360	11.6	90	2.2	12	2.9	2.2

KRISPROLLS

	Measure INFO/WEIGHT	per Measure KCAL	FAT	KCAL	PROT	CARB	FAT	FIBRE
Cracked Wheat, Original, Pagen*	1 Krisproll/13g	48	0.9	380	12	67	7	9
Swedish Toasts, Wholegrain, Pagen*	1 Toast/13g	51	0.8	390	11	67	6.5	8.5

KULFI

	Measure INFO/WEIGHT	per Measure KCAL	FAT	KCAL	PROT	CARB	FAT	FIBRE
Average	**1oz/28g**	**119**	**11.2**	**424**	**5.4**	**11.8**	**39.9**	**0.6**

KUMQUATS

	Measure INFO/WEIGHT	per Measure KCAL	FAT	KCAL	PROT	CARB	FAT	FIBRE
Raw	**1 Kumquat/20g**	**9**	**0.1**	**43**	**0.9**	**9.3**	**0.5**	**3.8**

K

LAGER

	Measure INFO/WEIGHT	per Measure		Nutrition Values per 100g / 100ml				
		KCAL	FAT	KCAL	PROT	CARB	FAT	FIBRE
1664, Alcohol Free, Kronenbourg*	1 Bottle/250ml	38	0	15	0	4	0	0
Alcohol Free, Becks*	1 Serving/275ml	55	0	20	0.7	5	0	0
Alcohol Free, Heineken*	1 Can/330ml	69	0	21	0	4.8	0	0
Amstel, Heineken*	1 Pint/568ml	227	0	40	0.5	3	0	0
Amstel, Pilsner, 3% , Heineken*	1 Serving/200ml	44	0	22	0	1.2	0	0
Average	*½ Pint/284ml*	*117*	*0*	*41*	*0.3*	*3.1*	*0*	*0*
Becks*	1 Can/275ml	113	0	41	0	3	0	0
Blanc, Kronenbourg*	½ pt/284ml	119	0	42	0	3.3	0	0
Budweiser, 66, Anheuser-Busch*	1 Bottle/330ml	102	0	31	0	0	0	0
Budweiser, Light, Anheuser-Busch*	1 Can/440ml	118	0	27	0.3	1.5	0	0
Budweiser, Zero Alcohol, Anheuser-Busch*	1 Can/330ml	46	0	14	0.1	3.3	0	0
Can, Carlsberg*	1 Can/440ml	141	0	32	0	2	0	0
Coors*	1 Can/440ml	154	0	35	0.2	2.7	0	0
Czech, Low Alcohol, M&S*	1 Bottle/500ml	20	0	4	0	0.4	0	0
Draught, Carling*	1 Pint/568ml	189	0	33	0	1.4	0	0
Export, Carlsberg*	1 Can/440ml	185	0	42	0.4	2.8	0	0.4
Export, Foster's*	1 Pint/568ml	210	0	37	0	2.2	0	0
Foster's*	1 Pint/568ml	193	0	34	0	3.1	0	0
German, Low Alcohol, Sainsbury's*	1 Bottle/330ml	92	0.3	28	0.4	5.9	0.1	0.1
Grolsch*	1 Sm Can/330ml	145	0	44	0	2.2	0	0
Heineken*, 5%, Heineken*	1 Bottle/250ml	110	0	44	0.4	3.4	0	0
Innis & Gunn*	1 Bottle/330ml	132	0	40	0.3	3.5	0	0
Light, Coors*	1 Pint/568ml	170	0	30	0.3	1.5	0	0
Light, Corona*	1 Bottle/330ml	105	0	32	1.5	0	0	0
Low Alcohol	*1 Can/440ml*	*44*	*0*	*10*	*0.2*	*1.5*	*0*	*0*
Perlenbacher, 0% Alcohol, Lidl*	1 Bottle/330ml	69	0	21	0	5.2	0	0
Pils, Holsten*	1 Can/440ml	167	0	38	0.3	2.4	0	0
Pilsner, Efes*	1 Can/500ml	226	0	45	0	7.6	0	0
Pilsner, Rheinbacher, Aldi*	1 Can/500ml	135	0	27	0	0	0	0
Premier, Kronenbourg*	½ Pint/284ml	136	0	48	0	0	0	0
Premium	*1 Can/440ml*	*260*	*0*	*59*	*0.3*	*2.4*	*0*	*0*
Premium, French, Biere Speciale, Tesco*	1 Serving/250ml	105	0	42	0.3	3.3	0	0
Premium, Light, Amstel*	1 Can/355ml	95	0	27	0	1.4	0	0
Premium, San Miguel*	1 Bottle/330ml	148	0	45	0.3	3.7	0	0
Shandy, Traditional Style, Asda*	1 Serving/200ml	44	0	22	0	4.6	0	0
Skinny Brands*	1 Bottle/330ml	89	0.3	27	0	0.9	0.1	0
Stella Artois*	1 Can/550ml	220	0	40	0.4	3.1	0	0
Tuborg Green, Carlsberg*	1 Serving/200ml	78	0	39	0.5	2.5	0	0
Vier, Becks*	1 Bottle/275ml	110	0	40	0	3	0	0

LAMB

	Measure INFO/WEIGHT	per Measure		Nutrition Values per 100g / 100ml				
		KCAL	FAT	KCAL	PROT	CARB	FAT	FIBRE
Breast, Lean, Roasted, Average	*1 Serving/100g*	*273*	*18.5*	*273*	*26.7*	*0*	*18.5*	*0*
Chops, Minted, Average	*1 Chop/100g*	*260*	*15.1*	*260*	*25.9*	*5.1*	*15.1*	*0.3*
Cutlets, Neck, Raw, Lean & Fat, Weighed with Bone	*1 Pack 210g*	*359*	*31.7*	*171*	*8.8*	*0*	*15.1*	*0*
Diced, From Supermarket, Healthy Range, Average	*½ Pack/200g*	*277*	*8.9*	*138*	*24.6*	*0.1*	*4.5*	*0*
Grill Steak, Average	*1oz/28g*	*70*	*4.7*	*250*	*20.2*	*4.4*	*16.9*	*0.4*
Lambless, Pieces, Tender, Alt*	½ Pack/160g	248	9.4	155	22	1.9	5.9	3.4
Leg, Joint, Raw, Average	*1 Joint/510g*	*858*	*45.5*	*168*	*20.9*	*1.4*	*8.9*	*0.2*
Leg, Roasted, Lean & Fat, Average	*1oz/28g*	*66*	*3.8*	*237*	*28.6*	*0*	*13.6*	*0*
Leg, Roasted, Lean, Average	*1oz/28g*	*58*	*2.7*	*206*	*29.9*	*0*	*9.6*	*0*
Loin, Chop, Grilled, Lean & Fat, Weighed with Bone	*1 Serving/100g*	*193*	*14*	*193*	*16.8*	*0*	*14*	*0*
Loin, Chops, Raw, Lean & Fat, Weighed with Bone	*1 Serving/100g*	*216*	*17.9*	*216*	*13.7*	*0*	*17.9*	*0*
Mince, Average	*1oz/28g*	*58*	*4.2*	*207*	*17.6*	*0.5*	*14.8*	*0*
Mince, Extra Lean, Sainsbury's*	1 Serving/225g	324	11.9	144	24.1	0	5.3	0.1

	Measure INFO/WEIGHT	per Measure KCAL	FAT	Nutrition Values per 100g / 100ml KCAL	PROT	CARB	FAT	FIBRE
LAMB								
Neck Fillet, Lean, Raw	**1 Serving/100g**	**232**	**17.6**	**232**	**18.4**	**0**	**17.6**	**0**
Rack, Raw, Lean & Fat	**1oz/28g**	**79**	**6.7**	**283**	**17.3**	**0**	**23.8**	**0**
Rack, Raw, Lean Only, Weighed with Bone	**1oz/28g**	**21**	**1.1**	**73**	**8.6**	**0**	**4**	**0**
Rack, Roasted, Lean	**1oz/28g**	**63**	**3.6**	**225**	**27.1**	**0**	**13**	**0**
Rack, Roasted, Lean & Fat	**1oz/28g**	**102**	**8.4**	**363**	**23**	**0**	**30.1**	**0**
Shank, in Minted Gravy, Asda*	1 Shank/267g	465	24.6	174	18	4.1	9.2	0.5
Shank, with Mint Gravy, Oakhurst, Aldi*	1 Shank/266g	357	11.7	134	22	1.1	4.4	0.5
Shanks, Harissa, Slow Cooked, Waitrose*	1 Shank/222g	492	28.1	222	26.5	0.5	12.7	0.5
Shoulder, Cooked, Lean & Fat	**1oz/28g**	**84**	**6.3**	**301**	**24.4**	**0**	**22.5**	**0**
Shoulder, Fillet, Average	**1oz/28g**	**66**	**5.1**	**235**	**17.6**	**0**	**18.3**	**0**
Shoulder, Raw, Average	**1oz/28g**	**70**	**5.7**	**248**	**16.8**	**0**	**20.2**	**0**
Shoulder, Roasted, Whole, Lean	**1oz/28g**	**61**	**3.4**	**218**	**27.2**	**0**	**12.1**	**0**
Steak, Leg, Raw, Average	**1 Steak/150g**	**169**	**5.5**	**112**	**20**	**0**	**3.6**	**0**
Steak, Minted, Average	**1 Steak/125g**	**212**	**9**	**170**	**22.7**	**3.4**	**7.2**	**0.9**
Steak, Raw, Average	**1 Steak/140g**	**190**	**7.6**	**136**	**21.7**	**0.2**	**5.4**	**0**
Stewing, Raw, Lean & Fat	**1oz/28g**	**57**	**3.5**	**203**	**22.5**	**0**	**12.6**	**0**
Stewing, Stewed, Lean & Fat	**1oz/28g**	**78**	**5.6**	**279**	**24.4**	**0**	**20.1**	**0**
LANGOUSTINE								
Fishmongers, Frozen, Tesco*	½ Pack/229g	262	5.3	114	23	0.1	2.3	0.5
Wholetail, Shelled, Scottish, Bannerman's Seafoods*	½ Bag/170g	129	0.7	76	18	0.1	0.4	0.5
LARD								
Average	**1oz/28g**	**249**	**27.7**	**891**	**0**	**0**	**99**	**0**
LASAGNE								
Al Forno, Aldi*	1 Pack/400g	556	26	139	10	9.3	6.5	1.5
Al Forno, Serves 2, Cook*	½ Pack/370g	585	29.2	158	10	11.1	7.9	1.3
Al Forno, The Best, Morrisons*	1 Pack/393g	515	20	131	10.9	9.9	5.1	1.1
Al Forno, TTD, Sainsbury's*	1 Pack/338g	449	18.6	133	7.6	12.4	5.5	1.6
Beef, & Chunky Vegetable, HL, Tesco*	1 Pack/360g	356	8.9	99	6.5	12	2.5	1.2
Beef, & Pancetta, Al Forno, Luxury, Iceland*	1 Pack/423g	838	50.4	198	10.8	11.5	11.9	0.7
Beef, & Smoked Bacon, Waitrose*	½ Pack/350g	606	36.4	173	9.4	10.1	10.4	1
Beef, COU, M&S*	1 Pack/365g	358	7.3	98	6.6	12.7	2	1.2
Beef, Counted, Morrisons*	1 Pack/350g	266	5.4	76	6.2	8.8	1.5	1.1
Beef, Low Fat, Well & Good, Co-Op*	1 Pack/360g	310	6.5	86	7.1	10	1.8	0.8
Beef, Oven Cooked, Slim Cook, Tesco*	1 Pack/453g	344	4.1	76	5.6	10.8	0.9	1.3
Beef, Ready Meal, Average	**1 Serving/400g**	**553**	**24**	**138**	**8.2**	**12.7**	**6**	**1.4**
Beef, Thrive, Waitrose*	1 Pack/232g	306	13.4	132	8.2	11.2	5.8	0.9
Butternut Squash, & Lentil, Love Your Veg!, Sainsbury's*	1 Pack/369g	310	10.3	84	3.2	10.3	2.8	2.8
Butternut Squash, Lean Cuisine*	1 Pack/311g	340	6	109	5.5	17.7	1.9	1
Family, Big Value Pack, Iceland*	¼ Pack/237g	322	14	136	5	15.9	5.9	1.4
for Two, Charlie Bigham's*	½ Pack/345g	545	32.1	158	7	9.5	9.3	0
Lakto-ove-vegetarisk, (swe), Quorn*	1 Pack/350g	350	8.8	100	4.5	14	2.5	1.5
Lentil, Kirstys*	1 Lasagne/357g	282	8.6	79	4.3	12.1	2.4	3.9
Mushroom Bolognese, Wicked Kitchen, Tesco*	1 Pack/370g	355	12.2	96	2.7	12.8	3.3	2.4
Mushroom, & Spinach, Waitrose*	1 Pack/400g	373	14	93	3.1	12.3	3.5	1.3
My Mamma's, Gino D'Acampo*	1 Pack/525g	735	36.2	140	7.2	12	6.9	0.9
Oven Baked, Plant Based, Asda*	1 Pack/365g	361	7.3	99	4.6	14	2	2.7
Sheets, Dry Weight, Tesco*	1 Serving/75g	300	1.1	400	13.2	80.9	1.5	4.9
Sheets, Dry, Average	**1 Sheet/20g**	**70**	**0.3**	**349**	**11.9**	**72.1**	**1.5**	**2.9**
Sheets, Egg, Dry WEight, Napolina*	1 Sheet/17g	63	0.6	369	14	69	3.5	2.4
Sheets, Wholewheat, Sainsbury's*	1 Serving/63g	216	1.4	346	12.7	64.8	2.3	7.8
Steak, 1264, Parsley Box*	1 Pack/270g	348	15.1	129	7	12	5.6	1.1
Triple Layered, Plant Chef, Tesco*	1 Serving/415g	532	17.8	128	8.5	12.5	4.3	2.6
Vegetable, Healthy Range, Average	**1 Serving/400g**	**318**	**8.2**	**80**	**3.5**	**11.8**	**2.1**	**1.5**

L

	Measure INFO/WEIGHT	per Measure KCAL	FAT	Nutrition Values per 100g / 100ml KCAL	PROT	CARB	FAT	FIBRE
LASAGNE								
Vegetable, Ready Meal, Average	**1 Serving/400g**	**408**	**17.6**	**102**	**4.1**	**12.4**	**4.4**	**1**
Vegetarian, Meat Free, Quorn*	½ Pack/250g	251	8.8	109	4.5	13.1	3.8	2.5
LAVERBREAD								
Average	**1oz/28g**	**15**	**1**	**52**	**3.2**	**1.6**	**3.7**	**0**
LEEKS								
Boiled, Average	**1oz/28g**	**6**	**0.2**	**21**	**1.2**	**2.6**	**0.7**	**1.7**
Creamed, Frozen, Waitrose*	1 Serving/225g	115	5.4	51	1.8	5.5	2.4	0
Raw, Unprepared, Average	**1 Leek/166g**	**64**	**1.5**	**39**	**2.8**	**5.1**	**0.9**	**3.9**
LEMON								
Fresh, Raw, Average	**1 Slice/5g**	**1**	**0**	**18**	**0.9**	**2.9**	**0.3**	**2.1**
Peel, Raw, Average	**1 Tbsp/6g**	**3**	**0**	**47**	**1.5**	**16**	**0.3**	**10.6**
Zest, Average	**1 Tsp/2g**	**2**	**0**	**100**	**0**	**25**	**0**	**0**
LEMON CURD								
Average	**1 Tbsp/15g**	**44**	**0.7**	**294**	**0.7**	**62.9**	**4.7**	**0.1**
Luxury, Average	**1 Tsp/7g**	**23**	**0.6**	**326**	**2.8**	**59.7**	**8.4**	**0.1**
Passionfruit, & Lemon, Scarlett & Mustard*	1 Tsp/5g	16	0.5	323	4.2	52.5	10.8	0
Thursday Cottage*	1 Tbsp/15g	54	1.8	363	3.5	59	12	0
LEMON SOLE								
Fillets, Raw, Average	**1 Serving/220g**	**177**	**2.8**	**81**	**17**	**0.2**	**1.3**	**0.3**
Goujons, Average	**1 Serving/150g**	**359**	**18.3**	**239**	**13.9**	**18.5**	**12.2**	**1**
Grilled, Average	**1oz/28g**	**27**	**0.5**	**97**	**20.2**	**0**	**1.7**	**0**
in Breadcrumbs, Average	**1 Fillet/142g**	**322**	**17.4**	**228**	**13.7**	**15.7**	**12.3**	**1**
LEMONADE								
7 Up, Free, Britvic*	1 Bottle/500ml	10	0	2	0	0	0	0
7 Up, Zero, Britvic*	1 Can/330ml	6	0	2	0.1	0.1	0	0
7-Up, Light, Britvic*	1 Can/330ml	4	0	1	0.1	0.2	0	0
Average	**1 Glass/250ml**	**52**	**0.2**	**21**	**0.1**	**5**	**0.1**	**0.1**
Cloudy, Ben Shaws*	½ Bottle/250ml	58	0.2	23	0.1	5.4	0.1	0
Cloudy, Diet, Asda*	1 Serving/200ml	6	1	3	0.5	0.5	0.5	0.5
Cloudy, Diet, Sparkling, M&S*	1 Serving/250ml	8	0.2	3	0.1	0.1	0.1	0.1
Diet, Average	**1 Glass/250ml**	**4**	**0.1**	**2**	**0.1**	**0.2**	**0**	**0**
Diet, Premium, Tesco*	1 Glass/250ml	8	0	3	0	0.4	0	0
Diet, Traditional Style, Tesco*	1 Glass/200ml	6	0	3	0	0.8	0	0
Passion Fruit, Tesco*	1 Can/250ml	10	0	4	0.1	0.4	0	0
Pink, No Added Sugar, Tesco*	1 Glass/250ml	8	0.2	3	0.1	0.3	0.1	0.1
Pink, Zero Calories, Lucozade*	1 Bottle/380ml	8	0	2	0.1	0.1	0	0
Raspberry, & Rose, Tesco*	1 Glass/250ml	5	0.2	2	0.1	0.2	0.1	0.1
Raspberry, Freshly Squeezed, Deluxe, Lidl*	1 Serving/200ml	54	1	27	0.1	5.3	0.5	0.5
Raspberry, R White*	1 Can/330ml	56	0	17	0	3.9	0	0
Rhubarb, Rose, & White Tea, Tesco*	1 Can/250ml	8	0	3	0	0.2	0	0
Schweppes*	1 Can/150ml	27	0	18	0	4.2	0	0
Slimline, Schweppes*	1 Glass/300ml	6	0	2	0	0	0	0
Still, Freshly Squeezed, M&S*	½ Bottle/250ml	100	0.5	40	0.1	9	0.2	0.5
Still, Freshly Squeezed, TTD, Sainsbury's*	1 Serving/200ml	60	1	30	0.5	7.4	0.5	0.5
Still, Morrisons*	1 Bottle/330ml	79	0.3	24	0.2	5.6	0.1	0.1
LEMSIP								
Beechams*	1 Sachet/3g	11	0	387	0	100	0	0
LENTILS								
& Red Kidney Beans, Cajun Style, Merchant Gourmet*	1 Pack/250g	292	8.5	117	5.7	12	3.4	7.7
Black Beluga, Ready to Eat, Merchant Gourmet*	1 Serving/63g	92	0.8	147	10.9	20.5	1.2	5.2
Cakes, Veggie, Beetroot, Kallo*	1 Cake/9g	40	1.1	424	25	51	12	6
French Inspired, Good Grains, Worldwide Foods, Aldi*	½ Pack/125g	149	3	119	7.2	15	2.4	5.2
Good Grains, Aldi*	1 Pack/250g	242	5.2	97	6.6	10	2.1	5

L

	Measure INFO/WEIGHT	per Measure KCAL	FAT	Nutrition Values per 100g / 100ml KCAL	PROT	CARB	FAT	FIBRE
LENTILS								
Green & Brown, Dried, Boiled in Salted Water, Average	**1 Tbsp/30g**	**32**	**0.2**	**105**	**8.8**	**16.9**	**0.7**	**3.8**
Green or Brown in Water, Tinned, Average	**½ Can/132g**	**131**	**0.8**	**99**	**8.1**	**15.4**	**0.6**	**3.8**
Green or Brown, Dried, Average	**1 Serving/50g**	**150**	**0.8**	**301**	**22.8**	**49.8**	**1.5**	**9.6**
Micro Grain, Delicious, Asda*	½ Pack/125g	123	2.3	98	6.8	11	1.8	4.9
Puy, Green, Dry, Average	**1 Serving/100g**	**306**	**1.4**	**306**	**24.7**	**49.5**	**1.4**	**10.3**
Red, Boiled in Unsalted Water, Average	**1oz/28g**	**28**	**0.1**	**102**	**7.6**	**17.5**	**0.4**	**2.6**
Sprouted, Raw, Average	**1 Serving/80g**	**85**	**0.4**	**106**	**9**	**22.1**	**0.5**	**0**
Wholegrain, & Edamame, COOK!, M&S*	½ Pack/145g	252	7	174	7.8	20.6	4.8	8.7
LETTUCE								
Average, Raw	**½ Cup/28g**	**4**	**0.1**	**13**	**1**	**1.7**	**0.3**	**1.1**
Lamb's, Average	**1 Serving/80g**	**12**	**0.2**	**14**	**1.4**	**1.6**	**0.2**	**1**
Little Gem, Average	**1 Lettuce/90g**	**14**	**0.4**	**15**	**0.8**	**1.8**	**0.5**	**0.7**
Radicchio, Red, Raw, Average	**1 Head/220g**	**29**	**0.2**	**13**	**1.4**	**1.6**	**0.1**	**3**
Romaine, Average	**1 Serving/80g**	**12**	**0.4**	**15**	**0.9**	**1.7**	**0.5**	**0.7**
Romaine, Hearts, Average	**1 Serving/80g**	**12**	**0.4**	**16**	**0.9**	**1.7**	**0.6**	**1**
Romaine, Sweet, Average	**1 Serving/80g**	**12**	**0.4**	**16**	**0.9**	**1.6**	**0.6**	**0.8**
Round, Average	**1 Serving/80g**	**10**	**0.2**	**13**	**1.4**	**2.2**	**0.2**	**1.1**
LILT								
Fruit Crush, Coca-Cola*	1 Can/330ml	66	0	20	0	4.6	0	0
Fruit Crush, Zero, Coca-Cola*	1 Can/330ml	12	0	4	0	0.3	0	0
Zero, Coca-Cola*	1 Can/330ml	10	0	3	0	0.3	0	0
LIME								
Peel, Raw	**1 Tbsp/6g**	**3**	**0**	**47**	**1.5**	**16**	**0.3**	**10.6**
Raw, Flesh Only, Average	**1 Lime/71g**	**18**	**0.1**	**25**	**0.6**	**8.8**	**0.2**	**2.4**
Zest, Average	**1 Tsp/2g**	**2**	**0**	**100**	**0**	**25**	**0**	**0**
LINGUINE								
Chicken, & Mushroom, Eat Well, M&S*	1 Pack/370g	359	8.5	97	9	9.2	2.3	1.7
Cooked	**1 Serving/100g**	**133**	**0.7**	**133**	**5.1**	**26.3**	**0.7**	**1.1**
Dry, Average	**1 Serving/100g**	**352**	**2.2**	**352**	**13.1**	**70**	**2.2**	**2.8**
Fresh, Dry, Average	**1 Pack/250g**	**681**	**6.5**	**272**	**12.3**	**51.7**	**2.6**	**4**
Prawn, King, & Chilli, Specially Selected, Aldi*	1 Serving/388g	466	13.6	120	5.5	16	3.5	1.4
Prawn, King, Fresh Ideas, Morrisons*	1 Pack/390g	343	5.1	88	5.3	12.5	1.3	2.4
Prawn, with Tomatoes, Chef Select, Lidl*	1 Pack/380g	383	4	101	4.3	17.4	1	2
Seafood, with Prawns, Scallops, Salmon, & Cod, M&S*	1 Pack/368g	379	11.8	103	7.8	10.1	3.2	1.2
Spinach, & Prawn, G&B, Asda*	1 Pack/371g	338	6.7	91	4	14	1.8	1.7
LINSEEDS								
Average	**1 Tsp/5g**	**23**	**1.7**	**464**	**21.7**	**18.5**	**33.5**	**26.3**
LION BAR								
Milk, Duo, Nestle*	1 Pack/60g	296	13.7	493	5.3	65.7	22.8	1.4
Mini, Nestle*	1 Bar/16g	80	3.6	486	4.6	67.7	21.7	0
Nestle*	1 Bar/52g	248	11.2	478	6.5	64.6	21.6	0
Peanut, Nestle*	1 Bar/40g	195	10	488	8.1	57.1	25	2.3
White, Nestle*	1 Bar/40g	194	8.8	484	5.7	65.2	22.1	0.4
LIQUEURS								
Amaretto, Average	**1 Pub Shot/25ml**	**97**	**0**	**388**	**0**	**60**	**0**	**0**
Chambord*	1 Serving/35ml	79	0	225	0	29.3	0	0
Cointreau, Specialite De France	**1 Serving/37ml**	**80**	**0**	**215**	**0**	**8.5**	**0**	**0**
Cream, Average	**1 Shot/25ml**	**81**	**4**	**325**	**0**	**22.8**	**16.1**	**0**
Grand Marnier*	1 Pub Shot/35ml	94	0	268	0	22.9	0	0
High Strength, Average	**1 Shot/25ml**	**78**	**0**	**314**	**0**	**24.4**	**0**	**0**
Kirsch, Average	**1 Shot/25ml**	**67**	**0**	**267**	**0**	**20**	**0**	**0**
LIQUORICE								
Allsorts, Average	**1 Sm Bag/56g**	**195**	**2.9**	**349**	**3.7**	**76.7**	**5.2**	**2**

L

	Measure INFO/WEIGHT	per Measure KCAL	FAT	Nutrition Values per 100g / 100ml KCAL	PROT	CARB	FAT	FIBRE
LIQUORICE								
Catherine Wheels, Barratt*	1 Wheel/22g	65	0.1	290	3.8	67.2	0.3	0.7
Catherine Wheels, Sainsbury's*	1 Wheel/17g	49	0.1	286	3.8	67.2	0.3	0.7
Filled, Klene*	1 Serving/20g	65	0.1	324	3.6	77	0.4	0
Panda*	1 Bar/32g	109	0.2	340	3.8	78	0.5	0
Raspberry, All Natural, Panda*	1 Bar/32g	98	0.1	307	3.6	72	0.4	0.9
Raspberry, Soft Eating, Rj's Licorice Ltd*	1 Stick/40g	139	0.6	347	3.1	79	1.4	0
Shapes, Average	**1oz/28g**	**78**	**0.4**	**278**	**5.5**	**65**	**1.4**	**1.9**
Sweet, Sugar Free, Dominion, Aldi*	1/3 Pack/25g	56	0.1	224	0.5	77	0.5	6.3
LIVER								
Calves, Fried	**1oz/28g**	**49**	**2.7**	**176**	**22.3**	**0**	**9.6**	**0**
Calves, Raw	**1oz/28g**	**29**	**1**	**104**	**18.3**	**0**	**3.4**	**0**
Chicken, Cooked, Simmered, Average	**1 Serving/100g**	**167**	**6.5**	**167**	**24.5**	**0.9**	**6.5**	**0**
Chicken, Fried, Average	**1oz/28g**	**47**	**2.5**	**169**	**22.1**	**0**	**8.9**	**0**
Chicken, Raw, Average	**1oz/28g**	**26**	**0.6**	**92**	**17.7**	**0**	**2.3**	**0**
Lamb's, Braised, Average	**1 Serving/100g**	**220**	**8.8**	**220**	**30.6**	**2.5**	**8.8**	**0**
Lamb's, Fried, Average	**1oz/28g**	**66**	**3.6**	**237**	**30.1**	**0**	**12.9**	**0**
Lamb's, Raw, Average	**1 Serving/125g**	**171**	**7.8**	**137**	**20.3**	**0**	**6.2**	**0**
Ox, Raw	**1oz/28g**	**43**	**2.2**	**155**	**21.1**	**0**	**7.8**	**0**
Pig's, Raw	**1oz/28g**	**32**	**0.9**	**113**	**21.3**	**0**	**3.1**	**0**
Pig's, Stewed	**1 Serving/70g**	**132**	**5.7**	**189**	**25.6**	**3.6**	**8.1**	**0**
Veal, Deluxe, Lidl*	1 Slice/150g	188	5.2	125	19.6	3.8	3.5	0
LIVER & BACON								
& Onions, Cook*	1 Portion/280g	372	21.3	133	11.8	4.3	7.6	0.5
Meal for One, M&S*	1 Pack/452g	430	16.7	95	7	8	3.7	1.2
Mini, Frozen, Waitrose*	1 Pack/250g	277	12	111	5.6	10.6	4.8	1.3
with Fresh Mashed Potato, Waitrose*	1 Pack/400g	416	17.2	104	7.3	9	4.3	1.3
with Mash, Colcannon, Asda*	1 Pack/400g	344	10.4	86	6.6	8.6	2.6	0.8
with Mash, Serves 1, Classic, Sainsbury's*	1 Pack/450g	448	18.7	103	6.4	8.6	4.3	2.5
LIVER SAUSAGE								
Average	**1 Slice/10g**	**22**	**1.5**	**216**	**15.3**	**4.4**	**15.2**	**0.2**
LOBSTER								
Boiled, Average	**1oz/28g**	**29**	**0.4**	**103**	**22.1**	**0**	**1.6**	**0**
Dressed, Canned, John West*	1 Can/43g	45	2.1	105	13	2	5	0
Raw, Average	**1 Serving/100g**	**92**	**1.4**	**92**	**18.7**	**0.3**	**1.4**	**0**
LOGANBERRIES								
Raw	**1oz/28g**	**5**	**0**	**17**	**1.1**	**3.4**	**0**	**2.5**
LOLLIPOPS								
Assorted, Co-Op*	1 Lolly/10g	40	0	400	0	97	0	0
Chupa Chups*	1 Lolly/12g	47	0	388	0	95	0.3	0
Cola, Chupa Chups*	1 Lollipop/12g	47	0	393	0	97	0	0
Double, Swizzels*	1 Lolly/50g	20	0	41	0	7	0	0
Drumsticks, Swizzels*	1 Lolly/12g	50	0.7	413	0.4	87.9	6.1	0
Refreshers, Bassett's*	1 Lolly/6g	25	0	417	0	108.3	0	0
LOQUATS								
Raw	**1 Med/16g**	**5**	**0**	**30**	**0.3**	**7.6**	**0.1**	**1.1**
LOZENGES								
Blackcurrant Flavour, Fishermans Friend, Lofthouses*	1 Lozenge/1g	3	0	251	0.1	97.2	1.3	0
Honey, Lemon, Echinacea, Herb, Ricola*	1 Lozenge/4g	15	0	385	0	95	0	0
Original Extra Strong, Fishermans Friend, Lofthouses*	1 Lozenge/1g	4	0	382	0.3	94.9	0	0.5
Original, Victory V*	1 Lozenge/3g	9	0	350	0	91	0	0
LUCOZADE								
Apple Blast, Lucozade*	1 Serving/200ml	70	0	35	0	8.4	0	0
Energy, Citrus Chill, Lucozade*	1 Serving/250ml	92	0	37	0	8.9	0	0

L

	Measure INFO/WEIGHT	per Measure KCAL	FAT	Nutrition Values per 100g / 100ml KCAL	PROT	CARB	FAT	FIBRE
LUCOZADE								
Energy, Original, GlaxoSmithKline UK Limited*	1 Bottle/380ml	141	0	37	0	8.9	0	0
Orange Energy Drink, GlaxoSmithKline UK Limited*	1 Bottle/500ml	350	0	70	0	17.2	0	0
Orange, Sport Lite, GlaxoSmithKline UK Limited*	1 Serving/500ml	50	0	10	0	2	0	0
Orange, Zero, Lucozade*	1 Bottle/380ml	15	0	4	0.1	0.5	0	0
Raspberry Sport Body Fuel, GlaxoSmithKline UK Limited*	1 Bottle/500ml	140	0	28	0	6.4	0	0
Zero Calories, Lucozade*	1 Serving/250ml	10	0	4	0.1	0.5	0	0
LUNCHEON MEAT								
Pork, Average	**1oz/28g**	**81**	**6.8**	**288**	**13.3**	**4**	**24.3**	**0**
Slices, Eastmans, Tesco*	2 Slices/25g	47	3.4	189	14.2	2.4	13.6	0.1
LYCHEES								
Fresh, Raw, Flesh Only	**1oz/28g**	**16**	**0**	**58**	**0.9**	**14.3**	**0.1**	**0.7**
in Syrup, Average	**1oz/28g**	**19**	**0**	**69**	**0.4**	**17.7**	**0**	**0.4**
Raw, Weighed with Skin & Stone	**1oz/28g**	**6**	**0**	**22**	**0.3**	**5.5**	**0.1**	**0.2**

L

	Measure INFO/WEIGHT	per Measure KCAL	FAT	Nutrition Values per 100g / 100ml KCAL	PROT	CARB	FAT	FIBRE
M&M'S								
Caramel, Crunchy, Limited Edition, M&M's, Mars*	1 Pack/36g	172	6.6	478	3.7	73.5	18.4	0
Crispy, Mars*	1 Serving/36g	179	8.8	498	4.1	63.9	24.4	2.7
Mars*	1 Pack/45g	218	9.7	485	5	68	21.5	0
Mini, Mars*	1 Pack/36g	176	8.4	489	6.3	63.6	23.2	0
Mix, Mars*	1 Serving/43g	214	10.2	503	7.7	63	24	0
Peanut Butter, Mars*	1 Pack/46g	240	14	520	8.7	56.3	30.3	2.2
Peanut, M&M's, Mars*	1 Serving/45g	230	11.6	516	10	58	26	0
Salted Caramel, M&M's, Mars*	1 Serving/36g	172	6.5	474	4.4	71	18	0
MACADAMIA NUTS								
Plain, Average	**1 Pack/100g**	**750**	**77.6**	**750**	**7.9**	**4.8**	**77.6**	**5.3**
Roasted, Salted, Average	**6 Nuts/10g**	**75**	**7.8**	**748**	**7.9**	**4.8**	**77.6**	**5.3**
MACARONI								
Dry, Average	**1oz/28g**	**99**	**0.5**	**354**	**11.9**	**73.5**	**1.7**	**2.6**
GF, Dry, Free From, Morrisons*	1 Serving/75g	258	0.8	344	5.6	77.1	1.1	1.9
MACARONI CHEESE								
& Mushroom, Vegan, Waitrose*	1 Pack/260g	320	13.5	123	4	14.1	5.2	2.1
As Prepared, Pasta n Sauce, Batchelors*	½ Pack/181g	214	3.4	118	4.9	19.9	1.9	0.6
Bites, Mac N Cheese, Crispy, M&S*	½ Pack/100g	255	13.8	255	7.9	23.9	13.8	1.6
Black Truffle, Pasta Evangelists*	1 Serving/349g	565	37.7	162	6.6	9.5	10.8	0
Butternut Cauli, Plant Chef, Tesco*	1 Pack/450g	518	11.2	115	3.6	18.6	2.5	1.8
Canned	**1oz/28g**	**39**	**1.8**	**138**	**4.5**	**16.4**	**6.5**	**0.4**
Cashew Mac, Plant Kitchen, M&S*	1 Pack/350g	532	25.2	152	5.3	15	7.2	2.8
Mac & Greens, Vegan, Allplants*	1 Serving/410g	570	23.4	139	6.8	13	5.7	3.2
Ready Meal, Average	**1 Serving/400g**	**580**	**25.5**	**145**	**6**	**15.8**	**6.4**	**1**
Rice, GF, Amy's Kitchen*	1 Pack/257g	416	18.2	162	6.3	18	7.1	0.4
Triple, Finest, Tesco*	1 Pack/400g	645	22.2	174	7.3	22	6	1.4
with Bacon, Microwaved, Iceland*	1 Pack/344g	499	17.6	145	5.8	18.5	5.1	1.2
with Ham, & Cauliflower, Cook*	1 Pack/300g	306	9.6	102	6.5	12.7	3.2	1.7
with Pancetta, Crispy, Deluxe, Lidl*	½ Pack/368g	769	38.3	209	8.9	19.2	10.4	1.7
MACAROONS								
Coconut, Mini, Sainsbury's*	1 Macaroon/22g	100	5.3	445	3.9	51.6	23.4	6.3
Coconut, Tesco*	1 Macaroon/33g	143	6.3	432	4.5	58	19	5.5
French, Average	**1 Serving/60g**	**225**	**11**	**375**	**6.7**	**46.7**	**18.3**	**3.3**
MACKEREL								
Atlantic, Raw, Average	**1 Fillet/75g**	**154**	**10.4**	**205**	**18.6**	**0**	**13.9**	**0**
Fillets, Honey Smoked, Sainsbury's*	1 Pack/280g	1016	80.9	363	20.5	5.1	28.9	0.5
Fillets, in Brine, Average	**1 Can/88g**	**206**	**15.3**	**234**	**19.4**	**0**	**17.4**	**0**
Fillets, in Mustard Sauce, Average	**1 Can/125g**	**274**	**19.4**	**219**	**14.1**	**5.4**	**15.5**	**0**
Fillets, in Olive Oil, Average	**1 Serving/50g**	**149**	**12.2**	**298**	**18.5**	**1**	**24.4**	**0**
Fillets, in Spicy Tomato Sauce, Average	**1oz/28g**	**56**	**3.9**	**199**	**14.3**	**3.8**	**14**	**0**
Fillets, in Sunflower Oil, Average	**1 Can/94g**	**262**	**20.6**	**279**	**20.2**	**0.2**	**21.9**	**0.2**
Fillets, in Tomato Sauce, Average	**1 Can/125g**	**251**	**18.3**	**200**	**14.3**	**2.7**	**14.7**	**0**
Fillets, Smoked, Average	**1 Fillet/75g**	**251**	**21.1**	**334**	**19.7**	**0.5**	**28.2**	**0.3**
Fillets, Smoked, Skinless, Average	**1 Fillet/65g**	**215**	**17**	**330**	**20.9**	**2.8**	**26.1**	**0.4**
Fillets, Smoked, Sweet Chilli, Market St, Morrisons*	½ Pack/93g	295	21.6	317	19.6	6.4	23.2	2.1
Fried in Blended Oil	**1oz/28g**	**76**	**5.5**	**272**	**24**	**0**	**19.5**	**0**
Grilled	**1oz/28g**	**67**	**4.8**	**239**	**20.8**	**0**	**17.3**	**0**
King, Raw	**1 Fillet/198g**	**208**	**4**	**105**	**20.3**	**0**	**2**	**0**
Raw with Skin, Weighed with Bone, Average	**1oz/28g**	**64**	**4.7**	**227**	**18.9**	**0**	**16.8**	**0**
Smoked, Peppered, Average	**1oz/28g**	**87**	**7**	**310**	**20.4**	**0.3**	**25.2**	**0.2**
MADRAS								
Beef, Canned, Cooked, Morrisons*	1 Can/401g	570	33.3	142	11.7	4.7	8.3	1
Beef, Tesco*	1 Pack/460g	616	37.7	134	10.6	4.5	8.2	1.2

	Measure INFO/WEIGHT	per Measure KCAL	FAT	Nutrition Values per 100g / 100ml KCAL	PROT	CARB	FAT	FIBRE
MADRAS								
Chicken, M&S*	1 Pack/400g	492	25.2	123	12.7	2.7	6.3	2.2
Chicken, M&S*	1 Pack/400g	472	23.2	118	12.9	2.5	5.8	1.9
Chicken, Sainsbury's*	1 Pack/400g	532	29.6	133	11	4.5	7.4	1.9
Chicken, Taste of India, Tesco*	½ Pack/215g	275	14.2	128	10.2	5.7	6.6	2.7
Chicken, Waitrose*	1 Pack/400g	672	42	168	14.6	3.7	10.5	1.8
MAGNUM								
Almond, Mini, Wall's*	1 Mini/55g	155	9.4	281	3.9	27	17	0
Almond, Vegan, Wall's*	1 Magnum/90g	248	16.2	276	2.2	26	18	0
Almond, Wall's*	1 Magnum/73g	243	14.6	332	4.8	32	20	0
Caramel, Double, Mini, Wall's*	1 Mini/50g	174	10	348	3.2	37	20	0
Caramel, Double, Wall's*	1 Magnum/73g	246	14.6	338	3.2	36	20	0
Chocolate, Double, Mini, Wall's*	1 Mini/50g	182	11.5	365	4	33	23	0
Chocolate, Double, Wall's*	1 Magnum/69g	248	15.9	359	4.1	33	23	0
Classic, Mini, Wall's*	1 Mini/50g	168	11	336	3.7	31	22	0
Classic, Vegan, Wall's*	1 Magnum/90g	234	14.3	261	1.3	27	16	0
Classic, Wall's*	1 Magnum/79g	244	15	309	3.6	29	19	1.2
Dark, Mini, Wall's*	1 Mini/50g	165	11	329	3.8	29	22	0
Double Coconut, Wall's*	1 Magnum/88g	239	14.1	272	3.2	27	16	0
Espresso, Black, Mini, Wall's*	1 Mini/50g	159	10.5	317	3.7	29	21	0
Espresso, Black, Wall's*	1 Magnum/82g	237	15.6	289	3.4	27	19	0
Honeycomb, & Almond, Wall's*	1 Magnum/73g	243	15	333	4.5	32.9	20.6	0
Honeycomb, Wall's*	1 Magnum/78g	240	13.2	308	3.6	35	17	0
Mint, Mini, Wall's*	1 Mini/50g	165	10.5	330	4.2	30	21	0
Mint, Wall's*	1 Magnum/78g	244	14	313	3.1	33	18	0
Peanut Butter, Double, Wall's*	1 Magnum/73g	245	15.3	336	4.2	32	21	0
Pistachio, Wall's*	1 Magnum/75g	250	15.8	333	4.2	30	21	0
Raspberry, Double, Mini, Wall's*	1 Mini/50g	170	10	339	3	36	20	0
Raspberry, Pink, Mini, Wall's*	1 Mini/50g	166	11.5	332	2.9	31	23	0
Raspberry, Pink, Wall's*	1 Magnum/73g	239	15.3	328	2.9	30	21	0
Ruby, Mini, Wall's*	1 Magnum/43g	136	7.7	317	5	34	18	0
Strawberry, & White, Wall's*	1 Magnum/88g	250	13.2	284	3	34	15	0
White Chocolate, & Cookies, Wall's*	1 Magnum/90g	285	16.2	317	4	34	18	0
White, Mini, Wall's*	1 Mini/55g	137	8.3	248	2.8	26	15	0
White, Wall's*	1 Magnum/79g	239	14.2	303	3.5	33	18	0
MAKHANI								
Chicken, Co-Op*	1 Pack/380g	467	16.3	123	8.7	12	4.3	1.5
Chicken, Morrisons*	½ Pack/175g	301	18.6	172	9.8	8.4	10.6	2
Chicken, Sainsbury's*	½ Pack/199g	313	21.3	157	12.2	2.9	10.7	2.5
Chicken, Tikka, Waitrose*	1 Pack/400g	560	30.4	140	14	3.8	7.6	2.1
MALTESERS								
MaltEaster, Chocolate Bunny, Mars*	1 Bunny/29g	157	9	541	7.1	57	31	0
Mini Bunnies, Mars*	1 Bunny/12g	64	3.6	534	8	53.5	30.2	0
Teasers, Mars*	1 Teaser/9g	48	2.8	538	7.3	57.2	30.8	0
Truffles, Mars*	1 Truffle/9g	51	3.2	565	6.7	53	36	0
MANDARIN ORANGES								
in Juice, Average	*1oz/28g*	*11*	*0*	*39*	*0.7*	*9*	*0*	*0.5*
in Light Syrup, Average	*1 Can/298g*	*201*	*0.1*	*68*	*0.6*	*16*	*0*	*0.1*
Segments, Canned, in Juice, Morrisons*	1 Can/298g	101	0	34	0.7	7.7	0	0.3
Weighed with Peel, Average	*1 Sm/50g*	*14*	*0*	*27*	*0.7*	*6.2*	*0.1*	*0.9*
MANGE TOUT								
Boiled in Salted Water	*1oz/28g*	*7*	*0*	*26*	*3.2*	*3.3*	*0.1*	*2.2*
Raw, Average	*1 Serving/80g*	*25*	*0.2*	*31*	*3.5*	*4*	*0.2*	*1.1*
Stir-Fried in Blended Oil	*1oz/28g*	*20*	*1.3*	*71*	*3.8*	*3.5*	*4.8*	*2.4*

	Measure INFO/WEIGHT	per Measure KCAL	FAT	Nutrition Values per 100g / 100ml KCAL	PROT	CARB	FAT	FIBRE
MANGO								
Dried, Average	**1 Serving/50g**	**174**	**0.5**	**347**	**1.4**	**83.1**	**1**	**4.9**
in Syrup, Average	**1oz/28g**	**22**	**0**	**80**	**0.3**	**20.5**	**0**	**0.9**
Ripe, Raw, Weighed with Skin & Stone, Average	**1 Mango/225g**	**60**	**0.2**	**27**	**0.3**	**6.5**	**0.1**	**1.2**
Ripe, Raw, without Peel & Stone, Flesh Only, Average	**1 Mango/207g**	**118**	**0.4**	**57**	**0.7**	**14.1**	**0.2**	**2.6**
Sliced, Canned, in Light Syrup, Del Monte*	½ Can/210g	141	0	67	0.5	16	0	1.4
Slices, Canned, in Juice, Tesco*	¼ Can/106g	41	0.1	39	0.4	8.6	0.1	0.8
MARINADE								
Peri Peri, Hot, Nando's*	1 Serving/20g	9	0.6	43	0.9	2.4	2.8	0
Peri Peri, Lemon & Herb, Nando's*	1 Serving/20g	13	0.7	63	0.5	5.9	3.6	0
Peri Peri, Mango & Lime, Nando's*	1 Serving/20g	32	1.2	159	0.7	26.9	5.9	0
Peri Peri, Medium, Nando's*	1 Serving/20g	16	0.8	82	1.4	8.1	4.2	0
Peri Peri. & Hot & Spicy, Brooklea, Aldi*	½ Pack/18g	58	0.9	329	5.3	60	5	12
Peri-Peri, Coat & Cook, Hot , Nando's*	1 Sachet/120g	113	7.9	94	1.9	4.9	6.6	0
Peri-Peri, Coat & Cook, Lemon & Herb, Nando's*	1 Sachet/120g	86	5.8	72	0.5	5.6	4.8	0
Sweet Chilli, Lime, Lemongrass, The Grill, M&S*	1 Bottle/250g	602	11.2	241	0.4	48.3	4.5	3
Tandoori, Oven Bake, Pataks*	½ Pack/60g	65	4.1	109	3	7.9	6.8	0
Tandoori, Spice, Patak's*	1 Tbsp/15g	15	0.4	99	3.5	10.1	2.7	5.9
Tikka, Oven Bake, Patak's*	1 Sachet/120g	120	7	100	2.7	7.6	5.8	0
MARJORAM								
Dried	**1 Tsp/1g**	**2**	**0**	**271**	**12.7**	**42.5**	**7**	**0**
MARMALADE								
Lemon & Lime, Average	**1 Tbsp/15g**	**40**	**0**	**267**	**0.2**	**66.4**	**0.1**	**0.4**
Lemon with Shred, Average	**1 Tbsp/15g**	**37**	**0**	**248**	**0.2**	**61.6**	**0**	**0.6**
Lime with Shred, Average	**1 Tbsp/15g**	**39**	**0**	**261**	**0.2**	**65**	**0.1**	**0.4**
Mandarin, Tangy, Bonne Maman*	1 Tbsp/15g	36	0	239	0.3	59	0.1	0.8
Merry Christmas, Cottage Delight*	1 Tbsp/15g	43	0	286	0.4	69.8	0.1	0
Olde English, Thick Cut, Hartley's*	1 Tbsp/15g	39	0	261	0.3	64.6	0.1	0
Onion, Red, Stokes*	1 Tbsp/15g	37	0	244	1.2	57.2	0.1	1.3
Orange & Ginger, Average	**1 Tbsp/15g**	**40**	**0**	**264**	**0.2**	**65.7**	**0.1**	**0.3**
Orange & Tangerine, Tiptree, Wilkin & Sons*	1 Tbsp/15g	40	0	268	0	67	0	0
Orange with Shred, Average	**1 Tbsp/15g**	**39**	**0**	**263**	**0.2**	**65.2**	**0**	**0.3**
Orange, Fine Cut, Maribel, Lidl*	1 Tbsp/15g	36	0	238	0.1	58.1	0.2	0.7
Orange, Med Cut, Tiptree, Wilkin & Sons*	1 Tbsp/15g	41	0	273	0	67	0	0
Orange, Reduced Sugar, Average	**1 Tbsp/15g**	**26**	**0**	**170**	**0.4**	**42**	**0.1**	**0.6**
Orange, Seville, Dark, Specially Selected, Aldi*	1 Tbsp/15g	41	0.1	271	0.5	66	0.6	0.5
Orange, Shredless, Average	**1 Tbsp/15g**	**39**	**0**	**261**	**0.2**	**65**	**0**	**0.1**
Orange, Sweet, Bonne Maman*	1 Tbsp/15g	36	0	241	0.3	59	0.1	1.2
Oxford, Original, Frank Cooper*	1 Tbsp/15g	38	0.1	255	0.4	62	0.4	0
Tangy, Fine Cut, Grandessa, Aldi*	1 Tbsp/15g	44	0.1	293	0.7	70	0.9	0.9
Thick Cut, Maribel*	1 Tbsp/15g	36	0	240	0.2	58.3	0.1	1.5
MARMITE*								
Yeast Extract, Marmite*	1 Tsp/9g	23	0	260	34	30	0.5	3.5
MARROW								
Boiled, Average	**1oz/28g**	**3**	**0.1**	**9**	**0.4**	**1.6**	**0.2**	**0.6**
Raw	**1oz/28g**	**2**	**0**	**6**	**0.3**	**1.2**	**0.1**	**0.3**
MARS								
Bar, Duo, Mars*	1 Pack/79g	355	13.3	450	4.3	69.3	16.9	0
Bar, from Multipack, Mars*	1 Bar/39.4g	177	6.6	448	4.4	69.3	16.7	0
Bar, Funsize, Mars*	1 Bar/18g	80	2.8	443	3.9	70.7	15.7	0
Bar, Protein, Mars*	1 Bar/57g	200	4.6	351	33	39	8.1	0
Bar, Snacksize, Mars*	1 Bar/34g	151	5.7	448	4.3	69	17	0
Bar, Standard, Single, Mars*	1 Bar/51g	228	8.5	448	4.4	69.3	16.7	0

	Measure INFO/WEIGHT	per Measure KCAL	FAT	Nutrition Values per 100g / 100ml KCAL	PROT	CARB	FAT	FIBRE
MARSHMALLOWS								
Average	*1 Mallow/5g*	*16*	*0*	*327*	*3.9*	*83.1*	*0*	*0*
Chocolate Mallows, Cadbury*	1 Mallow/13g	56	2.2	435	4.7	64.7	17.4	0.8
Double Chocolate, Mallow & Marsh*	1 Serving/35g	135	4.2	385	6.9	66.1	12.1	0
Fat Free, Tesco*	1 Mallow/7g	24	0	339	3.4	80.8	0.2	0.5
No Added Sugar, Sainsbury's*	1 Mallow/2g	5	0	206	3.3	77	0.1	0
Pink & White, Co-Op*	1 Mallow/7g	24	0	340	3	82	0	0
Pink & White, Waitrose*	1 Mallow/8g	26	0	327	3.8	77.4	0.1	0.5
Raspberry & Cream, Sainsbury's*	1 Mallow/7g	23	0	330	4.1	78.5	0	0.5
Soft Mallow Pieces, Mr Mallo*	1 Pack/80g	273	0	341	4.2	81	0	0
Tesco*	1 Serving/25g	82	0	329	2.9	78.9	0.1	0.5
Vegan, Dandies*	2 Mallows/28g	96	0	343	0	86	0	0
MARZIPAN								
Chocolate, M&S*	1 Marzipan/10g	47	2.2	470	7.6	58.3	22.1	3.8
Eggs, in Dark Chocolate, Favorina, Lidl*	1 Egg/20g	91	4	454	6.1	62.2	19.9	4.9
Fruits, Almond, M&S*	1 Sweet/12g	52	2	432	5.6	63.4	16.3	4.6
Plain, Average	*1oz/28g*	*115*	*4*	*412*	*5.8*	*67.5*	*14.2*	*1.7*
MASALA								
Aubergine, Microwaved, Waitrose*	½ Pack/125g	120	8.8	96	1.7	5	7	3.4
Beef, Coconut, Indian, Waitrose*	½ Pack/150g	232	15.6	155	10.2	4	10.4	2
Chicken, Chilli, Waitrose*	1 Pack/350g	378	17.8	108	11.4	3.3	5.1	1.9
Fish, Meal Kit, Aldi*	½ Pack/168g	260	15.3	155	10	6.7	9.1	2.5
Prawn Mango, Waitrose*	½ Pack/175g	175	11.2	100	5.8	4.3	6.4	1.3
Vegetable, Indian, Sainsburys*	1 Pack/300g	273	17.7	91	2.2	5.5	5.9	3.7
MASH								
Carrot, & Swede, Frozen, Microwaved, Iceland*	1 Serving/80g	23	0.4	29	1.1	3.6	0.5	2.7
Carrot, Swede, & Potato, Waitrose*	½ Pack/224g	110	4	49	0.9	5.9	1.8	2.8
Pea, & Mint, M&S*	1 Serving/151g	134	5.6	89	4.6	6.8	3.7	5.1
Root Vegetable, Tesco*	½ Pack/203g	136	2.4	67	1.5	11.6	1.2	1.8
MAYONNAISE								
Average	*1 Tsp/5g*	*35*	*3.8*	*690*	*0.9*	*1.6*	*75.5*	*0*
Avocado Oil, Vegan, Hunter & Gather*	1 Tsp/5g	27	3	545	2.6	0.7	59.8	0.2
Extra Light, Average	*1 Tbsp/33g*	*34*	*2*	*102*	*0.7*	*10.5*	*6.2*	*0.8*
Garlic, Retail, Average	*1 Tsp/11g*	*44*	*4.4*	*403*	*1.2*	*8.6*	*40.3*	*0*
Reduced Calorie, Average	*1 Tsp/6g*	*18*	*1.7*	*301*	*0.7*	*8.9*	*29*	*0.1*
Vegan, Heinz*	1 Tbsp/15g	98	10.8	654	0	3.9	72	0
Vegan, Hellmann's*	1 Serving/15g	98	10.8	654	0.5	3.9	72	0
Veganaise, Sriracha, Follow Your Heart*	1 Tbsp/15g	75	7.8	503	1.8	7.5	52	0
Vegenaise, Organic, Follow Your Heart*	1 Tbsp/15g	93	10	622	0.8	3.6	67	0
Winiary*	1 Tbsp/15ml	106	11.4	704	1.5	2.9	76.3	0
with a Spark of Chilli, Hellmann's*	1 Tbsp/15ml	41	4	276	0.8	7.5	27	0.3
MEAL REPLACEMENT								
Banana, Vegan, Purition*	1 Serving/40g	183	11.2	457	37.5	10.9	28	16.9
Berry Yoghurt Muesli, Exante Diet*	1 Sachet/54g	200	6.5	371	31	31	12	6.8
Breakfast Shake, Chocolate, Be Fast*	1 Bottle/250ml	200	3.8	80	3.3	12	1.5	2.5
Diet, Vegan, Chocolate Silk, The Protein Works*	1 Scoop/30g	110	1.1	365	74	4.5	3.6	10
Drink, Banana, Ready to Drink, Huel*	1 Bottle/500g	400	19	80	4	6.7	3.8	1.4
Drink, Berry, Ready To Drink, Huel*	1 Bottle/500ml	400	18.5	80	4	6.8	3.7	1
Lemon, Bar, Exante Diet*	1 Bar/59g	220	6	373	30.5	37.7	10.1	6.3
Mac & Cheeze, Hot & Savoury, Huel*	1 Serving/102g	400	11	392	24.5	46.1	10.8	6.2
Madras, Hot & Savoury, Huel*	1 Serving/95g	400	13	421	26.3	41	13.7	13.7
Mango, & Passion Fruit, Lighter Life*	1 Pack/40g	154	4.3	385	33.5	31.2	10.8	10.5
Pasta, Green Pesto Flavoured, The 1;1 Diet*	1 Sachet/54g	202	3.3	374	24.1	53.7	6.1	4.6
Pie, Cottage, Country, New You Plan*	1 Pack/49g	176	4	359	33.3	32.1	8.2	11.7

	Measure INFO/WEIGHT	per Measure KCAL	FAT	Nutrition Values per 100g / 100ml KCAL	PROT	CARB	FAT	FIBRE

MEAL REPLACEMENT

	Measure INFO/WEIGHT	KCAL	FAT	KCAL	PROT	CARB	FAT	FIBRE
Porridge, Cinnamon, Pot, Exante Diet*	1 Pot/60g	214	4.7	357	29.3	33	7.8	15
Porridge, Mixed Berry, CWP*	1 Pack/54g	200	2.6	370	23.1	56.1	4.9	4.4
Protein Blend, Myprotein*	1 Serving/50g	196	6.5	392	34	34	13	0
Ready to Drink, Chocolate, Huel*	1 Bottle/500ml	400	19	80	4	6.5	3.8	1.6
Ready to Drink, Vanilla, Huel*	1 Bottle/500ml	400	18.5	80	4	6.8	3.7	1.2
Shake, Abnormal*	1 Shake/95g	300	6.4	316	27.4	34.7	6.7	9
Shake, All-in-One, Vegan, Dark Chocolate Berry, Bulk*	2 Scoops/60g	216	1.9	360	48.2	31.8	3.2	5.6
Shake, Banana, Body design*	1 Serving/55g	206	2.1	375	32.7	49.6	3.8	6.6
Shake, Cafe Latte, As Sold, Shake That Weight*	1 Shake/34g	129	3	379	36.2	36.5	8.7	5.1
Shake, Caramel Shake, Exante Diet*	1 Shake/50g	201	6.5	402	36	30	13	7.1
Shake, Caramel, As Sold, Shake That Weight*	1 Sachet/34g	131	2.9	385	36.8	37.7	8.6	4.6
Shake, Chocolate, Diet Now*	1 Sachet/34g	137	4	404	27.6	42.8	11.9	6.7
Shake, Chocolate, Fullstop.*	1 Shake/70g	256	8.1	365	23.9	31.4	11.6	19.5
Shake, Chocolate, Mediterranean Style, Fast 800*	1 Serving/50g	198	9.8	397	46.1	9.8	19.6	14.7
Shake, Chocolate, Mo Protein *	1 Bottle/310ml	155	0.6	50	8.4	3.5	0.2	0.3
Shake, Chocolate, Nutrition, For Goodness Shakes*	1 Bottle/315ml	132	0.9	42	6.4	3.1	0.3	0.7
Shake, Coconut Latte, Exante Diet*	1 Pack/53g	205	6.4	386	32	33	12	6.5
Shake, Coffee Flavour, Huel*	1 Serving/100g	400	13	400	30	37	13	7.7
Shake, Coffee, Original, Fast 800*	5 Scoops/50g	200	8.2	399	44.2	13.6	16.3	14.8
Shake, Ensure Max Protein, Vanilla, Abbott Nutrition*	1 Shake/330ml	150	1.5	45	9.1	1.8	0.4	0.9
Shake, Latte, Smooth, Great Shape, Asda*	1 Bottle/330ml	208	6.9	63	5.5	4.8	2.1	1.6
Shake, Lemon Cheesecake, Exante*	1 Serving/51g	201	6.6	394	33.5	34.7	13	8.2
Shake, Mango, Made Up, Diet Now*	1 Sachet/250ml	224	4	90	7.2	11.1	1.6	1
Shake, Mixed Berry, Diet Now*	1 Sachet/34g	138	3.6	405	26.6	47.7	10.6	5.9
Shake, Salted Caramel Infusion, Made Up, Slim Fast*	1 Serving/290ml	238	3.2	82	6.9	9.9	1.1	2.6
Shake, Salted Caramel, Exante Diet*	1 Pack/52g	203	6.5	390	32.7	32.7	12.5	6.7
Shake, Strawberry, As Sold, Shake That Weight*	1 Sachet/34g	128	2.9	377	35.7	35.7	8.5	7.4
Shake, Strawberry, Delight, Great Shape, Asda*	1 Serving/330ml	198	6.3	60	5.1	5.1	1.9	1.2
Shake, Strawberry, Fast 800*	1 Glass/50ml	199	8.1	398	44.6	9.9	16.2	13.9
Shake, Vanilla, As Sold, Shake That Weight*	1 Sachet/34g	132	3.3	389	32.7	38.9	9.8	7.2
Shake, Vanilla, Fast 800*	1 Glass/50ml	199	8.1	398	44.6	9.9	16.2	13.9
Shake, Vanilla, Fast800*	1 Serving/50g	196	9.5	392	44	12.6	19	13.1
Shake, Vanilla, Herbalife*	2 Scoops/25g	90	1	360	36	52	4	12
Shake, Vegan, Coffee, Fast 800*	1 Scoop/10g	40	1.4	396	39	14.8	13.7	17.8
Spaghetti Bolognese, As Sold, Shake That Weight*	1 Sachet/45g	161	3.9	358	34.3	30.9	8.6	9.7
Sweet & Sour, Hot & Savoury, Huel*	1 Serving/95g	400	13	421	25.3	40	13.7	14.7
Thai Green Curry, Hot & Savoury, Huel*	2 Scoops/94g	401	13.2	427	26	43	14	11
Ultra Slim, Ready to Drink, Vanilla, Tesco*	1 Carton/330ml	224	3	68	4.2	10.5	0.9	1.5
Vanilla Creme, Diet, The Protein Works*	1 Serving/70g	256	4.6	365	29	45.9	6.6	9.5

MEATBALLS

	Measure INFO/WEIGHT	KCAL	FAT	KCAL	PROT	CARB	FAT	FIBRE
Al Forno, Charlie Bigham's*	½ Pack/324g	532	32.4	164	7	11.5	10	1.1
Beef & Pork, in Rustic Tomato Sauce, Cook*	1 Pack/300g	375	21	125	9.5	6.9	7	1.8
Beef, & Pork, Italian Style, Extra Special, Asda*	½ Pack/170g	466	26	274	29.4	3.5	15.3	0.6
Beef, 10% Fat, Mini, Oven Cooked, Sainsbury's*	4 Meatballs/61g	103	4.7	169	22.9	2	7.7	0.5
Beef, 10% Fat, Oven Cooked, Sainsbury's*	3 Meatballs/87g	148	6.7	170	22.9	2	7.7	0.5
Beef, Aberdeen Angus, 12 Pack, Waitrose*	1 Meatball/36g	93	7.1	259	18	2.3	19.8	0.1
Beef, As Sold, Tesco*	1 Meatball/28g	78	6.2	277	16.6	2.3	22.3	0.9
Beef, Ashfield Farm, Aldi*	1 Meatball/20g	45	2.7	232	23	3.9	14	0.5
Beef, British, 50% Reduced Fat, Waitrose*	1 Meatball/15g	27	1.1	178	21.1	6.7	7.2	0.9
Beef, Carrot, & Onion, Tesco*	4 Meatballs/94g	179	10.4	190	16.8	4.8	11.1	1.7
Beef, Co-Op*	½ Pack/175g	388	28	222	17	2.7	16	0
Beef, Farm Foods*	1 Meatball/33g	90	6.8	273	18.9	1.8	20.7	0
Beef, Frozen, Iceland*	¼ Pack/150g	364	24.3	243	17.7	5.2	16.2	1.7

M

MEATBALLS

INFO/WEIGHT	Measure	per Measure KCAL	per Measure FAT	Nutrition Values per 100g / 100ml KCAL	PROT	CARB	FAT	FIBRE
Beef, Frozen, M&S*	¼ Pack/120g	304	23.9	253	18.1	0.1	19.9	0.5
Beef, Giant, Musclefood*	1 Meatball/58g	92	4.3	158	18	4.9	7.4	0
Beef, Irish, Platinum Prime, Aldi*	1 Meatball/20g	30	0.7	150	24.6	4.4	3.6	0.9
Beef, Italian Style, As Consumed, Morrisons*	3 Meatballs/104g	235	14.7	226	19.7	4.5	14.1	0.9
Beef, Lean, Oven Baked, Iceland*	1 Meatballs/19g	28	1.1	150	20.7	3.7	5.7	0.5
Beef, M&S*	6 Meatballs/150g	363	25.5	242	18.3	3.5	17	0.7
Beef, Mini, Oven Cooked, Finest, Tesco*	5 Meatballs/72g	149	8.2	207	21.8	4	11.4	0.8
Beef, Reduced Fat, Tesco*	4 Meatballs/93g	166	6.7	178	21.6	6.2	7.2	0.8
Beef, Sainsbury's*	1 Meatball/24g	59	4	251	19.6	4.8	16.9	0.5
Beef, Skinny, Mini, 24, M&S*	½ Pack/120g	132	2.9	110	17.9	4.3	2.4	0.5
Chicken, 5% Fat, British, Ashfield Farm, Aldi*	1 Meatball/27g	36	1.3	135	18	5.1	4.7	1
Chicken, in Barbecue Sauce, Fray Bentos*	½ Can/190g	232	11.8	122	4.3	14.3	6.2	0.8
Chicken, in Tomato Sauce, Average	**1 Can/392g**	**580**	**32.9**	**148**	**7.7**	**10.4**	**8.4**	**0**
Chicken, Mediterranean Inspired, Tesco*	3 Meatballs/64g	120	3.9	188	21.9	11.3	6.1	0.2
Chicken, Spanish Style, Ready to Cook, Asda*	½ Pack/179g	179	6.4	100	8.6	7.4	3.6	1.9
Italian Style, Tesco*	¼ Pack/135g	309	21.1	229	13.5	7.7	15.6	1.1
Lamb, Daylesford*	1/3 Pack/112g	203	13.7	181	17.6	0.2	12.2	0
Lamb, with Grilled Aubergine, Tweakd*	1 Serving/527g	794	48.3	151	9.7	6.6	9.2	1.4
Meat Free, Oven Baked, Plant Based, Asda*	6 Meatballs/118g	176	11.3	149	5.9	5.7	9.6	8
Meat Free, Plant Pioneers, Sainsbury's*	½ Pack/190g	304	12.5	160	15.2	6.7	6.6	6.7
Meat Free, Swedish, Dafgards *	6 Balls/87g	163	8.7	187	13	10	10	2.7
Meat-less, Shallow Fried, V Taste, Morrisons*	3 Balls/60g	85	2.5	141	7.8	16.2	4.2	3.7
No Beef, Meat Free, Richmond*	4 Balls/88g	166	7.7	189	1.6	9.6	8.7	3.6
Plant Based, Future Farm*	½ Pack/125g	248	13.8	198	12	13	11	1
Plant Based, Moving Mountains*	½ Pack/150g	394	29.4	263	11.7	6.8	19.6	6.5
Pork, & Beef, Swedish Style, Tesco*	1 Meatball/14g	34	2.5	245	14.3	6.5	17.7	2
Pork, al Forno, Deluxe, Lidl*	½ Pack/400g	620	28	155	7.7	14.3	7	2
Pork, Duchy Originals, Waitrose*	5 Meatballs/68g	184	12.6	270	21.7	4	18.6	0
Pork, Italian, Al Forno, Sainsbury's*	1 Pack/450g	644	23.8	143	6.1	17.6	5.3	1.4
Reduced Fat, Aldi*	3 Meatballs/90g	188	8.6	209	23	6.8	9.5	1.3
Russian, Large, Aida Food*	1 Meatball/50g	116	9	232	17	1.5	18	0
Swedish, Meat Free, Green Cuisine, Birds Eye*	1 Serving/81g	190	12.1	236	16	6.8	15	4.9
Swedish, Real, Kottbullar, Scandi Kitchen*	½ Pack/150g	256	16.5	171	14.3	1.9	11	0
Tomato, Spicy, Vegetarian, The Deli, Aldi*	3 Balls/63g	126	5.7	200	5.5	20	9.1	7.5
Turkey, 5% Fat, British, Tesco*	4 Meatballs/95g	126	2.7	132	22.7	2.9	2.8	2.4
Turkey, Small, Fine, Ingelsta*	1 Serving/90g	225	15.3	250	14	11	17	0
Turkey, with Seasoning, Sainsbury's*	3 Meatballs/79g	168	8.5	213	22.8	6	10.8	0.5
Vegan, Gro, Co-Op*	5 Balls/95g	144	7.4	152	14	3	7.8	6.2
Vegan, Meat Free, Plant Chef, Tesco*	1 Ball/26g	51	2	194	13.1	16.7	7.6	3.5
Vegan, No Bull, Iceland*	4 Balls/41g	78	3.6	190	13	12	8.8	5.8
Vegetable, Protein, Goodlife*	4 Balls/88g	187	9.8	212	15.2	10.6	11.1	4.5
Vegetable, Protein, with Spinach, & Kale, Goodlife*	4 Balls/88g	187	9.8	212	15.2	10.6	11.1	4.5
Vegetarian, Vivera*	½ Pack/100g	169	7.3	169	17	7.4	7.3	3.3
Vegetarian, Super Greens Balls, as Sold, Heck*	1 Ball/28g	43	0.5	153	6.5	30.3	1.8	5.4
Vegetarian, Swedish Style, Quorn*	½ Bag/150g	195	6.9	130	13.2	7.4	4.6	3
Vegetarian, Swedish, Frozen, Quorn*	¼ Pack/75g	98	3.5	130	13.2	7.4	4.6	3
Vegetarian, Tomato & Basil, Linda McCartney*	5 Meatballs/91g	199	12.2	219	12.8	9	13.4	5.7

MELBA TOAST

INFO/WEIGHT	Measure	per Measure KCAL	per Measure FAT	Nutrition Values per 100g / 100ml KCAL	PROT	CARB	FAT	FIBRE
Average	**1 Serving/3g**	**13**	**0.2**	**396**	**12**	**76**	**4.9**	**4.6**
Date, Walnut, & Sunflower Seeds, M&S*	1 Toast/8g	30	0.8	390	7.1	65.3	10	5

MELON

INFO/WEIGHT	Measure	per Measure KCAL	per Measure FAT	Nutrition Values per 100g / 100ml KCAL	PROT	CARB	FAT	FIBRE
Cantaloupe, Flesh Only, Average	**½ Melon/255g**	**87**	**0.5**	**34**	**0.8**	**8.2**	**0.2**	**0.9**
Cantaloupe, Weighed with Rind, Average	**1 Wedge/100g**	**18**	**0.2**	**18**	**0.4**	**4.2**	**0.2**	**0.4**

	Measure			Nutrition Values per 100g / 100ml				
	INFO/WEIGHT	KCAL	FAT	KCAL	PROT	CARB	FAT	FIBRE
MELON								
Galia	**1 Serving/240g**	**60**	**0.1**	**25**	**0.8**	**5.8**	**0**	**0.2**
Honeydew, Raw, Flesh Only, Average	**1 Avg Wedge/125g**	**45**	**0.2**	**36**	**0.5**	**9.1**	**0.1**	**0.8**
Matice, Average	**1 Avg Serving/80g**	**25**	**0.4**	**31**	**0.5**	**6.8**	**0.5**	**0.5**
Medley, Pre Packed, Average	**1 Pack/240g**	**66**	**0.3**	**27**	**0.6**	**6**	**0.1**	**0.5**
Snowball, Sweet, Tesco*	1 Serving/80g	25	0.1	31	0.5	6.8	0.1	0.4
MERINGUE								
Average	**1 Meringue/8g**	**30**	**0**	**379**	**5.3**	**95.4**	**0**	**0**
Balls, Classic Pops, Flower & White*	¼ Pot/38g	184	10.6	491	3.9	55.2	28.2	0
Coffee Fresh Cream, Asda*	1 Meringue/28g	109	4.7	396	3.8	57	17	0.3
Cream, Fresh, Sainsbury's*	1 Meringue/35g	142	5.1	407	3.5	65.4	14.6	0.5
Mini, The Pantry, Aldi*	3 Meringues/9g	31	0	347	5.2	81.6	0	0
Nests, Average	**1 Nest/16g**	**63**	**0**	**397**	**4.8**	**93.3**	**0.1**	**0.1**
Shells, Mini, TTD, Sainsbury's*	1 Shell/5g	19	0	386	4.8	91.2	0.5	0.5
Shells, Mini, Waitrose*	1 Shell/5g	19	0	386	4.8	91.2	0.2	0
Shells, Strawberry & Cream, Finest, Tesco*	2 Meringue Shells/7g	28	0	396	5.1	93	0.4	0
Toffee Cream, Tesco*	1 Meringue/30g	114	5	380	4.2	52.9	16.5	0
Toffee, Sticky, 239, Oakhouse Foods*	1 Serving/88g	341	16.7	387	4.6	50	19	0.9
MILK								
Almond, Barista, Rude Health*	1 Serving/200ml	116	4.2	58	1.8	8	2.1	0.6
Almond, Dark Chocolate, Alpro*	1 Serving/200ml	94	2.6	47	0.8	7.6	1.3	0.8
Almond, No Sugars, Alpro*	1 Serving/200ml	26	2.2	13	0.4	0	1.1	0.3
Almond, Organic, Bunalun*	1 Serving/200ml	52	4.8	26	0.9	1	2.4	0
Almond, Original, Alpro*	1 Serving/200ml	48	2.2	24	0.5	3	1.1	0.2
Almond, Original, Fresh, Alpro*	1 Serving/200ml	48	2.2	24	0.5	3	1.1	0.2
Almond, Original, Roasted, Alpro*	1 Serving/100ml	22	1.1	22	0.4	2.4	1.1	0.4
Almond, Sweetened, UHT, Tesco*	1 Serving/200ml	50	2.4	25	0.7	2.8	1.2	0
Almond, Unsweetened, Actileaf, Aldi*	1 Serving/200ml	40	3	20	0.5	1.3	1.5	0.5
Almond, Unsweetened, Breeze, Blue Diamond*	1 Serving/250ml	32	2.8	13	0.5	0.2	1.1	0.3
Almond, Unsweetened, Just Free, Lidl*	1 Serving/200ml	36	2.8	18	0.5	0.8	1.4	0
Almond, Unsweetened, Kirkland Signature, Costco*	1 Serving/200ml	25	2.1	12	0.4	0.4	1	0.4
Almond, Unsweetened, Morrisons*	1 Serving/100ml	18	1.5	18	0.8	0.1	1.5	0.4
Almond, Unsweetened, Organic, Alpro*	1 Serving/200ml	30	2.4	15	0.5	0	1.2	0.2
Almond, Unsweetened, Roasted, Alpro*	1 Serving/200ml	26	2.2	13	0.4	0	1.1	0.4
Almond, Unsweetened, Sainsbury's*	1 Serving/200ml	36	2.6	18	0.5	1.1	1.3	0
Almond, Unsweetened, Silk*	1 Serving/200ml	25	2	12	0.4	0.2	1	0.2
Almond, Unsweetened, Tesco*	1 Serving/100ml	18	1.1	18	0.4	1.3	1.1	0.4
Almond, Unsweetened, UHT, Morrisons*	1 Serving/100ml	14	1	14	0.6	0.6	1	0
Almond, Unsweetened, Unroasted, Alpro*	1 Serving/200ml	26	2.6	13	0.5	0	1.3	0.2
Alternative, Unsweetened, Mighty Pea *	1 Serving/200ml	64	4	32	3.3	0.1	2	0.1
Chocolate, 1% Fat, Cocio*	1 Serving/200ml	96	2	48	3.7	5.8	1	0
Chocolate, Flavoured, Morrisons*	1 Serving/330ml	236	6.2	72	3.5	9.8	1.9	0.6
Coconut, & Almond, Fresh, Alpro*	1 Serving/200ml	48	2.6	24	0.3	2.6	1.3	0
Coconut, Average	**1 Can/400ml**	**698**	**69.7**	**174**	**1.4**	**2.9**	**17.4**	**2.9**
Coconut, Barista, Alpro*	1 Serving/200ml	66	2.8	33	1.5	3.4	1.4	0.2
Coconut, Reduced Fat, Average	**1 Serving/100g**	**104**	**10**	**104**	**1**	**2.4**	**10**	**0.4**
Condensed, Semi Skimmed, Sweetened	**1oz/28g**	**75**	**0.1**	**267**	**10**	**60**	**0.2**	**0**
Condensed, Skimmed, Unsweetened, Average	**1oz/28g**	**30**	**1.1**	**108**	**7.5**	**10.5**	**4**	**0**
Condensed, Whole, Sweetened, Average	**1oz/28g**	**93**	**2.8**	**333**	**8.5**	**55.5**	**10.1**	**0**
Dried, Skimmed, Average	**1oz/28g**	**99**	**0.3**	**355**	**35.4**	**52.3**	**0.9**	**0**
Dried, Whole, Average	**1oz/28g**	**137**	**7.4**	**490**	**26.3**	**39.4**	**26.3**	**0**
Evaporated, Average	**1 Serving/85g**	**136**	**7.6**	**160**	**8.2**	**11.6**	**9**	**0**
Evaporated, Reduced Fat, Average	**1oz/28g**	**33**	**1.5**	**118**	**7.4**	**10.5**	**5.2**	**0**
Goats, Pasteurised	**1 fl oz/30ml**	**18**	**1**	**60**	**3.1**	**4.4**	**3.5**	**0**

MILK

MILK	Measure INFO/WEIGHT	per Measure KCAL	FAT	Nutrition Values per 100g / 100ml KCAL	PROT	CARB	FAT	FIBRE
Kefir, Bibi's Homemade*	1 Glass/210g	128	7.4	61	3.3	4.3	3.5	0
Mega, Low Fat, Irish Dairy, Clonbawn*	1 Serving/200ml	88	2	44	3.8	5	1	0.5
Oat, Cacao, Alpro*	1 Serving/200ml	88	3.4	44	0.5	6.2	1.7	0.7
Plant Based, for Tea, Alpro*	1 Serving/30ml	18	1.3	60	2.1	2	4.3	1.6
Powder, Full Cream, Two Cows*	1 Tbsp/15g	75	4.2	503	25	36.5	28.2	0
Rice, Organic, Provamel*	1 Serving/250ml	122	3.8	49	0.1	9.5	1.5	0
Semi Skimmed, Average	*1fl oz/30ml*	*15*	*0.5*	*49*	*3.4*	*5*	*1.7*	*0*
Semi Skimmed, Lactose Free, Asda*	1 Serving/200ml	96	3.2	48	3.6	4.9	1.6	0.5
Semi Skimmed, Lactose Free, Dairy Manor, Lidl*	1 Serving/200ml	82	3	41	3.1	3.4	1.5	0.5
Semi Skimmed, Long Life, Average	*1fl oz/30ml*	*15*	*0.5*	*49*	*3.4*	*5*	*1.7*	*0*
Skimmed, Average	*1 Pint/568ml*	*194*	*0.5*	*34*	*3.3*	*5*	*0.1*	*0*
Skimmed, Lactofree, Arla*	1 Serving/200ml	62	1	31	3.7	2.8	0.5	0
Skimmed, Uht, Average	*1fl oz/30ml*	*10*	*0*	*34*	*3.4*	*5*	*0.1*	*0*
Soya, Flavoured, Average	*1 Glass/250ml*	*100*	*4.2*	*40*	*2.8*	*3.6*	*1.7*	*0*
Soya, No Added Sugar, Unsweetened, Average	*1 Serving/250ml*	*85*	*4.8*	*34*	*3.3*	*0.9*	*1.9*	*0.4*
Soya, Strawberry, Alpro*	1 Serving/200ml	124	3.6	62	3.3	7.6	1.8	0.5
Soya, Sweetened, Average	*1 Glass/200ml*	*94*	*4.2*	*47*	*3.4*	*3.7*	*2.1*	*0.4*
Soya, Sweetened, Calcium Enriched, Average	*1 Glass/200ml*	*91*	*3.9*	*46*	*3.4*	*3.7*	*2*	*0.3*
Soya, Vanilla, Alpro*	1 Serving/200ml	108	3.4	54	3	6.5	1.7	0.5
Whole, Average	*1 Serving/200ml*	*134*	*7.8*	*67*	*3.3*	*4.7*	*3.9*	*0*
Whole, Lactose Free, Lactofree, Arla*	1 Serving/200ml	114	7	57	3.4	2.8	3.5	0

MILK DRINK

MILK DRINK								
Almond, Sweetened, Plant Kitchen, M&S*	1 Serving/200ml	58	4	29	1	1.5	2	0.6
Almond, Unsweetened, Plant Kitchen, M&S*	1 Serving/200ml	58	2.4	29	0.5	3.5	1.2	1
Banana, Breakfast, Fuel 10K*	1 Carton/330g	218	4.6	66	6.1	6.7	1.4	1
Banana, High Protein, Nurishment*	1 Can/400g	396	12	99	5	13.5	3	0
Barista, Mylk, Dairy Free, Rebel Kitchen*	1 Serving/200ml	112	6.4	56	0.5	6.4	3.2	0.1
Breakfast, Chocolate, Protein, Fuel 10K*	1 Carton/330ml	208	3.3	63	6.1	6.9	1	1
Chocolate Coconut, Free From, Tesco*	1 Serving/250ml	125	5.4	49	0.4	6.8	2.1	0.7
Chocolate, High Protein, Nurishment*	1 Can/400g	384	10.8	96	5	12.9	2.7	0
Coconut, Plant Kitchen, M&S*	1 Serving/200ml	58	3.8	29	0.2	2.2	1.9	1
Kefir, Honey, & Ginger, Bio-tiful Dairy*	1 Bottle/250ml	161	6.8	64	2.9	7.1	2.7	0
Kefir, Natur, Nestle*	1 Glass/250ml	98	3.8	39	3	3.3	1.5	0
Kefir, Nature, Bio, Molkerei Biebermann*	1 Pot/150g	111	5.2	74	4.6	6	3.5	0
Kefir, Organic, Arla*	1 Serving/100ml	59	3	59	3.4	3.9	3	0
Kefir, Organic, Bio-tiful Dairy*	1 Serving/250g	145	7.5	58	3.2	4.6	3	0
Kefir, Pomegranate, & Blueberry, Light & Free, Danone*	1 Bottle/265ml	69	1.1	26	2.9	4.4	0.4	0
Kefir, Vanilla, Bio-tiful Dairy*	1 Serving/250ml	150	6.5	60	2.9	5.9	2.6	0
Kvarg, Pro+, Raspberry & Vanilla, Lindahls, Nestle*	1 Serving/250ml	144	1.8	55	8.7	3.4	0.7	0
Original, Mars*	1 Serving/330g	284	6.9	86	3.1	13.7	2.1	0
Soya, Chocolate, Low Sugar, Alpro*	1 Glass/150ml	102	3.2	68	3.3	8	2.1	2.2
Strawberry Flavoured, Goodness for Kids, Tesco*	1 Bottle/330ml	248	5.6	75	4	9.9	1.7	0.4
Strawberry, Flavoured, Asda*	1 Bottle/330ml	211	3.6	64	3.6	10	1.1	0.5
Strawberry, High Protein, Nurishment*	1 Can/400g	424	11.2	106	5	15.1	2.8	0
Vanilla, Breakfast, Protein, Fuel 10K*	1 Carton/330ml	218	4.6	66	6.1	6.7	1.4	1
Vanilla, High Protein, Nurishment*	1 Can/400g	396	12	99	5	13.5	3	0

MILK SHAKE

MILK SHAKE								
Banana Flavour, Frijj*	1 Bottle/500ml	325	4.5	65	3.7	10.5	0.9	0
Banana, Mix, As Prepared, Morrisons*	1 Serving/216ml	158	3.5	73	3.4	11.3	1.6	0
Chocolate Flavoured, Fresh, Thick, Frijj*	1 Bottle/500ml	350	5	70	3.5	11.7	1	0
Chocolate, Asda*	1 Serving/250ml	198	9.2	79	4.4	7	3.7	0.4
Chocolate, Belgian, M&S*	1 Bottle/300ml	360	14.4	120	4.2	14.6	4.8	0.7
Chocolate, Dry, Cadbury*	1 Serving/14g	54	0.9	387	7.7	64	6.3	21

	Measure INFO/WEIGHT	per Measure KCAL	FAT	Nutrition Values per 100g / 100ml KCAL	PROT	CARB	FAT	FIBRE
MILK SHAKE								
Chocolate, Fudge, Cowbelle, Aldi*	1 Serving/100ml	74	1.3	74	4.5	11	1.3	0.5
Chocolate, High Protein, For Goodness Shakes*	1 Bottle/475g	214	1.4	45	5.3	5.3	0.3	0.6
Chocolate, M&M's, Mars*	1 Serving/50g	196	8.3	392	42.6	9	16.6	15.8
Chocolate, Protein, Plant-Based, Ensure*	1 Bottle/330ml	180	6	55	6.1	4.2	1.8	1.5
Chocolate, Protein, Ufit*	1 Bottle/310ml	170	3.1	55	7.1	3.6	1	1.2
Chocolate, Sainsbury's*	1 Serving/100ml	66	1.2	66	3.6	10.2	1.2	0
Powder, Made Up with Semi-Skimmed Milk	**1 Serving/250ml**	**172**	**4**	**69**	**3.2**	**11.3**	**1.6**	**0**
Powder, Made Up with Whole Milk	**1 Serving/250ml**	**218**	**9.2**	**87**	**3.1**	**11.1**	**3.7**	**0**
Thick, Milky Way, Mars*	1 Bottle/440ml	282	4.8	64	3.4	10	1.1	0.7
Vanilla, High Protein, Ufit*	1 Serving/500ml	290	0.5	58	10	3.7	0.1	1
White Chocolate, Ufit*	1 Bottle/330ml	155	0.3	47	7.6	3.6	0.1	1
MILKY BAR								
Buttons, Nestle*	1 Pack/14g	78	4.6	543	10.6	53.1	31.7	0
Crunchies, Nestle*	1 Pack/30g	168	10.4	560	7	54.9	34.7	0
Egg, White Chocolate, Nestle*	1 Egg/65g	353	20.6	543	10.6	53.1	31.7	0
Funsize, Mars*	1 Bar/17g	75	2.7	449	3.8	71.8	16.3	0.6
Mini Eggs, Nestle*	1 Pack/90g	443	18.5	492	7	69.4	20.6	0
Munchies, Nestle*	1 Serving/70g	392	24.3	560	7	54.9	34.7	0.1
Nestle*	1 Sm Bar/13g	68	4	547	7.3	58.4	31.7	0
MILKY WAY								
Fun Size, Mars*	1 Bar/17g	75	2.7	447	3.8	71.6	16.2	0
Mars*	1 Bar/22g	96	3.3	446	3.9	72.4	15.5	0.6
MINCEMEAT								
Average	**1oz/28g**	**77**	**1.2**	**274**	**0.6**	**62.1**	**4.3**	**1.3**
MINSTRELS								
Galaxy, Mars*	1 Serving/39g	196	8.6	498	5.2	69.1	21.9	0
MINT								
Dried, Average	**1 Tsp/5g**	**14**	**0.2**	**279**	**24.8**	**34.6**	**4.6**	**0**
Fresh, Average	**2 Tbsp/3.2g**	**1**	**0**	**43**	**3.8**	**5.3**	**0.7**	**0**
MINTS								
Butter Mintoes, M&S*	1 Sweet/9g	35	0.6	391	0	84	6.8	0
Butter Mintoes, Tesco*	1 Sweet/7g	30	0.5	431	0.1	91.1	7.3	0.5
Creams, Bassett's*	1 Sweet/11g	40	0	365	0	91.8	0	0
Curiously Strong, M&S*	1 Sweet/1g	4	0	390	0.4	97.5	0	0
Extra Strong, Peppermint, Trebor*	1 Sweet/2g	10	0	395	0.3	98.5	0	0
Glacier, Fox's*	1 Sweet/5g	19	0	386	0	96.4	0	0
Humbugs, Co-Op*	1 Sweet/8g	34	0.6	425	0.6	89.9	7	0
Humbugs, M&S*	1 Sweet/9g	37	0.4	407	0.6	91.1	4.4	0
Humbugs, Tesco*	1 Sweet/9g	37	0.2	409	0.3	95.9	2.6	0.5
Imperials, Co-Op*	1 Sweet/3g	12	0	395	0.3	98	0.2	0
Imperials, M&S*	1 Sweet/3g	12	0	391	0	97.8	0	0
Imperials, Sainsbury's*	1 Sweet/3g	10	0	374	0	92.1	0	0
Imperials, Tesco*	1 Sweet/3g	12	0	397	0.6	98.7	0	0
Mint Assortment, M&S*	1 Sweet/7g	26	0.5	375	0.4	78.2	6.9	0
MIRIN								
Rice Wine, Sweetened, Average	**1 Tbsp/15ml**	**35**	**0**	**231**	**0.2**	**41.6**	**0**	**0**
MISO								
Average	**1oz/28g**	**57**	**1.7**	**203**	**13.3**	**23.5**	**6.2**	**0**
Paste, Mellow Yellow, Yutaka*	1 Serving/17g	26	0.8	156	9.7	19	4.8	4.5
White, Sweet, Organic, Clearspring*	1 Tbsp/15g	26	0.6	171	7.7	26	4	0.6
MIXED HERBS								
Average	**1 Tsp/5g**	**13**	**0.4**	**260**	**13**	**37.5**	**8.5**	**6.7**

	Measure INFO/WEIGHT	per Measure KCAL	FAT	Nutrition Values per 100g / 100ml KCAL	PROT	CARB	FAT	FIBRE
MOLASSES								
Average	**1 Tsp/5g**	**13**	**0**	**266**	**0**	**68.8**	**0.1**	**0**
MONKEY NUTS								
without Shell, Average	**1oz/28g**	**158**	**13.4**	**565**	**25.6**	**8.2**	**48**	**6.3**
MONKFISH								
Grilled	**1oz/28g**	**27**	**0.2**	**96**	**22.7**	**0**	**0.6**	**0**
Raw, Average	**1 Serving/150g**	**114**	**2.2**	**76**	**14**	**0**	**1.5**	**0**
MOUSSAKA								
Allplants*	1 Serving/420g	365	7.1	87	4.1	12	1.7	2.6
Beef, & Lamb, Waitrose*	1 Pack/323g	387	19.4	120	6.2	9.5	6	1.5
Beef, BGTY, Sainsbury's*	1 Pack/400g	300	10.4	75	6.1	6.8	2.6	1.2
for Two, Charlie Bigham's*	1 Serving/327g	425	27.8	130	6.1	6.9	8.5	0
Lamb, BGTY, Sainsbury's*	1 Pack/400g	296	10.4	74	5	6.1	2.6	3
Lamb, Cook*	1 Serving/380g	593	30.8	156	8.3	11.9	8.1	1.3
Lamb, Finest, Tesco*	½ Pack/334g	513	36.5	154	6.4	6.6	10.9	1.5
Lamb, Gastropub, M&S*	1 Pack/409g	528	31.5	129	6.2	7.5	7.7	2.2
Lamb, Oven Baked, Luxury, Iceland*	1 Pack/424g	903	58.9	213	9.8	11.3	13.9	1.7
Lamb, Serves 2, TTD, Sainsbury's*	½ Pack/400g	546	33.7	141	7.2	8	8.7	1.2
Meal to Share, M&S*	½ Pack/300g	417	27.3	139	6.7	7	9.1	1.2
Vegetarian, Quorn*	1 Pack/400g	364	16.4	91	3.6	9.8	4.1	1.2
Veggie, Meal to Share, M&S*	½ Pack/300g	303	16.5	101	3.3	8.6	5.5	1.9
Voussaka, Vegan, Waitrose*	1 Pack/365g	401	20.8	110	3.6	9.9	5.7	2.4
MOUSSE								
Aero Chocolate, Nestle*	1 Pot/58g	101	3	174	4.8	27.3	5.1	1.1
Apricot, Lite, Onken*	1 Pot/150g	156	2.2	104	4.6	18	1.5	0.3
Banoffee, COU, M&S*	1 Pot/70g	102	1.5	145	2.9	28.8	2.1	1.5
Birthday Cake, Halo Top*	1 Pot/100g	153	7.2	153	6.5	13.6	7.2	3.1
Blackcurrant, Bonne Maman*	1 Pot/70g	116	5.3	166	2.6	20.8	7.6	2
Blackcurrant, Onken*	1 Pot/150g	210	10.2	140	5.2	14.6	6.8	0
Cappuccino, Essential, Waitrose*	1 Pot/100g	279	16.7	279	4.2	27.7	16.7	0.5
Caramel, Meringue, Cadbury*	1 Pot/65g	181	6.7	277	4.6	42.4	10.3	1
Cherry, & Kirsch, Finest, Tesco*	1 Pot/100g	195	11.6	195	2.7	19.6	11.6	0.5
Chocolat au Lait, Carrefour*	1 Pot/60g	104	4.2	174	5.1	22	7	1.5
Chocolat Noir, Carrefour*	1 Pot/60g	100	3.9	166	5.8	20	6.5	2.7
Chocolate	**1 Pot/60g**	**83**	**3.2**	**139**	**4**	**19.9**	**5.4**	**0**
Chocolate, & Hazelnut, Onken*	1 Pot/125g	171	7.5	137	3.3	17.8	6	0
Chocolate, & Mint, COU, M&S*	1 Pot/70g	84	1.8	120	6.2	18.7	2.5	1
Chocolate, & Orange, COU, M&S*	1 Pot/70g	77	1.8	110	5.9	16	2.6	0.9
Chocolate, Bubbly, Aero, Nestle*	1 Pot/58g	93	3	159	5	23.1	5.1	0
Chocolate, Low Fat, Danette, Danone*	1 Pot/60g	73	1.1	121	5.1	20.8	1.9	1.5
Chocolate, Milk, with Ganache, Gu*	1 Pot/70g	274	19.6	391	6.6	29	28	1.3
Chocolate, Minty, Bubbly, Dessert, Aero, Nestle*	1 Pot/58g	108	5.9	186	4.6	18.9	10.2	0.3
Chocolate, Plain, Low Fat, Nestle*	1 Pot/120g	71	0.9	59	2.4	10.4	0.8	0
Chocolate, Pot, Halo Top*	1 Pot/100g	143	4.3	143	5.7	18.2	4.3	5.4
Chocolate, Pot, Plant Kitchen, M&S*	1 Pot/90g	288	19.4	320	3.5	26.5	21.6	2.8
Chocolate, Wispa, Cadbury*	1 Pot/45g	88	3.6	195	6	25.6	8	1.7
Lemon, COU, M&S*	1 Pot/70g	91	1.8	130	3.1	23.7	2.5	0.6
Lemon, Low Fat, Morrisons*	1 Pot/63g	99	5.8	158	3.7	15.4	9.3	0.3
Lemon, Sicillian, Deluxe, Lidl*	1 Pot/100g	210	12.4	210	2.6	22	12.4	0.5
Lemon, Ski, Nestle*	1 Pot/60g	77	2.8	128	3.8	17.8	4.6	0
Lemon, Tesco*	1 Pot/60g	91	4.9	152	3.8	15.4	8.2	0.4
Mango, & Passion Fruit, Finest, Tesco*	1 Pot/100g	239	15.7	239	3.7	18.4	15.7	0.7
Raspberry, Ripple, Value, Tesco*	1 Pot/47g	70	2.9	149	2.1	21.3	6.1	0.1
Rhubarb, Bonne Maman*	1 Pot/70g	120	5.3	171	2.4	22.8	7.6	1

	Measure INFO/WEIGHT	per Measure		Nutrition Values per 100g / 100ml				
		KCAL	FAT	KCAL	PROT	CARB	FAT	FIBRE
MOUSSE								
Rolo, Nestle*	1 Pot/50g	80	3	158	4.7	21.6	5.9	0
Strawberry, Asda*	1 Pot/64g	107	5.8	167	3.5	18	9	0.2
Strawberry, COU, M&S*	1 Pot/70g	90	1.3	128	4.5	23.2	1.8	0.3
Strawberry, Iceland*	1 Pot/100g	158	8.5	158	2.8	16.9	8.5	0.5
Strawberry, Ski, Nestle*	1 Pot/60g	73	2.9	121	3.9	15.4	4.9	0
Strawberry, Tesco*	1 Pot/60g	97	4.6	162	2.7	20.2	7.7	0.5
Summer Fruits, Light, Muller*	1 Pot/149g	143	0.6	96	4.3	18.7	0.4	0
Toffee, M&S*	1 Pot/90g	180	7.2	200	4.5	27.6	8	0.6
White Chocolate, Finest, Tesco*	1 Pot/92g	436	34.5	474	3.9	30.2	37.5	0
MUFFIN								
All Butter, English, Morrisons*	1 Muffin/65g	168	1.5	258	8.7	49.1	2.3	2.9
All Butter, M&S*	1 Muffin/65g	175	4.7	270	10.3	40.8	7.3	2.1
Ancient Grain, Rankin Selection*	1 Muffin/70g	212	3.6	303	10.7	49.4	5.2	7.8
Bacon, & Cheddar Cheese, Mini, M&S*	1 Muffin/20g	52	3	260	11.1	19.5	14.8	2.4
Blueberry, American Style, Aldi*	1 Muffin/85g	344	17.3	405	4.3	51.2	20.3	0
Blueberry, American Style, Sainsbury's*	1 Muffin/72g	256	13.1	355	5.1	42.7	18.2	1.9
Blueberry, Asda*	1 Muffin/77g	273	13.1	353	5	45	17	1.3
Blueberry, Bakery, Tesco*	1 Muffin/82g	307	13.1	374	4.3	52.2	16	1.9
Blueberry, Big, Asda*	1 Muffin/105g	342	11.2	326	7.5	49.8	10.7	2.3
Blueberry, Filled, Bakery in Store, M&S*	1 Muffin/103g	381	18.5	370	5	46.7	18	1
Blueberry, GF, Genius*	1 Muffin/95g	352	16.2	370	3.6	51	17.1	1.6
Blueberry, M&S*	1 Muffin/75g	255	12.6	340	4.9	41.9	16.8	1.3
Blueberry, Waitrose*	1 Muffin/65g	239	9.2	367	4.7	55.2	14.2	1.7
Caramel, Cadbury*	1 Muffin/116g	535	30.3	461	5.9	50.8	26.1	0
Caramel, Salted, Filled, Tesco*	1 Muffin/82g	320	15.5	390	4.7	49.5	18.9	1.6
Cheddar, & Spinach, Mini, Higgidy*	1 Muffin/22g	62	3.5	280	12.6	21.7	15.7	1.9
Cheddar, Farmhouse, Hovis*	1 Muffin/65g	163	4.2	251	11.6	35.4	6.5	2.5
Cheese, & Black Pepper, Finest, Tesco*	1 Muffin/72g	191	5.4	266	12.4	35.6	7.5	3
Cheese, TTD, Sainsbury's*	1 Muffin/69g	200	6	290	11.5	40.2	8.7	2.4
Chocolate Chip, Double, Co-Op*	1 Muffin/60g	246	12.6	410	6	49	21	3
Chocolate Chip, Double, Mini, Asda*	1 Muffin/19g	76	3.7	400	7.4	48.5	19.6	2.7
Chocolate Chip, Double, Tesco*	1 Muffin/100g	360	17.9	360	6.1	44.9	17.9	5.4
Chocolate Chip, Mini, Asda*	1 Muffin/22g	77	2.9	349	7	51	13	2.1
Chocolate Chip, Mini, BGTY, Sainsbury's*	1 Muffin/30g	130	6.7	434	5.5	52.1	22.5	0.8
Chocolate Chip, Mini, Essential, Waitrose*	1 Muffin/27g	108	5.1	399	5.9	49.8	19	2.5
Chocolate Chip, Mini, Tesco*	1 Muffin/25g	108	5.6	436	5	52.5	22.5	1.6
Chocolate, Double, Mini, M&S*	1 Muffin/32g	133	6.9	416	5.4	49.8	21.7	1.1
English, Egg, Cheese, & Sausage, From Restaurant	**1 Muffin/165g**	**487**	**30.9**	**295**	**13.1**	**18.8**	**18.7**	**0**
English, Kingsmill*	1 Muffin/75g	167	1.4	222	9.7	40.4	1.8	2.6
English, Tesco*	1 Muffin/72g	158	1.1	219	8.4	41.7	1.5	2.7
English, White, Butter, Waitrose*	1 Muffin/62g	166	2.2	266	10	47.7	3.5	1.9
Halloween, Asda*	1 Muffin/84g	346	16.8	412	4.8	53	20	1.3
Lancashire, Oven Bottom, Sheldons*	1 Muffin/65g	166	1.6	255	9.8	47.2	2.5	1.9
Lemon & Poppy Seed, Waitrose*	1 Muffin/121g	460	23.1	380	4.3	46.8	19.1	1.8
Lemon Curd, Patisserie, TTD, Sainsbury's*	1 Muffin/108g	418	20.9	386	5.4	47.1	19.3	1.4
Lemon Curd, Sicilian, Finest, Tesco*	1 Muffin/110g	402	17.5	366	5.1	49.9	15.9	1.4
Lemon Drizzle, Filled, Bakery in Store, M&S*	1 Muffin/121g	440	20	365	5.3	49.1	16.6	0.9
Mini, Tesco*	1 Muffin/28g	120	6.3	428	6.4	50	22.6	1.2
Muesli, Breakfast, Love Life, Waitrose*	1 Muffin/68g	216	6.2	318	9.1	50	9.1	3.4
Multiseed, Butter, TTD, Sainsbury's*	1 Muffin/70g	208	6.2	297	10.9	40.8	8.9	5.2
Oven Bottom, Asda*	1 Muffin/65g	175	1.8	269	9	51	2.7	2.1
Oven Bottom, Warburton's*	1 Muffin/63g	173	2.7	274	10.4	49.4	4.3	2.3
Plain, Co-Op*	1 Muffin/60g	135	1.1	225	11.2	41.3	1.9	2.4

MUFFIN

	Measure INFO/WEIGHT	per Measure KCAL	FAT	Nutrition Values per 100g / 100ml KCAL	PROT	CARB	FAT	FIBRE
Plain, English, Asda*	1 Muffin/66g	158	1.5	241	9.3	45	2.3	2.4
Plain, Prepared From Recipe, Average	**1 Muffin/57g**	**169**	**6.5**	**296**	**6.9**	**41.4**	**11.4**	**2.7**
Raspberry, Cream, Sainsbury's*	1 Muffin/90g	314	19.8	349	3.9	33.8	22	1.3
Sourdough, Toasting, Specially Selected, Aldi*	1 Muffin/68g	158	1.3	232	9.5	43	1.9	3.2
Toasting, Village Bakery, Aldi*	1 Muffin/68g	158	1.1	232	9.3	43	1.6	3.4
Toasting, Warburton's*	1 Muffin/64g	138	1	216	8.9	41.4	1.6	2.9
White, Tesco*	1 Muffin/72g	173	2.3	240	11.3	41.6	3.2	2.8
Wholemeal, Sainsbury's*	1 Muffin/65g	146	1.5	225	11.1	37.1	2.3	5.5
Wholemeal, Tesco*	1 Muffin/65g	130	1.3	200	12.6	32.9	2	5.7

MULBERRIES

Raw	**1oz/28g**	**10**	**0**	**36**	**1.3**	**8.1**	**0**	**0**

MULLET

Grey, Grilled	**1oz/28g**	**42**	**1.5**	**150**	**25.7**	**0**	**5.2**	**0**
Red, Grilled	**1oz/28g**	**34**	**1.2**	**121**	**20.4**	**0**	**4.4**	**0**

MUNCHIES

Original, Tube, Nestle*	1 Pack/55g	266	12.3	487	5.4	64.6	22.5	1.4

MUSHROOMS

Breaded, Average	**3 Mushroom/51g**	**77**	**2.9**	**152**	**4.3**	**20.8**	**5.7**	**0.6**
Breaded, Garlic, Average	**3 Mushroom/50g**	**92**	**4.9**	**183**	**5.2**	**18.7**	**9.7**	**1.7**
Button, Raw, Average	**1 Serving/50g**	**7**	**0.2**	**15**	**2.3**	**0.5**	**0.4**	**1.2**
Chestnut, Average	**1 Med/5g**	**1**	**0**	**13**	**1.8**	**0.4**	**0.5**	**0.6**
Chinese, Dried, Raw	**1oz/28g**	**80**	**0.5**	**284**	**10**	**59.9**	**1.8**	**0**
Closed Cup, Average	**1 Handful/30g**	**4**	**0.2**	**14**	**1.8**	**0.4**	**0.5**	**1.1**
Common, Boiled in Salted Water, Average	**1oz/28g**	**3**	**0.1**	**11**	**1.8**	**0.4**	**0.3**	**1.1**
Common, Fried, Average	**1oz/28g**	**44**	**4.5**	**157**	**2.4**	**0.3**	**16.2**	**1.5**
Common, Raw, Average	**1 Serving/80g**	**18**	**0.3**	**22**	**3.1**	**3.3**	**0.3**	**1**
Creamed, Average	**1oz/28g**	**23**	**1.5**	**82**	**1.3**	**6.8**	**5.5**	**0.5**
Dried	**1oz/28g**	**45**	**1.7**	**159**	**21.8**	**4.8**	**6**	**13.3**
Enoki, Average	**1 Serving/80g**	**34**	**0**	**42**	**3**	**7**	**0**	**3**
Flat, Large, Average	**1 Mushroom/52g**	**10**	**0.3**	**20**	**3.3**	**0.5**	**0.5**	**0.7**
Garlic, Average	**½ Pack/150g**	**159**	**14**	**106**	**2.1**	**3.7**	**9.3**	**1.7**
Oyster, Average	**1 Serving/80g**	**10**	**0.2**	**13**	**1.4**	**1.4**	**0.2**	**1.1**
Portobello, Raw, Average	**1 Mushroom/50g**	**7**	**0.2**	**14**	**1.8**	**0.4**	**0.5**	**1.1**
Shiitake, Cooked	**1oz/28g**	**15**	**0.1**	**55**	**1.6**	**12.3**	**0.2**	**0**
Shiitake, Dried, Raw	**1oz/28g**	**83**	**0.3**	**296**	**9.6**	**63.9**	**1**	**0**
Sliced, Average	**1oz/28g**	**3**	**0.1**	**12**	**1.8**	**0.4**	**0.3**	**1.1**
Steak, No Bull, Iceland*	1 Steak/80g	109	7.2	136	4.1	6.8	9	6.3
Straw, Canned, Drained	**1oz/28g**	**4**	**0.1**	**15**	**2.1**	**1.2**	**0.2**	**0**
Stuffed, Fire Pit, Tesco*	1 Mushroom/85g	90	4.6	106	6.1	7.5	5.4	1.7
Stuffed, Garlic & Cream Cheese, The Best, Morrisons*	2 Mushrooms/200g	298	15.2	149	5.9	13.3	7.6	1.8
Stuffed, Garlic, Cream Cheese, Herb, Breadcrumbs, Aldi*	½ Pack/92g	105	4.7	114	5.1	11	5.1	2.5
Stuffed, with Garlic & Cheese, Tesco*	1 Mushroom/85g	132	7.9	155	5.8	11.2	9.3	1.9

MUSSELS

Boiled, Flesh Only, Average	**1 Mussel/2g**	**2**	**0.1**	**104**	**16.7**	**3.5**	**2.7**	**0**
Boiled, Weighed in Shell, Average	**1 Mussel/7g**	**2**	**0.1**	**28**	**4.5**	**0.9**	**0.7**	**0**
Pickled, Drained, Average	**1oz/28g**	**32**	**0.6**	**112**	**20**	**1.5**	**2.2**	**0**
Raw, Weighed in Shell, Average	**1oz/28g**	**7**	**0.2**	**23**	**3.4**	**1**	**0.7**	**0**

MUSSELS IN

Garlic Butter Sauce, Average	**½ Pack/225g**	**179**	**11.5**	**80**	**6.4**	**2**	**5.1**	**0.2**
Oil, Smoked, Canned, Drained, John West*	1 Can/60g	117	7.3	196	19.9	1.6	12.2	0
Scottish, in White Wine & Cream, Waitrose*	½ Pack/129g	110	4.3	85	6.6	6.8	3.3	0.6
Seasoned White Wine Sauce, Bantry Bay*	1 Serving/450g	270	9	60	6.3	4.1	2	0.1
Tomato Sauce, Cooked, Italiamo, Lidl*	1 Pack/350g	438	34.3	125	7.3	1.9	9.8	0

	Measure INFO/WEIGHT	per Measure		Nutrition Values per 100g / 100ml				
		KCAL	FAT	KCAL	PROT	CARB	FAT	FIBRE
MUSSELS IN								
White Wine Sauce, Sainsbury's*	½ Pack/250g	215	10.2	86	6.4	5.6	4.1	0.7
MUSTARD								
American, Average	**1 Tsp/5g**	**5**	**0.2**	**102**	**4.4**	**10.5**	**5**	**2.5**
Coarse Grain, Average	**1 Tsp/5g**	**7**	**0.4**	**141**	**7.7**	**8.4**	**8.3**	**5.9**
Dijon, Average	**1 Tsp/5g**	**8**	**0.6**	**163**	**7.4**	**7.7**	**11.3**	**1.1**
English, Average	**1 Tsp/5g**	**9**	**0.4**	**173**	**6.8**	**19.2**	**7.6**	**1.2**
French, Average	**1 Tsp/5g**	**5**	**0.3**	**106**	**5.4**	**8.1**	**5.6**	**1.8**
German Style, Sainsbury's*	1 Serving/10g	9	0.6	92	5.5	2.8	6.5	0
Honey, Colman's*	1 Tsp/6g	12	0.5	208	7.4	24	8.2	0
Horseradish, Sainsbury's*	1 Tsp/5g	6	0.4	128	5.8	8.3	7.1	3.9
Hot Dog, Sainsbury's*	1 Tsp/5g	8	0.2	160	4	22.3	5	5
Powder, Average	**1 Tsp/3g**	**15**	**0.9**	**452**	**28.9**	**20.7**	**28.7**	**0**
Smooth, Average	**1 Tsp/8g**	**11**	**0.7**	**139**	**7.1**	**9.7**	**8.2**	**0**
Whole Grain, Average	**1 Tsp/8g**	**11**	**0.8**	**140**	**8.2**	**4.2**	**10.2**	**4.9**
MUSTARD CRESS								
Raw	**1oz/28g**	**4**	**0.2**	**13**	**1.6**	**0.4**	**0.6**	**1.1**

	Measure INFO/WEIGHT	per Measure KCAL	FAT	Nutrition Values per 100g / 100ml KCAL	PROT	CARB	FAT	FIBRE
NACHOS								
Beef, Chilli, Asda*	1 Serving/200g	208	10	104	10	4.7	5	0.8
Chilli Con, Co-Op*	1 Pack/380g	448	8.4	118	3.9	19	2.2	2.8
Chilli Con, Vegan, Gro, Co-Op*	1 Pack/380g	448	8.4	118	3.9	19	2.2	2.8
Chilli, Sainsbury's*	½ Pack/250g	695	32.2	278	10.9	29.5	12.9	1.3
Kit, Old El Paso*	½ Pack/260g	598	26	230	4	31	10	0
with Cheese, From Restaurant, Average	**1 Nacho/16g**	**49**	**2.7**	**306**	**8**	**32.2**	**16.8**	**0**
NASI GORENG								
Asian, Stir Fried, Waitrose*	1 Pack/391g	501	12.1	128	7.7	16.5	3.1	1.8
Indonesian, Asda*	1 Pack/360g	778	22.7	216	7.4	32.3	6.3	1.3
Slimming World*	1 Pack/550g	495	3.3	90	6.8	13.5	0.6	1.6
Taste Malaysia, M&S*	1 Pack/400g	664	28	166	5.9	19.5	7	0.7
Vitasia, Lidl*	1 Bowl/250g	438	11	175	7.3	25.8	4.4	1.1
NECTARINES								
Fresh, Raw, Weighed with Stone, Average	**1 Med/140g**	**50**	**0.1**	**36**	**1.2**	**8**	**0.1**	**1.1**
NESQUIK								
Chocolate Flavour, Powder, Dry Weight, Nesquik, Nestle*	1 Serving/15g	56	0.5	372	3	82.9	3.1	6.5
Strawberry Flavour, Powder, Dry Weight, Nesquik, Nestle*	1 Serving/15g	59	0	393	0	98.1	0	0
NETTLES								
Raw, Average	1 Serving/80g	34	0.1	42	2.7	7	0.1	6.9
NIK NAKS								
Cream 'n' Cheesy, KP Snacks*	1 Bag/34g	196	13	575	5.2	52.7	38.1	0.2
Nice 'n' Spicy, KP Snacks*	1 Bag/30g	171	11.5	571	4.6	51.6	38.4	1.6
Rib 'n' Saucy, Golden Wonder*	1 Bag/25g	143	9.4	571	4.5	53.7	37.6	0.5
Scampi 'n' Lemon, KP Snacks*	1 Bag/25g	143	9.4	573	4.9	53.1	37.5	0.1
NOODLES								
Bacon, Dry Supernoodles, Weight, Batchelors*	1 Pack/100g	526	23.6	526	9.4	69.2	23.6	1.6
BBQ Beef, Instant, Made Up, Sainsbury's*	1 Pack/245g	422	18.2	172	3.7	21.6	7.4	2
Beef, BBQ, Instant, Cooked, Aldi*	1 Serving/324g	515	19.4	159	3.7	21.9	6	1.1
Beef, BBQ, Made Up, Supernoodles, Batchelors*	½ Pack/150g	250	11.1	167	3.2	21.3	7.4	1
Beef, Chilli, Ramen, M&S*	1 Pack/484g	532	17.4	110	8.1	11.9	3.6	0.8
Beef, Oriental, GFY, Asda*	1 Pack/400g	372	6.8	93	7.4	12.1	1.7	1.7
Beef, Udon, Shanghai, M&S*	1 Pack/350g	452	14.3	129	7.2	15.1	4.1	1.6
Chicken Curry, As Sold, Shake That Weight*	1 Pack/45g	171	5	380	31.1	35.2	11	7.7
Chicken, Chinese, Fresh Ideas, Morrisons*	1 Pack/389g	354	7	91	6.3	11.6	1.8	1.8
Chicken, Instant, As Prepared, Maggi*	1 Pack/308g	271	10.5	88	1.9	12.1	3.4	0.6
Chicken, Instant, Made Up, Aldi*	1 Pack/280g	414	15.4	148	3	21	5.5	0.8
Chicken, Made Up, Supernoodles, Batchelors*	1 Serving/150g	264	11.8	176	3.1	23	7.9	0.4
Chicken, Oriental Style, Instant, Cooked, Koka*	1 Pack/485g	393	16.5	81	1.9	10.4	3.4	0.5
Chicken, Oriental, Slim Choice, Sainsbury's*	1 Pack/490g	333	5.4	68	6.8	6.9	1.1	1.9
Chicken, Pad Thai, Waitrose*	1 Pack/400g	588	24	147	6.6	15.5	6	2.6
Chicken, Peri Peri, Super Noodles, Batchelors*	1 Pack/290g	440	18.8	152	3.1	19.5	6.5	1.3
Chicken, Pot, Made Up, Super Noodles, Batchelors*	1 Pot/265g	353	14.9	133	2.5	17.7	5.6	0.9
Chicken, Snack Stop, Made Up, Mug Shot*	1 Pack/233g	175	1.2	75	2.3	14	0.5	1.2
Chicken, Soy, Ginger, Slimming World, Iceland*	1 Pack/550g	478	3.8	87	8.1	11.2	0.7	2
Chilli Chicken Cashew, Box Ingredients Only, Gousto*	1 Serving/317g	532	13.6	168	13.3	18	4.3	2.4
Chow Mein, Made Up, Supernoodles, Batchelors*	½ Pack/150g	262	11.8	175	3	23	7.9	0.4
Chow Mein, Newgate Express, Pot, Aldi*	1 Pot/78g	235	8.6	301	10.8	56.4	11	3
Cup, Soba, Teriyaki, As Sold, Nissin *	1 Pot/90g	193	8.4	214	5	26.2	9.3	0
Curry, Instant, Vitasia, Lidl*	1 Pack/108g	124	5.3	115	2.5	15.3	4.9	0
Curry, Mild, Dry Weight, Supernoodles, Batchelors*	½ Pack/50g	260	11.7	520	9.4	67.8	23.4	1.4
Curry, Singapore, Made Up, Naked Noodle Snack Pot*	1 Pot/329g	270	2	82	2.9	15.7	0.6	0.9
Duck, Hoisin, My Goodness, Sainsbury's*	1 Pack/363g	418	18.5	115	7.2	9.2	5.1	1.8
Duck, Shredded, Hoisin, G&B, Asda*	1 Pack/367g	396	6.2	108	5.8	17	1.7	1.8

	Measure INFO/WEIGHT	per Measure		Nutrition Values per 100g / 100ml				
		KCAL	FAT	KCAL	PROT	CARB	FAT	FIBRE
NOODLES								
Egg, Boiled	**1oz/28g**	**17**	**0.1**	**62**	**2.2**	**13**	**0.5**	**0.6**
Egg, Coconut, & Lemongrass, Waitrose*	½ Pack/121g	176	6.2	145	3.6	19.9	5.1	2.7
Egg, Dry, Average	**1 Block/63g**	**218**	**1.2**	**348**	**12.1**	**70.1**	**1.9**	**2.6**
Egg, Fine Thread, Dry, M&S*	1 Serving/63g	220	0.6	350	14.3	71.6	0.9	5.1
Egg, Fine, Blue Dragon*	1 Serving/100g	356	1.7	356	13.8	70	1.7	3.4
Egg, Fine, Dry Weight, Sharwood's*	1 Block/63g	216	1.3	346	12	70	2.1	2.5
Egg, Fine, Fresh, M&S*	1 Pack/275g	330	6.1	120	4.4	20.7	2.2	1.5
Egg, Fine, Morrisons*	¼ Pack/184g	232	0.9	126	4.6	24.8	0.5	1.9
Egg, Fine, Sainsbury's*	1 Nest/150g	256	2.7	171	6	31.8	1.8	1.8
Egg, Fine, Waitrose*	¼ Pack/63g	221	1.6	353	15	67.3	2.6	3.8
Egg, Tossed in Sesame Oil, Asda*	½ Pack/150g	174	10.5	116	2.3	11	7	0.6
Fried, Average	**1oz/28g**	**43**	**3.2**	**153**	**1.9**	**11.3**	**11.5**	**0.5**
Glass, Dry Weight	**1 Serving/100g**	**351**	**0.1**	**351**	**0.1**	**86.1**	**0.1**	**0.5**
Instant, Beef, As Prepared, Asda*	½ Pack/125g	180	7	144	3.1	20	5.6	1.7
Instant, Curry Flavour, As Sold, Asda*	½ Pack/43g	159	5.9	369	9.4	47.2	13.6	8.9
Instant, Curry, HFC, Tesco*	1 Pack/176g	246	9.2	140	3.3	18.5	5.2	3.1
Instant, MR.Noodles *	1 Pack/86g	380	12	442	11.6	67.4	14	2.3
Instant, Spicy Goreng, Hot Heads, Maggie*	1 Pack/119g	547	23.8	460	20	62	20	0
Konjac, Diet, Active Foods, Bulk Powders*	1 Pack/200g	12	1	6	0.5	3.5	0.5	3
Konjac, Raw, Asian Cuisine, Clean Foods*	1 Serving/100g	6	0	6	1	0	0	3.6
Laksa, Chicken, & Black Noodles, Thrive, Waitrose*	1 Pack/369g	406	10.3	110	8.7	11.6	2.8	1.6
Lost the Pot, Sweet Chilli, Pot Noodle*	1 Pack/92g	132	4.6	144	3.1	19.2	5	0.9
Medium, Straight To Wok, Tesco*	1 Pack/300g	441	5.1	147	5.5	26.3	1.7	2.6
Mi Goreng, Fried, Instant, Indo Mie*	1 Pack/80g	400	19.4	500	9.6	59.7	24.2	2.3
Mushroom, Teriyaki, Gro, Co-Op*	1 Pack/380g	338	6.5	89	3.2	15	1.7	1.1
Nest, Medium, Cooked, Waitrose*	1 Nest/63g	88	0.3	139	5	28.6	0.5	0.6
No Beef, Shanghai, Bowl, Plant Kitchen, M&S*	1 Pack/350g	466	11.2	133	6.1	19.1	3.2	1.5
Pad Kaprao, Thai Taste*	½ Pack/110g	261	5.2	237	6.3	42	4.7	1.4
Pad Thai, Allplants*	1 Serving/387g	507	18.6	131	4.9	16	4.8	2.5
Pad Thai, Chicken, Scratch*	1 Pack/380g	273	6.1	72	7.4	7.9	1.6	1.3
Pad Thai, Chicken, Waitrose*	½ Pack/100g	170	7.2	170	6.5	18.4	7.2	2.5
Pad Thai, GF, Amy's Kitchen*	1 Pack/268g	407	8.8	152	4.1	26	3.3	1.1
Pad Thai, Ribbon, Ready to Wok, Sharwood's*	1 Serving/150g	206	1.7	137	5	26.3	1.1	1
Pad Thai, Rice, M&S*	½ Pack/137g	246	4	179	3.7	33.4	2.9	2.3
Pea, with Garlic Dressing, High Protein, M&S*	½ Pack/211g	323	5.9	153	8.5	22.4	2.8	2
Plain, Boiled	**1oz/28g**	**17**	**0.1**	**62**	**2.4**	**13**	**0.4**	**0.7**
Plain, Dry	**1oz/28g**	**109**	**1.7**	**388**	**11.7**	**76.1**	**6.2**	**2.9**
Plain, Straight to Wok, Asda*	½ Pack/150g	232	0.8	155	6.2	31	0.5	2.2
Pork, Spiced, Asian Style, Super Quick, Hello Fresh*	1 Serving/337g	421	16.8	125	8	13	5	0
Pork, Spicy BBQ, Snack Pot, Tesco*	1 Pot/263g	276	4.5	105	4	17.7	1.7	1.4
Pork, Tonkotsu, Cup, Made Up, Nissin*	1 Cup/350g	322	13.3	92	2.6	11.3	3.8	0
Posh Noodles, Ramen, Creamy Malaysian Laksa, BOL*	1 Pot/345g	376	10.3	109	3.2	16.1	3	2.4
Posh Noodles, Teriyaki Udon, Sweet & Sticky, BOL*	1 Pot/360g	392	6.8	109	3.3	18.8	1.9	1.6
Prawn, Chilli, King, Finest, Tesco*	1 Pack/400g	340	8	85	4	11.9	2	0.9
Prawn, King, Laksa, Slimming World*	1 Pack/550g	346	3.8	63	4.5	8.8	0.7	1.5
Prawn, King, Singapore, Free From, Tesco*	1 Pack/338g	352	11.8	104	3.8	13.8	3.5	1.2
Prawn, Laksa, Diet Chef Ltd*	1 Pack/270g	173	5.4	64	3.1	8.1	2	0.8
Prawn, Tiger, Stir Fry, Tesco*	1 Pack/400g	596	14.8	149	6	23	3.7	2.7
Prawn, Zingy, M&S*	1 Pack/365g	310	4.4	85	4.1	13.8	1.2	1.1
Protein, Stir Fried, Morrisons*	½ Pack/143g	294	4.7	206	10.9	32	3.3	2.2
Protein, Super Sesame, Pot, Itsu*	1 Pot/315g	211	6	67	6.8	4	1.9	2.7
Ramen, Chicken, Microwaved, G&B, Asda*	1 Pack/316g	240	7.6	76	6.9	6.1	2.4	1.2
Ramen, Demae, Nissin*	1 Pack/500g	430	18	86	2.1	10.7	3.6	3

	Measure INFO/WEIGHT	per Measure KCAL	FAT	Nutrition Values per 100g / 100ml KCAL	PROT	CARB	FAT	FIBRE

NOODLES

	Measure INFO/WEIGHT	KCAL	FAT	KCAL	PROT	CARB	FAT	FIBRE
Rice, Chilli Chicken, Pot, As Sold, Itsu*	1 Pot/63g	219	2.2	348	8.4	69.8	3.5	2.5
Rice, Chow Mein, Pot, As Prepared, Free From, Asda*	1 Pot/376g	286	1.9	76	1.5	17	0.5	1
Rice, Cooked	**1 Cup/176g**	**192**	**0.4**	**109**	**0.9**	**24.9**	**0.2**	**1**
Rice, Pad Thai, Peanut, M&S*	1 Pack/275g	492	8	179	3.7	33.4	2.9	2.3
Rice, Satay, Pot, As Prepared, Itsu*	1 Pot/314g	229	3.5	73	1.7	14	1.1	0.7
Rice, Singapore Style, Morrisons*	½ Pack/166g	266	3.3	160	2.8	32.1	2	1.4
Rice, Singapore, Cooked, Tesco*	½ Pack/150g	224	2.7	149	2.6	30.1	1.8	0.9
Rice, Singapore, Market St, Morrisons*	¼ Pack/90g	192	6.2	214	3.5	33.4	6.9	1.9
Rice, Stir Fry, Tesco*	½ Pack/190g	304	10.8	160	2	24.8	5.7	1
Rice, Sweet Chilli, Ilumi*	1 Pot/375g	292	1.1	78	1.6	17	0.3	0.5
Rice, Vermicelli, Mama*	1 Serving/45g	166	0.4	370	7	81	1	0
Rice, Waitrose*	½ Pack/115g	175	0.8	152	3.1	33	0.7	0.8
Satay, Tesco*	1 Pot/200g	314	11	157	5.2	21.1	5.5	0.9
Singapore, BGTY, Sainsbury's*	1 Pack/369g	317	10	86	7.2	8.2	2.7	2.1
Singapore, Cook*	1 Serving/275g	289	5.8	105	5.7	16.6	2.1	1.6
Singapore, Dry Weight, Blue Dragon*	1 Serving/82g	276	5.2	337	5.7	63	6.4	2.2
Singapore, Sainsbury's*	1 Pack/450g	540	18	120	6.4	13.3	4	2.7
Singapore, Style, Asda*	1 Pack/400g	688	32	172	7	18	8	1
Singapore, Style, Sainsbury's*	½ Pack/150g	320	10.8	214	3.2	33.2	7.2	1.3
Singapore, with Chicken, G&B, Asda*	1 Pack/365g	383	5.5	105	5.4	17	1.5	1
Singapore, with Chicken, Pork, Egg, & Prawns, M&S*	1 Pack/400g	520	20.4	130	6	14.5	5.1	1.2
Soba, Clearspring*	1 Serving/75g	263	2	351	16	64	2.7	3.5
Soba, Japanese, Dry, Yutaka*	1 Serving/63g	218	0.8	349	12	70	1.2	5
Straight to Wok, Rice, Amoy*	1 Pack/150g	174	0.2	116	1.6	27.4	0.1	0
Straight to Wok, Singapore, Amoy*	1 Serving/150g	206	3.3	137	6.4	21.6	2.2	2.8
Straight to Wok, Thread, Fine, Amoy*	1 Pack/150g	237	3.9	158	5	28.7	2.6	0
Swede, Swoodles, Tesco*	1 Pack/250g	32	0.2	13	0.3	2.3	0.1	0.7
Sweet & Sour, Cup Shotz, Aldi*	1 Pack/63g	67	0.4	107	2.7	22	0.6	1
Sweet Chilli, Ready to Eat, Tesco*	½ Pack/100g	137	3.3	137	3.9	22.1	3.3	1.4
Teriyaki, Plant Chef, Tesco*	1 Pack/350g	336	8.8	96	1.9	15.2	2.5	2.6
Thai, Fastpot, Lighter Life*	1 Pot/55g	206	4.2	374	25.7	44.8	7.6	11.5
Thai, Style, Sainsbury's*	1 Pack/340g	381	7.8	112	3.3	19.4	2.3	0.7
Thai, Style, Snack, Cupshotz, Aldi*	1 Pack/55g	215	2.8	391	11.4	71.4	5.1	6.9
Turkey, Sweet Chilli, Box Ingredients Only, Gousto*	1 Serving/381g	549	13.7	144	11.3	16.4	3.6	1.8
Udon, Aubergine, Sticky Miso, Sainsbury's*	1 Pack/400g	448	11.2	112	2.6	18.2	2.8	1.7
Udon, Cooked, Just Cook, Sainsbury's*	½ Pack/129g	213	3.6	165	5.1	28.9	2.8	2.3
Udon, Fresh, M&S*	½ Pack/138g	213	1.9	155	4.4	30.4	1.4	1.8
Udon, Japanese, Sainsbury's*	1 Serving/150g	210	2.7	140	3.9	27.1	1.8	1.2
Udon, Teriyaki, Allplants*	1 Serving/365g	420	14.6	115	3.8	15	4	2.3
Udon, Yasai Yaki, Allplants*	½ Pack/380g	494	24.3	130	4.4	12	6.4	2.1
Vermicelli, Rice, Dry Weight, Ko-Lee*	1 Serving/50g	180	0	360	6.6	81	0	2
Wheat, High Protein, Tesco*	1 Pack/300g	459	3.3	153	9.4	25.4	1.1	1.8
Wholewheat, Cooked Weight, Sharwoods*	1 Portion/161g	215	1.5	134	5	24.8	0.9	2.7
Wholewheat, Dry, Sharwoods*	1 Portion/63g	224	1.4	356	13	66.2	2.3	9.2
Wholewheat, Dry, Tesco*	¼ Pack/66g	227	0.9	342	14.2	64.2	1.4	7.7
Wholewheat, Straight to Wok, Asda*	½ Pack/152g	225	1.2	148	4.9	29	0.8	2.8

NOUGAT

	Measure INFO/WEIGHT	KCAL	FAT	KCAL	PROT	CARB	FAT	FIBRE
Average	**1 Sm Bar/28g**	**108**	**2.4**	**384**	**4.4**	**77.3**	**8.5**	**0.9**
Blueberry, Almond, Deluxe, Lidl*	½ Bar/38g	142	1.5	379	1.8	83.2	3.9	0
Italian, Soft, Mixed Berry, Waitrose*	1 Bar/100g	435	11.1	435	3.9	78	11.1	3.5
Raspberry & Orange Hazelnut, Thorntons*	1 Sweet/9g	39	1.8	433	4.8	60	20	2.2

NUGGETS

	Measure INFO/WEIGHT	KCAL	FAT	KCAL	PROT	CARB	FAT	FIBRE
Chicken Style, Vegan, The Vegetarian Butcher*	½ Pack/90g	213	11.4	237	9.6	18.8	12.7	5

	Measure INFO/WEIGHT	per Measure KCAL	FAT	Nutrition Values per 100g / 100ml KCAL	PROT	CARB	FAT	FIBRE
NUGGETS								
No Chicken, Vegan, Plant Menu, Aldi*	4 Nuggets/80g	238	12.8	297	14	23	16	3.2
Nuggets, Vegan, Crispy, Quorn*	4 Nuggets/76g	144	6.3	190	9.4	17	8.3	4.5
NUT ROAST								
Average	**1 Serving/200g**	**704**	**51.4**	**352**	**13.3**	**18.3**	**25.7**	**4.2**
Butternut, Almond, & Pecan, Plant Kitchen, M&S*	½ Pack/220g	334	14.1	152	5	14.3	6.4	8.5
Cashew, Quinoa, & Carrot, Deluxe, Lidl*	¼ Pack/88g	252	16.5	286	12.5	14.2	18.7	5.5
Cheese, Melting, Sainsbury's*	1 Nut Roast/140g	364	20.6	260	9.2	19.6	14.7	6.4
Four, Waitrose*	1 Serving/163g	386	23.8	237	5.8	18.8	14.6	3.4
Hazelnut, Cashew, & Cranberry, Deluxe, Lidl*	1/3 Pack/117g	345	21.6	295	12	17.5	18.5	5.4
Kale, & Broccoli, Vegetarian, Tesco*	½ Pack/122g	226	12.1	185	5.9	13.7	9.9	8.8
Lentil, Average	**1oz/28g**	**62**	**3.4**	**222**	**10.6**	**18.8**	**12.1**	**3.8**
Lentil, Red Pepper, & Almond, Vegan, Deluxe, Lidl*	1 Roast/175g	352	17.5	201	8.2	15	10	8.5
Nut, & Cranberry, The Best, Morrisons*	1 Pack/400g	976	52.8	244	5.8	23.7	13.2	3.5
Sweet Potato, & Maple Carrot, Loaf, Sainsbury's*	¼ Loaf/100g	202	12.4	202	9.3	9.6	12.4	7.5
Vegan, GF, Clive's*	1 Serving/140g	261	11.8	186	4	21.5	8.4	4.3
Vegan, Good Health, Waitrose*	½ Pack/143g	315	19.7	220	11.3	7.6	13.8	9.9
NUTMEG								
Ground, Average	**1 Tsp/3g**	**16**	**1.1**	**525**	**5.8**	**45.3**	**36.3**	**0**
NUTS								
Cashew, Shots, Asda*	1 Pack/6g	35	2.9	583	18	18	48	3.2
Cashews & Peanuts, Honey Roasted, Average	**1 Serving/50g**	**290**	**21.4**	**579**	**21.6**	**26.6**	**42.9**	**4.2**
Chilli, & Lime, Punchy, Graze*	1 Serving/29g	173	13.6	598	22	22	47	7.4
Mixed	**1 Pack/40g**	**243**	**21.6**	**607**	**22.9**	**7.9**	**54.1**	**6**
Mixed, Almonds, Brazil, Hazel & Walnuts, M&S*	1 Serving/25g	168	16	670	16	4.8	64	5.4
Mixed, Roasted, & Salted, Tesco*	1 Serving/25g	160	13.9	641	20.4	10.7	55.6	8
Mixed, Roasted, Salted, Waitrose*	1 Pack/200g	1252	116.8	626	13.7	11.3	58.4	4.4
Mixed, Roasted, Tesco*	1 Pack/55g	335	26.8	609	23.4	15.1	48.8	7.8
Peanuts, & Cashews, Jumbo, Clancy*	½ Pack/75g	464	38.2	619	25	13	51	6.8
Selection, Roasted, M&S*	1 Pack/150g	903	74.4	602	24.9	9.5	49.6	9.2
Veggie Burst , Aldi*	1 Pack/25g	140	10	562	30	18	40	4.1
NUTS & RAISINS								
Mixed, Average	**1 Serving/30g**	**144**	**10.2**	**481**	**14.1**	**31.5**	**34.1**	**4.5**
Mixed, Grazin', Holland & Barrett*	1 Pack/200g	888	62	444	8.8	34	31	3.4
Peanuts, Mixed, Average	**1 Pack/40g**	**174**	**10.4**	**435**	**15.3**	**37.5**	**26**	**4.4**
Peanuts, Posh, & Ritzy Raisins, Holland & Barrett*	1 Pack/40g	152	6.2	379	8	54.5	15.4	3
Yoghurt Coated, Waitrose*	1 Serving/50g	264	18.4	527	10.9	38.2	36.7	3

	Measure	per Measure		Nutrition Values per 100g / 100ml				
	INFO/WEIGHT	KCAL	FAT	KCAL	PROT	CARB	FAT	FIBRE

OAT CAKES

Black Pepper, Savour Bakes, Aldi*	1 Oatcake/10g	45	1.8	450	10	57	18	9.5
Cheese, Nairn's*	1 Oatcake/8g	39	2.2	473	13.6	44.7	26.6	7.2
Fine Milled, Nairn's*	1 Oatcake/8g	35	1.7	449	10.5	52.6	21.8	8.6
Fruit, & Seed, On the Go, Nairn's*	1 Oatcake/13g	57	2	437	9.6	60.2	15.5	9.2
Herb & Pumpkin Seed, Nairn's*	1 Oatcake/10g	43	2.1	426	12.2	46.8	21.1	13
Highland, Walkers*	1 Oatcake/12g	54	2.5	451	10.3	56	20.6	6.7
Oatmeal, Rough, Nairn's*	1 Oatcake/11g	45	1.8	431	10.2	58.6	17.3	8
Oatmeal, Rough, Organic, Nairn's*	1 Oatcake/10g	45	1.7	437	10	57.6	16.1	10.6
Orkney, Thick, Stockan's*	1 Oatcake/25g	122	4.6	489	9.8	68	18.2	6.8
Orkney, Thin, Stockan's*	1 Oatcake/13g	65	2.9	501	10.4	62.4	22	6
Retail, Average	*1 Oatcake/13g*	*57*	*2.4*	*441*	*10*	*63*	*18.3*	*2*
Rough with Olive Oil, Paterson's*	1 Oatcake/13g	55	2.1	440	11.7	54.7	17	0
Rough, Crumbly, M&S*	1 Oatcake/13g	58	2.6	463	9.8	56.5	20.5	6.4
Rough, Sainsbury's*	1 Oatcake/10g	47	2	454	9.8	55.4	19.2	10
Rough, Scottish, Rivercote, Lidl*	1 Oatcake/11g	49	2	448	11	55.8	18.2	8.7
Rough, Scottish, Tesco*	1 Oatcake/10g	45	1.9	435	11.4	55.3	18.4	8
Seeded, Scottish, Rivercote, Lidl*	1 Oatcake/11g	48	2.1	461	11	54.9	19.9	9.1
Super Seeded, Organic, Nairns*	1 Oatcake/10g	44	1.9	444	13.4	50.2	19	9.2
Three Seed, Organic, Island Bakery*	1 Oatcake/8g	34	1.8	421	9.7	44	22	0
Traditional, M&S*	1 Oatcake/11g	49	2	445	11	59.3	18.3	6.6

OAT DRINK

Barista Edition, Oatly*	1 Serving/200ml	118	6	59	1	6.6	3	0.8
Milk, Acti-Leaf, Aldi*	1 Serving/250ml	120	3.8	48	0.5	7.7	1.5	0.7
Milk, Barista Blend, Califia*	1 Serving/200ml	110	6	55	0.7	5.7	3	0.8
Nordic, Jord*	1 Serving/100ml	49	1.5	49	1.2	7.1	1.5	0
Nordic, Organic, Jord*	1 Serving/100ml	54	1.5	54	0.8	8.8	1.5	0
Oat Milk, Barista Blend, Califa Farms*	1 Serving/200ml	110	6	55	0.7	5.7	3	0.8
Oat Milk, Barista, Organic, Rude Health*	1 Serving/200ml	116	4.8	58	0.7	7.8	2.4	0.9
Oat Milk, GF, Barista, Alpro*	1 Serving/200ml	122	6.2	61	0.3	7.9	3.1	0
Oat Milk, Organic, Healthy, Oatly*	1 Serving/250ml	100	1.2	40	1	6.7	0.5	0.8
Oat Milk, Unsweetened, Just Free, Lidl*	1 Serving/200ml	74	2.4	37	0.4	5.6	1.2	0.9
Oat, & Barley, Jord*	1 Serving/100ml	49	1.4	49	1.1	7.6	1.4	0
Oat, Original, Alpro*	1 Serving/200ml	88	3	44	0.3	6.8	1.5	1.4
Oatmilk, Tesco*	1 Serving/200ml	118	6	59	1	7	3	1
Semi Skimmed, Oatly*	1 Serving/100ml	46	1.5	46	1	6.6	1.5	0.8
Skinny, Oatly*	1 Serving/200ml	74	1	37	1	6.6	0.5	0.8
Whole, Oatly*	1 Serving/150ml	86	4.2	57	1	6.6	2.8	0.8

OCTOPUS

Raw	*1oz/28g*	*18*	*0.3*	*66*	*14.1*	*0*	*1*	*0*

OIL

Avocado, Olivado*	1 Tsp/5ml	40	4.4	802	0	0	88	0
Butter Flavour, Spray, Fry Light*	1 Spray/0.2m	1	0.1	516	0	0.3	53.4	0
Chilli, Average	*1 Tsp/5ml*	*41*	*4.6*	*824*	*0*	*0*	*91.5*	*0*
Coconut, Average	*1 Tsp/5ml*	*45*	*5*	*899*	*0*	*0*	*99.9*	*0*
Cod Liver, Average	*1 Capsule/1g*	*9*	*1*	*900*	*0*	*0*	*100*	*0*
Corn, Average	*1 Tsp/5ml*	*43*	*4.8*	*864*	*0*	*0*	*96*	*0*
Evening Primrose, Average	*1 Serving/1g*	*9*	*1*	*900*	*0*	*0*	*100*	*0*
Fish, Average	*1 Serving/1g*	*9*	*1*	*900*	*0*	*0*	*100*	*0*
Flax Seed, Average	*1 Tbsp/15ml*	*124*	*13.9*	*829*	*0*	*0*	*92.6*	*0*
Garlic, Infuse, Fry Light*	1 Spray/0.2ml	1	0.1	507	0	0.4	52.9	0
Grapeseed, Average	*1 Tsp/5ml*	*43*	*4.8*	*866*	*0*	*0*	*96.2*	*0*
Groundnut, Average	*1 Tsp/5ml*	*41*	*4.6*	*824*	*0*	*0*	*91.8*	*0*
Hazelnut, Average	*1 Tsp/5ml*	*45*	*5*	*899*	*0*	*0*	*99.9*	*0*

	Measure INFO/WEIGHT	per Measure KCAL	FAT	Nutrition Values per 100g / 100ml KCAL	PROT	CARB	FAT	FIBRE
OIL								
MCT, Pure, C8, Ketosource*	1 Tbsp/15ml	135	15	899	0	0	100	0
Mustard, Average	**1 Serving/100g**	**884**	**100**	**884**	**0**	**0**	**100**	**0**
Olive, Average	**1 Tsp/5ml**	**43**	**4.7**	**855**	**0**	**0**	**94.9**	**0**
Olive, Extra Virgin, Average	**1 Tsp/5ml**	**42**	**4.7**	**848**	**0**	**0**	**94.5**	**0**
Olive, Garlic, Average	**1 Tbsp/15ml**	**127**	**14.1**	**848**	**0**	**0**	**94.3**	**0**
Olive, Mild, Average	**1 Tbsp/15ml**	**129**	**14.4**	**862**	**0**	**0**	**95.7**	**0**
Olive, Spray, Average	**10 Sprays/2ml**	**10**	**1.1**	**508**	**0**	**0**	**54.6**	**0**
Palm, Average	**1 Tsp/5ml**	**45**	**5**	**899**	**0**	**0**	**99.9**	**0**
Peanut, Average	**1 Tsp/5ml**	**45**	**5**	**899**	**0**	**0**	**99.9**	**0**
Rapeseed, Average	**1 Tbsp/15ml**	**130**	**14.4**	**864**	**0**	**0**	**96**	**0**
Rice Bran, Average	**1 Tbsp/14g**	**120**	**13.6**	**884**	**0**	**0**	**100**	**0**
Sesame, Average	**1 Tsp/5ml**	**45**	**5**	**892**	**0.1**	**0**	**99.9**	**0**
Sunflower, Average	**1 Tsp/5ml**	**43**	**4.8**	**869**	**0**	**0**	**96.6**	**0**
Truffle, Fussels*	1 Tsp/5ml	45	5	901	0.1	0.1	99.1	0
Vegetable, Average	**1 Tbsp/15ml**	**129**	**14.3**	**858**	**0**	**0**	**95.3**	**0**
Walnut, Average	**1 Tsp/5ml**	**45**	**5**	**899**	**0**	**0**	**99.9**	**0**
OKRA								
Boiled in Unsalted Water, Average	**1 Serving/80g**	**22**	**0.7**	**28**	**2.5**	**2.7**	**0.9**	**3.6**
Raw, Average	**1 Serving/80g**	**18**	**0.6**	**23**	**2.1**	**2.2**	**0.7**	**3**
Stir-Fried in Corn Oil, Average	**1 Serving/80g**	**215**	**20.9**	**269**	**4.3**	**4.4**	**26.1**	**6.3**
OLIVES								
Black, Pitted, Average	**½ Jar/82g**	**135**	**13.3**	**164**	**1**	**3.5**	**16.2**	**3.1**
Green, Chimichurri, Tesco*	1 Serving/30g	46	4.7	155	1.1	1.1	15.6	2.8
Green, Garlic Stuffed, Asda*	1 Olive/3g	6	0.6	174	1.8	3.5	17	0
Green, Lemon & Coriander, Co-Op*	1 Pack/65g	90	9.1	139	1.1	1.3	14	2.9
Green, Pimento Stuffed, with Gouda & Cumin, Unearthed*	1 Serving/30g	65	6	217	6.6	1	20	2.6
Green, Pitted, Average	**1 Olive/3g**	**4**	**0.4**	**130**	**1.1**	**0.9**	**13.3**	**2.5**
Green, Pitted, with Chilli Peppers, Crespo*	1 Pack/70g	132	13.2	189	1.1	0.1	18.9	6.9
Green, Stuffed with Almonds, Pitted, Waitrose*	1 Serving/50g	90	8.4	180	3.8	3.2	16.9	2.5
Halkidiki, Stuffed with Garlic, Tesco*	¼ Pack/40g	66	6.7	164	1.3	0.3	16.8	3
Kalamata, in Brine, Drained, Finest, Tesco*	1 Serving/30g	79	8.3	264	1.5	1.2	27.7	1.9
Kalamata, Pitted, Gaea*	1 Serving/15g	26	2.8	172	0.9	2.1	18.7	0
Marinated, Mixed, M&S*	1 Serving/20g	33	3	165	1.6	6.5	14.9	3
Mixed, Mediterranean, Morrisons*	1 Serving/30g	74	7.7	248	1	1.6	25.8	2.9
Mixed, with Mature Cheddar, Tesco*	1/5 Pack/44g	77	7.6	174	3	0.7	17.1	2.6
Spanish, Chimichurri, Specially Selected, Aldi*	¼ Pot/35g	56	5.6	159	1.1	1.4	16	3.1
Spanish, Trio, Sainsbury's*	1/5 Pot/60g	90	7.7	150	1.1	5.1	12.8	5.4
OMELETTE								
Cheese & Mushroom, Apetito*	1 Serving/320g	486	25	152	6.2	14.4	7.8	1.9
Cheese, 2 Egg, Average	**1 Omelette/180g**	**479**	**40.7**	**266**	**15.9**	**0**	**22.6**	**0**
Cheese, HFC, Tesco*	1 Omelette/95g	214	16.4	226	13.2	4.1	17.3	0.6
Ham & Mushroom, Farmfoods*	1 Omelette/120g	200	16.7	167	8.7	1.8	13.9	0.1
Mushroom & Cheese, Tesco*	1 Omelette/120g	248	21.5	207	9.8	1.6	17.9	0.2
Plain, 2 Egg	**1 Omelette/120g**	**229**	**19.7**	**191**	**10.9**	**0**	**16.4**	**0**
Potato, Spanish, Waitrose*	1 Pack/500g	710	40	142	6.9	9.5	8	0.5
Potato, with Chorizo, Sol & Mar, Lidl*	¼ Omelette/125g	238	15	190	9.8	10	12	1.2
Spanish	**1oz/28g**	**34**	**2.3**	**120**	**5.7**	**6.2**	**8.3**	**1.4**
Spanish Tortilla, Potato, with Onion, Unearthed*	¼ Pack/125g	181	8.9	145	5.2	15	7.1	1.8
ONION POWDER								
Average	**1 Tsp/2g**	**7**	**0**	**341**	**10.4**	**79.1**	**1**	**15.2**
ONION RINGS								
Battered, Co-Op*	1 Ring/13g	30	1.1	227	3.2	34	8.3	2.7
Battered, Diggers*	1 Ring/20g	40	1.8	200	2.9	26.5	9.2	0

O

| | Measure | per Measure | | Nutrition Values per 100g / 100ml | | | | |
	INFO/WEIGHT	KCAL	FAT	KCAL	PROT	CARB	FAT	FIBRE
ONION RINGS								
Battered, Free From, Tesco*	3 Rings/63g	190	9.5	303	3.1	37.3	15.2	2.1
Battered, Mini, Frozen, Tesco*	4 Rings/34g	87	3.9	259	4.2	32.8	11.6	3.3
Battered, Sainsbury's*	1 Ring/12g	32	1.4	265	3.8	34.4	11.6	4.1
Beer Battered, Frozen, Tesco*	3 Rings/75g	213	10	284	4.6	36	13.3	0.8
Beer Battered, M&S*	1 Serving/70g	151	6.5	216	2.7	29.6	9.3	1.4
Beer Battered, Mash Direct*	½ Pack/100g	283	10.3	283	2.6	23.9	10.3	2.7
Breaded & Fried, From Restaurant	*1 Ring/12g*	*40*	*2.2*	*332*	*4.5*	*37.7*	*18.7*	*0*
Oven Crisp Batter, Tesco*	1 Ring/17g	44	1.9	259	4.1	34.4	11.2	2.1
ONIONS								
Baked	*1oz/28g*	*29*	*0.2*	*103*	*3.5*	*22.3*	*0.6*	*3.9*
Boiled in Unsalted Water	*1oz/28g*	*5*	*0*	*17*	*0.6*	*3.7*	*0.1*	*0.7*
Crispy, Top Taste*	1 Serving/10g	59	4.4	590	6	40	44	0
Dried, Raw, Average	*1oz/28g*	*88*	*0.5*	*313*	*10.2*	*68.6*	*1.7*	*12.1*
Flakes, Dried, Average	*1 Tbsp/15g*	*52*	*0.1*	*349*	*9*	*83.3*	*0.5*	*9.2*
Fried, Average	*1oz/28g*	*46*	*3.1*	*164*	*2.3*	*14.1*	*11.2*	*3.1*
Pickled, Average	*1 Onion/15g*	*3*	*0*	*19*	*0.7*	*4.1*	*0.1*	*0.6*
Raw, Average	*1 Med/180g*	*69*	*0.4*	*38*	*1.2*	*7.9*	*0.2*	*1.3*
Red, Raw, Average	*1 Med/180g*	*66*	*0.4*	*37*	*1.2*	*7.9*	*0.2*	*1.5*
Spring, Raw, Average	*1 Med/15g*	*4*	*0.1*	*24*	*1.9*	*2.9*	*0.5*	*1.4*
ORANGES								
Blood, Average	*1 Orange/140g*	*82*	*0*	*58*	*0.8*	*13.3*	*0*	*2.5*
Extract, Valencian, Dr Oetker*	1 Tsp/5g	900	100	900	0	0	100	0
Fresh, Weighed with Peel, Average	*1 Med/220g*	*97*	*0.5*	*44*	*0.9*	*10.8*	*0.2*	*3.2*
Fresh, without Peel, Average	*1 Med/154g*	*97*	*0.5*	*63*	*1.3*	*15.5*	*0.3*	*4.5*
Peel Only, Raw, Average	*1 Tbsp/6g*	*6*	*0*	*97*	*1.5*	*25*	*0.2*	*10.6*
OREGANO								
Dried	*1 Tsp/1g*	*3*	*0.1*	*306*	*11*	*49.5*	*10.3*	*0*
Fresh	*1 Tsp/1.3g*	*1*	*0*	*66*	*2.2*	*9.7*	*2*	*0*
OSTRICH								
Fillet, Steak, Pre Grilled, The Lions Kingdom*	1 Steak/125g	158	2	126	26.1	1	1.6	0
OVALTINE*								
Chocolate, Light, Dry Weight, Ovaltine*	1 Serving/20g	75	1.2	376	4.7	74	5.9	0
Chocolate, Light, Sachet, Ovaltine*	1 Sachet/25g	96	1.5	384	7.4	73	5.9	4.7
Hi Malt, Light, Instant Drink, Ovaltine*	1 Sachet/20g	72	1.2	358	9.1	67.1	5.9	2.8
Original, Light, Dry Weight, Ovaltine*	1 Serving/25g	103	2.4	412	12	69	9.5	2.9
Powder, Made Up with Whole Milk, Ovaltine*	1 Mug/227ml	220	8.6	97	3.8	12.9	3.8	0
OXTAIL								
Raw	*1oz/28g*	*18*	*1.1*	*65*	*7.6*	*0*	*3.8*	*0*
Stewed, Bone Removed	*1oz/28g*	*68*	*3.8*	*243*	*30.5*	*0*	*13.4*	*0*
OYSTERS								
Raw, Shelled, Shucked	*1 Oyster/14g*	*9*	*0.2*	*65*	*10.8*	*2.7*	*1.3*	*0*

O

	Measure INFO/WEIGHT	per Measure KCAL	FAT	Nutrition Values per 100g / 100ml KCAL	PROT	CARB	FAT	FIBRE
PAELLA								
Chicken, & Chorizo, Calorie Controlled, Morrisons*	1 Pack/299g	284	5.7	95	7.6	10.8	1.9	2
Chicken, & Prawn, King, BFY, M&S*	1 Pack/390g	429	10.1	110	8.6	12.1	2.6	1.9
Chicken, & Chorizo, Gold Standard Nutrition*	1 Pot/350g	416	13	119	9.3	12.8	3.7	1
Chicken, & Chorizo, Microwaved, Finest, Tesco*	½ Pack/350g	424	8	121	6.8	17.7	2.3	0.9
Chicken, & Chorizo, Rice Pot, Tesco*	1 Pack/330g	469	10.6	142	5.5	22	3.2	1.4
Chicken, & Chorizo, SlimWell, Aldi*	1 Pack/500g	430	3.5	86	5.7	13	0.7	2.4
Chicken, & Chorizo, The City Kitchen*	1 Pack/379g	428	9.9	113	7.5	14.5	2.6	1
Chicken, & Chorizo, Weight Watchers, Heinz*	1 Meal/399g	395	6.8	99	6.8	13	1.7	2.1
Chicken, & Prawn, Ancient Grain, Eat Well, M&S*	1 Pack/390g	433	10.5	111	7.6	12.8	2.7	2.4
Chicken, & Prawn, BGTY, Sainsbury's*	1 Pack/368g	383	8.8	104	8.2	11.4	2.4	1.9
Chicken, & Prawn, Slim Choice, Sainsbury's*	1 Pack/500g	425	3	85	6.2	13.1	0.6	1.3
Chicken, & Prawn, Slim Cook, Tesco*	1 Pack/500g	380	3	76	6.2	10.5	0.6	2.3
Chicken, & Vegetable, Well & Good, Co-Op*	1 Pack/380g	365	5.4	96	5.5	14.5	1.4	1.5
Chorizo, Spanish, Twist'd Flavour Co.*	1 Serving/125g	159	4.6	127	4	18	3.7	1.9
Prawn, King, & Chicken, The Best, Morrisons*	½ Pack/399g	519	19.6	130	5.9	14.7	4.9	1.7
Seafood, & Chicken, What's Cooking, Lidl*	½ Pack/375g	326	4.5	87	5.1	14	1.2	0
Vegetable, Chunky, Love Your Veg!, Sainsbury's*	1 Pack/382g	367	8	96	2.4	16.1	2.1	1.6
Vegetable, Wicked Kitchen, Tesco*	1 Pack/300g	276	10.5	92	1.7	12.4	3.5	1.9
PAIN AU CHOCOLAT								
Almond, The Delicatessen, Tesco*	1 Pain/100g	406	22	406	0	45	22	0
Average	**1 Pastry/60g**	**253**	**13.7**	**422**	**8**	**45.8**	**22.8**	**3.1**
GF, Schar*	1 Pain/65g	225	9.8	346	3.7	46	15	5.8
Mini, Asda*	1 Pastry/23g	96	5.5	420	8	43	24	3.3
Mini, M&S*	1 Pain/22g	92	5.2	419	9.8	40.2	23.5	3.5
PAIN AU RAISIN								
Takeaway, Average	**1 Pastry/100g**	**313**	**13.2**	**313**	**5.2**	**43**	**13.2**	**1.3**
Twist, Extra Special, Asda*	1 Pastry/110g	421	20.9	383	7	46	19	2.5
PAK CHOI								
Raw, Average	**1 Leaf/14g**	**2**	**0**	**11**	**1.3**	**1.9**	**0.2**	**0.9**
PAKORA								
Aloo, Bite Size, Shazans*	1 Pakora/20g	21	0.3	104	4.1	19	1.6	2.7
Bhaji, Onion, Fried in Vegetable Oil	**1oz/28g**	**76**	**4.1**	**271**	**9.8**	**26.2**	**14.7**	**5.5**
Bhajia, Potato Carrot & Pea, Fried in Vegetable Oil	**1oz/28g**	**100**	**6.3**	**357**	**10.9**	**28.8**	**22.6**	**6.1**
Bhajia, Vegetable, Retail	**1oz/28g**	**66**	**4.1**	**235**	**6.4**	**21.4**	**14.7**	**3.6**
Carrot, & Potato, Waitrose*	1 Pakora/55g	136	9.2	248	5.3	16.8	16.7	4.9
Chicken, Chilled, Asda*	½ Pack/185g	411	18.5	222	17	15	10	1.8
Chicken, Indian, Sainsbury's*	½ Pack/45g	95	3.3	211	27.7	7.8	7.4	1
Chicken, Indian, Waitrose*	1 Pakora/25g	45	1.5	181	21.9	8.5	6.1	2.3
Chicken, M&S*	½ Pack/50g	96	4	192	25.2	2.2	8.1	4.6
Chicken, Taste of India, Tesco*	1 Pack/150g	345	10.8	230	26.6	13.8	7.2	1.8
Chicken, with Raita Dip, Morrisons*	½ Pack/122g	312	20.9	255	15	9	17.1	2.3
Vegetable, Bite Size, Shazans*	1 Pakora/20g	63	2	314	6.1	49.3	10.2	6.5
Vegetable, Mrs Unis Spicy Foods Ltd*	½ Pack/100g	240	10.2	240	5.7	23.2	10.2	5.6
PANCAKE								
Blueberry, Kingsmill*	1 Pancake/28g	71	1.7	255	6.6	42.4	6.2	1.6
Blueberry, Lighter Life*	1 Pack/40g	151	4.4	378	32	31	11	10
Blueberry, Tesco*	1 Pancake/75g	195	3.1	260	4.8	49.5	4.1	2
Buttermilk, Aldi*	1 Pancake/40g	115	5.2	288	6.5	36	13	0.9
Buttermilk, Genesis*	1 Serving/100g	219	3.7	219	4.9	41	3.7	1.1
Buttermilk, Giant , Village Bakery, Aldi*	1 Pancake/65g	146	1.8	225	6.7	42	2.8	1.7
Buttermilk, Large, Tesco*	1 Pancake/65g	176	3.9	270	6.7	46.8	6	1.2
Buttermilk, Sainsbury's*	1 Pancake/40g	120	5.8	300	6.6	35.3	14.4	1.3
Buttermilk, The Best, Morrisons*	1 Pancake/65g	154	3.4	237	6.4	40.6	5.2	1.3

P

	Measure INFO/WEIGHT	per Measure KCAL	FAT	Nutrition Values per 100g / 100ml KCAL	PROT	CARB	FAT	FIBRE
PANCAKE								
Golden Syrup, GF, Free From, Morrisons*	1 Pancake/35g	89	0.6	255	4.4	54.6	1.8	1.6
Lemon, M&S*	1 Pancake/70g	183	4.1	261	5.9	45.1	5.9	1.8
Plain, Prepared From Recipe, Average	*1 Pancake/38g*	*86*	*3.7*	*227*	*6.4*	*28.3*	*9.7*	*0*
Protein, Ormo*	1 Pancake/45g	102	1.8	226	11.7	34.2	4.1	2.6
Raisin & Lemon, Asda*	1 Serving/30g	92	2.4	304	6	52	8	1.4
Raisin & Lemon, Sainsbury's*	1 Pancake/35g	95	1.5	272	6.3	51.8	4.4	2.2
Ready Made, Average	*1 Sm/30g*	*77*	*1.9*	*258*	*6.1*	*44.2*	*6.4*	*1.7*
Savoury, Made with Skimmed Milk, Average	*1 Pancake/77g*	*192*	*11.3*	*249*	*6.4*	*24.1*	*14.7*	*0.8*
Scotch	*1 Pancake/50g*	*146*	*5.8*	*292*	*5.8*	*43.6*	*11.7*	*1.4*
Syrup & Sultana, Kingsmill*	1 Pancake/36g	102	1.7	287	5.7	54.7	4.7	1.7
Vegetable Roll	*1 Roll/85g*	*185*	*10.6*	*218*	*6.6*	*21*	*12.5*	*0*
Wholegrain, Origianl, Griddle*	1 Pancake/40g	90	3	225	6.8	32.8	7.5	5.5
with Syrup, American Style, Large, Tesco*	1 Pancake/38g	102	1.3	268	5.1	54.2	3.4	0.9
PANCETTA								
Average	*½ Pack/65g*	*212*	*18.7*	*326*	*17*	*0.1*	*28.7*	*0*
Smoked, Diced, Dulano, Lidl*	1 Pack/125g	378	31.2	302	18	1	25	0.5
Smoked, Diced, Tesco*	¼ Pack/33g	96	7.9	291	18.5	0.3	24	0
Smoked, Diced, Tesco*	1 Pot/65g	205	16.9	315	20	0.3	26	0
PANINI								
Cheese, Tesco*	1 Panini/100g	249	9.1	249	10.5	31.3	9.1	3.1
Chicken, Arrabiata, Ginsters*	1 Panini/200g	489	16.8	245	12.8	29.4	8.4	2.4
Ham, & Cheese, Ginsters*	1 Panini/200g	567	25.6	283	13.3	28.7	12.8	1.6
Mozzarella, & Tomato, M&S*	1 Serving/176g	484	28.5	275	11.3	21.3	16.2	2.1
Tuna, & Sweetcorn, Tesco*	1 Serving/250g	559	16.4	224	12	29.3	6.6	1.4
PANNA COTTA								
BGTY, Sainsbury's*	1 Pot/150g	150	2.8	100	2.4	18.2	1.9	1.4
Caramel, Sainsbury's*	1 Serving/120g	319	15.1	266	4	31.8	12.6	0.7
Caramelon, Milbona, Lidl*	1 Pot/90g	152	8.1	169	2.4	19.5	9	0
Raspberry, COU, M&S*	1 Pot/140g	146	3.5	104	2.6	17.5	2.5	0.6
Raspberry, Hotel Chocolat*	1 Serving/30g	162	11.2	541	6	45.6	37.4	0
Sainsbury's*	1 Pot/100g	304	15.7	304	3	41.5	15.7	4
Strawberry, COU, M&S*	1 Pot/145g	145	3.8	100	2.6	15.7	2.6	0.8
PAPAYA								
Dried, Pieces, Nature's Harvest*	1 Serving/50g	178	0	355	0.2	85.4	0	2.6
Raw, Flesh Only, Average	*1 Serving/140g*	*37*	*0.1*	*26*	*0.4*	*6.6*	*0.1*	*1.2*
PAPPARDELLE								
Beef, Deluxe, Lidl*	1 Serving/400g	472	9.6	118	5.7	17.6	2.4	1.6
Beef, Ragu, Slow Cooked, M&S*	½ Pack/400g	512	22	128	7	12	5.5	1.1
Egg, Dry, Average	*1 Serving/100g*	*364*	*3.7*	*364*	*14.1*	*68.5*	*3.7*	*2.1*
Egg, Fresh, Cooked, No.1, Waitrose*	1 Serving/180g	331	3.1	184	6.3	35.2	1.7	1.5
Italian, Fresh, Waitrose *	1/3 Pack/117g	182	1.8	156	5.9	29.1	1.5	1.2
Nduja Meatballs, M&S*	1 Pack/400g	612	24	153	7.1	17.3	6	0.9
PAPRIKA								
Average	*1 Tsp/2g*	*6*	*0.3*	*289*	*14.8*	*34.9*	*13*	*0*
PARATHA								
Average	*1 Paratha/80g*	*258*	*11.4*	*322*	*8*	*43.2*	*14.3*	*4*
Roti, Plain, Crown Farms*	1 Slice/80g	250	10	312	5	46.2	12.5	1.2
PARCELS								
Feta, & Spinach, Filo, Sainsbury's*	1 Parcel/27g	83	5.6	307	5.8	23.8	20.7	1.8
Feta, & Herb, M&S*	1 Pack/104g	256	12.6	246	7.7	25.6	12.1	2
Goats Cheese, & Caramelised Onion, Asda*	1 Parcel/22g	71	4.2	325	6.6	30	19	2.3
Mac & Cheese, Bacon Wrapped, Stacks, M&S*	1 Parcel/20g	55	3.6	277	14.5	13.2	17.8	1.1
Pea, Minted, Sainsbury's*	1 Pack/150g	402	19.4	268	1.8	28.7	12.9	4

	Measure INFO/WEIGHT	per Measure KCAL	FAT	Nutrition Values per 100g / 100ml KCAL	PROT	CARB	FAT	FIBRE
PARCELS								
Salmon, Iceland*	1 Parcel/140g	365	21.1	261	10.3	20.7	15.1	0.6
Salmon, Smoked, Scottish, Waitrose*	1 Parcel/60g	133	10	221	15.6	2.3	16.6	0.5
Spinach, & Feta, Sainsbury's*	1 Parcel/35g	99	5.7	282	6.5	26.5	16.3	1.9
Tomato, & Mozzarella, Pastries, M&S*	1 Pastry/24g	66	3.3	273	7.3	28.6	13.8	2.1
Vegetable, Katsura, Crispy, M&S*	1 Pack/100g	281	13.7	281	5.6	32.8	13.7	2
PARSLEY								
Dried	**1 Tsp/1g**	**2**	**0.1**	**181**	**15.8**	**14.5**	**7**	**26.9**
Fresh, Average	**1 Tbsp/3.8g**	**1**	**0**	**27**	**2.4**	**2.2**	**1**	**4**
Root, Raw, Average	**1 Avg Root/33g**	**18**	**0.2**	**55**	**2.3**	**12.3**	**0.6**	**4.3**
PARSNIP								
Boiled, Average	**1 Serving/80g**	**53**	**1**	**66**	**1.6**	**12.9**	**1.2**	**4.7**
Honey Glazed, Roast, Baked, Aunt Bessie's*	1 Serving/100g	158	12	158	1.1	8.6	12	5.1
Honey Glazed, Roast, Deluxe, Lidl*	1 Serving/100g	134	5.7	134	1.4	17.2	5.7	4
Honey Roast, Oven Baked, Iceland*	1 Serving/100g	164	7.5	164	2	19.3	7.5	5.4
Honey Roasted, Tesco*	½ Pack/142g	159	5	112	1.2	16.8	3.5	4.2
Raw, Unprepared, Average	**1 Serving/100g**	**62**	**1**	**62**	**1.7**	**11.6**	**1**	**4.3**
PARTRIDGE								
Meat Only, Roasted	**1 Partridge/260g**	**551**	**18.7**	**212**	**36.7**	**0**	**7.2**	**0**
PASSATA								
Cherry Tomato, Mutti*	1 Serving/100g	51	1.2	51	1.6	7.6	1.2	0
Fina, Biona Organic*	1 Serving/100ml	34	0.2	34	1.4	5.8	0.2	1.7
Italian, Rustica, TTD, Sainsbury's*	1 Bottle/430g	155	6.9	36	1.1	3.7	1.6	1
Italian, with Onion & Garlic, Classic, Sainsbury's*	¼ Carton/125g	29	0.6	23	1.3	3.6	0.5	1.2
Italian, with Onion, & Garlic, Sainsbury's*	1 Pack/390g	117	2	30	1.9	4.3	0.5	1.5
Tomato, Garlic, Specially Selected, Aldi*	¼ Jar/175g	75	0.9	43	1.6	8.4	0.5	1.2
Tomato, Napolina*	½ Carton/196g	55	0.4	28	1.7	4.3	0.2	1.1
Tomato, with Garlic & Herb, Italian, Tesco*	½ Carton/250g	55	0.5	22	1.2	2.9	0.2	1.8
PASSION FRUIT								
Curd, Specially Selected, Aldi*	1 Tbsp/15g	49	1.9	327	2.4	49.2	12.5	0.1
Raw, Fresh, Average	**1 Fruit/18g**	**7**	**0.1**	**36**	**2.6**	**5.8**	**0.4**	**3.3**
Weighed with Skin, Average	**1 Fruit/30g**	**7**	**0.1**	**22**	**1.6**	**3.5**	**0.2**	**2**
PASTA								
Alphabet Shapes, Dry, Sainsbury's*	1 Serving/70g	223	1	319	10.2	65	1.4	2.8
Arrabiata, Roasted Vegetable, Low Fat, Co-Op*	1 Pack/380g	391	7.6	103	3.3	17	2	1.7
Beefy Bolognese, Pot Pasta, Pot Noodle*	1 Pot/268g	252	5.1	94	3.3	15	1.9	1.6
Bolognese, Bowl, COU, M&S*	1 Serving/282g	330	9.6	117	9.4	11.2	3.4	1.9
Bolognese, British Beef, Little Dish*	1 Pack/200g	192	5.2	96	4.8	12.7	2.6	1.3
Bucatini, Piccoli, No 14. Dry Weight, De Cecco*	1 Serving/60g	211	0.9	351	14	69	1.5	2.9
Butternut Mac, Oven Baked, Plant Based, Asda*	1 Pack/349g	391	5.2	112	3.7	20	1.5	1.8
Cajun Chicken, Island Salads*	1 Pasta/250g	211	9.9	84	3.1	9.2	4	0
Cappelletti, Prosciutto, Italian, Sainsbury's*	½ Pack/200g	362	9.4	181	9.6	23.9	4.7	2.2
Cavatoni, Dry, Italiamo, Lidl*	1 Serving/60g	213	1	355	11	73	1.6	2.3
Cheese & Broccoli, Made Up, Pasta n Sauce, Batchelors*	½ Pack/183g	212	3.1	116	4.4	20.4	1.7	0.7
Cheese Feast, Fully Loaded, Sainsbury's*	½ Pack/283g	382	13.3	135	6.2	15.6	4.7	2.7
Cheese, Leek, & Ham, Pasta n Sauce, Batchelors*	½ Pack/184g	235	3.9	128	5	21.9	2.1	0.7
Cheese, Three, Melt, Co-Op*	½ Pack/400g	632	21	158	7	20	5.2	1.2
Chicken, & Chorizo, Average	**1 Pack/400g**	**174**	**5.7**	**174**	**10.1**	**20.3**	**5.7**	**1.5**
Chicken, & Mushroom, Made Up, Mug Shot*	1 Serving/260g	221	3.6	85	2.2	15.7	1.4	0.5
Chicken, & Bacon, Italian, Iceland*	1 Pack/400g	492	11.6	123	6.8	16.9	2.9	1
Chicken, & Veg, What's Cooking, Lidl*	1 Serving/400g	368	9	92	7.5	9	2.2	0
Chicken, Arrabiata, COU, M&S*	1 Pack/350g	361	4.6	103	8.5	13.5	1.3	1.4
Chicken, Arrabiata, Tesco*	1 Pack/430g	486	6.4	113	7.4	16.5	1.5	2
Conchiglie, Cooked, Cucina, Aldi*	1 Serving/150g	216	0.9	144	5	29	0.6	1.3

PASTA

INFO/WEIGHT	KCAL	FAT	KCAL	PROT	CARB	FAT	FIBRE
Conchiglie, Dry Weight, Cucina, Aldi*	1 Serving/60g	188	0.6	314	11	63	1	2.9
Farfalle, Spinach, Cooked Weight, Tesco*	1 Serving/170g	300	1.2	176	5.8	35.7	0.7	2.2
Feta, & Semi Dried Tomato, No Mayonnaise, Tesco*	1 Pack/289g	494	19.4	171	5.5	21.4	6.7	1.4
Fettuccine, Edamame, & Mung Bean, Cooked, Aldi*	¼ Pack/158g	183	4	116	16	3	2.5	8.3
Fusilli, High Protein, Dry Weight, Morrisons*	1 Serving/75g	312	1.9	416	29.3	66.5	2.5	6
Girasoli, Butternut Squash, & Sage, Morrisons*	½ Pack/165g	296	7.9	179	5.8	27.2	4.8	2
Girasoli, Ricotta, & Spinach, Creamy, Aldi*	½ Pack/155g	312	15.5	201	7.1	19	10	2.2
Green Pea, GF, Dry, Free From, Morrisons*	1 Serving/75g	262	1.1	349	18.5	61.1	1.5	9.1
Ham, & Mushroom, Melt, Italian, Morrisons*	½ Pack/387g	631	21.7	163	7.5	20.3	5.6	0.9
Itailan Style, with Peppers, Morrisons*	1 Pack/550g	902	42.4	164	3.4	19.4	7.7	1.5
King Prawn Alfredo, Luxury, Iceland*	1 Pack/437g	620	25.3	142	6	15.7	5.8	1.8
Linguine, Cooked Weight, Sainsbury's*	1 Serving/200g	318	1.4	159	5.2	32.3	0.7	1.4
Mac & Greens, Vegan, Waitrose*	1 Pack/380g	437	17.1	115	3.2	13.7	4.5	3.7
Macaroni, Butternut Cauli Mac, Plant Chef, Tesco*	1 Pack/377g	434	9.4	115	3.6	18.6	2.5	1.8
Macaroni, GF, Free From, Morrisons*	1 Serving/50g	86	0.3	172	2.8	38.6	0.6	0.9
Margherite, Basil, & Pinenut, TTD, Sainsbury's*	½ Pack/125g	259	10.9	207	7.8	23.5	8.7	1.5
Medaglioni, Dry Weight, Vemondo, Lidl*	½ Pack/125g	276	5.7	221	6.8	36	4.6	0
Melt, Double Pepperoni, Iceland*	1 Pack/400g	544	17.6	136	5.2	17.5	4.4	2.9
Mezzelune, Spinach & Ricotta, The Best, Morrisons*	½ Pack/125g	235	8.1	188	6.3	25.4	6.5	1.2
Mezzelune, Sweet Potato, & Chilli, Bonsan*	1 Pack/250g	692	16.2	277	7.9	45.8	6.5	3.2
Mezzi, Dry Weight, TTD, Sainsbury's*	1 Serving/60g	191	0.7	318	12.4	62.8	1.2	3
Orzo, & Slow Roasted Tomato, Lidl*	½ Pack/105g	128	2	122	3.5	21.5	1.9	2.3
Orzo, Cooked Weight, TTD, Sainsbury's*	1 Serving/200g	318	1.2	159	6.2	31.4	0.6	1.5
Orzo, Cooked, Finest, Tesco*	1 Serving/170g	289	0.8	170	6.8	33.9	0.5	1.2
Orzo, Dry, Average	**1 Serving/100g**	**348**	**1.5**	**348**	**12.4**	**71.9**	**1.5**	**3**
Orzo, E Funghi, Orogel*	½ Pack/340g	220	7.3	65	1.6	8.8	2.2	1.8
Penne, Chickpea, Dry Weight, Pro Fusion*	1 Serving/60g	215	3.7	359	20	52	6.1	8.5
Pesto, Wicked Kitchen, Tesco*	1 Pack/225g	459	22.7	204	5.4	22	10.1	1.8
Pesto, with Semi Dried Tomatoes, Tesco*	1 Pack/225g	432	18.2	192	5.6	23.4	8.1	1.7
Red Lentil, Cooked Weight, Love Life, Waitrose*	1 Serving/180g	293	1.3	163	12.6	24.4	0.7	4.5
Rigatoni, Mezzi, Cooked Weight, TTD, Sainsbury's*	1 Serving/200g	318	1.2	159	6.2	31.4	0.6	1.5
Roasted Mushroom, & Mascarpone, M&S*	1 Pack/400g	676	29.6	169	5.5	19.7	7.4	1
Rotolo, Beef, & Pancetta, Deluxe, Lidl*	½ Pack/376g	703	39.8	187	8.2	13.8	10.6	1.7
Sacchettini, with Black Truffle, Deluxe, Lidl*	½ Pack/125g	362	7.2	290	9.3	48.9	5.8	0
Sausage, in Tomato & Basil Sauce, Sainsbury's*	1 Pack/393g	471	14.1	120	4.6	16.5	3.6	1.5
Shapes, Cooked, Smart Price, Asda*	1 Serving/175g	257	1.2	147	4.6	30	0.7	1.7
Shapes, Dry, Smart Price, Asda*	1 Serving/75g	265	1.3	353	11	72	1.7	4.1
Southern Fried Chicken, Tesco*	1 Pack/300g	522	22.8	174	5.8	19.7	7.6	1.9
Soy Bean, Organic, As Sold, Slendier*	1 Serving/50g	58	1.4	117	15	3.3	2.9	7.9
Tagliatelle, As Cooked, Essential, Waitrose*	¼ Pack/204g	346	3.5	170	6.4	31.5	1.7	1.5
Tomato, & Basil, Cooked, BGTY, Sainsbury's*	1 Pack/325g	354	2.9	109	4.1	20.1	0.9	2.1
Tomato, & Basil, Microwaved, Counted, Morrisons*	1 Pack/333g	270	1.3	81	3.2	15.2	0.4	1.8
Tomato, & Chorizo, Micro Pasta, Asda*	1 Pack/200g	356	7.2	178	6.5	28	3.6	4.7
Tuna, & Sweetcorn, Tesco*	½ Pot/150g	253	11.6	169	6.5	17.9	7.7	0.9
Wholewheat, Cooked, Tesco*	1 Serving/200g	284	1.8	142	5.7	27.9	0.9	4.5

PASTA BAKE

INFO/WEIGHT	KCAL	FAT	KCAL	PROT	CARB	FAT	FIBRE
Bacon & Leek, Average	**1 Serving/400g**	**633**	**32.3**	**158**	**6.7**	**14.8**	**8.1**	**1.3**
Beef, Bolognese, Meal to Share, M&S*	½ Pack/400g	700	30.8	175	9.3	16.6	7.7	1.2
Cheese, & Tomato, Italiano, Tesco*	1 Bake/300g	354	12.6	118	3.9	16.1	4.2	1
Cheese, 3, Tesco*	1 Serving/400g	580	12.8	145	6.3	21.7	3.2	2.3
Cheese, 3, Veg Packed, Gousto*	1 Serving/457g	649	25.1	142	7.6	15.5	5.5	1.2
Chicken, & Bacon, Average	**1 Serving/400g**	**627**	**28.7**	**157**	**9**	**13.7**	**7.2**	**1.6**
Chicken, Bacon & Mushroom, Average	**1 Serving/400g**	**632**	**29.2**	**158**	**7.8**	**15.1**	**7.3**	**2.3**

	Measure INFO/WEIGHT	per Measure KCAL	FAT	Nutrition Values per 100g / 100ml KCAL	PROT	CARB	FAT	FIBRE
PASTA BAKE								
Chicken, Pesto, & Mozzarella, Meal to Share, M&S*	½ Pack/400g	632	24.4	158	8.3	16.7	6.1	1.3
Mac 'n' Greens, Vegan, Slimming World*	1 Pack/550g	473	1.1	86	3.6	16.1	0.2	3
Meat Feast, Average	**1 Serving/400g**	**601**	**21.4**	**150**	**5.8**	**19.2**	**5.4**	**1.4**
Pepperoni, Tesco*	1 Pack/436g	575	16.1	132	6.1	17.8	3.7	1.6
Sausage, Average	**1 Serving/400g**	**591**	**24**	**148**	**5.5**	**17.7**	**6**	**1.9**
Tomato, & Mozzarella, Average	**1 Serving/400g**	**500**	**12.4**	**125**	**5.3**	**17.3**	**3.1**	**1.5**
Tomato, & Mascarpone, Iceland*	1 Pack/413g	491	13.6	119	4.1	17.4	3.3	1.6
Tomato, Creamy, Dolmio*	1 Serving/125g	141	9	113	2.3	8.4	7.2	0
Tomato, Inspired Cuisine, Aldi*	1 Pack/600g	774	21	129	7.8	16	3.5	2.3
Tuna, & Sweetcorn, Average	**1 Pack/400g**	**423**	**22.4**	**106**	**5**	**8.6**	**5.6**	**1.9**
Vegetable, Chargrilled, M&S*	½ Pack/400g	568	19.6	142	4.9	18.9	4.9	1.3
Vegetable, M&S*	1 Pack/350g	396	13.3	113	4.4	14.5	3.8	1.4
PASTA QUILLS								
Dry, Average	**1 Serving/75g**	**256**	**0.9**	**342**	**12**	**72.3**	**1.2**	**2**
GF, Salute*	1 Serving/75g	269	1.4	359	7.5	78	1.9	0
PASTA SALAD								
Cheese, Average	**1 Serving/370g**	**782**	**56.8**	**211**	**5.5**	**12.8**	**15.4**	**1.2**
Chicken, & Bacon, Caesar, Asda*	1 Pack/300g	552	30	184	6.9	16	10	1.2
Chicken, & Bacon, Caesar, Tesco*	1 Pack/265g	418	18.3	158	11.5	12.1	6.9	0.7
Chicken, & Bacon, Layered, Eat n go*	1 Pack/380g	395	18.2	104	5.5	9	4.8	1.6
Chicken, Bacon, & Sweetcorn, M&S*	1 Pack/380g	680	33.1	179	8.2	16.1	8.7	1.7
Chicken, Piri Piri, Asda*	1 Pack/320g	333	9	104	6	13	2.8	2
Chicken, Spicy, Asda*	1 Pack/309g	346	7.1	112	5.3	17	2.3	1.2
Chicken, Spicy, On the Go, Sainsbury's*	1 Pot/300g	455	10.8	152	6.4	22.7	3.6	1.5
Feta, & Slow Roasted Tomato, M&S*	1 Pack/190g	306	11.4	161	5.6	20	6	2.2
Goats Cheese, & Mixed Pepper, Sainsbury's*	1 Pack/200g	366	18.8	183	6.4	18.2	9.4	1.5
Ham, & Cheese, Asda*	½ Pack/160g	213	10.7	133	4.9	12	6.7	1.8
Italian, & Spinach, M&S*	1 Pack/200g	458	20	229	7.4	26.5	10	1.8
Orzo, & Roasted Tomatoes, M&S*	1 Pack/200g	230	3.2	115	3.7	20	1.6	2.9
Orzo, Specially Selected, Aldi*	1 Pack/210g	328	10.5	156	4	23	5	0.8
Pesto, & Pine Nut, Asda*	1 Serving/125g	306	13.8	245	6.7	29	11	3.7
Pesto, Spicy Chilli, Sainsbury's*	¼ Pot/63g	170	12.3	272	3.8	20.1	19.6	1.6
Prawn, Co-Op*	1 Pack/281g	323	14.6	115	4.5	12	5.2	1.8
Prawn, Growers Selection, Asda*	1 Pack/380g	365	9.1	96	5.1	13	2.4	1.2
Prawn, Morrison's*	1 Pack/250g	528	35.5	211	3.7	16.5	14.2	1.1
Salmon, Honey Roast, Scottish, M&S*	1 Pot/205g	285	13.3	139	6.3	12.9	6.5	1.7
Spinach, & Pine Nut, Sainsbury's*	½ Pot/100g	226	11.6	226	6.4	23	11.6	2.2
Tomato, & Basil, Sainsbury's*	1 Serving/83g	121	3.4	145	3.7	22.7	4.1	1.6
Tuna, & Sweetcorn, Meadow Fresh, Lidl*	½ Pack/190g	272	19	143	17.5	31.2	10	3
Tuna, & Sweetcorn, On the Go, Sainsbury's*	1 Pack/300g	492	17.1	164	5.9	21.6	5.7	1.4
Tuna, Jane Plan*	1 Pack/220g	242	7.7	110	6.9	12	3.5	0.8
PASTA SAUCE								
Amatriciana, M&S*	1 Jar/340g	425	32.3	125	3.4	6.3	9.5	2.9
Arrabbiata, Finest, Tesco*	½ Pot/175g	93	3.2	53	1.8	7	1.8	0.6
Arrabbiata, Fresh, Tesco*	½ Pot/175g	84	3.2	48	0.8	6.7	1.8	0.9
Arrabbiata, Waitrose*	1/3 Jar/116g	67	3.7	58	1.3	5.2	3.2	1.7
Artichoke, Sacla*	½ Pot/95g	249	21.8	262	1.9	9.2	23	5.3
Bacon, Smoky, Loyd Grossman*	½ Jar/175g	142	8.4	81	3	6.1	4.8	0.8
Basilico, Healthier Choice, Mr Organic*	1 Jar/350g	528	3.5	151	1.7	5.6	1	1.5
Beef Bolognese, Pouch, Dolmio*	1 Pack/170g	144	5.1	85	7.8	5.9	3	1.4
Bolognese, Baresa, Lidl*	¼ Jar/125g	55	0.5	44	1.6	7.6	0.4	1.6
Bolognese, Cucina, Aldi*	1 Serving/100g	37	0.5	37	0.9	7	0.5	0.9
Bolognese, Garlic & Onion, Intense, Dolmio*	1 Jar/500g	210	1	42	1.7	7.4	0.2	1.8

P

PASTA SAUCE

	Measure INFO/WEIGHT	per Measure KCAL	FAT	Nutrition Values per 100g / 100ml KCAL	PROT	CARB	FAT	FIBRE
Bolognese, Napolina*	½ Jar/175g	89	1.9	51	1.9	6.4	1.1	3.8
Bolognese, One Stop*	¼ Jar/125g	49	0.9	39	1.5	6	0.7	1.7
Bolognese, Smooth, Hidden Vegetables, Dolmio*	1 Portion/125g	60	1	48	1.4	7.7	0.8	1.9
Bolognese, Specially Selected, Aldi*	1 Jar/340g	187	9.2	55	1.5	5.5	2.7	1.1
Bolognese, Tesco*	1 Serving/100g	41	0.7	41	1.4	6.6	0.7	1.3
Bolognese, Tomato, & Herb, Sainsbury's*	1 Jar/500g	280	7	56	2	7.9	1.4	2
Bolognese, Waitrose*	¼ Jar/125g	79	5.2	63	1.2	4.4	4.2	1.5
Bolognese, with Beef, Tesco*	½ Pack/175g	170	10	97	5.6	4.7	5.7	2.1
Cacciatore, Fresh, Sainsbury's*	½ Pot/150g	152	8.8	101	5.4	8.1	5.9	1.5
Carbonara, Asda*	½ Pot/175g	359	29.8	205	7	6	17	0.1
Carbonara, Co-Op*	½ Pot/150g	270	25.5	180	3	4	17	0.1
Carbonara, Creamy, Dolmio Express, Dolmio*	1 Pack/150g	166	13.2	111	3.3	4.7	8.8	0.1
Carbonara, Creamy, Stir in Sauce, Dolmio*	1 Serving/75g	98	8	130	3.3	5.2	10.6	0.2
Cheddar Cheese, As Sold, Aldi*	1 Jar/340g	428	39.1	126	1.5	3.8	11.5	0.5
Cheese, Four, Classico*	1 Serving/125g	60	1	48	1.6	8	0.8	1.6
Cheese, Four, Sainsbury's*	1 Serving/150g	296	25.5	197	6.6	4.5	17	0.8
Cheese, Three, Co-Op*	1 Pack/300g	405	27	135	6	6	9	0.1
Cherry Tomato, Italian, Authentic, Mr Organic*	1 Serving/87g	55	2.4	63	1.7	7	2.7	2
Chunky Vegetable, Co-Op*	¼ Jar/125g	48	0.6	38	1.5	6.9	0.5	0.5
Mediterranean, Fresh, Waitrose*	1 Pot/350g	214	13.6	61	1.4	5	3.9	2.4
Mushroom, Chunky, Cucina, Aldi*	1 Jar/500g	200	2.5	40	1.6	7.4	0.5	1.3
Mushroom, Tesco*	1/6 Jar/120g	48	0.6	40	1.2	6.9	0.5	1.5
Napoletana, M&S*	½ Jar/170g	126	7.8	74	1.9	4.5	4.6	3.7
Napoletana, Sainsbury's*	½ Pot/150g	126	8.4	84	1.9	6.6	5.6	1.9
Parmesan, & Romano, Chunky, Ragu*	1 Serving/129g	80	2.5	62	2.3	10.1	1.9	1.6
Puttanesca, Loyd Grossman*	½ Jar/175g	117	6	67	1.4	5.5	3.4	0.7
Roasted Red Pepper, Sacla*	1 Jar/190g	357	34.2	188	1	5.1	18	0.9
Sun-Dried Tomato, Stir In, Cucina, Aldi*	½ Pot/75g	77	5	103	2	8	6.7	1.2
Sweet Pepper, Sainsbury's*	¼ Jar/125g	53	0.9	43	1.1	7.4	0.7	1.2
Sweet Pepper, Tesco*	½ Pot/77g	47	1.8	61	1.3	8.2	2.4	0.7
Toamto, & Basil, M&S*	½ Pack/175g	163	11.8	93	1.6	5.9	6.8	1.4
Tomato, & Basil, Dolmio*	1 Serving/170g	95	3.6	56	1.4	7.9	2.1	0
Tomato, & Basil, Loyd Grossman*	½ Jar/175g	107	6	61	1.5	5.8	3.4	0.8
Tomato, & Basil, Morrisons*	½ Jar/140g	76	0.7	54	1.7	10.1	0.5	1.3
Tomato, & Chilli, Pour Over, M&S*	1 Jar/330g	231	12.5	70	1.3	7.6	3.8	1.8
Tomato, & Garlic, Roasted, Loyd Grossman*	½ Jar/175g	133	5.6	76	2	9	3.2	1.4
Tomato, & Mascarpone, Sainsbury's*	½ Pot/150g	137	9.9	91	2.1	5.9	6.6	1.2
Tomato, & Onions, Original, Morrisons*	1 Serving/125g	51	1.4	41	1.4	6.3	1.1	1.2
Tomato, & Basil, Chef Select, Lidl*	½ Pack/175g	68	2.3	39	1.2	4.6	1.3	2
Tomato, & Basil, Fresh, Co-Op*	1 Pot/300g	135	4.8	45	1.6	4.5	1.6	3.3
Tomato, & Basil, Inspired Cuisine, Aldi*	½ Pot/175g	96	3.5	55	1.7	7	2	1
Tomato, & Basil, Morrisons*	½ Pot/175g	110	5.1	63	1.8	6.4	2.9	2.1
Tomato, & Basil, Stir In, Dolmio*	1 Pack/150g	114	9.2	76	2.3	8.2	6.1	1.7
Tomato, & Basil, Stir In, Morrisons*	½ Pack/78g	59	3.7	76	0.9	6.7	4.7	1.2
Tomato, & Basil, Tesco*	1 Serving/175g	89	3.7	51	1.1	6.3	2.1	1.1
Tomato, & Garlic, Asda*	¼ Jar/125g	52	0.6	42	1.6	7.8	0.5	0.6
Tomato, & Herb, HFC, Tesco*	¼ Jar/110g	36	0.8	33	0.8	5.5	0.7	0.8
Tomato, & Mascarpone, M&S*	½ Pot/175g	180	12.4	103	1.9	7.4	7.1	0.8
Tomato, & Mushroom, Morrisons*	¼ Jar/125g	42	0.5	34	1.1	6.1	0.4	1
Tomato, Basil, & Cream, Albert Heijn*	½ Pack/113g	88	5.6	78	2	5.5	5	0
Tomato, Creamy, Pasta Bake, Co-Op*	1 Serving/125g	165	12.5	132	1.8	7.6	10	0.5
Tomato, Creamy, Pasta Bake, Morrisons*	¼ Jar/125g	118	8	94	1	8	6.4	0.3
Tomato, Lasagne, Cucina, Aldi*	1 Jar/500g	165	2.5	33	1.2	6.3	0.5	0.8

	Measure INFO/WEIGHT	per Measure KCAL	FAT	Nutrition Values per 100g / 100ml KCAL	PROT	CARB	FAT	FIBRE
PASTA SAUCE								
Tomato, Onion, & Garlic, Baresa, Lidl*	1 Jar/500g	240	2.5	48	2.1	7.8	0.5	1.8
Tomato, Smooth, Cucina, Aldi*	1 Jar/500g	275	4.5	55	1.8	7	0.9	1.2
Tomato, with Basil Pesto, Rich, Express, Dolmio*	1 Pack/170g	146	10	86	2	6.2	5.9	0
Toscana, Deluxe, Lidl*	1 Jar/350g	343	21.7	98	3.9	6.3	6.2	0
Vegetable, Chargrilled, Stir-In, Sainsbury's*	½ Pot/75g	67	3.5	89	1.7	8.5	4.7	2.8
Vegetable, Roasted, Sainsbury's*	½ Pot/151g	103	5.9	68	1.6	6.7	3.9	0.4
PASTA SHELLS								
Dry, Average	**1 Serving/75g**	**265**	**1.5**	**353**	**11.1**	**71.8**	**2**	**2**
Egg, Fresh, Average	**1 Serving/125g**	**344**	**3.6**	**275**	**11.5**	**49.8**	**2.8**	**3.4**
PASTA TWISTS								
Dry, Average	**1oz/28g**	**99**	**0.4**	**354**	**12.2**	**71.8**	**1.5**	**2.2**
Wheat & GF, Glutafin*	1 Serving/75g	262	1.5	350	8	75	2	0.1
PASTE								
'Nduja, Cooks' Ingredients, Waitrose*	1 Tbsp/15g	80	7.6	536	15.7	2.4	50.8	3.3
Beef, Princes*	1 Thin Spread/7g	16	1.2	231	15.2	0.1	17.4	0
Beef, Sainsbury's*	1 Jar/75g	142	9.9	189	16	1.5	13.2	1.4
Chicken, Hunter's*	1 Serving/25g	54	4	214	14	2.7	16	0.5
Chicken, Sutherlands*	1 Serving/18g	31	2	170	12.5	4.4	11.2	0
Chilli, Sainsbury's*	1 Tsp/6g	5	0.4	82	1	2.9	5.8	7.3
Chipotle, Chilli, Tesco*	1 Tsp/5g	8	0.2	158	2.8	23.3	4.8	5.2
Crab, Sainsbury's*	1 Spread/5g	6	0.2	115	16.5	1.7	4.7	0.5
Harissa, Rose, M&S*	1 Tsp/5g	8	0.6	166	2.4	6.9	12.7	7.1
Salmon, & Haddock, Sainsbury's*	1 Tbsp/17g	21	0.9	123	14.3	4.4	5.1	1.3
Sardine, & Tomato, Princes*	1 Thin Spread/7g	11	0.7	164	13.1	6.3	9.6	0
Sardine, & Tomato, Sainsbury's*	1 Mini Pot/35g	60	3.8	170	16.9	1.2	10.8	1.3
Tamarind, M&S*	¼ Jar/30g	38	0	125	0.9	30.1	0.1	0.5
Tamarind, Sainsbury's*	1 Serving/9g	19	0.2	214	2.9	45	2	2.3
Tuna Mayo, Asda*	1 Pot/75g	137	9	183	16	3.2	12	0.6
PASTILLES								
Fruit, 30% Less Sugar, Rowntree's*	1 Sweet/3g	9	0	312	6.5	62	0.1	16.2
Fruit, Average	**1 Tube/33g**	**108**	**0**	**327**	**2.8**	**84.2**	**0**	**0**
Fruit, Rowntree's*	1 Tube/53g	186	0	351	4.4	83.7	0	0
Lamb, Picard*	½ Pack/100g	248	15	248	11	16	15	2.9
PASTRAMI								
Beef, Average	**1 Serving/40g**	**51**	**1.4**	**128**	**23.1**	**1.1**	**3.6**	**0.2**
Style, Vegan, Slices, Squeaky Bean*	1 Pack/100g	223	6.5	223	31	5.9	6.5	7.9
Turkey, Average	**½ Pack/35g**	**38**	**0.5**	**107**	**21.8**	**1.7**	**1.5**	**0.5**
PASTRY								
Apricot, Danish, Bakery in Store, M&S*	1 Pastry/130g	347	15	267	5.4	34.6	11.5	1.8
Bridie, Bells*	1 Bridie/100g	327	20	327	7	29	20	0
Cannoli, Pistachio, GF, Diforti*	1 Cannoli/40g	222	13.6	556	7.6	53	34	2.2
Case, From Supermarket, Average	**1 Case/230g**	**1081**	**58.9**	**470**	**5.8**	**55.9**	**25.6**	**1.2**
Cheese, & Spinach, Lattice, Aldi*	1 Serving/138g	406	26.2	294	7	24	19	2.2
Choux, Cooked, Average	**1oz/28g**	**91**	**5.5**	**325**	**8.5**	**29.8**	**19.8**	**1.2**
Churros, with Chocolate Dip, Plant Kitchen, M&S*	1 Churro/19g	76	4.8	398	4	38.2	25.2	1.2
Cinnamon Swirls, Bake it Fresh, Jus-Rol*	1 Swirl/45g	162	7.1	360	6.2	47.7	15.7	1.6
Cinnamon Swirls, Danish Selection, Tesco*	1 Swirl/35g	151	8.8	432	6.4	43.5	25.2	2.8
Cream Horn, Fresh, Asda*	1 Horn/50g	207	12	414	4.9	43	24	2
Danish, Raisin Whirl, Sainsbury's*	1 Pastry/90g	364	18.8	405	4.5	48.3	20.9	2.7
Feta, & Spinach, Rich & Creamy, Tesco*	½ Pack/65g	177	10.3	273	8.1	23.3	15.9	2.2
Feta, Herb, & Spinach, Tesco*	2 Pastries/65g	168	8.3	258	7.4	27.2	12.8	2.3
Filo, Average	**1 Sheet/45g**	**137**	**1.2**	**304**	**9**	**61.4**	**2.7**	**0.9**
Flaky, Cooked, Average	**1oz/28g**	**157**	**11.4**	**560**	**5.6**	**45.9**	**40.6**	**1.8**

P

	Measure INFO/WEIGHT	per Measure KCAL	FAT	Nutrition Values per 100g / 100ml KCAL	PROT	CARB	FAT	FIBRE

PASTRY

	Measure INFO/WEIGHT	KCAL	FAT	KCAL	PROT	CARB	FAT	FIBRE
Halloumi, Filo, Waitrose*	1 Pastry/32g	98	5.3	306	11.2	26.6	16.6	1.6
Horn, Filled with Jam, & Cream, M&S*	1 Horn/54g	218	12.3	404	3.9	45.6	22.8	0.6
Jambons, Fajita Chicken, Golden Bake*	1 Jambon/104g	280	17.7	269	7.3	22	17	1.5
Pains Au Lait, La Boulangere, Lidl*	1 Roll/35g	124	4.2	355	8.6	52	12	2.5
Prawn, Roses, Finest, Tesco*	1 Rose/17g	52	3.1	303	10.7	23.4	18.1	1.8
Puff, Block, Tesco*	1 Block/500g	2095	137	419	6.1	35.4	27.4	3.2
Puff, Frozen, Average	*1 Serving/47g*	*188*	*12*	*400*	*5*	*29.2*	*25.6*	*0*
Puff, GF, Jus-Rol*	1 Serving/50g	170	9.8	341	2.5	36.8	19.6	4
Quorn, Roll, Ginsters*	1 Roll/100g	299	18.8	299	8.2	21	18.8	6.2
Shortcrust, Cooked, Average	*1oz/28g*	*146*	*9*	*521*	*6.6*	*54.2*	*32.3*	*2.2*
Shortcrust, Raw, Average	*1oz/28g*	*127*	*8.1*	*453*	*5.6*	*44*	*29.1*	*1.3*
Slices, Cream, Cream Cake Selection, Tesco*	1 Slice/65g	249	12.4	383	4	48.3	19	1.2
Spring Roll Wrapper, Blue Dragon*	1 Wrapper/11g	37	0.1	337	5.8	77.4	0.5	0.1
Sweet Heart, All Butter, Brompton House*	1 Pastry/11g	59	3.5	539	5.9	56	32	1.6
Twists, Chocolate, All Butter, M&S*	1 Twist/71g	280	15.1	394	7.6	41.4	21.3	3.1
Twists, Sea Salt, & Pepper, M&S*	1 Twist/9g	44	2.2	491	10.2	56.3	24.2	3.4
Vanilla Slice, Frozen, Tesco*	1 Slice/38g	136	6	359	4.7	48.9	15.8	1.5

PASTY

	Measure INFO/WEIGHT	KCAL	FAT	KCAL	PROT	CARB	FAT	FIBRE
Beef, Iceland*	1 Pasty/130g	324	16.2	249	5.5	26.8	12.5	1.8
Cauliflower, Curried, Wicked Kitchen, Tesco*	1 Pasty/150g	361	19.5	241	4.1	26.2	13	1.1
Cheese, & Onion, Average	*1 Pasty/150g*	*435*	*27.6*	*290*	*7.3*	*24.5*	*18.4*	*1.4*
Chicken, Tikka, Asda*	1 Pasty/30g	103	6	343	8	31	20	2.3
Cornish, Average	*1 Pasty/160g*	*450*	*27.7*	*281*	*7*	*24.2*	*17.3*	*1.6*
Cornish, Frozen, Baked, Ginsters*	1 Pasty/130g	343	20.4	264	6.6	23.2	15.7	1.9
Cornish, Large, Ginsters*	1 Pasty/180g	500	32.8	278	6.4	21.4	18.2	0
Cornish, Mini, Sainsbury's*	1 Pasty/70g	280	20.1	400	7.3	28.1	28.7	1.5
No Beef, Vegan, Mae's Kitchen, Aldi*	1 Pasty/170g	420	25.5	247	5.9	20	15	3
No Bull, Meat Free, Vegan, Oven Baked, Iceland*	1 Pasty/190g	431	22.6	227	5.5	23.3	11.9	2.5
Quorn, Vegan, Ginsters*	1 Pasty/180g	436	23.8	242	6.4	23.1	13.2	2.7
Vegan, Waitrose*	1 Pasty/130g	346	20.3	266	7.7	22.3	15.6	2.6
Vegetable	*1oz/28g*	*77*	*4.2*	*274*	*4.1*	*33.3*	*14.9*	*1.9*
Vegetable, Moroccan, Ginsters*	1 Pasty/180g	409	22.5	227	3.8	23.6	12.5	2.4

PATE

	Measure INFO/WEIGHT	KCAL	FAT	KCAL	PROT	CARB	FAT	FIBRE
Ardennes, BGTY, Sainsbury's*	1 Serving/30g	59	4.5	197	12.3	3.2	15	0.5
Ardennes, Essential, Waitrose*	1 Serving/30g	95	7.9	318	12.7	7.1	26.4	0.5
Ardennes, Reduced Fat, Essential, Waitrose*	¼ Pack/43g	103	7.5	242	14.4	6	17.7	0.5
Ardennes, with Bacon, Tesco*	½ Pack/85g	241	20.6	284	11.4	5.1	24.2	1.1
Brussels, 25% Less Fat, Morrisons*	¼ Pack/43g	106	8.8	249	14.2	0.7	20.6	0
Brussels, Co-Op*	1 Serving/15g	51	4.6	340	11	4	31	2
Brussels, M&S*	1 Spread/7g	23	2.1	323	9.9	1.9	30.5	0.5
Brussels, Reduced Fat, Warren & Sons, Lidl*	1 Serving/35g	71	5.2	204	12	5	15	0.7
Brussels, Sainsbury's*	1 Pack/170g	663	64.9	390	10.6	1.1	38.2	0.1
Brussels, Sainsbury's*	1/5 Pack/34g	95	8.4	279	9.3	4.7	24.8	0.5
Brussels, Smooth, Eastmans, Tesco*	1/5 Pack/35g	87	9.2	249	9.6	4.6	26.2	0.5
Brussels, Smooth, Reduced Fat, Asda*	1 Serving/50g	94	6.5	187	12	5.5	13	0.5
Brussels, Smooth, Spreadable, Sainsbury's*	1 Serving/30g	97	8.7	323	10.7	4.7	29	0
Brussels, with Caramelised Shallots, The Best, Morrisons*	1 Serving/30g	91	7.5	304	8.8	10.7	25	0.5
Brussels, with Mushrooms, Wild, The Best, Morrisons*	1 Serving/30g	92	7.9	308	9.7	7.2	26.3	1.8
Chicken Liver, Smooth, M&S*	¼ Pack/42g	108	9	255	7.8	8	21.2	0.5
Chicken, Liver, Parfait, Specially Selected, Aldi*	1 Portion/85g	278	26.4	327	11	2.1	31	0.6
Chicken, Liver, Parfait, Waitrose*	1 Pack/100g	258	22.9	258	7.5	4.8	22.9	1.1
Chicken, Liver, with Madeira Jelly, Waitrose*	½ Pack/40g	100	8.7	251	6.4	6.8	21.7	1.4
De Campagne, M&S*	1 Serving/30g	47	2.7	158	13.6	5.4	8.9	0.9

	Measure INFO/WEIGHT	per Measure KCAL	FAT	Nutrition Values per 100g / 100ml KCAL	PROT	CARB	FAT	FIBRE
PATE								
De Campagne, Sainsbury's*	1 Serving/55g	129	10	235	16.3	1.4	18.2	0
De Campagne, Waitrose*	¼ Pack/40g	145	13.1	362	13.1	3.2	32.7	1.1
Duck, & Armagnac, Cottage Delight*	1 Serving/45g	113	9.2	252	15	2.1	20.4	0
Duck, & Orange, Smooth, M&S*	1 Serving/30g	94	7.9	315	7.7	11.5	26.4	0.5
Duck, Liver, with Port, TTD, Sainsbury's*	1/5 Pack/30g	71	5.6	238	8.2	8.3	18.8	1.3
Farmhouse, Co-Op*	1 Serving/57g	148	11.9	261	14	4.3	21	0
Farmhouse, with Mushrooms, Sainsbury's*	1 Serving/30g	76	6.8	252	11.3	1.2	22.5	0.5
Garlic, & Herb, Yeast, Tartex*	1 Serving/30g	69	5.4	230	7	10	18	0
Mackerel, Smoked	**1oz/28g**	**103**	**9.6**	**368**	**13.4**	**1.3**	**34.4**	**0**
Mackerel, Tesco*	1 Serving/29g	102	9.5	353	14.3	0.5	32.6	0
Mushroom, Coarse, Roasted, M&S*	1 Serving/30g	57	4.8	190	3.4	8	15.9	0.7
Mushroom, Roasted, Sainsbury's*	1 Serving/50g	74	5.9	149	3.1	7.2	11.8	0.8
Mushroom, Sainsbury's*	½ Pot/58g	85	6.7	147	3.9	5.8	11.6	0
Mushroom, Vegan, Suma*	1 Serving/50g	115	9.1	230	8.3	5.8	18.2	4.8
Mushroom, Wild, Yeast, GranoVita*	1 Serving/50g	106	8.5	213	10	5	17	0
Pork, & Garlic, Tesco*	¼ Pack/40g	111	9	276	9.6	8.6	22.5	0.5
Pork, Hyperu*	1 Serving/28g	104	9.8	372	10	4.3	35	0
Salmon, Sainsbury's*	½ Pack/50g	102	7.2	204	12.6	5.9	14.3	0.7
Salmon, Smoked, Coarse, M&S*	1 Serving/30g	61	4.4	202	14.4	2.9	14.7	0.6
Salmon, Smoked, Waitrose*	1 Serving/38g	70	4.7	185	16.8	1.3	12.4	0.5
Salmon, Smoked, with Gin, Castle MacLellan*	½ Pack/50g	124	9.2	247	10.2	8.7	18.5	0
Trout, Smoked, Waitrose*	1 Serving/34g	59	3.7	176	18.3	0.6	11.1	0
Tuna, Coarse, M&S*	½ Pack/57g	136	10.5	239	14.8	3.3	18.5	0.6
Vegetable	**1oz/28g**	**48**	**3.8**	**173**	**7.5**	**5.9**	**13.4**	**0**
PATTY								
Chicken, Spicy, Boca*	1 Patty/71g	130	5	183	15.5	18.3	7	2.8
Lamb, Curried, Island Delight*	1 Patty/140g	451	28	322	6.4	28	20	1.4
Lamb, Jamaican, Port Royal*	1 Patty/130g	352	17.4	271	7.2	30.5	13.4	0
Vegetable, Jamaican, Patty, Island Delight*	1 Patty/140g	423	22.4	302	5.2	35	16	0
Vegetarian, Jamaican, Port Royal*	1 Patty/130g	315	13.8	242	12.5	24.1	10.6	0
PAVLOVA								
Base, Cooks' Ingredients, Waitrose*	1 Serving/17g	62	0	366	4.8	91.2	0.2	0
Maltesers, Mars*	1 Serving/50g	205	8.1	410	3.6	61.7	16.2	0
Mini, Morrisons*	1 Piece/4g	17	0	396	5.8	92	0.5	0
Raspberry, Individual, M&S*	1 Serving/65g	133	1.6	205	4	41.8	2.4	0.2
Raspberry, M&S*	1 Serving/84g	193	8.1	230	2.3	33.3	9.6	0.3
Raspberry, Tesco*	1 Serving/65g	191	8.4	294	2.7	41.8	12.9	1.1
Sticky Toffee, Sainsbury's*	1 Serving/60g	249	9.8	415	3.7	63.1	16.4	0.9
PAW-PAW								
Raw, Fresh	**1oz/28g**	**10**	**0**	**36**	**0.5**	**8.8**	**0.1**	**2.2**
Raw, Weighed with Skin & Pips	**1oz/28g**	**6**	**0**	**20**	**0.3**	**5**	**0.1**	**1.3**
PEACH								
Dried, Average	**1 Pack/250g**	**472**	**1.6**	**189**	**2.6**	**45**	**0.6**	**6.9**
in Fruit Juice, Average	**1oz/28g**	**13**	**0**	**47**	**0.5**	**11.2**	**0**	**0.7**
in Light Syrup, Canned, As Sold	**1 Serving/100g**	**66**	**0**	**66**	**0.4**	**15.9**	**0**	**1**
Raw, Stoned, Average	**1oz/28g**	**9**	**0**	**33**	**1**	**7.6**	**0.1**	**1.5**
Raw, Weighed with Stone, Average	**1 Peach/125g**	**39**	**0.1**	**31**	**1**	**7.2**	**0.1**	**1.3**
Slices in Fruit Juice, Average	**1 Serving/100g**	**49**	**0**	**49**	**0.6**	**11.6**	**0**	**0.5**
PEANUT BUTTER								
Creamy, Pics*	2 Tbsp/30g	178	14.1	594	21.9	25	46.9	6.2
Crunchy, Natural, No Added Sugar or Salt, Average	**1 Tbsp/15g**	**91**	**7.3**	**606**	**27.6**	**12.2**	**48.4**	**7**
Dark, Roasted, Crunchy, Whole Earth*	1 Tbsp/15g	89	6.9	594	28.9	10.3	46.3	8.3
Extra Smooth, Skippy*	1 Tbsp/15g	87	6.5	581	27	17.1	43.3	7.8

	Measure INFO/WEIGHT	per Measure KCAL	FAT	Nutrition Values per 100g / 100ml KCAL	PROT	CARB	FAT	FIBRE
PEANUT BUTTER								
High Protein, Mayver's*	1 Tbsp/15g	84	6.3	562	32	13	42	9.1
Marmite, Crunchy, Marmite*	1 Tbsp/15g	86	6.8	574	28	12	45	7.9
Powder, Chocolate, PPB*	1 Serving/12g	45	0.7	375	45.1	28.4	6	13.9
Powdered, Original, PPD*	1 Serving/12g	48	1.1	398	47.6	26	9.4	9.8
Powdered, The Original, Pb2*	1 Tbsp/15g	69	1.7	462	46.2	38.5	11.5	7.7
Salted Date, Yumello*	1 Tbsp/15g	84	7.2	558	22.6	19.6	47.7	8.5
Smooth, Average	*1 Tbsp/15g*	*93*	*8.1*	*623*	*22.6*	*13.1*	*53.7*	*5.4*
Smooth, Reduced Fat, 30%, Morrisons*	1 Tbsp/15g	84	5.6	562	18	36.3	37.2	5
Smooth, Unsalted, Biona Organic*	1 Tbsp/15g	89	7.4	594	25.8	16.1	49.2	8.5
Whole Nut, Crunchy, Average	**1 Tbsp/15g**	**91**	**8**	**606**	**24.9**	**7.7**	**53.1**	**6**
PEANUTS								
BBQ, Crispy, Coated, Tesco*	1 Serving/25g	144	10	574	16.2	35.5	39.8	4.7
Chilli, Average	*½ Pack/50g*	*303*	*25.3*	*605*	*28.2*	*9.3*	*50.6*	*6.8*
Chocolate, Milk, Sainsbury's*	1 Pack/180g	1013	65.2	563	15.5	35.5	36.2	7
Crispy, Tesco*	1/8 Bag/25g	144	10	574	16.2	35.5	39.8	4.7
Crunchy, BBQ Coated, M&S*	1 Serving/30g	169	11.6	564	15.1	36.6	38.5	5.1
Dry Roasted, Average	*1 Serving/20g*	*117*	*9.8*	*587*	*25.7*	*11.5*	*48.8*	*6.5*
Dry Roasted, KP Snacks*	1 Serving/30g	178	14.1	594	30	7.2	47	8.6
Honey Roasted, Average	*1oz/28g*	*169*	*13.2*	*605*	*26.8*	*23.6*	*47*	*5.5*
Marmite, Graze*	1 Punnet/36g	208	16.2	579	28	12	45	8.3
Plain, Average	*10 Whole/10g*	*59*	*5*	*592*	*24.7*	*11*	*50*	*6.3*
Red Skin, BuyWholeFoodsOnline*	1 Serving/30g	169	13.8	563	25.6	12.5	46	0
Roast, Salted, Average	*10 Whole/12g*	*74*	*6.3*	*614*	*27.8*	*7.9*	*52.4*	*4.9*
Salted, Average	*10 Whole/6g*	*37*	*3.1*	*609*	*27*	*8.3*	*52*	*5.4*
Wasabi Coated, Alesto, Lidl*	1 Serving/30g	153	9.4	511	14.1	40.6	31.5	4.5
PEARL BARLEY								
Boiled	*1oz/28g*	*34*	*0.1*	*123*	*2.3*	*28.2*	*0.4*	*3.8*
Cooked, Average	*1 Serving/150g*	*184*	*0.7*	*123*	*2.3*	*28.2*	*0.4*	*3.8*
Raw, Average	*1oz/28g*	*99*	*0.3*	*352*	*9.9*	*77.7*	*1.2*	*15.6*
PEARS								
Abate Fetel, Average	*1 Med/133g*	*48*	*0.1*	*36*	*0.4*	*8.3*	*0.1*	*2.2*
Asian, Nashi, Raw, Average	*1 Lge/209g*	*80*	*0.4*	*38*	*0.5*	*9.7*	*0.2*	*3.3*
Comice, Raw, Weighed with Core	*1 Med/170g*	*56*	*0*	*33*	*0.3*	*8.5*	*0*	*2*
Conference, Average	*1 Lge/209g*	*88*	*0.2*	*42*	*0.3*	*10.1*	*0.1*	*2*
Dried, Average	*1 Pear Half/16g*	*33*	*0.1*	*204*	*1.9*	*48.4*	*0.5*	*9.7*
in Fruit Juice, Average	*1 Serving/225g*	*102*	*0.1*	*45*	*0.3*	*10.9*	*0*	*1.2*
in Syrup, Average	*1oz/28g*	*16*	*0*	*58*	*0.2*	*14.4*	*0.1*	*1.4*
Prickly, Raw, Fresh	*1oz/28g*	*8*	*0.1*	*30*	*0.4*	*7*	*0.2*	*0*
Raw, Weighed with Core, Average	*1 Med/166g*	*58*	*0.2*	*35*	*0.3*	*8.4*	*0.1*	*1.3*
William, Raw, Average	*1 Med/170g*	*58*	*0.2*	*34*	*0.4*	*8.3*	*0.1*	*2.2*
PEAS								
British, with a Taste of Chilli, M&S*	1 Serving/80g	75	3.8	94	4.4	5.4	4.8	5.6
Dried, Boiled in Unsalted Water, Average	*1oz/28g*	*31*	*0.2*	*109*	*6.9*	*19.9*	*0.8*	*5.5*
Dried, Raw, Average	*1oz/28g*	*85*	*0.7*	*303*	*21.6*	*52*	*2.4*	*13*
Edible Podded, Raw	*1 Cup/63g*	*25*	*0.1*	*39*	*2.6*	*7.1*	*0.2*	*2.4*
Frozen, Average	*1 Serving/85g*	*62*	*0.8*	*73*	*6*	*9.7*	*1*	*4.5*
Frozen, Boiled, Average	*1 Serving/75g*	*51*	*0.7*	*68*	*6*	*9.4*	*0.9*	*5.1*
Garden, Canned with Sugar & Salt, Average	*1 Serving/90g*	*59*	*0.6*	*66*	*5.3*	*9.3*	*0.7*	*5.1*
Garden, Canned, No Sugar Or Salt, Average	*1 Can/80g*	*36*	*0.3*	*45*	*4.4*	*6*	*0.4*	*2.8*
Garden, Frozen, Average	*1 Serving/90g*	*66*	*1*	*74*	*6.3*	*9.8*	*1.1*	*3.3*
Garden, Minted, Average	*1 Serving/80g*	*59*	*0.9*	*74*	*6.3*	*9.7*	*1.1*	*5.9*
Marrowfat, Average	*1 Sm Can/160g*	*134*	*0.9*	*84*	*6.1*	*13.7*	*0.6*	*3.7*
Mushy, Average	*1 Can/200g*	*173*	*1*	*86*	*6.2*	*14.4*	*0.5*	*2.2*

	Measure INFO/WEIGHT	per Measure KCAL	FAT	Nutrition Values per 100g / 100ml KCAL	PROT	CARB	FAT	FIBRE
PEAS								
Processed, Canned, Average	**1 Sm Can/220g**	**162**	**1.6**	**74**	**5.6**	**11.3**	**0.7**	**3.4**
Roasted, Chocolate, & Salted Caramel, Brave*	1 Serving/30g	129	5.1	431	16	44	17	16
Roasted, Sea Salt, & Vinegar, Brave*	1 Pack/35g	134	3.8	383	19	41	11	19
Roasted, Sour Cream, & Chive, Brave*	1 Pack/35g	132	3.8	377	20	41	11	20
Snow	**1 Serving/80g**	**24**	**0.2**	**29**	**3.3**	**3.9**	**0.2**	**2.1**
Sugar Snap, Average	**1 Serving/80g**	**27**	**0.2**	**33**	**3.2**	**4.8**	**0.2**	**1.4**
Wasabi, Average	**1 Serving/28g**	**114**	**3.8**	**406**	**15.2**	**54**	**13.7**	**8.6**
with Leeks & Pancetta, Finest, Tesco*	½ Pack/122g	146	7.4	120	6.3	7.6	6.1	4.6
PEASE PUDDING								
Canned, Re-Heated, Drained	**1oz/28g**	**26**	**0.2**	**93**	**6.8**	**16.1**	**0.6**	**1.8**
PECAN NUTS								
Average	**3 Nuts/6g**	**42**	**4.2**	**692**	**10**	**5.6**	**70.1**	**4.7**
Roasted, Salted, Waitrose *	1 Serving/25g	183	18.2	733	11.2	3.9	72.7	9.1
PENNE								
Brown Rice, GF, Pasta, Waitrose*	¼ Pack/125g	250	2.1	200	4.1	41	1.7	1.9
Cooked, Average	**1 Serving/185g**	**244**	**1.3**	**132**	**4.7**	**26.7**	**0.7**	**1.1**
Dry, Average	**1 Serving/100g**	**352**	**1.9**	**352**	**12.4**	**71.3**	**1.9**	**2.7**
Egg, Fresh, Average	**1 Serving/125g**	**352**	**4**	**282**	**11.1**	**52.2**	**3.2**	**2**
Free From, Tesco*	1 Serving/100g	340	2	340	8	72.5	2	2.5
Fresh, Dry, Average	**1 Serving/125g**	**222**	**2.4**	**178**	**7.3**	**32.2**	**1.9**	**1.6**
GF, Dry Weight, Free From, Tesco*	1 Serving/75g	266	0.8	355	7	78.4	1	2
Rigate, Dry Weight, Average	**1 Serving/90g**	**318**	**1.6**	**353**	**12.3**	**72.1**	**1.8**	**1.8**
PEPERAMI*								
Beef, Bars, Peperami*	1 Bar/20g	69	3.4	345	26	22	17	0
Hot, Peperami*	1 Stick/23g	112	9.9	497	22	3.2	44	1.2
Lunchbox Minis, 30% Less Fat, Peperami*	1 Stick/10g	40	3.1	400	26	5.5	31	3
Original, Peperami*	1 Stick/25g	126	11	504	24	2.5	44	0.1
Tender, Peperami*	1 Serving/20g	64	2.2	322	39	16.5	11	0
PEPPER								
Black, Freshly Ground, Average	**1 Tsp/2g**	**5**	**0.1**	**255**	**11**	**64.8**	**3.3**	**26.5**
Cayenne, Ground	**1 Tsp/2g**	**6**	**0.3**	**318**	**12**	**31.7**	**17.3**	**0**
White	**½ Tsp/1g**	**3**	**0**	**296**	**10.4**	**68.6**	**2.1**	**26.2**
PEPPERCORNS								
Black, Schwartz*	1 Tsp/2g	11	0.4	529	13	68.7	22.5	27
Green, Average	**1 Tsp/10g**	**4**	**0.1**	**44**	**1.6**	**5.3**	**0.8**	**4.7**
PEPPERONI								
Asda*	1 Slice/6g	26	2.2	434	26	1.6	36	0
Danish, Slices, Asda*	1 Slice/5g	25	2.3	493	18	1.8	46	0.6
for Pizza, Slices, Tesco*	6 Slices/20g	97	9.2	485	15.6	2.2	45.9	0.1
Sliced, Tesco*	1 Slice/5g	20	1.7	402	20	2.4	34.7	0
Sliced, Waitrose*	1 Slice/2g	8	0.7	425	23.7	0.1	36.6	0
Spicy, Dulano, Lidl*	1 Piece/5g	24	2.2	474	14.4	2.5	45	0.5
Spicy, Sliced, Ocado*	6 Slices/32g	130	11.8	407	18	0.5	37	0
PEPPERS								
Cherry Bell, Stuffed, Cream Cheese, Morrisons*	¼ Pack/37g	98	8.3	264	2.4	12.6	22.3	1.6
Cherry, Hot, Stuffed with Ricotta, Waitrose*	1 Pack/135g	185	10.3	137	5.4	10.5	7.6	2.7
Cherry, with Goats Cheese, Stuffed, Eat Well, M&S*	½ Pack/60g	91	5.7	152	4.7	10.5	9.5	2.8
Chilli, Dried, Flakes, Average	**1 Tsp/3g**	**13**	**0.4**	**425**	**16**	**56**	**15**	**44**
Chilli, Green, Raw, Unprepared, Average	**1 Med/13g**	**4**	**0**	**29**	**1.5**	**6.9**	**0.1**	**1.1**
Chilli, Red, Raw, Unprepared, Average	**1 Med/45g**	**13**	**0.1**	**29**	**1.5**	**6.9**	**0.1**	**1.1**
Green, Boiled in Salted Water	**1oz/28g**	**5**	**0.1**	**18**	**1**	**2.6**	**0.5**	**1.8**
Green, Raw, Unprepared, Average	**1 Med/160g**	**20**	**0.4**	**13**	**0.7**	**2.2**	**0.3**	**1.3**
Jalapeno, Raw	**1 Pepper/14g**	**4**	**0.1**	**28**	**1.2**	**5.4**	**0.6**	**2.6**

	Measure INFO/WEIGHT	per Measure KCAL	per Measure FAT	Nutrition Values per 100g / 100ml KCAL	PROT	CARB	FAT	FIBRE
PEPPERS								
Mixed Bag, From Supermarket, Average	**1oz/28g**	**7**	**0.1**	**25**	**1**	**4.4**	**0.4**	**1.7**
Orange, Sweet, Raw, Average	**1oz/28g**	**8**	**0.1**	**30**	**1.8**	**5**	**0.3**	**1.5**
Red, & Yellow, Flame Seared, M&S*	½ Pack/88g	24	0.9	27	0.8	3.1	1	1
Red, Boiled in Salted Water	**1oz/28g**	**10**	**0.1**	**34**	**1.1**	**7**	**0.4**	**1.7**
Red, Raw, Unprepared, Average	**½ Med/80g**	**21**	**0.3**	**27**	**0.8**	**5.3**	**0.3**	**1.3**
Stuffed, Cream Cheese, Sweet, Aldi*	1 Serving/60g	92	7.2	154	3.7	6.9	12	2.1
Stuffed, Goats Cheese, Finest, Tesco*	1/3 Jar/61g	91	5.1	149	4.5	12.8	8.4	2.1
Stuffed, with Rice Based Filling, Average	**1oz/28g**	**24**	**0.7**	**85**	**1.5**	**15.4**	**2.4**	**1.3**
Stuffed, with Vegetables, Cheese Topping, Average	**1oz/28g**	**31**	**1.9**	**111**	**3.4**	**9.8**	**6.7**	**1.5**
Yellow, Raw, Unprepared, Average	**1 Med/160g**	**35**	**0.3**	**22**	**1**	**4.4**	**0.2**	**1.4**
PERCH								
Raw, Atlantic	**1oz/28g**	**26**	**0.5**	**94**	**18.6**	**0**	**1.6**	**0**
PESTO								
Bail, Cucina, Aldi*	¼ Jar/48g	217	21.6	452	4.2	6.9	45	1.7
Basil, Bright & Green, Waitrose*	¼ Jar/48g	217	22.5	453	4.5	2.3	46.9	1.6
Basil, Finest, Tesco*	½ Pack/65g	278	27.4	428	7.9	3.6	42.2	0.9
Basil, Fresh, Sainsbury's*	1 Tbsp/15g	60	5.8	403	9.6	3.7	38.6	1.3
Black Olive, Wicked Kitchen, Tesco*	1 Serving/48g	159	14.9	331	2.6	9	31.1	2.5
Green, Average	**1 Tbsp/20g**	**103**	**9.5**	**517**	**20.4**	**2**	**47.5**	**0**
Green, Basil, Free From, Tesco*	¼ Jar/47g	198	18.6	422	3.7	11.6	39.7	1.5
Green, Free From, Asda*	¼ Jar/48g	172	17.1	362	2.9	6	36	1.1
Green, Reduced Fat, Tesco*	¼ Jar /49g	96	9.5	195	2.6	0.7	19.4	3.4
Pesto, Green, Baresa, Lidl*	¼ Jar/48g	173	17.1	364	4.1	4.8	35.9	2.6
Red, Asda*	½ Jar/100g	248	23	248	2.6	6.5	23	2.2
Red, Morrisons*	1 Tbsp/15g	47	4.4	311	5.7	6.6	29	5.9
Red, Rosso, Sundried Tomato, Finest, Tesco*	¼ Jar/47g	166	16.1	353	4	5.6	34.3	3.2
Sauce, Green, Lighter, Sainsbury's*	¼ Jar/47g	98	8.8	207	4.1	4.1	18.5	4.1
Sauce, Sun Dried Tomato, Extra Special, Asda*	¼ Jar/48g	159	15.7	334	3.4	4.8	33	2
Tomato, & Chilli, Tesco*	¼ Jar/47g	190	18.2	400	4	8.6	38.3	2.6
Tomato, Mezzetta*	2 Tbsp/30g	130	13	433	6.7	6.7	43.3	3.3
Tomato, Reduced Fat, No. 15, Sacla*	1 Tbsp/15g	29	2.6	194	3.2	7.5	17	1.9
Tomato, Sun Dried, Filippo Berio*	1 Tbsp/15g	73	6.3	484	7.3	18	42	0
PETIT POIS								
& Baby Carrots, Canned, Drained, Average	**½ Can/122g**	**58**	**0.8**	**47**	**2.9**	**7**	**0.7**	**3.2**
& Sweetcorn, M&S*	1 Serving/80g	65	1.3	81	5.5	9.2	1.6	4.1
Canned, Drained, Average	**1 Sm Can/200g**	**125**	**1**	**63**	**4.8**	**8.9**	**0.5**	**2.6**
Fresh, Frozen, Average	**1 Serving/80g**	**51**	**0.8**	**63**	**5.4**	**7.1**	**1**	**4.8**
with Leeks, & Pancetta, Waitrose*	½ Pack/110g	168	11	153	6	7.5	10	4.3
PHEASANT								
Meat Only, Roasted	**1oz/28g**	**62**	**3.4**	**220**	**27.9**	**0**	**12**	**0**
Meat Only, Roasted, Weighed with Bone	**1oz/28g**	**32**	**1.7**	**114**	**14.5**	**0**	**6.2**	**0**
PHYSALIS								
Raw, without Husk, Average	**5 Fruits/30g**	**16**	**0.2**	**53**	**1.9**	**11.2**	**0.7**	**0.4**
PICCALILLI								
Haywards*	1 Serving/28g	18	0.2	66	0.6	12	0.7	0.7
Heinz*	1 Serving/10g	10	0.1	99	1	20.5	0.6	0.6
Morrisons*	1 Serving/50g	38	0.4	75	1.6	15	0.7	0.6
Mustard, Asda*	1 Tbsp/15g	11	0.1	73	0.5	16	0.5	1.3
Mustard, Tesco*	1 Tbsp/15g	9	0.1	60	0.9	12.9	0.5	0.2
Original, Bartons*	1 Tbsp/15g	7	0.1	48	0.8	10.4	0.4	0
Tracklements*	1 Serving/30g	32	0.6	106	3.7	15.8	2.1	2.8
Waitrose*	1 Tbsp/15g	12	0.3	81	0.8	14.3	1.9	1.5

	Measure INFO/WEIGHT	per Measure KCAL	FAT	Nutrition Values per 100g / 100ml KCAL	PROT	CARB	FAT	FIBRE
PICKLE								
Banana Habanero , Mr Vikkis*	¼ Jar/55g	122	3.4	222	1.4	42.4	6.1	0
Branston, Original, Crosse & Blackwell*	1 Serving/12g	19	0.1	157	0.5	34	0.7	1.8
Branston, Sm Chunk, Squeezy, Crosse & Blackwell*	1 Serving/15g	19	0	127	0.9	29.8	0.2	1.1
Branston, Smooth, Squeezy, Crosse & Blackwell*	1 Serving/15g	19	0	127	0.9	29.8	0.2	1.1
Brinjal, Patak's*	1 Tsp/16g	61	4	381	2.1	34.5	24.8	0
Cornichons, Cocktail, Pickled, M&S*	1 Cornichon/5g	2	0	39	0.8	6.8	0.6	1.5
Cornichons, Freshona, Lidl*	1 Serving/50g	18	0.2	35	1.2	5.5	0.3	0
Cucumber, Dill Or Kosher Dill, Average	**1 Lge Pickle/135g**	**16**	**0.2**	**12**	**0.6**	**2.6**	**0.1**	**1.1**
Garlic, Patak's*	1 Tsp/16g	42	3	261	3.6	20	18.5	1.6
Ginger, Mothers Recipe*	1 Spoon/15g	30	1.4	201	2	28	9	3
Hot Chilli Jam, What A Pickle*	1 Tsp/8g	14	0	178	0.6	44	0.1	1.2
Lime, Hot, Patak's*	1 Tsp/16g	31	3	194	2.2	4	18.7	0.4
Lime, Oily	**1 Serving/39g**	**70**	**6.1**	**178**	**1.9**	**8.3**	**15.5**	**0**
Mild Mustard, Heinz*	1 Tbsp/10g	13	0.1	129	2.2	25.7	1.3	0.9
Red Cabbage, Asda*	1 Serving/50g	16	0	32	1.6	6	0.1	0
Sandwich, Tesco*	1 Tbsp/15g	16	0	108	0.6	25.2	0.2	1.4
Sweet	**1 Tsp/10g**	**14**	**0**	**141**	**0.6**	**36**	**0.1**	**1.2**
Tangy, Sandwich, Heinz*	1 Tsp/10g	13	0	134	0.7	31.4	0.2	0.9
PICNIC								
Cadbury*	1 Bar/38g	182	8.7	479	7.3	60	23	2.5
PIE								
Aloo Gobi, GF, Clive's*	1 Pie/235g	486	29.3	207	3	19.2	12.5	0
Apple, & Blackberry, Co-Op*	1 Serving/138g	338	15.2	245	3	33	11	2
Apple, & Blackberry, Shortcrust, M&S*	1 Serving/142g	469	17.8	330	4.3	50.2	12.5	1.1
Apple, & Blackberry, 494, Oakhouse Foods Ltd*	1 Serving/151g	310	10.9	205	1.9	33	7.2	1.1
Apple, Bramley, 2 Pack, 753, Oakhouse Foods Ltd*	1 Serving/150g	326	11.6	217	1.8	35.5	7.7	1
Apple, Bramley, Individual, Mr Kipling*	1 Pie/60g	210	7.9	351	3.4	54	13.2	1.4
Apple, Bramley, Individual, Sainsbury's*	1 Pie/54g	165	5	307	3.6	52.2	9.3	1.3
Apple, Bramley, Individual, Tesco*	1 Pie/60g	221	7.6	362	4	57.5	12.5	1.9
Apple, Commercially Prepared	**1 Slice/125g**	**296**	**13.8**	**237**	**1.9**	**34**	**11**	**1.6**
Apple, GF, Genius *	1 Pie/160g	387	17.8	242	1	38	11.1	3.3
Apple, Pastry Top & Bottom	**1oz/28g**	**74**	**3.7**	**266**	**2.9**	**35.8**	**13.3**	**1.7**
Apple, Prepared From Recipe, Average	**1oz/28g**	**74**	**3.5**	**265**	**2.4**	**37.1**	**12.5**	**0**
Apple, Shortcrust, Made Without Wheat, M&S*	¼ Pie/129g	317	9.9	246	3	40.1	7.7	2.3
Apple, with Custard	**1 Serving/217g**	**353**	**18.8**	**163**	**2.4**	**25.2**	**8.7**	**1.1**
Arabian Chickpea, Clive's*	1 Pie/237g	504	26	213	4.4	21.5	11	5
Banoffee, 2 Pack, 966, Oakhouse Foods*	1 Serving/128g	384	15.7	300	2.3	44.7	12.3	0.8
Banoffee, Mini, Waitrose*	1 Pie/26g	115	5.8	444	3.3	57	22.5	1.2
Banoffee, Tesco*	1/6 Pie/83g	217	11.2	261	2.6	31.5	13.5	1.5
Beef, Mince, Round, Munro The Butchers *	1 Round/523g	1271	51.3	243	13.7	24.4	9.8	1.3
Beef, Minced, & Cheesy Mash, Tesco*	½ Pack/368g	294	7.4	80	2.4	12.6	2	1
Beef, Minced, Aberdeen Angus, Shortcrust, M&S*	1 Pie/171g	435	26.6	255	9.3	19.3	15.6	3
Caramel, Crumble, Extra Special, Asda*	1 Pie/45g	179	6.7	402	3.4	63	15	2.3
Cauliflower, & Mushroom, Wicked Kitchen, Tesco*	1 Pie/381g	583	32.4	153	3.6	14.2	8.5	2.8
Cheddar, Vintage, Cauliflower, & Spinach, Deluxe, Lidl*	1 Pie/225g	613	38.1	272	6.2	25.8	16.9	0
Cheese, & Onion, Oven Baked, Average	**1 Serving/200g**	**654**	**40**	**327**	**8.2**	**30.4**	**20**	**1.2**
Cheese, & Potato	**1oz/28g**	**39**	**2.3**	**139**	**4.8**	**12.6**	**8.1**	**0.7**
Cherry, Bakery, Tesco*	1/6 Pie/87g	240	9.7	276	2.6	40.5	11.2	1.3
Cherry, Morello, Sainsbury's*	1/6 Pie/92g	258	10.2	281	2.6	41.7	11.1	2.3
Cherry, Morello, Waitrose*	1 Slice/75g	211	7.6	281	3.3	43.4	10.2	1.4
Chicken Curry, Chip Shop, Oven Baked, Iceland*	1 Pie/132g	365	22.1	277	8.5	21.5	16.8	2.8
Chicken, & Asparagus, Tesco*	1 Serving/170g	468	28.7	275	8.3	22.4	16.9	0.8
Chicken, & Gravy, Just, Fray Bentos*	½ Pie/215g	267	7.3	124	5.6	17.2	3.4	0.6

P

PIE

	Measure INFO/WEIGHT	per Measure KCAL	FAT	Nutrition Values per 100g / 100ml KCAL	PROT	CARB	FAT	FIBRE
Chicken, & Gravy, Roast, Deep Fill, Tesco*	¼ Pie/157g	358	16	228	9.7	23.7	10.2	1.5
Chicken, & Gravy, Shortcrust Pastry, Tesco*	1 Pie/250g	618	34.5	247	6.8	23.9	13.8	1
Chicken, & Ham, Deep Filled, Sainsbury's*	1 Pie/210g	594	37.2	283	8	23	17.7	1
Chicken, & Leek, & Bacon, Deluxe, Lidl*	1/3 Pie/171g	511	30.8	299	11	22	18	2.7
Chicken, & Leek, & Ham, Morrisons*	¼ Pie/137g	393	23.9	286	10.1	21.7	17.4	1
Chicken, & Leek, LC, Tesco*	1 Pie/350g	298	5.6	85	6.6	10.3	1.6	1.3
Chicken, & Leek, M&S*	1oz/28g	70	4.2	250	10.1	18.8	15.1	1.1
Chicken, & Mushroom, Average	**1 Serving/200g**	**540**	**31.7**	**270**	**8**	**23.8**	**15.9**	**1**
Chicken, & Bacon, Potato Topped, Finest, Tesco*	½ Pack/364g	429	16	118	7.9	11.1	4.4	1.2
Chicken, & Bacon, Tesco*	1 Pie/131g	295	14.1	225	8.9	22.3	10.8	1.4
Chicken, & Gravy, Chef Select, Lidl*	1/3 Pie/183g	518	30.9	283	10	21.4	16.9	2.6
Chicken, & Gravy, Classic, Waitrose*	1 Pie/200g	552	31.4	276	8.8	24.4	15.7	1.3
Chicken, & Gravy, GF, Genius *	1 Pie/160g	422	22.2	264	7.4	26	13.9	2.3
Chicken, & Leek, Filo , COU, M&S*	1 Pack/150g	160	2.8	107	10	12.1	1.9	0.8
Chicken, & Vegetable, Crestwood, Aldi*	1 Pie/140g	350	21	250	8.2	19	15	2.1
Chicken, & Vegetable, Frozen, Tesco*	1 Pie/129g	282	14.4	219	7.2	21.6	11.2	1.4
Chicken, Bacon, Smoked, & Leeks, TTD, Sainsbury's*	1 Pack/378g	491	25.7	130	8.4	8.2	6.8	1.5
Chicken, Creamy, Potato Topped, Gousto*	1 Serving/639g	460	9.6	72	6.5	8.7	1.5	1.3
Chicken, Deep Filled, Puff Pastry, Sainsbury's*	1 Pie/210g	538	31.9	256	10	19.9	15.2	3.1
Chicken, Ham Hock, & Leek, Finest, Tesco*	1 Pie/250g	562	28	225	9.2	21.2	11.2	1.3
Chicken, Ham Hock, Wiltshire, & Leek , TTD, Sainsbury's*	¼ Pie/138g	348	18.6	252	10.4	21.4	13.5	1.5
Chicken, Individual, Ready Made, Average	**1 Pie/155g**	**392**	**22.3**	**253**	**9.5**	**20.9**	**14.4**	**1.6**
Chicken, Leek, & Smoked Bacon, Gastropub, M&S*	½ Pie/250g	693	46.5	277	13	13.5	18.6	1.7
Chicken, Leek, & Wholegrain Mustard, Deluxe, Lidl*	1/3 Pie/167g	427	22.8	255	8.7	23.3	13.6	2.5
Chicken, Meat Free, Birds Eye*	1 Pie/155g	400	20.2	258	7.3	27	13	1.8
Chicken, Portobello, & Chestnut Mushroom, Pieminister*	1 Pie/270g	591	29.4	219	9.6	19.5	10.9	0
Chicken, Shortcrust Pastry, Individual, M&S*	1 Pie/150g	363	18.6	242	12.4	19.4	12.4	1.6
Chicken, Shortcrust, Oven Baked, Birds Eye*	1 Pie/155g	417	23.1	271	8.4	25	15	1.2
Chilli Roasted Sweet Potato, & Feta, Higgidy*	½ Pack/250g	715	44.2	286	6.3	26.9	17.7	2.1
Cod, & Haddock, Smoked, COU, M&S*	1 Pack/400g	320	9.6	80	6.1	9	2.4	1.2
Cottage, 1, Waitrose*	1 Pack/400g	580	30.4	145	8.2	10.3	7.6	1.6
Cottage, 1010, Parsley Box*	1 Pack/270g	329	16.5	122	6.1	10	6.1	1.5
Cottage, As Sold, Donald Russell*	1 Serving/440g	541	32.5	123	7.2	6.6	7.4	0.8
Cottage, Calorie Controlled, Love Life, Waitrose*	1 Pack/320g	253	4.5	79	4.5	11.3	1.4	1.6
Cottage, Calorie Counted, Asda*	1 Pack/350g	243	4.9	80	4.1	11	1.6	1.9
Cottage, Chilled, 400g, Quorn*	1 Pack/380g	315	8	83	3.4	11	2.1	3
Cottage, Classic, Allplants*	1 Serving/490g	431	3.9	88	5.3	13	0.8	3.2
Cottage, Classic, Co-Op*	1 Pack/400g	372	14	93	5.6	9.3	3.5	1
Cottage, Classic, Iceland*	1 Serving/364g	411	19.3	113	6	9.4	5.3	2
Cottage, Comforting, Gousto*	1 Serving/637g	631	26.1	99	7.3	9	4.1	2
Cottage, Frozen, 400g, Quorn*	1 Pack/400g	396	14	99	4.2	11	3.5	4
Cottage, Hearty, Aldi*	½ Pack/400g	476	18	119	9	10.2	4.5	0.7
Cottage, Honest Value, Co-Op*	1 Pie/350g	252	6.7	72	0	0.1	1.9	0
Cottage, Inspired Cuisine, Aldi*	1 Pack/427g	401	12.8	94	6.8	9.5	3	1.3
Cottage, Kershaws*	1 Pack/375g	388	5.6	103	3.3	17.8	1.5	2.6
Cottage, Kirstys*	1 Pack /388g	299	11.3	77	6	7.6	2.9	1.9
Cottage, Lentil, with Sweet Potato & Carrot, Kirstys*	1 Meal/396g	222	3.6	56	1.9	8.7	0.9	2.1
Cottage, Low Fat, Well & Good, Co-Op*	1 Pack/400g	332	10	83	2.8	11	2.5	2.4
Cottage, Meat Free, Morrisons*	1 Pack/337g	239	4.4	71	2.5	10.9	1.3	3
Cottage, Plant Kitchen, M&S*	1 Pack/400g	436	15.2	109	4.2	13.8	3.8	1.6
Cottage, Plant Pioneers, Sainsbury's*	1 Pack/370g	285	7	77	2.9	11.1	1.9	1.8
Cottage, Retail, Average	**1 Pack/400g**	**399**	**15.7**	**100**	**5.5**	**10.5**	**3.9**	**1.3**
Cottage, Slim Cook, Tesco*	1 Pack/443g	381	9.7	86	9.2	6.3	2.2	2

PIE

INFO/WEIGHT	Measure	per Measure KCAL	per Measure FAT	KCAL	PROT	CARB	FAT	FIBRE
Cottage, Vegan, Oven Baked, Slimming World*	1 Pack/500g	320	0.5	64	4.2	9.7	0.1	3.5
Cottage, Veggie, Meal for One, M&S*	1 Pack/400g	356	12.8	89	2.4	11.9	3.2	1.7
Cottage, with Ale Gravy, The Best, Morrisons*	1 Pack/391g	481	21.5	123	8.1	9.6	5.5	1.4
Cottage, with Real Ale Gravy, The Best, Morrisons*	1 Pack/391g	481	21.5	123	8.1	9.6	5.5	1.4
Cottage, with Red Wine, & Cheddar Crumb, Sainsbury's*	1 Pack/375g	488	23.3	130	6.8	10.2	6.2	3.3
Cottage, with Sweet Potato Mash, Mini, Kirstys*	1 Pack/250g	184	6.9	74	5.7	7.2	2.8	1.8
Courgette, Feta, & Spinach, Free From, Sainsbury's*	1 Pie/170g	405	26.2	238	4.2	20	15.4	1.4
Cumberland, Classic, Sainsbury's*	1 Pack/353g	438	18.7	124	5.7	12.3	5.3	2
Cumberland, Meal for One, M&S*	1 Pie/400g	472	18.8	118	7.3	11	4.7	1.2
Cumberland, Mini, 314, Oakhouse Foods Ltd*	1 Serving/214g	257	9.2	120	6.8	11.4	4.3	1.5
Cumberland, Oven Cooked, Morrisons*	1 Pack/439g	404	14.9	92	6.2	8.5	3.4	1.2
Cumberland, Serves 1, Classic, Sainsbury's*	1 Pack/353g	438	18.7	124	5.7	12.3	5.3	2
Cumberland, Waitrose*	1 Pack/328g	269	10.5	82	3.8	9	3.2	1.1
Fish	**1 Serving/250g**	**262**	**7.5**	**105**	**8**	**12.3**	**3**	**0.7**
Fruit, Pastry Top & Bottom	**1oz/28g**	**73**	**3.7**	**260**	**3**	**34**	**13.3**	**1.8**
Gammon, & Leek, 4232, Wiltshire Farm Foods*	1 Serving/449g	602	31	134	5.7	11	6.9	0
Homity, Chunk Of Devon*	1 Pie/250g	548	31.5	219	6.8	18.5	12.6	0
Key Lime, Vegan, Feed Me *	1 Pot/90g	352	19.7	391	1.5	47.6	21.9	0
Lemon Meringue	**1 Portion/120g**	**383**	**17.3**	**319**	**4.5**	**45.9**	**14.4**	**0.7**
Lentil, & Olive, Greek, Clive's*	1 Pie/235g	477	25.4	203	4.5	20	10.8	0
Meat, & Potato, Hollands*	1 Pie/179g	385	18.4	215	5.5	24	10.3	0
Mince, All Butter, Average	**1 Pie/65g**	**251**	**8.9**	**386**	**4**	**60.2**	**13.8**	**2.4**
Mince, All Butter, Crumble Topped, Finest, Tesco*	1 Mince Pie/44g	185	5.8	420	4.1	69.3	13.2	3.4
Mince, All Butter, Mini, Average	**1 Pie/20g**	**78**	**2.8**	**389**	**4.3**	**61.6**	**13.8**	**2.8**
Mince, All Butter, Puff Pastry, Average	**1 Pie60g**	**228**	**10.5**	**381**	**4.3**	**51.1**	**17.4**	**2.2**
Mince, Frangipane, Specially Selected, Aldi*	1 Pie/46g	191	9.2	415	5.7	52	20	2.8
Mince, Free From, Sainsbury's*	1 Pie/58g	226	7.5	393	2.3	64	13	2.5
Mince, Iced Top, Asda*	1 Pie/55g	220	7.7	399	2.8	63	14	4.7
Mince, Iced Top, Mini, Mr Kipling*	1 Pie/29g	118	4.3	403	3.3	63.5	14.7	1.8
Mince, Individual, Average	**1 Pie/65g**	**260**	**11**	**400**	**4.2**	**56.3**	**17**	**1.6**
Mince, Rum, Pineapple, & Coconut, TTD, Sainsbury's*	1 Pie/52g	203	6.5	387	3.3	64.5	12.3	2.7
Mince, Vegan, & GF, Holland & Barrett*	1 Pie/60g	217	7.8	361	2.3	60	13	2.6
Mushroom, Country, Fry's *	1 Pie/350g	335	16.6	96	2.4	10	4.7	1.4
Mushroom, Creamy, & Kale, Higgidy*	1 Pie/250g	625	36.5	250	4.6	25.1	14.6	2.2
Mushroom, Plant Kitchen, M&S*	1 Pie/200g	450	24.6	225	4.2	23.9	12.3	1.1
No Pork, Snack, Plant Pioneers, Sainsbury's*	1 Pie/65g	229	13.1	352	9.7	31.9	20.1	2.2
No-Pork, Mini, Higgidy*	1 Pie/44g	166	9.5	377	7.4	37.2	21.5	3
Parsnip, & Portobello Mushroom, Deluxe, Lidl*	1 Pie/190g	475	26.8	250	3.9	25.6	14.1	2.7
Pork, & Egg, M&S*	¼ Pie/110g	411	31	374	10.9	18.4	28.2	1.5
Pork, & Festive Fruit Stuffing, Morrisons*	1 Pie/28g	94	5.7	336	12.5	24.9	20.3	2
Pork, & Pickle, Mini, Sainsbury's*	1 Pie/50g	177	11.5	354	9.5	26.2	23	2.1
Pork, & Pickle, Snack, Sainsbury's*	1 Pie/65g	246	15.8	379	8.9	29.9	24.4	2.3
Pork, BBQ, Mini, Tesco*	1 Pie/50g	198	13.2	396	10.7	28.2	26.3	1.9
Pork, Bitesize, Tesco*	1 Pie/25g	98	6.5	393	10.8	28.1	26.1	1.5
Pork, Cheese & Pickle, Mini, Tesco*	1 Pie/49g	191	12.8	389	9.2	29.3	26.1	1.2
Pork, Cheese, & Pesto, Waitrose*	1 Pie/25g	99	6.5	395	11.2	28.3	25.9	1.8
Pork, Cheese, & Pickle, Mini, Morrisons*	1 Pie/50g	228	14.9	456	9	36.9	29.8	2
Pork, Cheese, & Pickle, Snack, Morrisons*	1 Pie/75g	326	22.1	435	9.8	31.4	29.5	2.4
Pork, Individual	**1 Pie/75g**	**272**	**19.3**	**363**	**10.8**	**23.7**	**25.7**	**0.9**
Pork, Lattice, Large, Market St, Morrisons*	1 Pie/450g	1742	132.8	387	7.9	21.6	29.5	1.8
Pork, Mini, Retail, Average	**1 Mini/50g**	**198**	**13.7**	**396**	**10.8**	**26.4**	**27.4**	**2.4**
Pork, Sliced	**1 Slice/100g**	**380**	**29.9**	**380**	**10.2**	**18.7**	**29.9**	**0**
Rhubarb, Lattice, Individual, Baked by Us, Morrisons*	1 Pie/135g	433	19.2	321	3.9	43.4	14.2	2

P

PIE

	Measure INFO/WEIGHT	per Measure KCAL	FAT	Nutrition Values per 100g / 100ml KCAL	PROT	CARB	FAT	FIBRE
Rhubarb, Shortcrust Pastry, Bakery, Tesco*	1 Slice/87g	219	9.3	251	3.1	34.8	10.7	1.7
Roasted Celeriac, & Butter Bean, Allplants*	1 Serving/485g	441	12.6	91	4.6	11	2.6	3.6
Sausage, & Mash, Tesco*	½ Pack/365g	288	5.1	79	2.3	13.7	1.4	1.2
Sausage, Leek, & Cider, Pukka Pies Ltd*	1 Pie/213g	488	27.5	229	5.1	22.4	12.9	1.3
Scotch, Co-Op*	1 Pie/132g	408	24.9	309	7.3	27.3	18.9	1.5
Shepherd's, Average	*1oz/28g*	*31*	*1.7*	*112*	*6*	*9.3*	*5.9*	*0.7*
Shepherd's, Vegetarian, Average	*1 Serving/400g*	*371*	*14.6*	*93*	*4*	*10.4*	*3.6*	*2.5*
Shepherds, Vegan, Slimming World*	1 Pack/500g	320	0.5	64	4.2	9.7	0.1	3.5
Spinach, Feta, & Pine Nut, Higgidy*	1 Pie/265g	684	47.4	258	9.2	15.6	17.9	1.5
Spinach, Twist, Filo Pastry, Alesis*	¼ Pie/100g	250	12.5	250	6.5	26.8	12.5	2.3
Squash, Spinach, & Feta Pie, Mud*	1 Pie/270g	821	48.6	304	5.1	32	18	0
Steak & Gravy, Shortcrust Pastry, Asda*	1 Pie/208g	541	31.2	260	10	24	15	0
Steak & Gravy, Shortcrust, Sainsbury's*	1 Pie/200g	592	29.6	296	9.1	30.9	14.8	1.7
Steak & Kidney, Donald Russell*	1 Pie/260g	549	33	211	7.8	17.3	12.7	0
Steak & Kidney, Fray Bentos*	½ Pie/213g	329	16.2	155	7	14.5	7.6	0.5
Steak, & Ale with Chips & Gravy	*1 Serving/400g*	*825*	*42.2*	*206*	*7.2*	*20.5*	*10.6*	*0.5*
Steak, & Ale, Average	*1 Pie/200g*	*507*	*28.7*	*253*	*9.8*	*21.1*	*14.4*	*1.3*
Steak, & Kidney, Individual	*1 Pie/200g*	*646*	*42.4*	*323*	*9.1*	*25.6*	*21.2*	*0.9*
Steak, & Gravy, Chef Select, Lidl*	1 Pie/200g	588	35.8	294	8.7	23.7	17.9	1.4
Steak, & Gravy, Puff Pastry Topped, Oven Baked, Asda*	1 Pie/150g	419	23.9	280	8.3	25	16	1.5
Steak, & Horseradish, Frozen, Deluxe, Lidl*	1 Pie/194g	650	42.5	335	10.9	22.6	21.9	2.1
Steak, & Mushroom, 474, Oakhouse Foods*	1 Serving/420g	416	17.6	99	5.2	9.6	4.2	1
Steak, & Old Peculiar Ale, Deluxe, Lidl*	1 Serving/167g	426	22.4	255	9.1	23.3	13.4	2.4
Steak, & Red Wine Gravy, Finest, Tesco*	½ Pie/250g	650	32	260	12.3	22.9	12.8	1.6
Steak, & Red Wine, GF, Made Without Wheat, M&S*	1 Pie/180g	522	31.7	290	10.3	21.7	17.6	1.8
Steak, & Red Wine, Shortcrust Topped, Cook*	1 Serving/295g	496	24.2	168	11.6	10.5	8.2	1.2
Steak, & Stilton, TTD, Sainsbury's*	1 Pie/250g	615	31	246	12.1	20.4	12.4	2.2
Steak, Aberdeen Angus, Top Crust, Waitrose*	½ Pie/280g	476	24.1	170	10	13.4	8.6	4.1
Steak, Puff Pastry, Average	*¼ Pie/100g*	*259*	*14.5*	*259*	*9.4*	*21.8*	*14.5*	*1.9*
Steak, Shortcrust, Average	*¼ Pie/100g*	*253*	*14.1*	*253*	*9.9*	*21.6*	*14.1*	*1.4*
Sweet Potato, & Feta, with Pumpkin Seeds, Higgidy*	1 Pie/270g	756	49.4	280	7.2	22.9	18.3	2.1
Sweet Potato, Feta, & Sunflower Seed, Deluxe, Aldi*	1 Pie/250g	660	42.8	264	6.3	19	17.1	1.6
Vegan Minced Steak, & Onion, Pukka Pie*	1 Pie/214g	539	29.7	252	6.7	24.3	13.9	1.7
Vegan, Gro, Co-Op*	1 Pie/50g	175	10	350	8.7	33	20	1.9
Vegetable	*1oz/28g*	*42*	*2.1*	*151*	*3*	*18.9*	*7.6*	*1.5*
Vegetable Balti, Fray Bentos*	½ Pie/213g	285	13.2	134	2.8	17.6	6.2	1
Vegetable, Rainbow, Plant Kitchen, M&S*	1 Pie/220g	367	15.8	167	5.4	16.6	7.2	7.2
Vegetable, Retail, Average	*1 Serving/200g*	*348*	*19*	*174*	*3.7*	*18.6*	*9.5*	*1.1*
Vegetarian, Chicken Style, & Mushroom, Quorn*	1 Pie/235g	588	33.2	250	5.5	23.7	14.1	3
Vegetarian, Deep Country, Linda McCartney*	1 Pie/166g	413	23.6	249	5.2	24.9	14.2	2.6
Vegetarian, Mince & Potato, Quorn*	1 Pie/200g	388	16	194	6.5	22.5	8	3
Vegetarian, Mushroom & Ale, Linda McCartney*	1 Pie/200g	439	23.5	219	4.1	25	11.7	1.2
Vegetarian, Steak, Meat Free, Quorn*	1 Pie/235g	439	18.8	187	5.6	22	8	2

PIGEON

	Measure INFO/WEIGHT	per Measure KCAL	FAT	Nutrition Values per 100g / 100ml KCAL	PROT	CARB	FAT	FIBRE
Meat Only, Roasted, Average	*1 Pigeon/115g*	*215*	*9.1*	*187*	*29*	*0*	*7.9*	*0*
Meat Only, Roasted, Weighed with Bone, Average	*1oz/28g*	*12*	*0.5*	*41*	*6.4*	*0*	*1.7*	*0*

PIKELETS

	Measure INFO/WEIGHT	per Measure KCAL	FAT	Nutrition Values per 100g / 100ml KCAL	PROT	CARB	FAT	FIBRE
Buttermilk, Waitrose*	1 Pikelet/28g	54	0.2	192	7.1	37.7	0.8	2.6
Sainsbury's*	1 Pikelet/24g	55	0.3	230	7.6	45.1	1.4	3.3
Tesco*	1 Pikelet/27g	52	0.3	193	6.6	38.1	1	2.4

PILAF

	Measure INFO/WEIGHT	per Measure KCAL	FAT	Nutrition Values per 100g / 100ml KCAL	PROT	CARB	FAT	FIBRE
Beef, with Tomatoes, & Green Beans, Hello Fresh*	1 Serving/448g	667	20	149	7.6	19.9	4.5	0.2
Bulgur Wheat, Sainsbury's*	1 Pack/381g	347	11.1	91	3.9	12.3	2.9	6.3

	Measure INFO/WEIGHT	per Measure KCAL	FAT	Nutrition Values per 100g / 100ml KCAL	PROT	CARB	FAT	FIBRE
PILAF								
Chicken, Co-Op*	1 Pack/550g	891	45.7	162	8.9	12	8.3	1.8
Chicken, Middle Eastern Inspired, Waitrose*	½ Pack/275g	639	28.9	232	13.2	19.9	10.5	2.7
with Tomato, Average	**1oz/28g**	**40**	**0.9**	**144**	**2.5**	**28**	**3.3**	**0.4**
PILCHARDS								
Fillets in Tomato Sauce, Average	**1 Can/120g**	**158**	**7.8**	**132**	**16.2**	**2.2**	**6.5**	**0.1**
Fillets in Virgin Olive Oil, Glenryck*	1 Serving/92g	223	14.4	242	23.3	2	15.7	0
in Brine, Drained, Glenryck*	1/3 Can/93g	167	10.4	180	19.7	1	11.2	1
in Hot Chilli Sauce, Glenryck*	1 Tin/155g	219	13.2	141	15.2	1	8.5	1
PIMMS*								
& Lemonade, Premixed, Canned, Pimms*	1 Can/250ml	160	0	64	0	8.4	0	0
25% Volume, Pimms*	1 Serving/50ml	80	0	160	0	5	0	0
PINE NUTS								
Average	**1 Tbsp/8g**	**56**	**5.5**	**695**	**15.7**	**3.9**	**68.6**	**1.9**
PINEAPPLE								
Caribbean Style, in Dark Chocolate, Lidl*	1 Piece/26g	111	3.3	426	2.4	74.3	12.6	2.8
Chunks, Average	**1 Serving/100g**	**66**	**0.1**	**66**	**0.5**	**15.5**	**0.1**	**0.3**
in Juice, Canned, Average	**1 Can/106g**	**57**	**0**	**53**	**0.3**	**12.9**	**0**	**0.6**
Pieces, Chunky, Dried, Holland & Barrett *	1 Piece/25g	90	0.1	359	0.5	89	0.5	1.2
Raw, Flesh Only, Average	**1 Med Slice/80g**	**40**	**0.1**	**50**	**0.5**	**13.1**	**0.1**	**1.4**
PISTACHIO NUTS								
Chilli, & Lime, Morrisons*	1 Pack/55g	334	27.6	608	25.6	8.8	50.1	9.5
Raw, Average, without Shells	**1 Serving/20g**	**111**	**8.9**	**557**	**20.6**	**28**	**44.4**	**10.3**
Roasted & Salted, without Shells, Average	**1 Serving/25g**	**152**	**13.6**	**608**	**19.6**	**9.9**	**54.5**	**6.1**
Salted, Roasted, Weighed with Shell	**1 Serving/100g**	**331**	**30.5**	**331**	**9.8**	**4.5**	**30.5**	**3.4**
Salted, Roasted, without Shells	**1 Serving/100g**	**601**	**55.4**	**601**	**17.9**	**8.2**	**55.4**	**6.1**
Squares, 180 Snacks*	1 Pistachio Square/7g	36	2.4	520	16	44	35	8
PIZZA								
'Nduja, & Burrata, Sourdough Base, No.1, Waitrose*	¼ Pizza/129g	284	10.6	220	8.9	26.5	8.2	2.1
American Hot, Carlos, Aldi*	½ Pizza/139g	338	12.1	243	10	30	8.7	2.6
American, Classic, Oven Cooked, Pizza Express*	½ Pizza/122g	335	13.2	274	12.8	30.3	10.8	2.3
American, Hot, Thin & Crispy, Stonebaked, Aldi*	½ Pizza/149g	357	16.4	240	9.7	25	11	2.8
Arrabiata, Vegan, Plant Menu, Aldi*	½ Pizza/170g	428	13.9	252	8.3	35	8.2	4.1
Bacon, & Mushroom, Thin & Crispy, Sainsbury's*	½ Pizza/150g	396	15.9	264	12.9	29.2	10.6	1.7
BBQ Chick'n, Plant Based, Gro, Co-Op*	1 Pizza/264g	529	16	200	7.2	27.6	6.1	3.6
BBQ Chicken, Stonebaked, Asda*	½ Pizza/348g	738	16.7	212	11	29	4.8	3.6
BBQ Meat Feast, Sourdough, Carlos, Aldi*	1 Slice/45g	127	5.4	282	14	29	12	1.8
BBQ Meat Feast, Stuffed Crust, Carlos, Aldi*	½ Pizza/250g	622	18.8	249	9.9	34	7.5	2.4
Beef, Chilli, Classic Crust, Tex Mex, Tesco*	½ Pizza/260g	655	26.5	252	10.9	27.9	10.2	2.5
Buffalo Chicken, Fully Loaded, Iceland*	¼ Pizza/168g	420	13.4	251	9.5	34	8	2.4
Buffalo Mozzarella, & Tomatoes, Finest, Tesco*	1 Pizza/207g	502	16.7	243	10.5	31.1	8.1	2.3
Cajun Chicken, Stonebaked, Chef Select, Lidl*	½ Pizza/160g	330	8	206	10.8	27.9	5	2.9
Caprino Verde, Specially Selected, Aldi*	½ Pizza/193g	490	21.2	254	9.4	27	11	2.9
Carbonara, Romana, Supermarket, Pizza Express*	½ Pizza/182g	486	17.8	267	12.2	31.2	9.8	2.5
Cauliflower, Spicy, Stonebaked, Plant Menu, Aldi*	½ Pizza/170g	406	13.8	239	6.8	33	8.1	4
Cehese & Tomato, 1319, Oakhouse Foods Ltd*	1 Serving/356g	904	26	254	8.9	37.1	7.3	1.9
Chargrilled Veg, Stone Baked, Tesco*	½ Pizza/162g	337	10.4	208	10.2	26.4	6.4	1.9
Chargrilled Vegetable & Basil Pesto, Sourdough, Asda*	1 Serving/239g	468	15.5	196	8.1	25	6.5	2
Chargrilled Vegetable, & Olive, Sainsbury's*	½ Pizza/97g	201	4.9	208	9.5	29.7	5.1	2.7
Cheese & Tomato, Average	**1 Serving/300g**	**711**	**35.4**	**237**	**9.1**	**25.2**	**11.8**	**1.4**
Cheese & Tomato, Baguette, Tesco*	1 Baguette/125g	275	8.5	220	11	28	6.8	2.8
Cheese & Tomato, Deep Pan, Goodfella's*	¼ Pizza/102g	259	10.8	253	11.5	29.6	10.5	3.7
Cheese & Tomato, Mini, M&S*	1 Pizza/95g	233	5.5	245	10	38.7	5.8	1.6
Cheese & Tomato, Retail, Frozen	**1oz/28g**	**70**	**3**	**250**	**7.5**	**32.9**	**10.7**	**1.4**

P

PIZZA

INFO/WEIGHT	Measure	per Measure KCAL	FAT	Nutrition Values per 100g / 100ml KCAL	PROT	CARB	FAT	FIBRE
Cheese & Tomato, Thin & Crispy, Essential, Waitrose*	½ Pizza/112g	306	10.6	273	14.3	30.7	9.5	3.5
Cheese & Tomato, Thin & Crispy, Sainsbury's*	1 Serving/135g	344	10	255	14.9	32.2	7.4	5
Cheese & Tomato, Thin & Crispy, Waitrose*	1 Pizza/280g	658	28.3	235	12.3	23.6	10.1	2.3
Cheese & Tomato, Thin, HFC, Tesco*	½ Pizza/144g	361	9.6	250	10.9	35.5	6.7	2.3
Cheese & Tomato, Mini, Co-Op*	1 Pizza/91g	259	7.5	285	10	41	8.2	2.8
Cheese & Tomato, Mini, Iceland*	½ Pizza/89g	251	10.8	282	11.7	30.8	12.1	1.8
Cheese & Tomato, Thin & Crispy, M&S*	¼ Pizza/116g	314	12.3	271	12.3	30.7	10.6	1.8
Cheese Feast, Deep Crust, Carlos, Aldi*	1 Pizza/155g	432	14.9	279	9.7	37.3	9.6	2.1
Cheese Feast, Light, Deep Dish, Chicago Town*	1 Pizza/144g	375	10.9	261	12	35	7.6	1.9
Cheese Feast, Stuffed Crust, Asda*	½ Pizza/204g	521	18.8	255	13	29	9.2	2.2
Cheese Feast, Stuffed Crust, Iceland*	½ Pizza/227g	624	22.9	275	13.4	31.2	10.1	2.8
Cheese Feast, Thin Crust, Chilled, Tesco*	½ Pizza/175g	467	22.4	267	14.7	23.4	12.8	2.5
Cheese Medley, Tiger Crust, Chicago Town*	1 Pizza/298g	992	47.7	333	14	32	16	1.5
Cheese Meltdown, Thin & Crispy, 10", Asda*	1 Pizza/287g	723	28.7	252	12	28	10	1.7
Cheese, & Garlic, Tesco*	½ Pizza/102g	304	11.7	298	9.2	38.1	11.5	2.4
Cheese, & Tomato, Lidl*	1 Pizza/120g	190	5.3	158	10.4	17.9	4.4	2.5
Cheese, & Tomato, Snack, Asda*	1 Pizza/110g	302	9.1	275	10	38	8.3	2.7
Cheese, Big 5, Classic Crust, Co-Op*	½ Pizza/225g	610	22.5	271	11	33	10	2.6
Cheese, Four, Deep Dish, Chicago Town*	1 Pizza/148g	433	17.8	292	12	33	12	0
Cheese, Four, Finest, Tesco*	½ Pizza/230g	575	21.2	250	12.1	29.8	9.2	1.3
Cheese, Four, Stonebaked, Thin, Carlos, Aldi*	½ Pizza/176g	498	17.4	283	13	34	9.9	2.8
Cheese, Four, Thin & Crispy, Iceland*	½ Pizza/148g	354	12.6	239	10.7	29.1	8.5	1.6
Cheese, Stuffed Crust, Takeaway, Tesco*	½ Pizza/203g	521	17.7	256	11.5	31.8	8.7	2.5
Cheese, Thick Crust, From Restaurant, Average	*1 Pizza/976g*	*2655*	*107.3*	*272*	*12*	*31.3*	*11*	*1.8*
Cheese, Thin Crust, From Restaurant, Average	*1 Pizza/627g*	*1906*	*98.3*	*304*	*14.2*	*26.5*	*15.7*	*2*
Cheezeburger, Deep Dish, Chicago Town*	1 Pizza/162g	431	17.8	266	6.6	35	11	1.7
Chicken Arrabbiata, Spicy, Wood Fired, M&S*	½ Pack/224g	522	19.5	233	13.3	24.5	8.7	1.7
Chicken Arrabiata, Spicy, Ultra Thin, M&S*	½ Pack/87g	216	8.4	248	12.6	26.8	9.7	1.7
Chicken Tikka, Ultra Thin, Iceland*	½ Pizza/159g	404	15.9	254	11.9	27.6	10	2.7
Chicken, & Chorizo, 12", TTD, Sainsbury's*	½ Pizza/290g	702	20.9	242	12.2	32.1	7.2	2.6
Chicken, & Sweetcorn, Stonebaked, Tesco*	1 Serving/177g	354	9.6	200	11.9	26	5.4	2
Chicken, & Vegetable, Stone Baked, GFY, Asda*	½ Pizza/161g	349	3.7	217	13	36	2.3	1.7
Chicken, & Bacon, Stonebaked, Tesco*	½ Pizza/147g	376	14.7	256	13	27.1	10	2.5
Chicken, & Bacon, Stuffed, Chicago Town*	1 Pack/640g	1747	64	273	11	33	10	1.7
Chicken, BBQ, M&S*	½ Pizza/210g	430	11.8	205	11.6	27.5	5.6	1.8
Chicken, BBQ, Stonebaked, Tesco*	½ Pizza/158g	285	9.5	180	10.5	20.9	6	3.9
Chicken, BBQ, Thin & Crispy, Sainsbury's*	½ Pizza/167g	399	12.4	238	11.4	30.4	7.4	2.2
Chicken, Cajun Style, Stonebaked, Tesco*	1 Pizza/561g	1318	55	235	11.9	24.8	9.8	1.4
Chicken, Cajun, Sainsbury's*	½ Pizza/146g	285	2.6	195	12.9	31.8	1.8	2.6
Chicken, Chargrilled, Iceland*	1 Pizza/381g	804	25.5	211	12.3	25.4	6.7	2
Chicken, Chargrilled, Thin & Crispy, Asda*	1 Pizza/373g	780	18.6	209	9	32	5	1.6
Chicken, Club, Deep Dish, Chicago Town*	1 Pizza/153g	391	13.5	255	11	32	8.8	0.9
Chicken, Fajita, Musclefood*	1 Pizza/220g	315	9.5	143	10	15	4.3	2.6
Chicken, Garlic, Thin & Crispy, Stonebake, Sainsbury's*	½ Pizza/160g	386	17.3	241	10.7	25.2	10.8	3.5
Chicken, Hot & Spicy, Deep Pan, Tesco*	½ Pizza/222g	423	7.3	191	10.5	30	3.3	2.1
Chicken, Piri Piri, Classic Crust, Takeaway, Tesco*	1 Pizza/550g	1196	38.4	217	10.3	28.3	7	2.4
Chicken, Romano, Goodfella's*	½ Pizza/189g	447	17.6	236	11	26	9.3	0
Chicken, Spicy, Thin & Crispy, Morrisons*	½ Pizza/144g	330	8.8	229	11.4	30.8	6.1	2.7
Chicken, Stone Baked, Goodfella's*	½ Pizza/171g	407	15	238	13	26	8.8	1.9
Chicken, Sweet Chilli, BGTY, Sainsbury's*	½ Pizza/138g	276	2.3	200	13	33.2	1.7	2.1
Chicken, Sweet Chilli, Extra Thin, Morrison's*	½ Pizza/146g	301	7.9	206	10.7	27.9	5.4	1.7
Chicken, Tomato, & Ricotta, Sainsbury's*	1 Pizza/215g	482	14.4	224	12.7	27	6.7	2.4
Chilli Salsiccia, Wood Fired, Irresistible, Co-Op*	1 Pizza/235g	639	21.9	272	12	34	9.3	1.2

PIZZA

INFO/WEIGHT	Measure	per Measure KCAL	per Measure FAT	Nutrition Values per 100g / 100ml KCAL	PROT	CARB	FAT	FIBRE
Cured Meats, Italian, Wood Fired, M&S*	½ Pizza/209g	550	24.7	263	13.5	25	11.8	1.4
Delizioza, Trattoria Alfredo*	1 Pizza/330g	729	28	221	10	25	8.5	0
Double Pepperoni, Spicy, Iceland*	½ Pizza/171g	394	14	231	9.4	28.5	8.2	2.8
Double Pepperoni, Thin & Crispy, Stonebaked, Co-Op*	1 Slice/40g	106	4	266	11	31	10	2.5
Double Pepperoni, Tiger Crust, Chicago Town*	½ Pizza/160g	538	27.2	336	13	31	17	1.5
Falafel, Vegan, Stonebaked, Goodfellas *	½ Pizza/182g	397	12.7	218	6.4	30	7	0
Feta, Mascarpone, & Caramelised Onion, M&S*	½ Pizza/240g	612	28.1	255	9.8	26.9	11.7	1.6
Fiorentina, Classic, Supermarket, Pizza Express*	1 Pack/200g	420	13.8	210	8.9	26.9	6.9	2.3
Four Cheese, & Balsamic Red Onion, Finest, Tesco*	½ Pizza/210g	559	24.2	266	10.4	29.1	11.5	1.9
French Bread, Slice, Stouffers*	1 Slice/138g	369	18.4	267	10	26.7	13.3	1.3
Funghi, Dr Oetker*	½ Pizza/183g	449	21.9	246	8	25	12	1.6
Funghi, Ristorante, Dr Oetker*	1 Pizza/365g	847	43.4	232	7.6	22.5	11.9	1.8
Garlic Mushroom, & Spinach, M&S*	½ Pizza/222g	521	22.2	235	8.9	26.4	10	1.7
Goats Cheese, & Red Onion, Tesco *	½ Pizza/210g	559	24.2	266	10.4	29.1	11.5	1.9
Ham & Cheese, Snack, Asda*	1 Pack/114g	287	8.2	252	11	34	7.2	2.4
Ham, & Mushroom, Average	**1 Serving/250g**	**533**	**16**	**213**	**10.5**	**28.4**	**6.4**	**2.1**
Ham, & Pineapple, Average	**1 Serving/250g**	**555**	**16.8**	**222**	**11**	**29.2**	**6.7**	**2.1**
Ham, & Mushroom, Deep Pan, Oven Baked, Iceland*	1/3 Pizza/100g	245	7.3	245	11.1	32.2	7.3	2.9
Hawaiian, Stonebaked, Cucina, Aldi*	½ Pizza/165g	326	5.6	198	9.5	32	3.4	1.6
Hawaiian, Thin Crust, Tesco*	½ Pizza/192g	365	9.4	190	10.3	25.6	4.9	1.8
Hoisin Pork, The Best, Morrisons*	½ Pizza/211g	499	15.4	236	10.6	30.9	7.3	1.9
Jackfruit, BBQ, Aldi*	½ Pizza/180g	418	13.7	232	6.6	32	7.6	3.9
King Prawn, Garlic & Chilli, No.1, Waitrose*	¼ Pizza/124g	273	9.1	220	10.8	27	7.3	1.6
La Reine, Oven Cooked, Supermarket, Pizza Express*	½ Pack/130g	280	8.1	215	11.3	27.3	6.2	2.5
Margherita, Average	**1 Slice/108g**	**239**	**8.6**	**239**	**11**	**30.5**	**8.6**	**1.2**
Margherita, Classic, Supermarket, Pizza Express*	½ Pizza/127g	312	10.8	245	10	31.5	8.5	1.4
Margherita, GF, Free From, Sainsbury's*	½ Pizza/150g	430	18.6	287	8.5	33.3	12.4	3.9
Margherita, GF, Supermarket, Pizza Express*	½ Pizza/134g	341	13	254	9	31.3	9.7	2.6
Margherita, Sourdough, Pizzeria, Crosta & Mollica*	½ Pizza/201g	462	14.7	230	10	30	7.3	2.3
Margherita, Sourdough, Wood Fired, Plant Kitchen, M&S*	1/3 Pizza/115g	252	11.3	219	6	25.6	9.8	2
Margherita, Thin & Crispy, Stonebaked, Co-Op*	½ Pizza/147g	350	10.6	238	11	31	7.2	2.6
Margherita, Thin Crust, Takeaway, Goodfella's*	½ Pizza/206g	594	26.7	289	13	29	13	0
Margherita, Thin, Stonebaked, Goodfella's*	½ Pizza/170g	419	18.7	246	11	25	11	1.5
Margherita, Three Cheezly, Vegan, One Planet*	½ Pizza/214g	445	10.9	208	5.6	35.8	5.1	2.2
Margherita, Vegan, Plant Chef, Tesco*	¼ Pizza/65g	164	5.7	254	6	35.8	8.9	3.5
Margherita, with Pesto, Oven Baked, The Best, Morrisons*	½ Pizza/212g	531	17.6	251	10.3	32	8.3	3.3
Margherita, Wood Fired, Irresistible, Co-Op*	1 Slice/70g	181	7	258	9.9	30	10	3.4
Meat Feast, Deep & Loaded, Sainsbury's*	½ Pizza/298g	818	30	275	13.2	32.7	10.1	2.6
Meat Feast, Deep Pean, Sainsbury's*	½ Pizza/193g	492	16.8	255	11.9	31.2	8.7	2
Meat Feast, Mega, Asda*	½ Pizza/428g	1044	33.8	244	9.5	33.6	7.9	3.2
Meat Feast, Sourdough, Morrisons*	½ Pizza/177g	469	20.5	265	13.7	24.3	11.6	4.1
Meat Feast, Stone Baked Thin, Goodfella's*	1 Pizza/341g	897	34.1	263	13	29	10	2.6
Meat Feast, Stuffed Crust, Takeaway, Oven Baked, Asda*	½ Pizza/213g	561	20.9	263	14	29	9.8	1.6
Meat Feast, Thin & Crispy, Asda*	½ Pizza/183g	410	14.6	224	11	27	8	1.4
Meat Feast, Thin & Crispy, Stonebaked, Co-Op*	½ Pizza/167g	399	13	239	11	30	7.8	2.3
Meat Feast, Thin Crust, Tesco*	½ Pizza/178g	430	20.2	242	13.6	21.3	11.4	2.3
Meats, Italian, Finest, Tesco*	½ Pizza/217g	449	8.5	207	13.6	29.4	3.9	1.3
Meaty, Mega, Deep Dish, Chicago Town*	1 Pizza/157g	442	18.9	281	11	31	12	0
Mediterranean Vegetable, Flatbread, Kirsty's Kitchen*	1 Pizza/202g	436	16.2	216	2.8	32	8	2.1
Melt, Pepperoni, Nutrisystem*	1 Melt/108g	220	6	204	11.1	29.6	5.6	0
Mini, Party, Tesco*	1 Pizza/11g	26	1.1	248	11.4	28.6	10.5	1.9
Mozzarella, & Basil, Sourdough, Carlos, Aldi*	¼ Pizza/83g	218	7.8	261	12	31	9.3	2
Mozzarella, & Sunblush Tomato, 12", TTD, Sainsbury's*	½ Pizza/251g	638	17.8	254	12.4	35	7.1	2.6

PIZZA

	Measure INFO/WEIGHT	per Measure KCAL	FAT	KCAL	PROT	CARB	FAT	FIBRE
Mozzarella, Italian, & Basil, Ultra-Thin, Wood Fired, M&S*	1 Pack/173g	420	20.1	243	11.1	22.7	11.6	1.8
Mozzarella, Ristorante, Dr Oetker*	½ Pizza/184g	472	23.9	257	10	25	13	0
Mushroom, & Truffle, Sourdough, No.1, Waitrose*	¼ Pizza/120g	334	16.5	279	9.1	28.7	13.8	2
Mushroom, & Roasted Pepper, Allplants*	1 Pizza/353g	660	22.9	187	1.3	32.7	6.5	3.7
Mushroom, Garlic, Thin Crust, Tesco*	½ Pizza/163g	340	14.6	209	11	21.1	9	3.6
Mushroom, Vegan, Plant Chef, Tesco*	¼ Pizza/73g	180	6.5	246	5.6	34.7	8.9	2.5
New Yorker, Stuffed Crust, Iceland*	1/3 Pizza/176g	445	21.5	253	11	24	12.2	1.6
Oval, Thin & Crispy, Waitrose*	1 Oval/142g	358	10.1	252	12.9	33	7.1	2
Pancetta, Mushroom, & Mascarpone, Crosta & Mollica*	½ Pizza/223g	580	26.8	260	11	26	12	1.8
Pepperoni, Average	**1 Serving/250g**	**671**	**28.4**	**269**	**11.8**	**29.6**	**11.4**	**2.1**
Pepperoni, Deep & Crispy, Iceland*	1 Serving/175g	490	21	280	11.9	31.1	12	1.8
Pepperoni, Double, Deep Pan, Asda*	¼ Pizza/80g	223	8.8	280	12	32	11	2.1
Pepperoni, Double, Deep Pan, Chicago Town*	½ Pizza/199g	575	23.9	289	12	32	12	0
Pepperoni, Double, Iceland*	½ Pizza/154g	471	22.3	306	13	29.8	14.5	1.9
Pepperoni, Double, Stonebaked, Asda*	½ Pizza/151g	407	18.2	269	12	28	12	1.2
Pepperoni, Double, Stuffed Crust, Oven Baked, Iceland*	½ Pizza/216g	616	23.1	285	13.1	33.2	10.7	2
Pepperoni, Double, Thin & Crispy, Sainsbury's*	½ Pizza/174g	470	20	270	11.2	29.5	11.5	1.9
Pepperoni, Flatbread, Asda*	1 Pizza/237g	670	23.7	283	11	35	10	2.7
Pepperoni, GF, Kirsty's Kitchen*	½ Pizza/150g	317	12.3	211	4	29	8.2	2.8
Pepperoni, Hand Stretched, Stone Baked, Sainsbury's*	1 Pizza/298g	852	31.3	286	13	33.3	10.5	3
Pepperoni, Hot & Spicy, Stuffed Crust, Asda*	1 Pizza/245g	666	30	272	13.9	26.5	12.2	2.4
Pepperoni, Loaded, Tomato Stuffed Crust, Chicago Town*	¼ Pizza/150g	433	16.5	288	11	35	11	1.8
Pepperoni, Mini, Tesco*	1 Serving/22g	71	3.7	323	11.8	30.5	16.8	2.7
Pepperoni, Reg Crust, From Restaurant, Average	**1 Pizza/959g**	**2445**	**94**	**255**	**14.3**	**28**	**9.8**	**0**
Pepperoni, Salame, Ristorante, Dr Oetker*	½ Pizza/165g	465	23.2	281	10	28	14	0
Pepperoni, Snack, Co-Op*	1 Pizza/103g	296	10.3	287	12	35	10	2.6
Pepperoni, Spicy, Meat'zza, M&S*	½ Pizza/155g	431	34.3	278	12	6.7	22.1	1.9
Pepperoni, Stone Baked, Tesco*	½ Pizza/140g	399	17.5	285	12.7	29.1	12.5	2.8
Pepperoni, Stone Baked, Thin Crust, Asda*	1 Pizza/289g	754	34.7	261	12	26	12	1.8
Pepperoni, Stonebaked, Chef Select, Lidl*	¼ Pizza/85g	209	7.4	246	11.1	29.5	8.7	2.4
Pepperoni, Stonebaked, Pizzeria, Waitrose*	1/3 Pizza/121g	390	16.5	323	13.6	35.1	13.7	2.6
Pepperoni, Thin & Crispy, Sainsbury's*	½ Pizza/139g	393	18.3	282	12.5	27.6	13.1	1.8
Pepperoni, Thin & Crispy, Essential, Waitrose*	½ Pizza/133g	380	18	286	12.3	28.8	13.5	1
Pepperoni, Thin & Crispy, HFC, Tesco*	½ Pizza/148g	383	13.2	258	10.6	32.8	8.9	2.4
Pepperoni, Thin & Crispy, M&S*	½ Pizza/165g	459	20.5	278	12	28.9	12.4	1.4
Pepperoni, Thin, Stone Baked, Goodfella's*	½ Pizza/159g	432	19.1	271	13	27	12	2.2
Pesto Chicken, Stonebaked, The Best, Morrisons*	¼ Pizza/106g	245	6.8	231	10.4	31.6	6.4	2.8
Philly Cheese Steak, Co-Op*	½ Pizza/241g	599	21.7	249	11	30	9	2.5
Pocket, Margherita, Oven Cooked, Morrisons*	¼ Pack/48g	130	4.8	271	7.3	36.3	10.1	2.8
Pollo, ad Astra, Supermarket, Pizza Express*	½ Pizza/144g	315	8.7	218	11.3	28.9	6	1.8
Pollo, Primavera, Wood Fired, Ultra Thin, M&S*	1 Pizza/185g	414	15.9	224	10.4	25.3	8.6	1.9
Pollo, Ristorante, As Sold, Dr Oetker*	½ Pizza/183g	408	16.5	223	8.8	25.7	9	1.8
Pork, Pulled, BBQ, Fully Loaded, Takeaway, Sainsbury's*	½ Pizza/262g	691	26.7	264	10.5	31.4	10.2	2.2
Prawn, King, Garlic, Wood Fired, Finest, Tesco*	½ Pizza/222g	471	14.7	212	10.4	26.8	6.6	2.1
Prosciutto Cotto, Mushroom, & Mascarpone, Co-Op*	½ Pizza/227g	513	17	226	11	27	7.5	2.4
Prosciutto, Dr. Oetker (swe)*	1/3 Pizza/110g	251	10.9	228	9.9	24	9.9	1.7
Prosciutto, Gino D'acampo*	½ Pizza/207g	506	20.6	245	8.7	29	10	2
Quattro Formaggi, Ristorante, Dr Oetker*	½ Pizza/170g	457	23.8	269	10.8	24.1	14	1.6
Roasted Vegetable, & Houmous, Plant Based, Asda*	½ Pizza/188g	360	7.1	192	5.9	32	3.8	4.1
Salami, & Ham, Pizzeria, Waitrose*	½ Pizza/205g	443	13.7	216	10.1	28.7	6.7	1.8
Salami, & Pepperoni, Waitrose*	½ Pizza/190g	578	30.8	304	13.4	23.9	16.2	2.1
Salami, Mozzarella, Pesto, Dr. Oetker (swe)*	1 Pizza/360g	914	50.4	254	9	23	14	1.7
Salami, Napoli Diavolo, Pizza, Wood Fired, M&S*	½ Pizza/244g	549	24.9	225	10.8	21.7	10.2	1.7

	Measure INFO/WEIGHT	KCAL	FAT	Nutrition Values per 100g / 100ml KCAL	PROT	CARB	FAT	FIBRE
PIZZA								
Salami, Ultra Thin Italian, Tesco*	1 Serving/263g	692	25.5	263	12	31.9	9.7	1
Salami, Ventricina, Truly Irresistible, Co-Op*	½ Pizza/230g	577	19.6	251	8.5	34	8.5	2.6
Selection, Slices, M&S*	1 Serving/52g	120	4.1	230	9.4	30.3	7.8	1.9
Sloppy Giuseppe, Supermarket, Pizza Express*	½ Pizza/151g	333	10.9	220	10	28.1	7.2	1.6
Spicy Chicken, Thin & Crispy, Sainsbury's*	1/3 Pizza/128g	276	6.9	216	10.9	30	5.4	2
Spicy Salami, & Red Chill, Finest, Tesco*	½ Pizza/187g	484	18.5	259	12.4	31.7	9.9	1.4
Spinach & Ricotta, Carlos, Aldi*	½ Pizza/170g	362	14.4	213	9.1	24	8.5	2.6
Spinach, & Ricotta, Thin Crust, Italian, Tesco*	½ Pizza/190g	365	16.7	192	9.6	18.7	8.8	1.9
Spinach, & Mushrooms, Vegan, Vemondo, Lidl*	1 Pizza/390g	573	10.5	147	4.9	24.4	2.7	0
Spinach, & Ricotta, Chef Select, Lidl*	½ Pizza/160g	339	10.6	212	9.8	26.6	6.6	3.7
Spinach, & Ricotta, Irresistible, Co-Op*	¼ Pizza/105g	270	11.5	258	9.5	30	11	2.2
Spinach, & Ricotta, Stonebaked, M&S*	½ Pizza/253g	543	17.4	215	8	29.2	6.9	2.1
Sub, Cheese & Tomato, Ovenbaked, Asda*	1 Baguette/122g	277	8.3	227	11	29	6.8	2.7
Sub, Pepperoni Pizza, Ovenbaked, Asda*	1 Baguette/122g	272	9.3	223	11	26	7.6	3.1
The Big Cheese, The Pizza Company*	1 Serving/142g	374	15.3	264	11.7	28.8	10.8	2.4
The Pepperoni Party, The Pizza Company*	¼ Pizza/143g	396	18	277	11.6	28.1	12.6	2.2
The Whole Hog, Deep & Loaded, M&S*	½ Pizza/345g	823	33.4	239	12.3	24.9	9.7	1.5
Tomato, Mozzarella, & Pesto, Momenti, Dr Oetker*	1 Pizza/182g	422	14.9	232	8.5	30	8.2	2.3
Triple Meat, Party Pizza, Tostino's*	½ Pizza/149g	340	17	228	6.7	24.8	11.4	1.3
Truffle, Salsiccia, Truly Irresistible, Co-Op*	½ Pack/97g	296	12.6	305	13	33	13	1.2
Vegan, Alfredo, Lidl*	1 Pizza/390g	573	10.5	147	4.9	24.3	2.7	0
Vegan, Hacendado*	1 Pizza/400g	724	21.2	181	6.4	26	5.3	2.5
Vegan, No Cheese, Houmous Style Sauce, Iceland*	½ Pizza/140g	346	18.2	247	6.1	24	13	4.7
Vegetable, & Peppers, Fire Roasted, Waitrose*	½ Pizza/235g	442	16.7	188	9.8	21.3	7.1	2.7
Vegetable, & Pesto, Chargrilled, Specially Selected, Aldi*	½ Pizza/305g	756	29	248	9.2	30	9.5	2.9
Vegetable, Average	**1 Avg Slice/70g**	**133**	**3.7**	**190**	**8.2**	**27.5**	**5.2**	**2.4**
Vegetable, Deep Pan, Co-Op*	1 Pizza/425g	829	29.8	195	8	25	7	2
Vegetable, Extra Thin, Morrisons*	1 Serving/176g	385	17.1	219	8.3	22.9	9.7	3.4
Vegetable, Frozen, HL, Tesco*	1 Pizza/400g	604	10.8	151	8.1	23.5	2.7	4.4
Vegetable, GFY, Asda*	¼ Pizza/94g	141	2.7	150	7	24	2.9	3.7
Vegetable, Mediterranean, Stonebaked, Carlos, Aldi*	½ Pizza/173g	323	8.7	187	7.5	26.6	5	2.9
Vegetable, Mediterranean, Thin & Crispy, Tesco*	½ Pizza/179g	350	10.7	195	7.1	27.3	6	2.1
Vegetable, Romano, Goodfella's*	½ Pizza/195g	419	15	215	9	26	7.7	0
Vegetable, Salsa, Spicy, Stonebaked, Vegan, Goodfella's*	½ Pizza/181g	385	11.4	213	5.8	32	6.3	2.9
Vegetable, Thin & Crispy, Iceland*	½ Pizza/150g	345	11	230	9.8	29.9	7.3	2.9
Vegetable, Thin & Crispy, Sainsbury's*	½ Pizza/193g	419	13.3	217	8	29.7	6.9	2
Veggie Feast, Thin Crust, Stonebaked, Asda*	½ Pizza/168g	360	13.6	214	7.9	26	8.1	3.1
Veggie, Very, Stonebaked, M&S*	½ Pizza/274g	537	15.9	196	7.9	27	5.8	2.1
PIZZA BASE								
Deep Pan, Italian, Sainsbury's*	1 Base/220g	684	11	311	7	59.5	5	1.4
Deep Pan, Napolina*	1 Base/260g	757	7.8	291	7.9	58	3	0.2
Dough, Ready Rolled, Tesco*	1 Base/400g	1248	22.4	312	10	54	5.6	2.9
GF, Schar*	1 Pizza/150g	436	5.2	291	3	60	3.5	4.7
Italian, Classic, Sainsbury's*	1 Base/150g	452	7.2	301	7.6	57	4.8	1.5
Light & Crispy, Napolina*	1 Base/150g	436	4.5	291	7.9	58	3	0.2
Low Carb, Thin & Crispy, Lizza*	1 Base/100g	233	11	233	22	2.4	11	19
M&S*	1 Base/150g	418	8.1	279	9.2	47.5	5.4	1.9
Mini, Napolina*	1 Base/75g	218	2.2	291	7.9	58	3	0.2
Original, Dough, Frozen, Northern Dough Co. *	1 Base/220g	451	2.9	205	7.1	39.4	1.3	3.4
Thin & Crispy, Sainsbury's*	1 Base/150g	504	7.8	336	9.9	62.3	5.2	4.3
Wholemeal, Multiseed, Dough It Yourself*	1 Base/200g	544	9.4	272	12.4	49.1	4.7	0
PLAICE								
Fillets, in Breadcrumbs, Average	**1 Serving/150g**	**331**	**17.9**	**221**	**12.8**	**15.5**	**11.9**	**0.8**

	Measure INFO/WEIGHT	per Measure KCAL	FAT	Nutrition Values per 100g / 100ml KCAL	PROT	CARB	FAT	FIBRE
PLAICE								
Fillets, Lightly Dusted, Average	**1 Fillet/113g**	**188**	**9.2**	**166**	**12.9**	**10.4**	**8.2**	**0.6**
Fillets, Raw, Average	**1oz/28g**	**24**	**0.4**	**87**	**18.2**	**0**	**1.5**	**0**
Goujons, Baked	**1oz/28g**	**85**	**5.1**	**304**	**8.8**	**27.7**	**18.3**	**0**
Goujons, Fried in Blended Oil	**1oz/28g**	**119**	**9**	**426**	**8.5**	**27**	**32.3**	**0**
Grilled	**1oz/28g**	**27**	**0.5**	**96**	**20.1**	**0**	**1.7**	**0**
in Batter, Fried in Blended Oil	**1oz/28g**	**72**	**4.7**	**257**	**15.2**	**12**	**16.8**	**0.5**
Steamed	**1oz/28g**	**26**	**0.5**	**93**	**18.9**	**0**	**1.9**	**0**
PLANTAIN								
Boiled in Unsalted Water	**1oz/28g**	**31**	**0.1**	**112**	**0.8**	**28.5**	**0.2**	**1.2**
Raw, Average	**1 Med/179g**	**218**	**0.7**	**122**	**1.3**	**31.9**	**0.4**	**2.3**
Ripe, Fried in Vegetable Oil	**1oz/28g**	**75**	**2.6**	**267**	**1.5**	**47.5**	**9.2**	**2.3**
PLUMS								
Average, Stewed without Sugar	**1oz/28g**	**8**	**0**	**30**	**0.5**	**7.3**	**0.1**	**1.3**
Dried, in Port, Chocolate Covered, Hotel Chocolat*	2 Plums/20g	80	6.4	401	4.5	40	32	9.8
Fresh, Raw, Weighed without Stone, Average	**1 Plum/66g**	**24**	**0.1**	**36**	**0.6**	**8.6**	**0.1**	**1.9**
Weighed with Stone, Average	**1 Plum/90g**	**31**	**0.1**	**34**	**0.5**	**8.1**	**0.1**	**1.8**
Yellow, Waitrose*	1 Plum/50g	20	0	39	0.6	8.8	0.1	1.5
POLLOCK								
Alaskan, Morrisons*	1 Pack/450g	558	5.4	124	28.2	0	1.2	0
Fillet, Breaded, Skinless & Boneless, Savers, Morrisons*	1 Fillet/142g	311	11.5	219	13.1	22.9	8.1	1
Fillets, Breaded, HFC, Tesco*	1 Fillet/128g	269	8.2	210	14.6	22.4	6.4	2.1
White Fish, Fillets, Basics, Sainsbury's*	1 Fillet/74g	62	0.4	84	20.4	0	0.5	0
POLO								
Fruits, Nestle*	1 Tube/37g	142	0	383	0	96	0	0
Mints, Original, Nestle*	1 Sweet/2g	8	0	402	0	98.2	1	0
Spearmint, Nestle*	1 Tube/35g	141	0.4	402	0	98.2	1.1	0
POMEGRANATE								
Raw, Fresh, Flesh Only, Average	**1 Sm Fruit/86g**	**59**	**0.3**	**68**	**1**	**17.2**	**0.3**	**0.6**
Raw, Weighed with Rind & Skin, Average	**1 Sm Fruit/154g**	**59**	**0.3**	**38**	**0.5**	**9.6**	**0.2**	**0**
POMELO								
Fresh, Raw, Weighed with Skin & Seeds	**100 Grams/100g**	**11**	**0.1**	**11**	**0.2**	**2.5**	**0.1**	**0**
Raw, Flesh Only, Average	**1 Fruit/340g**	**129**	**0.1**	**38**	**0.8**	**9.6**	**0**	**1**
POP TARTS								
Chocolate, Kellogg's*	1 Pop Tart/50g	198	8.5	396	5	136	17	2
Cookies 'n' Creme, Kellogg's*	1 Pop Tart/50g	190	5	380	4	70	10	2
Frosted Blueberry, Mini Crisps, Kellogg's*	1 Pop Tart/23g	100	2.5	435	4.4	78.3	10.9	0
Frosted Brown Sugar Cinnamon, Kellogg's*	1 Pop Tart/50g	210	7	420	6	68	14	2
Frosted Chocolate Fudge, Kellogg's*	1 Pop Tart/52g	200	5	385	5.8	71.2	9.6	1.9
Frosted Hot Fudge Sundae, Kellogg's*	1 Pop Tart/48g	190	4.5	396	4.2	70.8	9.4	2.1
Frosted Raspberry, Kellogg's*	1 Pop Tart/52g	200	5	385	3.8	73.1	9.6	1.9
Strawberry Sensation, Kellogg's*	1 Pop Tart/50g	198	5.5	395	4	70	11	2
POPCORN								
Air Popped, Plain, Average	**1 Sm Bag/17g**	**66**	**0.8**	**387**	**12.9**	**77.9**	**4.5**	**14.5**
Butter, Microwave, Act II*	1 Bag/90g	425	16.2	472	9	69	18	9
Butter, Microwave, Butterkist*	1 Bag/70g	305	12.7	436	8.5	55.2	18.1	9.6
Butter, Microwave, Popz*	1 Serving/100g	480	27.5	480	7.5	51.1	27.5	9.2
Butter, Toffee, Belgian Milk Chocolate Coated, M&S*	1 Pack/100g	505	25	505	6.5	60.4	25	4.1
Butterfly, Sweet & Salty, Sainsbury's*	1 Pack/14g	68	3.5	487	8.4	52	24.7	11.6
Caramel Crunch, The Gourmet Popcorn Co. *	1 Serving/25g	105	2	421	2.5	84.4	8.2	0
Caramel, & Espresso, The British Popcorn Co.*	½ Pack/15g	72	3.7	483	5.7	56	24.7	7
Caramel, Salted, Butterkist*	1 Serving/20g	83	1.9	417	3.4	77.7	9.5	3.5
Chocolate, & Pecan, M&S*	1 Pack/27g	130	5.2	480	3.3	72.9	19.3	3.6
Coconut, & Vanilla, The Foodie Market, Aldi*	1 Serving/27g	130	6.2	483	9.2	57	23	8.2

POPCORN

INFO/WEIGHT	Measure	per Measure KCAL	FAT	Nutrition Values per 100g / 100ml KCAL	PROT	CARB	FAT	FIBRE
Cookie, Tesco*	1 Serving/25g	113	3.3	452	3.3	79	13.2	1.8
Corn Triangles, Popped, Sweet & Salty, M&S*	1/3 Pack/23g	98	2.3	427	6.4	76.3	10	3.1
Cotton Candy, American Style, Epic*	1 Pot/150g	766	41.7	511	6.1	59.7	27.8	7
Maple, Shapers, Boots*	1 Bag/20g	94	3.6	469	12	59	18	10
Original, Cracker Jack*	1 Pack/35g	148	3	424	5.6	81.9	8.5	5.6
Peanut Butter, & Almond, Propercorn*	1 Serving/25g	115	5	460	12.9	50.2	20.2	12.9
Peanut Butter, The Foodie Market, Aldi*	1 Pack/27g	133	6.5	493	12	53	24	8.3
Peanut, & Almond, Smooth, Propercorn*	1 Serving/25g	115	5	460	12.9	50.2	20.2	12.9
Plain, Oil Popped, Average	**1 Bag/74g**	**439**	**31.7**	**593**	**6.2**	**48.7**	**42.8**	**0**
Popping Corn, Average	**1 Serving/30g**	**112**	**1.3**	**375**	**10.9**	**73.1**	**4.3**	**12.7**
Salt & Vinegar, Snack-A-Jacks, Quaker*	1 Sm Pack/13g	47	1.3	360	12	55	9.9	14
Salted Caramel, Propercorn*	1 Serving/20g	97	4.6	484	4.7	61.8	22.9	5.9
Salted, Blockbuster*	1 Bowl/25g	99	2.9	397	10.6	62.2	11.7	8.6
Salted, Cineworld, Munchbox*	1 Serving/55g	235	9.1	427	9.6	52.7	16.6	14.4
Salted, Crunch Corn, Propercorn*	1 Serving/30g	140	7.9	468	5	52.1	26.4	12.2
Salted, Diet Chef Ltd*	1 Pack/23g	107	3.8	465	10.5	66.6	16.6	14
Salted, Light, Microwave, Act II*	1 Pack/85g	336	6.5	395	10.6	71	7.6	15.8
Salted, Lightly, Popping Corn, Graze*	1 Punnet/28g	127	7	454	8	44	25	13
Salted, Lightly, Sea, Propercorn*	1 Bag/10g	44	1.7	436	8.6	56.7	16.9	11
Salted, Lightly, The Foodie Market, Aldi*	1 Pack/27g	127	5.7	471	11	56	21	7.6
Salted, Microwave, Popz*	1 Serving/20g	101	6	504	7	51.5	30	9.2
Salted, Microwave, Propercorn*	1 Pack/20g	84	3.8	418	8.5	47.4	19.1	11.4
Salted, Microwave, Snaktastic, Lidl*	1 Pack/100g	483	23	483	10.7	53	23	10.8
Salted, Microwave, Sunsnacks*	1 Pack/100g	498	22.9	498	10.7	51.3	22.9	10.8
Salted, Spar*	1 Serving/20g	97	4.9	483	8.5	50.8	24.5	12.8
Salted, Variety Pack, Tesco*	1 Bag/11g	57	3.4	522	7.6	48.3	31.3	8.5
Salted, Variety, Asda*	1 Bag/11g	54	2.8	489	8.3	52	25	510
San Carlo*	1 Serving/20g	97	5	485	9.5	50	25	11
Sea Salt, Metcalfe's Food Co*	1 Sm Pack/17g	82	4	480	9.7	47.2	23.4	11.7
Smart Food*	1 Serving/50g	290	18.2	579	12.9	49.4	36.5	8.6
Sour Cream & Black Pepper, Propercorn*	1 Bag/20g	88	3.7	440	10.8	50.1	18.3	15.9
Sweet & Salty, Microwave, Butterkist*	1 Pack/70g	298	14.1	425	8.2	48.5	20.2	8.4
Sweet & Salt, Metcalfe's Food Co*	1 Bag/17g	82	4.1	481	8.1	53.4	23.8	10.3
Sweet & Salted, Co-Op*	1 Bag/25g	111	4	443	6.4	62	16	11
Sweet & Salted, Mackie's*	1 Bag/100g	486	25.3	486	4.4	52	25.3	16.7
Sweet & Salted, Maize & Grain*	1 Serving/18g	89	4.4	495	7.6	59.1	24.6	3.5
Sweet & Salted, Snackrite, Aldi*	1 Serving/30g	141	6	471	7.1	62	20	7.5
Sweet & Salty, Bloom's*	1 Portion/28g	138	7	492	4	58.6	25	8.5
Sweet & Salty, Corn, Proper*	1 Pack/14g	63	2.5	451	5.4	63.2	18	10.8
Sweet & Salty, M&S*	1 Bag/15g	73	3.7	488	7.7	55.4	24.4	7.8
Sweet & Salty, Propercorn*	1 Bag/14g	63	2.5	451	5.4	63.2	18	10.8
Sweet & Salty, Tesco*	1/4 Bag/27g	132	6.3	488	6.3	60	23.4	6.1
Sweet 'n' Salted, Big Night In*	1 Serving/50g	232	9.2	464	5	65	18.3	9.7
Sweet, & Salted, Snaktastic, Lidl*	1 Serving/25g	122	5.8	486	7.7	59	23	6.3
Sweet, & Salted, The Foodie Market, Aldi*	1 Bag/27g	120	4.2	444	9.3	63	15.6	7.4
Sweet, Asda*	1 Bag/13g	63	2.9	483	5.3	62	22	7.7
Sweet, Butterkist, Butterkist*	1 Pack/120g	612	29.8	510	2.8	68.5	24.8	5.6
Sweet, Cinema Style, Basics, Sainsbury's*	1 Handful/20g	90	4.4	450	5.9	57.5	21.8	11.1
Sweet, Cinema Style, Butterkist*	1 Bag/85g	447	22	526	5.2	65.2	25.9	5.8
Sweet, Coconut & Vanilla, Propercorn*	1 Bag/25g	122	5.5	486	6	61.6	22.1	7.7
Sweet, Deli, Passions, Aldi*	1 Bag/27g	121	4.2	448	7	74.8	15.6	10.7
Sweet, Microwave, Butterkist*	1 Pack/70g	316	15.4	452	7	53	22	7.2
Sweet, Propercorn*	1 Pack/20g	93	3.7	464	5.8	65.5	18.5	6.3

	Measure INFO/WEIGHT	per Measure KCAL	FAT	Nutrition Values per 100g / 100ml KCAL	PROT	CARB	FAT	FIBRE
POPCORN								
Toffee, Butterkist*	1 Sm Bag/50g	212	4.7	424	3.1	80.1	9.4	3.2
Toffee, Sainsbury's*	1 Serving/50g	208	6.4	415	1.8	73.8	12.7	3.3
Toffee, Snack Pack, Butterkist*	1 Bag/25g	106	2.4	424	3.1	80.1	9.4	3.2
Toffee, Snaktastic, Lidl*	1 Serving/25g	106	2.1	424	2.4	82.8	8.4	2.8
POPPADOMS								
Balti, Mini, Vitasia, Lidl*	½ Bag/30g	153	9.5	510	18.4	34.3	31.6	7.4
Chilli, Cumin, Sharwoods*	1 Poppadom/9g	37	2	432	15.9	35.5	23.4	7.9
Fried in Vegetable Oil, Takeaway, Average	*1 Poppadom/13g*	*65*	*5*	*501*	*11.5*	*28.3*	*38.8*	*5.8*
Garlic & Coriander, Ready to Eat, Sharwood's*	1 Poppadom/9g	39	1.9	438	18.4	43	21.4	6.5
Mango Chutney Flavour, Mini, M&S*	1 Poppadom/25g	130	8.3	518	13.1	39.9	33	4.5
Plain, Ready to Eat, Average	*2 Poppadom/16g*	*68*	*2.8*	*427*	*19.8*	*46.6*	*17.3*	*6.6*
Spicy, Cook to Eat, Sharwood's*	1 Poppadom/12g	30	0.1	257	20.2	43	0.5	13
Spicy, COU, M&S*	1 Pack/26g	84	0.6	325	23.5	51.9	2.4	8.1
POPPETS*								
Chocolate Raisins, Poppets*	1 Pack/35g	140	4.7	401	4.9	65.4	13.3	0
Orangy, Milk Choc, Poppets*	1 Pouch/130g	585	17.2	450	2	79	13.2	0.6
Toffee, Milk Chocolate, Poppets*	1 Box/100g	491	23	491	5.3	68	23	0
PORK								
& Stuffing, Sliced, Asda*	1 Slice/53g	79	2.7	148	23	2.2	5.1	0.7
Belly, Fresh, Raw, Weighed with Skin, Average	*1 Serving/100g*	*518*	*53*	*518*	*9.3*	*0*	*53*	*0*
Belly, Roasted, Lean & Fat	*1oz/28g*	*82*	*6*	*293*	*25.1*	*0*	*21.4*	*0*
Belly, Slices, Woodside Farms, Tesco*	1 Slice/125g	382	33.5	306	15.9	0.1	26.8	0.3
Diced, Lean, Average	*1oz/28g*	*31*	*0.5*	*109*	*22*	*0*	*1.8*	*0*
Escalope, Average	*1 Escalope/75g*	*108*	*1.7*	*144*	*31*	*0*	*2.2*	*0*
Escalope, Lean, Healthy Range, Average	*1 Escalope/75g*	*80*	*1.5*	*106*	*22*	*0*	*2*	*0*
Gyros, Eridanous, Lidl*	1 Serving/125g	185	8.8	148	19	2	7	0
Ham, Hock, Raw, Weighed with Bone, Fat & Skin	*100g*	*124*	*5*	*124*	*18.4*	*0*	*5*	*0*
Joint with Crackling, Ready to Roast, Average	*1 Joint/567g*	*1283*	*80.1*	*226*	*24.2*	*0.8*	*14.1*	*0*
Joint, Ready to Roast, Average	*½ Joint/254g*	*375*	*18*	*148*	*19.2*	*2.3*	*7.1*	*0.2*
Kebabs, Maple BBQ, Sticky, Co-Op*	1 Kebab/100g	174	9.5	174	17	4.5	9.5	0.7
Leg, Joint, Healthy Range, Average	*1 Serving/200g*	*206*	*4.4*	*103*	*20*	*0.6*	*2.2*	*0*
Loin, Applewood Smoked, Asda*	1 Slice/15g	18	0.5	122	21.8	0.5	3.6	0
Loin, Chop, Raw, Lean & Fat, Boneless	*1 Avg Chop/185g*	*287*	*12.8*	*155*	*21.6*	*0*	*6.9*	*0*
Loin, Chop, Raw, Lean Only, Boneless	*1 Avg Chop/155g*	*197*	*5.3*	*127*	*22.4*	*0*	*3.4*	*0*
Loin, Chops, Boneless, Grilled, Average	*1oz/28g*	*83*	*4.1*	*298*	*27*	*0*	*14.6*	*0*
Loin, Chops, Grilled, Lean	*1oz/28g*	*52*	*1.8*	*184*	*31.6*	*0*	*6.4*	*0*
Loin, Chops, Raw, Lean & Fat, Weighed with Bone	*1 Chop/130g*	*248*	*19.9*	*191*	*13.2*	*0*	*15.3*	*0*
Loin, Joint, Roast, Lean	*1oz/28g*	*51*	*1.9*	*182*	*30.1*	*0*	*6.8*	*0*
Loin, Joint, Roasted, Lean & Fat	*1oz/28g*	*71*	*4.3*	*253*	*26.3*	*0*	*15.3*	*0*
Loin, Roast, Slices, The Deli, Aldi*	1 Slice/20g	25	0.8	126	21	2.1	3.9	0.5
Loin, Roasted, Prime Cut, Slices, Tesco*	1 Slice/21g	26	0.7	123	23	0.2	3.2	0.5
Loin, Steak, Cajun, Smoky, Cooked, Tesco*	½ Pack/151g	340	22.8	225	19.1	2.7	15.1	1.1
Loin, Steak, Fried, Lean	*1oz/28g*	*53*	*2*	*191*	*31.5*	*0*	*7.2*	*0*
Loin, Steak, Fried, Lean & Fat	*1oz/28g*	*77*	*5.2*	*276*	*27.5*	*0*	*18.4*	*0*
Loin, Steak, Grilled, Sainsbury's*	1 Steak/68g	169	10.6	248	26.2	0.7	15.5	0.8
Loin, Steak, Hoisin, Grilled, Iceland*	1 Steak/61g	160	8.3	263	28.6	6.2	13.6	0.5
Loin, Steak, Lean, Raw, Average	*1 Serving/175g*	*345*	*19.6*	*197*	*22.7*	*0*	*11.2*	*0.4*
Loin, Steak, Pepper Crusted, M&S*	½ Pack/150g	189	6	126	22.5	1	4	1
Loin, Steaks, Maple BBQ, Fire Pit, Tesco*	1 Steak/76g	210	13.3	277	23.4	5	17.6	2
Loin, Steaks, Memphis BBQ, Ashfield Farm, Aldi*	½ Pack/220g	598	35.2	272	28	4.5	16	0.5
Loin, with Rind, Uncooked, Average	*1 Serving/100g*	*246*	*18.8*	*246*	*19.3*	*0*	*18.8*	*0*
Medallions, Average	*1 Medallion/125g*	*140*	*2.6*	*112*	*22.6*	*0*	*2*	*0*
Mince, Lean, Healthy Range, Average	*1 Pack/400g*	*504*	*20.2*	*126*	*19.8*	*0.4*	*5*	*0.3*

	Measure INFO/WEIGHT	per Measure KCAL	FAT	Nutrition Values per 100g / 100ml KCAL	PROT	CARB	FAT	FIBRE
PORK								
Mince, Raw	**1oz/28g**	**46**	**2.7**	**164**	**19.2**	**0**	**9.7**	**0**
Mince, Stewed	**1oz/28g**	**53**	**2.9**	**191**	**24.4**	**0**	**10.4**	**0**
N'Duja, Average	**1 Serving/40g**	**208**	**20**	**515**	**10**	**6.2**	**49.4**	**0.5**
Patties, Breakfast, Frozen, Oakhurst, Aldi*	1 Pattie/45g	132	9.4	293	25	1.6	21	0.5
Pulled, BBQ, British, The Jolly Hog*	½ Pack/196g	350	14.7	178	16.2	11.2	7.5	0.5
Pulled, BBQ, Iceland*	½ Pack/195g	372	17.9	191	20.7	6.3	9.2	0.5
Pulled, Birchwood, Lidl*	½ Pack/128g	196	6.1	153	17.7	9.5	4.8	0
Pulled, Slow Cooked, M&S*	½ Pack/85g	143	4.8	168	17.6	11.5	5.7	0.2
Pulled, Vegetarian, Linda McCartney*	1 Pack/300g	567	25.8	189	19.5	6.2	8.6	0
Raw, Lean, Average	**1oz/28g**	**42**	**1.2**	**151**	**28.6**	**0**	**4.1**	**0**
Rissole, Low Fat, Oh So Lean*	1 Rissole/50g	89	1.2	178	16.6	10.4	2.3	0
Roast, Lean Only, Average	**1oz/28g**	**34**	**0.9**	**121**	**22.7**	**0.3**	**3.3**	**0**
Roast, Slices, Average	**1 Slice/30g**	**40**	**1.4**	**134**	**22.7**	**0.4**	**4.5**	**0**
Saltimbocca, Cook with, M&S*	½ Pack/143g	207	9.6	145	19.6	1.5	6.7	0.1
Saucisson Sec, Slices, Tesco*	3 Slices/15g	53	4.1	355	26	0.6	27.4	1.1
Shoulder, Boneless, Average	**1 Piece/430g**	**127**	**3.4**	**127**	**22.5**	**0**	**3.4**	**0**
Shoulder, Whole, Lean & Fat, Raw, Average	**100g**	**236**	**18**	**236**	**17.2**	**0**	**18**	**0**
Shoulder, Whole, Lean Only, Roasted	**1 Serving/150g**	**345**	**20.3**	**230**	**25.3**	**0**	**13.5**	**0**
Steak, Lean & Fat, Average	**1oz/28g**	**61**	**3.8**	**219**	**23.8**	**0**	**13.7**	**0.1**
Steak, Lean, Stewed	**1oz/28g**	**49**	**1.3**	**176**	**34.6**	**0**	**4.6**	**0**
Stir Fry Strips, Lean, Healthy Range, Average	**¼ Pack/113g**	**118**	**2.3**	**104**	**21.3**	**0**	**2**	**0**
Tenderloin, Lean, Boneless, Raw, Average	**1 Serving/100g**	**109**	**2.2**	**109**	**21**	**0**	**2.2**	**0**
PORK CRACKLING								
BBQ, Low & Sow, The Snaffling Pig Co.*	1 Bag/14g	87	6.6	621	43.9	0.5	47.5	0
Teasingly Hot Chilli, Mr Tubs*	1 Pot/55g	386	34.6	701	33	1	62.9	0
PORK DINNER								
Roast, 1303, Oakhouse Foods Ltd*	1 Serving/400g	412	15.2	103	7.3	8.9	3.8	2.1
Roast, Birds Eye*	1 Pack/340g	410	12	121	7.6	14.7	3.5	1.6
Roast, Luxury, 1310, Oakhouse Foods*	1 Pack/500g	545	23.5	109	7.4	8.2	4.7	1.3
Roast, Mini, 1003, Oakhouse Foods*	1 Pack/240g	223	8.9	93	7	7	3.7	1.5
PORK IN								
Gravy, Baby Potatoes, Carrots, & Savoy Cabbage, M&S*	1 Pack395g	288	9.9	73	6.2	5.7	2.5	1.6
Mustard & Cream, Chops	**1oz/28g**	**73**	**6**	**261**	**14.5**	**2.4**	**21.6**	**0.3**
PORK SCRATCHINGS								
Crispy Strips, Mr Porky*	1 Bag/20g	102	5.7	508	62.4	0.6	28.4	0
Crunch, Lightly Seasoned, Openshaws*	1 Bag/30g	147	7.3	491	64.3	3.4	24.2	0
Crunch, Mr Porky*	1 Pack/25g	129	6.9	515	65.7	0.6	27.7	0
Crunch, Traditional Black Country*	1 Bag/25g	138	8.9	554	57.8	0.4	35.7	0
Hand Cooked, Mr Porky*	½ Pack/33g	212	17.1	653	44.3	0.4	52.7	0
KP Snacks*	1 Pack/20g	125	9.6	624	47.3	0.5	48.1	0.5
Original, Mr Porky*	1 Pack/17g	107	8.7	646	42.5	0.4	52.7	0
Pn, Proteinium*	1 Bag/30g	156	7.9	520	69.7	0.1	26.2	0
Puffs, Original Salted, The Curators*	1 Serving/22g	118	6.1	536	71.1	0.1	27.8	0.7
Puffs, Sea Salt & Cider Vinegar, The Curators*	1 Bag/22g	109	5.5	494	66.9	1	25.2	0.5
Puffs, Smoky Bacon, The Curators*	1 Bag/22g	106	4.6	484	73.6	2	21.1	0.5
Puffs, Spicy BBQ, The Curators*	1 Pack/25g	128	7.1	513	60.3	10	28.4	1
PORT								
Average	**1 Serving/50ml**	**78**	**0**	**157**	**0.1**	**12**	**0**	**0**
White, Average	**1 Glass/125ml**	**182**	**0**	**146**	**0.1**	**11**	**0**	**0**
POT NOODLE*								
Beef & Tomato, King, Made Up, Pot Noodle*	1 Pot/420g	543	19.8	129	3.3	18.5	4.7	1.1
Beef & Tomato, Made Up, Pot Noodle*	1 Pot/320g	426	14.7	133	3.4	19.4	4.6	1.3
Bombay Bad Boy, King, Made Up , Pot Noodle*	1 Pot/420g	542	19.7	129	3.3	18.5	4.7	1.1

P

	Measure INFO/WEIGHT	per Measure KCAL	FAT	Nutrition Values per 100g / 100ml KCAL	PROT	CARB	FAT	FIBRE

POT NOODLE*

	Measure INFO/WEIGHT	KCAL	FAT	KCAL	PROT	CARB	FAT	FIBRE
Bombay Bad Boy, Made Up, Pot Noodle*	1 Pot/320g	415	15.3	130	3.3	18.4	4.8	1.1
Chicken & Mushroom, King, Made Up, Pot Noodle*	1 Pot/420g	545	19.3	130	3.3	18.8	4.6	1
Chicken & Mushroom, Made Up, Pot Noodle*	1 Pot/305g	430	18	141	3	19	5.9	1
Chilli Beef, Made Up, Pot Noodle*	1 Pot/305g	384	14.6	126	3	17.7	4.8	0.8
Chow Mein Chinese, Made Up, Pot Noodle*	1 Pot/320g	416	14.7	130	3.2	19	4.6	1.3
Curry, Original, King, Made Up, Pot Noodle*	1 Pot/420g	507	18.1	121	2.6	17.9	4.3	1
Curry, Original, Made Up, Pot Noodle*	1 Pot/320g	431	15	135	3.1	20	4.7	1.2
Curry, Spicy, Made Up, Pot Noodle*	1 Pot/300g	393	14.4	131	2.9	19.1	4.8	1.1
Jerk Chicken Flavour, Made Up, Pot Noodle*	1 Pot/303g	433	17.9	143	3.2	18	5.9	1
Piri Piri Chicken, Made Up, Pot Noodle*	1 Pot/307g	430	15.4	140	3	20	5	0
Sweet & Sour, Made Up, Pot Noodle*	1 Pot/305g	436	17.1	143	2.6	20	5.6	1.2

POTATO BOMBAY

	Measure INFO/WEIGHT	KCAL	FAT	KCAL	PROT	CARB	FAT	FIBRE
Average	½ Pack/150g	176	10.2	117	2	13.7	6.8	1.2

POTATO CAKES

	Measure INFO/WEIGHT	KCAL	FAT	KCAL	PROT	CARB	FAT	FIBRE
Average	1 Cake/70g	127	1.2	180	3.8	37.5	1.7	2.4
Bubble & Squeak, Dragonfly*	1 Cake/100g	145	2.6	145	1.8	28.5	2.6	1.2
Bubble & Squeak, Rosti, Morrisons*	1 Rosti Cake/78g	136	6.2	175	1	23.5	8	2.8
Fried, Average	1oz/28g	66	2.5	237	4.9	35	9	0.8
Grilled, Asda*	1 Cake/45g	90	0.9	200	4.2	40	1.9	2.9

POTATO SALAD

	Measure INFO/WEIGHT	KCAL	FAT	KCAL	PROT	CARB	FAT	FIBRE
& Egg, with Mayonnaise, Tesco*	½ Tub/150g	115	8.5	77	2.9	3.1	5.7	1.2
& Yoghurt, Meadow Fresh, Lidl*	1 Portion/50g	72	4	144	1.8	15.4	8	1.8
Charlotte, Extra Special, Asda*	1/3 Pack/92g	119	7.9	130	1.3	11	8.6	2.3
Charlotte, TTD, Sainsbury's*	½ Pack/150g	212	14.1	141	2	11	9.4	2
From Restaurant, Average	1/3 Cup/95g	108	5.7	114	1.5	13.5	6	0
Reduced Calorie, Pre Packed	1oz/28g	27	1.1	97	1.3	14.8	4.1	0.8
Vegan, Plant Kitchen, M&S*	1 Serving/50g	87	7	174	1.9	9.4	13.9	1.9
Vegan, Sainsbury's*	¼ Pot/75g	139	10.4	185	1.7	12.2	13.9	2.1
with Mayonnaise, Retail	1oz/28g	80	7.4	287	1.5	11.4	26.5	0.8

POTATO SKINS

	Measure INFO/WEIGHT	KCAL	FAT	KCAL	PROT	CARB	FAT	FIBRE
Bacon, & Cheese, Oven Baked, Supermarket, TGI Friday's*	2 Potato Skins/78g	125	4	160	3.2	24.2	5.1	2.3
Cheese & Bacon, Loaded, Asda*	½ Pack/125g	275	15	220	13	15	12	3.3
Cheese, & Bacon, Sainsbury's*	1 Skin/97g	154	6.6	159	6.9	16.2	6.8	2.9
Cheese, & Chive, Mini, Co-Op*	1 Skin/28g	48	2.3	172	7.1	15	8.2	3.8
Cheese, & Chive, Oven Baked, Asda*	1 Pack/245g	392	15.7	160	5.9	18	6.4	3
Cheese, & Jalapeno, Bannisters*	1 Skin/65g	92	4.1	142	5.9	14.1	6.3	2.4
with Sour Cream	1 Serving/275g	541	34.6	197	7.2	13.8	12.6	2.2

POTATO WAFFLES

	Measure INFO/WEIGHT	KCAL	FAT	KCAL	PROT	CARB	FAT	FIBRE
Dunnes Stores*	1 Waffle/50g	71	2.2	142	1.9	22.3	4.5	2.4
Frozen, Cooked	1oz/28g	56	2.3	200	3.2	30.3	8.2	2.3
Hash Brown, Four Seasons, Aldi*	2 Hash Browns/55g	126	7.2	230	2.6	25	13	2.2
Hash Brown, McCain*	3 Waffles/81g	129	7	159	2	17.3	8.6	2.4
Hash Brown, Oven Baked, Iceland*	1 Waffle/48g	132	7.1	275	3.3	30.3	14.8	3.6
Hashbrown, Birds Eye*	3 Waffles/79g	129	6.9	163	2	18	8.7	2.4
Potato, & Carrot, Mini, Oven Baked, Asda*	1 Serving/60g	124	3.8	205	3.2	32	6.3	3.3
Sweet Potato, Birds Eye*	1 Waffle/59g	150	9.4	255	2.2	24	16	2.9
Uncooked, Average	1 Waffle/62g	113	5.1	182	2.4	24.4	8.3	1.8

POTATO WEDGES

	Measure INFO/WEIGHT	KCAL	FAT	KCAL	PROT	CARB	FAT	FIBRE
Dirty, Carlos, Aldi*	1 Pack/450g	688	25.6	153	4.5	20	5.7	1.8
Fiery & Filthy, Wicked Kitchen, Tesco*	½ Pack/219g	285	7.2	130	2.1	21.5	3.3	3.1
Frozen, Average	1 Serving/120g	145	4.1	121	2	20.5	3.4	2.2
Garlic, & Rosemary, Frozen, Jumbo frozen*	1/3 Pack/200g	276	8.8	138	2.5	21	4.4	2.3
Jacket, Oven Baked, McCain*	1 Serving/100g	161	4.2	161	2.5	27	4.2	2.8

	Measure			Nutrition Values per 100g / 100ml				
	INFO/WEIGHT	KCAL	FAT	KCAL	PROT	CARB	FAT	FIBRE
POTATO WEDGES								
Lightly Spiced, Four Seasons, Aldi*	1 Serving/120g	196	5.1	163	3	27	4.2	2.6
Maris Piper, Aldi*	1 Serving/100g	189	7.8	189	2.3	26	7.8	2.6
Southern Fried, Oven Baked, Iceland*	1 Serving/100g	190	6.2	190	2.9	28.4	6.2	4.3
Spicy, Asda*	1 Serving/100g	145	5.7	145	1.8	21.8	5.7	2.1
Spicy, Lutosa*	1 Serving/160g	245	7.2	153	2.2	25	4.5	2.5
Spicy, Oven Cooked, Green Isle*	1 Serving/150g	339	15	226	3.4	28	10	3.4
Sweet Potato, Spiced, Allplants*	1 Serving/130g	240	8.3	185	2.4	28	6.4	3.4
with Sour Cream Dip, Waitrose *	½ Pack/201g	273	8.2	136	2.8	20.2	4.1	3.7
POTATOES								
Alphabites, Captain Birds Eye, Birds Eye*	9 Bites/56g	75	3	134	2	19.5	5.3	1.4
Anya, Raw, TTD, Sainsbury's*	1 Serving/100g	75	0.3	75	1.5	17.8	0.3	1.1
Apache, Albert Bartlett & Sons Ltd*	1 Serving/175g	278	17.3	159	2.4	14	9.9	6.5
Baby, Boiled, Finest, Tesco*	1 Serving/176g	125	0.2	71	1.8	14.9	0.1	1.8
Baby, Raw, Linroyale*	1 Serving/100g	65	0.3	65	1.4	14.1	0.3	0
Baby, Salad, Boiled with Skins, Garden Of Elveden*	1 Serving/100g	64	0.1	64	1.9	14.9	0.1	13.8
Baby, with Herbs & Butter, Morrisons*	1 Serving/100g	94	2.3	94	1.9	14.6	2.3	1.9
Baby, with Herbs, & Butter, Sainsbury's*	½ Pack/193g	145	3.5	75	2.8	11.1	1.8	1.9
Baked, & Cheese, Waitrose*	½ Pack/215g	232	4.9	108	3.6	16.8	2.3	3.2
Baked, Flesh & Skin, Average	**1 Med/200g**	**218**	**0.2**	**109**	**2.3**	**25.2**	**0.1**	**2.4**
Baked, Flesh Only, Weighed with Skin, Average	**1oz/28g**	**20**	**0**	**72**	**1.5**	**16.6**	**0.1**	**1.2**
Baked, in Microwave, Flesh & Skin, Average	**1oz/28g**	**29**	**0**	**105**	**2.4**	**24.1**	**0.1**	**2.3**
Baked, in Microwave, Flesh Only, Average	**1oz/28g**	**28**	**0**	**100**	**2.1**	**23.3**	**0.1**	**1.6**
Baked, in Microwave, Skin Only, Average	**1oz/28g**	**37**	**0**	**132**	**4.4**	**29.6**	**0.1**	**5.5**
Baked, Mature Cheddar Cheese, M&S*	½ Pack/206g	225	6.6	109	3.6	16.9	3.2	1
Baked, Skin Only, Average	**1oz/28g**	**55**	**0**	**198**	**4.3**	**46.1**	**0.1**	**7.9**
Baked, Tuna & Sweetcorn, Average	**1 Serving/300g**	**273**	**6.8**	**91**	**5**	**12.6**	**2.2**	**0.9**
Baked, with Cheese & Butter, Tesco*	1 Potato/214g	212	4.2	99	3	16.4	2	1.9
Baking, Raw, Average	**1 Med/250g**	**198**	**0.2**	**79**	**2.1**	**18**	**0.1**	**1.6**
Boiled with Skin	**1 Potato/125g**	**98**	**0.1**	**78**	**2.9**	**17.2**	**0.1**	**3.3**
Boiled, Average	**1 Serving/120g**	**86**	**0.1**	**72**	**1.8**	**17**	**0.1**	**1.2**
Bombay, for Two, Sainsbury's*	½ Pack/144g	155	9	108	1.8	9.8	6.3	2.2
Charlotte, Average	**1 Serving/184g**	**139**	**0.5**	**76**	**1.6**	**17.4**	**0.2**	**3.3**
Dauphinoise, Average	**1 Serving/200g**	**335**	**23.9**	**168**	**2.2**	**12.8**	**12**	**1.5**
Desiree, Average	**1 Serving/200g**	**152**	**0.4**	**76**	**2.2**	**16.4**	**0.2**	**0.6**
Fritters, Crispy, Oven Baked, Birds Eye*	1 Fritter/20g	29	1.6	145	2	16.3	8	1.2
Hasselback, Average	**1 Serving/175g**	**182**	**1.6**	**104**	**1.9**	**22**	**0.9**	**2.9**
Jersey Royal, Canned, Average	**1 Can/186g**	**116**	**0.2**	**62**	**1.4**	**14**	**0.1**	**1.2**
Jersey Royal, New, Raw, Average	**1oz/28g**	**21**	**0.1**	**75**	**1.6**	**17.2**	**0.2**	**1.5**
Lattices, Tesco*	¼ Pack/103g	221	8.4	215	3	29.8	8.2	5.2
Maris Piper, Raw, Average	**1 Serving/200g**	**151**	**0.4**	**75**	**2**	**16.5**	**0.2**	**1.4**
Mash, Creamy, Maris Piper, Extra Special, Asda*	½ Pack/200g	202	10	101	1.3	12	5	2.3
Mash, Creamy, Morrisons*	½ Pack/216g	190	5	88	1.9	14.2	2.3	1.3
Mashed, Bubble & Squeak, Tesco*	½ Pack/157g	116	1.9	74	1.9	13.2	1.2	1.7
Mashed, Cheddar, Cheesy & Smooth, Tesco*	½ Pack/210g	227	9.2	108	3.4	13.3	4.4	0.9
Mashed, From Restaurant, Average	**1/3 Cup/80g**	**66**	**1**	**83**	**2.3**	**16.1**	**1.2**	**0**
Mashed, From Supermarket, Healthy Range, Average	**1 Serving/200g**	**160**	**3.1**	**80**	**1.8**	**14.6**	**1.6**	**1.3**
Mashed, Home Prepared with Whole Milk	**1 Cup/210g**	**162**	**1.2**	**77**	**1.9**	**17.6**	**0.6**	**2**
Mashed, Made Up with Water, Average	**1 Serving/180g**	**118**	**0.3**	**66**	**1.7**	**14.5**	**0.2**	**1.3**
Mashed, Truffle, Gastropub, M&S*	½ Pack/225g	270	11.7	120	1.8	15.9	5.2	1.2
Mashed, with Cream & Butter, Ultimate, M&S*	½ Pack/225g	268	13.7	119	2.5	12.8	6.1	1.2
New, Average	**1 Serving/100g**	**75**	**0.3**	**75**	**1.5**	**17.8**	**0.3**	**1.1**
New, Baby, Canned, Average	**1 Can/120g**	**69**	**0.2**	**58**	**1.4**	**12.9**	**0.2**	**1.4**
New, Baby, Raw, Average	**1 Avg Serving/180g**	**135**	**0.5**	**75**	**1.7**	**17.1**	**0.3**	**1.6**

	Measure INFO/WEIGHT	per Measure KCAL	FAT	Nutrition Values per 100g / 100ml KCAL	PROT	CARB	FAT	FIBRE
POTATOES								
New, Peeled, Canned, in Water, Drained, Sainsbury's*	1 Can/180g	112	0.9	62	1.4	13	0.5	1.5
New, with Herb Dressing, Morrisons*	½ Pack/146g	114	1.6	78	1.7	14.3	1.1	1.9
Pan Fried, Aldi*	1 Serving/250g	182	2	73	2.7	13.7	0.8	0
Parmentier, Tesco*	1 Pack/400g	504	14.4	126	2	20.7	3.6	1.6
Potato, Colcannon, M&S*	½ Pack/200g	210	11.8	105	1.5	10.5	5.9	1.9
Raw, Peeled, Flesh Only	**1 Serving/100g**	**75**	**0.2**	**75**	**2**	**17.3**	**0.2**	**1.4**
Red, Flesh Only, Average	**1 Serving/300g**	**218**	**0.4**	**72**	**2**	**16.4**	**0.2**	**1.2**
Roast, Dry, No Oil, No fat	**1 Med/60g**	**47**	**0.1**	**79**	**2.7**	**18**	**0.1**	**1.6**
Roast, Frozen, Average	**1 Med/60g**	**90**	**3**	**149**	**2.6**	**23.5**	**5**	**1.4**
Roast, in Lard, Average	**1 Med/60g**	**89**	**2.7**	**149**	**2.9**	**25.9**	**4.5**	**1.8**
Roast, in Oil, Average	**1 Med/60g**	**89**	**2.7**	**149**	**2.9**	**25.9**	**4.5**	**1.8**
Roast, New, Rosemary, Ainsley Harriott*	1 Serving/150g	133	4	89	2	16	2.7	1.3
Roast, Roasties, Frozen, Cooked, Aunt Bessie's*	1 Serving/125g	162	6.1	130	1.9	18	4.9	2.3
Roast, with Goose Fat, TTD, Sainsbury's*	½ Pack/185g	216	4.4	117	2.7	21.1	2.4	3
Roasties, Crispy & Fluffy, Frozen, Aunt Bessie's*	1 Serving/100g	103	1.9	103	2	18	1.9	2.4
Roasting, Average	**1 Serving/150g**	**202**	**5.2**	**135**	**2.5**	**23.4**	**3.5**	**1.6**
Rosemary, & Garlic, M&S*	½ Pack/193g	154	3.9	80	1.4	13.5	2	1.3
Scallops, Battered, Deep Fried, Average	**1 Scallop/67g**	**216**	**14.5**	**323**	**5.4**	**27.3**	**21.6**	**0**
Smiles, Weighed Frozen, McCain*	½ Pack/228g	406	16.2	178	2.1	24.9	7.1	2.8
White, Raw, Flesh & Skin	**1 Lge/369g**	**284**	**0.3**	**77**	**2**	**17.5**	**0.1**	**2.2**
White, Raw, Weighed with Skin, Flesh Only, Average	**1 Med/213g**	**153**	**0.3**	**72**	**1.9**	**16.1**	**0.2**	**1.2**
POUSSIN								
Meat & Skin, Raw, Average	**1oz/28g**	**57**	**3.9**	**202**	**19.1**	**0**	**13.9**	**0**
Spatchcock, British, Waitrose*	½ Poussin/225g	364	20.2	162	19	1.2	9	0
POWERADE								
Berry & Tropical Fruit, Coca-Cola*	1 Bottle/500ml	90	0	18	0	4.1	0	0
Isotonic, Sports Drink, Coca-Cola*	1 Bottle/500ml	120	0	24	0	5.6	0	0
PRAWN COCKTAIL								
Asda*	1 Pot/170g	371	30.6	218	8.9	3.9	18	0
Best Ever, M&S*	1 Serving/85g	251	22.3	295	10.8	4.1	26.2	0.5
BGTY, Sainsbury's*	½ Pot/85g	119	7.9	140	9.1	4.7	9.3	0.5
Delicious, Boots*	1 Pack/250g	285	6.5	114	5.5	17	2.6	1.2
Fishmonger, Aldi*	1 Pot/170g	266	18.8	156	8.1	6	11	0.6
International Seafood Co, Morrisons*	½ Pot/90g	316	30.6	351	8.3	3	34	0
King, Extra Special, Asda*	1 Pack/204g	474	22.5	232	8.9	23	11	1.8
LC, Tesco*	1 Pot/140g	210	16	150	7.5	4.3	11.4	1.3
Lobster & Prawn, Posh, Christmas, M&S*	1 Cocktail/90g	244	21.6	271	11.2	2.4	24	0.3
Reduced Fat, 30%, Tesco*	½ Pot/85g	122	8	143	10.6	3.6	9.4	0.6
Reduced Fat, Good Health, Waitrose*	½ Pot/100g	208	16.5	208	10.9	3.6	16.5	0.5
Reduced Fat, Lighthouse Bay, Lidl*	1 Serving/50g	60	3.4	120	9.1	5.6	6.7	0.5
Reduced Fat, M&S*	1 Pack/200g	296	20	148	9.9	4.5	10	0.5
PRAWN CRACKERS								
Asda*	1 Serving/25g	134	8.8	535	2	53	35	0
M&S*	1 Bag/50g	262	15.6	525	2.8	57.4	31.3	0.8
Meal for Two, Meal Box, Tesco*	½ Pack/23g	127	8	554	2	57.3	35	1.1
Ready to Eat, Sharwood's*	½ Bag/30g	154	8.1	514	2	64.6	27.1	1.7
Sainsbury's*	1 Serving/25g	134	7.8	534	2.1	60.8	31.3	0.6
Side, Asda*	½ Pack/40g	199	10	498	1.5	67	25	1.1
Snackrite, Aldi*	1 Pack/25g	136	8	546	2.6	61	32	1.1
Snaktastic, Lidl*	1 Serving/15g	80	4.6	533	2.1	61.2	31	0.5
Sweet Chilli, Thai Dragon, Aldi*	1 Serving/20g	95	4	475	1.6	71	20	0
Thai Sriracha, Three Tigers*	1 Bag/60g	319	18.2	531	1.8	61.9	30.4	1.4

	Measure INFO/WEIGHT	per Measure KCAL	FAT	Nutrition Values per 100g / 100ml KCAL	PROT	CARB	FAT	FIBRE
PRAWN TOAST								
from Chinese Selection, Ken Hom, Tesco*	1 Toast/14g	50	3.8	364	11	17.1	27.4	2.6
Mini, Oriental Selection, Party, Iceland*	1 Toast/15g	52	3.6	345	10.5	22	23.9	2.1
Oriental Snack Selection, Sainsbury's*	1 Toast/20g	57	2.5	283	9.4	31.7	12.3	3.8
Oven Baked, Asda*	1 Toast/24g	89	6.5	372	9	22	27	2.2
Oven Cooked, Sainsbury's*	½ Pack/59g	237	17.7	401	11.8	19.7	30	2.7
Sesame Prawn, Toasted Triangles, M&S*	1 Pack/220g	616	39.6	280	12.4	17.3	18	2
Waitrose*	2 Pieces/70g	250	16.8	357	11.4	22.8	24	2.1
PRAWNS								
Boiled	**1 Prawn/3g**	**3**	**0**	**99**	**22.6**	**0**	**0.9**	**0**
Breaded, Coconut, Oven Baked, Sainsbury's*	½ Pack/84g	214	10.7	255	12.3	22.3	12.7	1.4
Cold Water, Ready to Eat, Waitrose*	1 Pack/175g	121	0.9	69	16.1	0.5	0.5	0.5
Cooked & Peeled, Average	**1oz/28g**	**21**	**0.2**	**77**	**17.6**	**0.2**	**0.6**	**0**
Hot & Spicy, Average	**1 Serving/170g**	**461**	**26.9**	**271**	**9.4**	**22.8**	**15.8**	**2.2**
Icelandic, Raw, Average	**1oz/28g**	**30**	**0.4**	**106**	**22.7**	**0**	**1.6**	**0**
Jumbo, Tempura, Oven Baked, Iceland*	1 Prawn/11g	40	2.5	362	12.6	26.6	22.7	0.8
King, Breaded	**1 Prawn/13g**	**33**	**1.8**	**260**	**15.1**	**17.8**	**14**	**1.2**
King, Cooked, Organic, M&S*	½ Pack/75g	61	0.8	81	17.9	0.4	1	0.4
King, Garlic Butter, Sainsbury's*	½ Pack/80g	95	4.3	119	17.4	0.5	5.4	0.5
King, Hot & Spicy, in Breadcrumbs, Tesco*	1 Prawn/10g	27	1.5	273	12	21	15.3	1.5
King, in Tomato, & Garlic Sauce, Iceland*	½ Pack/116g	128	8	110	10.2	1.2	6.9	1
King, Jumbo, Cooked & Peeled, Finest, Tesco*	½ Pack/75g	60	0.4	80	18.4	0.4	0.5	0.1
King, Large, Peeled, Cooked, Honduran, Eat Well, M&S*	½ Pack/70g	64	0.8	91	19.3	0.3	1.2	0.7
King, Marinated, with Semi Dried Tomatoes, & Basil, M&S*	1 Pack/135g	251	18.6	186	11.2	4	13.8	0.5
King, Raw, Average	**1 Bag/200g**	**145**	**1.9**	**72**	**15.8**	**0.2**	**1**	**0.1**
King, Sweet & Sour, Tesco*	½ Pack/193g	147	0.8	76	12.3	5.2	0.4	1.3
King, Tails, Sea Spray, Iceland*	½ Pack/85g	95	0.8	112	7.6	18.1	0.9	0.6
King, Tandoori, Average	**1 Prawn/59g**	**33**	**0.6**	**55**	**5.7**	**5.9**	**1.1**	**0.7**
North Atlantic, Peeled, Cooked, Average	**1oz/28g**	**22**	**0.3**	**80**	**17.5**	**0**	**1.1**	**0**
North Atlantic, Raw, Average	**1oz/28g**	**17**	**0.1**	**62**	**14.4**	**0**	**0.4**	**0**
Panko Breaded, Fishmonger, Aldi*	1 Serving/100g	267	12.2	267	11.7	26.2	12.2	0.5
Piri Piri, with Peppers, M&S*	½ Pack/115g	102	1.7	89	13.5	5	1.5	0.8
Sesame, Rainbow Layer Pot, M&S*	1 Pot/270g	324	14.6	120	6.3	9.2	5.4	4.6
Tempura, with Sweet Chilli, M&S*	1 Serving/100g	221	10.8	221	9.9	20.5	10.8	1.2
Tiger, Cooked & Peeled, Average	**1 Pack/180g**	**151**	**2**	**84**	**18.4**	**0.1**	**1.1**	**0**
Tiger, Jumbo, Average	**1 Serving/50g**	**39**	**0.2**	**78**	**18.2**	**0.3**	**0.5**	**0**
Tiger, Raw, Average	**1 Prawn/30g**	**19**	**0.2**	**64**	**14.2**	**0**	**0.7**	**0**
PRAWNS WITH								
Chilli, Coriander & Lime, King, Waitrose*	1 Pack/140g	143	3.2	102	19.9	0.5	2.3	0.6
Chorizo, & Lentils, Cook*	1 Pot/315g	246	5.4	78	5.7	8.2	1.7	3.3
Ginger & Spring Onion, Sainsbury's*	1 Pack/300g	198	9.3	66	4.7	4.7	3.1	0.3
King, with a Creamy Cocktail Sauce, M&S*	1 Pack/120g	278	23.3	232	12.6	1.3	19.4	1.1
King, with Garlic Butter, M&S*	1 Serving/100g	165	9	165	12.5	9.1	9	0.5
Orzo, Harissa, Hello Fresh*	1 Serving/358g	584	14.3	163	9	23	4	0
PRESERVE								
Bramble, Seedless, Mackays*	1 Tbsp/15g	40	0	269	0.3	66.8	0.1	0
Curd, Passion Fruit, The Cherry Tree*	1 Tbsp/15g	54	2.8	359	3.5	44.2	18.5	0
Ginger Shred, Robertsons*	1 Tbsp/15g	40	0	267	0.1	66	0	0
Ginger, Asda*	1 Tbsp/15g	39	0.1	261	0.5	63	0.5	1.7
Ginger, Stem, Curd, Woolliss & Son Ltd*	1 Tbsp/15g	51	1.3	343	2.6	65	8.4	0
Red Currant Jelly, Tiptree, Wilkin & Sons*	1 Tbsp/15g	40	0	264	0	66	0	0
Rhubarb & Ginger, Mackays Ltd*	1 Tbsp/15g	40	0	269	0.3	66.7	0	0
Rhubarb, Harbinger, Single Variety Co.*	1 Tsp/5g	11	0	212	0.6	48	0	0
Three Berry, Scottish, Mackays*	1 Tbsp/15g	41	0	272	0.4	67.6	0	0

P

	Measure INFO/WEIGHT	per Measure KCAL	FAT	Nutrition Values per 100g / 100ml KCAL	PROT	CARB	FAT	FIBRE
PRETZELS								
Bavarian, Bakery Instore, Lidl*	1 Pretzel/85g	251	5	295	9.4	50.6	5.9	0
Bites, Rock Salt, Indie bay snacks *	1 Pack/26g	99	1.1	381	13.1	71.2	4.2	3.1
Bites, Spelt, Dark Chocolate, Indie Bay*	1 Bag/31g	149	7.3	480	11.9	50.7	23.7	0
Bites, Spelt, Easy Cheesy, Indie Bay*	1 Pack/26g	99	1.2	380	12.9	70.1	4.6	3.1
Jumbo, Tesco*	1 Serving/50g	194	3.4	388	9.7	71.9	6.8	5.4
Mini, M&S*	1 Pack/45g	194	6	430	10.4	66.6	13.4	4.9
Pieces, Jalapeno, Snyders*	1 Pack/125g	590	23.3	472	7.1	67.4	18.6	3.2
Plain, Bakery, Tesco*	1 Pretzel/108g	316	5.8	293	9.5	50.3	5.4	2.7
Salted Caramel, Tesco*	1 Serving/25g	104	1.9	416	9.8	75.2	7.6	3.6
Salted, Average	**1 Serving/30g**	**114**	**0.8**	**380**	**10.3**	**79.8**	**2.6**	**3**
Salted, Mini, M&S*	1 Pack/25g	96	0.5	382	10.9	78	2.1	3.9
Soft, Cinnamon Sugar, Auntie Anne's*	1 Pretzel/112g	380	1	339	7.1	75	0.9	1.8
Soft, Salted, Original, Auntie Anne's*	1 Pretzel/112g	310	1	277	7.1	58	0.9	1.8
Sour Cream & Onion, M&S*	1 Serving/30g	136	4.4	455	11	70.9	14.5	0.7
Sour Cream & Chive, Baked, Penn State*	1 Bag/22g	94	2.1	426	9.5	74	9.5	2.9
Sour Cream & Chive, Christmas Trees, Snackrite, Aldi*	1 Serving/25g	106	2.2	422	10	74	8.9	3
Sticks, Salted, Co-Op*	1 Serving/15g	60	0.6	397	11	77	4.3	3.6
Superseeds, Crunchy, Indie Bay*	1 Pack/26g	106	2.9	408	18.7	54.7	11.3	6.4
Thins, Salted, M&S*	¼ Pack/20g	83	1.8	414	9	72	9.2	3.6
Turkey, Emmental, & Avocado, Finest, Tesco*	1 Pretzel/192g	487	21.9	254	13.1	23.9	11.4	1.6
Wheat, GF, Trufree*	1 Bag/60g	282	12	470	0.5	72	20	0.7
PRINGLES*								
Barbecue, Pringles*	1 Serving/50g	266	18	533	4.9	48	36	5.1
BBQ Spare Rib, Rice Infusions, Pringles*	1 Pack/23g	108	5.3	469	5.1	60	23	2.6
Cheese & Onion, Pringles*	1 Serving/25g	132	8.5	528	4.1	50	34	3.4
Hot & Spicy, Pringles*	1 Serving/25g	132	8.5	530	4.6	49	34	3.7
Light, Original, Pringles*	1 Serving/25g	121	6.2	484	4.3	59	25	3.6
Light, Sour Cream & Onion, Pringles*	1 Serving/25g	122	6.2	487	4.7	57	25	3.6
Margarita Pizza, Classic Takeaways, Pringles*	1 Serving/25g	134	8	538	3.9	53	32	2.6
Minis, Original, Pringles*	1 Pack/23g	118	6.9	514	5.1	55	30	3.7
Minis, Sour Cream & Onion, Pringles*	1 Pack/23g	118	6.7	511	5.2	56	29	3.5
Original, Pringles*	1 Serving/25g	130	8.5	522	3.8	51	34	2.6
Prawn Cocktail, Pringles*	1 Serving/25g	130	8	518	4.1	53	32	2.5
Salt & Vinegar, Pringles*	1 Serving/25g	128	8	512	3.9	52	32	2.4
Sour Cream & Onion, Pringles*	1 Serving/30g	154	9.6	515	4.2	51	32	2.9
Texas BBQ Sauce, Pringles*	1 Serving/25g	132	8.5	527	4.2	50	34	3.5
PROFITEROLES								
12 Chocolate, Waitrose*	3 Profiteroles/65g	284	21.4	437	6	28.7	33	0.4
Asda*	1 Serving/64g	218	17.2	343	5	20	27	0
Black Forest, Tesco*	1 Profiterole/19g	71	4.3	374	4.9	37.4	22.6	0.7
Chocolate Orange, Tesco*	1 Profiterole/17g	67	4.5	393	5.2	32.8	26.5	1.2
Chocolate, 8 Pack, Co-Op*	¼ Pack/112g	330	17.9	295	6	31	16	2
Chocolate, Double, Finest, Tesco*	½ Pack/51g	182	11.7	357	6	30.3	23	1.9
Chocolate, Sainsbury's*	1/6 Pot/95g	192	8.5	202	5.4	25.1	8.9	0.8
Chocolate, Stack, Sainsbury's*	¼ Pack/76g	311	19.5	409	5.3	39.3	25.6	2
Chocolate, Tesco*	4 Profiteroles/59g	202	16.1	343	5.2	18.5	27.4	1
Choux & Chocolate Sauce, Tesco*	1 Serving/77g	295	22	386	5.1	26.9	28.7	0.5
Classic French, Sainsbury's*	1 Serving/90g	284	15.5	316	6.6	33.7	17.2	0.1
Dessert, Lovetts*	1 Pot/80g	207	9.4	259	5.9	29.6	11.7	1.9
Filled with Cream, Stack, Fresh, M&S*	1 Serving/75g	303	22.8	404	5.6	26.3	30.4	1.5
Hazelnut, Praline , Partytime, Lidl*	3 Profiteroles/54g	228	15.9	422	5.4	32.8	29.4	2.2
in a Pot, Waitrose*	1 Pot/80g	207	11.3	259	6.3	25.6	14.1	2.9
Savoury with Cheese & Chive, CBY, Asda*	¼ Pack/15g	95	7.7	634	9.1	32.1	51.3	3.5

INFO/WEIGHT	Measure	per Measure		Nutrition Values per 100g / 100ml				
		KCAL	FAT	KCAL	PROT	CARB	FAT	FIBRE
PROFITEROLES								
Strawberry Cream Filled, Jumbo bakery *	1 Profiterole/25g	99	6.7	395	4.4	34.2	26.9	0.3
Waitrose*	4 Profiteroles/75g	269	17.9	359	4.8	31.1	23.9	0.7
PROSECCO								
11%, Average	*1 Sm Glass/125ml*	*103*	*0*	*82*	*0*	*1.7*	*0*	*0*
12%, Average	*1 Sm/125ml*	*112*	*0*	*89*	*0*	*1.4*	*0*	*0*
Extra Dry, M&S*	1 Glass/125ml	85	0	68	0	0	0	0
PRUNES								
Dried, Average	*1 Prune/7g*	*11*	*0*	*158*	*2.5*	*36.4*	*0.4*	*5.8*
in Apple Juice, Average	*1 Serving/90g*	*76*	*0.1*	*84*	*0.8*	*19.8*	*0.1*	*1.4*
in Fruit Juice, Average	*1oz/28g*	*24*	*0*	*86*	*0.9*	*20.9*	*0.2*	*2.9*
in Syrup, Average	*1oz/28g*	*25*	*0*	*89*	*0.9*	*21.5*	*0.2*	*2.6*
Soft Eating, M&S*	1 Serving/30g	65	0.2	217	1.7	49.1	0.7	3.9
Soft, Pitted, Mamiaa, Aldi*	1 Pouch/70g	52	0.4	74	0.6	15	0.5	3.6
Stewed with Sugar	*1oz/28g*	*29*	*0.1*	*103*	*1.3*	*25.5*	*0.2*	*3.1*
Stewed without Sugar	*1oz/28g*	*23*	*0.1*	*81*	*1.4*	*19.5*	*0.3*	*3.3*
PUDDING								
Banoffee, Sticky, Allplants*	1 Serving/85g	246	12.8	289	3	35	15	1.9
Beef, & Onion, Minced, Hollands*	1 Pudding/165g	353	19	214	6.5	20.6	11.5	0
Black Forest, Brilliant, Graze*	1 Punnet/37g	97	3.3	262	4	40	9	2
Bread, Retail Average	*1 Slice/120g*	*301*	*8*	*251*	*8.4*	*41.8*	*6.7*	*0.5*
Cherry Bakewell, Freaks Of Nature*	1 Pudding/100g	322	16.4	322	4.6	36.9	16.4	2.6
Chocolate Brownie, Classic, Co-Op*	¼ Pack/100g	429	25	429	6.1	44	25	2.4
Chocolate, Brownie, Waitrose*	1 Serving/98g	391	24.8	399	4.5	37.7	25.3	1
Chocolate, Colombian, Pot, Pots & Co*	1 Pot/65g	196	12.3	301	4.2	27.8	18.9	0
Chocolate, Dark, Colombian, Lighter, Pots & Co*	1 Pot/65g	195	12.5	300	4.3	26.4	19.3	0
Chocolate, Fudge, Hot, Freaks Of Nature*	1 Pudding/100g	279	10.5	279	2.7	42.5	10.5	1.9
Chocolate, Ganache, Mini Pot, Gu*	1 Pot/45g	199	16.6	442	3.3	26.4	36.8	2.3
Chocolate, High Protein, Nutrii*	1 Pot/150g	120	2.2	80	10	6.1	1.5	0
Chocolate, M&S*	¼ Pudding/76g	265	12	350	4.1	48	15.8	2.1
Chocolate, Melt in The Middle, Frozen, Waitrose*	1 Pudding/90g	310	14.4	344	6.7	41.4	16	3.5
Chocolate, Melt in The Middle, Mini, Tesco*	1 Pudding/20g	85	5.9	427	7.5	30.2	29.5	5.5
Chocolate, Melt-in-the-Middle, OGGS*	1 Pud/80g	277	11.9	346	4.5	44	14.9	1.7
Chocolate, Melting Middle, Hot, Puds, Gu*	1 Pud/100g	409	26.9	409	6	36	26.9	2.7
Chocolate, Melting Middle, M&S*	1 Pudding/155g	510	27.8	330	5.8	36.2	18	3.1
Chocolate, No Moo, Iceland*	1 Pudding/80g	298	18.4	372	5.6	35	23	0.8
Chocolate, Protein, Lindahls, Nestle*	1 Pot/140g	104	0.8	74	10	6.8	0.6	0.7
Chocolate, Steamed, Aunty's*	1 Pudding/95g	298	5.9	314	4.2	52.8	6.2	2
Eve's, Average	*1oz/28g*	*67*	*3.7*	*241*	*3.5*	*28.9*	*13.1*	*1.4*
Fondant, Chocolate Peanut, Allplants*	1 Serving/92g	363	23	395	8.3	32	25	2.9
Jam, Roly Poly, Sainsbury's*	¼ Pack/81g	291	11.5	359	4.4	53.3	14.2	0.5
Liegeois, Zott*	1 Pot/175g	163	4.2	93	1.2	16.4	2.4	0
Mango, & Passion Fruit, Pot, Pots & Co*	1 Po/65g	150	7.9	231	1.2	28.8	12.2	0
Mango, Mandarin, & Passion Fruit, Gu*	1 Pud/77g	157	8.5	204	2.1	22	11	0.5
Pease, Canned, Forsight*	1/3 Can/138g	134	1	97	6	15.9	0.7	1.7
Pease, Durham Foods *	1/3 Pack/70g	66	0.4	95	5.9	16.8	0.5	1.6
Protein, Fitness, Myq*	1 Pot/150g	110	2.1	73	10.3	5	1.4	0
Queen of Puddings	*1oz/28g*	*60*	*2.2*	*213*	*4.8*	*33.1*	*7.8*	*0.2*
Roly Poly, Jam, Aunt Bessie's*	1 Serving/75g	278	9	370	3.6	62	12	1.4
Souffle, Hot Chocolate, Gu*	1 Pot/65g	298	23.5	458	6	24.1	36.2	2.5
Sponge, Lemon, Mr Kipling*	1 Pudding/100g	379	16.9	379	3.1	53.3	16.9	0.7
Sponge, Spotted Dick, Asda*	1 Pudding/95g	401	21.9	422	4.4	489	23	1.7
Steak & Kidney, Meaty Puds, Fray Bentos*	1 Pack/400g	856	44	214	6.6	22.7	11	0.8
Steak & Kidney, Waitrose*	1 Pudding/190g	426	20.1	224	8.9	22.6	10.6	1

P

PUDDING

INFO/WEIGHT	Measure	per Measure		Nutrition Values per 100g / 100ml				
		KCAL	FAT	KCAL	PROT	CARB	FAT	FIBRE
Sticky Toffee, 626, Oakhouse Foods Ltd*	1 Serving/150g	468	18	312	2.4	48.6	12	1
Sticky Toffee, Cartmel*	1 Individual/150g	543	27.3	362	3.4	50	18.2	1
Sticky Toffee, Co-Op*	¼ Pudding/100g	355	20	355	3	40	20	0.7
Sticky Toffee, Deluxe, Lidl*	½ Pudding/225g	806	36	358	2.5	50	16	2.1
Sticky Toffee, Donald Russell*	1 Pudding/140g	511	22.4	365	2.7	54	16	0.3
Sticky Toffee, Extra Special, Asda*	¼ Pudding/100g	378	18	378	1.9	52	18	1.8
Sticky Toffee, Gro, Co-Op*	1 Pudding/95g	252	6.7	265	0.9	48	7.1	3
Sticky Toffee, Gu*	1 Pudding/85g	277	14.5	326	2.3	40.5	17.1	1.4
Sticky Toffee, Irresistible, Co-Op*	1 Serving/100g	335	14	335	2.1	48	14	3.7
Sticky Toffee, M&S*	1 Pud/115g	431	18.9	375	4	51.8	16.4	2.2
Sticky Toffee, OGGS*	1 Pud/80g	276	11.9	346	4.5	43.8	14.9	1.7
Sticky Toffee, Plant Kitchen, M&S*	¼ Pack/119g	381	8.9	321	3.4	58.5	7.5	2.9
Sticky Toffee, Puree, Wiltshire Farm Foods*	1 Pack/155g	277	17	179	1.4	19	11	0
Sticky Toffee, Tesco*	1 Serving/110g	287	14.7	261	3.3	31.8	13.4	0.7
Strawberry, Jelly Pud, with Devon Custard, Ambrosia*	1 Pot/150g	129	1.2	86	0.7	19.4	0.8	0
Suet, Average	*1oz/28g*	*94*	*5.1*	*335*	*4.4*	*40.5*	*18.3*	*0.9*
Summer Fruits, Eat Well, M&S*	1 Pudding/135g	128	0.7	95	1.7	20.8	0.5	3
Summer, Layered, Individual, Waitrose*	1 Pudding/150g	150	0.8	100	2.1	21	0.5	1.5
Summer, Layered, Waitrose*	¼ Pudding/101g	95	0.5	94	2.1	19.3	0.5	2
Syrup, M&S*	1 Serving/105g	370	10.5	352	3.9	61.7	10	0.8
Torte, Cheeky Little Chocolate, Gu*	1 Pud/50g	211	14.6	422	5.7	31.6	29.1	1.8
Vanilla, Protein, Everest*	1 Pack/200g	140	3	70	10	4.1	1.5	0

PUMPKIN

INFO/WEIGHT	Measure	per Measure		Nutrition Values per 100g / 100ml				
		KCAL	FAT	KCAL	PROT	CARB	FAT	FIBRE
Boiled in Salted Water	*1oz/28g*	*4*	*0.1*	*13*	*0.6*	*2.1*	*0.3*	*1.1*
Potimarron, Raw, Average	*1 Serving/80g*	*21*	*0.1*	*26*	*1*	*6.5*	*0.1*	*1.9*
Puree, Baking Buddy*	1 Serving/53g	22	0	42	1.7	6.7	0	2.5

	Measure INFO/WEIGHT	per Measure KCAL	FAT	Nutrition Values per 100g / 100ml KCAL	PROT	CARB	FAT	FIBRE
QUAVERS								
Cheese, Walkers*	1 Bag/20g	107	6	534	2.7	62.5	30.1	1.1
Prawn Cocktail, Walkers*	1 Pack/16g	84	4.6	524	3.6	64	28.6	1.8
Salt & Vinegar, Walkers*	1 Pack/16g	84	4.6	522	1.9	64	28.6	1.1
QUESADILLA								
Beef, Mexican, Aldi*	1 Quesadilla/150g	345	17.1	230	14.8	16.8	11.4	0
Chicken, from Restaurant, Average	**1 Serving/300g**	**867**	**46.7**	**289**	**15.6**	**22.2**	**15.6**	**1.7**
Feta, & Sweet Potato, Hello Fresh*	1 Serving/434g	434	14	100	3.5	13.6	3.2	1.6
Meal Kit, Mexican, Asda *	¼ Pack/119g	281	4.3	236	6.9	44	3.6	1.1
Meal Kit, Toasted Cheese, Old El Paso*	1 Quesadilla/63g	135	2.1	215	6.6	38.4	3.4	2.2
QUICHE								
Asparagus, & Mushroom, Tesco*	½ Quiche/200g	474	32.8	237	5.1	17.2	16.4	1.2
Asparagus, & Vegetable, Herby Summer, Higgidy*	1 Quiche/400g	848	50	212	5.9	18.9	12.5	2.7
Bacon, & Cheese, Sainsbury's*	¼ Quiche/100g	237	15	237	7	18.6	15	0.7
Bacon, & Leek, Morrisons*	1 Quiche/400g	1224	87.6	306	8.3	18.4	21.9	0.8
Bacon, Cheese, & Tomato, Asda*	1/3 Pack/133g	345	22.6	259	6.5	20	17	0.7
Bacon, Leek & Mushroom, M&S*	¼ Quiche/100g	245	16.4	245	6.9	17.2	16.4	1.3
Bacon, Maple, & Extra Mature Cheddar, Finest, Tesco*	¼ Quiche/105g	282	18.7	269	10.4	16.4	17.8	0.6
Bacon, Mushroom, & Leek, Slice, M&S*	1 Slice/60g	138	8.8	230	8.2	16	14.7	0.8
Bacon, Smoked, & Mature Cheddar, Higgidy*	1/6 Quiche/67g	176	11.7	262	9.5	17.4	17.4	1.1
Balsamic Onion, & Cheddar, Mature, Aldi*	¼ Quiche/100g	298	18	298	8.4	24	18	2
Balsamic Onion, Sweet, Higgidy*	¼ Quiche/100g	292	18.5	292	9.2	22.6	18.5	1.3
Brie, & Bacon, Waitrose*	¼ Quiche/100g	271	17.4	271	8.9	19.1	17.4	1.1
Brie, & Winter Spiced Chutney, Higgidy*	¼ Quiche/100g	246	15.5	246	7.4	19.7	15.5	1.4
Broccoli, & Cheddar, Crustless, Oven Baked, Asda*	1 Quiche/150g	296	18	197	7.4	14	12	1.9
Broccoli, & Cheddar, Family, Oven Baked, Asda*	1/3 Quiche/133g	325	20	244	6.5	21	15	1.5
Broccoli, & Tomato, Tesco*	¼ Quiche/100g	222	13	222	7	18.7	13	1.1
Broccoli, Cheese, & Tomato, M&S*	1/3 Quiche/133g	293	18.2	220	6.2	17	13.7	1.7
Broccoli, Spinach, & Ricotta, Waitrose*	¼ Quiche/100g	223	14.6	223	8.2	13.8	14.6	1.7
Broccoli, Tesco*	1 Serving/100g	249	17.2	249	6	17.6	17.2	1.4
Broccoli, Tomato, & Cheese, Crestwood, Aldi*	¼ Quiche/100g	212	12	212	5.9	19	12	1.8
Broccoli, Tomato, & Cheese, Sainsbury's*	¼ Quiche/100g	214	12.7	214	5.6	18.5	12.7	2
Butternut, Kale, & Chilli, Crustless, Tesco*	1 Quiche/160g	345	22.8	216	8.7	12.3	14.3	1.7
Cauliflower, Cheese, Higgidy*	½ Quiche/200g	540	37.2	270	9	17.4	18.6	1.5
Cheddar Cheese, & Bacon, Reduced Fat, Crustless, Tesco*	1 Quiche/160g	270	13.3	169	8.8	14.5	8.3	0.6
Cheddar, & Bacon, Crustless, Crestwood, Aldi*	¼ Quiche/85g	242	16	285	12.9	15.3	18.8	0.6
Cheddar, & Bacon, Crustless, Tesco*	¼ Quiche/85g	195	12.4	229	10.6	13.7	14.6	0.5
Cheddar, & Onion, Tesco*	¼ Quiche/100g	260	16.5	260	9.6	17.9	16.5	0.8
Cheddar, Vintage, & Broccoli, Jon Thorners*	1/3 Quiche/200g	556	34	278	12	16	17	0
Cheddar, Vintage, & Maple Bacon, Irresistible, Co-Op*	¼ Quiche/100g	268	18	268	8.7	18	18	1.3
Cheese, & Bacon, Crustless, Tesco*	¼ Quiche/85g	196	13.4	230	9.8	11.8	15.7	1.5
Cheese, & Broccoli, Morrisons*	1/3 Quiche/134g	338	22.4	253	7.1	18.4	16.8	1.7
Cheese, & Egg	**1oz/28g**	**88**	**6.2**	**314**	**12.5**	**17.3**	**22.2**	**0.6**
Cheese, & Leek, & Chive, Sainsbury's*	1/3 Quiche/125g	292	20.2	234	7.1	14.9	16.2	1.3
Cheese, & Onion, Caramelised Onion, Finest, Tesco*	¼ Quiche/100g	300	18.6	300	9.4	22.4	18.6	1.7
Cheese, & Onion, Retail, Average	**¼ Quiche/100g**	**262**	**17.8**	**262**	**8.4**	**17.1**	**17.8**	**1.3**
Cheese, & Tomato, Retail, Average	**¼ Quiche/100g**	**268**	**17.1**	**268**	**8**	**20.2**	**17.1**	**1.1**
Cheese, & Bacon, Crustless, Ovenbaked, Iceland*	¼ Quiche/85g	178	11.8	209	9.5	11.4	13.9	0.5
Cheese, & Bacon, Eastmans, Tesco*	¼ Quiche/100g	256	15.8	256	8.4	19.5	15.8	0.9
Cheese, & Broccoli, Co-Op*	¼ Quiche/100g	233	15	233	7.1	17	15	1.4
Cheese, & Pickle, Asda *	¼ Quiche/100g	255	14	255	7.9	23	14	0.9
Cheese, Pickle, & Tomato, Waitrose*	1 Quiche/400g	976	58.8	244	7.4	20	14.7	10
Goats Cheese, & Red Pepper, Morrisons*	1 Quiche/160g	450	29.9	281	7	20.7	18.7	1.1
Lorraine, Retail, Average	**¼ Quiche/100g**	**280**	**19.5**	**280**	**9**	**16.8**	**19.5**	**2**

Q

QUICHE

	Measure INFO/WEIGHT	per Measure KCAL	FAT	Nutrition Values per 100g / 100ml KCAL	PROT	CARB	FAT	FIBRE
Lorraine, Smoked Bacon & Cheese, M&S*	¼ Quiche/100g	270	18.4	270	9.7	16.4	18.4	1.6
Lorraine, Smoky Bacon, & Cheddar, Morrisons*	½ Quiche/262g	804	55.3	307	10.2	18.8	21.1	0.7
Mediterranean Style, Vegetable, Individual, Waitrose*	1 Quiche/155g	364	22.2	235	7.6	18.5	14.3	1.1
Mediterranean Vegetable, Waitrose *	1 Serving/100g	236	15.3	236	7.2	16.6	15.3	1.5
Mushroom	**1oz/28g**	**80**	**5.5**	**284**	**10**	**18.3**	**19.5**	**0.9**
Pea, Higgidy*	1 Serving/65g	161	10.3	248	8.5	18.4	15.8	1.7
Pea, Minted, & Bacon, Waitrose*	¼ Quiche/100g	253	14.9	253	8	21.1	14.9	1.4
Roasted Vegetable, Genius*	1 Quiche/160g	322	19.2	201	7.5	15.3	12	1.5
Salmon, & Spinach, Sainsbury's*	1/3 Quiche/125g	318	21.9	254	8.2	15.9	17.5	1
Salmon, & Spinach, Smoked, Little, Higgidy*	1 Quiche/155g	448	31.5	289	8.6	17.5	20.3	0.9
Salmon, & Spinach, with Cheddar Crumb, Higgidy*	¼ Quiche/100g	267	18	267	10	16.9	18	1.3
Salmon, & Broccoli, Jon Thorners*	¼ Quiche/100g	289	16.6	289	12.8	16.9	16.6	0
Salmon, & Broccoli, M&S*	½ Quiche/200g	432	26.6	216	7.6	15.9	13.3	1
Salmon, Broccoli, & Cheddar, TTD, Sainsbury's*	¼ Quiche/100g	257	17.4	257	7.2	17.1	17.4	1.3
Scotch Egg, Tesco*	1 Quiche/180g	494	31	274	10.7	18.7	17.2	1.2
Smoked Bacon, English, Higgidy*	¼ Quiche/100g	264	17.6	264	9.6	17.7	17.6	1.1
Spanish, 501, Oakhouse Foods Ltd*	1 Serving/117g	252	14.6	216	7.7	18.2	12.5	0.8
Spinach, & Ricotta, Tesco*	¼ Quiche/100g	237	14.9	237	5.8	19.9	14.9	1
Spinach, & Feta, Home Chef*	1 Quiche/200g	466	29	233	8.6	16.2	14.5	0
Spinach, & Red Pepper, Higgidy*	¼ Quiche/100g	246	16.4	246	8.2	17.1	16.4	1.6
Spinach, & Tomato, Higgidy*	1 Quiche/155g	426	28.7	275	10.2	19.2	18.5	2
Spinach, & Tomato, Vegan, Higgidy*	½ Pack/190g	460	27.7	242	4.2	24.4	14.6	2.9
Spinach, Edamame, & Kale, Crustless, Tesco*	1 Quiche/160g	350	22.2	219	8.7	13.9	13.8	2.2
Spinach, Feta, & Roasted Red Pepper, Higgidy*	¼ Quiche/100g	246	16.4	246	8.2	17.1	16.4	1.6
Spinach, Feta, & Roasted Tomato, Higgidy*	1 Quiche/155g	435	29.3	281	10.2	20	18.9	1.8
Squiche, Red Onion, & Brie, Mud*	1 Serving/125g	455	28.8	364	10	27	23	1.8
Swiss Gruyere, & Cheddar, Best Ever, M&S*	¼ Quiche/100g	274	18.2	274	13	13	18.2	1.2
Tomato, Mozzarella, & Pesto, Crustless, Morrisons*	¼ Quiche/85g	175	11.3	206	8.2	13	13.3	0.7
Tomato, Roasted, & Pesto, Higgidy*	¼ Quiche/100g	281	19.7	281	7.9	20	19.7	1.8
Vegetable, Mediterranean Style, Classic, Sainsbury's*	1 Quiche/400g	868	50.4	217	6.2	19.8	12.6	2.2

QUINCE

Average	**1 Avg fruit/209g**	**37**	**0.1**	**18**	**0.2**	**4.3**	**0.1**	**1.3**

QUINOA

& Bulgar Wheat, Mix, Cooked Weight, Morrisons*	1 Serving/80g	83	1	104	3.5	18.1	1.2	3.2
& Bulgar Wheat, Mix, Dry Weight, Morrisons*	1 Serving/30g	83	1	277	9.3	48.3	3.3	8.7
Bean, Zesty, Steam Bag, Microwaved, Iceland*	1 Bag/125g	174	7.4	139	6.1	13.6	5.9	3.5
Bio, Mix, Dry Weight, Provida*	1 Serving/45g	159	2.7	353	14	57	6	7
Cajun, Good Grains, Worldwide Foods, Aldi*	½ Pack/110g	185	3.5	168	7.7	24	3.2	6.4
Canned, Drained, Napolina*	½ Can/75g	94	1.3	125	4.2	21	1.7	4.4
Dry Weight, Average	**1 Serving/70g**	**258**	**4.2**	**368**	**14.1**	**64.2**	**6.1**	**7**
Mediterranean, Aldi*	1 Pack/125g	179	5.1	143	4.1	20.8	4.1	3.2
Puffed, Organic, As Sold, BuyWholeFoodsOnline*	1 Serving/50g	178	0.5	355	7	77	1	3
Red	**1 Serving/100g**	**358**	**6**	**358**	**12.9**	**62.2**	**6**	**9.7**
Tomato, & Olive, Microwaveable, Good Grains, Aldi*	½ Pack/125g	235	7.7	188	5.3	26.4	6.2	3.2
Tricolour, Cooked Weight, Sowans*	1 Serving/185g	222	3.5	120	4.4	21.3	1.9	2.8

	Measure			Nutrition Values per 100g / 100ml				
	INFO/WEIGHT	KCAL	FAT	KCAL	PROT	CARB	FAT	FIBRE
RABBIT								
Meat Only, Raw	**1oz/28g**	**38**	**1.5**	**137**	**21.9**	**0**	**5.5**	**0**
Meat Only, Raw, Weighed with Bone	**1 Serving/200g**	**164**	**6.6**	**82**	**13.1**	**0**	**3.3**	**0**
Meat Only, Stewed	**1oz/28g**	**32**	**0.9**	**114**	**21.2**	**0**	**3.2**	**0**
Meat Only, Stewed, Weighed with Bone	**1oz/28g**	**11**	**0.3**	**41**	**7.6**	**0**	**1.1**	**0**
RADISH								
Black, Raw, Average	**1 Lge/9g**	**1**	**0**	**16**	**1**	**3**	**0**	**2**
Red, Unprepared, Average	**1 Radish/8g**	**1**	**0**	**11**	**0.6**	**1.7**	**0.2**	**0.8**
White, Mooli, Raw	**1oz/28g**	**4**	**0**	**13**	**0.7**	**2.5**	**0.1**	**0**
RAISINS								
& Sultanas, Jumbo, M&S*	1 Serving/80g	212	0.4	265	2.4	62.4	0.5	2.6
& Sultanas, The Fruit Factory*	1 Box/14g	43	0.1	305	3	72.3	0.5	4
Chocolate, Bonds Of London*	1 Serving/30g	126	5.1	419	4.8	64	17	0
Chocolate, Milk, Mister Choc, Lidl*	1 Serving/40g	172	5.9	431	4.2	69.2	14.8	2.1
Lime Infused, Tangy, Nak'd*	1 Pack/25g	68	0	272	2.1	69.3	0	0
Milk Chocolate, Belgian, M&S*	½ Pack/63g	274	9.6	438	4.6	68.9	15.3	2.9
Mini, Snack, The Foodie Market, Aldi*	1 Box/14g	39	0.1	277	3	63	1	2.7
Raspberry, Chocolate, Super Nature*	1 Pack/40g	201	11.2	502	3	59	28	0
Ruby Chocolate, Holland & Barrett*	1 Serving/30g	134	6.6	448	4.6	60	22	1.2
Seedless, Average	**1 Serving/75g**	**215**	**0.4**	**287**	**2.2**	**68.5**	**0.5**	**3.2**
Yoghurt Coated, Fruit Bowl*	1 Pack/25g	114	4.8	455	2	67	19	3
Yoghurt Coated, Snack Bag, Asda*	1 Pack/25g	106	4	422	2.4	67	16	1
Yoghurt, Cranberry Foods Ltd*	1 Pack/50g	222	9.8	445	2.6	66.4	19.5	1.4
RAITA								
Plain, Average	**1oz/28g**	**16**	**0.6**	**57**	**4.2**	**5.8**	**2.2**	**0**
RASPBERRIES								
Freeze Dried, Honey Berry*	1 Tsp/2g	5	0	263	8.1	30.1	1.9	29.3
Fresh, Raw, Average	**1 Serving/80g**	**20**	**0.2**	**25**	**1.3**	**4.7**	**0.3**	**4.5**
Frozen, Average	**1 Serving/100g**	**27**	**0.3**	**27**	**1.3**	**4.7**	**0.3**	**4.5**
in Juice, Canned, Morrisons*	½ Can/150g	81	0.3	54	0.4	12	0.2	1.4
RATATOUILLE								
Average	**1oz/28g**	**23**	**2**	**82**	**1.3**	**3.8**	**7**	**1.8**
Canned, Freshona, Lidl*	¼ Can/188g	66	2.3	35	0.9	4.5	1.2	1.2
Vegetables, in Tomato Sauce, D'aucy*	½ Can/180g	79	3.4	44	1.2	4.8	1.9	1.5
RAVIOLI								
Asparagus, & Mozzarella, Dell'ugo*	½ Pack/125g	229	4.6	183	8.2	28	3.7	2.2
Beef	**1 Serving/300g**	**501**	**13.7**	**167**	**6.4**	**25**	**4.6**	**1.4**
Beef, & Red Wine, Italiano, Tesco*	½ Pack/200g	424	13	212	7.3	30	6.5	2.3
Butternut Squash, & Marjoram , M&S*	½ Pack/125g	336	15.5	269	8.9	29.2	12.4	2.5
Cheese, & Tomato, Canned, Sainsbury's*	½ Can/200g	170	2	85	3.5	15	1	0.9
Crab, & Crayfish, Dell'ugo*	½ Pack/125g	266	10.4	213	12.6	21.5	8.3	0.7
Gorgonzola, & Walnut, M&S*	½ Pack/125g	345	15.8	276	10.6	29.2	12.6	1.5
Lasagne, M&S*	½ Pack/125g	335	16.1	268	11.2	25.8	12.9	1.9
Parmesan, M&S*	½ Pack/125g	331	13.9	265	10.2	30.2	11.1	1.5
Spinach, & Ricotta, Deluxe, Lidl*	1 Pack/400g	419	12.2	105	3.8	14.6	3	2
Spinach, & Ricotta, Meal for One, M&S*	1 Serving/375g	555	22.1	148	5.1	17.6	5.9	1.8
Spinach, Vegan, Cooked, Waitrose*	½ Pack/159g	249	4.9	157	4.5	26.7	3.1	2.1
REDCURRANTS								
Raw, Average	**1oz/28g**	**6**	**0**	**20**	**1.1**	**4.3**	**0**	**3.3**
Raw, Stalks Removed	**1 Serving/100g**	**21**	**0**	**21**	**1.1**	**4.4**	**0**	**0**
RELISH								
Burger, Tangy, Asda*	1 Tbsp/15g	16	0.1	106	1.6	24	0.5	0.9
Burger, Tangy, Morrisons*	1 Tbsp/15g	16	0.1	110	1.2	25.2	0.4	0.3
Chilli, Slowly Reduced, Irresistible, Co-Op*	1 Tbsp/15g	30	0.1	202	0.6	48	0.6	1.4

R

	Measure INFO/WEIGHT	per Measure KCAL	FAT	Nutrition Values per 100g / 100ml KCAL	PROT	CARB	FAT	FIBRE
RELISH								
House, Supermarket, Gourmet Burger Kitchen*	1 Tbsp/15g	18	0.1	122	1.5	27	0.6	1.8
Jalapeno, & Tomato, Batts, Lidl*	1 Tbsp/15g	16	0	107	1.1	24.3	0.3	1.4
Onion, Sainsbury's*	1 Tbsp/15g	23	0.1	151	0.9	36	0.4	0.7
Pickle, Deli, New York, French's*	1 Tbsp/15g	14	0	92	1	21.1	0.1	1.6
Red Pepper, & Sweetcorn, Burger, Aldi*	1 Tbsp/15g	16	0.1	105	1.2	23	0.6	1.3
Sweet Onion, Californian, French's*	1 Tbsp/15g	21	0	140	0.9	33	0.2	1.2
Sweet Onion, Morrisons*	1 Tbsp/15g	17	0.1	115	1	26.5	0.4	0.9
Sweetcorn, American Style, Maryland, Tesco*	1 Tbsp/15g	15	0	101	1.1	23.9	0.1	0.9
Sweetcorn, Morrisons*	1 Tbsp/15g	15	0.1	97	0.9	21.7	0.5	0.9
Tomato, & Chilli, Devilish, Shaws*	1 Tbsp/15g	27	0.2	180	1	41.1	1	0
Tomato, Snap, Westcountry Spice*	1 Tbsp/15g	23	0.2	152	1.2	33	1.6	1.4
REVELS								
Mars*	1 Pack/35g	169	7.4	483	5.2	67.6	21	0
RHUBARB								
Canned, in Light Syrup, Princes*	1 Can/245g	86	0.2	35	0.5	7.4	0.1	1.2
Chunks, Frozen, Picard*	1 Serving/80g	11	0.4	14	1	1.4	0.5	2.3
In Juice, Canned, Drained, Average	**1 Serving/100g**	**46**	**0**	**46**	**0.5**	**10.8**	**0**	**0.8**
Raw, Average	**1 Serving/80g**	**17**	**0.2**	**21**	**0.9**	**4.5**	**0.2**	**1.8**
Stewed with Sugar, Average	**1oz/28g**	**32**	**0**	**116**	**0.4**	**31.2**	**0**	**2**
RIBENA*								
Blackcurrant Juice Drink, Ready Made, Ribena*	1 Carton/200ml	82	0	41	0	10.6	0	0
Blackcurrant, Diluted with Water, Ribena*	1 Serving/100ml	46	0	46	0	11.4	0	0
Blackcurrant, Original, Undiluted, Ribena*	1 Serving/50ml	108	0	216	0	53	0	0
Blackcurrant, Really Light, No Added Sugar, Ribena*	1 Carton/250ml	8	0	3	0	0.8	0	0
Light, Ribena*	1 Carton/288ml	26	0	9	0.1	2.1	0	0
Pineapple & Passion Fruit, Juice Drink, Ribena*	½ Bottle/250ml	103	0	41	0	9.9	0	0
Raspberry, Sparkling, Ribena*	1 Bottle/250ml	42	0	17	0.1	4	0	0
Strawberry Juice Drink, Ribena*	1 Carton/288ml	12	0	4	0	0.5	0	0
RIBS								
Beef, Boneless, in BBQ Sauce, Tesco*	½ Pack/109g	294	16.6	270	23.6	9	15.2	1.3
Peking, Taste of China, Tesco*	½ Pack/104g	222	12.4	214	16.4	10.1	12	0
Pork, Barbecue, Meat Only, Cooked, Average	**1 Serving/130g**	**360**	**23.4**	**275**	**21.4**	**7.2**	**17.9**	**0.3**
Pork, Chinese Style, Average	**1 Serving/300g**	**736**	**44.7**	**245**	**17.9**	**10**	**14.9**	**0.7**
Pork, Chops, Raw, Lean & Fat, Weighed with Bone	**1 Chop/130g**	**241**	**16.1**	**186**	**18.5**	**0**	**12.4**	**0**
Pork, Full Rack, Sainsbury's*	1 Serving/225g	567	38.7	252	18	6.5	17.2	0.9
Pork, Oriental, Sticky, Oven Cooked, Sainsbury's*	1 Serving/155g	452	25.5	292	22.6	11.8	16.5	2.4
Pork, Rack, Slow Cooked, Sweet BBQ, Morrisons*	½ Pack/158g	442	26.4	280	21	11.1	16.7	0.7
Pork, Salt & Chilli, Tesco*	½ Pack/99g	316	23.3	319	24.8	1.6	23.5	1
Pork, Smokey BBQ, Slow Cooked, Sainsbury's*	½ Pack/118g	298	14.4	253	23.9	11.3	12.1	1
Pork, Smoky BBQ, Rack, Tex Mex, Tesco*	½ Pack/158g	337	21.1	213	17.6	5.6	13.3	0.2
Pork, Spare, BBQ, Cooked, Iceland*	½ Pack/150g	290	16.8	193	16.5	6.2	11.2	1.1
Rack, Pork, BBQ Maple, Slow Cooked, Tesco*	1 Serving/112g	343	23.7	306	23	5.9	21.1	0.5
Spare, Barbecue, Chinese Style, Farmfoods*	1 Pack/400g	464	25.2	116	9.3	5.6	6.3	0.1
Spare, Cantonese, Mini, Sainsbury's*	1 Rib/38g	97	5	259	17.2	17.3	13.4	1
Spare, Chinese Style, Summer Eating, Asda*	1 Serving/116g	334	18.6	288	32	4.1	16	0.8
Veggie, BBQ, Sweet n Smoky, Ribz, Plant Power*	1 Serving/150g	244	8.8	163	10.4	14.9	5.9	3.2
RICE								
& Quinoa, M&S*	½ Pack/145g	190	4.6	131	3	21.3	3.2	2.4
Arborio, Dry, Average	**1 Serving/80g**	**279**	**0.6**	**348**	**7.1**	**78.3**	**0.8**	**0.8**
Basmati, & Wild, Cooked, Sainsbury's*	½ Pack/125g	150	0.8	120	3.1	25.7	0.6	1.3
Basmati, & Wild, Dry Weight, Tilda*	1 Serving/70g	244	0.3	349	9.4	77	0.5	1
Basmati, Boil in the Bag, Dry, Average	**1 Serving/50g**	**176**	**0.4**	**352**	**8.4**	**77.8**	**0.8**	**0.4**
Basmati, Brown, Dry, Average	**1 Serving/50g**	**177**	**1.5**	**353**	**9.5**	**71.8**	**3**	**2.2**

R

RICE

INFO/WEIGHT	Measure	per Measure KCAL	FAT	Nutrition Values per 100g / 100ml KCAL	PROT	CARB	FAT	FIBRE
Basmati, Cooked, Average	**1 Serving/140g**	**190**	**3.9**	**136**	**2.4**	**25.6**	**2.8**	**0.8**
Basmati, Dry Weight, Average	**1 Serving/60g**	**212**	**0.6**	**353**	**8.1**	**77.9**	**1**	**0.6**
Basmati, Indian, Dry, Average	**1 Serving/75g**	**260**	**0.7**	**346**	**8.4**	**76.1**	**0.9**	**0.1**
Basmati, Lemon & Herb, Steamed, Tilda*	1 Serving/125g	172	2.8	137	2.6	26.1	2.2	1.2
Basmati, Mexican, Spicy, Tilda*	½ Pack/125g	152	3.1	122	2.4	21.6	2.5	1.8
Basmati, Microwave, Cooked, Average	**1 Serving/125g**	**182**	**2.3**	**146**	**2.7**	**30**	**1.8**	**0**
Basmati, Peri Peri, Tilda*	1 Pack/250g	325	6.2	130	2.5	23.5	2.5	1.8
Basmati, White, Dry, Average	**1 Serving/75g**	**262**	**0.4**	**349**	**8.1**	**77.1**	**0.6**	**2.2**
Basmati, Wholegrain & Wild, Pouch, Tilda*	½ Pack/125g	160	2.6	128	3	23.4	2.1	1.7
Basmati, Wholegrain, Cooked, Tilda*	1 Serving/125g	161	2.6	129	2.8	23.3	2.1	3
Black, Dry Weight, Holland & Barrett*	1 Serving/60g	208	1.9	346	9.8	67.6	3.1	3.9
Brown, Basmati, Microwave Pouch, Sainsbury's*	1 Pouch/250g	340	3	136	3.2	27.6	1.2	0.9
Brown, Cooked, Average	**1 Serving/140g**	**173**	**1.5**	**123**	**2.6**	**26.6**	**1.1**	**0.9**
Brown, Dry, Average	**1 Serving/75g**	**266**	**2.3**	**355**	**7.5**	**76.2**	**3**	**1.4**
Brown, Long Grain, Dry, Average	**1 Serving/50g**	**182**	**1.4**	**364**	**7.6**	**76.8**	**2.8**	**2**
Brown, Short Grain, Dry, Average	**1 Serving/50g**	**176**	**1.4**	**351**	**6.8**	**77.6**	**2.8**	**1**
Brown, Whole Grain, Cooked, Average	**1 Serving/170g**	**223**	**1.9**	**132**	**2.6**	**27.8**	**1.1**	**1.2**
Brown, Whole Grain, Dry, Average	**1 Serving/40g**	**138**	**1.2**	**344**	**7.4**	**71.6**	**2.9**	**3**
Cauliflower, Frozen, Tesco*	1 Sachet/150g	36	0.3	24	1.8	2.1	0.2	3.2
Cauliflower, Fullgreen*	1 Pack/200g	40	0.4	20	1.5	4	0.2	2.5
Cauliflower, Microwaved, G&B, Asda*	½ Pack/200g	68	1.8	34	2.9	2.1	0.9	2.7
Chinese Style, Express, Uncle Ben's*	1 Pack/250g	392	5.5	157	3.4	30.9	2.2	0.4
Coconut, Lime, & Coriander, Waitrose*	½ Pack/125g	200	3.1	160	3.1	30.8	2.5	1.4
Egg Fried, Average	**1 Serving/300g**	**624**	**31.8**	**208**	**4.2**	**25.7**	**10.6**	**0.4**
Fried, Chicken, Takeaway, Iceland*	1 Pack/336g	631	18.1	188	7.5	26.5	5.4	1.5
Fried, Teriyaki Chicken, Waitrose*	1 Serving/250g	822	35	329	19.6	28	14	6
Garlic, Roasted, Express Rice, Uncle Ben's*	½ Pack/125g	190	2.6	152	3.2	30	2.1	0.9
Golden Veg, Micro, Asda*	½ Pack/125g	195	1.9	156	3.5	31.2	1.5	2.3
Golden Vegetable, Savoury Rice, Batchelors*	½ Pack/116g	157	0.8	135	3.9	27.5	0.7	1.6
Golden Vegetable, Savoury, Sainsbury's*	½ Pack/147g	189	0.9	129	2.9	27.1	0.6	2
Golden Vegetable, Special, Worldwide Foods, Aldi*	½ Pack/125g	181	2.1	145	3.7	27	1.7	3
Golden, Savoury, Steam Bags, Iceland*	1 Bag/149g	179	3.1	120	3.1	21.4	2.1	1.6
Jasmine, Long Grain, Cooked Weight, Tesco*	1 Serving/236g	321	2.4	136	2.5	29.1	1	0.5
Jasmine, Microwave, Tesco*	½ Pouch/125g	206	1.6	165	3.3	34.4	1.3	1
Jasmine, Thai, Microwave, Morrisons*	½ Pack/125g	222	2	178	3.1	37.3	1.6	0.8
Lemon, & Thyme, Uncle Ben's*	½ Pouch/125g	192	2.8	154	3.3	30	2.2	1
Long Grain, & Wild, Dry, Average	**1 Serving/75g**	**254**	**1.5**	**338**	**7.6**	**72.6**	**2**	**1.7**
Long Grain, American, Cooked, Average	**1 Serving/160g**	**229**	**2.8**	**143**	**3**	**28.8**	**1.8**	**0.2**
Long Grain, American, Dry, Average	**1 Serving/50g**	**175**	**0.5**	**350**	**7.2**	**77.1**	**1.1**	**0.6**
Long Grain, Dry, Average	**1 Serving/50g**	**169**	**0.5**	**337**	**7.4**	**75.5**	**1**	**1.7**
Long Grain, Microwavable, Cooked, Average	**1 Serving/150g**	**180**	**0.9**	**120**	**2.7**	**25.8**	**0.6**	**0.7**
Mexican Inspired, Micro, Tesco*	1 Bag/142g	184	2	130	3.2	25.5	1.4	1.1
Mexican Style, Micro, Asda*	½ Pouch/125g	185	2.9	148	3.5	27	2.3	2
Mexican Style, Microwave, Lidl*	½ Pack/125g	235	3.5	188	3	37	2.8	1.3
Mexican Style, Special, Worldwide Foods, Aldi*	½ Pack/181g	262	3.3	145	3.1	28	1.8	2.9
Mexican, M&S*	1 Serving/250g	368	5.5	147	3.3	27.5	2.2	2.2
Mushroom, Pilau, Indian, Sainsbury's*	1 Serving/100g	119	2.4	119	3	21.3	2.4	1.9
Onion Bhaji, Uncle Ben's*	½ Pack/125g	200	2.9	160	3.3	31	2.3	1.4
Pilau, Cooked, Average	**1 Serving/200g**	**349**	**8.8**	**174**	**3.5**	**30.3**	**4.4**	**0.8**
Pilau, Dry, Average	**1oz/28g**	**101**	**0.7**	**362**	**8.4**	**78.2**	**2.4**	**3.4**
Pudding, Dry Weight, Average	**1 Serving/100g**	**356**	**1.1**	**356**	**6.9**	**82**	**1.1**	**0.4**
Saffron, Cooked, Average	**1 Serving/150g**	**208**	**4.7**	**139**	**2.6**	**25.3**	**3.2**	**0.5**
Special Fried, Chinese Takeaway, Iceland*	1 Pack/350g	630	17.5	180	5.5	28.2	5	1.2

R

RICE

INFO/WEIGHT	Measure	per Measure KCAL	FAT	Nutrition Values per 100g / 100ml KCAL	PROT	CARB	FAT	FIBRE
Special Fried, Chinese Takeaway, Morrisons*	½ Pack/175g	256	8.6	146	6.1	18.7	4.9	1.4
Special Fried, M&S*	½ Pack/150g	300	12.3	200	6.7	24.2	8.2	1.2
Spicy Mexican, Microwave, Uncle Ben's*	½ Pouch/125g	199	3.8	159	3.8	28	3	1.5
Spinach, & Carrot, Pilau, Waitrose*	1 Pack/350g	466	8.4	133	3.1	24.8	2.4	1.2
Sticky, Omnipork, in Lotus Leaf, Omni Eat*	1 Pack/250g	302	6.2	121	5.7	18.9	2.5	1.6
Thai, Cooked, Average	*1 Serving/100g*	*136*	*1.8*	*136*	*2.5*	*27.4*	*1.8*	*0.3*
Thai, Dry, Average	*1 Serving/50g*	*174*	*0.2*	*348*	*7.1*	*78.9*	*0.4*	*0.9*
Thai, Fragrant, Dry, Average	*1 Serving/75g*	*272*	*0.5*	*363*	*7.2*	*82*	*0.7*	*0.3*
Thai, Glutinous, Sticky, White, Dry, Raw	*1 Serving/100g*	*370*	*0.6*	*370*	*6.8*	*81.7*	*0.6*	*2.8*
Tomato, & Basil, Tilda*	½ Pack/125g	154	3.1	123	2.1	22.4	2.5	1.1
Vegetable, Golden, Freshly Frozen, Asda*	1 Sachet/200g	238	2.6	119	3.2	23.6	1.3	1.3
Vegetable, Mediterranean, SteamFresh, Birds Eye*	1 Bag/190g	226	4.9	119	2.3	21	2.6	1.1
White, Cooked, Average	*1 Serving/140g*	*182*	*1.1*	*130*	*2.6*	*28.7*	*0.8*	*0.2*
White, Cooked, Frozen, Average	*1 Serving/150g*	*168*	*0.8*	*112*	*2.9*	*23.8*	*0.6*	*1.2*
White, Fried	*1oz/28g*	*37*	*0.9*	*131*	*2.2*	*25*	*3.2*	*0.6*
White, Long Grain, Dry Weight, Average	*1 Serving/50g*	*181*	*1*	*362*	*7.1*	*79.1*	*1.9*	*0.4*
White, Microwave, Cooked, Average	*½ Pack/125g*	*185*	*2.4*	*148*	*3.3*	*29.4*	*1.9*	*1.4*
Whole Grain, Dry, Average	*1 Serving/50g*	*171*	*1.2*	*342*	*8.2*	*72*	*2.3*	*4*
Wholegrain, & Freekeh, Sainsbury's*	½ Pack/125g	206	3.2	165	4.4	29.2	2.6	3.6
Wholegrain, Microwave Pouch, Average	*½ Pack/125g*	*191*	*2.1*	*153*	*3.3*	*29.7*	*1.7*	*3.1*
Wild, Cooked, Average	*1 Cup/164g*	*166*	*0.6*	*101*	*4*	*21.3*	*0.3*	*1.8*
with Mixed Vegetables, White & Wild, Steam Bag, Tesco*	1 Bag/150g	168	1.8	112	2.6	21.7	1.2	1.9
With Red Kidney Beans, Average	*1oz/28g*	*49*	*1*	*175*	*5.6*	*32.4*	*3.5*	*2.5*

RICE CAKES

INFO/WEIGHT	Measure	per Measure KCAL	FAT	Nutrition Values per 100g / 100ml KCAL	PROT	CARB	FAT	FIBRE
& Corn, Salt & Vinegar, Sainsbury's*	1 Rice Cake/9g	34	0.3	375	7.3	77	3.5	3.3
Apple, Organix*	3 Rice Cakes/6g	23	0.1	391	6.8	88	1.1	0.5
Asda*	1 Rice Cake/8g	31	0.2	386	8.7	81.1	3	2.8
Caramel, Flavour, Kallo*	1 Rice Cake/10g	38	0.5	383	6.2	78.9	4.8	3.9
Caramel, Free From, Tesco*	1 Rice Cake/11g	41	0.3	373	5.9	80.9	2.5	1.8
Caramel, Harvest Morn, Aldi*	1 Rice Cake/12g	46	0.2	385	5.6	87	1.5	1.8
Caramel, Jumbo, Snack-A-Jacks*	1 Rice Cake/13g	51	0.3	390	5.5	87	2.1	1.4
Caramel, Jumbo, Tesco*	1 Rice Cake/10g	34	0.3	340	7	74	3	5
Chocolate Covered, Thin, Kallo*	1 Rice Cake/11g	54	2.5	495	7.8	63	23	3.5
Chocolate Orange, Tesco*	1 Rice Cake/21g	95	4	453	5	62	19	7
Chocolate, Chip, Jumbo, Snack-A-Jacks*	1 Rice Cake/15g	62	1	410	6	81	7	1.7
Chocolate, Dark, Organic, Kallo*	1 Rice Cake/12g	57	2.9	471	6.8	57.2	24.1	7.4
Chocolate, Milk, Kallo*	1 Rice Cake/17g	83	3.7	486	7	65	22	0
Chocolate, Milk, Mini, Sainsbury's*	1 Pack/30g	138	5	459	7.8	67.9	16.8	2.9
Chocolate, Milk, Minis, Kids, Kallo*	1 Pack/14g	69	3.3	496	6.6	62.6	23.8	0
Chocolate, Milk, Sainsbury's*	1 Pack/38g	178	7	469	7.7	66.2	18.5	3.2
Corn, Salt & Vinegar, Co-Op*	1 Rice Cake/9g	33	0.5	367	8.9	75.6	5.6	5.6
Dark Chocolate, Minis, Kallo*	1 Pack/21g	102	4.8	486	6.2	61	23	5.2
Dark Chocolate, Morrisons*	1 Rice Cake/17g	80	3.3	473	6.5	65.1	19.5	4.5
Dark Chocolate, Rivercote, Lidl*	1 Rice Cake/17g	80	3.8	480	6.9	58.5	23	5.7
Home Bargains*	1 Rice Cake/17g	81	3	483	6.7	73	18	3
Idly, Average	*1 Idly/40g*	*59*	*0.4*	*149*	*4.1*	*30.8*	*1*	*1.3*
Lightly Salted, Tesco*	1 Rice Cake/7g	27	0.2	381	8.9	77.2	3.2	4.1
Low Fat, BGTY, Sainsbury's*	1 Rice Cake/7g	29	0.2	388	8.1	81.5	2.4	3.9
Milk Chocolate, & Salted Caramel, The Best, Morrisons*	1 Rice Cake/17g	85	3.6	487	5.9	67.4	20.9	2.6
Milk Chocolate, Mini, Snack Pack, Kallo*	1 Pack/23g	104	5	452	6.1	56.5	21.7	0
Multigrain, Harvest Morn, Aldi*	1 Rice Cake/8g	30	0.2	374	11	72	2.3	11
Multigrain, High Protein, M&S*	1 Rice Cake/8g	31	0.2	387	21.8	67.4	2.8	2.3
Pea, & Lentil, Protein, Sainsbury's*	1 Rice Cake/8g	31	0.2	370	21.6	60.6	2.5	9.3

R

RICE CAKES	Measure INFO/WEIGHT	per Measure KCAL	FAT	Nutrition Values per 100g / 100ml KCAL	PROT	CARB	FAT	FIBRE
Pear, & Berries, Tesco*	1 Rice Cake/2g	7	0	372	7.3	84	0.6	0.7
Salt & Vinegar, Asda*	1 Rice Cake/8g	30	0.2	353	9.1	72	2.6	3.4
Salt & Vinegar, Morrisons*	1 Rice Cake/9g	30	0.2	335	6.7	69.2	2.6	3.8
Salt & Vinegar, Snack-A-Jacks, Quaker*	1 Pack/22g	89	1.6	406	7	77.4	7.4	0.8
Salt & Vinegar, Tesco*	1 Rice Cake/12g	47	0.7	392	6.3	78	5.7	1.8
Salt, & Vinegar, Jumbo, Snack-A-Jacks*	1 Rice Cake/10g	41	0.6	391	7.4	75.4	5.7	1.6
Salt, & Vinegar, Jumbo, Tesco*	1 Rice Cake/9g	31	0.2	347	8.4	72.7	2.5	6
Salt, & Vinegar, Wholegrain, Tesco*	1 Rice Cake/9g	28	0.2	314	8.4	61.9	2.6	6
Salted Caramel, M&S*	1 Rice Cake/19g	90	3.7	474	6.8	66.8	19.5	2.6
Salted, Lightly, Thick Slice, Low Fat, Kallo*	1 Rice Cake/8g	28	0.2	372	8	78.7	2.8	5.1
Salted, Slightly, Organic, Thin Slice, Kallo*	1 Rice Cake/5g	17	0.1	372	8	78.7	2.8	5.1
Salted, Slightly, Thick Slice, Organic, Kallo*	1 Rice Cake/8g	28	0.2	372	8	78.7	2.8	5.1
Sea Salt, Harvest Morn, Aldi*	1 Rice Cake/8g	29	0.5	362	8.8	76.2	6.2	6.2
Sea Salt, Jacob's*	1 Rice Cake/5g	19	0.2	384	8.3	78	3.4	3.9
Sesame Seed, Organic, Kallo*	1 Rice Cake/7g	27	0.4	398	8.4	77	5.5	3.8
Sesame, No Added Salt, Thick Sliced, Organic, Kallo*	1 Rice Cake/10g	37	0.3	373	8	78	3.2	5.4
Sour Cream & Chive, Mini, Snack-A-Jacks, Quaker*	1 Pack/19g	78	1.8	411	7.4	74.2	9.5	1.6
Sour Cream, & Black Pepper, M&S*	1 Rice Cake/9g	39	1	432	7.1	75.8	10.8	1.6
Sweet & Salty, Tesco*	1 Rice Cake/9g	35	0.2	385	7	83.1	2.2	2.3
Sweet Chilli, Harvest Morn, Aldi*	1 Rice Cake/10g	47	1.7	452	7.2	67	16	4.4
Thin Slice, No Added Salt, Organic, Kallo*	1 Rice Cake/5g	19	0.1	372	8	78.7	2.8	5.1
Veggie, Lentil, & Pea, Kallo*	1 Rice Cake/9g	38	0.1	424	2.4	4.7	1.2	0.6
Wholegrain, Free From, Tesco*	1 Rice Cake/8g	31	0.3	393	7.8	81.7	3.2	3.1
Wholegrain, Lightly Salted, Kallo*	1 Rice Cake/7g	28	0.2	394	8.5	82.3	2.7	0
Yoghurt, & Strawberry, M&S*	1 Bag/25g	120	4.8	480	5.3	71.2	19.1	0.9
RICE PUDDING								
& Jam, Fat Free, Aunt Bessie's*	¼ Pack/131g	136	0.3	104	2.4	23	0.2	0.6
50% Less Fat, Asda*	½ Can/212g	180	1.7	85	3.3	16.2	0.8	0.2
830, Wiltshire Farm Foods*	1 Serving/160g	181	4.8	113	2.9	18	3	0
Apple, Ambrosia*	1 Pot/150g	125	2.3	104	2.7	18.8	1.9	0.5
Apple, Brooklea, Aldi*	1 Pot/180g	200	3.2	111	2.9	21	1.8	0.5
Canned, Average	*1oz/28g*	*25*	*0.7*	*89*	*3.4*	*14*	*2.5*	*0.2*
Canned, Light, Salco, Lidl*	1 Can/400g	316	2.8	79	2.8	15.1	0.7	0.5
Clotted Cream, Morrisons*	1 Pudding/145g	265	17.3	183	3.1	15.5	11.9	0.7
Clotted Cream, Waitrose*	1 Pot/150g	286	18	191	3.1	17.3	12	0.7
Creamed, Canned, Ambrosia*	1 Can/425g	382	8.1	90	3.1	15.2	1.9	0
Creamed, Pot, Ambrosia*	1 Pot/150g	156	3.8	104	3.3	17	2.5	0.1
Creamed, Value, Tesco*	1 Can/425g	348	3.4	82	3.2	15.5	0.8	0
Light, 30% Less Sugar, Ambrosia*	½ Can/200g	154	2.6	77	3.3	13	1.3	0.5
Light, Tesco*	½ Can/200g	152	1.6	76	2.8	14.4	0.8	0.1
Low Fat, Canned, Belbake, Lidl*	½ Can/200g	158	1.4	79	2.8	15.1	0.7	0.5
Low Fat, Muller Rice, Muller*	1 Serving/180g	182	4.7	101	3.4	16.1	2.6	0
Pot, Ambrosia*	1 Pot/125g	126	3.1	101	3.3	16.3	2.5	0
Raspberry, Low Fat, Muller Rice, Muller*	1 Pot/180g	189	4	105	3	18.4	2.2	0
Raspberry, Mullerice, Muller*	1 Pot/190g	201	4.4	106	3.2	18.2	2.3	0.5
Riz Au Lait, Bonne Maman*	1 Pot/100g	149	5.3	149	3.3	22	5.3	0.1
Stockwell & Co., Tesco*	½ Can/200g	162	1.6	81	3.1	15.3	0.8	0
Strawberry, Muller*	1 Pot/180g	191	4	106	3	18.6	2.2	0
Tesco*	1 Can/400g	376	6.8	94	3.1	16.3	1.7	0.6
Vanilla Custard, Mullerrice, Muller*	1 Pot/200g	230	5	115	3.4	19.8	2.5	0.3
RICE WINE								
Sake, Average	*1 Tbsp/15ml*	*20*	*0*	*134*	*0.5*	*5*	*0*	*0*

R

	Measure INFO/WEIGHT	per Measure KCAL	FAT	Nutrition Values per 100g / 100ml KCAL	PROT	CARB	FAT	FIBRE
RIGATONI								
Dry, Average	**1 Serving/80g**	**272**	**1.2**	**340**	**11.4**	**68.4**	**1.5**	**2.7**
RISOTTO								
aux Asperges, Vertes, Frozen, Picard*	½ Pack/250g	308	11	123	3.1	17	4.4	0.6
Balls, Green Vegetable, & Mozzarella, Sainsbury's*	1 Ball/50g	126	6.4	252	6.8	26	12.7	3
Butternut Squash, Free From, Sainsbury's*	1 Pack/400g	381	14.1	95	1.4	13.5	3.5	2.1
Butternut Squash, Fresh Ideas, M Kitchen, Morrisons*	1 Pot/350g	371	11.9	106	1.8	16.8	3.4	0.7
Butternut Squash, Kale, & Spelt, Tesco*	1 Pack/361g	347	8.7	96	3.4	14.1	2.4	2.4
Cherry Tomato, & Basil, Napolina*	1 Serving/320g	285	10.6	89	1.8	12.4	3.3	0
Chicken	**1 Serving/380g**	**494**	**17.4**	**130**	**7.2**	**15.2**	**4.6**	**1.3**
Chicken, & Mushroom, for Two, Charlie Bigham's*	1 Serving/350g	556	26.2	159	7.2	15.8	7.5	0
Chicken, & Asparagus, COU, M&S*	1 Pack/360g	320	4.3	89	7.7	11.7	1.2	0.5
Chicken, & Chorizo, Italian Inspired, Asda*	1 Pack/390g	515	14	132	8.3	16	3.6	0.8
Chicken, & Chorizo, Super, Bachelors *	½ Pack/130g	178	2	137	4.2	26.4	1.5	0.7
Chicken, & Lemon, WW*	1 Pack/320g	330	3.5	103	6	17	1.1	1.2
Chicken, & Mushroom, BFY, M&S*	1 Pack/380g	407	10.3	107	8.8	11.4	2.7	0.9
Chicken, & Mushroom, Chef Select, Lidl*	1 Pack/333g	330	9	99	6.6	11.5	2.7	1
Chicken, & Mushroom, Extra Special, Asda*	1 Pack/400g	532	16	133	5.8	18	4	0.7
Chicken, & Mushroom, Italian Inspired, Asda*	1 Pack/373g	403	10.8	108	6.6	14	2.9	0.5
Chicken, & Mushroom, Meal for One, M&S*	1 Pack/400g	468	13.2	117	8.1	13.3	3.3	0.8
Chicken, & Mushroom, Portobello, Finest, Tesco*	1 Pack/372g	454	12.3	122	8	14.2	3.3	1.2
Chicken, & Roast Red Pepper, Beautifully Balanced, Tesco*	1 Pack/380g	312	6.1	82	5.4	10.9	1.6	1.1
Courgette, & Pea, Vegan, Waitrose*	½ Pack/187g	172	6.2	92	3.2	11	3.3	2.7
Crab, & Pea, Lemony, Box Ingredients Only, Gousto*	1 Serving/310g	493	10.9	159	7.3	24.6	3.5	2.2
Green Bean, Asparagus & Pecorino, Finest, Tesco*	1 Pack/400g	460	15.6	115	4.4	15	3.9	1.5
Haddock, & Leek One-Pot, Easy, Gousto*	1 Serving/425g	480	8.1	113	6.9	17.5	1.9	1.8
Haddock, Smoked, Finest, Tesco*	1 Pack/396g	412	8.7	104	5.6	15.1	2.2	1
Mediterranean Inspired, Calorie Controlled, Tesco*	1 Pack/350g	294	0.5	84	3.9	16.8	0.1	1.2
Mixed Pepper, & Chive, Box Ingredients Only, Gousto*	1 Serving/332g	485	8.6	146	4.4	26.1	2.6	2.1
Mushroom, Calorie Counted, Tesco*	1 Pack/365g	339	8.4	93	3.4	14	2.3	1.4
Mushroom, Creamy, Co-Op*	1 Pack/401g	497	20	124	4.2	15	5	0.6
Mushroom, HL, Tesco*	1 Pack/366g	339	8.3	93	3.4	14	2.3	1.4
Mushroom, Plant Based, Asda*	1 Pack/400g	448	15.6	112	2.2	16	3.9	1.8
Mushroom, Risotto, Cook*	1 Serving/340g	530	23.5	156	4.2	19.7	6.9	0
Mushroom, Three, Allplants*	1 Serving/378g	507	19.3	134	4.2	17	5.1	1.9
Prawn, COU, M&S*	1 Pack/350g	378	7.7	108	4.3	17.3	2.2	0.8
Prawn, Pea & Mint, King, M&S*	½ Pack/300g	405	18.6	135	3.8	15.9	6.2	0.9
Pumpkin, & Feta, Woolworths*	1 Serve/350g	430	18.2	123	3.2	15.1	5.2	0
Red Pepper, & Italian Cheese, Roasted, M&S*	1 Pack/400g	500	13.2	125	2.9	20.4	3.3	1
Red Pepper, with Herb Rolled Goats Cheese, Gousto*	1 Serving/335g	469	10	140	4.4	23.5	3	1.8
Roasted Pumpkin, Pre-Mix, Belladotti*	1 Serving/58g	209	1.6	361	7.4	72.3	2.7	0
Seafood, Youngs*	1 Pack/350g	424	13	121	4.5	17.4	3.7	0.1
Squash, Orzo, Sumptuous, Orzotto, Jamie Oliver*	½ Pack/125g	169	3.9	135	5	19	3.1	5.6
Vegetable, Average	**1oz/28g**	**41**	**1.8**	**147**	**4.2**	**19.2**	**6.5**	**2.2**
Vegetable, Brown Rice, Average	**1oz/28g**	**40**	**1.8**	**143**	**4.1**	**18.6**	**6.4**	**2.4**
Vert, Serves 1, At Home, Cote*	1 Pack/374g	606	32.9	162	4.1	15.9	8.8	1.5
with Mushroom, & Garlic, Cucina, Aldi*	1 Serving/200g	214	3	107	2.6	20	1.5	1
ROCK SALMON								
Raw, Flesh Only, Average	**1oz/28g**	**43**	**2.7**	**154**	**16.6**	**0**	**9.7**	**0**
ROCKET								
Fresh, Raw, Average	**1 Serving/80g**	**12**	**0.4**	**16**	**0.8**	**1.7**	**0.5**	**1.2**
ROE								
Cod, Average	**1 Can/100g**	**96**	**2.8**	**96**	**17.1**	**0.5**	**2.8**	**0**
Cod, Hard, Coated in Batter, Fried	**1oz/28g**	**53**	**3.3**	**189**	**12.4**	**8.9**	**11.8**	**0.2**

R

	Measure INFO/WEIGHT	per Measure KCAL	FAT	Nutrition Values per 100g / 100ml KCAL	PROT	CARB	FAT	FIBRE
ROE								
Cod, Hard, Fried in Blended Oil	**1oz/28g**	**57**	**3.3**	**202**	**20.9**	**3**	**11.9**	**0.1**
Herring, Soft, Fried in Blended Oil	**1oz/28g**	**74**	**4.4**	**265**	**26.3**	**4.7**	**15.8**	**0.2**
Herring, Soft, Raw	**1oz/28g**	**22**	**0.1**	**78**	**18.2**	**0.5**	**0.4**	**0**
ROGAN JOSH								
Chicken, & Pilau Rice, Morrisons*	1 Pack/419g	528	13.8	126	7.4	15.2	3.3	2.9
Chicken, Breast, Chunks, Hot, Sainsbury's*	½ Pack/114g	143	2	126	23.6	3.9	1.8	1
Chicken, Munch*	1 Pack/197g	292	4.1	148	10.4	20.7	2.1	0
Chicken, with Pilau Rice, Farmfoods*	1 Pack/325g	354	6.8	109	5.3	17.1	2.1	0.4
Chickpea, & Kale, Tideford Organics*	1 Pot/300g	180	6.9	60	2.5	6.2	2.3	1.8
Lamb, Indian, Takeaway, CBY, Asda*	½ Pack/200g	218	12	109	8	5.1	6	1.4
Lamb, Indian, Waitrose*	½ Pack/175g	268	17.3	153	10	4.9	9.9	1.9
Lamb, Main for 2, Microwaved, Sainsbury's*	½ Pack/190g	230	11.4	121	12.4	3.6	6	1.6
Lamb, Sainsbury's*	1 Pack/400g	660	44.4	165	11.3	4.9	11.1	1.9
Lamb, Takeaway, Tesco*	½ Pack/192g	228	14	119	6.3	5.7	7.3	2.5
Prawn, COU, M&S*	1 Pack/400g	360	2.4	90	4.9	16.2	0.6	0.8
ROLL								
Bacon, Breakfast, Co-Op*	1 Roll/134g	355	11.7	265	17	29	8.7	1.8
Cheddar, & Onion Chutney, Veggie, Higgidy*	1 Roll/27g	93	5.5	345	8.6	33.3	20.4	1.6
Cheese, & Onion, Co-Op*	1 Roll/66g	195	11.9	295	7	26	18	2
Cheese, & Onion, Iceland*	1 Roll/67g	222	13.6	332	7.5	29.6	20.4	1.5
Cheese, & Onion, M&S*	1 Roll/25g	80	5.1	320	9.6	24.7	20.5	1.3
Cheese, & Onion, Tesco*	1 Roll/67g	203	12.1	305	7.3	28	18.1	1.9
Cheese, & Pickle, Sainsbury's*	1 Roll/136g	359	13.6	264	10.6	35.1	10	0
Cheese, & Bacon, Snack, Sainsbury's*	1 Roll/30g	95	5.3	318	9.9	28.5	17.8	2.4
Cheese, & Onion, Mini, Sainsbury's*	1 Roll/10g	29	1.5	292	6.9	30.6	15.4	1.9
Cheese, & Onion, Sainsbury's*	1 Roll/66g	190	9.8	288	6.9	30.6	14.8	2.5
Cornish, in Pastry, Pork Farms*	1 Roll/75g	226	15.1	301	6.6	24.5	20.1	0
Egg Mayo, & Cress, Fullfillers*	1 Roll/125g	266	11.8	213	10	25.7	9.4	0
Feta, & Red Pepper, Specially Selected, Aldi*	1 Roll/27g	103	6.7	387	8.9	31	25	3.3
Feta, & Red Pepper,, Veggie, Higgidy*	1 Roll/27g	97	6	360	9.3	32.3	22.3	2
Ham, & Salad, BGTY, Sainsbury's*	1 Roll/178g	292	3.4	164	10.8	25.9	1.9	0
Ham, & Salad, J D Gross, Lidl*	1 Roll/154g	293	9.2	190	7.7	29.1	6	1.9
Mushroom, Miso, Vegan, Higgidy*	1 Roll/27g	92	5.1	345	7.1	37.3	19	3.9
Ploughman's, Large, Ginsters*	1 Pack/140g	473	33.5	338	10.2	20.5	23.9	1.8
Pork, Stuffing, & Apple Sauce, Roast, Boots*	1 Roll/218g	602	26.2	276	10	32	12	1.8
Salmon, Oak Smoked, M&S*	1 Roll/55g	139	6.2	252	14.6	23.1	11.3	1.2
Sausage, Lincolnshire, COU, M&S*	1 Roll/175g	280	4.7	160	10	23.2	2.7	2.6
Tuna, Cheese Melt, Boots*	1 Roll/199g	612	35.8	308	13	23	18	1.2
Turkey, Salad, Northern Bites*	1 Roll/231g	323	8.3	140	8.6	19.6	3.6	3
Vegetable Samosa, & Mango Chutney, Vegan, Higgidy*	1 Roll/27g	86	4.7	318	4.9	36	17.4	2.7
ROLO								
Little, Nestle*	1 Pack/40g	196	9.4	491	4	65.5	23.5	0.5
Nestle*	1 Sweet/5g	24	1	478	4.4	68.2	20.4	1.1
ROOT BEER								
Average	**1 Can/330ml**	**135**	**0**	**41**	**0**	**10.6**	**0**	**0**
ROSEMARY								
Dried	**1 Tsp/1g**	**3**	**0.2**	**331**	**4.9**	**46.4**	**15.2**	**0**
Fresh	**1 Tsp/0.7g**	**1**	**0**	**99**	**1.4**	**13.5**	**4.4**	**0**
ROSTI								
Baskets, Vegetable Jalfrezi, Aldi*	1 Rosti/165g	279	12.1	169	3.2	21	7.3	2.2
Cheese, & Onion, Tesco*	1 Rosti/92g	202	10.9	220	5.1	21.6	11.9	3.2
Chicken, & Ham, The Best, Morrisons*	1 Pack/400g	496	20.8	124	7.8	11	5.2	1.1
Maris Piper & Onion, M&S*	1 Rosti/35g	77	4.2	219	1.9	24.7	12	2.4

R

	Measure INFO/WEIGHT	per Measure KCAL	FAT	Nutrition Values per 100g / 100ml KCAL	PROT	CARB	FAT	FIBRE
ROSTI								
Potato & Root Vegetable, COU, M&S*	1 Rosti/100g	85	2.7	85	1.6	13.3	2.7	1.5
Potato Cakes, Baby, M&S*	1 Rosti/23g	40	1.5	175	3.5	25.1	6.7	1.6
Potato, Fritters, Ikea*	1 Rosti/60g	68	1.2	114	2.9	19	2	0
Potato, McCain*	1 Rosti/95g	161	8.6	169	2.2	19.6	9.1	0
Sweet Potato, Tesco*	½ Pack/91g	258	16	283	2.7	26.2	17.6	4.4
ROULADE								
Chocolate, Finest, Tesco*	1 Serving/80g	222	4.5	277	3.4	53.2	5.6	2.3
Chocolate, Sainsbury's*	1 Serving/72g	264	15.7	367	5.7	36.9	21.8	1.8
Kir Royale, Boozy, Deluxe, Lidl*	1 Slice/73g	215	4.3	294	2.6	57.2	5.9	1
Peach, M&S*	1 Slice/47g	126	5.9	268	4.3	33.7	12.6	1.1
Turkey, with Pork, Leek, & Bacon Stuffing, M&S*	½ Pack/250g	382	14.5	153	20.6	4.4	5.8	0.3
RUM								
37.5% Volume	**1 Pub Shot/35ml**	**72**	**0**	**207**	**0**	**0**	**0**	**0**
40% Volume	**1 Pub Shot/35ml**	**78**	**0**	**222**	**0**	**0**	**0**	**0**
Clean R, Low Alcohol, 0.5%, Clean Co.*	1 Serve/50ml	12	0	24	0	5	0	0
Clean R, Low Alcohol, 1.2%, Clean Co.*	1 Serve/50ml	16	0	31	0	5	0	0
Malibu, 21% Volume, Pernod Ricard*	1 Pub shot/25ml	50	0	200	0	29	0	0
Non Alcoholic, STRYYK*	1 Serve/25ml	2	0	7	0	2.5	0	0
Spiced Gold, 28%, Captain Morgan*	1 Shot/25ml	50	0	201	0	1.3	0	0
Spiced, Original, 35%, Captain Morgan*	1 Shot/25ml	48	0	193	0	0.4	0	0
White	**1 Pub Shot/35ml**	**72**	**0**	**207**	**0**	**0**	**0**	**0**
RUSKS								
Reduced Sugar, Farleys *	1 Rusk/17g	70	1.5	409	7.9	73.8	8.5	2.8
Wheat, Crispy, Elite*	1 Rusk/10g	38	0.7	396	13.7	68.9	6.8	3.1

R

	Measure INFO/WEIGHT	per Measure KCAL	FAT	Nutrition Values per 100g / 100ml KCAL	PROT	CARB	FAT	FIBRE
SAAG								
Aloo, A Taste of India, Tesco*	½ Pack/150g	188	12.5	125	2.3	9.1	8.3	2.1
Aloo, M&S*	½ Pack/125g	121	7.1	97	1.6	8.7	5.7	2.1
Aloo, with Peas, Box Ingredients Only, Gousto*	1 Serving/382g	466	13.4	122	4.2	17.7	3.5	3.9
Chicken, Microwaved, Slimming World, Iceland*	1 Pack/500g	395	8	79	11.5	3.9	1.6	1.6
Chicken, Slim Choice, Sainsbury's*	1 Pack/476g	352	5.7	74	11.9	3.7	1.2	0.8
Chicken, SlimWell, Aldi*	1 Pack/480g	331	7.2	69	11	2.1	1.5	1.8
Chicken, with Gunpowder Potatoes, Tesco*	1 Pack/348g	369	15	106	6.7	8.3	4.3	3.9
Mixed Vegetable, Microwaved, Iceland*	1 Serving/379g	375	18.6	99	2.8	9.1	4.9	3.7
Paneer, Sainsbury's*	1 Pack/300g	441	32.7	147	7.1	3.9	10.9	2.5
Paneer, Tofu, Allplants*	1 Pack/361g	361	18.4	100	4.7	7.5	5.1	2.5
SAFFRON								
Average	**1 Tsp/1g**	**2**	**0**	**310**	**11.4**	**61.5**	**5.9**	**0**
SAGE								
Dried, Ground	**1 Tsp/1g**	**3**	**0.1**	**315**	**10.6**	**42.7**	**12.7**	**0**
Fresh	**1oz/28g**	**33**	**1.3**	**119**	**3.9**	**15.6**	**4.6**	**0**
SALAD								
3 Bean, with Mint Vinaigrette, M&S*	1 Pack/240g	278	10.6	116	6.5	5.3	4.4	14.8
Agretti, Raw, Average	**1 Serving/80g**	**14**	**0**	**17**	**1.8**	**2.2**	**0**	**2.3**
Alfresco, Sharing, Co-Op*	1 Serving/80g	21	0.4	26	1	4.6	0.5	0.9
Asian Inspired, Sainsbury's*	½ Pack/113g	98	6.8	87	1.9	4.9	6	3.2
Avocado, & Egg, Nourish Bowl, M&S*	1 Pack/285g	333	15.4	117	6.3	6.6	5.4	8.3
Avocado, & Feta, & Rice, Good to Go, Waitrose*	1 Pack/240g	350	13.4	146	3.4	18.4	5.6	4.1
Avocado, & Feta, Gourmet To Go, M&S*	1 Pack/320g	512	32	160	5.4	12.1	10	3.1
Avocado, & Feta, Side, Waitrose*	1 Pack/201g	285	17.5	142	4.4	10.3	8.7	2.6
Avocado, Feta, & Grain, M&S*	1 Pack/320g	531	28.8	166	5.5	13.9	9	3.6
Avocado, Kale, & Grains, Eat Well, M&S*	½ Pack/90g	108	4.5	120	4.3	11.9	5	5
Baby Leaf, & Beetroot, Bistro, M&S*	1 Pack/165g	41	0	25	2	3.6	0	2
Baby Leaf, & Rocket, Florette*	1 Serving/25g	5	0.1	20	2.1	0.9	0.5	2
Baby Leaf, & Rocket, Organic, Sainsbury's*	1 Pack/60g	9	0.3	15	1.8	1.1	0.5	1.6
Baby Leaf, Aldi*	1 Serving/50g	11	0	22	3.5	1	0.1	1.5
Baby Leaf, Italian Style, M&S*	1 Bag/65g	14	0.3	22	1.3	2.3	0.5	1.3
Baby Leaf, Peppery, Nature's Pick, Aldi*	1 Serving/75g	26	0.4	34	1.9	4.6	0.5	2.1
Baby Leaf, Seasonal, Morrisons*	½ Pack/50g	10	0.3	21	1.4	1.6	0.6	1.8
Babyleaf, Sainsbury's*	1 Pack/90g	17	0.4	19	1.7	1.7	0.5	1.1
Bean, Four, Sainsbury's*	½ Pot/125g	121	3.2	107	6.6	11.5	2.8	4.8
Bean, Mixed, Canned, in Vinaigrette, Sainsbury's*	½ Can/133g	144	1.1	108	6	16.7	0.8	5.1
Beet, Baby Leaf, & Seed, Salad Bowl, Bold, Morrisons*	½ Pack/85g	74	2.8	87	3.9	9.2	3.3	2.2
Beetroot, & Feta, Veggie Pot, Eat Well, M&S*	1 Pot/140g	182	10.5	130	4.4	8.9	7.5	4.7
Beetroot, & Lettuce, Asda*	1 Serving/30g	5	0	16	1.4	2.7	0	2.5
Beetroot, & Carrot, Baby Leaf, Morrisons*	½ Pack/60g	17	0.2	29	1.8	4	0.3	1.5
Beetroot, & Goats Cheese, Sainsbury's*	½ Pack/68g	72	4.9	106	5.1	4.5	7.2	1.2
Beetroot, & Tomato, Santini, M&S*	½ Pack/110g	58	1.8	53	1.3	7.8	1.6	1.1
Beetroot, Aldi*	1/3 Pot/100g	35	0.5	35	0.8	6.1	0.5	2.1
Beetroot, Baby Spinach, & Kale, Market St, Morrisons*	½ Pack/60g	14	0.2	24	2.6	1	0.3	3.6
Beetroot, Carrot, & Roasted Lentil, M&S*	1 Pack/230g	109	4.7	47	1.4	4.7	2	2.2
Beetroot, Goats Cheese, & Rocket, Tesco*	1 Pack/120g	72	3.4	60	2.7	5.3	2.8	1.4
Beetroot, Lambs Lettuce, & Red Chard, Bistro, Lidl*	1 Serving/80g	20	0.2	25	1.8	2.9	0.2	2.3
Beetroot, Lidl*	1 Serving/50g	30	0.4	59	1	11	0.8	2.1
Beetroot, Morrisons*	1 Tsp/10g	4	0	42	1.2	7	0.4	2.7
Beetroot, Rocket, & Feta, M&S*	1 Pack/140g	182	10.5	130	4.4	8.9	7.5	2.7
Beetroot, Rocket, & Feta, with Pumpkin Seeds, M&S*	1 Pot/140g	161	7.1	115	4.1	11.6	5.1	3.2
Beetroot, Tesco*	1 Tub/305g	143	2.7	47	1	7.7	0.9	2.2
Bistro, Asda*	1 Serving/180g	29	0	16	1.4	2.7	0	2.5

	Measure INFO/WEIGHT	per Measure KCAL	FAT	Nutrition Values per 100g / 100ml KCAL	PROT	CARB	FAT	FIBRE
SALAD								
Bistro, Florette*	1/3 Bag/46g	16	0.2	35	1.3	4.9	0.5	2.7
Bistro, Lidl*	1 Serving/160g	40	0.4	25	2.2	3.6	0.2	2.9
Black Quinoa, Asian Style, with Ponzu Dressing, Waitrose*	½ Pack/80g	110	3.1	138	4.3	19.8	3.9	3.3
Bowl, Essential, Waitrose*	1 Pack/330g	92	1.6	28	1.3	3.6	0.5	1.8
Broccoli, & Peanut, Finest, Tesco*	½ Pack/105g	196	9.2	187	6.9	18.4	8.8	3.3
Burrito, BBQ, Bowl, Allplants*	½ Pack/380g	543	12.2	143	4.2	21	3.2	5.3
Burrito, Specially Selected, Aldi*	1 Pot/220g	288	9.5	131	2.2	19	4.3	2.9
Butterhead, & Spinach, Waitrose*	½ Pack/70g	15	0.4	22	1.7	1.5	0.6	1.7
Butternut, Roasted, & Broccoli, M&S*	½ Pack/160g	160	6.2	100	2.9	11.9	3.9	2.6
Cabbage, with Green Peppers, Eridanous, Lidl*	1 Serving/100g	112	4.5	112	1	15	4.5	2.3
Caesar	**1 Serving/200g**	**352**	**27.8**	**176**	**4.8**	**8.1**	**13.9**	**0.7**
Caesar, Chicken, Shapers, Boots*	1 Pack/200g	205	5.8	102	8.2	10	2.9	1
Caesar, Kit, Tesco*	1 Pack/262g	404	31.7	154	3.4	7.3	12.1	1.2
Caesar, Kit, Waitrose*	1 Bag/250g	436	36.1	174	4.4	6.1	14.4	1.3
Caesar, M&S*	½ Pack/125g	214	15.9	171	4.2	9.2	12.7	1.3
Caesar, with Dressing, Croutons & Parmesan, M&S*	1 Serving/115g	190	15.5	165	4.3	6.4	13.5	1.4
Cauli-Caesar, Chargrilled, BOL Foods*	1 Jar/280g	356	17.6	127	3.7	12.7	6.3	2.4
Chciken, Oriental, Bowl, Tweakd*	1 Pack/260g	271	11.8	104	9.2	6.2	4.5	1.5
Cheese, & Onion, Market St, Morrisons*	1 Pack/260g	330	19.8	127	4.6	9.3	7.6	1.6
Chicken Caesar, with Caesar Dressing, Tesco*	1 Pack/185g	337	20	182	11.5	9.1	10.8	1.4
Chicken, & Mango, Spicy, Lidl*	1 Serving/260g	99	1.3	38	5	3.8	0.5	1.4
Chicken, Bacon, & Pasta, Caesar, Morrisons*	1 Pack/183g	307	14.6	168	10.3	13.3	8	0.8
Chicken, Bang Bang, The City Kitchen*	1 Pack/250g	352	12.7	141	7.5	15.8	5.1	1.1
Chicken, BBQ, Cobb, Eat Well, M&S*	1 Pack/305g	311	14.6	102	10	4.2	4.8	0
Chicken, Caesar, Chargrilled, Eat & Go, Aldi*	1 Pack/175g	294	16.4	168	12	8.9	9.4	1.2
Chicken, Chargrilled, High Protein, M&S*	1 Pack/270g	243	10	90	7.6	5	3.7	3.1
Chicken, Fajita, Naked, Inspired Cuisine, Aldi*	1 Pack/370g	426	6.7	115	8.5	15.4	1.8	1.4
Chicken, Harissa, & Grain, Eat & Go, Aldi*	1 Pack/242g	358	13.3	148	9.2	14	5.5	2.3
Chicken, Katsu, & Sticky Rice, M&S*	1 Pack/270g	367	11.3	136	6.4	17.7	4.2	0.8
Chicken, Mexican Inspired, Aldi*	1 Pack/230g	294	14	128	7	10	6.1	2.7
Chicken, Nourish Bowl, On the Go, Sainsbury's*	1 Pack/282g	415	23.1	147	8.4	8	8.2	4.1
Chicken, Piri Piri, Rice, & Bean, Waitrose*	1 Pack/176g	155	4	88	7.1	8.8	2.3	1.7
Chicken, Red Thai Style, Eat Well, M&S*	1 Pack/275g	264	12.4	96	5.6	6.1	4.5	4.4
Chicken, Spiced, & Mango, Asda*	1 Pack/225g	133	4	59	4.4	5.1	1.8	2.3
Chickpea, & Bean, Dahl, Waitrose*	½ Pack/95g	145	5.1	153	5.6	17.3	5.4	6.4
Chickpea, Curried, Asda*	1 Pack/230g	251	6	109	5.4	14	2.6	4.9
Chickpea, Dhal, Morrisons*	¼ Pack/53g	71	2.9	134	5.3	13.7	5.5	4
Classic, Asda*	1 Pack/185g	46	0.9	25	1.2	2.7	0.5	3.4
Coleslaw, Deli Style, Waitrose*	½ Pack/110g	99	8.1	90	1.1	4.5	7.4	1
Corn, Smokey Charred, Waitrose*	½ Pack/113g	108	2.6	96	2.7	15	2.3	2.4
Cous Cous, & Vegetable, Roasted, Waitrose*	1 Pack/220g	396	13.4	180	5.1	26.1	6.1	1.2
Cous Cous, Beetroot, & Feta, Asda*	1 Pack/275g	272	10.4	99	4	12	3.8	1.3
Cous Cous, Feta, The Deli, Aldi*	1 Pot/220g	323	16.1	147	3.3	16	7.3	1.5
Crayfish, & Mango, Sainsbury's*	1 Pack/310g	329	6.5	106	4.1	17	2.1	1.2
Crisp, Mixed, Morrisons*	1 Pack/230g	39	0.7	17	1	2.8	0.3	0
Crisp, Mixed, Tesco*	1 Pack/200g	40	0.6	20	1.1	3.2	0.3	2
Crunchy, & Crisp, Asda*	1 Pack/250g	55	1.5	22	0.8	3.3	0.6	1.4
Crunchy, Side, Florette*	1 Serving/80g	25	0.4	31	1.1	4	0.5	3.1
Deli, with New Potatoes, & Mustard Mayonnaise, M&S*	1 Pack/295g	298	18.6	101	6.4	3.5	6.3	2.4
Duck, & Herb, Crispy, M&S*	½ Pack/140g	378	25.6	270	20.7	3.7	18.3	1.4
Edamame, & Petit Pois, Finest, Tesco*	½ Pack/100g	108	4.3	108	6	9.3	4.3	3.9
Edamame, & Greens, Finest, Tesco*	1 Pack/200g	240	11	120	7.3	8.6	5.5	3.5
Edamame, & Sprouting Pea, Finest, Tesco*	1 Serving/100g	136	5.7	136	7.6	11.4	5.7	4.4

S

SALAD

INFO/WEIGHT	Measure	per Measure KCAL	FAT	Nutrition Values per 100g / 100ml KCAL	PROT	CARB	FAT	FIBRE
Edamame, Asda*	½ Pack/110g	90	3.3	82	5.9	4.8	3	5.9
Edamame, Rainbow, M&S*	½ Pack/85g	62	3.1	73	5.2	3.7	3.6	2.7
Egg, & Ham, with Salad Cream Dressing, M&S*	1 Pack/240g	149	7.2	62	4.9	3.2	3	1.2
Egg, & Spinach, Baby, Waitrose*	1 Pack/215g	167	13.5	78	3.5	1.8	6.3	1
Egg, & Avocado, Free Range, M&S*	1 Pack/225g	268	14.4	119	6.9	7.4	6.4	2.3
Egg, & Avocado, Grains, Waitrose*	1 Pack/260g	351	16.1	135	5.3	13.1	6.2	2.9
Egg, & Spinach, High Protein, M&S*	1 Pot/105g	130	8.1	124	11.9	1.7	7.7	0.5
Egg, Free Range, & Bacon, Side, Eat Well, M&S*	1 Pack/205g	242	16.2	118	9.8	1.6	7.9	0.6
English Garden, Tesco*	1 Serving/180g	22	0.4	12	0.7	1.8	0.2	0.7
Falafel, & Vegetables, with Tabbouleh, M&S*	1 Pack/335g	385	19.4	115	3.5	10.7	5.8	3.1
Falafel, & Rice, Mexican Inspired, Plant Chef, Tesco*	1 Pack/235g	256	5.9	109	4.2	15.5	2.5	3.8
Falafel, Bulgur Wheat & Houmous, Eat Well, M&S*	1 Pack/300g	375	15.3	125	4.1	13.2	5.1	4.8
Feta, & Sunblushed Tomato, M&S*	1 Serving/190g	361	21.1	190	5.5	17.2	11.1	2.1
Feta, & Beetroot, Co-Op*	1 Pack/250g	312	12.3	125	5.3	13	4.9	2.8
Feta, Tomato, & Olive, Amazon Fresh*	1 Pack/271g	260	19.5	96	3.2	4.3	7.2	0.7
Fine Cut, Sweet & Crunchy, Asda*	1 Serving/80g	25	0.4	31	1.1	3.9	0.5	4.4
Goats Cheese, & Lentil, M&S*	1 Pack/215g	316	10.3	147	6.9	17.4	4.8	3.3
Grain Bowl, Spiced Squash, Allplants*	1 Serving/370g	392	12.2	106	3.3	15	3.3	2.6
Grain, Mixed, Courgette, & Pea, Waitrose *	½ Pack/150g	242	6.8	161	4.8	23.8	4.5	2.9
Grain, Mixed, Deluxe, Lidl*	1 Pack/215g	275	9.2	128	4.1	15.3	4.3	5.8
Grain, Triple, Tesco*	1 Pack/225g	212	1.4	94	3.7	17.2	0.6	2.7
Grains, & Greens, Plant Kitchen, M&S*	½ Pack/145g	180	2.3	124	6.4	17.5	1.6	6.8
Greek	**1oz/28g**	**36**	**3.5**	**130**	**2.7**	**1.9**	**12.5**	**0.8**
Green Bean, Aldi*	½ Pack/80g	62	2.7	77	4.6	5	3.4	3.9
Green, Average	**1oz/28g**	**4**	**0.1**	**13**	**0.8**	**1.8**	**0.3**	**0.9**
Green, Mixed, Average	**1 Serving/100g**	**12**	**0.3**	**12**	**0.7**	**1.8**	**0.3**	**1**
Ham Hock, & Piccalilli, Waitrose*	1 Pack/240g	257	7.4	107	4.7	14	3.1	2.3
Ham Hock, Ploughmans, Waitrose*	1 Pack/185g	170	8.1	92	7.1	5.4	4.4	0.9
Ham, & Egg, Free Range, G&B, Asda*	1 Pack/250g	150	6.2	60	5.3	3.1	2.5	1.9
Hipster, Wicked Kitchen, Tesco*	½ Pack/100g	146	7.9	146	2.8	14	7.9	3.8
House, Bowl, Sainsbury's*	¼ Pack/83g	67	3.5	81	1.7	8.5	4.2	1.5
House, Side, Tesco*	1 Pack/120g	24	0.4	20	1.2	2.4	0.3	1.4
Italian Style, Peppery, Meadow Fresh, Lidl*	1 Bag/160g	30	1.4	19	2.3	0.5	0.9	1.8
Italian, Meadow Fresh, Lidl*	1 Serving/80g	19	0.2	24	2	2.2	0.3	2.2
Italian, Strong & Peppery, Sainsbury's*	1 Serving/80g	18	0.4	22	2.5	1	0.5	1.8
Italian, Tomato, Balsamic, & Italian Cheese, Sainsbury's*	½ Pack/80g	56	3.6	70	3.3	3.6	4.5	0.8
Italian, with Pesto Dressing, Tesco*	½ Pack/128g	205	14.9	160	6.8	6.1	11.6	1.9
Italiana, Freshcoolis*	1 Bag/100g	25	0.1	25	1.6	3.4	0.1	1.8
Katsu Inspired, Power Bowl, Plant Menu, Aldi*	1 Bowl/380g	361	8	95	3	14	2.1	3.1
King Prawn, & Mango, Bowl, Tesco*	1 Pack/228g	153	5	67	4.3	6.3	2.2	2.1
Lambs Lettuce, Sainsbury's*	1 Serving/80g	12	0.4	15	1.7	0.6	0.5	0.7
Large, Bowl, Sainsbury's*	1/6 Pack/52g	12	0.2	23	0.9	4.3	0.3	1.1
Lean & Green, Pure*	1 Salad/320g	278	14.7	87	6.8	4.4	4.6	1.6
Leaves, Meadow Fresh, Lidl*	1 Serving/80g	25	0.2	31	2.4	3.4	0.3	2.3
Leaves, Mixed, Little Leaves*	½ Bag/63g	12	0.3	19	2.5	1.2	0.5	1.8
Lettuce, Lambs, & Pea Shoot, Good Health, Waitrose*	1 Bag/100g	21	0.5	21	1.9	1.3	0.5	1.7
Mediterranean Style, Bowl, with Dressing, Sainsbury's*	1 Pack/155g	67	1.9	43	1.1	6	1.2	1.8
Mediterranean, Style, Asda*	½ Pack/135g	22	0	16	1	3	0	0
Mixed Leaf, Medley, Waitrose*	1 Serving/25g	4	0.1	15	0.8	1.7	0.5	1.4
Mixed Leaf, Tesco*	1 Serving/20g	3	0.1	14	0.9	1.6	0.4	0.9
Mixed Leaf, Tomato & Olive, Tesco*	1 Serving/170g	150	13.3	88	1	3.4	7.8	2
Mixed Leaf, with Beetroot, Earthy, Waitrose*	1 Bag/140g	34	0.6	24	1.5	3.6	0.4	2.1
Mixed Leaves, Carrot, Tomatoes, & Cucumber, Co-Op*	½ Pack/80g	22	0.6	27	1	3.7	0.7	0.9

SALAD

INFO/WEIGHT	Measure	per Measure KCAL	FAT	Nutrition Values per 100g / 100ml KCAL	PROT	CARB	FAT	FIBRE
Mixed Rice, Tesco*	1 Pack/215g	198	0.9	92	2.3	18.9	0.4	1.7
Mixed, Bowl, Waitrose*	¼ Pack/64g	9	0.3	14	0.8	1.6	0.5	1.4
Mixed, Medley, Bowl, Waitrose*	¼ Pack/60g	9	0.3	15	0.9	1.7	0.5	1
Mixed, Sweet & Crispy, Tesco*	1 Serving/200g	48	0.6	24	1	4.2	0.3	2
Mozzarella, Garden, Co-Op*	1 Pack/230g	204	13	89	4.8	4.1	5.6	1.6
New Potato, Tuna, & Egg, M&S*	1 Pack/340g	255	12.9	75	3.8	6.7	3.8	0.7
Noodle, Chicken, Hoisin, Well & Good, Co-Op*	1 Pack/244g	288	7.8	118	8.3	13	3.2	1.2
Noodle, Chicken, Sweet Chilli, Asda*	1 Pack/250g	268	5.2	107	7.3	14	2.1	1.2
Noodle, Coconutty, Meal for One, M&S*	1 Pack/300g	366	14.4	122	2.9	15.7	4.8	2
Noodle, Prawn, Sesame, M&S*	1 Pack/220g	242	8.1	110	5.6	12.9	3.7	1.5
Noodle, Slaw, Bang Bang, M&S*	1 Pack/180g	211	9.2	117	4.2	12.5	5.1	2.3
Octopus, Drained, Medusa*	1 Serving/100g	163	11	163	15	1.6	11	0
Onion Bhaji, & Rice, Beautifully Balanced, Tesco*	1 Pack/255g	309	8.7	121	4.1	16.8	3.4	3.4
Pea Shoot, & Baby Leaf, Sainsbury's*	1 Serving/80g	20	0.4	25	3	1.6	0.5	0.8
Pea Shoot, Mild, Asda*	1 Serving/80g	20	0.4	25	2.5	2.4	0.5	2.1
Pea Shoot, Oaklands, Lidl*	1 Pack/80g	23	0.7	29	3.3	0.9	0.9	2
Ploughmans, Pot, M&S*	1 Pot/170g	301	21.8	177	5.2	8.8	12.8	2.8
Poke, King Prawn, Taiko Foods*	1 Bowl/293g	331	10	113	3.8	15.9	3.4	1.4
Polish, Dega*	1 Serving/80g	119	7.7	149	1.7	13	9.6	0
Potato, Baby, & Free Range Egg, Asda*	1 Pack/270g	159	7.6	59	1.9	5.9	2.8	1.2
Potato, Jersey Royal, Pea, & Mint, M&S*	½ Pack/125g	112	4	90	2.3	11.5	3.2	2.9
Protein Power Bowl, Allplants*	1 Serving/421g	530	21.5	126	6.3	12	5.1	3.4
Purple Grain, Nourish, Morrisons*	½ Pack/118g	126	3.2	107	3.2	15.4	2.7	4
Quinoa, & Kale, Supergreen, Asda*	½ Pot/135g	232	10	172	6.4	16	7.4	8.9
Quinoa, & Supergreen, Eat Well, M&S*	1 Pack/180g	180	10.4	100	4.3	5	5.8	5.3
Quinoa, Tomato, Red Pepper, & Mango, Lidl*	1 Pot/210g	191	4.2	91	2.6	14.1	2	2.5
Rainbow, Feta, & Beetroot, Layered, M&S*	1 Pack/265g	339	18	128	4.2	10.3	6.8	4.3
Rainbow, Morrisons*	½ Bowl/72g	20	0.1	27	1.4	3.7	0.2	2.5
Rainbow, Nature's Pick, Aldi*	½ Pack/75g	21	0.4	28	1.1	3.9	0.5	1.5
Rainbow, Side, Waitrose*	1 Pack/120g	30	0.6	25	1.4	3.2	0.5	2
Rainbow, Tesco*	¼ Pack/80g	21	0.2	26	1.2	3.8	0.2	1.9
Ranch, Kit, Morrisons*	¼ Pack/73g	107	7.1	147	4.7	9.2	9.7	1.8
Ribbon, Asda*	1 Pack/115g	33	0.6	29	1.6	4.3	0.5	0.5
Rice Bowl, Smoked Salmon, Teriyaki, Boots*	1 Pack/195g	308	8.4	158	5.4	24	4.3	1.4
Rice Noodle, The Deli, Aldi*	1/3 Pack/62g	62	2.7	101	1.4	12.2	4.4	3.1
Rocket, & Parmesan, Wild, Italian, Sainsbury's*	1 Serving/50g	88	7.4	177	7.5	3.4	14.8	0.5
Romaine, Premium, Marketside*	1 Serving/80g	14	0	18	1.2	3.5	0	2.4
Root Vegetable, & Grains, Co-Op*	½ Pack/150g	148	4.5	99	3.3	13.3	3	3.1
Rose Verde, Side, M&S*	½ Pack/80g	16	0.3	20	1	2.4	0.4	1.3
Rose Verde, Side, M&S*	½ Pack/80g	16	0.3	20	1	2.4	0.4	1.3
Rose Verde, Side, M&S*	½ Pack/80g	16	0.3	20	1	2.4	0.4	1.3
Salmon, Honey & Ginger, G&B, Asda*	1 Pack/380g	445	11	117	6.1	15	2.9	2.8
Salmon, Lime, & Miso, with Sticky Rice, M&S*	1 Pack/285g	396	13.4	139	5.3	18.2	4.7	1.4
Salmon, Moroccan Style, Light Lunch, John West*	1 Pack/220g	299	11.7	136	11.7	8.8	5.3	3.4
Salmon, Oak Smoked, Aldi*	1 Pack/129g	254	5.8	197	5	8.6	4.5	1.3
Salmon, Scandi, Bowl, Tweakd*	1 Pack/300g	442	32.4	147	6.3	5	10.8	2
Side, Garden, with Cherry Tomatoes, Waitrose*	1 Pack/170g	25	0.7	15	0.8	2	0.4	1.3
Side, Simple, with Dressing, Tesco*	½ Pack/83g	69	5.4	83	1.2	4.2	6.5	1.6
Side, Sweet & Crisp, Tesco*	1 Pack/128g	65	2.4	51	3.7	3.9	1.9	1.6
Simple, Bowl, Sainsbury's*	1 Bowl/130g	26	0.6	20	1.2	3	0.5	1.2
Simple, Bowl, Tesco*	1 Bowl/135g	32	0.4	24	1.3	2.9	0.3	2.1
Simple, with Sour Cream, & Chive, Tesco*	1 Pack/165g	139	10.9	84	1.2	4.2	6.6	1.5
Slaw, Apple, Celery, & Walnut, M&S*	½ Pack/100g	171	13.5	171	2.1	9.4	13.5	1.8

	Measure INFO/WEIGHT	per Measure		Nutrition Values per 100g / 100ml				
		KCAL	FAT	KCAL	PROT	CARB	FAT	FIBRE
SALAD								
Slaw, Rainbow, Japanese, BOL Foods*	1 Jar/300g	279	6.3	93	4.2	12.9	2.1	3.1
Super Green, M&S*	1 Pack/190g	167	7.4	88	5.1	6.7	3.9	3
Super Zucca, with Chicken, Zizzi*	1 Serving	693	25	693	50	53	25	0
Superbowl, Tweakd*	1 Serving/580g	710	30.2	122	3.3	13.6	5.2	2.4
Superfood, Punchy, Nourish, Morrisons*	½ Pack/50g	10	0.2	21	2.4	1.1	0.3	2.3
Sweet & Crispy, M&S*	1 Serving/140g	49	1.4	35	1.7	4.7	1	1.6
Sweet & Crisp, Asda*	1 Serving/80g	26	0.4	32	1.5	4.4	0.5	2.3
Sweet & Crispy, Bowl, Sainsbury's*	½ Pack/110g	118	11.2	107	1	2	10.2	1.8
Sweet & Crunchy, Bowl, Sainsbury's*	¼ Pack/85g	42	0.6	49	1.6	8.2	0.7	2
Sweet & Crunchy, Side, Eat Well, M&S*	1 Pack/145g	48	0.9	33	1.5	4.3	0.6	2.3
Sweet Leaf, Fully Prepared, Fresh, Sainsbury's*	¼ Pack/75g	12	0.1	16	0.8	3	0.1	2.1
Sweet Pepper, Market St, Morrisons*	1 Pack/140g	41	0.4	29	0.9	4.5	0.3	2.2
Sweet Potato, & Red Pepper, Deli, M&S*	1 Serving/250g	113	5.6	45	0.8	5.6	2.2	0.9
Sweet Potato, Piri Piri, & Qunioa, M&S*	1 Pack/200g	278	9.4	139	4	17	4.7	6.3
Sweet Potato, Skinny, M&S*	1 Serving/70g	69	2.9	99	2	12	4.2	2.6
Sweet, & Crunchy, Co-Op*	1 Pack/160g	27	1.1	17	1	3.7	0.7	0.9
Tabbouleh, & Dill Carrot, Pickled, Waitrose*	1 Pack/299g	266	11.4	89	3	8.7	3.8	3.8
Tabbouleh, Aldi*	1 Serving/70g	42	1	60	0	1.1	1.4	0
Tomato, & Mozzarella, Waitrose*	1 Pack/180g	313	25.7	174	6.4	3.9	14.3	1.8
Tomato, & Onion	**1oz/28g**	**20**	**1.7**	**72**	**0.8**	**4**	**6.1**	**1**
Tomato, Cherry, Tesco*	1 Pack/210g	136	9.4	65	0.9	4.2	4.5	1.1
Tuna, & Potato, Beautifully Balanced, Tesco*	1 Pack/258g	124	1.8	48	5.7	3.6	0.7	2.1
Tuna, Bowl, Fresh, Asda*	1 Serving/160g	184	11.2	115	8	5	7	0
Tuna, French Style, Light Lunch, John West*	1 Pack/220g	218	6.2	99	7.5	9.8	2.8	2.5
Tuna, French, Fisherman*	1 Tin/230g	317	14	138	8.9	10.2	6.1	0
Tuna, Italian Style, Light Lunch, John West*	1 Pack/220g	205	5.7	93	7.3	9.8	2.6	0.5
Tuna, Mediterranean Style, Light Lunch, John West*	1 Pack/220g	211	4.2	96	8.5	10	1.9	2.4
Tuna, Mediterranean Style, Nixe, Lidl*	1 Pack/220g	254	5.5	116	10	12	2.5	2.8
Tuna, Mexican Style, Lunch On The Go, John West*	1 Pack/252g	290	5.5	115	9.7	13	2.2	2
Tuna, Mexican Style, Nixe, Lidl*	1 Pack/220g	277	9	126	10.6	11.5	4.1	0.5
Tuna, with Pickled Cucumber, Mr Freed's*	½ Pack/63g	190	16.7	301	15.4	0.4	26.5	0
Tuna, with Rice, Nixe, Lidl*	1 Pack/220g	308	14.3	140	8.9	11.3	6.5	0.5
Tuna, with Spicy Tomato Sauce, Jane Plan*	1 Pack/220g	224	7	102	7	10	3.2	2.8
Vegetable, Mixed, without Dressing, From Restaurant	**1 ½ Cups/207g**	**33**	**0.1**	**16**	**1.2**	**3.2**	**0.1**	**2.1**
Vitality Mix, Superfood, Florette*	½ Bag/60g	14	0	23	1.8	1.7	0	2.3
Waldorf, Average	**1 Serving/100g**	**193**	**17.7**	**193**	**1.4**	**7.5**	**17.7**	**1.3**
Watercress, Spinach & Rocket, Prepared , Tesco*	½ Pack/40g	10	0.3	26	2.5	1.1	0.8	2
Watercress, Spinach & Rocket, Waitrose*	1 Bag/145g	30	1.2	21	2.2	1.2	0.8	1.5
Watercress, Spinach, & Rocket, Meadow Fresh, Lidl*	½ Bag/40g	10	0.2	24	2.5	1.5	0.5	1.8
Wheatberries, Lentils, & Green Vegetables, Waitrose*	½ Pack/150g	218	7	145	5.9	16.5	4.7	6.4
Wheatberry, & Grains, Lidl*	1 Serving/108g	176	6.7	164	5.5	22.1	6.2	4.9
Wholefood, Super Nutty, M&S*	1 Pack/200g	330	17.4	165	6.6	12.8	8.7	4.7
SALAD CREAM								
Average	**1 Tbsp/15g**	**50**	**4.2**	**335**	**1.7**	**18.6**	**27.8**	**0.1**
Free From, Tesco*	1 Tbsp/15g	31	2.2	205	0.7	16.6	15	0.3
Reduced Calorie, Average	**1 Tbsp/15g**	**19**	**1.2**	**130**	**1**	**12.9**	**7.9**	**0.2**
Vegan, GranoVita*	1 Tbsp/15g	37	3.4	247	0.9	9.9	22.6	0
Vegan, Heinz*	1 Tbsp/15g	45	3.5	299	0.9	20.5	23.1	0
SALAD DRESSING								
Caesar, Vegan, Plant Menu, Aldi*	1 Tbsp/15ml	65	6.8	432	0.8	5	45	1.1
Chilli & Lime, Heinz*	1 Tbsp/15ml	24	2.1	163	0.4	7.5	14.6	0
Garlic, & Herb, Creamy, Knorr*	1 Tbsp/15ml	22	2	148	0.1	7	13.2	0.1
Greek, Light, Knorr*	1 Tbsp/15ml	9	0.6	61	0.1	5	4.2	0.3

S

	Measure INFO/WEIGHT	per Measure KCAL	FAT	Nutrition Values per 100g / 100ml KCAL	PROT	CARB	FAT	FIBRE
SALAD DRESSING								
Maple, & Mustard, Dunnes Stores*	1 Tbsp/15ml	53	4.8	356	0.9	15	32	0.9
Soy, Sesame, & Ginger, Susan's*	1 Tbsp/15ml	9	0.9	60	0	1	6	0
SALAMI								
Average	**1 Slice/5g**	**18**	**1.3**	**360**	**28.4**	**1.8**	**26.2**	**0**
Calabrian, Salsiccia, Piccante, No.1, Waitrose*	1 Serving/30g	117	8.8	390	30.3	0.5	29.5	0.7
Danish, Average	**1 Serving/17g**	**89**	**8.8**	**524**	**13.2**	**1.3**	**51.7**	**0**
German, Average	**1 Serving/60g**	**200**	**16.4**	**333**	**20.3**	**1.6**	**27.3**	**0.1**
German, Peppered, Average	**3 Slices/25g**	**86**	**6.8**	**342**	**22.2**	**2.5**	**27.1**	**0.2**
Milano, Average	**1 Serving/70g**	**278**	**22.6**	**397**	**25.9**	**0.9**	**32.2**	**0**
Milano, Italian, Reduced Fat, M&S*	1 Slice/5g	13	0.7	252	30	0.5	14.4	0.1
Napoli, Average	**1 Slice/5g**	**17**	**1.3**	**342**	**27.1**	**0.8**	**25.5**	**0**
SALMON								
Chestnut Smoked, Scottish, No.1, Waitrose*	½ Pack/50g	88	4.6	176	22.8	0.6	9.1	0.5
Cooked, Prepacked, Average	**1 Fillet/93g**	**180**	**11.1**	**194**	**21.8**	**0**	**11.9**	**0**
Fillet, Hot Smoked, Honey Roast, Market St, Morrisons*	1 Fillet/90g	273	18.9	303	24.3	4	21	0.3
Fillet, Sockeye, Wild Caught, Finest, Tesco*	1 Fillet/106g	176	7.8	166	24.3	0.1	7.4	0.7
Fillets, Boneless, Skin-On, Fresh, Cooked, Average	**1 Sm Fillet/120g**	**265**	**17.1**	**221**	**23.2**	**0.2**	**14.2**	**0.1**
Fillets, Hot Smoked, Sweet Chilli, Waitrose*	1 Fillet/72g	178	9.9	247	26.2	4.5	13.8	0.5
Fillets, Hot Smoked, Teriyaki, M&S*	1 Fillet/90g	209	12.2	232	21	6.5	13.5	0.5
Fillets, in Teriyaki Marinade, Good Health, Waitrose*	1 Fillet/91g	176	9.2	193	23	2.1	10.1	0.9
Fillets, Lightly Smoked, Scottish, Waitrose*	1 Serving/175g	382	26.6	218	18.7	1.3	15.2	0.6
Fillets, Raw, Average	**1 Sm Fillet/120g**	**227**	**14**	**189**	**20.9**	**0.1**	**11.7**	**0.1**
Fillets, Raw, Skin-On, Average	**1 Avg Fillet/120g**	**214**	**13.9**	**179**	**18.3**	**0.2**	**11.6**	**0.2**
Fillets, Red Thai Marinade, Infused, Fishmonger, Aldi*	1 Fillet/110g	189	12.1	172	17	1.4	11	0.5
Fillets, Sweet Chilli, Hot Smoked, Ready to Eat, Tesco*	1 Fillet/90g	211	12.4	234	22.7	4.6	13.8	0.4
Fillets, Traditionally Smoked, Finest, Tesco*	1 Fillet/113g	226	13.3	200	23.4	0	11.8	0
Flakes, Honey Roast, Average	**1oz/28g**	**56**	**3**	**198**	**24**	**1.9**	**10.7**	**0.2**
Flakes, Sweet Chilli, M&S*	½ Pack/70g	143	4.6	204	24.5	11.7	6.6	0.6
Goujons, Average	**1 Pack/150g**	**321**	**16.4**	**214**	**16.4**	**12.4**	**11**	**1.1**
Gravadlax, Cured with Salt, Sugar & Herbs	**1 Serving/100g**	**119**	**3.3**	**119**	**18.3**	**3.1**	**3.3**	**0.4**
Grilled	**1oz/28g**	**60**	**3.7**	**215**	**24.2**	**0**	**13.1**	**0**
Hot Smoked, Average	**1 Serving/62g**	**103**	**4.4**	**166**	**24**	**0.9**	**7.2**	**0.1**
Mild Oak Smoked, Average	**1 Slice/25g**	**46**	**2.5**	**182**	**22.6**	**0.1**	**10.2**	**0**
Pink in Brine, Average	**1 Sm Can/105g**	**129**	**5.5**	**122**	**18.8**	**0**	**5.3**	**0**
Pink, Canned, Average	**1 Serving/125g**	**162**	**7.2**	**130**	**19.5**	**0.1**	**5.8**	**0.1**
Poached, Average	**1 Serving/90g**	**176**	**10.5**	**195**	**22.5**	**0.2**	**11.7**	**0.3**
Red in Brine, Average	**1oz/28g**	**42**	**2.2**	**149**	**19.7**	**0**	**7.8**	**0**
Red, Average	**½ Can/90g**	**141**	**7.4**	**156**	**20.4**	**0.1**	**8.2**	**0.1**
Ribbons, Oak Smoked, M&S*	1 Serving/100g	207	9.7	207	27.9	1.9	9.7	0.6
Smoked, Average	**1 Serving/70g**	**126**	**7**	**179**	**21.9**	**0.5**	**10**	**0.1**
Smoked, Infused with Lemon & Pepper, Fishmonger, Aldi*	½ Pack/50g	86	4.4	173	23	0.5	8.8	0.5
Smoked, Trimmings, Average	**1 Serving/55g**	**101**	**5.7**	**184**	**22.8**	**0.2**	**10.3**	**0**
Steaks	**1 Serving/100g**	**180**	**11**	**180**	**20.2**	**0**	**11**	**0**
Steamed	**1oz/28g**	**55**	**3.6**	**197**	**20.1**	**0**	**13**	**0**
SALMON EN CROUTE								
1322, Oakhouse Foods*	1 Serving/335g	874	58	261	8.6	16.8	17.3	1.6
Retail, Average	**1oz/28g**	**81**	**5.3**	**288**	**11.8**	**18**	**19.1**	**0**
Scottish, with Creamy Sauce, Oven Cooked, Sainsbury's*	1 En Croute/190g	608	39.1	320	10.8	22.5	20.6	0.9
SALSA								
Beetroot, Love Beets*	1 Serving/80g	75	0.2	94	1.2	20	0.3	2.9
Chipotle, Smokey, M&S*	¼ Pack/51g	37	0.4	73	1.8	13.2	0.8	3
Chunky, Sainsbury's*	½ Pot/84g	43	1.4	51	1.1	7.8	1.7	1.2
Cool, Sainsbury's*	¼ Pot/58g	30	1.2	52	1.4	6.3	2.1	1.1

S

	Measure INFO/WEIGHT	per Measure KCAL	FAT	Nutrition Values per 100g / 100ml KCAL	PROT	CARB	FAT	FIBRE
SALSA								
Fajita, Carrefour*	1 Tbsp/15g	6	0	42	1	8.5	0	1.2
Mild, Original, Old El Paso*	1 Sachet/144g	60	0.7	42	1.6	9	0.5	0
Original from Dinner Kit, Old El Paso*	1 Jar/226g	71	0.7	32	1.2	6	0.3	0
Red, Medium, M&S*	¼ Jar/49g	34	1.5	69	1.4	8.3	3	1.8
Spicy Mango & Lime, Morrisons*	½ Pot/85g	62	0.3	73	1	15.9	0.4	1.3
Spicy Red Pepper, Fresh, Waitrose*	½ Pot/85g	27	0.8	32	1.9	4.1	0.9	1.6
Tomato, & Mango, Holy Moly*	1 Serving/30g	20	0.1	68	1.3	14	0.2	0
Tomato, Chunky, Tesco*	1 Pot/170g	68	2.2	40	1.1	5.9	1.3	1.1
Tomato, Cool, Asda*	1 Pot/215g	84	1.1	39	1.4	6.4	0.5	1.5
Tomato, Onion, Coriander & Chilli, Fresh, Waitrose*	1 Tub/170g	110	5.3	65	1.3	8	3.1	1.2
Tomato, Sun Ripened, Tesco*	1 Serving/40g	46	1.7	115	5	14.2	4.2	4.6
SALT								
Alternative, Reduced Sodium, Losalt*	½ Tsp/1g	0	0	0	0	0	0	0
Kosher, Average	**1 Tsp/5g**	**0**	**0**	**0**	**0**	**0**	**0**	**0**
Rock, Average	**¼ Tsp/1g**	**0**	**0**	**0**	**0**	**0**	**0**	**0**
Table, Average	**1 Tsp/5g**	**0**	**0**	**0**	**0**	**0**	**0**	**0**
SAMBUCA								
Average	**1 Pub Shot/35ml**	**122**	**0**	**348**	**0**	**37.2**	**0**	**0**
SAMOSAS								
Chicken, Indian, Waitrose*	1 Samosa/50g	124	7.2	248	7.8	21	14.4	1.8
Chicken, Premier*	1 Slice/110g	272	14.3	247	5.9	25.7	13	0
Chicken, Tikka, Indian, Sainsbury's*	1 Samosa/55g	131	5.5	237	9.4	25	10	4.6
Indian Style Selection, Co-Op*	1 Samosa/21g	50	2.7	240	5	27	13	3
Lamb, Premier*	1 Slice/110g	260	11.8	236	6	28	10.7	0
Meat, Takeaway, Average	**1 Samosa/110g**	**299**	**19**	**272**	**11.4**	**18.9**	**17.3**	**2.4**
Punjabi, Cofresh*	1 Samosa/50g	81	5	162	2	16	10	3
Vegetable, Average	**1 Samosa/110g**	**258**	**12.8**	**235**	**4.8**	**26.9**	**11.6**	**2.5**
SANDWICH								
All Day Breakfast, Tesco Classic*	1 Pack/374g	636	29.9	170	8	14.5	8	3
Bacon, & Egg, Sainsbury's*	1 Pack/160g	384	17.8	240	13	22	11.1	1.8
Bacon, & Egg, Tesco*	1 Pack/213g	494	19.6	232	14.8	21.6	9.2	1.8
Bacon, Lettuce & Tomato, Select & Go, Lidl*	1 Pack/178g	368	12.8	207	11	23.1	7.2	2.7
Beef, & Pate, M&S*	1 Pack/188g	310	7.3	165	11.2	21.6	3.9	2.4
Beef, & Horseradish, Tesco*	1 Pack/175g	364	9.6	208	13.2	25.7	5.5	1.6
Beef, Med Rare, & Stilton, Finest, Tesco*	1 Pack/201g	461	15.3	229	13.5	25.8	7.6	1.9
BLT, Asda*	1 Pack/172g	325	11.9	189	9.9	21.8	6.9	4.6
BLT, Boots*	1 Pack/176g	371	11.6	211	10	26	6.6	2.8
BLT, Classic, Waitrose*	1 Pack/181g	347	13	192	9.1	21.5	7.2	2.2
BLT, on Fibre Enriched Bread, Co-Op*	1 Pack/182g	377	12.2	207	12	22	6.7	4.5
Brie, & Cranberry, Morrisons*	1 Pack/178g	438	20.3	246	10.4	24.4	11.4	2.2
Brie, & Grape, Finest, Tesco*	1 Pack/209g	527	31.6	252	8.5	20.6	15.1	1.5
Brie, & Bacon, with Chilli Relish, Waitrose*	1 Pack/219g	525	27.1	240	11.6	19.4	12.4	2.1
Cheddar, & Tomato, Red, Tesco*	1 Pack/165g	474	23.8	287	9.2	29.2	14.4	1.9
Cheddar, Cheese, Farmhouse, & Celery, M&S*	1 Pack/200g	482	25.4	241	11.1	19.4	12.7	2.1
Cheese & Onion, Spar*	1 Pack/147g	393	17.9	268	11.1	27.2	12.2	2.3
Cheese Triple, Tesco*	1 Pack/247g	630	29.6	255	8.8	26.8	12	2.1
Cheese, & Ham, Smoked, Co-Op*	1 Pack/167g	334	8.4	200	15	24	5	2
Cheese, & Onion, Tesco*	1 Pack/172g	505	28.3	294	10.2	24.5	16.5	3.3
Cheese, & Pickle, Tesco*	1 Pack/140g	400	19.3	286	12.7	27.8	13.8	1.4
Cheese, & Tomato, Co-Op*	1 Pack/155g	365	18.5	235	10.6	21.8	11.9	1.9
Cheese, & Tomato, Organic, M&S*	1 Pack/165g	559	35.3	339	11.8	24.8	21.4	1.9
Cheese, & Onion, Soft Oatmeal Bread, M&S*	1 Pack/170g	497	30.1	292	10.3	21.9	17.7	2.1
Cheese, & Pickle, On Malted Bread, Waitrose*	1 Pack/148g	433	21	293	12.3	27.6	14.2	2.7

S

SANDWICH

	Measure INFO/WEIGHT	per Measure KCAL	FAT	Nutrition Values per 100g / 100ml KCAL	PROT	CARB	FAT	FIBRE
Cheese, & Red Onion, Co-Op*	1 Pack/150g	411	21	274	11	24	14	2.7
Cheese, & Smoked Ham, Tesco*	1 Pack/167g	412	18	247	14.8	21.7	10.8	1.7
Cheese, Cheddar, on White, Asda*	1 Pack/147g	418	20.5	285	13	27	14	1.6
Chicken Salad, Deep Filled, Eat & Go, Aldi*	1 Pack/209g	362	9.6	173	12	20	4.6	2.4
Chicken Salad, on Malted Bread, Morrisons*	1 Pack/212g	367	7.2	173	13.9	20.6	3.4	2
Chicken Salad, Tesco*	1 Pack/226g	369	8.6	163	12.6	18.5	3.8	2.4
Chicken, & Avocado, Black Pepper Mayo, Waitrose*	1 Pack/213g	392	12.4	184	9.8	21.8	5.8	2.5
Chicken, & Avocado, Roast, on Soft Malted Bread, M&S*	1 Pack/200g	412	14.2	206	11.2	23	7.1	2.7
Chicken, & Avocado, Roast, Tesco*	1 Pack/173g	360	13.3	208	12.1	21.4	7.7	2.4
Chicken, & Bacon, & Avocado, M&S*	1 Pack/242g	508	28.3	210	10.7	15.8	11.7	3.2
Chicken, & Bacon, Deep Filled, Co-Op*	1 Pack/166g	556	33.2	335	16	23	20	3
Chicken, & Bacon, Tesco*	1 Pack/195g	486	24.2	249	14.3	20	12.4	2.7
Chicken, & Chorizo, with Red Pepper Sauce, Tesco*	1 Pack/186g	394	13.2	212	13	23.1	7.1	1.8
Chicken, & Sweetcorn, Malted Bread, Sainsbury's*	1 Pack/193g	370	9.8	192	12.3	22.9	5.1	2.6
Chicken, & Avocado, Tesco*	1 Pack/174g	347	9.9	199	10.9	24.1	5.7	3.6
Chicken, & Bacon, Caesar, Triple, Morrisons*	1 Pack/279g	713	32.3	256	12.2	25	11.6	1.2
Chicken, & Chorizo, Lidl*	1 Pack/176g	392	13.6	223	11.8	25.5	7.7	2.3
Chicken, & Mayo, Deli Club, Tesco*	1 Pack/183g	384	10.8	210	15.5	22.8	5.9	2.1
Chicken, & Stuffin', Vegan, Gro, Co-Op*	1 Pack/194g	466	16.5	240	11	28	8.5	3.6
Chicken, & Stuffing, Asda*	1 Pack/190g	393	10.3	207	13	25	5.4	1.9
Chicken, & Stuffing, Lidl*	1 Pack/169g	338	7.9	200	12.9	25.3	4.7	2.6
Chicken, Roast, Mozzarella, & Pesto, Tesco*	1 Pack/231g	468	18.4	203	11.8	20	8	1.8
Chicken, Salad, Lighter, On the Go, Sainsbury's*	1 Pack/201g	321	5	160	12.3	21.2	2.5	1.7
Chicken, Tikka, & Mango Chutney, Tesco*	1 Pack/201g	352	4.8	175	11.6	25.4	2.4	2.6
Crayfish, & Rocket, Finest, Tesco*	1 Pack/178g	365	10.5	205	9.8	27.5	5.9	2.1
Egg & Cress, on Malted Bread, Tesco*	1 Pack/178g	352	11.4	198	9.3	24.8	6.4	2.2
Egg & Cress, with Mayo, on Malted Bread, Co-Op*	1 Pack/169g	390	20.3	231	9	20	12	3.1
Egg Mayo, Boots*	1 Pack/160g	379	17.6	237	9.4	24	11	1.9
Egg Mayo, Free Range, Asda*	1 Pack/178g	311	10.1	175	9.3	21.5	5.7	2.1
Egg Mayonnaise, & Cress, Co-Op*	1 Pack/159g	405	24	255	8.8	20.8	15.1	1.9
Egg Mayonnaise, Double, Tesco*	1 Pack/189g	412	19.3	218	10.3	20.4	10.2	1.5
Egg Mayonnaise, Tesco*	1 Pack/188g	397	15.6	211	8.9	24.5	8.3	1.1
Egg, & Avocado, & Chilli Chutney, M&S*	1 Pack/209g	368	15.1	176	7.7	18.3	7.2	3.5
Egg, & Bacon, Handmade, Tesco*	1 Pack/217g	489	20.4	225	13.4	20.8	9.4	2
Egg, & Cress, BGTY, Sainsbury's*	1 Pack/145g	268	7.5	185	9.1	25.4	5.2	2.7
Egg, & Cress, Co-Op*	1 Pack/159g	398	23.8	250	9	21	15	2
Egg, & Cress, Free Range, Sainsbury's*	1 Pack/185g	359	13	194	9.8	21.8	7	2.3
Egg, & Ham, Deli Club, Tesco*	1 Pack/220g	433	15.4	197	11.4	20.5	7	2.7
Egg, & Salad, on Softgrain Bread, HL, Tesco*	1 Pack/197g	290	4.7	147	7	23.6	2.4	1.7
Egg, & Tomato & Salad Cream, M&S*	1 Pack/214g	402	14.8	188	7.8	22.6	6.9	2
Egg, & Watercress, GF Seeded Bread, Eat Well, M&S*	1 Pack/192g	382	16.9	199	8	20.6	8.8	2.9
Egg, & Watercress, Eat Well, M&S*	1 Pack/190g	355	10.8	187	9.8	22.9	5.7	2.4
Ham, & Cheese, & Pickle, Average	**1 Pack/220g**	**524**	**25.1**	**238**	**12.2**	**21.6**	**11.4**	**2.5**
Ham, & Egg, Honey Roast, Tesco*	1 Pack/192g	355	9.8	185	12.8	20.6	5.1	2.5
Ham, & Mustard Mayo, Smoked, Oatmeal Bread, M&S*	1 Pack/150g	282	6.4	188	13.2	23.2	4.3	2
Ham, & Mustard, Tesco*	1 Pack/147g	437	27.9	297	10.6	20.8	19	1.2
Ham, & Cheese, Co-Op*	1 Pack/170g	396	14.1	233	13.6	24.8	8.3	2.5
Ham, & Cheese, Morrisons*	1 Pack/183g	273	4.6	149	12.5	19.2	2.5	4.1
Ham, Cheese, & Coleslaw, Tesco*	1 Pack/185g	370	12.2	200	10.4	23.3	6.6	2.8
Ham, Smoked, & Mustard Mayonnaise, M&S*	1 Pack/163g	334	10.1	205	13	23.2	6.2	2.4
New Delhi Inspired, Wicked Kitchen, Tesco*	1 Pack/192g	297	2.9	155	6.5	25.5	1.5	6.9
No Tuna, & Sweetcorn, Plant Pioneers, Sainsbury's*	1 Pack/185g	335	6.8	181	6.7	28.2	3.7	4
Prawn Mayo, on Fibre Enriched Malted Bread, Co-Op*	1 Pack/179g	322	9.3	180	9.3	23	5.2	2.4

	Measure INFO/WEIGHT	per Measure KCAL	FAT	Nutrition Values per 100g / 100ml KCAL	PROT	CARB	FAT	FIBRE
SANDWICH								
Prawn Mayo, on Oatmeal Bread, On the Go, Sainsbury's*	1 Pack/176g	329	8.8	187	10.6	23.9	5	1.9
Prawn Mayonnaise, Morrisons*	1 Pack/157g	234	3.9	149	9	22.7	2.5	3
Prawn Mayonnaise, on Oatmeal Bread, Tesco*	1 Pack/181g	338	10.1	187	10.2	22.9	5.6	2.1
Prawn Mayonnaise, Soft Malted Brown Bread, M&S*	1 Pack/200g	354	12.8	177	9.2	19.8	6.4	2.7
Prawn, & Salmon, Smoked, M&S*	1 Pack/445g	1135	63.6	255	11.7	19.3	14.3	1.4
Roast Chicken, & Salad, on Malted Brown, M&S*	1 Pack/237g	363	6.4	153	11.5	19.1	2.7	2.9
Roasted Vegetables & Avocado, Red Pepper Bread, M&S*	1 Pack/184g	311	8.1	169	6	24.6	4.4	3.5
Salmon, & Cucumber, M&S*	1 Pack/168g	329	13.9	196	11	19.5	8.3	2.6
Salmon, & Soft Cheese, Smoked, Waitrose*	1 Pack/180g	416	18	231	11.5	22.6	10	2.2
Salmon, & Cream Cheese, Smoked, Sainsbury*	1 Pack/168g	408	17.5	243	11.7	24.5	10.4	2.2
Salmon, & Cucumber, Good to Go, Waitrose*	1 Pack/185g	316	9.2	171	12.1	18	5	2.8
Salmon, & Cucumber, on Wholemeal Bread, Morrisons*	1 Pack/166g	302	8.8	182	10.5	21.4	5.3	3.2
Sausage, Bacon, & Egg, Triple, Tesco*	1 Pack/265g	591	21.5	223	10.9	25.2	8.1	2.6
Seafood, Medley, M&S*	1 Pack/227g	468	28.1	206	7.2	16.3	12.4	3.5
Smoked Ham, & Cheddar, Tesco*	1 Pack/168g	414	18.1	247	14.8	21.7	10.8	1.7
Steak	**1 Serving/204g**	**459**	**14.1**	**225**	**14.9**	**25.5**	**6.9**	**0**
Sub, Tuna, & Salad, From Restaurant, Average	**1 Serving/256g**	**584**	**28**	**228**	**11.6**	**21.6**	**10.9**	**0**
Sweet Chilli Chicken, no Mayo, Tesco*	1 Pack/175g	317	6.7	181	9.6	26.4	3.8	1.7
Tofu, Fiery, & Slaw, Wicked Kitchen, Tesco*	1 Pack/236g	425	11.6	180	6.5	26.4	4.9	2.3
Tuna & Cucumber, on Oatmeal Bread, Waitrose*	1 Pack/199g	304	4.8	153	11.8	20.1	2.4	2.1
Tuna & Cucumber, Tesco*	1 Pack/184g	328	7.4	178	11.8	22.6	4	2.1
Tuna Mayo, Essential, Waitrose*	1 Pack/133g	283	7.4	213	13.3	25.9	5.6	2.9
Tuna Mayonnaise, & Cucumber, Finest, Tesco*	1 Pack/183g	387	15	211	10.6	22.5	8.2	2.2
Tuna Mayonnaise, Sainsbury's*	1 Pack/150g	314	9.9	209	11.4	24.5	6.6	2.8
Tuna, & Cucumber, BGTY, Sainsbury's*	1 Pack/178g	268	3.2	151	11.3	22.3	1.8	3.1
Tuna, & Cucumber, On the Go, Sainsbury's*	1 Pack/196g	284	5.5	145	9.6	19.4	2.8	2.1
Tuna, & Sweetcorn, Loved by Us, Co-Op*	1 Pack/200g	380	9.2	190	11.7	24.1	4.6	2.4
Tuna, & Sweetcorn, Malted Bread, Asda*	1 Pack/202g	365	10.7	181	11	21	5.3	2.5
Tuna, & Sweetcorn, on Malted Bread, Sainsbury's*	1 Pack/200g	362	9.2	181	11.9	21.8	4.6	2.4
Tuna, & Cucumber, Calorie Controlled, Tesco*	1 Pack/180g	268	3.1	149	10.5	22	1.7	1.8
Tuna, & Sweetcorn, on Malted Bread, Co-Op*	1 Pack/185g	337	8.5	182	12	22	4.6	2.6
Tuna, & Sweetcorn, on Malted Bread, Tesco*	1 Pack/178g	329	9.8	185	9.7	22.8	5.5	2.6
Turkey, & Cranberry, COU, M&S*	1 Pack/180g	279	3.1	155	12.1	22.8	1.7	2.9
Turkey, & Trimmings, Christmas, Tesco*	1 Pack/209g	476	16.5	228	12.5	25.5	7.9	2.3
Turkey, & Trimmings, Light Choices, HL, Tesco*	1 Pack/154g	256	4.3	166	10.1	24.1	2.8	2.2
Turkey, & Stuffing, GF, Tesco*	1 Pack/171g	343	15.2	201	11.4	15.6	8.9	6.2
Turkey, Mango, & Houmous, Aldi*	1 Pack/165g	291	8.1	176	9.1	22.4	4.9	3.9
SANDWICH FILLER								
Cheese & Onion, Reduced Fat, Supermarket, Average	**1 Serving/100g**	**227**	**18.1**	**227**	**11.8**	**4.4**	**18.1**	**1.7**
Cheese & Onion, Supermarket, Average	**1 Serving/100g**	**405**	**38.6**	**405**	**10.2**	**4.1**	**38.6**	**1.3**
Cheese, & Onion, Double Cheese, Tesco*	1 Serving/50g	102	7.4	205	12.9	4.5	14.9	0.6
Chicken & Bacon with Sweetcorn, Sainsbury's*	1 Serving/60g	123	9.4	205	12	4	15.7	0.9
Chicken Tikka , Meadow Fresh, Lidl*	½ Pot/100g	170	10.5	170	11.8	6.7	10.5	0.5
Chicken, & Bacon, The Deli, Aldi*	½ Pot/105g	284	24.2	270	14	2	23	0.5
Chicken, & Stuffing, Meadow Fresh, Lidl*	½ Pot/100g	298	23.5	298	11.5	9.6	23.5	1.1
Chicken, Coronation, Deli, Meadow Fresh, Lidl*	1 Serving/30g	78	5.7	261	12	9.8	19	1.2
Chicken, Coronation, Tesco*	1 Serving/50g	108	7.1	217	12.1	10	14.2	0.7
Coronation Chicken, Sainsbury's*	¼ Tub/60g	183	14.8	305	12.1	8.9	24.6	1.2
Egg & Bacon, Fresh, Tesco*	1 Serving/45g	112	9	248	12.7	4.2	20.1	0.6
Egg Mayonnaise, BGTY, Sainsbury's*	1 Serving/63g	71	4.1	113	10.2	3.4	6.5	0.1
Egg Mayonnaise, Country Fresh, Aldi*	¼ Pack/50g	106	8.9	211	9.8	2.9	17.8	0
Egg Mayonnaise, Meadow Fresh, Lidl*	½ Pack/100g	261	24.3	261	8.5	2.1	24.3	0
Prawn Marie Rose, Sainsbury's*	1 Serving/60g	121	10.6	201	8.1	2.5	17.6	0.9

	Measure INFO/WEIGHT	per Measure KCAL	FAT	Nutrition Values per 100g / 100ml KCAL	PROT	CARB	FAT	FIBRE
SANDWICH FILLER								
Prawn Mayonnaise, Deli, Asda*	1 Serving/50g	170	16.5	339	9	1.6	33	0.4
Seafood Cocktail, Asda*	1 Serving/50g	104	8.5	207	4.8	9	17	0.5
Seafood Cocktail, Sainsbury's*	1 Serving/55g	99	6.9	180	5.9	10.6	12.6	0.5
Smoked Salmon & Soft Cheese, M&S*	1 Pack/170g	450	40.6	265	11.1	4.9	23.9	0
Tuna & Sweetcorn, Reduced Fat, Supermarket	**1 Serving/100g**	**119**	**5.4**	**119**	**11.5**	**5.8**	**5.4**	**1.2**
Tuna & Sweetcorn, in Mayonnaise, Asda*	1 Serving/50g	66	3.4	131	8.3	8	6.9	0.9
Tuna & Sweetcorn, Tesco*	1 Serving/54g	127	9.8	235	8.6	8.1	18.1	0.6
SANDWICH SPREAD								
Heinz*	1 Tbsp/10ml	22	1.3	220	1	24	13	1
Light, Heinz*	1 Tbsp/10g	16	0.9	161	1.1	18.2	9.2	0.9
SARDINES								
Fillets, with Lemon & Herb Dressing, Morrisons*	1 Can/100g	109	4.9	109	14.3	1.5	4.9	1
Grilled	**1oz/28g**	**55**	**2.9**	**195**	**25.3**	**0**	**10.4**	**0**
in Brine, Canned, Drained	**1oz/28g**	**38**	**2.1**	**136**	**17**	**0**	**7.6**	**0**
in Oil, Canned, Drained	**1oz/28g**	**51**	**3.2**	**180**	**19.1**	**0**	**11.6**	**0**
in Spring Water, Portuguese, Sainsbury's*	1 Can/90g	176	10.5	195	21.3	1.2	11.6	0.5
in Tomato Sauce, Canned	**1oz/28g**	**45**	**2.8**	**162**	**17**	**1.4**	**9.9**	**0**
Raw, Whole with Head	**1oz/28g**	**22**	**1.2**	**78**	**9.7**	**0**	**4.3**	**0**
SATAY								
Chicken with Peanut Sauce, Waitrose*	1 Pack/250g	492	27	197	18.9	6	10.8	0.5
Chicken, 12 Mini, Taste Original*	1 Stick/10g	21	1.3	217	19.9	3.1	13.6	1.2
Chicken, Indonesian, Mini, Sainsbury's*	1 Stick/10g	17	0.7	171	23	4	7	0.7
Chicken, Sticks, Asda*	1 Stick/20g	43	2.8	216	18	4.5	14	0
Chicken, with Peanut Dip, Sainsbury's*	1 Pack/90g	171	10	190	15.4	6.3	11.1	1.5
Satay, Spicy, with Noodles, G&B, Asda*	1 Pack/365g	336	9.1	92	6.5	10	2.5	1.3
SATSUMAS								
Fresh, Raw, Flesh Only, Average	**1 Sm/56g**	**21**	**0**	**37**	**0.9**	**8.6**	**0.1**	**1.3**
Weighed with Peel, Average	**1 Sm/60g**	**16**	**0**	**26**	**0.6**	**6.1**	**0.1**	**0.6**
SAUCE								
Aioli, Garlic, Leon*	1 Jar/245g	1333	137.7	544	0.8	8.3	56.2	0.7
Aioli, Garlic, Vegan, Heinz*	1 Tbsp/15g	95	10.2	636	0.2	4	68.3	0
Aioli, Garlic, Vegan, Leon*	1 Tbsp/15g	85	8.8	565	0.6	8.1	58.7	0.9
Apple, Bramley, M&S*	1 Tsp/5g	4	0	84	0.1	19.2	0.5	1.2
Apple, Bramley, Sainsbury's*	1 Tsp/15g	17	0	111	0.2	27.2	0.1	1.8
Apple, Everyday Value, Tesco*	1 Tbsp/15g	15	0	105	0.1	24.8	0.1	0.5
Apple, Hak*	1 Tbsp/15g	7	0	47	0.3	10	0.3	2
Arrabiata, Italian, Tesco*	½ Pot/175g	74	0.9	42	1.1	7.9	0.5	1
Arrabiata, M&S*	½ Jar/170g	85	6.3	50	1.8	2	3.7	0.7
aux Cepes, marius*	1 Serving/55g	125	12.9	227	2.1	4.4	23.4	0
Bacon & Tomato, Smoked, Stir in, Dolmio*	½ Tub/75g	74	4.2	98	4.6	7.2	5.6	1.3
Balti, Cooking, Asda*	¼ Jar/125g	64	1.9	51	0.9	7.8	1.5	1.1
Balti, Loyd Grossman*	½ Jar/175g	180	11.7	103	1.3	8.4	6.7	1.7
Balti, Morrisons*	¼ Jar/112g	69	3.4	62	1	6.9	3	1.7
Barbecue, Sweet, Heinz*	1 Tbsp/15g	27	0	181	0.9	44	0.2	0
Barbeque, Cook in, Homepride*	1 Can/500g	375	7.5	75	0.7	14.6	1.5	0.6
BBQ, Bold Spicy Texas, Bulls-Eye*	1 Serving/20g	27	0	135	1.1	31	0	0
BBQ, Jerk, Reggae Reggae, Levi Roots*	1 Jar/310g	375	0.3	121	1.1	28.8	0.1	0.5
BBQ, Korean, Kalbi-Bulgogi, Jayone*	1 Tbsp/15g	36	0.5	242	4.5	49	3.2	0
BBQ, Reduced Sugar, & Salt, Tesco*	1 Tbsp/15g	11	0.1	71	0.4	15.9	0.5	0.6
BBQ, Roasted Onion, Heinz*	1 Tbsp/15ml	25	0	169	1.3	37	0.2	0
BBQ, Smoky, Asda*	1 Tbsp/15g	14	0.1	93	1.3	21	0.5	1.2
BBQ, Sticky, Spread & Bake, Heinz*	¼ Jar/78g	131	0.5	168	1	39.6	0.6	1.2
BBQ, The Grill House, M&S*	¼ Bottle/75g	123	1	164	2	35.5	1.3	1.1

SAUCE

	INFO/WEIGHT	KCAL	FAT	KCAL	PROT	CARB	FAT	FIBRE
Bearnaise, Sainsbury's*	1 Tbsp/15g	59	6.2	393	0.6	5	41	0
Bechamel, M&S*	1 Jar/425g	480	34.8	113	2.1	7	8.2	1.6
Bechamel, Plant Kitchen, M&S*	1 Jar/410g	377	32.4	92	0.7	3.9	7.9	1.1
Biryani, Reduced Fat, Waitrose*	1 Serving/115g	55	1.8	48	1.8	5.7	1.6	1.9
Black Bean, & Red Pepper, Sharwood's*	½ Jar/213g	132	3	62	1.9	10.5	1.4	1.2
Black Bean, Canton, Stir Fry, Blue Dragon*	½ Pack/60g	53	1.2	88	2.8	14.8	2	1.5
Black Bean, Stir Fry, Amoy*	½ Pack/60g	58	1.9	96	2.3	14.1	3.2	0.9
Black Bean, Stir Fry, Asda*	1 Pouch/120g	125	2.8	104	1.6	19	2.3	0.7
Black Bean, Stir Fry, Sharwood's*	1 Jar/195g	127	0.6	65	2.3	12.9	0.3	0
Bolognese, Dolmio*	1 Serving/100g	33	0.2	33	1.5	6.3	0.2	1.3
Bolognese, Morrisons*	1/5 Jar/145g	52	1	36	1.2	5.6	0.7	1.2
Bolognese, Smart Price, Asda*	¼ Jar/110g	44	1	40	0.1	7.6	0.9	0.5
Bolognese, Vegan, Sacla*	1 Jar/350g	259	13.3	74	3.2	6.2	3.8	1.1
Bone Marrow, Heston from Waitrose, Waitrose*	½ Pack/100g	188	9.6	188	19	6.1	9.6	0.6
Bouillabaisse, M&S*	½ Pouch/100g	132	11.8	132	1.8	4.3	11.8	0.7
Brandy Flavour, Bird's*	1 Serving/115g	101	1.6	88	2.7	16.2	1.4	0.5
Bread, Made with Semi-Skimmed Milk	**1 Serving/45g**	**42**	**1.4**	**93**	**4.3**	**12.8**	**3.1**	**0.3**
Brown, Bottled	**1 Tsp/6g**	**6**	**0**	**99**	**1.1**	**25.2**	**0**	**0.7**
Buldak, Extremely Hot, Chicken Flavour, Samyang*	1 Tsp/5g	12	0.4	250	4	33.3	8	2.5
Burger, Heinz*	1 Tbsp/15g	56	5.3	372	0.9	12	35.5	0
Butter Chicken, Lidl*	1 Jar/350g	438	29.1	125	1.8	10	8.3	1.4
Butter Chicken, Patak's*	½ Jar/225g	279	20.2	124	1.2	9.1	9	0
Butter Chicken, Tesco*	¼ Jar/125g	134	10.4	107	0.8	6.9	8.3	0.8
Caesar, Dressing, Florette*	1 Tbsp/15g	45	4.6	302	1.4	2.8	31	0.3
Calabrese, Deluxe, Lidl*	1 Jar/350g	336	22	96	2.8	6.8	6.3	0
Caramel Drizzle , Nestle*	1 Tbsp/15g	47	1.2	311	7.3	53	7.8	0
Caramel, Salted, Finest, Tesco*	¼ Pot/65g	266	8.5	409	3.2	69	13.1	1.2
Caramel, Sea Salt, Ghirardelli *	2 Tbsp/30g	120	0	400	0	92	0	0
Carbonara, Pot, Tesco*	½ Pot/175g	194	13.8	111	4.8	4.8	7.9	0.6
Casserole, Sausage, Morrisons*	¼ Jar/125g	51	0.1	41	0.8	9	0.1	0.2
Ch**se, Vegan, Sacla*	1 Jar/350g	374	33.9	107	0.7	4.3	9.7	0
Cheese, Made with Semi-Skimmed Milk	**1 Serving/60g**	**107**	**7.6**	**179**	**8.1**	**9.1**	**12.6**	**0.2**
Cheese, Made with Whole Milk	**1 Serving/60g**	**118**	**8.8**	**197**	**8**	**9**	**14.6**	**0.2**
Chilli & Garlic, Blue Dragon*	1 Serving/30ml	26	0.1	85	1.1	19.7	0.2	0
Chilli Con Carne, Homepride*	½ Jar/250g	145	1.2	58	1.6	11.1	0.5	1.6
Chilli Con Carne, Hot, Asda*	1 Jar/500g	285	3	57	1.9	11	0.6	0.9
Chilli Con Carne, Hot, Uncle Ben's*	1 Jar/500g	295	3	59	2.3	10.9	0.6	1.7
Chilli Con Carne, Mild, Sainsbury's*	½ Jar/250g	122	1.2	49	1.7	9.4	0.5	0.5
Chilli, Con Carne, Mexican, Co-Op*	¼ Jar/128g	82	0.8	64	2.6	10	0.6	3.2
Chilli, Cooking, Medium, Fiesta, Aldi*	¼ Jar/125g	60	0.6	48	2.3	7.3	0.5	2.7
Chilli, Extra Hot, Crucials*	1 Tbsp/15g	7	0.2	45	0.9	6.4	1.3	2.1
Chilli, Extra Hot, Maggi*	1 Tbsp/15g	16	0	107	0.7	25.3	0	1.4
Chilli, Hot, Cooking, Asda*	¼ Jar/125g	71	0.7	57	1.9	11	0.6	0.9
Chilli, Hot, Mexican, Morrisons*	¼ Jar/125g	72	0.6	58	2.2	11.2	0.5	2
Chilli, Hunan Smoky, Cooking, Sharwoods*	1 Pack/230g	168	1.2	73	1.2	15.5	0.5	1.3
Chilli, Korean, Hot & Fiery, Stir Fry, Yogi Yo*	1 Sachet/100g	219	0.8	219	3.2	48.5	0.8	0
Chilli, Korean, Stir Fry, Yogi Yo*	½ Sachet/50g	82	0.2	165	1.6	37.9	0.5	0
Chilli, Tomato Based, Bottled, Average	**1 Tbsp/15g**	**16**	**0**	**104**	**2.5**	**19.8**	**0.3**	**5.9**
Chinese, Stir Fry, Ashfield Farm, Aldi*	½ Pack/87g	80	2.5	92	1.4	15	2.9	0.8
Chocolate, Dessert, M&S*	1 Dtsp/11g	35	1	330	2.1	59.3	9.4	1.9
Chow Mein, Stir Fry, Asda*	½ Pack/85g	101	6.3	119	0.8	12	7.4	0.6
Chow Mein, Stir Fry, Blue Dragon*	1 Sachet/120g	127	1.3	106	0.9	23	1.1	0.4
Coconut, & Lemon Grass, Tesco*	½ Pack/90g	74	5.3	82	1.3	5.4	5.9	1.2

SAUCE

	Measure INFO/WEIGHT	per Measure KCAL	FAT	Nutrition Values per 100g / 100ml KCAL	PROT	CARB	FAT	FIBRE
Coronation, Stokes*	1 Tbsp/15g	85	7.9	568	1.7	20.7	52.9	0.2
Coronation, The Garlic Farm*	1 Tsp/5g	33	3.4	655	1.8	6.9	68.9	0
Cranberry Jelly, Morrisons*	1 Tsp/12g	23	0	189	0.2	47	0	0.1
Cranberry, & Clementine, Aldi*	1 Tbsp/15g	30	0	198	0	48.2	0	1.9
Cranberry, Sainsbury's*	1 Tsp/15g	26	0.1	170	0.5	41.5	0.5	0.5
Cranberry, Tesco*	1 Tsp/15g	23	0	156	0.1	38.8	0	0.9
Creamy, Vegan, Waitrose*	½ Pot/175g	159	10.8	91	1.6	7	6.2	2.3
Curry, Asda*	1 Tbsp/15g	62	2.1	414	13	59	14	1.3
Curry, Basics, Sainsbury's*	¼ Jar/110g	70	2.8	64	0.7	9.7	2.5	0.9
Curry, Chinese Style, Tesco*	¼ Jar/125g	59	0.5	47	0.4	10.3	0.4	0.5
Curry, Cook in, Homepride*	½ Can/250g	170	6.2	68	0.8	10.5	2.5	0.7
Curry, HFC, Tesco*	¼ Jar/110g	53	0.8	48	0.7	9.4	0.7	0.6
Curry, Hubbards, Sainsbury's*	¼ Jar/110g	68	2.4	62	0.8	9	2.2	1.4
Curry, Katsu, Pouch, Yo!*	½ Pouch/50g	98	5.8	197	1.6	21.1	11.5	1.3
Curry, Korma, Patak's*	½ Jar/225g	328	23.6	146	1.2	10.5	10.5	0
Curry, Medium, Uncle Ben's*	1 Jar/500g	330	10	66	0.9	10.9	2	0
Curry, Mild & Creamy, Cooking, Asda*	¼ Jar/125g	114	5.9	91	1	11	4.7	0.8
Dessert, Strawberry, & Phizzecco, Waitrose*	1 Serving/15g	28	0.1	187	0.7	44.2	0.6	0.8
Dhansak, Sharwood's*	1 Jar/445g	668	34.7	150	4.7	15.2	7.8	1.4
Diane, COOK!, M&S*	1 Tub/180g	180	15.5	100	2.7	2.2	8.6	1.1
Dill & Lemon, Delicate for Fish, Schwartz*	1 Pack/300g	387	34.2	129	1.1	5.6	11.4	0.5
Dill, Original, John Ross Jr. Ltd*	1 Tbsp/15g	42	2.5	279	2.9	28	16.9	0
for Meatballs, Cucina, Aldi*	¼ Jar/125g	39	0.6	31	1.1	5.7	0.5	1
Garlic, & Herb, Crucials*	1 Tsp/5ml	18	1.9	364	1.1	4.5	37.9	0.7
Garlic, Creamy, Sainsbury's*	1 Tbsp/15g	44	4.3	296	0.5	7.6	29	1.5
Garlic, Heinz*	1 Tbsp/15g	60	5.4	398	2.2	15	36	0.3
Garlic, Peri Peri, Medium, Nando's*	1 Serving/20g	10	0.6	49	0.8	4.2	3	0.8
Garlic, Turkish Style, Heinz*	1 Tbsp/15g	56	5.2	371	1.9	11	35	0
Goan, Spicy, Sainsbury's*	½ Jar/137g	104	4.7	76	1.5	8.5	3.4	2.7
Hoisin, & Plum, Stir Fry, HL, Tesco*	1 Serving/250g	148	3.2	59	2.1	9.7	1.3	1.3
Hoisin, & Garlic, Blue Dragon*	1 Pouch/120g	176	1.8	147	1.5	31.5	1.5	0
Hoisin, Rich & Fruity, Tesco*	1 Serving/29g	48	0.4	166	1.7	36.4	1.3	0.8
Hoisin, Sharwood's*	1 Tbsp/15g	32	0	211	2.7	49.5	0.3	0.1
Hoisin, Slimming World*	1 Pot/350g	130	1.4	37	1.8	5.9	0.4	1.4
Hoisin, Stir Fry, Aldi*	½ Pack/87g	138	3.1	159	1.2	30	3.6	0.7
Hoisin, Stir Fry, Amoy*	½ Pouch/60g	66	1.4	110	2.1	20.3	2.3	0.1
Hoisin, Stir Fry, Asda*	½ Pack/63g	54	0.4	86	0.6	18	0.6	3.1
Hoisin, Stir Fry, Tesco *	½ Pouch/60g	58	0.8	96	1.5	19.4	1.3	0.5
Hoisin, Stokes*	1 Jar/330g	874	6.3	265	2.3	58.5	1.9	0
Hollandaise, Fresh, Average	**1 Pack/150g**	**342**	**32.4**	**228**	**2.4**	**6.1**	**21.6**	**0**
Honey & Mustard, Chicken Tonight, Knorr*	¼ Jar/125g	132	6.6	106	1	12.6	5.3	1.8
Honey Mustard, Bunlimited*	1 Tbsp/15g	30	2.4	201	0.7	13.8	15.7	0
Honey, Soy, & Miso, Sachets, Yo! Sushi*	1 Serving/50g	88	0	176	2.2	38	0.1	7.1
Horseradish, & Mustard, Hella, Wicked Kitchen, Tesco*	1 Tbsp/15ml	16	0.7	105	3.8	10.9	4.5	2.9
Horseradish, Colman's*	1 Tbsp/15g	16	0.9	104	1.2	7.7	6.2	2.9
Horseradish, Creamed, Waitrose*	1 Tbsp/16g	30	1.6	185	2.4	19.6	9.9	2.3
Horseradish, Finest, Tesco*	1 Tsp/5g	16	1.4	325	2.7	14.1	28.1	2.2
Horseradish, Hot, Morrisons*	1 Serving/20g	31	1.5	157	2.2	19.1	7.7	1.7
Horseradish, Hot, Tesco*	1 Tsp/5g	12	0.8	233	1.8	17.4	16.9	2.1
Hot Pepper, Original, Squeezy Bottle, Encona*	1 Tsp/5ml	1	0	21	0.9	1.1	0.9	0
Hot, Pineapple, Barnfathers*	1 Serving/10ml	4	0	43	0.6	7.8	0	0
Jalfrezi, Average	**1 Sm Jar/350g**	**326**	**23.7**	**93**	**1.3**	**6.7**	**6.8**	**1.6**
Karahi, Hot, Cookie, Irresistible, Co-Op*	1/3 Jar/120g	136	8	113	2.5	9.1	6.7	2.9

	Measure INFO/WEIGHT	per Measure KCAL	FAT	Nutrition Values per 100g / 100ml KCAL	PROT	CARB	FAT	FIBRE
SAUCE								
Katsu Curry, Blue Dragon*	1 Serving/100g	240	2	240	1	54	2	1
Katsu Curry, Japanese, Sharwood's*	½ Pouch/125g	79	3.6	63	1.1	7.7	2.9	0.8
Katsu Curry, Tesco*	1 Pack/180g	169	13	94	1.2	5.2	7.2	1.7
Katsu, Curry, Sainsbury's*	½ Jar/170g	138	7.1	81	1.7	8.5	4.2	1
Katsu, Spice & Simmer, Taste of Japan, Asda*	1/3 Jar/115g	142	9.1	123	1.3	11	7.9	1
Ketjap Manis, Cooks' Ingredients, Waitrose*	1 Serving/25ml	30	0.1	122	1.2	27.9	0.5	0.5
Kicap Manis, Malay Taste*	1 Tbsp/15ml	36	0.1	237	1.3	55.9	0.9	0
Korma, 2 Step, Sainsbury's*	½ Jar/180g	216	13.3	120	1.6	10.5	7.4	2.6
Korma, 30% Less Fat, Sharwoods*	¼ Jar/105g	101	6.2	96	1.1	9.2	5.9	0.9
Korma, Cooking Sauce, Waitrose*	1 Jar/350g	696	51.8	199	3.4	12.2	14.8	1.8
Korma, Cooking, Asda*	¼ Jar/122g	131	7.8	107	1.5	10	6.4	1.1
Korma, Cooking, Free From, Tesco*	1 Jar/500g	405	21.5	81	0.8	9.3	4.3	1
Korma, Curry, Uncle Ben's*	1 Jar/500g	630	42	126	1.4	11.1	8.4	0
Korma, Dunnes Stores*	1 Jar/300g	435	36	145	2.1	8.1	12	0.9
Korma, Mild Curry, BFY, Morrisons*	¼ Jar/118g	150	7.2	127	1.3	16.8	6.1	1.5
Korma, Milk, Morrisons*	¼ Jar/112g	172	13.5	153	1.7	8.4	12	2.3
Korma, Tesco*	¼ Jar/125g	192	14.6	154	2.4	9.9	11.7	1.3
Korma, Tiger Khan Gold*	1 Jar/340ml	520	42.5	153	4.8	7.8	12.5	0
Lasagne, White, Baresa, Lidl*	1 Jar/470g	794	71.9	169	0.6	7	15.3	0.5
Lasagne, White, Sainsbury's*	¼ Jar/119g	130	11.4	109	0.8	4.5	9.6	0.5
Lemon Chicken, Uncle Ben's*	1 Jar/450g	315	1.4	70	0.3	16.2	0.3	0.3
Madras, Aldi*	1 Serving/113g	68	2.3	60	1.5	9	2	0
Madras, Hot, Cooking, Sainsbury's*	¼ Jar/125g	81	33.6	65	1	8.6	27	1
Madras, Hot, Patak's*	¼ Jar/113g	92	5.4	82	1.5	7	4.8	0
Madras, Sharwood's*	¼ Jar/105g	84	4.7	80	1.5	7.2	4.5	2.1
Makhani, Butter, M&S*	½ Jar/170g	291	22.6	171	1.9	10	13.3	1.9
Marie Rose, Irresistible, Co-Op*	1 Tbsp/15g	63	5.8	423	1.4	16	39	12
Marie Rose, The Best, Morrisons*	1 Tbsp/15g	64	5.8	428	2	18.2	38.5	0.1
Meatball, Moroccan Style, Alfez*	¼ Jar/112g	110	4.9	98	1.3	13.1	4.4	0.5
Mint Jelly, Tesco*	1 Tbsp/15g	34	0	224	0.3	55.2	0.1	0.7
Mint, Asda*	1 Tbsp/15g	13	0.1	88	0.9	19	0.6	2
Mint, Bramwells, Aldi*	1 Serving/30g	28	0.2	93	0.5	21	0.5	0
Mint, British, Finest, Tesco*	1 Tbsp/15g	12	0	77	0.9	17.3	0.2	1.2
Mint, Crucials*	1 Tbsp/15g	9	0	63	0.8	13.8	0.3	1.2
Mint, Reduced Sugar, Tesco*	1 Tbsp/15g	12	0.1	81	1.8	16.2	0.5	2.1
Mint, Sainsbury's*	1 Dtsp/10g	13	0	126	2.5	28.7	0.1	4
Mint, Value, Tesco*	1 Serving/10g	4	0	41	1.1	9	0.1	1.8
Mushroom, Creamy, Chicken Tonight, Knorr*	¼ Jar/125g	100	7.4	80	0.8	5.7	5.9	0.6
Mushroom, Creamy, Cooking, Sainsbury's*	¼ Jar/114g	72	4.6	63	0.5	5.9	4	0.5
Mustard, & Dill, for Gravadlax, No.1, Waitrose*	1 Sachet/20g	56	3.1	281	3.1	31.6	15.3	2.4
Olive, & Tomato, Asda*	1 Jar/340g	374	28.9	110	1.6	5.7	8.5	2
Oyster & Spring Onion, Stir Fry, Blue Dragon*	1 Sachet/120g	134	0	112	1.5	26.3	0	0
Pad Thai, M&S*	1 Sachet/125g	120	1	96	2.8	18.5	0.8	1.3
Pad Thai, Stir Fry, Morrisons*	1 Pack/120g	142	5.2	118	2.2	17.4	4.3	0.4
Panang, Thai, Seasoned Pioneers*	1 Pack/400g	440	31.2	110	1.6	8.3	7.8	1.6
Parsley, Fishmongers, Morrisons*	½ Pack/90g	112	8.9	124	2.1	6.2	9.9	0.9
Parsley, Fresh, Microwaved, Sainsbury's*	1/3 Pot/100g	78	5.4	78	1.7	5.3	5.4	0.5
Parsley, Tesco*	½ Jar/89g	85	5.1	95	2.8	8.1	5.7	1.1
Pasta Bake, Tomato & Herb, Homepride*	¼ Jar/121g	126	8.8	104	1.8	7.2	7.3	1
Pasta Bake, Tuna, Homepride*	½ Jar/250g	208	13	83	1.4	7.6	5.2	0.9
Peanut Satay, Dipping, Tesco*	½ Jar/45g	68	3.1	151	4.6	16.5	6.9	2.2
Peanut Satay, Stir Fry, Amoy*	1 Pack/120g	217	11.9	181	5.2	16.9	9.9	2.5
Peanut, Sainsbury's*	1 Sachet/70g	185	9.2	264	1.9	34.7	13.1	1.6

S

SAUCE

	Measure INFO/WEIGHT	per Measure KCAL	FAT	Nutrition Values per 100g / 100ml KCAL	PROT	CARB	FAT	FIBRE
Pepper, As Prepared, Colman's*	1 Portion/75ml	89	4.7	119	4.7	11	6.3	0
Pepper, Creamy, As Sold, Schwartz*	1 Serving/85g	71	5.8	83	1.3	4	6.8	0.5
Peppercorn, GF, Tesco*	½ Pot/90g	54	4.2	60	1.9	2.3	4.7	0.2
Peppercorn, Slimming World*	½ Pack/175g	72	0	41	2.9	6.2	0	2.2
Peppercorn, Waitrose*	1 Serving/60g	64	4.7	107	4.1	4.5	7.9	0.5
Perinaise, Hot, Squeezy Bottle, Nando's*	1 Tbsp/15ml	49	4.4	327	0.5	14	29	0
Perinaise, Mild, Squeezy Bottle, Nando's*	1 Serving/15g	46	4.2	309	0.3	13	28	0
Pesto, Red, Italian Inspirations, Co-Op*	1 Tbsp/15g	45	4	298	4.7	8.1	27	2.5
Pizza, Margherita, M&S*	3 Tbsp/45g	35	0.7	78	2	13.6	1.5	0.9
Pizza, Mutti*	1 Can/400g	144	2	36	1.6	5.4	0.5	0
Pizza, Tomato & Herb, Tesco*	½ Jar/100g	51	1.6	51	1.7	6.5	1.6	1.9
Plum, & Hoisin, Gressingham Foods*	1 Tbsp/15g	33	0.1	220	1.1	52.3	0.7	0.2
Plum, & Hoisin, Rich & Vibrant, Waitrose*	½ Pack/70g	99	0.4	141	1.6	32.1	0.5	1.1
Plum, & Hoisin, Stir Fry, Morrisons*	½ Pack/90g	103	0.1	114	0.6	27.6	0.1	0.1
Plum, Dipping, M&S*	1 Tbsp/15g	34	0	228	0.1	56.2	0.2	0.3
Plum, Sticky, Stir Fry, Blue Dragon*	1 Serving/60g	145	0.2	242	0.1	35.6	0.3	0
Pomme Frite, Benedicta*	1 Serving/15g	47	4.4	315	0.9	12.1	29.2	0
Pomodoro, TTD, Sainsbury's*	½ Pot/175g	152	10.7	87	1.8	5.3	6.1	1.8
Prawn Cocktail, Morrisons*	1 Portion/15ml	81	8.5	540	1.4	5.5	56.9	1.1
Ragu, Tomato, & Jackfruit, Tideford Organics*	1 Pack/300g	126	3.6	42	1.5	5.7	1.2	1.1
Red Hot, Buffalo Wings, Bramwells, Aldi*	1 Tbsp/15g	8	0.4	53	1.5	4.6	2.6	2.5
Red Hot, Fire Roasted Jalapeno, Franks*	1 Tsp/5g	1	0	24	0.8	4.1	0.3	1
Red Hot, Wings, Buffalo, Franks*	1 Tbsp/15g	4	0.2	30	0.8	2	1.5	2.5
Red Pepper, & Chilli, M&S*	½ Pack/75g	63	3.6	84	1.6	7.7	4.8	1.9
Red Pepper, M&S*	1 Pot/180g	270	17.3	150	0.8	14.3	9.6	1.7
Redcurrant, Colman's*	1 Tsp/12g	44	0	368	0.7	90	0	0
Roasted Vegetables, with Olives, M&S*	½ Tub/175g	164	11.6	94	1.6	6.5	6.6	1.2
Rogan Josh, Deluxe, Lidl*	1/3 Jar/116g	122	7.3	105	2.3	8.8	6.3	1.9
Rogan Josh, Kashmiri, Pasco*	1 Jar/350g	578	47.2	165	1.3	8.9	13.5	0
Rogan Josh, Low Fat, Tesco*	¼ Jar/125g	38	0.6	31	0.9	4.9	0.5	1.4
Rogan Josh, Medium, Sharwood's*	½ Jar/210g	151	7.6	72	1.4	8.6	3.6	0.5
Rogan Josh, Patak's*	¼ Jar/173g	112	5	65	1.2	8	2.9	0
Rogan Josh, Sizzle, Spice, Patak's*	1 Jar/360g	310	14.8	86	1.2	10	4.1	0
Rogan Josh, Spice & Simmer, Asda*	1/3 Jar/120g	101	5.6	84	1.3	8.3	4.7	1.5
Saag Masala, 2 Step Cooking, Sainsbury's*	½ Jar/178g	141	6.4	79	2.1	7.8	3.6	3.3
Saag Masala, Cooking, Specially Selected, Aldi*	1/3 Jar/120g	90	4.6	75	1.6	7.4	3.8	2.6
Salted Caramel, Dipping, Waitrose*	1 Tsp/5g	21	1.2	425	2.4	46.4	24.5	4.4
Salted Caramel, Jude's*	1 Tsp/7g	23	0.4	332	2	69.3	5.1	0
Satay, Blue Dragon*	1 Serving/25g	74	3	294	2	44	12	1
Satay, Dipping, Inspired Cuisine, Aldi*	1 Tbsp/15g	28	1.6	188	5	17	11	1.5
Satay, Stir Fry, Tesco*	1 Pack/120g	144	7.4	120	3.3	11.6	6.2	1.9
Satay, Tesco*	1 Jar/180g	265	14	147	4.7	10.9	7.8	7.1
Saucy, Heinz*	1 Serving/10g	43	4.1	432	0.9	14.7	40.8	0
Sausage Casserole, Cook in, Homepride*	½ Jar/250g	92	0.5	37	0.7	8	0.2	0.6
Seafood, Average	*1 Tsp/5g*	*20*	*1.9*	*410*	*1.4*	*15.4*	*38*	*0.2*
Shepherds Pie, Homepride*	¼ Pie/122g	50	0.6	41	1.3	7.6	0.5	1.2
Soy & Ginger, Sticky, Sainsbury's*	¼ Jar/38g	54	0.8	143	1.7	29	2.2	0.5
Soy, & Garlic, Stir Fry, Fresh Tastes, Asda*	1 Pack/180g	175	6.7	97	1.7	14.1	3.7	0.5
Soy, & Chilli, M&S*	½ Pack/75g	70	0.1	93	0.9	21.9	0.1	0.5
Soy, & Garlic, Stir Fry, Asda*	½ Pack/85g	89	3	105	0.9	17	3.5	0.5
Soy, Average	*1 Tsp/5ml*	*3*	*0*	*64*	*8.7*	*8.3*	*0*	*0*
Soy, Dark, Average	*1 Tsp/5g*	*4*	*0*	*84*	*4*	*16.7*	*0.1*	*0.2*
Spanish Chicken, Batts, Lidl*	½ Jar/250g	122	4.8	49	1.3	5.9	1.9	1.4

	Measure INFO/WEIGHT	per Measure KCAL	FAT	Nutrition Values per 100g / 100ml KCAL	PROT	CARB	FAT	FIBRE

SAUCE

	Measure INFO/WEIGHT	KCAL	FAT	KCAL	PROT	CARB	FAT	FIBRE
Spanish Chicken, Chicken Tonight, Knorr*	¼ Jar/125g	68	2	55	1.6	7.3	1.6	2.3
Spanish Style Chicken, Cooking, Lidl*	¼ Jar/125g	66	1.4	53	1.8	8.1	1.1	1.7
Spare Rib, Lee Kum Kee*	2 Tbsp/38g	80	1	211	2.6	39.5	2.6	2.6
Sriracha, Tabasco*	1 Tbsp/15ml	18	0	121	2.1	27	0	0
Sriracha, Thai Style, Oh So Delish, Aldi*	1 Pack/26g	109	3.4	420	11	60	13	9.3
Stir Fry, Chinese Style, Fresh, Just Cook, Sainsbury's*	½ Pouch/87ml	88	3.7	101	1.3	14.1	4.3	0.5
Stir Fry, Chow Mein, 30% Less Sugar, Sharwoods*	½ Pouch/60g	49	0.8	81	1.2	15.9	1.4	0.5
Stir Fry, Chow Mein, Amoy*	½ Pouch/60g	82	3.1	137	1.6	21.1	5.1	0.1
Stir Fry, Katsu, Aromatic, Blue Dragon*	1 Serving/60g	62	2.7	104	1	15	4.5	0
Stir Fry, Pad Thai, Passage To India *	¼ Pack/50g	55	0.2	110	1.1	25.1	0.3	0
Stir Fry, Sichuan Style, Hot & Spicy, Lee Kum Kee*	1 Jar/360g	457	19.1	127	3.6	13	5.3	0
Stir Fry, Singapore Curry, Amoy*	1 Pack/120g	84	4.3	70	0.9	7.8	3.6	1.3
Stir Fry, Sweet Chilli, & Garlic, Sainsbury's*	½ Pack/60g	65	0.3	108	0.5	25.8	0.5	0.5
Stir Fry, Sweet Chilli, Morrisons*	½ Pouch/60g	84	0.2	140	0.3	34	0.3	0.5
Stir Fry, Szechuan, Tomato, Blue Dragon*	1 Sachet/120g	143	3.2	119	1	22.4	2.7	0
Stir Fry, Vegetarian, Lee Kum Kee*	1 Serving/40g	53	0.2	133	1.3	32	0.5	0
Stroganoff, Cooking Sauce, Lloyd Grossman*	½ Pack/165g	203	14.8	123	1.6	8.6	9	0.7
Stroganoff, Cooking, Loyd Grossman*	½ Pack/165g	203	14.8	123	1.6	8.6	9	0.7
Stroganoff, Creamy, M&S*	1 Pouch/200g	190	15.2	95	0.6	4.6	7.6	1.8
Sun-Dried Tomato, & Basil, Stir in, M&S*	½ Pot/75g	106	9.2	141	1.4	3.9	12.3	4.7
Sweet & Sour, Take-Away	**1oz/28g**	**44**	**1**	**157**	**0.2**	**32.8**	**3.4**	**0**
Sweet & Sour, Stir Fry, Pouch, Average	**1 Pouch/120g**	**148**	**2.3**	**124**	**0.8**	**25.7**	**1.9**	**1**
Sweet Chilli & Garlic, Stir Fry & Dipping, Tesco*	½ Jar/95ml	78	0	82	0.3	20.1	0	0.1
Sweet Chilli, & Garlic, 30% Less Sugar, Sharwoods*	1 Pouch/60g	61	0.8	101	0.9	21.5	1.3	0.5
Sweet Chilli, & Garlic, Stir Fry, Pouch, Asda*	½ Pouch/60g	71	0	118	0.5	29	0	0.6
Sweet Chilli, Aromatic & Sweet, Waitrose*	½ Pouch/70g	58	0.4	83	0.9	18.1	0.5	1
Sweet Chilli, Dipping, M&S*	1 Tbsp/15g	34	0.1	225	0.9	53.2	0.7	0.6
Sweet Chilli, Dipping, Morrisons*	1 fl oz/30ml	64	0.6	212	0.4	47.3	2.1	1
Sweet Chilli, Dipping, Taste of Asia, Lidl*	1 Tbsp/15g	30	0	203	0.5	49.3	0.2	1.1
Sweet Chilli, Heinz*	1 Serving/25g	38	0.1	150	0.3	36.5	0.4	6.4
Sweet Chilli, Hot, Squeezy, Blue Dragon*	1 Serving/10ml	18	0.1	184	0.5	43.6	0.6	1.3
Sweet Chilli, Szuchuan Inspired, Tesco*	¼ Jar/126g	106	0.5	84	0.4	19.2	0.4	1
Sweet Chilli, Thai, Blue Dragon*	1 Serving/15g	28	0.1	188	0.5	45.5	0.6	0
Sweet Chilli, Thai, Encona*	1 Tbsp/15g	23	0	154	0.3	37	0.2	0
Sweet Curry, Eazy Squirt, Heinz*	1 Serving/10ml	12	0	124	0.7	29	0.3	0.5
Sweet Pepper, Stir in, Dolmio*	½ Pot/75g	77	4.6	103	1.4	9.6	6.2	1.6
Sweet, & Sour, Ben's Original*	½ Jar/225g	158	1.1	70	0.5	16	0.5	0.8
Szechuan Style, Stir Fry, Fresh Ideas, Tesco*	1 Sachet/50g	114	4.8	228	1.9	33.4	9.7	0.1
Szechuan, Spicy Tomato, Stir Fry, Blue Dragon*	½ Sachet/60g	59	1.8	98	1.3	15.8	3	0.9
Taco, Ireland, Tesco*	1 Serving/15g	41	3.6	273	1.4	13.6	23.7	0
Taco, Mild, No Added Sugar (SWE), Santa Maria*	1 Jar/230g	78	0	34	1.4	6	0	0
Tartare	**1oz/28g**	**84**	**6.9**	**299**	**1.3**	**17.9**	**24.6**	**0**
Teriyaki, Asda*	1 Serving/98g	99	0.1	101	2.1	23	0.1	0
Teriyaki, Deliciously Versatile, M&S*	1 Tbsp/15g	19	0.2	127	2.6	25.7	1.3	0
Teriyaki, Lee Kum Kee*	1 Serving/15g	27	0	178	2.2	42.4	0	0.5
Teriyaki, Pouch, Tesco*	½ Sachet /90g	89	0.8	99	0.7	21.9	0.9	0.1
Teriyaki, Rich & Savoury, Waitrose*	1 Serving /70g	122	0.4	174	0.5	42.6	0.5	0.5
Teriyaki, Sainsbury's*	1 Tbsp/15ml	31	0.1	209	1.6	49.2	0.5	1.8
Teriyaki, Sticky, Sainsbury's*	¼ Bottle/71g	81	0.4	113	1.1	26.3	0.5	1
Teriyaki, Stir Fry, Blue Dragon*	1 Pack/120g	131	0.2	109	0.9	25.9	0.2	0
Teriyaki, Stir Fry, Tesco*	½ Pack/90g	101	0.7	112	1.8	24.2	0.8	0.6
Teriyaki, Tesco*	1 Tsp/5ml	8	0	161	4	36	0.1	0
Thai Green Curry, Stir Fry, Market St, Morrisons*	½ Pack/90g	98	6	109	1.2	10.6	6.7	0.9

SAUCE	Measure INFO/WEIGHT	per Measure KCAL	FAT	Nutrition Values per 100g / 100ml KCAL	PROT	CARB	FAT	FIBRE
Thai Green Style, M&S*	½ Pack/75g	76	4.6	101	1.5	9.4	6.2	1
Thousand Island, The Skinny Food Co.*	1 Serving/15ml	2	0.1	13	0.5	2.3	0.5	2.1
Tikka Masala, Ready Made, Average	*1 Sm Jar/350g*	*422*	*28.8*	*121*	*2*	*9.6*	*8.2*	*1.2*
Tomato & Cheese, Pasta Bake, Dolmio*	¼ Jar/125g	70	1.5	56	2.1	9.1	1.2	1.2
Tomato & Mushroom, Pasta, Cucina, Aldi*	¼ Jar/125g	59	0.6	47	2	8.2	0.5	1.4
Tomato & Basil, for Meatballs, Dolmio*	¼ Jar/125g	48	0.2	38	1.5	6.9	0.2	1.3
Tomato & Basil, Italian, Fresh, Asda*	½ Tub/175g	107	5.7	60	1.5	6.1	3.2	0.6
Tomato & Basil, Italian, Sainsbury's*	½ Pot/175g	88	3	50	1.9	6.2	1.7	1
Tomato, & Bacon, Pasta Bake, Aldi*	¼ Jar/123g	107	6.8	87	1.5	7.4	5.5	0.9
Tomato, & Basil, Low FODMAP, Bay's Kitchen*	1 Jar/260g	148	8.1	57	1.3	6.3	3.1	1.1
Tomato, & Basil, No Added Sugar, Lloyd Grossman*	½ Jar/175g	96	3.9	55	1.5	6.9	2.2	0.8
Tomato, & Basil, Rich & Herby, M&S*	½ Pot/175g	124	6.1	71	1.8	7.4	3.5	1.5
Tomato, & Basil, Stir In, Baresa, Lidl*	½ Pack/75g	67	4.6	89	1.5	6.3	6.1	1.2
Tomato, & Chorizo, Stir in, Morrisons*	½ Pot/78g	68	4.1	87	2.4	7.3	5.2	0.5
Tomato, & Mascarpone, Vegan, Waitrose*	½ Pot/50g	49	3.4	98	1.9	7.3	6.7	0.5
Tomato, & Red Pepper, Extra Special, Asda*	½ Pot/175g	96	2.3	55	1.3	8.6	1.3	1.6
Tomato, Heinz*	1 Tbsp/17g	18	0	103	0.9	24.1	0.1	0.7
Tomato, Smooth, Tesco*	1 Jar/200g	60	0.8	30	1.4	5.5	0.4	1.5
Vindaloo, Hot, Patak's*	1 Jar/540g	518	34.6	96	1.5	6.4	6.4	0
Watercress, Sainsbury's*	1 Serving/100g	87	6.4	87	2.8	4.2	6.4	0.5
White, Savoury, Made with Semi-Skimmed Milk	*1oz/28g*	*36*	*2.2*	*128*	*4.2*	*11.1*	*7.8*	*0.2*
White, Savoury, Made with Whole Milk	*1oz/28g*	*42*	*2.9*	*150*	*4.1*	*10.9*	*10.3*	*0.2*
White, Vegan, Sacla*	1 Jar/350g	382	31.8	109	0.7	6.1	9.1	0
Worcestershire, Average	*1 Tsp/5g*	*3*	*0*	*65*	*1.4*	*15.5*	*0.1*	*0*
Yoghurt, & Mint, Crucials*	1 Tbsp/15g	58	5.9	387	1.3	6.4	39.5	0.4
SAUCE MIX								
Beef Bourguignon, Colman's*	1 Pack/40g	136	0.8	340	7	72	2	3
Beef Stroganoff, Colman's*	1 Pack/40g	140	3.6	350	11.6	56.1	8.9	2.7
Bolognese, As Prepared, Morrisons*	¼ Pack/283g	280	4	99	7.5	13.3	1.4	1.4
Bread, As Sold, M&S*	¼ Pack/18g	64	1.2	368	11.4	62.4	6.9	5.5
Bread, Made Up, Colman's*	1 Serving/75ml	70	1.5	95	5	14	2	0.6
Cheese, Made Up with Skimmed Milk	*1 Serving/60g*	*47*	*1.4*	*78*	*5.4*	*9.5*	*2.3*	*0*
Chicken Chasseur, Schwartz*	1 Pack/40g	126	1.8	316	9.6	59.1	4.6	6.8
Chilli Con Carne, Asda*	1 Sachet/50g	157	0.8	314	7	68	1.6	2.5
Chilli Con Carne, Recipe Mix, Schwartz*	1 Pack/41g	133	1.5	324	8.2	60.8	3.6	0
Chip Shop Curry, Dry Weight, Bisto*	1 Dtsp/9g	38	1.6	427	3.4	63.5	17.7	1.3
Dauphinoise Potato Bake, Schwartz*	1 Pack/40g	161	10.5	402	6.8	34.7	26.3	15.8
Hollandaise, Colman's*	1 Pack/28g	104	3.1	372	6.4	61.6	11.1	1.8
Hollandaise, Made Up, Schwartz*	1 Serving/79g	58	2	73	3.9	8.7	2.5	0
Lemon Butter for Fish, Schwartz*	1 Pack/38g	136	3	357	6.1	65.3	8	5.8
Mushroom, Wild, Schwartz*	½ Sachet/15g	55	1.2	368	10.5	61.5	8.1	2.8
Paprika For Chicken, So Juicy, Maggi*	1 Pack/34g	91	1.4	267	8.8	45.5	4	7.1
Parsley & Chive for Fish, Schwartz*	1 Pack/38g	150	4.3	394	9.4	61.8	11.4	3.5
Parsley, Creamy, Made Up, Schwartz*	1 Serving/79g	59	2	75	4.2	8.7	2.5	0.3
Parsley, Elmwood, Co-Op*	1 Pack/21g	15	0.5	72	3.7	9.1	2.2	0.5
Parsley, Made Up, Bisto*	1 Serving/50ml	43	2.5	86	1	9.6	5	1
Pepper, Dry, Bisto*	1 Tbsp/15g	74	4.2	494	4.2	55.1	28	2.4
Peppercorn, Made Up with Water, CBY, Asda*	1 Serving/63ml	52	3.9	84	0.7	5.4	6.2	1.7
Peppercorn, Mild, Creamy, Schwartz*	1 Pack/25g	88	2.2	352	13.8	55	8.6	5
Peri-Peri, Medium, Nando's*	1 Serving/20g	9	0.7	45	0.7	1.1	3.4	0
Sausage Casserole, Schwartz*	1 Pack/35g	116	0.8	330	10	63.2	2.2	8.8
Savoury Mince, Schwartz*	1 Sachet/35g	115	0.7	329	14	62.5	2.1	1.8
Shepherd's Pie, Schwartz*	1 Pack/38g	118	0.9	311	8.2	60.3	2.3	11.1

S

	INFO/WEIGHT	KCAL	FAT	KCAL	PROT	CARB	FAT	FIBRE
SAUCE MIX								
Spaghetti Bolognese, Colman's*	1 Pack/40g	120	0.4	300	8.9	64.1	0.9	5.2
Spaghetti Bolognese, Schwartz*	1 Pack/40g	114	0.6	285	9.2	59	1.6	7
Spaghetti Carbonara, Schwartz*	1 Pack/32g	135	6.4	421	10.4	49.4	20.1	7.2
Stroganoff, Beef, Schwartz*	1 Pack/35g	125	3.6	358	15.6	50.8	10.3	4.4
Stroganoff, Mushroom, Schwartz*	1 Pack/35g	121	3.1	345	10.9	52.4	8.9	5.9
White, Made Up with Semi-Skimmed Milk	***1oz/28g***	***20***	***0.7***	***73***	***4***	***9.6***	***2.4***	***0***
White, Made Up with Skimmed Milk	***1oz/28g***	***17***	***0.3***	***59***	***4***	***9.6***	***0.9***	***0***
SAUERKRAUT								
Average	***1oz/28g***	***3***	***0***	***11***	***1.1***	***1.6***	***0***	***0.9***
Garlic, & Dill, Raw, Vadasz*	1 Serving/50g	10	0.2	20	1.2	2	0.5	2.4
with Ginger, & Lemon, Organic, Raw Vibrant Living*	1 Serving/30g	6	2.5	21	1	3.5	8.2	0
SAUSAGE								
Beef, Average	***1 Sausage/60g***	***151***	***11.1***	***252***	***14.5***	***7***	***18.5***	***0.6***
Bierwurst, Slices, German Sausage Selection, Sainsbury's*	1 Slice/3g	7	0.6	232	14.6	1.1	18.8	0.5
Bockwurst, Average	***1 Sausage/45g***	***114***	***10.4***	***253***	***10.8***	***0.8***	***23***	***0***
Bratwurst, Unearthed*	1 Sausage/90g	245	21.6	272	13	1	24	0
Chicken, Berlinki, Morliny*	1 Sausage/50g	91	6.5	182	15	1	13	0
Chicken, British, Tesco*	1 Sausage/57g	99	4.4	175	17.2	8.4	7.8	1.1
Chicken, Chipolatas, Italian, Grilled, Ashfield Farm, Aldi*	1 Chipolata/34g	50	2.4	146	16	3.9	7	0.9
Chicken, Italia, Grilled, Heck*	1 Sausage/34g	49	0.9	145	28.5	2.4	2.6	0
Chipolata, Average	***1 Chipolata/28g***	***81***	***6.5***	***291***	***12.1***	***8.7***	***23.1***	***0.7***
Chipolata, Chicken, Italian, Grilled, Heck*	2 Chipolatas/59g	76	2.3	129	21.5	1.6	3.9	0
Chipolata, Chicken, Paprika, Heck*	2 Chipolatas/60g	78	2	130	22	2.4	3.4	0
Chipolata, Chicken, Simply, Grilled, Heck*	2 Chipolatas/58g	77	2.3	133	22.2	1.8	3.9	0
Chipolata, Chicken, Tomato, & Basil, M&S*	2 Chipolatas/68g	116	7.1	170	14.2	3.7	10.4	2.4
Chipolata, Premium, Average	***1 Chipolata/80g***	***187***	***13.8***	***234***	***14.8***	***4.7***	***17.3***	***1.2***
Chipolatas, Chicken, TTD, Sainsbury's*	2 Chipolatas/49g	75	3.6	154	16.8	4.9	7.3	1
Chipolatas, Vegan, Italia, Pan Fried, Heck*	2 Chipolatas/54g	49	0.6	90	6.6	9.2	1.1	8.9
Chorizo Style, Bangrs, Grilled, Wicked Kitchen, Tesco*	2 Sausages/99g	152	4	154	11.5	15.2	4	5.8
Chorizo, Average	***1 Serving/80g***	***250***	***19.4***	***313***	***21.1***	***2.6***	***24.2***	***0.2***
Chorizo, Lean, Average	***1 Sausage/67g***	***131***	***9.2***	***195***	***15.7***	***2.3***	***13.7***	***0.8***
Cocktail, Average	***1 Sausage/7g***	***23***	***1.9***	***323***	***12.1***	***8.6***	***26.7***	***0.9***
Cocktail, Plant Based, This Isn't Pork, This*	1 Sausage/15g	20	0.3	130	1.1	16	2.3	7
Cocktail, Vegan, Plant Pioneers, Sainsbury's*	½ Pack/70g	202	9.9	288	23.1	13.9	14.2	6.3
Cocktail, Veggie, Gosh!*	1 Serving/40g	96	5.1	241	6.4	21	12.9	7.2
Cumberland, Average	***1 Sausage/57g***	***167***	***13***	***293***	***13.8***	***8.6***	***22.8***	***0.8***
Cumberland, Vegetarian, Cauldron Foods*	1 Sausage/46g	75	4	163	14	6.5	8.6	2
Frankfurter, Dulano, Lidl*	1 Frankfurter/35g	97	8.8	278	11.2	2	25	0
Frankfurters, Turkey, Mini, Dulano, Lidl*	½ Pack/80g	204	17.6	255	13	1	22	0.6
Garlic, Average	***1 Slice/11g***	***25***	***2***	***227***	***15.7***	***0.8***	***18.2***	***0***
Honey, & Mustard, Dinky, M&S*	1 Sausage/15g	42	3.1	277	15.1	8.2	20.1	1.1
Irish, Average	***1 Sausage/40g***	***119***	***8.3***	***298***	***10.7***	***17.2***	***20.7***	***0.7***
Lincolnshire, Average	***1 Sausage/42g***	***122***	***9.1***	***291***	***14.6***	***9.2***	***21.8***	***0.6***
Lincolnshire, Vegetarian, Grilled, Linda McCartney*	1 Sausage/50g	104	5.8	209	13.6	10.2	11.5	5
Lorne, Average	***1 Sausage/25g***	***78***	***5.8***	***312***	***10.8***	***16***	***23.1***	***0.6***
Meat Free, Green Cuisine, Birds Eye*	1 Sausage/60g	126	7.2	210	16	6.4	12	6
Meat Free, Richmond*	2 Sausage/79g	115	4.3	145	8.8	14	5.4	3.6
Meat Free, The Meatless Farm Co*	1 Sausage/50g	117	8	234	14.4	6.8	15.9	3.2
Meat Free, Vegan, Plant Menu, Aldi*	1 Sausage/36g	73	5	203	10	6.9	14	3.7
Mediterranean Style, Vegetable, PlantLife, Waitrose*	2 Sausages/83g	113	5.1	136	8.3	8.3	6.1	7.5
Merguez	***1 Merguez/55g***	***165***	***14.3***	***300***	***16***	***0.6***	***26***	***0***
Patties, Breakfast, Iceland*	1 Pattie/48g	125	8.8	261	20.2	3.5	18.3	1
Patties, Plant Based, Meatless Farm*	1 Patty/60g	138	8.6	230	17.1	6.1	14.3	3.3

S

	Measure INFO/WEIGHT	per Measure KCAL	FAT	Nutrition Values per 100g / 100ml KCAL	PROT	CARB	FAT	FIBRE

SAUSAGE

	Measure INFO/WEIGHT	KCAL	FAT	KCAL	PROT	CARB	FAT	FIBRE
Pigs In Blankets, Cooked, Sainsbury's*	1 Roll/15g	42	2.8	280	3.1	11.2	18.5	1
Plant Based, Patties, Breakfast, Classic, Beyond Meat*	2 Patties/58g	180	12	310	19	10.3	20.7	3.4
Plant Based, Vegan, Moving Mountains*	1 Sausage/56g	140	7.6	250	14	6.7	13.6	5.6
Polish Kabanos, Sainsbury's*	1 Sausage/25g	92	7.6	366	23	0.1	30.4	0.1
Pork & Beef, Average	*1 Sausage/45g*	*133*	*10.2*	*295*	*8.7*	*13.6*	*22.7*	*0.5*
Pork & Herb, Average	*1 Sausage/75g*	*231*	*19.5*	*308*	*13.2*	*5.4*	*26*	*0.4*
Pork & Tomato, Grilled, Average	*1 Sausage/47g*	*127*	*9.7*	*273*	*13.9*	*7.5*	*20.8*	*0.4*
Pork & Apple, Average	*1 Sausage/57g*	*146*	*10.7*	*256*	*14.5*	*7.5*	*18.8*	*1.9*
Pork, & Caramelised Onion, Grilled, Finest, Tesco*	2 Sausages/94g	291	22.8	309	13.5	9	24.2	0.7
Pork, Average	*1 Sausage/45g*	*139*	*11.2*	*309*	*11.9*	*9.8*	*25*	*0.8*
Pork, Battered, Thick, Average	*1oz/28g*	*126*	*10.2*	*448*	*17.3*	*21.7*	*36.3*	*2*
Pork, Extra Lean, Average	*1 Sausage/54g*	*84*	*3.7*	*155*	*17.3*	*6.1*	*6.8*	*0.8*
Pork, Frozen, Fried	*1oz/28g*	*88*	*6.9*	*316*	*13.8*	*10*	*24.8*	*0*
Pork, Frozen, Grilled	*1oz/28g*	*81*	*5.9*	*289*	*14.8*	*10.5*	*21.2*	*0*
Pork, Garlic & Herb, Average	*1 Sausage/76g*	*203*	*16.5*	*268*	*12*	*6*	*21.8*	*1.2*
Pork, Premium, Average	*1 Sausage/74g*	*191*	*13.6*	*258*	*14.9*	*8.3*	*18.4*	*1*
Pork, Reduced Fat, Chilled, Grilled	*1 Sausage/45g*	*104*	*6.2*	*230*	*16.2*	*10.8*	*13.8*	*1.5*
Pork, Reduced Fat, Healthy Range, Average	*1 Sausage/57g*	*86*	*3.4*	*151*	*15.6*	*9*	*6*	*0.9*
Pork, Skinless, Average	*1oz/28g*	*81*	*6.6*	*291*	*11.7*	*8.2*	*23.6*	*0.6*
Pork, Thick, Average	*1 Sausage/39g*	*115*	*8.7*	*296*	*13.3*	*10*	*22.4*	*1*
Premium, Chilled, Fried	*1oz/28g*	*77*	*5.8*	*275*	*15.8*	*6.7*	*20.7*	*0*
Premium, Chilled, Grilled	*1oz/28g*	*82*	*6.3*	*292*	*16.8*	*6.3*	*22.4*	*0*
Red Pepper, & Butternut Squash, The Deli, Aldi*	1 Sausage/42g	50	0.6	118	4.8	18	1.4	6.8
Sausoyges, No Pork, Plant Kitchen, M&S*	1 Sausage/45g	67	2.8	149	15.6	5.6	6.2	4.4
Saveloy, Unbattered, Takeaway, Average	*1 Saveloy/65g*	*192*	*14.5*	*296*	*13.8*	*10.8*	*22.3*	*0.8*
Shroomdog, Cumberland, Plant Pioneers, Sainsbury's*	2 Sausages/88g	128	4	145	7.6	16.1	4.6	4.6
Shroomdogs, Chorizo, Plant Pioneers, Sainsbury's*	2 Sausages/66g	104	4.4	158	6	16	6.6	5.3
Smoked, Average	*1 Sausage/174g*	*588*	*52.2*	*338*	*13*	*4*	*30*	*0*
Turkey & Chicken, Average	*1 Sausage/57g*	*126*	*8.2*	*222*	*14.4*	*8.2*	*14.6*	*1.8*
Turkey, Average	*1 Sausage/57g*	*90*	*4.6*	*157*	*15.7*	*6.3*	*8*	*0*
Turkey, Caramelised Onion, Butchers Choice, Asda*	2 Sausages/115g	145	4.5	126	13	8.7	3.9	0.9
Turkey, Caramelised Red Onion, Sainsbury's*	2 Sausages/104g	165	6.5	158	18.3	6.9	6.2	0.5
Vegan, Bangers, Herby, Grilled, Plant Chef, Tesco*	2 Sausages/92g	157	7.8	171	16.9	4	8.5	5.6
Vegan, Breakfast, Grilled, Heck*	2 Sausages/77g	112	6	146	5.5	8.1	7.8	10.3
Vegan, Cumberland Style, Bangers, Plant Chef, Tesco*	2 Sausages/103g	175	7.7	170	8.6	15.6	7.5	3
Vegan, Naked Glory*	2 Sausages/73g	111	4.1	152	9.9	14	5.6	3.9
Vegan, Vemondo, Lidl*	1 Sausage/45g	96	5	213	6.1	19	11	6.9
Vegetarian, Chorizo Puppies, Plant Kitchen, M&S*	2 Sausages/90g	164	10.9	182	6.7	7.5	12.1	7.9
Vegetarian, Chorizo, & Red Pepper, Linda McCartney*	2 Sausages/90g	142	5.8	158	14.1	8.1	6.4	6.2
Vegetarian, Cocktail, Quorn*	1 Sausage/15g	31	1.7	206	12.4	11.6	11.3	4.3
Vegetarian, Outrageously Succulent, Linda McCartney*	2 Sausages/84g	129	5.2	153	18.6	2.3	6.2	6.6
Vegetarian, Quorn*	1 Sausage/40g	79	4.5	198	11.2	10.6	11.1	5.5
Veggie, Square, Simon Howie*	1 Sausage/68g	134	6.1	197	10.4	20.7	8.9	0
Wiejska, Polish, Sainsbury's*	1/8 Pack/50g	78	4.5	157	18.7	0.4	9	0.5
Wild Boar	*1 Sausage/85g*	*220*	*17*	*259*	*16.5*	*1.2*	*20*	*0*
with Vegetables, & Pork, Morrisons*	1 Sausage/43g	74	3.2	171	11.7	13	7.4	2.9

SAUSAGE & MASH

	Measure INFO/WEIGHT	KCAL	FAT	KCAL	PROT	CARB	FAT	FIBRE
2 British Pork & Rich Onion Gravy, M&S*	1 Pack/400g	340	6.8	85	5.7	12.2	1.7	1.3
Bangers, Microwaved, Iceland*	1 Pack/500g	455	16.5	91	3	11.4	3.3	1.8
Classic Kitchen, Tesco*	1 Pack/450g	510	23.2	113	4	12	5.1	1.3
Cumberland, Finest, Tesco*	1 Pack/387g	712	46.8	184	7.5	10.2	12.1	1.6
Cumberland, Good Choice, Iceland*	1 Pack/460g	580	27.1	126	5.3	12.2	5.9	1.8
Frozen, HFC, Tesco*	1 Pack/380g	371	8.4	98	3.3	15.5	2.2	1.4

	Measure INFO/WEIGHT	per Measure		Nutrition Values per 100g / 100ml				
		KCAL	FAT	KCAL	PROT	CARB	FAT	FIBRE
SAUSAGE & MASH								
Inspired Cuisine, Aldi*	1 Pack/435g	491	22.6	113	4.8	11	5.2	1.4
LC, Tesco*	1 Pack/400g	360	8.8	90	4.4	11.8	2.2	1.4
Shroomdogs, Plant Pioneers, Sainsbury's*	1 Pack/384g	353	8.1	92	3	14.1	2.1	1.9
with Onion Gravy, Bangers, British Classic, Sainsbury's*	1 Pack/450g	562	30.6	125	4.8	9.9	6.8	2.6
SAUSAGE MEAT								
Pork, Average	**1oz/28g**	**96**	**8.2**	**344**	**9.9**	**10.2**	**29.4**	**0.6**
Pork, with Black Pepper, & Nutmeg, Waitrose*	1/6 Pack/57g	141	10.2	247	16.7	4.5	17.9	0.8
SAUSAGE ROLL								
Artisan, Mini, Donald Russell*	1 Roll/58g	176	12.4	303	11.8	14.7	21.3	2.6
Bacon, & Cheddar, Smoked, M&S*	1 Roll/45g	167	10.7	372	13.8	24.9	23.8	1.4
Best Ever, M&S*	1 Roll/80g	235	14.9	294	11.1	19.5	18.6	2.2
Cheese, & Bacon, Tesco*	1 Roll/60g	181	10.7	301	9.1	25.4	17.8	1.7
Chicken Style, Vegan, Fry's*	1 Roll/80g	274	16	342	10.6	31	20	4.1
Cocktail, Average	**1 Roll/15g**	**57**	**3.7**	**378**	**8.9**	**29.4**	**24.9**	**1.9**
Crestwood, Aldi*	1 Roll/97g	312	18.4	322	8.5	27	19	1.9
Dinky, Hand Crafted, M&S*	1 Roll/15g	55	3.6	369	11.5	25.5	24.1	2.2
Eastmans, Tesco*	1 Roll/60g	179	9.6	299	7.5	30	16	2.6
Jumbo, Iceland*	1 Roll/117g	302	14.7	258	10.1	24.6	12.6	2.9
Jumbo, Sainsbury's*	1 Roll/145g	456	26.3	314	9.5	27.2	18.1	2.3
Linda McCartney*	1 Roll/51g	145	8.2	287	10.9	22.7	16.2	3.8
Meat Free, Mini, Frys*	1 Roll/22g	73	3.7	325	12	31	16.3	3.3
Meat Free, No Porkies, Oven Baked, Iceland*	1 Roll/90g	271	15.6	301	9.3	25.1	17.3	4.2
Mini, Greggs, Iceland*	1 Roll/26g	72	4.4	277	7.8	23	17	0
Mini, Linda McCartney*	1 Roll/14g	41	2.2	293	11.3	23.7	15.8	5.2
Mini, M&S*	1 Roll/30g	112	8.2	373	9.5	21.7	27.2	1.6
Mini, Waitrose*	1 Roll/35g	124	9.2	353	13	16.1	26.3	1
No Pork, Vegan, Plant Menu, Aldi*	1 Roll/60g	169	7.8	281	7.1	33	13	4.1
No Sausage, Vegan, Mini, Plant Pioneers, Sainsbury's*	1 Roll/30g	84	4	279	6.3	31	13.4	4.6
No Sausage, Vegan, Plant Menu, Aldi*	1 Roll/90g	284	17.1	316	8.2	27	19	3.9
Pork, & Cranberry, Higgidy*	1 Roll/26g	106	6.4	402	8.3	39.1	24.1	2
Pork, Allcroft's*	1 Roll/50g	166	9.7	331	9.8	28.2	19.4	2
Pork, Bowyers*	1 Roll /45g	147	8.4	326	7	31.7	18.6	2.4
Pork, British, Handcrafted, Mini, M&S*	1 Roll/18g	71	5	392	11.6	22.8	27.8	2
Pork, Cocktail, Mini, M&S*	1 Roll/42g	152	9.9	361	11.1	25.5	23.5	1.6
Pork, Finest, Tesco*	1 Roll/47g	174	11.5	371	12.2	24.9	24.4	1.5
Pork, Handcrafted, M&S*	1 Roll/80g	271	18.1	339	10.8	22.4	22.6	1.4
Pork, Mini, Tesco*	1 Roll/10g	37	2.2	374	10.2	32.6	22.1	1.9
Pork, Morrisons*	1 Roll/70g	195	9	278	9.6	31.2	12.8	1.5
Pork, TTD, Sainsbury's*	1 Roll/65g	242	16.8	372	11.5	22.9	25.8	1.1
Puff Pastry	**1 Roll/60g**	**230**	**16.6**	**383**	**9.9**	**25.4**	**27.6**	**1**
TTD, Sainsbury's*	1 Roll/27g	103	7	383	12.3	23.9	26.1	1.4
Vegan, Mae's Kitchen, Aldi*	1 Roll/90g	284	17.1	316	8.2	27	19	3.9
Vegan, Naughty vegan*	1 Roll/105g	333	18.9	317	8.9	28.2	18	3
Vegan, No Pork, Plant Kitchen, M&S*	1 Roll/60g	180	10.9	300	9.7	22.8	18.2	3.7
Vegetarian, 3 Pack, Quorn*	1 Roll/70g	193	10.5	276	12	21	15	3.3
Vegetarian, Chilled, Quorn*	1 Roll/70g	181	8.8	259	10.1	24.5	12.5	3.9
Vegetarian, Chilled, Single Pack, Quorn*	1 Roll/130g	292	12.1	225	12.3	21.2	9.3	3.8
SCALLOPS								
& Prawns, King, in Creamy Lobster Sauce, Sainsbury's*	1 Dish/112g	204	14.4	182	12.3	4	12.9	0.5
Coquilles St Jacques, M&S*	1 Serving/150g	177	9.2	118	6.5	8.9	6.1	0.9
Raw, Bay or Sea with Roe, Average	**1 Scallop/15g**	**13**	**0.1**	**88**	**16.8**	**2.4**	**0.8**	**0**
Roeless, Extra Large, Arctic Royal*	½ Pack/150g	58	0.8	39	8.5	0.1	0.5	0
Steamed, Average	**1oz/28g**	**33**	**0.4**	**118**	**23.2**	**3.4**	**1.4**	**0**

S

	Measure INFO/WEIGHT	per Measure KCAL	FAT	Nutrition Values per 100g / 100ml KCAL	PROT	CARB	FAT	FIBRE
SCAMPI								
& Chips, with Peas	**1 Serving/490g**	**822**	**43.6**	**168**	**10.1**	**11.3**	**8.9**	**1.2**
Bites, Vegetarian, Linda McCartney*	½ Pack/125g	279	11.5	223	14.7	18.3	9.2	3.7
Breaded, Baked, Average	**½ Pack/255g**	**565**	**27.4**	**222**	**10.7**	**20.5**	**10.7**	**1**
Breaded, Fried in Oil, Average	**1 Serving/100g**	**237**	**13.6**	**237**	**9.4**	**20.5**	**13.6**	**0**
Fish, Bites, Fishmonger, Aldi*	¼ Pack/109g	245	10.6	225	9.7	24	9.7	1.4
Fishless, Vegan, Oven Baked, Quorn*	½ Pack/89g	175	8.2	197	8.3	25	9.2	11
Fries, Smiths*	1 Pack/27g	132	6.3	489	10	59.3	23.3	0.7
Tails, Breaded, Oven Baked, Whitby Seafoods*	1 Serving/100g	207	7.7	207	10	23	7.7	3
White Tail, Aldi*	½ Pack/125g	256	9.6	205	10	23	7.7	2.4
Whole Tail, Breaded, Oven Baked, Asda*	½ Pack/150g	314	12.2	209	11	23	8.1	0.8
Whole, Extra Large, Whitby Seafoods*	½ Bag/125g	151	0.8	121	9.4	20	0.6	1.7
Wholetail, Breaded, Fresh, Waitrose*	1 Serving/81g	176	7.9	217	13.6	17.9	9.7	1.7
Wholetail, Deluxe, Lidl*	½ Pack/101g	262	12.1	259	12.5	23.9	12	2.9
Wholetail, in Breadcrumb Coating, Morrisons*	½ Pack/113g	244	8.7	216	11	24.5	7.7	2.5
Wholetail, Jumbo, Chilled, Whitby Seafoods*	½ Pack/100g	201	7	201	9.6	24.2	7	1.4
Wholetail, Jumbo, Gastro, Youngs*	½ Pack/115g	238	9.5	207	11.3	21.1	8.3	1.3
SCONE								
All Butter, & Cherry, Finest, Tesco*	1 Scone/70g	245	7.2	349	7.1	56	10.3	1.9
Cheese, Average	**1 Scone/40g**	**145**	**7.1**	**363**	**10.1**	**43.2**	**17.8**	**1.6**
Cherry, & Almond, Cheeky Little Rascal, Bettys*	1 Scone/50g	218	9	437	6.4	61	18	0
Cherry, M&S*	1 Scone/60g	202	7.3	337	6.9	49.7	12.2	1.9
Clotted Cream, Cornish, TTD, Sainsbury's*	1 Scone/70g	269	12.7	384	8.4	46.6	18.2	2.1
Cream, Mini, Co-Op*	1 Scone/24g	86	4.1	360	6.8	44	17	1.1
Devon, M&S*	1 Scone/59g	225	9.6	380	7.1	50.8	16.2	1.5
Fresh Cream with Strawberry Jam, Tesco*	1 Scone/88g	299	12.9	340	6.3	44.7	14.7	1.8
Fruit, Average	**1 Scone/40g**	**126**	**3.9**	**316**	**7.3**	**52.9**	**9.8**	**0**
Orange, & Sultana, Cheeky Little Rascal, Bettys*	1 Scone/50g	202	7	403	5.1	63	14	0
Plain, Average	**1 Scone/40g**	**145**	**5.8**	**362**	**7.2**	**53.8**	**14.6**	**1.9**
Potato, Average	**1 Scone/40g**	**118**	**5.7**	**296**	**5.1**	**39.1**	**14.3**	**1.6**
Red Berry, Mixed, Finest, Tesco*	1 Scone/110g	344	9.5	313	7.8	50.1	8.6	1.9
Specially Selected, Aldi*	1 Scone/65g	226	6.2	347	8.9	55	9.5	2.5
Strawberry, Fresh Cream, BGTY, Sainsbury's*	1 Scone/50g	154	5.6	309	5.1	47	11.2	1.1
Wholemeal	**1 Scone/40g**	**130**	**5.8**	**326**	**8.7**	**43.1**	**14.4**	**5.2**
Wholemeal, Fruit	**1 Scone/40g**	**130**	**5.1**	**324**	**8.1**	**47.2**	**12.8**	**4.9**
SEA BASS								
Butterflied, Fishmonger, Aldi*	1 Pack/180g	284	13.1	158	23	0.5	7.3	0.5
Cooked, Dry Heat, Average	**1 Fillet/100g**	**124**	**2.6**	**124**	**23.6**	**0**	**2.6**	**0**
Fillet, Boneless, Waitrose*	1 Fillet/90g	160	9.1	178	21.3	0.5	10.1	0.5
Fillet, Lemon & Pepper, Tesco*	½ Pack/82g	180	12.4	220	19.4	1	15.1	1.7
Fillets, Caramelised Ginger & Lime Butter, Sainsbury's*	1 Fillet/115g	258	18.1	224	19.9	0.5	15.7	0.5
Fillets, Large, Frozen, Iceland*	1 Fillet/140g	235	13.7	168	20	0	9.8	0
Fillets, Lemon & Herb, Market St, Morrisons*	½ Pack/90g	197	12.2	219	23.3	0.5	13.6	0.6
Fillets, Mediterranean Inspired, Tesco*	1 Fillet/151g	239	12.4	158	19.5	1.1	8.2	1.1
Fillets, with Butter, Cooked, Tesco*	1 Fillet/86g	189	13	220	19.4	1	15.1	1.7
Fillets, With Rocket Pesto Butter, Waitrose*	½ Pack/95g	220	15.4	232	20.1	1.2	16.2	0.5
Fillets, with Soy, Chilli, & Ginger, Pan Fried, Sainsbury's*	1 Fillet/82g	159	8.5	193	24.4	0.5	10.3	0.9
Raw, Fillet, Average	**1 Fillet/95g**	**108**	**3.4**	**113**	**20.3**	**0**	**3.5**	**0.1**
SEA BREAM								
Butterflied, Pan Fried, Sainsbury's*	1 Fillet/116g	252	13.9	217	25	1.6	12	0.6
Fillet, Cooked, Dry Heat, Average	**1 Serving/100g**	**124**	**3**	**124**	**24**	**0**	**3**	**0**
Fillets, Raw, Average	**1oz/28g**	**27**	**0.8**	**96**	**17.5**	**0**	**2.9**	**0**
Fillets, with Rocket Pesto Butter, Waitrose*	1 Fillet/87g	220	15.4	253	22.7	0.5	17.7	0.5
Roasted, with Norfolk Potatoes, At Home, Cote*	1 Pack/528g	702	43.3	133	9.6	4.5	8.2	0.8

S

	Measure INFO/WEIGHT	per Measure KCAL	FAT	Nutrition Values per 100g / 100ml KCAL	PROT	CARB	FAT	FIBRE
SEAFOOD								
& Prawn Cocktail, Deli Filler, Waitrose*	½ Tub/100g	199	15.5	199	5.8	9	15.5	0.5
Cocktail, Average	*1oz/28g*	*24*	*0.4*	*87*	*15.6*	*2.9*	*1.5*	*0*
Mix, Cooked, Iceland*	1 Pack/500g	440	7	88	15.1	3.8	1.4	0.1
Mix, Skellig Bay, Aldi*	½ Pack/125g	174	6.6	139	23	0.5	5.3	0.5
Selection, Fresh, Tesco*	1 Pack/234g	187	2.3	80	17.7	0.1	1	0
Selection, Ready to Eat, Asda*	1 Pack/240g	230	5.8	96	12	6.5	2.4	0.5
Selection, Sainsbury's*	½ Pack/100g	75	1	75	15.2	1.3	1	0.5
Shells, Waitrose*	1 Shell/60g	86	4.7	143	16.2	1.6	7.9	0
SEAFOOD STICKS								
& Prawns, Market St, Morrisons*	1 Pack/190g	384	28.7	202	7.9	7.1	15.1	2.6
Average	*1 Stick/15g*	*16*	*0*	*106*	*8*	*18.4*	*0.2*	*0.2*
SEASONING MIX								
Beef Casserole, Newgate, Lidl*	1 Pack/43g	140	0.9	325	5.5	67.9	2.2	5.7
Chicken Casserole, Bramwells*	1 Pack/40g	125	0.7	312	9.1	63	1.7	3.9
Chicken Kebab, Sachet, Colman's*	1 Sachet/30g	97	3	323	11	41	9.9	14
Chicken Supreme, As Sold, Erin*	1 Sachet/40g	157	4.4	392	12.1	61	11	3.2
Chilli Con Carne, Bisto*	4 Dtsp/76g	302	12.9	397	5.4	53.2	17	4.9
Cottage Pie, GF, Schwartz*	1 Pack/30g	91	0.6	302	10.2	59	1.9	0
Fajita, Schwartz*	1 Serving/5g	14	0.2	278	7.5	55	4.2	0
Fajitas, Smoky BBQ, Old El Paso*	1 Pack/35g	110	0.5	313	6.3	67.2	1.3	3.5
Fish Pie, Colman's*	1 Pack/20g	65	0.3	326	9.8	64	1.4	3.6
Katsu, Street Food, Schwartz*	1 Pack/15g	44	0.6	294	10.9	49.9	3.8	0
Lamb Hot Pot, Colman's*	¼ Pack/10g	32	0.2	320	12	61	1.5	4
Lemon & Herb, for Chicken, Cook in Bag, Average	*1 Bag/34g*	*121*	*1.9*	*356*	*10.8*	*63.7*	*5.5*	*4.1*
Mediterranean, for Chicken, Cook in Bag, Average	*1 Bag/33g*	*99*	*0.7*	*302*	*10.6*	*56.6*	*2*	*7*
Mexican Chicken, As Sold, So Juicy, Maggi*	1 Pack/40g	123	1.7	308	7.4	57.2	4.2	6
Mexican, Street Food, Schwartz*	½ Pack/7g	20	0.3	287	11.1	39.1	4.3	0
Paprika, for Chicken, Cook in Bag, Average	*1 Bag/34g*	*96*	*1.3*	*283*	*12.3*	*45.8*	*4*	*8.1*
Potato Wedges, Garlic & Herb, Schwartz*	1 Pack/38g	106	1.9	278	11.4	47.1	4.9	11.7
Shepherds Pie, Colman's*	1 Pack/50g	158	0.8	315	12	60	1.6	5.4
Spaghetti Bolognese, Bramwells, Aldi*	1 Sachet/44g	132	2	300	10.9	57.3	4.6	7.3
Taco, Old El Paso*	¼ Pack/9g	30	0.4	334	5.5	69	4	0
Tikka Masala, Slow Cook, As Sold, Schwartz*	½ Sachet/18g	49	0.8	279	9.6	43.9	4.8	10.9
SEAWEED								
Baby, Organic, Numami *	1 Serving/10g	28	0.4	275	16.6	41.3	3.7	52
Laverbread, Selwyn's*	1 Serving/10g	3	0	28	3.3	1.3	0.4	0
Nori, Dried, Raw	*1oz/28g*	*38*	*0.4*	*136*	*30.7*	*0*	*1.5*	*44.4*
Seaveg, Crispies, Clearspring*	1 Pack/4g	18	1.2	462	30	0.1	31	31
Snacks, Crispy, Wasabi, Bibigo*	1 Serving/5g	31	2.4	598	19.6	25.7	46.8	0
Wakame, Dried, Raw	*1oz/28g*	*20*	*0.7*	*71*	*12.4*	*0*	*2.4*	*47.1*
SEED MIX								
3, Toasted, Tesco*	1 Serving/25g	141	11.5	562	26	1.4	45.9	19.8
Chia & Flaxseed, Sprinkles, Tesco*	1 Serving/26g	135	9.2	518	24.2	15.9	35.3	20.2
Choccy Ginger, Munchy Seeds*	1 Pack/25g	120	7.8	481	9.1	44	31	3.4
Flaxseed, Sunflower, Pumpkin, & Chia, & Goji, Linwoods*	1 Serving/20g	104	7.4	518	19	8	37	18
Four, Whitworths*	1 Serving/25g	141	11.8	565	26.8	1.4	47.2	14.5
Linseed, Fruity, Mix, Alesto, Lidl*	1 Serving/30g	154	11.1	512	17.5	18.3	37	17.8
Omega Mix, Bare Nature*	1 Serving/35g	209	17.8	598	25.2	3.5	51	12
Omega, Morrisons*	¼ Pack/25g	138	11.4	554	20.9	15	45.6	6.4
Omega, Munchy Seeds*	1 Bag/25g	153	12.4	613	28.4	13.1	49.7	2.2
Pumpkin, & Sunflower, Holland & Barrett*	1 Serving/30g	171	13.8	570	22	17	46	5.6
Seven, Tamari Mix, Munchy Seeds*	1 Serving/30g	172	14.4	575	22	18	48	8
Super Seeds, Salad Topper, Good4U*	1 Serving/25g	144	11.2	575	30	7	45	10

S

	Measure INFO/WEIGHT	per Measure KCAL	FAT	Nutrition Values per 100g / 100ml KCAL	PROT	CARB	FAT	FIBRE
SEED MIX								
The Foodie Market, Aldi*	1 Serving/30g	172	13.8	575	23	12	46	8.7
Warm Cinnamon, Munchy Seeds*	1 Pack/25g	129	9	516	16	34	36	6.3
SEEDS								
Chia, Artisan Grains*	1 Serving/10g	44	3.1	436	20	2	31	37.9
Chia, Bio, Chia Direct*	1 Tbsp/15g	69	4.7	460	21.2	3.8	31.4	33.7
Chia, Black, The Chia Co*	1 Tbsp/15g	67	5.2	447	20	45	35	37
Chia, Clever, Holland & Barrett*	1 Tbsp/15g	74	4.6	490	18	6	31	38
Chia, Milled, Mix, Natural Selection*	1 Tbsp/15g	80	6.3	530	24	5.4	42	19
Chia, Milled, Organic, Linwoods*	1 Tbsp/15g	65	4.5	435	24	2.6	30	29
Chia, Organic, BuyWholeFoodsOnline*	1 Tbsp/15g	65	4.6	436	20	2	31	37.9
Chia, Organic, Sevenhills Wholefoods*	1 Tbsp/15g	66	4.3	437	22.1	6.7	28.8	31.3
Chia, Sainsbury's*	1 Tbsp/15g	62	3.8	414	21.8	8.6	25	33.6
Chia, Tesco*	1 Tbsp/15g	64	4.3	428	22.3	2.6	28.8	34.7
Chia, The Foodie Market, Aldi*	1 Tbsp/15g	66	4.6	442	17	7.7	31	34
Chia, White, The Chia Co*	1 Tbsp/15g	67	4.7	447	20.7	4.7	31.3	37.3
Chironji, Raw, Average	*1 Serving/10g*	*7*	*0.6*	*66*	*1.9*	*1.2*	*5.9*	*0.4*
Fiery, Graze*	1 Pack/34g	173	14.8	510	21.8	17.3	43.5	7.9
Flaxseed, Sunflower & Pumpkin, Milled, Linwoods*	1 Scoop/10g	54	4.9	542	22.7	2.4	49.1	16.2
Hemp, Hearts, Good Hemp*	1 Serving/30g	171	13.9	569	32.5	9.2	46.3	2.6
Hemp, Milled, Organic, Flax, & Chia Seed, Multiboost*	1 Serving/25g	124	9	496	24	1.6	36	28
Hemp, Shelled, Linwoods*	1 Serving/20g	123	10.4	617	35	1.1	52	2.1
Milled, with Flax, & Chia, Tesco*	1 Tbsp/15g	85	6.7	567	26.4	6.4	44.8	16.4
Mix, Four, Morrisons*	1 Serving/30g	174	13.5	580	25.9	15.6	45.1	3.9
Mixed, Cranberries, & Goji Berries, Sainsbury's*	1 Serving/10g	51	3.2	508	17	33.1	32.5	7.7
Mixed, Milled, with Freeze Dried Raspberries, Yum & Yay*	1 Serving/25g	132	10.4	530	24.3	3	41.8	22.4
Mixed, Wholesome, Love Life, Waitrose*	1 Serving/30g	166	13.6	554	21.3	15.5	45.2	8
Mixed, with Salted Caramel, Whitworths*	1 Serving/25g	148	11.9	591	26.8	10.7	47.6	6.4
Mustard, Average	*1 Tsp/3.3g*	*15*	*0.9*	*469*	*34.9*	*34.9*	*28.8*	*14.7*
Nigella, Average	*1 Tsp/5g*	*20*	*1.7*	*392*	*21.3*	*1.9*	*33.3*	*8.4*
Omega Mix, Grape Tree*	1 Serving/40g	225	17.6	563	20	23	44	16
Phool Makhana, Raw, Average	*1 Serving/10g*	*35*	*0*	*350*	*9.7*	*77*	*0.1*	*7.6*
Pomegranate, Lidl*	1 Pot/80g	49	0.2	61	1.2	11.8	0.2	3.4
Pomegranate, Nature's Pick, Aldi*	1 Pack/80g	49	0.5	61	1.2	11.8	0.6	3.4
Poppy, Average	*1 Tbsp/9g*	*47*	*3.9*	*533*	*18*	*23.7*	*44.7*	*10*
Pumpkin, & Sunflower, Toasted, Sainsbury's*	1 Serving/10g	64	5.6	643	28	1.9	56	9.8
Pumpkin, Average	*1 Tbsp/10g*	*57*	*4.6*	*568*	*27.9*	*13*	*45.9*	*3.8*
Pumpkin, Coated, Crunchy, Nutriliciousme*	1 Pack/30g	172	13.7	572	25.8	10.3	45.6	8.3
Pumpkin, Crunchy Coated, Nutrilicious*	1 Pack/30g	172	13.7	572	25.8	10.3	45.6	8.3
Quinoa, Paul's Finest*	1 Serving/10g	35	0.6	354	14.1	57.2	6.1	7
Sesame, Average	*1 Tsp/2g*	*12*	*1.1*	*610*	*22.3*	*3.6*	*56.4*	*7.8*
Sesame, Black, Sainsbury's*	1 Tsp/5g	30	2.6	593	21.4	1.8	52.6	13.6
Sesame, Snappy, Holland & Barrett*	1 Pack/300g	1794	174	598	18	0.9	58	7.9
Sunflower, Average	*1 Tbsp/10g*	*59*	*4.9*	*585*	*23.4*	*15*	*48.7*	*5.7*
SEMOLINA								
Average	*1oz/28g*	*98*	*0.5*	*348*	*11*	*75.2*	*1.8*	*2.1*
Pudding, Creamed, Ambrosia*	1 Can/425g	344	7.2	81	3.3	13.1	1.7	0.2
Pudding, Creamed, Co-Op*	1 Can/425g	382	8.5	90	4	15	2	0
SHALLOTS								
Pickled in Hot & Spicy Vinegar, Tesco*	1 Onion/18g	14	0	77	1	18	0.1	1.9
Pickled, Drained, Garners*	1 Shallot/15g	15	0.1	97	1	21.6	0.5	2.5
Raw, Average	*1 Serving/80g*	*16*	*0.2*	*20*	*1.5*	*3.3*	*0.2*	*1.4*
SHANDY								
Bitter, Original, Ben Shaws*	1 Can/330ml	89	0	27	0	6	0	0

S

	Measure INFO/WEIGHT	per Measure KCAL	FAT	Nutrition Values per 100g / 100ml KCAL	PROT	CARB	FAT	FIBRE
SHANDY								
Canned, Morrisons*	1 Can/330ml	36	0	11	0	1.8	0	0
Homemade, Average	**1 Pint/568ml**	**148**	**0**	**26**	**0.2**	**2.9**	**0**	**0**
Lager, 0.9%, Bavaria*	1 Can/330ml	76	0	23	0.1	5	0	0
Lemonade, Traditional Style, Tesco*	1 Can/330ml	63	0	19	0	4.7	0	0
Panache, Carrefour*	1 Bottle/250ml	68	0	27	0.5	6.3	0	0
SHARON FRUIT								
Average	**1oz/28g**	**19**	**0**	**68**	**0.7**	**17.3**	**0**	**1.5**
SHERRY								
Dry, Average	**1 Glass/120ml**	**139**	**0**	**116**	**0.2**	**1.4**	**0**	**0**
Medium	**1 Serving/50ml**	**58**	**0**	**116**	**0.1**	**5.9**	**0**	**0**
Sweet	**1 Serving/50ml**	**68**	**0**	**136**	**0.3**	**6.9**	**0**	**0**
SHORTBREAD								
All Butter, Deans*	1 Biscuit/15g	77	3.8	511	4.9	65.7	25.4	1.2
All Butter, Deluxe, Lidl*	1 Biscuit/20g	103	5.3	517	4.3	64.9	26.5	1
All Butter, Finger, Highland, TTD, Sainsbury's*	1 Biscuit/20g	103	5.5	515	4.6	61.8	27.4	1.2
All Butter, Fingers, Highland, Sainsbury's*	1 Biscuit/19g	97	4.9	509	4.4	64.1	25.7	1.8
All Butter, Giant, Fingers, Higland, Sainsbury's*	1 Biscuit/35g	182	10.1	520	4.8	59.4	28.8	1.8
All Butter, Petticoat Tails, Co-Op*	1 Biscuit/13g	68	3.8	520	5	60	29	2
All Butter, Round, Luxury, M&S*	1 Biscuit/20g	105	5.8	525	6.2	60	29	2
All Butter, Selection, Waitrose*	1 Biscuit/18g	95	11	527	5.3	58.3	61.1	3
All Butter, Trufree*	1 Biscuit/11g	58	3.1	524	2	66	28	0.9
All Butter, with Toffee, Scottish, M&S*	1 Biscuit/6g	32	1.7	515	5.7	61.9	26.9	1.2
Average	**1oz/28g**	**139**	**7.3**	**498**	**5.9**	**63.9**	**26.1**	**1.9**
Belgian Chocolate Chunk, Asda*	1 Biscuit/20g	106	6.2	531	7	56	31	1.8
Butter Enriched, Morrisons*	1 Biscuit/19g	95	4.8	500	5.8	62.1	25.3	1
Choc Chip, Fair Trade, Co-Op*	1 Biscuit/19g	100	6	526	5.3	57.9	31.6	2.6
Chocolate Chip, Jacob's*	1 Biscuit/17g	87	4.7	513	5.2	61.2	27.5	1.8
Chocolate Chunk, TTD, Sainsbury's*	1 Biscuit/22g	113	6.2	518	5.3	59.5	28.2	2.4
Chocolate, Belgian, Chunky, TTD, Sainsbury's*	1 Biscuit/70g	353	19	505	5.5	58.8	27.2	1.4
Clotted Cream, Finest, Tesco*	1 Biscuit/20g	109	6.4	543	5.2	58	32.2	1.7
Coffee, No.1, Waitrose*	1 Biscuit/15g	81	4.4	539	5.2	62.9	29.2	1.8
Demerara, Rounds, TTD, Sainsbury's*	1 Biscuit/22g	113	5.9	508	5.1	62.2	26.5	1.8
Finger, Tower Gate, Lidl*	1 Finger/17g	90	4.8	516	6.4	59.2	27.6	2.5
Fingers, Asda*	1 Finger/18g	93	5.1	519	5.8	60.3	28.3	18
Fingers, Clotted Cream, Paterson's*	1 Finger/15g	76	3.8	507	6.4	62.4	25.3	0
Fingers, Scottish, Finest, Tesco*	1 Finger/21g	104	5	498	5.1	65.5	23.9	2
Free From, Morrisons*	1 Biscuit/18g	92	4.7	511	6	61.8	26.3	1.4
Highlanders, Walkers Shortbread Ltd*	1 Biscuit/22g	113	5.9	514	5.2	61.7	26.9	1.9
Lavender, Waitrose*	1 Biscuit/10g	53	2.8	532	5.5	63.5	28	2
Millionaire, Salted Caramel, M&S*	1 Slice/55g	261	12.5	475	4	63	22.7	1.2
Mini Bites, Co-Op*	1 Biscuit/10g	53	3	530	7	59	30	2
Mini, Bites, Tesco*	1 Bite/12g	63	3.5	528	7.2	58.1	29.3	1.3
Oatflake, Sinclair Of Rhynie*	1 Biscuit/23g	112	6.6	486	4.6	53.6	28.8	2.2
Pecan All Butter, Sainsbury's*	1 Biscuit/18g	99	6.5	548	5.3	49.9	36.3	2.5
Petticoat Tails, All Butter, Highland, Sainsbury's*	1 Segment/11g	57	3.1	518	6	59.9	27.8	2.3
Pure Butter, GF, Walkers*	1 Biscuit/16g	83	4.4	518	3.6	63.5	27.4	1.3
Pure Butter, Scottie, Mini, Walkers*	1 Scottie/3g	15	0.8	509	5.8	63.3	25.3	2.3
Rings, Handbaked, Border*	1 Biscuit/17g	86	4.9	520	6.2	61.2	29.5	0
Rose Petal, & Chinese Tea, 1, Waitrose*	1 Biscuit/10g	53	2.9	527	5.8	59.6	29	2.1
Rounds, All Butter, Toffee & Pecan, M&S*	1 Biscuit/20g	111	7	553	4.7	54.1	34.9	2
Salted Caramel, Milk Choc Chunk, Walkers Shortbread Ltd*	1 Biscuit/21g	111	6.2	527	5.2	59.3	29.5	1.7
Salted Caramel, Cartwright And Butler*	1 Biscuit/22g	103	5.4	469	4.2	58.1	24.7	1.4
Salted Caramel, Scottish, Morrisons*	1 Biscuit/20g	106	6.1	530	5.5	57.5	30.5	2

	Measure INFO/WEIGHT	per Measure KCAL	FAT	Nutrition Values per 100g / 100ml KCAL	PROT	CARB	FAT	FIBRE
SHORTBREAD								
Stem Ginger, All Butter, Duchy, Waitrose*	1 Biscuit/13g	65	3.2	502	5	63.4	25	1.7
SHORTCAKE								
Bites, Mini, Sainsbury's*	1 Biscuit/12g	62	3.1	515	6.2	64.5	25.5	1.4
Caramel, Baked in the Tray, Tesco*	1 Slice/49g	247	13.2	504	3.4	61.6	26.9	1.1
Caramel, Milk, Slice, Cake & Eat It*	1 Biscuit/40g	202	10.9	505	5	60	27.2	1.2
Caramel, Mini, Thorntons*	1 Piece/14g	69	4.1	491	5	50.6	29.5	0
Caramel, Slice, Holly Lane, Aldi*	1 Slice/50g	252	14	503	5.4	57	28	1.7
Caramel, Slices, Sainsbury's*	1 Slice/33g	162	8.4	491	5.3	59.6	25.5	1.3
Squares, Caramel, Tesco*	1 Slice/25g	127	7.7	506	6.3	54.3	30.7	2.4
SHRIMP								
Boiled, Average	**1 Serving/60g**	**70**	**1.4**	**117**	**23.8**	**0**	**2.4**	**0**
Butterfly, Oven Crispy, Seapak*	7 Shrimp/84g	220	11	262	11.9	23.8	13.1	1.2
Frozen, Average	**1oz/28g**	**20**	**0.2**	**73**	**16.5**	**0**	**0.8**	**0**
in Tomato Sauce, Arbi*	1 Pack/300g	504	41.1	168	10	0.9	13.7	0.5
Medium, Raw, Wild gulf*	¼ Pack/112g	80	1	71	13.4	0.9	0.9	0
Panko Breaded, Kirkland Signature, Costco*	1 Shrimp/26g	62	3.4	240	12.7	17	13.2	1.1
Shredded, Jeeny's*	1 Pack/30g	81	0.3	269	30.1	35.2	0.9	0
SKATE								
Grilled	**1oz/28g**	**22**	**0.1**	**79**	**18.9**	**0**	**0.5**	**0**
in Batter, Fried in Blended Oil	**1oz/28g**	**47**	**2.8**	**168**	**14.7**	**4.9**	**10.1**	**0.2**
Raw, Edible Portion	**1oz/28g**	**18**	**0.1**	**64**	**15.1**	**0**	**0.4**	**0**
SKIPS								
Cheesy, KP Snacks*	1 Bag/17g	89	5	524	6.2	58.5	29.5	1
Prawn Cocktail, KP Snacks*	1 Bag/17g	92	5.4	543	4.7	57	32	2.4
SKITTLES								
Chewies, Mars*	1 Serving/44g	177	2.6	403	0	86.2	5.9	0
Giants, Skittles*	1/3 Pack/47g	191	2	406	0	91.4	4.2	0
Mars*	1 Pack/55g	223	2.4	406	0	90.6	4.4	0
Sweet Heat, Mars*	¼ Pack/49g	196	2.1	399	0	89.8	4.2	0
SLICES								
Bacon & Cheese, Pastry, Tesco*	1 Slice/165g	480	32	291	7.4	21.7	19.4	1
Bean, Cheesy, Pastry, Sainsbury's*	1 Slice/180g	524	28.3	291	7.5	25.9	15.7	3.4
Beef, Minced Steak & Onion, Tesco*	1 Slice/150g	424	27.2	283	8.7	21.3	18.1	1.6
Cheese & Onion, Pastry, Tesco*	1 Slice/150g	412	23.2	275	6.9	26	15.5	1.9
Chicken & Mushroom, Tesco*	1 Slice/165g	457	28.9	277	9.2	20.6	17.5	0.9
Chicken & Bacon, Wall's*	1 Slice/225g	576	33.5	256	10.5	19.9	14.9	0
Chicken & Mushroom, Ginsters*	1 Slice/180g	439	26.8	244	8.3	19.1	14.9	1.8
Chicken & Mushroom, Sainsbury's*	1 Slice/164g	427	26.5	259	7.3	21.3	16.1	1
Chicken Fajita, Puff Pastry, Sainsbury's*	1 Slice/165g	404	17.6	245	9.2	27	10.7	2
Chicken, & Bacon, Asda*	1 Slice/156g	416	21.9	266	10	24	14	1.4
Chicken, & Mushroom, Iceland*	1 Slice/130g	322	16.6	248	7	25.4	12.8	1.6
Custard, Iceland*	1 Slice/35g	121	5.1	345	4	49.4	14.5	0.5
Custard, Pastry, Tesco*	1 Slice/94g	266	10.7	283	3.2	41.6	11.3	0.9
Fresh Cream, Tesco*	1 Slice/75g	311	21	414	3.5	37.4	27.9	1
Minced Beef, & Onion, Puff Pastry, Dunnes Stores*	1 Slice/160g	446	30.4	279	6.8	23	19	1
Minced Steak & Onion, Sainsbury's*	1 Slice/165g	475	29.9	288	15.2	16	18.1	2.5
Steak, Large, Ginsters*	1 Slice/204g	516	30.6	253	10.9	17.9	15	0
Steak, Peppered, Ginsters*	1 Slice/180g	457	27	254	8.4	21.3	15	1.6
Steak, Puff Pastry, Sainsbury's*	1 Slice/150g	328	11.7	219	8.4	27.7	7.8	2.3
Steak, Puff Pastry, Tesco*	1 Slice/150g	387	22	258	8.5	22.1	14.7	1.6
Vanilla, Baked by Us, Morrisons*	1 Slice/103g	290	12.4	282	3	40	12	0.9
SLIM FAST*								
Bars, Chocolate Caramel Treat, Snack, Slim Fast*	1 Bar/26g	95	2.6	360	3.5	63	10	1.5

S

	Measure INFO/WEIGHT	per Measure KCAL	FAT	Nutrition Values per 100g / 100ml KCAL	PROT	CARB	FAT	FIBRE
SLIM FAST*								
Bars, Chocolate, Nutty, Nougat, Snack, Slim Fast*	1 Bar/25g	95	3	380	4	63	12	1.5
Bars, Heavenly Chocolate Delight, Snack, Slim Fast*	1 Bar/24g	95	3.2	390	5	58	13	7
Bars, Heavenly Chocolate, Crunch Snack, Slim Fast*	1 Bar/24g	95	3.2	390	5	58	13	7
Bars, Nutty Salted Caramel, Meal, Slim Fast*	1 Bar/60g	218	6.8	364	25.4	26.9	11.3	18.7
Bars, Summer Berry, Meal, Slim Fast*	1 Bar/60g	210	5	350	23.3	51.7	8.3	5.8
Chunky Chocolate, Shake, Ready to Drink, Slimfast*	1 Shake/325ml	204	5.2	63	4.6	6.6	1.6	1.5
Crackers, Cheddar Flavour Bites, Snack Bag, Slim Fast*	1 Pack/22g	92	2	417	9.6	72.8	9.2	2.5
Meal Replacement, Chocolate, Slim Fast*	1 Bar/60g	211	5.4	352	25	38.3	9	11.2
Milk Shake, Blissful Banana, Powder, Dry, Slim Fast*	2 Scoops/37g	131	2.4	359	13.4	60.2	6.7	11
Milk Shake, Chunky Chocolate, Powder, Dry, Slim Fast*	2 Scoops/37g	132	2.7	363	13.9	59	7.5	10.9
Milk Shake, Simply Vanilla, Powder, Dry, Slim Fast*	2 Scoops/37g	131	2.4	360	13.4	60.9	6.5	11
Milk Shake, Summer Strawberry, Powder, Dry, Slim Fast*	2 Scoops/37g	139	2.4	380	13.5	60.1	6.6	11.1
Milk Shake, Caramel Temptation, Powder, Dry, Slim Fast*	1 Serving/37g	139	2.2	380	14	62	6	11
Noodles, Chicken Tikka Masala, Box, Slim Fast*	1 Box/250g	81	2.2	33	2.3	2.7	0.9	2.5
Noodles, Spicy Thai, Slim Fast*	1 Box/240g	70	3.1	29	0.9	2.4	1.3	2.4
Pretzels, Sour Cream & Chive, Snack Bag, Slim Fast*	1 Pack/23g	99	2.2	432	9.7	74.9	9.5	4.1
Tortillas, Barbecue Flavour, Snack Bag, Slim Fast*	1 Bag/22g	96	2.6	435	6.5	73.9	11.8	3.6
SMARTIES								
Mini Eggs, Nestle*	5 Eggs/17g	85	3.5	499	3.9	73.5	20.4	2.8
Mini, Treat Size, Smarties, Nestle*	1 Carton/14g	68	2.8	471	5	68.1	19.6	1
Nestle*	1 Tube/40g	188	7.1	469	3.9	72.5	17.7	2.4
SMOOTHIE								
Almond, & Banana, Allplants*	1 Serving/140g	302	14.1	216	6.5	24.2	10.1	4.4
Almond, & Berry, Allplants*	1 Serving/140g	186	6.2	133	6.5	18	4.4	3.4
Apple, Pear, Ginger, & Oats, Ikea*	1 Bottle/250ml	88	0	35	0.7	8	0	0
Berry Beets, Mindful Chef*	1 Serving/140g	55	0.6	39	1.1	5.6	0.4	4.4
Berry Light, Super Smoothie, Innocent*	1 Serving/150ml	54	0.1	36	0.5	8.5	0	1.2
Berry Set Go, Innocent*	1 Bottle/330ml	142	0	43	0	11	0	0
Berry, & Beetroot, Sachet, M&S*	1 Sachet/110g	65	0.2	59	1.2	12.1	0.2	2.2
Berry, & Mango, Allplants*	1 Serving/140g	106	1.5	76	1.2	16	1.1	2.8
Berry, Dry Weight, Lighter Life*	1 Scoop/20g	71	1.2	354	17	48	5.8	20
Blackberries & Blueberries, Innocent*	1 Bottle/250ml	120	0.2	48	0.5	12	0.1	2.1
Blackcurrant, & Blueberry, Asda*	1 Serving/250ml	125	1.2	50	0.5	12	0.5	0.6
Blue Spark, Super Smoothie, Innocent*	1 Serving/150ml	81	0	54	0.3	12	0	1
Bolt from the Blue, Innocent*	1 Serving/150ml	62	0	41	0	10	0	0
Breakfast Oats, Mindful Chef*	1 Pack/140g	158	2.8	113	2.5	19.1	2	3
Cacao, & Black Cherry, Super Smoothie, Innocent*	1 Serving/248ml	154	0	62	0.8	14	0	0.9
Carrot, Mango, & Turmeric, Plant Kitchen, M&S*	1 Bottle/250ml	165	2.2	66	0.7	13.5	0.9	0.4
Cherries, & Strawberries,, Just For Kids, Innocent*	1 Carton/180ml	92	0	51	0.4	11	0	1.3
Cucumber, & Melon, Mindful Chef*	1 Serving/140g	34	0.7	24	1.4	2.7	0.5	1.6
Cucumber, Avocado, & Lime, M&S*	1 Bottle/250ml	148	3.5	59	0.4	10.4	1.4	1.4
Enliven, The Juice Company, Aldi*	1 Serving/100ml	61	0.5	61	0.4	13.3	0.5	0.5
Ginger, Boost Me, Swisse me*	1 Pack/119g	83	2.1	70	0.6	12	1.8	1.8
Green, Lean, Mindful Chef*	1 Pack/140g	78	0.8	56	1.3	10	0.6	2.5
Guava, Pineapple, & Apple, Innocent*	1 Serving/250ml	140	1.2	56	1	13	0.5	1.1
Kefir, Cacao, Bio-tiful Dairy*	1 Bottle/250ml	162	6.8	65	3.1	6.8	2.7	0
Kefir, Raspberry, Bio-tiful Dairy*	1 Bottle/250ml	162	6.8	65	3	7.2	2.7	0
Kiwi, & Cucumber, Lean, Naked Juice Co*	1 Bottle/350ml	98	0	28	0.2	6.9	0	0
Magnificent Mango, Innocent*	1 Bottle/250ml	136	0	54	0.4	12	0	1.4
Mango, & Greens, Allplants*	1 Serving/140g	102	1.1	73	1.8	15	0.8	2.7
Mango, Avocado, Pear, & Matcha, Super, M&S*	1 Glass/150ml	117	0.9	78	0.7	15	0.6	0.5
Mango, Pineapple, & Passion Fruit, Eat Well, M&S*	1 Bottle/250g	170	1.2	68	0.5	14.9	0.5	0.9
Mangoes & Passion Fruits, Pure Fruit, Innocent*	1 Bottle/250ml	135	0	54	0.4	12	0	1.4

SMOOTHIE

	Measure INFO/WEIGHT	per Measure KCAL	FAT	Nutrition Values per 100g / 100ml KCAL	PROT	CARB	FAT	FIBRE
Mixed Berry, CBY, Asda*	1 Glass/250ml	143	0	57	0.6	12.6	0	1.6
Orange, Banana, Mango, Morning Boost, Tropicana*	1 Serving/250ml	125	0	50	0.1	9.2	0	2.3
Orange, Energiser, Mindful Chef*	1 Serving/140g	76	0.4	54	0.8	11.1	0.3	2.1
Orange, Mango, & Passionfruit, On the Go, Sainsbury's*	1 Serving/150g	84	0.8	56	0.5	12.8	0.5	0.7
Oranges, Mangoes & Pineapples For Kids, Innocent*	1 Carton/180ml	94	0.2	52	0.7	11.7	0.1	0.9
Peaches & Passionfruit, for Kids, Innocent*	1 Carton/180ml	95	0	53	0.6	14.7	0	0.9
Pear, Kiwi, Kale, & Fennel, Waitrose*	1 Serving/150ml	64	0	43	0.5	9.8	0	0.9
Pineapple, Apple, & Carrot, Innocent*	1 Carton/180ml	94	0	52	0.6	12	0	0.3
Pineapple, Banana & Coconut, CBY, Asda*	1 Glass/250ml	178	2.8	71	0.7	13.6	1.1	1
Pineapples, Bananas & Coconuts, Innocent*	1 Bottle/250ml	172	2.8	69	0.7	13.6	1.1	1
Pomegranates, Blueberries & Acai, Special, Innocent*	1 Serving/250ml	170	0.5	68	0.6	15.6	0.2	0.8
Power to the Purple, 40, Innocent*	1 Sm Bottle/330g	132	1.6	40	0	10	0.5	0.5
Protein Superfood, Mango & Banana, PhD Nutrition*	1 Serving/130g	175	7.7	135	15.4	4.2	5.9	1.4
Raspberry & Blueberry, Plus, Tesco*	1 Serving/100ml	59	0.3	59	2.6	11.6	0.3	0.5
Revitalise, The Juice Company, Aldi*	1 Serving/150ml	75	0.5	50	0.4	12	0.3	0.5
Strawberries & Bananas, Pure Fruit, Innocent*	1 Bottle/250ml	132	0.2	53	0.7	13.1	0.1	1.3
Strawberry & Banana, Tesco*	1 Bottle/250ml	112	0.5	45	0.6	10.1	0.2	0.8
Strawberry, & Banana, Ready Made, Asda*	1 Glass/150ml	90	0	60	0.7	13	0	1.8
Summer Sunrise, Mindful Chef*	1 Pack/140g	78	0.3	56	0.9	11.6	0.2	1.8
Super Berry, M&S*	1 Bottle/150g	94	0.8	63	1	13.1	0.5	1
Super Green, Mindful Chef*	1 Pack/140g	99	4.5	71	1.6	7.7	3.2	2.4
Super, Gut Health, M&S*	1 Bottle/250ml	195	0.5	78	1	16.9	0.2	2.5
Super, Power, M&S*	1 Bottle/250ml	388	2.8	155	2.2	10.5	1.1	0.7
Super, Protect, M&S*	1 Bottle/250ml	190	7	76	0.8	11.4	2.8	0.8
Tropical, Light, Innocent*	½ Bottle/150ml	60	0.8	40	0.8	8.7	0.5	1.1
Vanilla Bean, M&S*	1 Bottle/500ml	450	13	90	3.3	13.9	2.6	0
Vitamin Bundle, Innocent*	1 Bottle/300ml	135	0	45	0	11	0	0.5
Watermelon, & Raspberry, Lean, Naked Juice Co*	1 Bottle/360ml	97	0	27	0.2	6.6	0	0

SMOOTHIE MIX

Banana, Kale & Mango, As Sold, Iceland*	1 Sachet/150g	90	0.4	60	1.1	12.2	0.3	2.3
Beautiful Berries, My Goodness, Sainsbury's*	1 Serving/80g	39	0.4	49	1	8.9	0.5	3.7
Berry, Banana, Frozen, Sainsbury's*	1 Serving/80g	43	0.4	54	0.8	10.3	0.5	3.1
Berry, Frozen, Love Life, Waitrose*	1 Serving/80g	31	0	39	1.1	7.2	0	2.9
Breakfast, Love Smoothies*	1 Sachet/120g	238	4.9	198	6.8	28.2	4.1	6.5
Carrot Kick, Sainsbury's*	1 Serving/80ml	39	0.4	49	0.7	10	0.5	2.1
Detox Zing, Love Smoothies*	1 Bag/120g	68	0.4	57	1.1	11.3	0.3	2.2
Detox, Pack'd*	1 Pouch/140g	69	0.7	49	2.3	11	0.5	2.2
Energy, Pack'd*	1 Pouch/140g	85	0.8	61	1.4	14	0.6	3.3
Gorgeous Greens, Asda*	1 Serving/80g	34	0.4	43	1.2	7.8	0.5	1.2
Grape Escape, Love Smoothies*	1 Serving/120ml	74	0.4	62	0.7	13	0.3	2.3
Green, Four Seasons, Aldi*	1 Serving/100g	47	0.6	47	1.6	8.1	0.6	1.6
Greens, Glowing, My Goodness, Sainsbury's*	1 Serving/80g	47	2.1	59	2.1	5.5	2.6	2.6
Mango, & Pineapple, Totally Tropical, Asda*	1 Serving/80g	44	0.4	55	0.6	12	0.5	2.1
Melange Vert, Lidl*	1 Sachet/150g	60	0.3	40	0.5	8.1	0.2	0
Orange, Lidl*	1 Pack/148g	61	0.3	41	2	8.1	0.2	0
Strawberry & Banana, Frozen, Love Life, Waitrose*	1 Serving/80g	37	0.3	46	0.7	8.2	0.4	3.4
Strawberry, & Banana, Frozen, Iceland*	1 Serving/80g	51	0.2	64	0.9	13.2	0.3	2.6
Strawberry, Blueberry, & Banana, Lidl*	1 Pack/150g	82	0.6	55	1	9.9	0.4	2.6
Summer Fruits, & Banana, Frozen, Asda*	1 Serving/80g	41	0.4	51	1	10	0.5	1.4
Tropical, Frozen, Love Life, Waitrose*	1 Serving/80g	45	0.2	57	0.7	11.8	0.3	1.9
Tropical, Lidl*	1 Serving/75g	39	0.2	52	0.5	11.4	0.2	0.8
Very Berry, Sainsbury's*	1 Serving/80g	39	0.4	49	0.9	9.2	0.5	3.1
Vitality, Pack'D*	1 Pouch/140g	97	1.4	69	1.1	13	1	1.8

	Measure INFO/WEIGHT	per Measure KCAL	FAT	Nutrition Values per 100g / 100ml KCAL	PROT	CARB	FAT	FIBRE
SMOOTHIE MIX								
Yellow Frozen, Morrisons*	1 Portion/80g	41	0.2	51	0.5	10.9	0.2	1.9
SNACKS								
Amaretti, & Almond, Chocolate Curiosities, Graze*	1 Punnet/32g	171	12.2	535	17	33	38	9.4
Apple, Grape, Pineapple, & Cheese, Waitrose*	½ Pack/110g	152	8.8	138	6.1	9.9	8	1.2
Balls, Cotton Candy , Herr's*	1 Serving/28g	160	10	571	3.6	53.6	35.7	3.6
BBq Chilli Crunch, Co-Op*	1 Serving/30g	156	9.3	520	12	45	31	4.9
Bean, Crunch, Chilli, Graze*	1 Punnet/30g	135	5.7	451	17	48	19	9.2
Boondi, Regal Snacks*	1 Serving/15g	81	5.4	542	8.2	44.4	36.3	0
Box, Smokehouse BBQ, Crunch, Graze*	1 Pack/31g	137	4.6	441	9.9	60	15	7.3
Chakri, Cofresh*	1 Serving/40g	204	10.4	510	9	60	26	5
Cheddar, Popped, British, Barbers*	1 Pack/20g	122	10.2	611	37	0	51	0
Cheese Savouries, Morrisons*	1 Serving/25g	130	7.5	520	11.3	49.2	30	3.8
Cheese Savouries, Tesco*	1 Serving/25g	133	7.8	531	11.3	50	31.3	2.1
Chickpea Mix, Crunchy, Salt & Vinegar, Co-Op*	1 Pack/30g	127	6.6	422	16	37	22	17
Chili & Lime, Nutty Protein Power, Punchy, Graze*	1 Punnet/41g	245	19.7	597	22	21	48	8.3
Choccy Wonders, Almond, & Coconut, Graze*	1 Punnet/36g	189	14.8	524	12	21	41	20
Choccy Wonders, Banana & Peanut, Graze*	1 Punnet/37g	186	12.6	503	13	29	34	17
Choccy Wonders, Pretzel & Hazelnut, Graze*	1 Punnet/31g	160	10.8	516	13	32	35	16
Chocolate, Dark, Cherry, & Pecan Mix, Co-Op*	1 Serving/30g	131	6.9	438	4.4	51	23	4.5
Chorizo, Cheddar, & Toasts, Bodega*	1 Pack/64g	240	14.5	375	21.4	20.7	22.7	0
Classic, Aperitivo, Mix, Aldi*	1 Serving/25g	125	6.5	500	16	49	26	0
Cocoa Paradise , Graze*	1 Punnet/28g	140	8.7	501	4.8	50	31	6.8
CocoTop, Organic, Tiana*	1 Tub/50g	292	20.6	583	6.9	46.2	41.3	25.5
Cookies, Lemon Almond, & Tea, Graze*	1 Punnet/24g	103	4.3	428	6.8	55	18	3.2
Corn, Giant, Sweet Red Pepper, Sainsbury's*	1 Pack/35g	160	5.6	457	5.7	70	16	5.4
Corn, Original, Mister Corn*	1 Serving/30g	145	6.3	482	7.6	63	21	5.5
Crunch, Sea Salted, Lightly, Graze*	1 Serving/31g	128	4	413	16	53	13	11
Dexter the Dog, Morrisons*	1 Bag/15g	78	4.3	522	2.8	61.6	29	2
Dip Dip Hooray, Graze*	1 Serving/25g	134	8.5	535	18	33	34	9.1
Focaccia, Baby, Bo*	1 Serving/30g	146	7	487	10	63.3	23.3	3.3
Grilled Cheese Crunch, Graze*	1 Punnet/27g	150	10.5	555	18	35	39	7.4
Honey Roast Crunch, Graze*	1 Punnet/30g	133	4.2	443	12	62	14	8.8
Honey, Sesame, Chinese Style, Graze*	1 Punnet/30g	46	2.7	153	7.9	8.6	9	3.1
Hot Pepper Kick, M&S*	1 Pack/110g	557	29	506	15.4	48.8	26.4	6
Lion, Lightly Salted, Sainsbury's*	1 Pack/15g	78	4.4	522	2.8	61.6	29	2
Lotus Seeds, Popped, Caramel, Karma Bites*	1 Pack/25g	105	3.2	421	5.3	76.3	12.6	1.5
Lotus Seeds, Popped, Peri-Peri, Karma Bites*	1 Pack/25g	100	5.1	398	9.2	68.8	20.4	2
Lotus Seeds, Popped, Wasabi, Karma Bites*	1 Pack/25g	100	5.1	400	9.2	68.7	20.5	2
Macaron, Coconut, White Chocolate, Graze*	1 Punnet/29g	162	11.6	557	9.8	43	40	5.4
Mini C's, Cheese, GF, Schar*	1 Serving/30g	137	5.1	457	7.3	67	17	3.5
Mix, Sweet & Salty, Reese's*	½ Pack/28g	139	7.6	496	12.4	54.7	27.1	0
Mumbai Street Mix, Sensations, Walkers*	1 Serving/30g	167	11	556	14.3	40.8	36.5	3.7
Nut Mix, Acti-Snack*	1 Pack/40g	250	21.4	625	22.7	17.9	53.4	8.8
Nutty Protein Mix, Snacking Essentials*	1 Serving/25g	150	12.4	600	22.6	12.9	49.5	6
Pea Snaps, Sweet Chilli, & Lemon, Yushoi*	1 Pack/21g	90	3.2	429	17.1	48.1	15.2	12.9
Peanut Butter, Protein, Power, Graze*	1 Punnet/27g	136	8.1	503	22	33	30	6.2
Poppy Seed, & Onion, Bagel Crunch, Graze*	1 Punnet/37g	207	14.1	560	18	35	38	4.1
Pretzel, & Peanut, Chocolate Curiosities, Graze*	1 Pack/36g	177	9.4	492	17	44	26	9
Pretzel, Sweet Mustard, Graze*	1 Punnet/25g	129	7.2	517	14	48	29	4.1
Protein Mix, Bare Nature*	1 Serving/30g	156	9.7	519	32.6	19.9	32.4	8.9
Protein Mix, Salt & Pepper, Co-Op*	1 Pack/38g	196	12.9	517	32	16	34	8.1
Protein Mix, Veggie, Sainsbury's*	¼ Pack/30g	142	7.9	473	29.2	22.1	26.3	15.5
Protein Power, Veggie, Alesto, Lidl*	1 Serving/28g	134	7.3	479	30.3	25.5	26	10.7

SNACKS

	Measure INFO/WEIGHT	per Measure KCAL	FAT	KCAL	PROT	CARB	FAT	FIBRE
Rice, Sushi Mix, Mitsuba*	1 Serving/30g	124	2.3	412	9	75.5	7.7	2.1
Salt & Pepper, Combo Mix, Sainsbury's*	1 Serving/30g	143	6.4	476	4.3	65.5	21.2	3.1
Salt & Vinegar, Crunch, Graze*	1 Punnet/28g	124	4.8	444	16	51	17	12
Sesame Sticks, Suma*	1 Serving/25g	120	7.5	480	18.1	39	30	4.9
Slightly Salted, Baked Pea Sticks, Yushoi *	1 Pack/21g	88	3.2	419	19.4	43.1	15.4	15.5
Smoky Barbecue, Crunch, Retail, Graze*	1 Pack/31g	137	5	443	11	57	16	7.9
Smoky Paprika Crunch, Tesco*	1 Pack/45g	171	3.2	381	23.4	46.8	7.1	18
Sour Cream & Onion, Lentil Curls, Passions Deli, Aldi*	1 Pack/20g	91	3.4	454	11	63	17	3.6
Soy & Balsamic Vinegar, Baked Pea Sticks, Yushoi *	1 Serving/21g	88	2.9	417	18.6	47.9	13.7	13.5
Sweet & Salty, Veggie Protein Power, Graze*	1 Punnet/30g	162	10.2	539	25	30	34	8.2
Sweet Chilli, Crunch, Graze*	1 Punnet/31g	139	5.3	448	15	55	17	9.9
Sweet Chilli, with Lemon, Baked Pea Sticks, Yushoi *	1 Pack/21g	90	3.2	428	17.4	48.1	15.3	13.1
Sweet Memphis BBQ, Veggie Protein Power, Graze*	1 Pack/38g	193	10.3	509	17	44	27	5.3
Teddy Faces, Snackrite, Aldi*	1 Bag/19g	93	4.4	490	3.4	66	23	1.5
Texan Style BBQ Crunch, Lidl*	1 Pack/31g	130	3.2	419	8.9	69	10.4	7
Thai Sriracha Mix, Natural Selection*	1 Pack/26g	109	3.4	420	11	60	13	9.3
Thai Sweet Chilli, Weight Watchers*	1 Bag/22g	87	2	395	34.6	38.6	9.1	10.9
Triple Berry Fusion, Graze*	1 Punnet/36g	122	0.3	340	2.2	82	0.9	4.5
Veggie Caesar, Graze*	1 Punnet/24g	115	4.6	478	17	52	19	9.4

SNAILS

	Measure INFO/WEIGHT	per Measure KCAL	FAT	KCAL	PROT	CARB	FAT	FIBRE
in Garlic Butter, Average	**6 Snails/50g**	**219**	**20.8**	**438**	**9.7**	**8**	**41.5**	**1**
Raw, Average	**1 Snail/5g**	**4**	**0.1**	**90**	**16.1**	**2**	**1.4**	**0**

SNAPPER

	Measure INFO/WEIGHT	per Measure KCAL	FAT	KCAL	PROT	CARB	FAT	FIBRE
Red, Fried in Blended Oil	**1oz/28g**	**35**	**0.9**	**126**	**24.5**	**0**	**3.1**	**0**
Red, Weighed with Bone, Raw	**1oz/28g**	**12**	**0.2**	**42**	**9.2**	**0**	**0.6**	**0**

SNICKERS

	Measure INFO/WEIGHT	per Measure KCAL	FAT	KCAL	PROT	CARB	FAT	FIBRE
99Kcal, Mars*	1 Bar/20g	99	5.1	502	8.4	58	26	0
Crispy, Mars*	1 Serving/20g	97	4.6	483	7.1	61	23	0
Mars*	1 Single/48g	245	13.4	510	9.5	54.3	27.9	1.3
Peanut Butter, Creamy, Mars*	1 Bar/18g	95	5.3	519	10	51	29	48
Peanut Butter, Crunchy, Snickers*	1 Bar/26g	130	7	500	11.5	57.7	26.9	3.8
Peanut Butter, Hi-Protein, Mars*	1 Bar/57g	225	8.6	394	35	35	15	0
Protein, Mars*	1 Bar/51g	199	7.1	391	35.6	36.1	13.9	0
White, Mars*	1 Bar/49g	241	11.8	491	9	59	24	0

SOLE

	Measure INFO/WEIGHT	per Measure KCAL	FAT	KCAL	PROT	CARB	FAT	FIBRE
Dover, on the Bone, Pan Fried, Sainsbury's*	1 Fillet/200g	190	2.2	95	19.4	1.5	1.1	0.5
Fillet, Yellowfin, Dusted, Garlic & Herb, Lidl*	1 Fillet/116g	184	7.3	159	15.1	10.3	6.3	0.5
Fillet, Yellowfin, Lightly Dusted, Northern Catch, Aldi*	1 Fillet/114g	171	4.6	150	20	7.6	4	2.5
Fillets, Lemon & Pepper, Co-Op*	1 Fillet/113g	232	13	205	11	13	12	0.8
Fillets, Lightly Dusted, Salt, & Black Pepper, Co-Op*	1 Fillet/113g	220	12.4	195	12	11	11	1
Yellow Fin, Fillets, Lemon & Parsley, Tasty Catch, Aldi*	1 Fillet/115g	193	8.3	168	15	10	7.2	1
Yellow, Fillet, Lightly Dusted, As Consumed, Morrisons*	1 Fillet/124g	218	8.5	176	14	13.9	6.9	1
Yellowfin, Fillets, Ocean Trader, Lidl*	1 Fillet/106g	153	6.1	144	14.5	8.1	5.8	0.5
Yellowfin, Lightly Dusted, Garlic & Herb Crumb, Aldi*	1 Fillet/113g	177	6.8	157	16	9.7	6	0.7

SOPOCKA

	Measure INFO/WEIGHT	per Measure KCAL	FAT	KCAL	PROT	CARB	FAT	FIBRE
Sliced, Cured, Pork Loin	**1 Serving/100g**	**101**	**2.9**	**101**	**17.8**	**0.8**	**2.9**	**0**

SORBET

	Measure INFO/WEIGHT	per Measure KCAL	FAT	KCAL	PROT	CARB	FAT	FIBRE
Blackcurrant, Yorvale Ltd*	1 Serving/100g	120	0.2	120	0	28.8	0.2	0
Damson, Mary's farmhouse*	1 Scoop/50g	42	0	85	0.3	21	0	0
Exotic Fruit, Sainsbury's*	1 Serving/75g	90	1.5	120	1.2	24.1	2	0
Granita, al Limone, Grom*	2 Scoops/100g	116	0.5	116	0.5	28.5	0.5	0
Jamaican Me Crazy, Ben & Jerry's*	1 Serving/100g	130	0	130	0.2	32	0	0.4
Lemon	**1 Scoop/60g**	**79**	**0**	**131**	**0.9**	**34.2**	**0**	**0**

S

INFO/WEIGHT	Measure	per Measure		Nutrition Values per 100g / 100ml				
		KCAL	FAT	KCAL	PROT	CARB	FAT	FIBRE

SORBET

Mandarin Orange, Yorvale Ltd*	1 Serving/100g	125	0.2	125	0.1	30.5	0.2	0
Mango, Tesco*	1 Scoop/50g	57	0.4	113	0.5	25.6	0.8	0.8
Mango, Waitrose*	1 Pot/100g	90	0	90	0.1	22.1	0	0.6
Orange, Del Monte*	1 Sorbet/500g	625	0.5	125	0.2	32.1	0.1	0
Passion Fruit, Yorvale Ltd*	1 Serving/100g	109	0.2	109	0.1	26.6	0.2	0
Raspberry & Blackberry, Fat Free, M&S*	1 Sorbet/125g	140	0	112	0.4	27.5	0	0.6
Raspberry, Gelatelli, Lidl*	1 Serving/50g	62	0.2	124	0.2	29.1	0.3	1.2
Raspberry, Haagen-Dazs*	½ Cup/105g	120	0	114	0	28.6	0	1.9
Raspberry, Sainsbury's*	1 Scoop/50ml	54	0.2	109	0.5	25	0.5	0.5
Raspberry, Tesco*	1 Scoop/64g	73	0.3	114	0.2	26.8	0.5	0.5
Watermelon, Lidl*	1 Scoop/50g	38	0.2	77	0.3	17.7	0.4	0.3

SOUFFLE

Cheese	**1oz/28g**	**71**	**5.4**	**253**	**11.4**	**9.3**	**19.2**	**0.3**
Lemon, Finest, Tesco*	1 Pot/80g	270	20.5	338	2.9	24.1	25.6	0.2
Ricotta & Spinach, M&S*	1 Serving/120g	186	13.3	155	8	6.2	11.1	2.1
Strawberry, M&S*	1 Serving/95g	171	10.1	180	1.6	19.5	10.6	0.9

SOUP

Almond, Deluxe, Lidl*	1 Serving/280g	409	40	146	1.4	2.1	14.3	1.4
Asparagus, Chef's Selection, Knorr*	1 Serving/250ml	76	3	30	0.7	4.4	1.2	0.2
Asparagus, Cream of, Canned, M&S*	½ Can/200g	108	7.2	54	0.9	4.3	3.6	0.2
Asparagus, in a Cup, Made Up, Sainsbury's*	1 Sachet/224ml	139	4.9	62	1.3	8.8	2.2	0.7
Asparagus, with Croutons, Aldi*	1 Sachet/229ml	96	3.7	42	0.5	6.5	1.6	0.5
Bacon, & Bean, Smoked, Diet Chef Ltd*	1 Pack/300g	162	3.3	54	2.8	8.2	1.1	2.1
Bacon, & Bean, Three, Smoked, Chunky, Baxters*	1 Can/400g	232	4.8	58	2.9	8.8	1.2	1.8
Bacon, & Lentil, CBY, Asda*	½ Pot/300g	177	4.2	59	3.8	7.2	1.4	1.2
Bacon, Smoked, & Kale, Sainsbury's*	1 Pot/600g	366	21	61	1.4	5.7	3.5	0.8
BBQ Bean, Smoky, Canned, Love Your Veg!, Sainsbury's*	½ Can/200g	112	1.4	56	2.6	8.3	0.7	2.8
Bean, & Vegetable, Three, LC, Tesco*	½ Can/200g	110	0.6	55	2.6	9.7	0.3	1.9
Bean, & Veg, Stew, Mighty, Big Soup, Heinz*	1 Can/500g	355	4.5	71	3	11.8	0.9	3
Bean, & Vegetable, Chunky, Sainsbury's*	1 Can/400g	268	4	67	3.5	9.3	1	3.6
Bean, Butter, & Chorizo, Meal, Sainsbury's*	1 Pot/400g	257	9.6	64	3.9	5.6	2.4	2.3
Bean, Chilli, Mexican, Tesco*	1 Carton/600g	270	6.6	45	2.2	6.4	1.1	1.9
Bean, Hearty, Italian Inspired, Love Life, Waitrose*	½ Pot/300g	151	6.6	50	1.5	5.2	2.2	1.8
Bean, Italian Style, Tesco*	1 Can/300g	153	3.6	51	2.8	7.3	1.2	1.1
Bean, Mexican, Fresh, Morrisons*	½ Pot/300g	171	3.9	57	2.1	8.3	1.3	1.9
Bean, Tuscan, Chunky, Love Life, Waitrose*	½ Can/200g	101	1	50	2.6	7.6	0.5	2.3
Bean, Tuscan, Slimming World, Iceland*	½ Pot/250g	100	0.5	40	2.6	5.1	0.2	3.7
Bean, Tuscan, Tesco*	1 Can/400g	212	2.8	53	2.8	7.7	0.7	2.4
Beef & Vegetable, Chunky, Canned, Sainsbury's*	1 Can/400g	212	6.8	53	4.2	4.6	1.7	1.2
Beef Chilli, Chunky, Canned, Morrisons*	½ Can/200g	123	1.8	62	5	6.9	0.9	2.7
Beef, & Mushroom, Big Soup, Heinz*	1 Can/515g	216	2.6	42	2.3	7	0.5	0.7
Beef, & Tomato, Cup a Soup, Made Up, Batchelors*	1 Serving/252g	83	1.6	33	0.6	6.3	0.6	0.4
Beef, & Vegetable, Big Soup, Heinz*	1 Can/400g	212	4	53	3.5	7.5	1	0.9
Beef, & Vegetable, Chunky, Eat Smart, Morrisons*	½ Can/200g	94	2	47	3.5	5.3	1	1.5
Beef, & Vegetables, Chunky, Newgate, Lidl*	1 Tin/400g	232	3.2	58	3.6	8.2	0.8	1.8
Beef, Broth, Big Soup, Heinz*	1 Can/400g	184	2.8	46	2.5	7	0.7	0.9
Beef, Broth, Classic, Heinz*	1 Can/400g	180	2	45	1.9	7.6	0.5	0.8
Beef, Chilli, Chunky, Asda*	1 Can/400g	212	4	53	4.2	5.7	1	2.4
Beef, Fiery, Pho, Vietnamese, Naked Soup*	1 Pack/300g	108	2.1	36	0.9	6.5	0.7	0
Beetroot, Carrot, & Apple, Waitrose*	1 Pot/350g	105	3.2	30	0.7	4.2	0.9	1.1
Beetroot, Curly Kale, with Quinoa, Tideford Organics*	½ Pack/300g	87	2.1	29	0.8	4.2	0.7	1.1
Black Bean, Mexican, Extra Special, Asda*	½ Pot/263g	194	10.8	74	2.3	7	4.1	1.7
Bone Broth, Mushroom, & Barley, Super Good, Baxters*	1 Can/400g	168	6.4	42	1.4	5.2	1.6	0.8

S

SOUP

	Measure INFO/WEIGHT	per Measure KCAL	per Measure FAT	KCAL	PROT	CARB	FAT	FIBRE
Bread, with Fruit Mix, Estonia, Tartu Mill*	1 Serving/50g	162	0.4	323	4.7	70.6	0.9	6.7
Broccoli, & Stilton, Classics, Fresh, Tesco*	½ Pot/300g	156	10.8	52	2.4	1.8	3.6	1.5
Broccoli, & Stilton, Cup Soup, Ainsley Harriott*	1 Sachet/230g	99	2.1	43	0.9	7.8	0.9	0.2
Broccoli, & Stilton, Fresh, Sainsbury's*	½ Pot/300ml	141	9.9	47	2.7	1.8	3.3	1.5
Broccoli, & Spinach, Souper, M&S*	½ Pot/300g	102	3.9	34	2.1	2.7	1.3	1.6
Broccoli, & Stilton, Canned, Sainsbury's*	1 Can/400g	180	10.4	45	1.5	3.9	2.6	0.5
Broccoli, & Stilton, Canned, Tesco*	½ Can/200g	100	5	50	1.8	4.9	2.5	0.5
Broccoli, Pea, & Basil, Soupologie*	½ Pot/300g	124	6.2	41	2.4	2.7	2.1	1.4
Broccoli, Salmon & Watercress, Stay Full, Baxters*	1 Can/400g	244	8.8	61	3.3	5.8	2.2	2.4
Broth, Savoury, Lighter Life*	1 Pack/6g	18	0.6	301	13.6	37.9	9.6	4.4
Butternut Squash, & Bacon, Smoked, Aldi*	½ Can/200g	122	8	61	1.8	4.2	4	0.5
Butternut Squash, & Chilli, Sainsbury's*	½ Pot/300g	112	7.2	37	0.7	3.1	2.4	0.2
Butternut Squash, & Tarragon, Waitrose*	½ Pot/300g	123	6.6	41	0.8	4.5	2.2	1
Butternut Squash, & Chickpea, Spiced, Heinz*	½ Can/200g	69	1	35	1.1	6.3	0.5	1.2
Butternut Squash, & Lentil Dhansak, Plant Based, Baxters*	1 Can/380g	171	1.5	45	2.4	7.2	0.4	1.5
Butternut Squash, & Tarragon, Creamy, Waitrose*	½ Pot/300g	126	6.6	42	0.8	4.5	2.2	1
Butternut Squash, Bisque, Well Yes, Campbell's*	1 Can/450g	264	9.8	59	0.6	8.9	2.2	0.4
Butternut Squash, Fresh, Waitrose*	½ Pot/300g	153	8.7	51	0.5	5.8	2.9	0.8
Butternut Squash, M&S*	1 Serving/400g	132	3.2	33	0.6	5.3	0.8	1
Butternut Squash, New England, Skinnylicious, Glorious!*	½ Pot/300g	87	2.1	29	0.5	4.5	0.7	1.4
Butternut Squash, Smooth, Fresh, M&S*	½ Pot/300g	105	3.3	35	0.8	5	1.1	0.9
Butternut Squash, Soupreme, Aldi*	½ Pot/300g	60	3.3	20	0.5	1.5	1.1	1.5
Butternut Squash, Tesco*	½ Pot/300g	82	4.3	27	0.4	2.5	1.4	1.5
Butternut, & Sage, Crosse & Blackwell*	1 Can/400g	215	12.4	54	0.5	5.8	3.1	0.4
Butternut, Spiced, New Covent Garden Food Co*	½ Pack/280g	95	4.8	34	0.8	3.3	1.7	1.1
Carrot, & Butter Bean, Vegetarian, Baxters*	1 Can/400g	232	7.6	58	1.7	7.2	1.9	2.1
Carrot, & Coriander, Average	**1 Can/400g**	**167**	**8.6**	**42**	**0.6**	**4.8**	**2.2**	**1**
Carrot, & Coriander, Fresh, Tesco*	½ Pot/300g	99	4.8	33	0.6	2.9	1.6	2.2
Carrot, & Lentil, Weight Watchers*	1 Can/295g	87	0.3	29	1.3	5.5	0.1	0.7
Carrot, & Butternut, with Chilli, Soupologie*	1 Pack/600g	240	10.2	40	0.7	4.9	1.7	1.4
Carrot, & Lentil, Farmers Market, Heinz*	1 Serving/200g	84	0.3	42	1.7	7.8	0.2	0.9
Carrot, Ginger, & Butternut, Super, Chef Select, Lidl*	½ Pack/300g	111	4.2	37	1	4.4	1.4	1.3
Carrot, Red Lentil & Cumin, Organic, Waitrose*	1 Pack/350g	175	8.8	50	0.2	6.7	2.5	0.5
Carrot, Roasted, & Ginger, Re:nourish*	1 Bottle/500g	179	6	36	0.6	4.6	1.2	2.2
Carrot, Thai, Skinny, Aldi*	½ Pot/300g	90	4.8	30	0.5	3.3	1.6	0.6
Cauliflower Cheese, Kale, & Cheddar, Yorkshire Provender*	½ Pot/300g	192	12.6	64	2.5	3.4	4.2	0.6
Cauliflower, & Celeriac, Love Life, Waitrose*	1 Pot/350g	79	3.1	23	1.6	1.4	0.9	1.3
Cauliflower, & Wensleydale, Crosse & Blackwell*	1 Can/400g	184	8	46	1.6	5.3	2	0.4
Cauliflower, Chicken, & Turmeric, Waitrose*	1 Pot/400g	221	7.6	55	3	5.8	1.9	1.4
Cauliflower, Chickpea, & Turmeric, Indian, Glorious!*	½ Pot/300g	114	2.4	38	2	4.4	0.8	2.7
Cauliflower, Masala Spiced, Specially Selected, Aldi*	½ Can/200g	106	6.4	53	1.7	4.1	3.2	0.6
Cauliflower, Onion, & Potato, Soup of the Day, Heinz*	½ Carton/200g	76	3.2	38	1.4	4.4	1.6	1
Celeriac, Velvety, Waitrose*	½ Pot/300g	151	11.5	50	0.8	2.8	3.8	0.9
Chicken Arrabbiata, Meal, G&B, Asda*	1 Pot/380g	167	1.9	44	3.6	5.6	0.5	1.8
Chicken Bone, Broth, Borough Broth Co.*	1 Pack/324g	58	1.6	18	2.6	0.6	0.5	0.5
Chicken Flavour, Tasty, Complan*	1 Sachets/55g	243	8.6	442	15.8	59.6	15.6	0
Chicken Jambalaya, Spicy, Waitrose*	½ Pot/300g	156	4.2	52	3.8	5.1	1.4	1
Chicken Noodle, & Vegetable, Waitrose*	1 Can/400g	140	2.4	35	1.6	5.5	0.6	0
Chicken Noodle, Aromatic, Asda*	1 Can/395g	162	2	41	1.5	7.3	0.5	0.5
Chicken Noodle, Canned, Asda*	1 Can/400g	180	3.2	45	1.5	7.9	0.8	0.3
Chicken Noodle, Canned, Heinz*	1 Can/400g	128	1.2	32	1.3	6.1	0.3	0.2
Chicken Noodle, Canned, Sainsbury's*	½ Can/200g	80	1	40	1.6	6.9	0.5	0.7
Chicken Noodle, Chinese, Fresh, Asda*	½ Pot/300g	120	2.1	40	2.3	5.6	0.7	0.8

SOUP

	Measure INFO/WEIGHT	per Measure KCAL	FAT	Nutrition Values per 100g / 100ml KCAL	PROT	CARB	FAT	FIBRE
Chicken Noodle, Clear, Weight Watchers*	1 Can/295g	51	0.6	17	0.8	3.1	0.2	0.2
Chicken Noodle, Dry, Nissin*	1 Pack/85g	364	14.1	428	9.5	62	16.6	3.3
Chicken Noodle, Fresh, Sainsbury's*	½ Pot/300g	132	3.3	44	2.9	5.6	1.1	0.5
Chicken Noodle, Super Good, Baxters*	1 Can/400g	200	5.2	50	3.1	6.6	1.3	0.5
Chicken Noodle, Thai Green, Yorkshire Provender*	½ Pot/300g	159	6	53	2.9	5.6	2	0
Chicken Noodle, with Sweetcorn, Canned, M&S*	1 Can/400g	184	3.2	46	2.8	6.8	0.8	0.4
Chicken Tortilla, Fresh, Hyvee*	1 Cup/245g	210	11	86	4.9	6.9	4.5	0.4
Chicken, & Bean, Mexican Spiced, Eat Smart, Morrisons*	1 Can/400g	200	2	50	2.9	7.3	0.5	1.9
Chicken, & Leek, Cup a Soup, Made Up, Batchelors*	1 Serving/259g	96	4.7	37	0.5	4.7	1.8	0.7
Chicken, & Lentil, Spinach, & Cumin, Yorkshire Provender*	½ Pot/300g	159	4.8	53	3.9	4.6	1.6	2.1
Chicken, & Multigrain, Finest, Tesco*	½ Pot/298g	125	3.6	42	3.2	3.9	1.2	1.3
Chicken, & Mushroom, Grain Soup , Sainsbury's*	1 Pot/600g	332	14.5	55	3.8	4.4	2.4	0.5
Chicken, & Orzo, Tuscan, Glorious!*	½ Pot/300g	120	1.2	40	2.8	6.2	0.4	0.7
Chicken, & Sweetcorn, Fresh, Average	**1 Serving/300g**	**146**	**3.1**	**48**	**2.4**	**7.3**	**1**	**0.6**
Chicken, & Vegetable, Canned, Average	**1 Can/400g**	**192**	**8.5**	**48**	**2.5**	**4.6**	**2.1**	**0.8**
Chicken, & Barley, Broth, Heinz*	½ Can/200g	58	0.4	29	1.4	4.9	0.2	0.9
Chicken, & Bean, Mexican Inspired, Waitrose*	½ Pot/299g	245	11.1	82	3.8	7.3	3.7	1.9
Chicken, & Bean, Mexican Style, Slimzone, Asda*	½ Can/200g	90	1	45	2.8	6.6	0.5	1.8
Chicken, & Chorizo, Smoky, Waitrose*	½ Pot/300g	123	4.2	41	2.5	3.9	1.4	1.2
Chicken, & Chorizo, Spanish, Extra Special, Asda*	½ Pot/300ml	150	7.5	50	2.5	4.2	2.5	0.5
Chicken, & Grains, Chunky, Fresh, M&S*	½ Pot/300g	162	6	54	2.8	5.7	2	1.1
Chicken, & Leek, Canned, Duncan's, Aldi*	1 Can/400g	108	2.8	27	1.3	3.8	0.7	0.5
Chicken, & Multigrain, Crosse & Blackwell*	1 Can/391g	176	3.1	45	2	4.5	0.8	1.1
Chicken, & Mushroom, Chestnut, Fresh, Finest, Tesco*	1 Pot/600g	282	9.6	47	3	5.1	1.6	0.1
Chicken, & Noodle, Canned, Bramwells, Aldi*	1 Can/400g	148	3	37	1.4	5.5	0.8	1.2
Chicken, & Spelt, Broth, Deluxe, Lidl*	½ Pot/300g	141	3.3	47	3	5.6	1.1	1.5
Chicken, & Vegetable, Low Fat, Soupreme, Aldi*	½ Pot/303g	100	2.1	33	2	4.5	0.7	0.8
Chicken, & Vegetable, Meal Soup, Sainsbury's*	1 Pot/400g	268	9.6	67	3.8	7	2.4	1.3
Chicken, & Vegetable, Slimming World*	1 Carton/500g	170	2	34	3.7	3.3	0.4	1.1
Chicken, Arrabbiata, Hearty, Bowl, Sainsbury's*	1 Pack/400g	198	4	50	2.5	6.8	1	1.6
Chicken, Balti, Meal, Sainsbury's*	1 Pack/400g	242	7.1	61	3.9	6.3	1.8	1.8
Chicken, Broth, Favourites, Baxters*	1 Can/400g	164	2.8	41	1.6	7.2	0.7	0.7
Chicken, Chunky, Spicy Keralan, M&S*	½ Pot/300g	204	10.8	68	2.9	5.5	3.6	0.9
Chicken, Classic, New Covent Garden*	½ Carton/280g	151	7	54	3.7	4	2.5	0.5
Chicken, Cream of, Avonmore*	½ Carton/350g	238	16.4	68	1.8	4.4	4.7	0.2
Chicken, Cream Of, Bramwells, Aldi*	1 Can/400g	208	12	52	1.5	4.7	3	0.5
Chicken, Cream of, Canned, Sainsbury's*	1 Can/400g	216	12	54	1.9	4.5	3	0.5
Chicken, Cream of, Canned, Tesco*	1 Can/400g	192	12	48	2.5	2.8	3	0.1
Chicken, Cream of, Cup, As Prepared, Sainsbury's*	1 Sachet/226g	95	1.8	42	0.5	8.3	0.8	0.5
Chicken, Cream of, Knorr*	1 Serving/250ml	50	2	20	0.3	2.8	0.8	0
Chicken, Cream Of, No Added Sugar, Heinz*	½ Can/200g	106	6	53	1.6	4.9	3	0.1
Chicken, Cream of, Reduced Salt, Heinz*	1 Can/400g	216	12	54	1.7	4.9	3	0.1
Chicken, Cream of, Soupreme, Aldi*	1 Can/400g	228	15.2	57	1.8	3.8	3.8	0.4
Chicken, Cup A Soup, Knorr*	1 Sachet/170g	139	6.5	82	1.7	10	3.8	0.5
Chicken, Green Thai, Spiced, M&S*	½ Pot/300g	195	11.4	65	2	6.3	3.8	0.6
Chicken, Green Thai, Waitrose*	1 Pot/600g	462	30	77	4.4	3.5	5	1.6
Chicken, Hotpot, Chunky, Big Soup, Heinz*	½ Can/258g	126	3.1	49	2.3	7.4	1.2	0.8
Chicken, Jamaican Jerk, TTD, Sainsbury's*	½ Pot/300g	169	3.6	56	3.5	6.6	1.2	2.5
Chicken, Katsu, Naked, Hearty, Sainsbury's*	1 Pot/397g	258	11.9	65	2.1	6.5	3	1.6
Chicken, Keralan, Sainsburys*	½ Carton/300g	252	15.3	84	3.5	5.5	5.1	1.1
Chicken, Made Up, Cup a Soup, Batchelors*	1 Sachet/253g	91	5.1	36	0.6	4	2	0.5
Chicken, Miso, Noodle, Waitrose*	1 Pot/400g	268	8.8	67	5.9	5.9	2.2	0.9
Chicken, Moroccan Inspired, Finest, Tesco*	½ Pot/300g	156	3.3	52	3.7	4.9	1.1	4

S

SOUP

	Measure INFO/WEIGHT	per Measure KCAL	FAT	Nutrition Values per 100g / 100ml KCAL	PROT	CARB	FAT	FIBRE
Chicken, Moroccan Inspired, Love Life, Waitrose*	½ Pot/300g	136	2.4	45	2.7	6.1	0.8	1.4
Chicken, Moroccan Inspired, Morrisons*	½ Pot/300g	211	7.5	70	2.6	8.1	2.5	2.7
Chicken, Moroccan, Harira, Hearty, Baxters*	1 Can/400g	236	2.8	59	3.2	9.5	0.7	1.9
Chicken, Mulligatawny, Finest, Tesco*	½ Pot/300g	237	9.9	79	5	6.7	3.3	1
Chicken, Multigrain, Hearty, Waitrose*	½ Pot/300g	141	3	47	3.6	4.9	1	2.1
Chicken, Nduja, & Kale, TTD, Sainsbury's*	½ Pot/300g	153	5.4	51	3	4.8	1.8	2.1
Chicken, Peri Peri, Asda*	½ Can/197g	77	1.8	39	1.8	5.5	0.9	0.6
Chicken, Potato & Bacon, Big Soup, Heinz*	1 Can/515g	294	11.3	57	3	6.1	2.2	0.5
Chicken, Potato & Leek, Weight Watchers*	1 Can/295g	97	2.4	33	1.1	5.1	0.8	0.3
Chicken, Potato, & Bacon, Chunky, Tesco*	½ Can/200g	100	2.6	50	3.6	5.7	1.3	0.7
Chicken, Roast, Cream of, Crosse & Blackwell*	1 Can/400g	214	10.4	54	3.8	3.5	2.6	0.6
Chicken, Savers, Morrisons*	½ Can/200g	78	4.6	39	0.9	3.5	2.3	0.4
Chicken, Spiced, Coconut, & Wild Rice, Waitrose*	½ Pot/300g	267	12.9	89	4.2	7.7	4.3	1.3
Chicken, Thai Green Curry, Waitrose*	1 Pot/600g	456	26.4	76	2.7	5.9	4.4	0.9
Chicken, Thai Style, Canned, Soupreme, Aldi*	1 Can/400g	200	10.8	50	2.5	3.8	2.7	1.1
Chicken, Thai, Deluxe, Lidl*	½ Can/190g	129	6.8	68	1.6	7	3.6	1.5
Chicken, Thai, Fresh, Finest, Tesco*	½ Pot/300g	192	11.7	64	3	3.8	3.9	0.7
Chicken, The Kee Diet*	1 Pack/40g	161	4	402	25.5	40.2	10	8.2
Chicken, Tomato, & Grains, Tuscan, Glorious!*	½ Pack/300g	111	2.1	37	2	4.9	0.7	1.5
Chicken, Weight Watchers*	1 Can/295g	97	3	33	1.6	4.4	1	0
Chickpea, & Coconut, Indonesian Style, Lidl*	1 Pot/400g	340	22.8	85	1.4	5.2	5.7	3.3
Chickpea, Albert Heijn*	1 Pack/570ml	450	19.9	79	3	8	3.5	1.5
Chilli, Tomato, & Pasta, COU, M&S*	1 Serving/300g	150	5.7	50	1.3	7.2	1.9	0.9
Chipotle, & Bean, Mexican Inspired, Waitrose*	1 Can/396g	198	5.9	50	1.9	6.3	1.5	1.6
Chowder, Seafood, Waitrose*	1 Can/404g	226	11.3	56	2.2	5.6	2.8	0.6
Chowder, Smoked Haddock & Salmon, Cully & Sully*	1 Pack/400g	232	9.2	58	2.6	6.2	2.3	0.9
Chowder, Sweetcorn, Microwaved, Slimming World*	1 Pot/500g	160	2.5	32	1.1	5.3	0.5	0.7
Clear, Unox*	1 Serving/200g	72	2.8	36	2	3.6	1.4	0.5
Coconut, Corn, & Sweet Potato, Creamy, Bol*	½ Pot/300g	204	3.9	68	2.5	10.4	1.3	2.3
Coconut, Curry, Sri Lankan, Spiced, TTD, Sainsbury's*	½ Pot/300g	195	9.3	65	1.3	7.3	3.1	1.5
Coconut, Lime, & Chilli, Glorious!*	½ Tub/300g	168	2.4	56	3.4	6.7	0.8	4.1
Country Garden, Canned, Vegetarian, Baxters*	1 Can/400g	144	2	36	1	6.2	0.5	1
Courgette, & Parmesan, Fresh, Sainsbury's*	1 Pack/300ml	198	16.8	66	1.5	2.5	5.6	0.4
Crayfish, Deluxe, Lidl*	1 Serving/280g	174	11.8	62	1.3	4.5	4.2	0.5
Daal, Lentil, Bangalore, Glorious!*	1 Pot/600g	294	8.4	49	2	6.1	1.4	2.2
Dahl, Indian Spiced, Asda*	½ Pot/300g	138	3	46	2.2	5.8	1	2.6
Dahl, Lentil, Bangalore, Sainsbury's*	1 Serving/300g	117	2.7	39	1.7	4.7	0.9	2.3
Dhal, Lentil, Co-Op*	1 Pot/600g	324	11.4	54	2.1	6.1	1.9	1.8
Egyptian, Shorbet Lesan Asfour*	1 Cup/180g	100	3.3	56	5.5	3.9	1.8	0
Fish, Bouillabaise, Bistro, M&S*	1 Pack/820g	2665	18	325	10	4.3	2.2	1.3
Fish, Bouillabaise, Waitrose*	½ Pot/300g	102	3	34	2.2	3.5	1	1
Florida Spring Vegetable, Dry Weight, Knorr*	¼ Pack/12g	36	0.5	300	9.2	56.7	4.2	8.3
French Onion, & Gruyere , Fresh, TTD, Sainsbury's*	1 Pot/400g	216	10.4	54	2.2	4.7	2.6	1.3
French Onion, & Red Onion, Canned, Waitrose*	1 Can/400g	140	2.4	35	2.2	4.8	0.6	0.6
French Onion, Waitrose*	½ Pot/300g	105	3.3	35	1.2	4.8	1.1	0.6
Game, Royal, Favourites, Baxters*	1 Can/400g	152	0.8	38	1.8	6.9	0.2	0.3
Garden Pea, & Spinach, Protein Boosting, Power, BOL*	½ Pot/300g	180	4.2	60	5.9	2.4	1.4	7.1
Garden Vegetable, Fresh, Tesco*	½ Pot/300g	117	0.6	39	1.4	7.2	0.2	1.4
Gazpacho, Hacendada*	1 Serving/333ml	250	23.3	75	0.6	2.5	7	0
Golden Vegetable, Cup a Soup, Made Up, Batchelors*	1 Sachet/250ml	80	2.3	32	0.3	5.5	0.9	0.4
Green Veg, Broth, Chinese Style, Veg Pot, Naked Noodle*	1 Pot/300g	216	0.6	72	2.8	13.8	0.2	2
Green Vegetable, & Kale, British, Crosse & Blackwell*	1 Can/394g	130	1.2	33	1.6	5.1	0.3	1.8
Green, Superfood, Lighter Life*	1 Bowl/53g	203	5.5	383	25.9	42.6	10.3	8.2

S

	Measure INFO/WEIGHT	KCAL	FAT	Nutrition Values per 100g / 100ml KCAL	PROT	CARB	FAT	FIBRE
		per Measure		Nutrition Values per 100g / 100ml				

SOUP

	Measure INFO/WEIGHT	KCAL	FAT	KCAL	PROT	CARB	FAT	FIBRE
Haddock, Smoked, Chowder, M&S*	½ Pot/300g	141	6.6	47	2.1	4.3	2.2	0.6
Ham Hock, & Vegetable, Broth, Crosse & Blackwell*	1 Can/400g	158	2	40	2.7	5.7	0.5	0.8
Ham, Hock, & Sweetcorn, TTD, Sainsbury's*	1 Pack/600g	468	22.8	78	2.6	7.8	3.8	1.1
Highlander's Broth, Favourites, Baxters*	1 Can/400g	192	5.6	48	1.7	6.3	1.4	0.9
Hot & Sour	*1 Serving/233g*	*90*	*2.8*	*39*	*2.6*	*4.3*	*1.2*	*0.5*
Jackfruit, Bean, & Chipotle Chilli, Plant Based, Baxters*	1 Can/380g	201	1.1	53	2.8	8.6	0.3	2.4
Kotosoupa, with Noodles, Greek, Knorr*	½ Pack/505ml	106	2.5	21	0.8	4.2	0.5	0.5
Laksa, Chicken Coconut, with Noodles, Chef Select, Lidl*	1 Pack/380g	411	9.5	108	7.4	13.1	2.5	1.4
Laksa, Chicken Noodle, Cook*	1 Pack/300g	300	9	100	6.6	12.2	3	0.9
Lamb, & Vegetable, Big Soup, Heinz*	½ Can/200g	120	2.6	60	3	9.1	1.3	1.3
Lamb, Minted, Hot Pot, Big Soup, Heinz*	1 Can/500g	295	6.5	59	2.8	8.5	1.3	1
Leek, & Chicken, Knorr*	1 Serving/300ml	82	5.2	27	0.6	2.4	1.7	0.1
Leek, & Potato	*1oz/28g*	*15*	*0.7*	*52*	*1.5*	*6.2*	*2.6*	*0.8*
Leek, Potato, & Barber's Cheddar , TTD, Sainsbury's*	½ Pot/300g	201	11.1	67	2.6	5.4	3.7	0.9
Lentil, & Bacon, Canned, Sainsbury's*	½ Can/200g	110	1.8	55	3.1	8.2	0.9	0.9
Lentil, & Bacon, Canned, Tesco*	1 Serving/200g	96	1.4	48	3.2	7.2	0.7	0.5
Lentil, & Bacon, Chunky, Canned, M&S*	1 Can/400g	204	2.4	51	3.3	7.2	0.6	1.8
Lentil, & Bacon, Classic, Heinz*	1 Can/400g	232	5.6	58	2.7	8.4	1.4	0.7
Lentil, & Bacon, Favourites, Baxters*	1 Can/400g	208	2.8	52	3.4	7.3	0.7	0.8
Lentil, & Barley, Superbean, M&S*	1 Pack /600g	270	9	45	1.8	5.1	1.5	2.1
Lentil, & Ham, Red, Waitrose*	½ Pot/300g	147	3.3	49	3.9	5.8	1.1	2
Lentil, & Smoked Bacon, Fresh, Tesco*	1 Pack/600g	420	11.4	70	3.9	8.5	1.9	1.6
Lentil, & Vegetable, LC, Tesco*	1 Can/400g	188	0.8	47	2.5	8.8	0.2	1.1
Lentil, & Vegetable, Spicy, Chilled, M&S*	½ Serving/300g	150	2.4	50	2.7	8	0.8	1.1
Lentil, & Bacon, Canned, Classic, Morrisons*	1 Can/400g	220	4.4	55	3.4	7.5	1.1	0.8
Lentil, & Bacon, Smoked, New Covent Garden Soup Co*	½ Pack/280g	182	6.2	65	5.9	4.1	2.2	2.8
Lentil, & Red Pepper, Smoky, Plant Chef, Tesco*	1 Serving/400g	184	2	46	2.8	6.8	0.5	1.2
Lentil, & Spinach, Dahl, Tideford Organics*	½ Pot/300g	117	6.3	39	1.4	3.1	2.1	0.9
Lentil, & Vegetable, Vegetarian, Baxters*	1 Can/400g	160	0.8	40	1.9	7.4	0.2	1.2
Lentil, Asda*	½ Can/202g	89	0.4	44	2.6	8	0.2	0.7
Lentil, Classic, Heinz*	1 Can/400g	180	0.8	45	2.4	8.5	0.2	0.8
Lentil, Hearty, Biona Organic*	½ Jar/340g	163	0.7	48	2.7	8.1	0.2	1.6
Lentil, Maggi*	1 Serving/250ml	68	0.6	27	1.8	4.5	0.2	0.6
Lentil, Newgate, Lidl*	½ Can/200g	100	0.4	50	3.1	8.2	0.2	1.4
Lentil, Red, with Carrots, Potato & Onion, Asda*	1 Can/400g	192	0.8	48	1.4	10.2	0.2	1.2
Lentil, Scotty Brand*	1 Pot/550g	374	1.6	68	3.9	10.4	0.3	3.8
Lentil, Spicy, M&S*	1 Serving/100g	50	1.1	50	2.6	6.3	1.1	2.1
Lobster, Bisque, Waitrose*	½ Carton/300g	201	13.8	67	0.9	5.5	4.6	0.6
Mexican Bean Chilli, Re:nourish*	1 Bottle/500g	165	5.5	33	1.3	4.6	1.1	1.1
Mighty Mexican Style, Nourish, Morrisons*	1 Can/400g	200	2	50	2.9	7.3	0.5	1.9
Minestrone, & Smoked Bacon, Baxters*	1 Pot/350g	172	6	49	2.2	5.8	1.7	0.7
Minestrone, Canned, Average	*1 Can/400g*	*252*	*12*	*63*	*1.8*	*7.6*	*3*	*0.9*
Minestrone, Fresh, Average	*1 Carton/600g*	*244*	*4.9*	*41*	*1.7*	*6.8*	*0.8*	*1.2*
Minestrone, Italian, Cup, As Prepared, Ainsley Harriott*	1 Cup/223ml	92	1	41	0.7	8.4	0.4	0.4
Minestrone, Pack, Dry, Knorr*	1 Pack/61g	204	2.4	335	12	58.8	4	6.9
Minestrone, with Croutons in a Cup, Sainsbury's*	1 Sachet/225ml	88	1.4	39	0.6	7.5	0.6	0.6
Minestrone, with Croutons in a Mug, Tesco*	1 Sachet/23g	83	1.9	360	9	62.6	8.1	2.7
Minestrone, with Croutons, Cup a Soup, Batchelors*	1 Serving/254g	89	1.8	35	0.6	6.5	0.7	0.5
Minestrone, with Croutons, Dry, Soupreme, Aldi*	1 Serving/27g	94	1.7	349	7.6	65.3	6.4	4.4
Minestrone, with GF Pasta, Tideford*	1 Pot/600g	180	4.8	30	1.3	3.9	0.8	1.4
Miso, Paste, Wakame, Sachets, Yutaka*	1 Sachet/18g	18	0.6	100	7.1	16	3.6	0
Miso, Rainbow, Japanese, Skinny Soup, Glorious!*	½ Pot/300g	81	0.9	27	1.4	4.1	0.3	0.9
Miso, Wakama*	1 Sachet/8g	27	0.6	336	18.7	48.6	7.6	0

SOUP

INFO/WEIGHT	Measure	per Measure KCAL	FAT	Nutrition Values per 100g / 100ml KCAL	PROT	CARB	FAT	FIBRE
Miso, with Tofu, Instant, Kikkoman*	1 Sachet/10g	35	1	350	30	30	10	0
Moroccan Bean, Very Special, Wattie's*	1 Serving/265g	176	0.8	66	3.2	11.4	0.3	2
Moroccan, with Vegan Pieces, Quorn*	½ Pot/283g	136	1.7	48	4.2	4.4	0.6	3.7
Mulligatawny	*1 Serving/220g*	*213*	*15*	*97*	*1.4*	*8.2*	*6.8*	*0.9*
Multigrain, High Fibre, Waitrose*	1 Pot/400g	232	6	58	2.6	6.8	1.5	3.5
Mushroom, As Prepared, Mugshot *	1 Sachet/224g	103	2.7	46	0.4	8.2	1.2	0.2
Mushroom, Canned, HL, Tesco*	1 Can/400g	132	5.6	33	0.5	4.4	1.4	0.2
Mushroom, Cream of, Bramwells, Aldi*	½ Can/200g	106	5.8	53	1.3	5.4	2.9	0.5
Mushroom, Cream of, Canned, Tesco*	½ Can/200g	94	5.8	47	0.7	4.8	2.9	0.2
Mushroom, Cream of, Classics, Heinz*	1 Can/400g	208	11.2	52	1.5	5.2	2.8	0.1
Mushroom, Cream of, Condensed, Batchelors*	1 Can/295g	330	25.1	112	1.3	7.5	8.5	0.2
Mushroom, Cream Of, Tesco*	½ Can/200g	116	7.2	58	1.3	5	3.6	0.4
Mushroom, Fresh, Average	*1 Serving/300g*	*146*	*9.3*	*49*	*1.3*	*4*	*3.1*	*0.8*
Mushroom, Risotto, Grain, Meal Soup, Sainsbury's*	1 Pack/400g	257	11.2	64	2	7	2.8	1.5
Mushroom, Wild, Cup, As Prepared, Waitrose*	1 Serving/213g	98	3	46	0.6	7.5	1.4	0.5
Mushroom, with Croutons in a Cup, Waitrose*	1 Sachet/212g	102	4.2	48	0.6	6.8	2	0.5
Mushroom, with Croutons, Soup in a Mug, Tesco*	1 Serving/226ml	115	4.7	51	1	6.8	2.1	0.4
Noodle, Cantonese Hot & Sour, Baxters*	1 Serving/215g	133	2.8	62	1.4	11.1	1.3	0.5
Noodle, Chicken, Chilli, Ramen, Waitrose*	1 Pack/401g	325	8.8	81	7.7	7.1	2.2	1.3
Noodle, Cup, Shin, Nongshim*	1 Cup/75g	326	11.2	435	7	68	15	0
Noodle, No Chicken, Amy's Kitchen*	1 Can/400g	180	6	45	2.2	5.5	1.5	0.8
Noodle, Red Thai, Re:nourish*	1 Bottle/500g	200	10	40	0.7	4.8	2	0.6
Noodle, Seafood, Ramyun, Nongshim*	1 Pack/125g	522	16.2	418	8.3	67	13	0
Noodle, Sweet & Spicy, Cup Soup, Made Up, Tesco*	1 Sachet/220g	77	0.2	35	0.7	7.5	0.1	0.6
Onion, French	*1oz/28g*	*11*	*0.6*	*40*	*0.2*	*5.7*	*2.1*	*1*
Oxtail, Average	*1 Can/400g*	*163*	*4.5*	*41*	*2*	*5.8*	*1.1*	*0.4*
Oxtail, Canned	*1 Serving/220g*	*97*	*3.7*	*44*	*2.4*	*5.1*	*1.7*	*0.1*
Pancetta, & Lentil, Tuscan Style, Aldi*	1 Serving/200g	170	3.6	85	10	6.7	1.8	0
Pancetta, Barley, & Kale, Finest, Tesco*	½ Pot/302g	148	5.4	49	2.6	4.4	1.8	2.6
Parsnip, & Honey, Fresh, Sainsbury's*	½ Carton/300g	192	12.6	64	1.1	5.4	4.2	1.5
Parsnip, Spicy, Average	*1 Serving/400g*	*212*	*11.2*	*53*	*0.9*	*6*	*2.8*	*1.6*
Parsnip, Winter Spiced, Tideford Organics*	1 Pot/600g	216	8.4	36	0.9	4.5	1.4	1.1
Paste, Miso, White, Japanese, Organic, Clearspring*	1 Tbsp/15g	26	0.6	170	7	23	4.1	0
Pea, & Ham	*1 Serving/220g*	*154*	*4.6*	*70*	*4*	*9.2*	*2.1*	*1.4*
Pea, & Mint, Best of British, Crosse & Blackwell*	1 Can/400g	192	8.4	48	1.7	4.6	2.1	1.9
Pea, & Mint, Fresh, Co-Op*	½ Tub/300g	105	1.7	35	1.7	4.8	0.6	1.8
Pea, & Mint, Fresh, Finest, Tesco*	1 Serving/300g	165	7.2	55	1.3	6	2.4	1.5
Pea, & Mint, Fresh, M&S*	1 Serving/164g	49	0.2	30	1.8	6.3	0.1	1.5
Pea, & Mint, Fresh, Sainsbury's*	½ Pot/300g	102	2.7	34	1.4	5	0.9	1.9
Pea, & Mint, Fresh, Tesco*	½ Pot/300g	145	3.3	48	2.4	6	1.1	2.4
Pea, & Mint, Garden, Vegetarian, Baxters*	½ Can/200g	100	1.6	50	2.5	7.3	0.8	1.9
Pea, & Mint, Slimming World, Iceland*	1 Tub/500g	205	2	41	2.5	5.6	0.4	2.7
Pea, & Mint, with Leek, Fresh, Waitrose*	1 Serving/300g	123	4.5	41	1.7	4.4	1.5	1.5
Pea, & Leek, Soupologie*	1 Pack/600g	288	15.6	48	1.7	3.6	2.6	1.4
Pea, & Mint, Cup, Waitrose*	1 Cup/215ml	103	2.2	48	1.1	8.3	1	0.5
Pea, & Watercress, Daylesford*	½ Pack/250g	125	6.2	50	1.9	5	2.5	1
Pea, Basil, & Lemon, Re:nourish*	1 Serving/500g	205	4	41	2.1	5.3	0.8	3.4
Pea, Coconut, & Tumeric, Tideford Organics*	½ Pot/300g	99	3	33	1.6	3.5	1	1.6
Pea, Edamame, & Spinach, Canned, Waitrose*	1 Can/400g	172	3.6	43	2.4	5.5	0.9	1.4
Pea, Garden, & Ham, Bramwells, Aldi*	1 Can/400g	208	4	52	3.5	6.2	1	2.1
Pea, Hearty, & Wiltshire Cured Ham Hock, Waitrose*	½ Carton/300g	165	4.2	55	3.1	6.6	1.4	1.8
Pea, Minted, & Asparagus, Canned, TTD, Sainsbury's*	½ Can/200g	72	2.8	36	1.4	3.8	1.4	1.2
Pea, Split, Yellow, Simply Organic*	1 Pot/600g	354	3	59	4.3	10.4	0.5	2.6

SOUP

INFO/WEIGHT	Measure	per Measure KCAL	per Measure FAT	Nutrition Values per 100g / 100ml KCAL	PROT	CARB	FAT	FIBRE
Peas, & Greens, Soupreme, Aldi*	1 Pot/600g	306	7.2	51	1.7	7.5	1.2	1.8
Pepper, & Chorizo, Canned, Sainsbury's*	1 Can/400ml	172	4	43	7	2	1	0
Pepper, with Chilli, Italiamo, Lidl*	1 Can/390ml	222	9.4	57	0.6	7.6	2.4	1.3
Potage Brighton Surgele, Picard*	¼ Pack/250g	205	13.5	82	2.9	4.6	5.4	2
Potato, & Leek, in a Cup, As Prepared, Sainsbury's*	1 Serving/218ml	96	2.4	44	0.5	7.8	1.1	0.5
Potato, & Leek, Optifast, Nestle*	1 Pack/44g	172	4.8	392	36	34	11	6.5
Prawn, King, & Glass Noodles, Pho, pot	**1 Pot/642g**	**212**	**2.6**	**33**	**1.8**	**5.4**	**0.4**	**0.5**
Prawn, Tom Yum, Cook*	1 Portion/335g	231	3	69	3.5	10.8	0.9	0
Pumpkin, & Sweet Potato, Super-Licious, Baxters*	1 Pot/350g	168	7.4	48	0.9	5.9	2.1	0.8
Pumpkin, Creamy, Very Special, Heinz*	1 Sm Can/290g	188	5.5	65	1.3	9.9	1.9	1.1
Pumpkin, Spicy, Fresh, Sainsbury's*	½ Pot/300g	87	3	29	0.9	4.2	1	1.3
Quinoa, Kale, & Red Lentil, Organic, Amy's Kitchen*	1 Can/414g	244	9.9	59	1.6	7.8	2.4	1.6
Ramen, Classic, Broth, Brilliant, Itsu*	1 Serving/250ml	138	1.2	55	0.5	12	0.5	0.5
Ramen, Hot & Sour, Bowl, As Prepared, Morrisons*	½ Pack/386g	170	1.2	44	1.3	8.6	0.3	0.7
Red Lentil, Apricot, & Chilli, Tideford Organics*	1 Pot/600g	228	8.4	38	1.3	4.6	1.4	1
Red Lentil, Spicy, Waitrose*	1 Pot/600g	270	3.6	45	1.6	8	0.6	0.6
Red Pepper, & Wensleydale, Asda*	1 Carton /600g	306	12.6	51	2.5	5	2.1	0.8
Red Pepper, Canned, Morrisons*	½ Can/198g	117	5.7	59	1	6.7	2.9	1
Red Pepper, Roasted, & Tomato, Canned, Sainsbury's*	1 Can/400g	196	6	49	1	7.5	1.5	0.9
Red Pepper, Roasted, & Tomato, M&S*	1 Serving/150g	105	7.4	70	1.4	5	4.9	0.6
Red Pepper, Roasted, Fresh, Waitrose*	1 Pack/600g	172	9	29	0.8	3	1.5	1
Roasted Red Pepper, Classic, Morrisons*	½ Can/200g	117	5.8	59	1	6.7	2.9	1
Roasted Tomatoes, & Basil, Love Yourself Diet*	1 Pack/255g	139	9	55	1.6	4.3	3.5	0
Root Vegetable, Roasted, Waitrose*	1 Pot/350g	102	3.2	29	0.6	3.7	0.9	1.7
Sausage, & Vegetable, Big Soup, Heinz*	½ Can/200g	138	5	69	2.7	8.3	2.5	0.9
Scotch Broth, British, Sainsbury's*	1 Can/400g	156	4	39	1.7	5.3	1	1
Scotch Broth, Canned, Tesco*	½ Can/200g	85	2.6	42	1.3	5.9	1.3	0.8
Scotch Broth, Classic, Heinz*	1 Can/400g	156	2.4	39	1.4	6.7	0.6	0.6
Scotch Broth, Favourites, Baxters*	1 Can/400g	168	4	42	1.8	6.8	1	1.4
Scotch Broth, Scotty Brand*	½ Pot/275g	72	0.8	26	1.1	5.8	0.3	2.2
Seafood Chowder, Canned, TTD, Sainsbury's*	½ Can/200g	114	5.6	57	1.9	5.9	2.8	0.5
Shellfish, Felix*	1 Serving/350g	206	11.2	59	1.7	5.2	3.2	0
Spinach, & Green Lentil, Spiced, Asda*	½ Pot/250g	122	5	49	2.7	5	2	0
Spinach, & Olive, Italiamo, Lidl*	1 Can/400g	252	15.2	63	1.2	5.4	3.8	1.1
Spinach, Creme Fraiche, & Nutmeg, Organic, Waitrose*	½ Pot/300g	243	22.8	81	0.9	2.3	7.6	1.1
Split Pea, Organic, Amy's Kitchen*	1 Can/400g	172	1.6	43	2	7.8	0.4	2.4
Squash, & Red Pepper, Spiced, Sainsbury's*	½ Can/200g	78	2.6	39	0.6	5.7	1.3	1.1
Steak, & Potato, Angus, Big Soup, Heinz*	½ Can/250g	120	2	48	3.1	6.8	0.8	0.6
Steak, & Ale, Chunky, Asda*	1 Can/400g	188	4.4	47	3	5.9	1.1	0.6
Steak, & Vegetables, Big Soup, Heinz*	1 Can/498g	294	5	59	3.7	8.3	1	1
Sundried Tomato, & Grain, Cup a Soup, Batchelors*	1 Serving/226g	81	0.7	36	1.2	6.7	0.3	1.1
Super Chicken Noodle, Dry Pack, Knorr*	1 Serving/13g	45	0.7	345	14	59	5.4	2.1
Sweet Potato, & Cauliflower, Super Soup, Bol*	½ Pot/300g	162	3	54	2.5	7.9	1	2.2
Sweet Potato, & Coconut, Plant Chef, Tesco*	1 Can/400g	228	10.8	57	0.7	7	2.7	1.2
Sweet Potato, & Lentil, Dahl, Yorkshire Provender*	1 Pot/600g	330	16.2	55	2.6	6.9	2.7	0
Sweet Potato, & Red Chilli, Asda*	½ Pot/300g	144	5.4	48	0.5	7.1	1.8	0.8
Sweet Potato, Coconut & Chilli, TTD, Sainsbury's*	½ Pot/300g	176	5.7	59	0.9	8.5	1.9	1.8
Sweet Potato, Coconut, & Chilli, The Best, Morrisons*	½ Pot/300g	222	11.7	74	1	8	3.9	1.2
Sweet Potato, Coconut, & Rice, Fresh, Waitrose*	½ Pot/300g	218	10.5	73	1.5	7.7	3.5	2.1
Sweet Potato, Roasted, Coconut, & Chilli, Finest, Tesco*	½ Pot/298g	197	11.3	66	0.8	6.2	3.8	1.8
Sweet Potato, Sri Lankan, Plant Based, Baxters*	1 Can/380g	205	6.8	54	0.8	7.9	1.8	1.4
Sweetcorn, & Yellow Pepper, Blended, Heinz*	½ Can/200g	98	4.2	49	0.9	6.6	2.1	0.6
Szechuan, Hot & Sour, Made Up, Cup a Soup, Batchelors*	1 Serving/253g	76	0.5	30	0.4	6.7	0.2	0.5

SOUP

	Measure INFO/WEIGHT	per Measure KCAL	FAT	Nutrition Values per 100g / 100ml KCAL	PROT	CARB	FAT	FIBRE
Tarka Dahl, Canned, M&S*	1 Can/400g	224	4.4	56	1.9	8.6	1.1	1.8
Thai Chicken, & Lemongrass, Cup Soup, Ainsley Harriott*	1 Sachet/224g	101	3.4	45	0.6	7.3	1.5	0.1
Thai Green Curry, Vegetable, Heart, Bowl, Sainsbury's*	1 Pack/400g	256	10.8	64	0.8	8.3	2.7	1.6
Thai Green, Vegetable, Naked, Hearty, Sainsbury's*	1 Pot/400g	256	10.8	64	0.8	8.3	2.7	1.6
Thai, Dry Weight, Sachet, Knorr*	1 Sachet/35g	133	4.2	379	10	57	12	3.5
Three Bean, Chilli, Fresh, Tesco*	½ Pot/300g	129	0.3	43	3.3	6	0.1	2.2
Three Bean, Hearty, Nourish, Morrisons*	1 Can/400g	228	4	57	2.8	8.2	1	2.2
Tom Yum, Chicken, Cook*	1 Pack/280g	126	3.1	45	3.8	5.4	1.1	0.7
Tomato, & Basil, CBY, Asda*	½ Pot/297g	89	2.4	30	1	4.3	0.8	0.7
Tomato, & Basil, Cup, Co-Op*	1 Sachet/45g	158	1.8	350	2	76	4	4
Tomato, & Basil, Fresh, Finest, Tesco*	½ Pot/300g	219	14.7	73	1	6.3	4.9	0.6
Tomato, & Basil, Fresh, Low Fat, Sainsbury's*	½ Carton/300ml	75	1.8	25	1.1	4.1	0.6	0.7
Tomato, & Basil, Fresh, M Kitchen, Morrisons*	½ Pot/300g	115	3.6	38	1	5.5	1.2	0.7
Tomato, & Basil, Fresh, M&S*	½ Pot/300g	120	5.1	40	1	5	1.7	1.3
Tomato, & Basil, Italian Plum, Finest, Tesco*	1 Pot/600g	360	13.8	60	1.3	7.2	2.3	0.6
Tomato, & Basil, Italian Style, Co-Op*	1 Pack/500g	200	10	40	1	4	2	0.6
Tomato, & Basil, Italian, Vegetarian, Baxters*	1 Can/415g	170	3.7	41	1.4	5.7	0.9	0.6
Tomato, & Basil, M&S*	½ Pot/300g	105	4.2	35	0.7	4.5	1.4	1
Tomato, & Basil, Rich, Waitrose*	1 Serving/130g	53	1.3	41	1.3	6.3	1	0.7
Tomato, & Basil, Sun Dried, Heinz*	1 Serving/275ml	124	5.2	45	0.6	6.5	1.9	0.1
Tomato, & Brown Lentil, Healthy, Baxters*	1 Can/415g	199	0.8	48	2.6	9	0.2	2.7
Tomato, & Butter Bean, Classic, Heinz*	½ Can/200g	92	1.4	46	1.3	8.1	0.7	0.8
Tomato, & Lentil, Truly Irresistible, Co-Op*	½ Pot/300g	165	2.1	55	3.1	8	0.7	1.2
Tomato, & Red Pepper, Fire Roasted, Asda*	½ Tub/265g	114	6.9	43	0.7	4.1	2.6	1
Tomato, & Three Bean, Canned, BGTY, Sainsbury's*	½ Can/198g	113	1	57	3.4	8.7	0.5	2.2
Tomato, & Three Bean, Eat Smart, Morrisons*	1 Can/400g	228	4	57	2.8	8.2	1	2.2
Tomato, & Thyme, Organic, Duchy, Waitrose*	½ Pot/300g	140	8.9	47	1.2	3.3	3	1
Tomato, & Vegetable, Cup a Soup, Batchelors*	1 Serving/218g	107	2.6	49	1.1	8.5	1.2	0.6
Tomato, & Balsamic, Finest, Tesco*	½ Pot/300g	116	4.2	38	1.2	4.9	1.4	0.7
Tomato, & Basil, Bramwells, Aldi*	1 Can/400g	188	8.8	47	0.8	4.9	2.2	2.1
Tomato, & Basil, Canned, Sainsbury's*	1 Can/400g	228	11.2	57	1	6.5	2.8	0.8
Tomato, & Basil, Chef Select, Lidl*	½ Pot/300ml	99	2.4	33	1	4.7	0.8	1.7
Tomato, & Basil, Creamy, Cully & Sully*	1 Pot/400g	324	25.2	81	1	4.5	6.3	1
Tomato, & Basil, Fresh, Tesco*	1 Pot/600g	180	4.2	30	0.9	4.7	0.7	0.6
Tomato, & Basil, Jane Plan*	1 Pack/300g	159	8.4	53	0.9	5.6	2.8	1
Tomato, & Basil, M&S*	½ Pot/300g	99	2.4	33	1	5	0.8	1
Tomato, & Basil, New Covent Garden Food Co*	½ Carton/280g	112	4.5	40	1.2	5.4	1.6	0.9
Tomato, & Chorizo, Deluxe, Lidl*	½ Can/200g	168	8.8	84	2.7	8.2	4.4	0.5
Tomato, & Chorizo, Specially Selected, Aldi*	½ Can/200g	168	8.8	84	2.7	8.2	4.4	0.5
Tomato, & Lentil, Souper Spicy, Fresh, M&S*	½ Pot/300g	141	2.1	47	2.5	6.1	0.7	3.1
Tomato, & Mascarpone, Asda*	½ Carton/300g	228	13.2	76	2.8	6.1	4.4	0.4
Tomato, & Three Bean, Canned, Slimzone, Asda*	1 Can/400g	180	2	45	2.5	7.6	0.5	1.9
Tomato, Asda*	1 Can/400g	116	3.2	29	1	4.2	0.8	0.7
Tomato, Basil, Biona Organic*	½ Jar/340g	173	0.3	51	0.7	12.2	0.1	0.7
Tomato, Bean, & Kale, Chunky, Fresh, Waitrose*	½ Pot/300g	121	3.6	40	1.4	5.2	1.2	1.6
Tomato, Borlotti Bean & Kale, Fresh, M&S*	1 Pot/600g	318	10.2	53	2	6.3	1.7	2.1
Tomato, Cannellini Beans, & Garlic, Heinz*	½ Can/200g	110	2.2	55	2.4	9.1	1.1	2.4
Tomato, Cream of, Canned, Average	**1 Can/400g**	**208**	**12**	**52**	**0.8**	**5.9**	**3**	**0.7**
Tomato, Cream of, Fresh, Eat Well, M&S*	½ Pot/300g	165	8.4	55	1	5.9	2.8	1.3
Tomato, Cream of, Fresh, Sainsbury's*	1 Pot/600g	318	19.2	53	0.8	5.2	3.2	1.3
Tomato, Cream of, Fresh, Waitrose*	½ Pot/300g	168	8.1	56	0.9	6.6	2.7	0.6
Tomato, Cream of, In a Cup, As Prepared, Sainsbury's*	1 Sachet/224g	92	1.3	41	0.5	8.3	0.6	0.6
Tomato, Cream Of, Pot, Heinz*	1 Pot/280g	135	3.1	48	1.2	8	1.1	0.8

S

	Measure INFO/WEIGHT	per Measure KCAL	FAT	Nutrition Values per 100g / 100ml KCAL	PROT	CARB	FAT	FIBRE
SOUP								
Tomato, Cup, Made Up, Bramwells, Aldi*	1 Sachet/252g	83	1.8	33	0.5	5.8	0.7	0.5
Tomato, Gazpacho, Innocent*	1 Bowl/200g	80	4.6	40	0.6	2.8	2.3	2.4
Tomato, Mediterranean, Vegetarian, Baxters*	1 Can/400g	126	0.4	32	0.9	5.6	0.1	0.8
Tomato, Optifast, Nestle*	1 Pack/44g	172	4.8	392	36	34	11	6.5
Tomato, Organic, Auga*	1 Pack/400g	252	16	63	0.8	5.9	4	1.4
Tomato, Original, Cup a Soup, Batchelors*	1 Sachet/254g	104	2.3	41	0.6	7.3	0.9	0.5
Tomato, Plum, & Basil, Newgate, Lidl*	1 Can/400g	160	6.4	40	0.7	5.4	1.6	0.7
Tomato, Red Lentil & Pepper, CBY, Asda*	½ Pot/300g	177	3.3	59	3	8.8	1.1	0.9
Tomato, Red Pepper, & Lentil, Morrisons*	1 Pot/600g	372	12.6	62	2.2	7.4	2.1	2.3
Tomato, Smart Price, Asda*	1 Can/400g	184	7.6	46	0.6	6.5	1.9	0.9
Tomato, Spicy, Lentil, & Red Pepper, Fresh, Sainsbury's*	1 Pot/600g	390	7.8	65	3.7	8.8	1.3	1.8
Tomato, Spinach, & Lentil, Heinz*	½ Can/200g	85	1.4	43	1.7	7.7	0.7	1.1
Tomato, Stockwell & Co., Tesco*	1 Can/400g	192	6.4	48	0.5	7.5	1.6	0.5
Tomato, Vine Sun Dried, & Lentil, Finest, Tesco*	1 Pack/600g	366	14.4	61	2.6	6.4	2.4	1.5
Tomato, Weight Watchers*	1 Can/295g	76	1.5	26	0.7	4.6	0.5	0.3
Turkey, Broth, Canned, Baxters*	½ Can/208g	79	1.5	38	1.3	6.5	0.7	0.7
Vegetable Tagine, Slimming World*	1 Tub/500g	215	2	43	2.6	5.6	0.4	3.1
Vegetable, & Three Bean, Chunky, M&S*	1 Can/400g	228	3.6	57	3	7.7	0.9	3.1
Vegetable, Barley, Amy's Kitchen*	1 Can/400g	152	4.8	38	0.8	5.3	1.2	1.2
Vegetable, Canned	**1oz/28g**	**13**	**0.2**	**48**	**1.4**	**9.9**	**0.6**	**1.5**
Vegetable, Fresh, Average	**1 Serving/300g**	**118**	**4.1**	**40**	**1.4**	**5.4**	**1.4**	**1.3**
Vegetable, Instant, Cup, Average	**1 Pack/19g**	**69**	**2**	**362**	**8.7**	**57.1**	**10.5**	**5.5**
Vegetable, Red Thai, Super, Glorious!*	½ Carton/300g	165	4.8	55	2	7.2	1.6	2
Watercress, M&S*	½ Pot/300g	75	5.1	25	1.3	1.5	1.7	0.6
SOUP MIX								
Broccoli, & Stilton, Knorr*	1 Portion/225ml	101	7.2	45	0.8	3.1	3.2	0.5
Butternut Squash, & Red Pepper, Asda*	½ Pack/178g	57	0.9	32	1	6.1	0.5	1.4
Butternut Squash, & Sweet Potato, COOK!, M&S*	1 Pack/600g	360	1.2	60	1.1	12.3	0.2	2.3
Butternut Squash, Sainsbury's*	¼ Pack/150g	63	2.1	42	0.8	6.3	1.4	0.9
Country, Morrisons*	1 Serving/80g	82	0.6	102	6	13.7	0.8	7.8
Farmers, Asda*	½ Pack/252g	83	1.3	33	1.5	4.7	0.5	3.2
Leek & Potato, As Sold, G&B, Asda*	¼ Pack/125g	69	0.4	55	1.7	10.5	0.3	1.7
Potato, & Leek, Sainsbury's*	1 Serving/100g	31	0.5	31	1.4	5.5	0.5	1
Red Pepper, & Carrot, Nature's Pick, Aldi*	1 Serving/100g	16	0.5	16	1.4	1.8	0.5	0.8
Soup Mix, Winter, Sainsbury's*	¼ Pack/148g	34	0.7	23	0.5	3.7	0.5	0.6
Sweet Potato, Nature's Pick, Aldi*	1 Serving/100g	24	0.5	24	0.8	4.1	0.5	1.2
Vegetable, & Lentil, Boiled, Sainsbury's*	¼ Pack/150g	57	0.8	38	1.8	6.2	0.5	2.1
Vegetable, & Lentil, Cook with, M&S*	¼ Pack/150g	75	0.6	50	1.9	8.2	0.4	2.9
Vegetable, Asda*	½ Pack/250g	95	1.2	38	0.9	7.5	0.5	0.7
Vegetable, Dunnes Stores*	1 Pack/320g	70	1.6	22	1	3.4	0.5	2.1
Vegetable, Kit, Morrisons*	1 Pack/500g	220	3.5	44	1.2	6.6	0.7	3
Vegetable, with Croutons, Sainsbury's*	1 Serving/224ml	107	3.1	48	0.7	7.8	1.4	0.7
Winter, Broth, Morrisons*	1 Pack/600g	294	3.6	49	1.5	7.9	0.6	3.1
SOUTHERN COMFORT								
37.5% Volume	**1 Pub Shot/35ml**	**72**	**0**	**207**	**0**	**0**	**0**	**0**
SOYA								
Chicken, Drumsticks, Mini, Like Meat*	3 Drumsticks/90g	194	8.7	215	12	17	9.7	7.1
Chunks, Protein, Natural, Nature's Harvest*	1 Serving/50g	172	0.5	345	50	35	1	4
Chunks, Tree Of Life*	1 Serving/34g	123	0.3	361	52	36	1	0
Chunks, with Chilli, Coriander, & Soy Marinade, M&S*	1 Pack/175g	180	1.6	103	18.6	1.7	0.9	6.8
Schnitzel, Golden Crumbed, Fry's*	1 Schnitzels/80g	186	12	232	10.3	16	15	6.1
Schnitzel, Like Meat*	1 Pack/180g	436	21.6	242	11	19	12	6.5
Tenderstrips, Roast, Naked Glory*	½ Pack/120g	172	5.5	143	20	4.3	4.6	5.8

S

	Measure INFO/WEIGHT	per Measure KCAL	FAT	Nutrition Values per 100g / 100ml KCAL	PROT	CARB	FAT	FIBRE
SOYA								
Tenderstrips, Smoky BBQ , Naked Glory*	1 Serving/70g	80	0.3	115	18	8	0.4	5.1
Tenderstrips, Tikka, Vegetarian, Naked Glory*	1 Serving/70g	91	1.9	130	20	3.4	2.7	5
SPAGHETTI								
Bare Naked, Barenaked*	1 Serving/100g	17	0.1	17	0.3	0.9	0.1	3.4
Black Bean, Organic, Dry, Explore Asian*	1 Serving/56g	198	2	353	44	15	3.6	21
Canned, in Tomato Sauce, Asda*	½ Can/195g	127	1	65	1.7	13	0.5	1.1
Chilli Prawn, Cooked, BGTY, Sainsbury's*	1 Pack/375g	356	10.1	95	4.3	12.8	2.7	1.2
Cooked, Average	*1oz/28g*	*33*	*0.2*	*119*	*4.1*	*24.8*	*0.6*	*1.1*
Dry, Average	*1oz/28g*	*98*	*0.4*	*350*	*12.1*	*72.1*	*1.5*	*2.4*
Durum Wheat, Dry, Average	*1oz/28g*	*97*	*0.1*	*348*	*12.4*	*71.8*	*0.4*	*1.4*
Edamame, Organic, Dry, Explore Asian*	1 Serving/56g	204	2	365	45	18	3.6	20
Fresh, Cooked, Average	*1 Serving/125g*	*182*	*2.2*	*146*	*6.1*	*26.9*	*1.7*	*1.8*
Fresh, Dry, Average	*1 Serving/100g*	*278*	*3*	*278*	*10.8*	*53*	*3*	*2.2*
GF, Cooked Weight, Free From, Love Life, Waitrose*	1 Serving/180g	283	0.9	157	3.1	35.3	0.5	0.6
GF, Cooked, Free From, Morrisons*	1 Portion/75g	129	0.4	172	2.8	38.6	0.6	0.9
GF, Free From, Tesco*	1 Serving/75g	266	0.8	355	7	78.4	1	2
in Tomato Sauce, Canned	*1oz/28g*	*18*	*0.1*	*64*	*1.9*	*14.1*	*0.4*	*0.7*
Marinara	*1 Serving/450g*	*675*	*18.9*	*150*	*8*	*19*	*4.2*	*0.9*
Noodles, Dry Weight, The Skinny Food Co.*	1 Serving/70g	4	0	6	0	3.8	0	10
Prawn, Chilli, Waitrose*	1 Pack/360g	382	11.5	106	4.4	13.9	3.2	2
Tricolore, Dry, Italiamo, Lidl*	1 Serving/60g	210	0.7	350	12.5	70.5	1.2	0
Whole Wheat, Cooked, Average	*1oz/28g*	*32*	*0.3*	*113*	*4.7*	*23.2*	*0.9*	*3.5*
Whole Wheat, Dry, Average	*1 Serving/100g*	*324*	*2.6*	*324*	*13.5*	*62.2*	*2.6*	*8*
with Sausages, in Tomato Sauce, Heinz*	1 Can/400g	352	14	88	3.4	10.8	3.5	0.5
SPAGHETTI & MEATBALLS								
Beef, & Roasted Veg, M&S*	1 Pack/380g	365	8.4	96	5.6	12.5	2.2	1.7
Beef, with Spiced Tomato & Pepper Sauce, BFY, M&S*	1 Pack/380g	361	9.9	95	7.3	10	2.6	1.2
Discover The Choice*	1 Pack/450g	486	26.6	108	7.7	5.5	5.9	0.8
Shroomballs, Plant Pioneers, Sainsbury's*	1 Pack/387g	375	8.9	97	3.4	14.5	2.3	2.5
Taste of Italy, Tesco*	1 Pack/420g	479	15.1	114	7.2	12.4	3.6	1.7
Veggie, Plant Based, Asda*	1 Pack/378g	473	18.9	125	6.3	12	5	3
SPAM*								
25% Less Sodium, Spam*	2 Slices/180g	579	51.4	321	12.5	1.8	28.6	0
Pork & Ham, Chopped, Spam*	1 Serving/100g	289	24.3	289	15	3.2	24.3	0
SPICE MIX								
Baharat, Blends, Bart*	1 Pinch/1g	3	0.1	333	13.7	18.5	13.7	0
Biryani, Sachet, Schwartz*	1 Sachet/28g	89	2.9	318	15.4	29.8	10.4	21.6
Chilli Con Carne, Bramwells, Aldi*	¼ Sachet/13g	41	0.5	318	9.7	55	3.7	13
Creole, Seasoned Pioneers*	1 Tbsp/15g	47	0.8	313	8.3	43.2	5.2	15.1
Dukkha, Cooks' Ingredients, Waitrose*	1 Tsp/5g	17	0.8	349	18.3	30.7	17	19.6
for Fajitas, Old El Paso*	1 Pack/35g	107	2.1	306	9	54	6	0
for Mexican Fajitas, Discovery*	½ Pack/15g	34	1	230	8	35	6.5	17.5
Moroccan, Rub, Schwartz*	1 Serving/3g	9	0.3	309	15	36.4	11.4	19.5
Napoli, Spaghetti, Kania*	1 Serving/22g	68	0.3	311	7.1	63.5	1.4	0
Peri Peri, Lemon & Herb, Extra Mild, Bag & Bake, Nando's*	1 Serving/5g	14	0	276	4.4	59.7	1	0
Peri Peri, Medium, Bag & Bake, Nando's*	1 Bag/20g	57	0.2	286	4.6	60	1.2	0
Peri Peri, Pan Fry, Nando's*	1 Sachet/20g	21	1.3	105	3	7	6.5	5.5
Ras El Hanout, Al'fez*	1 Tsp/2g	4	0.2	217	9.8	25.7	8.3	17.5
Ras El Hanout, Blend, Finest, Tesco*	1 Tsp/5g	16	0.5	320	9.4	37.1	9.2	23.6
Rogan Josh, Authentic, Schwartz*	1 Pack/35g	108	3.5	309	11.1	30.3	10	26.7
Smokehouse BBQ, Wrap It, Schwartz*	¼ Pack/8g	24	0.2	317	8.1	59.2	3.2	9.5
Sriracha Seasoning, Schwartz*	1 Tsp/2g	5	0.1	261	6.5	44.6	4.3	0
Zaatar, Waitrose*	1 Serving/10g	42	3	416	14.7	8.2	30.2	26.1

	Measure INFO/WEIGHT	per Measure KCAL	FAT	Nutrition Values per 100g / 100ml KCAL	PROT	CARB	FAT	FIBRE
SPINACH								
Baby, Average	**1 Serving/90g**	**22**	**0.7**	**25**	**2.8**	**1.6**	**0.8**	**2.1**
Boiled or Steamed, Average	**1 Serving/80g**	**17**	**0.6**	**21**	**2.6**	**0.9**	**0.8**	**2.1**
Canned, Average	**1 Serving/80g**	**16**	**0.4**	**20**	**2.8**	**1.3**	**0.5**	**2.7**
Chopped, Tinned, TRS Wholesale Ltd*	1 Can/395g	122	2.4	31	3	1.8	0.6	3
Creamed, Hacendado*	1 Pack/450g	288	15.8	64	2.8	4.4	3.5	1.9
Creamed, with Macarpone, Finest, Tesco*	½ Pack/121g	94	6	78	4.1	2.8	5	2.7
Raw, Average	**1 Serving/80g**	**19**	**0.6**	**24**	**2.9**	**1.4**	**0.7**	**2.2**
SPIRALI								
Dry, Average	**1 Serving/50g**	**176**	**0.8**	**352**	**12.2**	**72.6**	**1.6**	**2.8**
SPIRITS								
40% Volume	**1 Shot/35ml**	**78**	**0**	**222**	**0**	**0**	**0**	**0**
Amaretti, Non Alcoholic, Lyre's*	1 Single/25ml	18	0	70	0	17	0	0
American Malt, Non Alcoholic, Lyre's*	1 Single/25ml	4	0	17	0	3.7	0	0
Aperitif, Dry, Non Alcoholic, Lyre's*	1 Single/25ml	4	0	15	0	2.9	0	0
Aperitif, Rosso, Non Alcoholic, Lyre's*	1 Single/25ml	15	0	59	0	14	0	0
Coffee Originale, Non Alcoholic, Lyre's*	1 Single/25ml	16	0	64	0	15	0	0
Dark Cane, Non Alcoholic, Lyre's*	1 Single/25ml	5	0	20	0	4.5	0	0
Dry London, Non Alcoholic, Lyre's*	1 Single/25ml	2	0	10	0	1.9	0	0
Italian Orange, Non Alcoholic, Lyre's*	1 Single/25ml	19	0	76	0	18	0	0
Italian Spritz, Non Alcoholic, Lyre's*	1 Single/25ml	20	0	80	0	20	0	0
Licor 43, Diego Zamora*	1 Single/25ml	76	0	304	0.2	36.6	0.1	0
Orange Sec, Non Alcoholic, Lyre's*	1 Single/25ml	15	0	61	0	15	0	0
Spiced Cane, Non Alcoholic, Lyre's*	1 Single/25ml	4	0	18	0	3.9	0	0
Spiced Citrus, Ultra Low Alcohol, Atopia*	1 Single/25ml	6	0	23	0	5	0	0
White Cane, Non Alcoholic, Lyre's*	1 Single/25ml	4	0	15	0	3.4	0	0
SPLIT PEAS								
Dried, Average	**1oz/28g**	**89**	**0.5**	**319**	**22.1**	**57.4**	**1.7**	**3.2**
Green, Dried, Average	**1 Serving/80g**	**261**	**1.3**	**326**	**22.5**	**45**	**1.6**	**20**
Yellow, Cooked, Average	**1 Serving/80g**	**101**	**0.7**	**126**	**9.3**	**15.4**	**0.9**	**9.8**
Yellow, Dry, Average	**1 Serving/40g**	**105**	**0.7**	**263**	**20.1**	**29.3**	**1.8**	**24.6**
SPONGE FINGERS								
Almond Fingers, Tesco*	1 Finger/46g	174	6.1	379	5.3	58.8	13.2	1.7
Boudoir, Sainsbury's*	1 Finger/5g	20	0.2	396	8.1	82.8	3.6	0.4
Tesco*	1 Finger/5g	19	0.2	386	7.6	80.6	3.7	1
Trifle, Average	**1 Sponge/24g**	**77**	**0.5**	**319**	**5.2**	**69.9**	**2.2**	**0.8**
SPONGE PUDDING								
Average	**1 Portion/170g**	**578**	**27.7**	**340**	**5.8**	**45.3**	**16.3**	**1.1**
Blackberry & Apple, HE, Tesco*	1 Pot/103g	159	1.4	155	3.1	32.6	1.4	0.7
Blueberry, & Lemon, Waitrose*	1 Pudding/105g	288	13.6	274	4.4	33.8	13	2.3
Cherry & Almond Flavour, Sainsbury's*	¼ Pudding/110g	334	15.7	304	3.5	40.3	14.3	0.7
Chocolate & Sauce, Co-Op*	1 Pack/225g	608	29.2	270	5	34	13	0.6
Chocolate, M&S*	1 Pudding/105g	401	24.3	382	5.7	36	23.1	3.5
Chocolate, Sainsbury's*	¼ Pudding/110g	464	28.3	422	5.4	42.3	25.7	0.8
Chocolate, Tesco*	1 Serving/115g	430	19.2	374	3.7	50.8	16.7	2.7
Chocolate, Trufree*	1 Serving/115g	374	17.2	325	2.5	44	15	2
Chocolate, Waitrose*	1 Pudding/110g	400	22.5	363	3.6	41.4	20.4	1.7
Golden Syrup, Co-Op*	1 Can/300g	945	39	315	2	47	13	0.6
Golden Syrup, Lyons*	1 Sponge/95g	351	14.2	369	3.2	55.3	14.9	0.6
Honey& Fig, M&S*	¼ Pudding/73g	225	12	310	3.6	34.8	16.6	3.4
Lemon, M&S*	1 Pudding/105g	326	16	310	4.3	39.4	15.2	2.3
Lemon, Waitrose*	1 Serving/105g	212	2.5	202	3.4	41.7	2.4	1.4
Milk Chocolate, Sticky Puds, Cadbury*	1 Pudding/95g	390	17.3	360	4.2	48.9	16	0.8
Mixed Berry, BGTY, Sainsbury's*	1 Pudding/110g	189	2.6	172	2.4	33.3	2.4	3.8

S

	Measure INFO/WEIGHT	per Measure KCAL	per Measure FAT	Nutrition Values per 100g / 100ml KCAL	PROT	CARB	FAT	FIBRE
SPONGE PUDDING								
Pear & Ginger, COU, M&S*	1 Pudding/100g	175	0.7	175	1.9	39.8	0.7	1.1
Raspberry, Tesco*	1 Serving/100g	377	14.5	377	3.2	58.2	14.5	0.7
Salted Caramel, Specially Selected, Aldi*	1 Pudding/115g	459	20.7	399	3.6	54	18	1
Salted Caramel, Tesco*	1 Pudding/115g	464	21.6	404	3.2	55.2	18.8	0.6
Syrup, BGTY, Sainsbury's*	1 Pudding/110g	338	4.5	307	2.8	64.6	4.1	0.4
Syrup, Finest, Tesco*	1 Pudding/115g	330	9	287	3.1	51.2	7.8	0.6
Syrup, GFY, Asda*	1 Sponge/105g	207	4.3	197	2	38	4.1	2.6
Syrup, Iceland*	1 Pudding/115g	462	18.6	402	3.9	59.3	16.2	1.7
Syrup, Individual, Tesco*	1 Pudding/110g	390	14.5	355	3.1	55.6	13.2	0.5
Syrup, Sainsbury's*	¼ Pudding/110g	408	13	371	2.7	63.5	11.8	0.4
Syrup, Value, Tesco*	1 Serving/100g	307	10.2	307	2.1	51.7	10.2	0.6
Toffee & Pecan	**½ Pudding/100g**	**395**	**18.4**	**395**	**4.3**	**52.3**	**18.4**	**1.4**
Treacle, Heinz*	1 Serving/160g	445	13	278	2.5	48.9	8.1	0.6
Treacle, Waitrose*	1 Pudding/105g	385	13.8	367	2.8	59.5	13.1	0.5
with Custard	**1 Serving/200g**	**521**	**24.9**	**261**	**4.8**	**34.1**	**12.4**	**0.9**
with Jam or Treacle	**1oz/28g**	**93**	**4**	**333**	**5.1**	**48.7**	**14.4**	**1**
SPOTTED DICK								
Average	**1 Serving/105g**	**343**	**17.5**	**327**	**4.2**	**42.7**	**16.7**	**1**
with Custard	**1 Serving/210g**	**438**	**15.6**	**209**	**3.4**	**31.5**	**7.4**	**1.3**
SPRATS								
Fried	**1oz/28g**	**116**	**9.8**	**415**	**24.9**	**0**	**35**	**0**
Raw	**1oz/28g**	**33**	**2.1**	**117**	**12.4**	**0**	**7.5**	**0**
SPREAD								
Aivar, Pelagonia *	1 Tbsp/20g	32	1.4	161	3.7	20	7	0
Almond, 100%, Sainsbury's*	1 Tbsp/20g	128	10.9	639	29.3	4.3	54.4	7.6
Average	**1 Thin Spread/7g**	**51**	**5.7**	**726**	**0.1**	**0.5**	**81**	**0**
Banoffee, Caramel, Sainsbury's*	1 Serving/15g	63	3.5	423	2.6	50	23.6	0.5
Biscoff, Smooth, Lotus*	1 Tbsp/15g	88	5.7	584	2.9	57	38.1	0.8
Butter Me Up, Light, Tesco*	1 Thin Spread/7g	24	2.7	350	0.3	0.5	38	0
Butter Style, Average	**1 Thin Spread/7g**	**44**	**4.8**	**627**	**0.7**	**1.1**	**68.9**	**0**
Chocolate, & Hazelnut, Gu*	1 Tsp/5g	31	2.4	619	5.9	41	47	3.7
Clover, Light, Dairy Crest Ltd*	1 Thin Spread/7g	32	3.4	456	1.3	2	49.2	0
Enriched Olive, Tesco*	1 Thin Spread/7g	38	4.1	540	0.2	1.2	59	0
Heart, Cholesterol Reducing, Dairygold	**1 Thin Spread/7g**	**24**	**2.5**	**338**	**0.7**	**2.8**	**36**	**0**
I Can't Believe It's Not Butter, Original, Unilever*	1 Thin Spread/7g	27	2.9	384	0.5	1.4	42	0
Lactofree Spreadable, Lactofree, Arla*	1 Thin Spread/7g	48	5.2	679	0.5	0.5	75	0
Light, Benecol*	1 Thin Spread/7g	23	2.4	326	0	2.7	35	0
Low Fat, Average	**1 Thin Spread/7g**	**27**	**2.8**	**390**	**5.8**	**0.5**	**40.5**	**0**
Nut Butter, Almond, Smooth, Pip & Nut*	1 Tbsp/15g	96	8.2	640	26.7	6	54.7	8
Nut Butter, Almond, Smooth, Whole Earth*	1 Tbsp/15g	94	8	628	30.6	26	53	9.1
Nut Butter, Mixed, Biona*	1 Tbsp/15g	91	7.6	604	22	10.5	50.8	8.4
Nut Butter, Praline, Nut Blend*	1 Tbsp/15g	93	7.6	617	20.2	19.9	50.4	11.5
Nut Butter, Soy, Wowbutter Foods*	1 Tbsp/15g	94	7	625	21.9	25	46.9	9.4
Olive Oil, Bertolli*	1 Serving/10g	53	5.9	532	0.5	0.5	59	0
Olive, Light, Tesco*	1 Thin Spread/7g	21	2.2	296	0.1	2.3	31.7	0.5
Olive, Reduced Fat, Waitrose*	1 Thin Spread/7g	29	3.2	412	0.5	1.3	45	0.5
Olive, Sainsbury's*	1 Thin Spread/7g	29	3.2	410	0.5	1	45	0.5
Olive, Tesco*	1 Thin Spread/7g	29	3.2	415	0.2	2	45	0.7
Orange, Thick Cut, St Dalfour*	1 Spread/11g	23	0	211	0.6	52	0.1	1.6
Plant Butter, Salted, Flora*	1 Thin Spread/7g	49	5.5	701	0.5	0.5	79	0
Plant Butter, Unsalted, Flora*	1 Thin Spread/7g	49	5.5	701	0.5	0.5	79	0
Pro Activ with Olive Oil, Flora*	1 Thin Spread/7g	22	2.4	315	0.5	0.5	35	0
Pro Activ, Light, Flora*	1 Thin Spread/7g	22	2.4	315	0.5	0.5	35	0

S

	Measure INFO/WEIGHT	per Measure KCAL	FAT	Nutrition Values per 100g / 100ml KCAL	PROT	CARB	FAT	FIBRE
SPREAD								
ProActiv, Buttery, Flora*	1 Thin Spread/7g	44	4.9	629	0.5	0.5	70	0
Reduced Fat, Average	*1 Thin Spread/7g*	*25*	*2.7*	*356*	*0.6*	*3*	*38*	*0*
Soft, Reduced Fat, Smart Price, Asda*	1 Thin Spread/7g	32	3.5	455	0.2	1	50	0
Spreadable, Salted, Tesco*	1 Thin Spread/7g	45	4.9	641	0.3	1.7	70.2	0.5
Sunflower, Average	*1 Thin Spread/7g*	*42*	*4.6*	*595*	*0.1*	*0.4*	*65.9*	*0.4*
Sunflower, Low Fat, Aldi*	1 Thin Spread/7g	26	2.7	366	0.2	5.7	38	0
Sunflower, Original, Aldi*	1 Thin Spread/7g	44	4.8	633	0.5	0.5	69	0.5
Tomato, & Basil, with Sunflower Seeds, Vemondo, Lidl*	1 Serving/30g	92	8.6	305	4	7	28.5	0
Vegan Block, Organic, Naturli*	1 Thin Spread/7g	47	5.2	670	0.5	0.5	75	0
Vegan, Spreadable, Organic, Naturli*	1 Thin Spread /7g	48	5.2	681	0.5	0.5	75	0
Vegetable, Soft, Tesco*	1 Thin Spread/7g	46	5.1	661	0.1	1	73	0
Vitalite, Dairy Free, Dairy Crest Ltd*	1 Thin Spread/7g	35	3.9	504	0	0	56	0
with Soya, Dairy Free, Pure Spreads*	1 Thin Spread/7g	40	4.4	569	0.5	1	63	0
with Sunflower, Dairy Free, Organic, Pure Spreads*	1 Thin Spread/7g	34	3.7	490	0.5	2.9	53.1	0
SPRING ROLLS								
Chicken, Katsu, Curry, Finest, Tesco*	1 Roll/28g	74	3.7	266	8.8	27.2	13.1	1.9
Chicken, Starter, Asda*	1 Roll/47g	119	6.1	253	11	21	13	2.7
Duck, Asda*	1 Roll/17g	46	2.1	267	7.1	30	12	3.4
Duck, Chinese Takeaway, Morrisons*	1 Roll/40g	97	4.4	243	7	27.8	11.1	2
Duck, Hoisin , Sainsbury's*	1 Roll/20g	57	3	287	5.9	30.6	15.3	1.8
Duck, Mini, Asda*	1 Roll/18g	47	1.9	259	8.7	32.8	10.3	1.9
Duck, Mini, Chef Select, Lidl*	1 Roll/20g	66	3.9	328	6.3	31.1	19.3	2.1
Duck, Party Bites, Sainsbury's*	1 Roll/20g	49	1.8	245	10.1	31.4	8.8	1
Duck, Party, Asda*	1 Roll/18g	47	2	259	7.1	32	11	3.1
Duck, Waitrose *	1 Roll/36g	92	4.4	256	8.2	26.8	12.1	3.6
From Restaurant, Average	*1 Roll/140g*	*344*	*14.8*	*246*	*11.1*	*23.2*	*10.6*	*0*
M&S*	1 Roll/36g	66	2.3	183	4.6	25.6	6.4	2.2
Mini Vegetable, Co-Op*	1 Roll/18g	40	1.6	220	4.1	30.9	9.1	2.7
Mini, Asda*	1 Roll/20g	35	0.6	175	3.5	33.6	3	1.9
Mini, Sainsbury's*	1 Roll/12g	27	1.2	221	4.2	28.7	9.9	1.6
No Duck, Hoisin, Vegan, Iceland*	1 Roll/20g	40	1.2	201	3.8	31.4	6.1	3.2
No Duck, Plant Chef, Tesco*	1 Roll/18g	43	1.6	239	4.9	33.3	9	2.8
No Duck, Plant Pioneers, Sainsbury's*	1 Roll/46g	90	3.8	195	2.7	25.6	8.3	3.3
No Duck, with Hoisin Dip, Plant Kitchen, M&S*	1 Roll/21g	45	1.1	211	5.7	34	5.3	2.4
Oriental Vegetable, Tesco*	1 Roll/60g	148	7.4	248	3.6	29.7	12.4	1.4
Prawn, Crispy, M&S*	1 Roll/34g	75	3.4	220	10	22.2	9.9	1.3
Thai, Sainsbury's*	1 Roll/30g	69	3.4	229	2.9	28.8	11.3	3.5
Vegetable, Asda*	1 Roll/62g	126	5.6	203	3.5	27	9	2.7
Vegetable, Asda*	1 Roll/18g	46	2.2	254	5.1	30	12	3.1
Vegetable, Cantonese, Large, Sainsbury's*	1 Roll/63g	130	6.3	205	3.6	25.3	9.9	1.5
Vegetable, Chilled, Tesco*	1 Roll/68g	149	7.6	221	4	25.9	11.3	1.6
Vegetable, Chinese Snack Selection, Waitrose*	1 Roll/18g	51	2.2	282	4.2	36.8	12.1	4.4
Vegetable, Chinese Takeaway, Sainsbury's*	1 Roll/59g	100	3.7	170	4	24.4	6.3	2.8
Vegetable, Co-Op*	1 Roll/50g	116	7	232	3.3	23	14	2.4
Vegetable, Iceland*	1 Roll/19g	35	1.3	183	3.3	26.1	6.6	2.8
Vegetable, M&S*	1 Roll/37g	80	3.6	215	4.3	27.8	9.6	2
Vegetable, Mini, Occasions, Sainsbury's*	1 Roll/24g	52	2.3	216	4.1	28.2	9.6	2.9
Vegetable, Mini, Party Food, M&S*	1 Roll/20g	40	1.6	200	3.7	26.2	8.1	2.7
Vegetable, Mini, Tesco*	1 Roll/16g	33	1.3	208	4	28.3	8.1	3
Vegetable, Sainsbury's*	1 Roll/53g	129	7	244	4.3	25.3	13.3	2.9
Vegetable, Zulekha*	1 Roll/20g	16	0.4	79	2	13	2	0
SPRITE*								
Sprite*	1 Bottle/500ml	70	0	14	0	3.3	0	0

S

	Measure INFO/WEIGHT	per Measure KCAL	FAT	Nutrition Values per 100g / 100ml KCAL	PROT	CARB	FAT	FIBRE
SPRITE*								
Zero, Lemon & Lime, Sprite*	1 Bottle/500ml	6	0	1	0	0	0	0
Zero, Sprite*	1 Can/330ml	3	0	1	0	0	0	0
SPRITZER								
Red Grape, Non-Alcoholic, Extra Special, Asda*	1 Bottle/750ml	330	0	44	0	11	0	0
Rose & Grape, Non Alcoholic, Extra Special, Asda*	1 Bottle/750ml	90	0	12	0	3	0	0
White Wine, Echo Falls*	1 Serving/125ml	78	0	39	0	0	0	0
with White Zinfadel, Echo Falls*	1 Serving/200ml	216	0	108	0	0	0	0
SQUASH								
Spaghetti, Baked	**1oz/28g**	**6**	**0.1**	**23**	**0.7**	**4.3**	**0.3**	**2.1**
Spaghetti, Including Pips & Rind, Raw	**1oz/28g**	**5**	**0.1**	**20**	**0.4**	**3.4**	**0.4**	**1.7**
Summer, All Varieties	**1 Sm/118g**	**21**	**0.2**	**18**	**1.2**	**3.8**	**0.2**	**1.2**
Winter, Acorn, Baked, Average	**1oz/28g**	**16**	**0**	**56**	**1.1**	**12.6**	**0.1**	**3.2**
Winter, Acorn, Raw, Average	**1oz/28g**	**9**	**0**	**30**	**0.6**	**6.8**	**0.1**	**1.7**
Winter, All Varieties, Flesh Only, Raw, Average	**1oz/28g**	**10**	**0**	**34**	**1**	**8.6**	**0.1**	**1.5**
SQUID								
Calamari, Breaded, Dunnes Stores*	½ Pack/125g	386	31.2	309	9.1	12	25	0.6
Calamari, Golden Battered, Oven Baked, Youngs*	½ Pack/125g	289	13.4	231	7.6	25.6	10.7	0.8
in Batter, Fried in Blended Oil, Average	**1oz/28g**	**55**	**2.8**	**195**	**11.5**	**15.7**	**10**	**0.5**
Raw, Average	**1oz/28g**	**23**	**0.5**	**81**	**15.4**	**1.2**	**1.7**	**0**
Rings, Salt & Pepper, Smokey, Sainsbury's*	1 Pack/100g	109	3.4	109	18.2	1.5	3.4	0.5
Salt & Pepper Chargrilled, Cooked, Tesco*	1 Pack/80g	78	2.3	98	17.9	0	2.9	0.1
Stuffed, Ready to Eat, Tricana *	1 Tin/120g	86	1.4	72	13.8	1.4	1.2	0
STAR FRUIT								
Average*	1oz/28g	9	0.1	31	0.5	7.1	0.3	1.3
STARBURST								
Fruit Chews, Tropical, Mars*	1 Tube/45g	168	3.3	373	0	76.9	7.3	0
Mars*	1 Pack/45g	182	3.3	405	0	83.9	7.3	0
STEAMED PUDDING								
Butterscotch, & Pecan, Aunty's*	1 Pudding/95g	293	6.8	308	3.8	53.2	7.2	1
Golden Syrup, Steamed, Aunty's*	1 Pudding/95g	278	3.9	293	3.3	57.3	4.1	0.8
Sticky Toffee, Steamed, Aunty's*	1 Pudding/95g	279	4.6	294	3.4	55.6	4.8	1
STEW								
Aubergine, & Split Pea, Allplants*	1 Serving/380g	429	17.9	113	4.5	12	4.7	2.7
Bean, Moroccan, V Taste, Morrisons*	1 Pack/301g	256	5.1	85	4	11.6	1.7	3.8
Beef & Dumplings	**1 Serving/652g**	**766**	**32.7**	**117**	**7.4**	**10.7**	**5**	**0.8**
Beef, Asda*	½ Can/196g	178	4.9	91	10	7	2.5	1.5
Beef, Canned, Asda*	1 Can/392g	353	13.7	90	8.9	5.3	3.5	0.9
Beef, Canned, Princes*	1 Serving/196g	145	5.1	74	8	4	2.6	1.5
Beef, Diet Chef Ltd*	1 Pack/270g	200	3.5	74	7.3	7.8	1.3	1.1
Beef, Meal for One, M&S*	1 Pack/440g	350	8.4	80	7	8.7	1.9	2
Beef, Minced, & Onion, Tesco*	1 Pack/300g	219	7.2	73	3.6	8.8	2.4	0.9
Beef, Value, Tesco*	1 Serving/200g	170	9.8	85	4	6.2	4.9	1
Brazilian, One Pot, Aldi*	1 Pot/381g	373	14.8	98	3.2	11	3.9	3.2
Chicken & Dumplings, Birds Eye*	1 Pack/320g	282	8.6	88	7	8.9	2.7	0.5
Chicken & Dumplings, Tesco*	1 Serving/450g	567	29.7	126	7.6	9.1	6.6	0.7
Chicken, & Dumplings, Oven Baked, Iceland*	1 Serving/467g	500	20.1	107	4.5	11.9	4.3	1.1
Chicken, & Vegetable, 1325, Oakhouse Foods Ltd*	1 Serving/400g	308	10	77	4.9	7	2.5	1.7
Chicken, Catalan, Ready Set Cook!, Aldi*	½ Pack/200g	214	2.2	107	15	7.4	1.1	3.7
Chicken, Morrisons*	1 Pack/400g	492	7.6	123	17.6	8.9	1.9	0.5
Chickpea, Moroccan, Allplants*	½ Pack/380g	551	20.1	145	4.8	17	5.3	3.9
Chilli Bean, Jamaican Style, Plant Menu, Aldi*	1 Pack/400g	468	14	117	3.4	16	3.5	4.3
Lamb, with Basmati Rice, Hello Fresh*	1 Serving/369g	336	1	91	3	19	0.3	0
Lentil & Vegetable, Organic, Simply Organic*	1 Pack/400g	284	6	71	3.5	11	1.5	1.3

	Measure INFO/WEIGHT	per Measure KCAL	FAT	Nutrition Values per 100g / 100ml KCAL	PROT	CARB	FAT	FIBRE
STEW								
Lentil, Moroccan, Plant Kitchen, M&S*	1 Pack/300g	282	6	94	3.5	14.2	2	2.5
Lentil, Moroccan, Plant Menu, Aldi*	1 Pack/300g	321	6	107	4.5	16	2	4.1
Moroccan, Vegetable, Slimfree, Aldi*	1 Pack/500g	155	2.5	31	1.2	4.7	0.5	1.9
Peri Peri, & Black Bean, Hello Fresh*	1 Serving/588g	759	29.4	129	7	13	5	0
Rainbow, Roots, & Vegetables, Gro, Co-Op*	1 Pack/400g	232	6.4	58	2.6	8.3	1.6	2.8
Roots, Hearty, Allplants*	½ Pack/380g	433	19.8	114	4.2	11	5.2	3
Sweet Potato, & Bean, Vegan, Waitrose*	½ Pack/220g	152	2.9	69	2.2	9.3	1.3	5.8
Sweet Potato, & Coconut, Piri Piri, Power Pot, BOL Foods*	1 Pot/450g	378	6.8	84	4.4	11.2	1.5	4.3
Tuscan Bean, Tasty Veg Pot, Innocent*	1 Pot/400g	320	7.6	80	3.1	12.5	1.9	3.6
Vegetable, Moroccan, Lidl*	1 Pack/500g	145	2	29	1.1	4	0.4	2.4
STIR FRY								
Baby Pak Choi, & Pepper, M&S*	1 Serving/110g	32	0.3	29	2.1	3.4	0.3	2
Beef, & Broccoli, Chinese, Box Ingredients Only, Gousto*	1 Serving/465g	498	17.7	107	8.4	10.8	3.8	2
Beef, BGTY, Sainsbury's*	½ Pack/125g	156	5.1	125	22	0.1	4.1	0
Beef, Chilli, Noodles, Musclefood*	1 Pack/235g	226	3.8	96	10	11	1.6	1.8
Beef, Chilli, Spicy, Musclefood*	1 Serving/353g	314	8.8	89	13.4	2.5	2.5	1.6
Beef, Steak, The Juicy Meat Co.*	½ Pack/140g	277	9.9	198	31.6	1.6	7.1	0.5
Beef, Teriyaki, Aldi*	½ Pack/196g	214	5.7	109	13	8.2	2.9	0.5
Beef, Teriyaki, M&Ss*	1 Pack/500g	375	3.5	75	10	7.1	0.7	0.1
Beef, Teriyaki, with Onions, Carrots, & Peppers, Waitrose*	1 Serving/210g	228	6.7	109	10.7	9.2	3.2	0.2
Broccoli, Tenderstem, Specially Selected, Aldi*	1/3 Pack/80g	26	0.4	32	2.4	3.6	0.5	2.7
Brown Rice, & Edamame Bean, Waitrose*	½ Pack/150g	204	6.1	136	5	17.3	4.1	4.8
Butternut Squash, & Edamame, Waitrose*	½ Pack/151g	74	1.5	49	3.1	6.2	1	1.6
Butternut Squash, Mangetout, & Chilli, Asda*	½ Pack/130g	79	3.5	61	1.6	5.8	2.7	3.5
Chicken Chow Mein, Fresh, HL, Tesco*	1 Pack/400g	312	4.8	78	5.7	11.4	1.2	1.3
Chicken, & Broccoli, Hello Fresh*	1 Serving/446g	651	22.3	146	10	15	5	0
Chicken, 387, Oakhouse Foods Ltd*	1 Pack/430g	404	2.6	94	8.4	12.9	0.6	1.8
Chicken, Chinese Style, Kit, Asda*	½ Pack/190g	160	1.9	84	12	6.6	1	0.5
Chicken, Chinese, Meal Kit, Aldi*	½ Pack/211g	278	8.6	132	16	7.6	4.1	1.2
Chicken, Fajita, Kit, Tesco*	½ Pack/230g	288	10.6	122	14.8	4.4	4.5	2.2
Chicken, Fajita, Musclefood*	1 Serving/358g	301	10.4	84	11.4	2	2.9	2.3
Chicken, Fajita, Ready Set Cook!, Aldi*	1 Pack/535g	749	30	140	18	3.6	5.6	0.8
Chicken, Naked, Musclefood*	1 Serving/350g	217	4.2	62	9.9	2.5	1.2	1
Chicken, Peri Peri, Meals in Minutes, Iceland*	½ Bag/343g	419	17.5	122	5.7	12.5	5.1	1.5
Chicken, Teriyaki, Tesco*	½ Pack/250g	315	13.5	126	13.5	5.7	5.4	0.5
Chicken, Thai, Musclefood*	1 Serving/336g	279	8.7	83	11.8	1.9	2.6	2.4
Chicken, Tikka, Biryani, Iceland*	½ Pack/351g	432	17.9	123	5.6	13.4	5.1	0.7
Chinese Chicken, As Consumed, Iceland*	½ Pack/371g	353	2.6	95	6.5	15.2	0.7	1
Chinese Prawn, Iceland*	1 Pack/340g	235	4.4	69	3.1	11.1	1.3	2.1
Chinese Style Rice with Vegetables, Tesco*	1 Serving/550g	495	13.8	90	2.2	14.8	2.5	0.3
Edamame Bean, & Broccoli, Asda*	1 Pack/320g	227	10.2	71	3.9	5.5	3.2	2.3
Edamame Bean, Oaklands, Lidl*	½ Pack/150g	70	2.4	47	3.5	3	1.6	3.3
Ginger, Bright & Colourful, Waitrose*	1 Serving/105g	32	0.5	31	1.9	4	0.5	2.2
Green Vegetable, M&S*	1 Pack/220g	165	13	75	3.1	2.5	5.9	2.2
Malaysian Peanut Satay, Kit, Street Kitchen*	1 Pack/255g	477	19.9	187	4.7	25	7.8	0
Meal Kit, Teriyaki Chicken, Go Cook, Asda*	½ Pack/267g	318	6.7	119	13	11	2.5	0.6
Mixed Pepper, Sainsbury's*	1 Pack/300g	188	12.9	70	1.5	4.6	4.8	1.2
Mixed Peppers, Co-Op*	1 Serving/150g	46	0.8	31	1.8	4	0.5	2.3
Mushroom, Asda*	1 Pack/320g	144	4.2	45	2.5	4.4	1.3	2.5
Mushroom, Morrisons*	¼ Pack/80g	25	0.4	31	2.1	3.5	0.5	2.1
Mushroom, Sweet & Crunchy, Stir Fried, Oaklands, Lidl*	1/3 Pack/86g	25	0.2	29	1.7	3.5	0.2	3.2
Mushroom, Tender, Waitrose*	1 Pack/400g	180	8	45	2.1	2.3	2	4.7
Oriental Style Pak Choi, M&S*	1 Pack/220g	165	12.5	75	2.2	3.5	5.7	2.4

STIR FRY

	Measure INFO/WEIGHT	per Measure KCAL	FAT	Nutrition Values per 100g / 100ml KCAL	PROT	CARB	FAT	FIBRE
Oriental Style, Vegetables, Sainsbury's*	1 Pack/300g	195	14.4	65	1.5	4.1	4.8	2.1
Oriental, Wokfresh, Birds Eye*	½ Pack/250g	65	1.2	26	1	4.2	0.5	2.5
Pork, Super Quick, Hello Fresh*	1 Serving/338g	531	13	157	9.4	20.9	3.8	0
Pork, Teriyaki, Noodle, with Mushrooms, Hello Fresh*	1 Serving/393g	444	15.7	113	7	11	4	0
Protein, Green Isle*	1 Serving/100g	185	11	185	7	12	11	6.2
Rice, Quinoa & Vegetable, Waitrose*	½ Pack/134g	199	7.8	148	5.4	15.6	5.8	6
Salmon, Teriyaki, Musclefood *	1 Serving/275g	475	15.4	173	12	17	5.6	2.2
Singapore, Noodle, Iceland*	½ Pack/346g	294	10.7	85	5.4	8.2	3.1	1.5
Sticky Veg Satay, Cook*	1 Pack/289g	335	9	116	3.5	18.9	3.1	1.2
Sweet Mixed Pepper, Waitrose*	½ Pack/150g	111	6.1	74	2.1	4.2	4.1	5.8
Teriyaki, Kit, Co-Op*	½ Pack/170g	104	0.8	61	1.6	12	0.5	1.6
Turkey, Thai, Noodle, Box Ingredients Only, Gousto*	1 Serving/390g	542	12.9	139	11.2	15.7	3.3	2
Vegetable & Mushroom, Asda*	½ Pack/160g	59	2.4	37	2.4	3.4	1.5	3.4
Vegetable Mix, As Consumed, Tesco*	½ Pack/128g	72	3	56	1.9	5.5	2.3	3
Vegetable Mix, Chinese Inspired, Tesco*	1 Pack/320g	166	9.3	52	1.5	3.8	2.9	2.3
Vegetable, & Bean Sprout, Tesco*	½ Bag/160g	94	5	59	2	4.5	3.1	2.7
Vegetable, & Beansprout, Tesco*	½ Pack/160g	95	5	59	2	4.5	3.1	2.7
Vegetable, & Beansprout, Tesco*	½ Pack/143g	86	4.6	60	2.1	4.3	3.2	2.6
Vegetable, Chop Suey, Chinese, Sharwood's*	1 Pack/310g	223	3.4	72	1.5	13.9	1.1	0.6
Vegetable, Oriental Mix, Tesco*	½ Pack/126g	88	4.4	70	2.6	5.7	3.5	2.7
Vegetable, Rainbow, Fresh Tastes, Asda*	½ Pack/225g	119	5	53	1.8	4.6	2.2	3.8
Vegetable, Ready Prepared, M&S*	½ Pack/150g	38	0.4	25	2.2	3.5	0.3	2.2
Vegetable, Thai Style, Tesco*	½ Pack/135g	42	0.7	31	2.3	4.2	0.5	2.1
Vegetables, Chinese, Ready to Cook, Morrisons*	¼ Pack/81g	25	0.3	31	1.7	4.2	0.4	2.1
Vegetables, Co-Op*	1 Serving/80g	29	0.4	36	1.8	5	0.5	2.7
Vegetables, Family, M&S*	¼ Pack/137g	48	0.7	35	2.1	4.4	0.5	2.3
Vegetables, Farm Stores, Asda*	½ Pack/160g	77	2.9	48	1.8	5.7	1.8	1.1
Vegetables, Mixed, Frozen, Tesco*	¼ Pack/150g	81	3.8	54	1.5	4.4	2.5	4
Vegetables, Superbright, Waitrose*	½ Pack/150g	129	7.2	86	3.5	4.3	4.8	5.6
Vegetables, Sweet & Crunchy, Stir Fried, Oaklands, Lidl*	1 Serving/87g	33	0.2	38	1.6	5.2	0.2	4.4

STOCK

	Measure INFO/WEIGHT	per Measure KCAL	FAT	Nutrition Values per 100g / 100ml KCAL	PROT	CARB	FAT	FIBRE
Beef, Cooks' Ingredients, Waitrose*	1 Jar/500g	110	2.5	22	3.2	0.9	0.5	0.5
Beef, Fresh, Sainsbury's*	¼ Pot/113g	27	0.6	24	5.1	0.5	0.5	0.5
Beef, Heston from Waitrose, Waitrose*	¼ Pack/125g	34	0.6	27	4.9	0.8	0.5	0.9
Beef, Made Up, Stock Pot, Knorr*	1 Serving/100ml	10	0.4	10	0.2	1	0.4	0
Beef, Pot, Made Up, Tesco*	¼ Pot/125ml	12	0.4	10	0.4	1.3	0.3	0.1
Beef, Rich Farm-Bred, Oxo*	1 Pack/320g	61	3.2	19	0.9	1.5	1	0.2
Beef, Rich, Stock Pot, Knorr*	1 Pot/28g	42	1.1	150	3	27	4	0.8
Beef, Slow Cooked, Finest, Tesco*	¼ Pouch/113ml	18	0.2	16	2	1.6	0.2	0
Bone Broth, Pure Beef, Powder, Honest And Good*	1 Tbsp/15g	64	0.6	430	99	1	4	0
Bouillon, Vegetable, Powder, Mix, Dry Weight, Asda*	1 Tsp/5g	13	0.5	260	10	35	10	10
Broth, Beef Bone, 10hr, Daylesford*	1 Serving/250ml	125	2.5	50	5.7	3.7	1	1.7
Chicken, Atkins & Potts*	1 Pack/350g	56	2.1	16	1.3	1.1	0.6	0.1
Chicken, Bone, Broth, Ossa*	1 Cup/250ml	28	1.2	11	2.6	0.2	0.5	0.5
Chicken, Concentrated, M&S*	1 Tsp/5g	16	0.9	315	25.6	12.2	18.1	0.8
Chicken, Cooks' Ingredients, Waitrose*	1 Pack/500ml	75	0.5	15	3.2	0.3	0.1	0.2
Chicken, Fresh, Finest, Tesco*	¼ Pouch/113ml	15	0.4	13	2	0.1	0.4	0.5
Chicken, Fresh, Pot, Sainsbury's*	¼ Pot/111g	21	0.6	19	4.1	0.5	0.5	0.5
Chicken, Fresh, Pot, Tesco*	1/3 Pot/100ml	19	1.2	19	1	1.1	1.2	0.1
Chicken, Fresh, Sainsbury's*	½ Pot/142ml	23	0.1	16	3.7	0.1	0.1	0.3
Chicken, GF, Stock Pot, As Sold, Knorr*	1 Stock Pot/28g	26	1.1	92	4.1	9.1	4	1
Chicken, Granules, Knorr*	1 Tsp/4.5g	10	0.2	232	13.1	36.5	3.7	0.4
Chicken, Home Prepared, Average	**1fl oz/30ml**	**7**	**0.3**	**24**	**3.8**	**0.7**	**0.9**	**0.3**

	Measure	per Measure		Nutrition Values per 100g / 100ml				
	INFO/WEIGHT	KCAL	FAT	KCAL	PROT	CARB	FAT	FIBRE
STOCK								
Chicken, Made Up, Stock Pot, Knorr*	1 Serving/125ml	15	0.3	12	0.2	1.6	0.2	0
Chicken, Organic, Pot, Kallo*	1 Pot/24g	30	2.6	124	4.2	1.2	11	0
Chicken, Rich & Savoury, Pot, As Sold, Tesco*	1 Pot/28g	48	1.6	171	7.1	22.8	5.7	1.4
Fish, Home Prepared, Average	*1 Serving/250ml*	*42*	*2*	*17*	*2.3*	*0*	*0.8*	*0*
Kaffir Lime, & Ginger, Pot, Knorr*	1 Pot/26g	16	0.2	62	6.5	6.3	0.6	2.2
Mushroom, Pot, As Sold, Knorr*	1 Pot/28g	41	0.8	148	2.8	28	2.7	1.6
Red Wine, Pot, As Sold, Oxo*	1 Pot/20g	22	0.1	111	0.8	25.6	0.5	2.8
Smoked Chilli, & Tomato, Pot, As Sold, Knorr*	1 Pot/26g	14	0.2	55	6	5.5	0.8	1.8
Vegetable, Cooks Ingredients, Waitrose*	1 Pouch/500ml	15	0.5	3	0.2	0.4	0.1	0.5
Vegetable, Fresh, COOK!, M&S*	¼ Pouch/125ml	15	0.1	12	0.3	2.5	0.1	0.1
Vegetable, Made Up, Stock Pot, Knorr*	1 Serving/125ml	8	0.6	6	0.5	0.5	0.5	0.5
Vegetable, Organic, Knorr*	1 Pot/26g	32	2.2	122	5.2	5.2	8.6	1.2
Vegetable, Organic, Pot, Kallo*	1 Pot/24g	23	1.5	96	1.5	7.5	6.1	0
Vegetable, Pot, As Prepared, Tesco*	¼ Pot/125ml	11	0.2	9	0.3	1.5	0.2	0.1
Vegetable, Pot, As Sold, Knorr*	1 Pot/33g	59	3	180	6	17	9	1.5
STOCK CUBES								
Beef, Dry Weight, Bovril*	1 Cube/6g	12	0.2	197	10.8	29.3	4.1	0
Beef, Dry Weight, Oxo*	1 Cube/6g	15	0.3	265	17.4	38.4	4.9	4.2
Beef, Knorr*	1 Cube/10g	31	2.3	310	5	19	23	0
Beef, Made Up, Oxo*	1 Cube/189ml	17	0.4	9	0.6	1.3	0.2	0.1
Beef, Meat Free, Dry Weight, Oxo*	1 Cube/6g	16	0.3	262	14.7	39.1	4.7	2.3
Beef, Organic, Kallo*	1 Cube/12g	25	1	208	16.7	16.7	8.3	0
Beef, Reduced Salt, Made Up, Oxo*	1 Cube/500ml	45	2.5	9	0.6	1.3	0.5	0.5
Beef, Tesco*	1 Cube/7g	17	0.2	260	9.7	48.9	2.8	1.3
Chicken	*1 Cube/6g*	*14*	*0.9*	*237*	*15.4*	*9.9*	*15.4*	*0*
Chicken, Dry, Average	*1 Cube/10g*	*29*	*1.8*	*293*	*7.3*	*25.5*	*18*	*0.4*
Chicken, Made Up, Average	*1 Pint/568ml*	*43*	*1*	*8*	*0.4*	*1.1*	*0.2*	*0.1*
Chicken, Reduced Salt, Dry, Oxo*	1 Cube/7g	22	0.3	321	14.6	54.9	3.9	2.8
Chicken, Reduced Salt, Prepared, Oxo*	1 Cube/500ml	50	2.5	10	0.5	1.7	0.5	0.5
Fish, Knorr*	1 Cube/10g	32	2.4	321	8	18	24	1
Fish, Sainsbury's*	1 Cube/11g	31	2.2	282	19.1	7.3	20	0.9
Garlic, & Herb, Organic, Made Up, Kallo*	1 Cube/500ml	35	2.5	7	0.1	0.6	0.5	0
Ham, Knorr*	1 Cube/10g	31	1.9	313	11.8	24.4	18.7	0
Lamb, Made Up, Knorr*	1 Serving/100ml	5	0.6	5	0.3	0.3	0.6	0.1
Mushroom, Organic, As Prepared, Kallo*	1 Cube/500ml	35	2.5	7	0.1	0.5	0.5	0
Vegetable, Average	*1 Cube/7g*	*18*	*1.2*	*253*	*13.5*	*11.6*	*17.3*	*0*
Vegetable, Low Salt, Organic, Made Up, Kallo*	1 Serving/500ml	50	3.5	10	0.3	0.7	0.7	0.2
STOVIES								
Chef Select, Lidl*	1 Pack/412g	346	3.7	84	4.6	13	0.9	2.9
Mckinley's *	1 Serving/390g	351	7.8	90	4.3	13.4	2	0.8
Scottish, Mcintosh Of Strathmore*	1 Pack/300g	231	6.3	77	4	10.8	2.1	2.4
STRAWBERRIES								
Dried, Urban Fresh Fruit*	1 Pack/35g	111	0.1	318	1.6	77	0.4	5.9
Fresh, Raw, Average	*1 Berry/12g*	*3*	*0*	*28*	*0.8*	*6*	*0.1*	*1.4*
Frozen, Average	*1 Serving/100g*	*30*	*0.2*	*30*	*0.8*	*6.3*	*0.2*	*1*
in Fruit Juice, Canned, Average	*1/3 Can/127g*	*58*	*0*	*46*	*0.4*	*11*	*0*	*1*
in Syrup, Canned, Average	*1 Serving/100g*	*63*	*0*	*63*	*0.4*	*15.2*	*0*	*0.6*
STROGANOFF								
Beef, & Rice, Charlie Bigham's*	1 Serving/395 g	675	34.8	171	8.5	13.1	8.8	0
Beef, & Rice, TTD, Sainsbury's*	1 Pack/410g	595	20.9	145	9.6	15.2	5.1	1.7
Beef, & Mushroom, Eat Well, M&S*	1 Pack/380g	452	11.4	119	7.7	14.2	3	2.4
Beef, & Mushroom, Jane Plan*	1 Pack/300g	339	15.3	113	5.3	10.7	5.1	1.2
Beef, Asda*	1 Serving/120g	276	20.4	230	16	3.3	17	0.6

S

	Measure INFO/WEIGHT	per Measure KCAL	FAT	Nutrition Values per 100g / 100ml KCAL	PROT	CARB	FAT	FIBRE
STROGANOFF								
Beef, Creamy, COOK!, M&S*	½ Pack/250g	292	17	117	10.3	3.5	6.8	0
Beef, Luxury, Iceland*	1 Pack/388g	528	13.6	136	8.2	17.5	3.5	0.9
Beef, Oven Baked, Slimming World*	1 Pack/500g	265	2.5	53	8.2	3.4	0.5	1.2
Beef, with Wild Rice, Extra Special, Asda*	1 Pack/389g	451	9.3	116	6	17	2.4	0.9
Chicken, with Rice, BGTY, Sainsbury's*	1 Pack/415g	448	5.4	108	7	17.1	1.3	1.1
Mushroom, & Rice, V Taste, Morrisons*	1 Pack/322g	386	15.1	120	3.5	14.4	4.7	2.9
Mushroom, 7535, Wiltshire Farm Foods*	1 Serving/421g	425	14.7	101	2.9	12	3.5	0
Mushroom, Creamy, Box Ingredients Only, Gousto*	1 Serving/327g	487	9.5	149	4.9	25.3	2.9	2
Mushroom, Eat Smart, Morrisons*	1 Pack/400g	312	4.4	78	2.6	14.3	1.1	1
Mushroom, Portobello, Charred, Finest, Tesco*	½ Pack/164g	207	14.9	126	3.9	6.1	9.1	2.2
Mushroom, Roasted, Plant Kitchen, M&S*	1 Pack/350g	248	14.3	71	2.9	5.4	4.1	0.5
Mushroom, with Rice, 1341, Oakhouse Foods Ltd*	1 Serving/398g	370	9.5	93	2.9	13.3	2.4	3
Mushroom, with Rice, BGTY, Sainsbury's*	1 Serving/450g	418	6.8	93	3.3	16.6	1.5	1
Pork, Classic Kitchen, Tesco*	½ Pack/222g	284	13.5	128	12.9	4.6	6.1	1.2
STRUDEL								
Apple with Sultanas, Tesco*	1/6 Strudel/100g	245	12	245	2.9	30.9	12	0.7
Apple, Apfelstrudel, Alpenfest*	1 Slice/125g	201	3.1	161	1.9	31.7	2.5	0
Apple, Co-Op*	1 Slice/100g	225	12	225	3	28	12	3
Apple, Dessert Menu, Aldi*	½ Strudel/94g	248	12.2	264	2.9	33	13	2.2
Apple, Ovenbaked, CBY, Asda*	1 Slice/100g	249	12	249	2.7	31.6	12	1.7
Apple, Sainsbury's*	1 Serving/90g	233	11.7	259	2.8	31.6	13	1.9
Apple, Tesco*	1 Serving/94g	226	11.6	241	2.6	28.9	12.4	1.7
Berry, Frozen, Tesco*	1 Serving/94g	220	9.9	234	2.7	31.2	10.5	1.9
Toaster, Strawberry, Pillsbury*	1 Strudel/55g	175	6.5	318	4.6	48.2	11.8	0.9
STUFFING								
Cranberry, & Orange, Plant Kitchen, M&S*	1 Serving/50g	81	3.4	162	5.7	15.9	6.8	7.1
Nut, & Thyme, Sainsbury's*	1 Serving/44g	64	1.4	146	4.6	22.7	3.2	4
Oatmeal, & Onion, Speyside Specialities*	1 Pack/440g	1518	74.5	345	8.2	40.8	16.9	0
Olde English Chestnut, Sainsbury's*	1 Serving/110g	216	12.8	196	9.4	13.5	11.6	2.1
Pork, Chestnut & Onion, Cooked, Finest, Tesco*	1/8 Pack/41g	108	6.9	263	12.9	13.6	16.8	2.4
Pork, Sage, & Onion, M&S*	¼ Pack/85g	186	12.7	219	11.7	8.5	14.9	2
Pork, Sausagemeat, Gourmet, Waitrose *	1 Serving/56g	137	10	245	15.9	4.8	17.8	0.8
Sage & Onion, for Chicken, Paxo*	1 Serving/50g	60	0.6	120	3.4	22.8	1.3	1.7
Sage & Onion, Quixo, Aldi*	1 Serving/45g	53	0.5	117	3.3	22	1.2	2
Sage, & Onion, Waitrose*	¼ Pack/56g	137	7.1	244	4.5	26.9	12.6	2.4
Sausagemeat, Sainsbury's*	1 Serving/100g	175	4.2	175	7	27	4.2	2.3
STUFFING BALLS								
British Pork, Sage & Onion, Cooked, Finest, Tesco*	1 Ball/25g	55	2.5	224	13.9	17.4	10.2	2.2
Pork, Sage, & Onion, Sainsbury's*	1 Ball/24g	63	4.4	258	12	11	18	2.2
Pork, Sausagemeat, Aunt Bessie's*	1 Ball/26g	55	2.1	212	7.2	27.3	8.2	3
Sage & Onion, Aunt Bessie's*	1 Ball/26g	60	1.6	229	5.5	39	6.3	3.1
STUFFING MIX								
Apple & Herb, Special Recipe, Sainsbury's*	1 Serving/41g	68	0.9	165	3.8	32.4	2.2	2.2
Cornbread, Stove Top, Kraft *	½ Cup/28g	100	1	357	10.7	71.4	3.6	3.6
Dry, Average	**1 Serving/25g**	**84**	**1**	**338**	**9.6**	**70.1**	**3.8**	**5.3**
Garlic, & Herb, Tesco*	1 Serving/50g	90	1.3	179	4.7	32.8	2.6	2.8
Mediterranean, Spicy, Veggie Fillers, As Cooked, Paxo*	1 Serving/110g	86	1.5	78	2.8	12.6	1.4	1.7
Sage & Onion, Asda*	1 Ball/30g	56	0.7	187	5.3	35	2.2	3.4
Sage & Onion, Co-Op*	1 Serving/28g	94	0.6	335	10	68	2	6
Sage & Onion, Prepared, Tesco*	1 Serving/100g	50	0.4	50	1.5	10.1	0.4	0.9
Sage & Onion, As Prepared, Newgate, Lidl*	1 Serving/45g	52	0.5	116	3.3	22.1	1.2	2
Sage & Onion, Dry Weight, Tesco*	1 Pack/170g	578	4.1	340	10.3	69.3	2.4	6.3
Sage & Onion, Dry, Asda*	1 Serving/11g	56	0.7	527	15.1	94.1	6.6	9.4

INFO/WEIGHT	Measure		Nutrition Values per 100g / 100ml				
	KCAL	FAT	KCAL	PROT	CARB	FAT	FIBRE
STUFFING MIX							
Sage & Onion, GF, Dry Weight, Mrs Crimble's*	1 Pack/150g	522	5.4	348	12.7	62.9	3.6	0
Sage & Onion, M&S*	1 Serving/30g	108	1	359	11.4	67.8	3.4	6
Sage & Onion, with Apple, Made Up, Paxo*	1 Serving/50g	69	0.8	138	3.8	26	1.6	2.2
Sage, & Onion, Kania, Lidl*	1 Serving/50g	56	0.8	113	3	21	1.5	1.8
Sage, & Onion, Sainsbury's*	1 Serving/50g	189	2.2	378	10.6	71	4.4	6
SUET							
Beef, Tesco*	1 Serving/100g	854	91.9	854	0.6	6.2	91.9	0.1
Vegetable, Average	**1oz/28g**	**234**	**24.6**	**836**	**1.2**	**10.1**	**87.9**	**0**
Vegetable, Light, Shredded, As Sold, Atora*	¼ Pack/50g	314	26.4	627	9.9	23.7	52.7	8.9
SUGAR							
Brown, Soft, Average	**1 Tsp/4g**	**15**	**0**	**382**	**0**	**96.5**	**0**	**0**
Brown, Soft, Light, Average	**1 Tsp/5g**	**20**	**0**	**393**	**0.2**	**97.8**	**0.1**	**0**
Caster, Average	**1 Tsp/5g**	**20**	**0**	**399**	**0**	**99.8**	**0**	**0**
Cubes, Silver Spoon*	1 Cube/4g	16	0	400	0	100	0	0
Dark Brown, Muscovado, Average	**1 Tsp/7g**	**27**	**0**	**380**	**0.2**	**94.8**	**0**	**0**
Dark Brown, Soft, Average	**1 Tsp/5g**	**18**	**0**	**369**	**0.1**	**92**	**0**	**0**
Demerara, Average	**1 Tsp/5g**	**18**	**0**	**368**	**0.2**	**99.2**	**0**	**0**
Golden, Unrefined, Average	**1 Tsp/4g**	**16**	**0**	**399**	**0**	**99.8**	**0**	**0**
Granulated, Organic, Average	**1 Tsp/4g**	**16**	**0**	**398**	**0.2**	**99.7**	**0**	**0**
Icing, Average	**1 Tsp/4g**	**16**	**0**	**394**	**0**	**102.2**	**0**	**0**
Light Or Diet, Average	**1 Tsp/4g**	**16**	**0**	**394**	**0**	**98.5**	**0**	**0**
Muscovado, Light, Average	**1 Tsp/5g**	**19**	**0**	**384**	**0**	**96**	**0**	**0**
White, Granulated, Average	**1 Tsp/5g**	**20**	**0**	**398**	**0**	**100**	**0**	**0**
SULTANAS							
Average	**1oz/28g**	**82**	**0.1**	**291**	**2.8**	**69.2**	**0.4**	**2**
SUNDAE							
Blackcurrant, Holly Lane, Aldi*	1 Sundae/47g	201	8.5	427	3.2	61	18	3.2
Blackcurrant, M&S*	1 Sundae/53g	212	10.2	400	3	54.2	19.2	1.9
Caramel, From Restaurant, Average	**1 Sundae/155g**	**304**	**9.3**	**196**	**4.7**	**31.8**	**6**	**0**
Chocolate & Vanilla, HL, Tesco*	1 Sundae/120g	193	3.1	161	2.8	31.5	2.6	0.6
Chocolate & Vanilla, Tesco*	1 Sundae/70g	140	6	199	2.8	27.5	8.6	0.5
Chocolate Brownie, Tesco*	1 Pot/136g	271	15	199	5.2	18.8	11	1.9
Chocolate Mint, COU, M&S*	1 Pot/90g	108	2.3	120	5.4	17.8	2.6	0.5
Chocolate Nut	**1 Serving/70g**	**195**	**10.7**	**278**	**3**	**34.2**	**15.3**	**0.1**
Chocolate, Sainsbury's*	1 Pot/140g	393	29.8	281	2.5	19.3	21.3	0.6
Chocolate, Triple, Sainsbury's*	1 Pot/125g	253	14.1	203	5.2	18.9	11.3	2.3
Ice Cream	**1 Serving/170g**	**482**	**15.4**	**284**	**5.9**	**45.3**	**9.1**	**0.3**
Strawberry & Vanilla, Tesco*	1 Serving/68g	120	3.9	177	2	29.5	5.7	0.1
Strawberry, & Raspberry, COU, M&S*	1 Pot/110g	154	4.1	140	3.1	23.3	3.7	0.4
Strawberry, M&S*	1 Sundae/45g	173	8	385	3.4	53.3	17.8	1
Toffee & Vanilla, Tesco*	1 Serving/70g	133	4.5	189	2.1	30.7	6.4	0.1
Toffee, Asda*	1 Serving/120g	322	19.2	268	2.1	29	16	0
Toffee, M&S*	1 Tub/130g	421	29.6	324	2.3	27.3	22.8	0.4
Toffee, Pot, Sainsbury's*	1 Pot/95g	140	4.5	147	3.3	22.5	4.7	0.5
Toffee, Sainsbury's*	1 Sundae/140g	378	27.2	270	3.1	20.2	19.4	0.9
Vanilla Caramel, Aldi*	1 Sundae/72g	159	7.4	221	2.6	29.2	10.3	0.7
SUPPLEMENT							
100% Plant Protein, Scitec Nutrition*	1 Scoop/40g	136	1.7	340	70	5	4.3	0
100% Whey Protein, Double Chocolate, Optimum Nutrition*	1 Serving/32g	120	1.5	374	77	4.3	4.7	2.3
Black Edition, Banana, Huel*	1 Scoop/45g	198	8.6	440	44	19	19	7.5
Black Edition, Chocolate, Huel*	1 Scoop/45g	180	7.6	400	40	17	17	8.2
Black Edition, Huel*	1 Scoop/45g	195	8.6	433	43	18	19	8.3
Black Edition, Salted Caramel, Huel*	1 Scoop/45g	200	9	444	44.4	17.8	20	7.9

S

SUPPLEMENT

	Measure INFO/WEIGHT	per Measure KCAL	FAT	Nutrition Values per 100g / 100ml KCAL	PROT	CARB	FAT	FIBRE
Black Edition, Strawberries & Cream, Huel*	1 Scoop/45g	200	9	444	45.6	17.8	20	7.8
Black Edition, Vanilla, Huel black edition *	1 Scoop/45g	199	9	442	44	29	20	7.3
Capsules, Dietary Fibre, Tony Ferguson*	3 Capsules/2g	5	0.1	242	4.1	28.6	4.1	65.3
Cognition, Organic Functional Blend , Naturya*	1 Serving/25g	84	2.2	335	12	40	9	25
Collagen, Bovine, Premium, Nutravita*	1 Serving/15g	54	0	360	93	0	0	0
Complete Protein, Strawberries & Cream, Huel*	1 Scoop/29g	105	1.1	362	69	11	3.8	5.5
Energy Gummies, High Five*	6 Gummies/26g	87	0.1	333	0	80	0.2	0
Fibre Boost, Well + Within*	1 Tsp/5g	10	0	209	3.4	86.6	0.7	78.8
Hemp, 85% Pure, Protein, Good Hemp*	1 Serving/25g	95	0.9	381	85	0.1	3.6	4.4
Hemp, Protein, Fibre, Boost, Good Hemp*	1 Serving/30g	88	2.1	292	28	14	6.9	50
Hydrogel, Caffeine, Energy +, Scitec Nutrition*	1 Gel Pack/55ml	100	0	182	0	45.4	0	0
Impact Whey Isolate, Unflavoured, Myprotein*	1 Scoop/25g	103	1.9	412	82	4	7.5	0
Impact Whey, Banana, Myprotein*	1 Pack/25g	99	1.6	395	77	7.1	6.2	0
Inulin, Powder, Organic, Real Food Source*	1 Spoon/10g	20	0	204	0	6	0	90
Inulin, Powder, Pure, SimplyGo*	1 Scoop/5g	10	0	210	0	8	0	89
Inulin, Pure, from Chicory, Natures Aid*	1 Serving/5g	10	0	208	0	8	0	88
Isohydro, Scitec Nutrition *	1 Scoop/15g	50	0	336	0	86.4	0	0
Konjac, Glucomannan, Capsules, BuyWholeFoodsOnline*	2 Capsules/1g	2	0	192	1.1	2.1	0.3	89.4
Pea Protein Isolate, Chocolate, PeakSupps*	1 Scoop/30g	101	0.9	337	75.5	5.9	3	2.3
Pea Protein, Rich Chocolate, Nuzest*	1 Scoop/25g	101	2.2	405	75.2	4.7	8.6	1.7
Pea Protein, Unflavoured, Pulsin*	1 Serving/10g	41	0.9	406	80	0	9.1	1.4
Pea Protein, Vanilla, Nuzest*	1 Scoop/10g	41	0.9	413	79.2	4.5	8.6	1.3
Pecan, & Cinnamon, Purition*	1 Serving/40g	190	13.2	475	36.7	6.8	33	16.5
Performent, Lean, PE Protein*	1 Scoop/25g	97	1.6	389	46	29.5	6.5	12
Plant Protein, Nutrilite*	1 Serving/10g	40	0.5	400	80	3.2	4.8	0
Portein Powder, Strawberry, Bulk*	1 Serving/30g	116	1.9	385	75.2	6.6	6.4	0.6
Powder, Clean Greens, Super U*	1 Tsp/5g	15	0.1	291	23.7	29.9	2.9	31.6
Powder, Psyllium Husk, Nkd Living*	1 Scoop/10g	19	0	187	2	4	0.5	78
Protein Powder, Collagen, Chocolate, Gonutro*	1 Serving/12g	61	3.5	508	45	4.7	29	15.9
Protein Powder, Hemp, 50%, BuyWholeFoodsOnline*	1 Scoop/20g	87	2.2	434	50	24	11	19
Protein Powder, Jersey Hemp*	1 Scoop/30g	116	5.4	387	47	2.3	18	12.7
Protein Powder, Overnight, Sport In Science*	1 Serving/35g	130	2	371	73	5.3	5.7	3.2
Protein Powder, Salted Caramel, Phd Smart Protein*	1 Scoop/30g	116	3	388	62	12	10	1
Protein Powder, The Fit, Innermost*	1 Scoop/10g	37	0.3	368	72.5	11.2	3	3.5
Protein Powder, Unflavoured, Genepro*	1 Scoop/7g	59	0.3	815	416.7	8.3	4.2	0
Protein Powder, Vanilla, Vegan, Bulk*	1 Scoop/35g	130	2.1	371	66	10	6.1	6.6
Protein Powder, Vegan, Salted Caramel, Misfits*	1 Serving/25g	93	1.8	372	66.4	6.4	7.2	9.2
Protein Shake, Coconut, Purition*	1 Serving/40g	192	12.8	480	41	7.8	32	17.2
Protein Shake, Macadamia & Vanilla, Purition*	1 Serving/40g	198	14	495	39.1	8.6	35	15.6
Protein Shake, Vegan Hemp, Chocolate, Purition*	1 Serving/40g	194	12.1	484	35.4	11.3	30.3	27.3
Protein, All Plant, Nutrilite*	1 Serving/30g	120	1.4	400	80	3.2	4.8	0
Protein, Hemp, Powder, Funktional Foods*	1 Tbsp/15g	54	1.6	362	49	10	11	13
Protein, Powder, Collagen, Chocolate, Myprotein*	1 Scoop/30g	106	0.2	352	81	47	0.6	1.8
Protein, Powder, Vegan, Misfits*	1 Serving/25g	76	0.1	304	61.2	13.2	0.3	2
Protein, Pro V-Gain, Vegan, Chocolate, Sci MX*	1 Scoop/15g	53	0.3	353	73	7.4	2.3	5.9
Protein, Pure Whey Isolate, Vanilla, Bulk Powders*	1 Scoop/30g	115	0.6	382	87	4	2	0
Protein, Smart, Peanut Butter Cup, PhD Nutrition*	1 Scoop/30g	116	3	388	62	12	10	1
Protein, Super Shake Powder, Pulsin*	1 Serving/30g	114	2.8	380	65.7	6	9.3	4.7
Protein, Superfood, Amazing Grass*	1 Scoop/29g	113	2.6	390	69	5.2	9	9
Protein, Superfood, Original, Amazing Supergrass*	1 Scoop/20g	85	2.4	427	68	9	12	4.7
Protein, Vegan, Chocolate Flavour, Wyldsson*	1 Serving/35g	128	2.1	367	57	14.9	5.9	14.6
Protein, Vegan, Peanut Butter, Motion *	1 Sachet/25g	97	2.2	388	68	14.8	8.8	7.3
Protein, Whey Isolate, R1 Protein*	1 Scoop/29g	109	0	377	85.6	3.4	0	0

	Measure INFO/WEIGHT	per Measure KCAL	FAT	Nutrition Values per 100g / 100ml KCAL	PROT	CARB	FAT	FIBRE
SUPPLEMENT								
Protein, Whey Protein, Vanilla, Everlast*	1 Scoop/10g	38	0.6	378	77.3	3.3	6	0
Psyllium Husks, Organic, BuyWholeFoodsOnline*	1 Tbsp/15g	45	0	300	0	10	0	70
Pyllium Husk, Organic, Just Natural*	1 Serving/10g	19	0.1	189	1.5	0.1	0.6	89
Shake, Chocolate, Protein, USN*	2 Scoops/100g	376	2.2	376	36	51	2.2	2.4
Shake, Complete Food, Banana Caramel, Bulk*	1 Serving/100g	400	12	400	30	37	12	9.6
Smoothie, Golden Milk, Purition*	1 Scoop/10g	48	3.2	480	39	9	32.5	18
Supergreens, Organic, Superfood Blend, Vegatox*	1 Tsp/5g	15	0.1	305	30.9	32.8	2.8	21.7
Tablet, Berocca*	1 Tablet/4.5g	5	0	109	0	5.7	0.1	0
Vanilla Shake, Michael Mosley*	1 Serving/50g	198	8	396	42.4	12.4	16	14
Vegan Diet Fuel, USN*	2 Scoops/55g	210	3.2	382	48	34	5.8	1.3
Vitality, Snacks, Plant Made*	1 Pack/10g	40	1	397	14.4	53	9.8	12
Whey Protein Concentrate, Natural, Unflavoured, Pulsin*	1 Serving/10g	41	0.7	407	80	6	7	0
Whey Protein, Cinnamon Donut Flavour, Per4m*	1 Scoop/30g	106	0.7	352	71	11.5	2.4	1
Whey Protein, Holland & Barrett*	1 Serving/24g	94	1.9	392	73.3	7.1	7.9	0
Whey Protein, Iso:Pro, Myprotein*	1 Scoop/25g	100	0.2	399	97	0	1	0.8
Whey Protein, Pure, Strawberry, Bulk Powders*	1 Scoop/30g	125	2.2	417	76.3	8.7	7.5	0.4
Whey Protein, Salted Caramel, Impact, Myprotein*	1 Serving/50g	205	3.6	410	79	7.1	7.2	0.2
Whey Protein, Simply, Chocolate, PE Nutrition*	1 Scoop/25g	82	1.1	330	67	5.3	4.5	0.4
Whey Protein, Strawberry, Natural, Impact, Myprotein*	1 Scoop/25g	98	1.8	391	73	7.3	7.1	0.8
Whey Protein, Ultra, Lean Muscle, Sci Mx*	1 Serving/45g	177	2.2	393	77	6.4	5	7.2
Whey, Protein, Banana, PBN*	1 Scoop/30g	119	1.7	397	78.6	7.1	5.8	0.7
SUSHI								
Big Boy Box, Tanpopo*	1 Pack/506g	906	16.7	179	6	31.6	3.3	0
California Rolls 8 Pack	*1 Pack/206g*	*354*	*9.3*	*172*	*5.1*	*27.5*	*4.5*	*1.4*
Californian Roll & Nigiri, Selection, M&S*	1 Pack/215g	355	5.8	165	7.1	28	2.7	1.1
Chicken, & Duck, Hoisin, Selection, Asda*	1 Pack/167g	278	4.5	166	5	30	2.7	1.3
Chicken, Katsu, & Tempura Rice, Tanpopo*	1 Pack/290g	803	53.9	277	7.6	21	18.6	0.6
Chicken, Katsu, Bento, Taiko Foods*	1 Pack/235g	526	26.1	224	6.2	25.1	11.1	0
Chicken, Katsu, Tesco*	1 Pack/76g	122	2.6	161	4.4	27.4	3.4	1.5
Classic, My Sushi, Lidl*	1 Pack/200g	328	42	164	4.7	31.5	21	0
Collection, Eat & Go, Aldi*	1 Pack/219g	324	5.5	148	4.9	26	2.5	1.3
Crispy Salmon, Roll, Taiko Foods*	1 Roll/29g	62	2.7	214	6.5	24.8	9.4	0
Dragon Roll, Firecracker Prawn, M&S*	1 Pack/166g	224	4.5	135	4.2	22.9	2.7	0.9
Dragon Roll, Katsu Chicken, M&S*	1 Pack/167g	241	3.3	144	5.1	25.8	2	1.2
Duck, & Chicken, Eat & Go, Aldi*	1 Pack/130g	206	2.6	158	4.7	30	2	1
Duck, Crispy, Roll, Taiko Foods*	1 Roll/30g	49	1.2	163	4.8	26.8	4	0
Fish & Vegetable, Co-Op*	1 Pack/143g	238	3.7	166	4.6	31	2.6	0.7
Fish Roll, Nigiri & Maki Selection, M&S*	1 Pack/210g	315	4.8	150	6.5	25.8	2.3	1
Fish Selection, Large, Tesco*	1 Pack/218g	365	6.8	167	5.3	29	3.1	0.9
Fish Selection, Morrisons*	1 Pack/152g	236	1.5	155	4	32	1	0.9
Fish, Selection, Asda*	1 Pack/153g	242	2.6	158	5.3	30	1.7	0.6
Fish, Snack Pack, On the Go, Sainsbury's*	1 Pack/96g	150	2.4	156	5.5	27.3	2.5	1.2
Fish, Snack, Tesco*	1 Pack/104g	159	2.6	153	4.5	28	2.5	1.5
Futomaki, Veg & Chive, Waitrose*	1 Pack/146g	169	4.5	116	2.6	19	3.1	1.6
Hosomaki, Vegan, Morrisons*	1 Pack/140g	220	1.7	158	3	33	1.2	1.5
Katsu Chicken, Snack, M&S*	1 Pack/63g	96	0.8	153	3.8	31	1.3	1.1
Mixed, Temari, & Rolls, Supermarket, Yo! Sushi*	1 Pack/381g	686	14.9	180	4.4	20.3	3.9	0.7
Naniwa, Box, Lidl*	1 Pack/190g	262	3.8	138	4.6	25	2	0.6
Nigiri, Mini, Taiko Foods*	1 Box/100g	147	1.7	147	4.9	27.4	1.7	0
Prawn, Cocktail, Roll, Taiko Foods*	1 Roll/29g	49	1.9	173	5.7	22.2	6.6	0.9
Rice Bowl, Smoked Salmon, Taiko Foods*	1 Bowl/321g	465	12.5	145	4.8	21.9	3.9	1.7
Rice Bowl, Sweet Chilli Chicken, Taiko Foods*	½ Bowl/167g	247	6	148	7.6	20.7	3.6	1.2
Roll, Selection, Ultimate, Supermarket, Yo! Sushi*	1 Pack/336g	642	20.2	191	4.8	10.8	6	0.8

	Measure INFO/WEIGHT	per Measure KCAL	FAT	Nutrition Values per 100g / 100ml KCAL	PROT	CARB	FAT	FIBRE
SUSHI								
Rolls, California, MSC, Taiko Foods*	1 Pack/135g	252	9.7	187	4.4	24	7.2	0
Rolls, Duck, Teriyaki, Taiko Foods*	1 Pack/131g	224	7.5	171	6	20.8	5.7	0
Rolls, Tuna, Crispy, Taiko Foods*	1 Roll/29g	47	1.1	163	5.9	25.8	3.8	0
Rolls, Veggie, Snack, Shapers, Boots*	1 Pack/66g	93	0.6	141	3.5	28.8	0.9	1.4
Salmon & Prawn, Nigiri, M&S*	1 Pack/125g	186	1.4	149	7	27.2	1.1	1
Salmon Avocado, Spicy, Roll, Taiko Foods*	1 Roll/30g	53	2.3	177	4.7	21.9	7.6	0
Salmon Rolls, Crispy, Asian Fusion, Waitrose*	1 Pack/176g	377	16.5	214	6.5	24.8	9.4	0
Salmon Wrap, Taiko Foods*	1 Pack/198g	317	10.7	160	5.1	22.3	5.4	0
Salmon, & King Prawn, Select & Go, Lidl*	1 Pack/275g	424	11.8	154	5.6	22.9	4.3	0.8
Salmon, & Prawn, Selection, Co-Op*	1 Pack/148g	241	3.8	163	5.2	29	2.6	0.7
Salmon, Avocado, Spicy, Taiko Foods*	1 Pack/180g	319	13.7	177	4.7	21.9	7.6	0
Salmon, Gochiso, Taiko Foods*	1 Pack/187g	327	11.2	175	5.3	24.2	6	0
Salmon, Smoked, & Tuna, Tesco*	1 Pack/136g	227	3.9	167	4.9	29.8	2.9	0.7
Salmon, Smoked, & Tuna, Tesco*	1 Pack/136g	218	4.4	160	5.9	26.6	3.2	0.7
Salmon, Smoked, Snack Pack, Tesco*	1 Pack/69g	114	1.9	165	5	29.1	2.7	0.9
Salmon, Smoked, Snack, Eat & Go, Aldi*	1 Pack/69g	106	1.4	153	5.8	26	2	0.7
Salmon, Teriyaki, Roll, Taiko Foods*	1 Roll/32g	49	1.5	156	5.1	22.4	4.8	0
Selection, Vegan, Supermarket, Yo! Sushi*	1 Pack/222g	400	6.4	180	4.1	12.1	2.9	0
Signature, Rolls, Taiko Foods*	1 Pack/380g	635	21.7	167	4.6	23.8	5.7	1.2
Simple Snack, Taiko Foods*	1 Pack/90g	126	1.8	140	3.3	26.8	2	0
Snack Box, with Soy Sauce, Eat Well, M&S*	1 Box/78g	115	1.1	147	4.5	28.8	1.4	0.6
Taiko, Fuji Set, Waitrose*	1 Pack/345g	507	11	147	5	24	3.2	1
Tokujo Maki, Taiko*	1 Box/266g	418	11.4	157	4.1	24.5	4.3	0
Tuna Rolls, Spicy, Panka*	1 Pack/167g	296	13	177	5	21.1	7.8	0.9
Vegan, Supermarket, Yo! Sushi*	1 Pack/127g	216	2.8	170	3.8	33.3	2.2	0
Vegetable Selection Pack, M&S*	1 Pack/154g	215	2.8	140	2.8	28.1	1.8	1.3
Vegetable, Box, Lidl*	1 Box/210g	353	10.8	168	4.7	24.6	5.1	2
Vegetable, Eat & Go, Aldi*	1 Pack/144g	216	1.9	150	2.6	32	1.3	1.1
Vegetable, Morrisons*	1 Pack/75g	126	2.9	168	3.4	29.2	3.9	1.4
Vegetable, Selection, Aldi*	1 Pack/149g	238	5.1	160	3.1	29	3.4	1.1
Vegetable, Selection, M&S*	1 Pack/132g	197	1.5	149	4	30.1	1.1	1.1
Vegetable, Taster, Co-Op*	1 Pack/68g	118	3.5	174	3.8	27.9	5.2	1
Vegetarian, Snack Selection, Tesco*	1 Pack/85g	106	2.8	125	3.7	20.1	3.3	0.6
Wrap, Tuna, MSC, Taiko Foods*	1 Wrap/100g	159	3.2	159	4.6	27.6	3.2	0
Yasai, Taiko Foods*	1 Pack/214g	315	4.7	147	3.4	27.9	2.2	0
Yo!, Bento Box, Sainsbury's*	1 Pack/208g	530	6.2	255	8.4	48.7	3	0.9
SWEDE								
Boiled, Average	**1oz/28g**	**3**	**0**	**11**	**0.3**	**2.3**	**0.1**	**0.7**
Raw, Flesh Only, Peeled	**1 Serving/100g**	**24**	**0.3**	**24**	**0.7**	**5**	**0.3**	**1.6**
Raw, Unprepared, Average	**1oz/28g**	**5**	**0.1**	**18**	**0.7**	**3.8**	**0.3**	**1.6**
SWEET & SOUR								
Chicken, & Noodles, Chinese Takeaway, Tesco*	1 Pack/350g	350	0.7	100	5.7	18.8	0.2	0.2
Chicken, Breaded, Fried, From Restaurant, Average	**6 Pieces/130g**	**346**	**18**	**266**	**13**	**22.3**	**13.8**	**0**
Chicken, Chinese Favourites Box, M&S*	½ Pack/125g	146	0.8	117	8.1	19.3	0.6	1.1
Chicken, Chinese Takeaway, Sainsbury's*	1 Pack/264g	515	16.9	195	13.1	21.3	6.4	1
Chicken, Crispy, with Sweet & Sour Sauce, Tesco*	½ Pack/165g	354	16.7	214	11.1	19.3	10.1	1
Chicken, in Batter, Cantonese, Chilled, Sainsbury's*	1 Pack/350g	560	21	160	8.9	22.4	6	0.9
Chicken, with Egg Fried Rice, Calorie Controlled, Tesco*	1 Pack/380g	380	3	100	6.9	15.5	0.8	1.6
Chicken, with Noodles, Steamed, HE, Tesco*	1 Pack/370g	289	0.7	78	8.3	10.8	0.2	0.6
Chicken, with Rice, 233, Oakhouse Foods Ltd*	1 Meal/400g	544	12	136	6.3	20.7	3	0.6
Chicken, with Rice, Chilled, BGTY, Sainsbury's*	1 Pack/400g	344	3.6	86	6	13.5	0.9	1
Chicken, with Rice, Weight Watchers, Heinz*	1 Pack/310g	360	3.1	116	5.2	21.2	1	0.4
No Chicken, with Fried Rice, Plant Pioneers, Sainsbury's*	1 Pack/375g	514	11.3	137	5.7	21	3	1.8

S

	Measure INFO/WEIGHT	per Measure KCAL	FAT	Nutrition Values per 100g / 100ml KCAL	PROT	CARB	FAT	FIBRE
SWEET & SOUR								
Pork	**1oz/28g**	**48**	**2.5**	**172**	**12.7**	**11.3**	**8.8**	**0.6**
Sweet & Sour, with Rice, Counted, Morrisons*	1 Pack/303g	358	2.1	118	6.7	20.4	0.7	1.4
Sweet & Sour, with Rice, Oh So Lean*	1 Pack/400g	106	0.8	27	0.8	5.8	0.2	0.5
with Long Grain Rice, Rice Time, Uncle Ben's*	1 Pot/300g	393	2.4	131	1.9	28.4	0.8	0.7
SWEET POTATO								
Baked, Flesh Only, Average	**1 Med/130g**	**150**	**0.5**	**115**	**1.6**	**27.9**	**0.4**	**2.8**
Boiled in Salted Water, Average	**1 Med/200g**	**168**	**0.6**	**84**	**1.1**	**20.5**	**0.3**	**2.3**
Garlic Roasted, As Sold, Strong Roots*	1 Serving/125g	142	5.1	114	1.9	15	4.1	4.7
Mash, Tesco*	½ Pack/200g	180	3.6	90	1.4	16	1.8	2.2
Mashed, Microwaved, Sainsbury's*	½ Pack/200g	144	3.2	72	1.2	12.3	1.6	1.6
Purple, Raw, Average	**1 Serving/80g**	**79**	**0.4**	**99**	**1.2**	**21.3**	**0.5**	**3**
Raw, Peeled, Average	**1 Sm/130g**	**112**	**0.1**	**86**	**1.6**	**20.1**	**0**	**2.1**
Raw, Unprepared, Average	**1 Potato/200g**	**174**	**0.6**	**87**	**1.2**	**21.3**	**0.3**	**3**
Steamed, Average	**1 Med/200g**	**168**	**0.6**	**84**	**1.1**	**20.4**	**0.3**	**2.3**
Wedges, Chilled, Cooked, Sainsbury's*	½ Pack/150g	150	3	100	1.7	17.1	2	3.4
Wedges, Eat Well, M&S*	½ Pack/150g	123	2.2	82	1.4	14.5	1.5	2.6
Wedges, Morrisons*	1 Serving/125g	190	6.5	152	1.5	23.4	5.2	2.9
Wedges, Sainsbury's*	1 Serving/125g	186	6.2	149	2.2	21.8	5	3.9
SWEETBREAD								
Lamb, Fried	**1oz/28g**	**61**	**3.2**	**217**	**28.7**	**0**	**11.4**	**0**
SWEETCORN								
Baby, Frozen, Average	**1oz/28g**	**7**	**0.1**	**24**	**2.5**	**2.7**	**0.4**	**1.7**
Boiled, Average	**1oz/28g**	**31**	**0.6**	**111**	**4.2**	**19.6**	**2.3**	**2.2**
Canned with Sugar & Salt, Average	**1 Lge Can/340g**	**369**	**4**	**108**	**3.2**	**21.5**	**1.2**	**1.9**
Frozen, Average	**1 Serving/80g**	**84**	**1.7**	**105**	**3.8**	**17.9**	**2.1**	**1.8**
No Sugar & Salt, Canned, Average	**½ Can/125g**	**99**	**1.3**	**79**	**2.7**	**15**	**1.1**	**1.6**
with Peppers, Canned, Average	**1 Serving/50g**	**40**	**0.2**	**79**	**2.6**	**16.4**	**0.3**	**0.6**
SWEETENER								
Calorie Free, Truvia*	1 Sachet/1.5g	0	0	0	0	99	0	0
Canderel*	1 Tbsp/2g	8	0	379	24.7	7	0	5.3
Canderel, Spoonful, Canderel*	1 Tsp/0.5g	2	0	384	2.9	93	0	0
Erythritol, 100%, Pure Via*	1 Tsp/5g	0	0	0	0	100	0	0
Granulated, Low Calorie, Splenda*	1 Tsp/0.5g	2	0	391	0	97.7	0	0
Granulated, Tesco*	1 Tsp/1g	4	0	383	1.8	94	0	0
Natural Syrup, Fruit, Dark, Sweet Freedom*	1 Tsp/5g	13	0	292	0	79	0	0
Silver Spoon*	1 Tablet/0.1g	0	0	325	10	71	0	0
Stevia, & Erythritol, Nkd Living*	1 Tsp/5g	0	0	0	0	99.5	0	0
Tablet, Average	**1 Tablet/0.1g**	**0**	**0**	**355**	**8.7**	**73**	**0**	**0.8**
Tablets, Low Calorie, Canderel*	1 Tablet/0.1g	0	0	342	13	72.4	0	0
Tablets, Splenda*	1 Tablet/0.1g	0	0	345	10	76.2	0	1.6
Xylosweet, Xylitol*	1 Serving/4g	10	0	240	0	100	0	0
SWEETS								
Almonds, Sugared, Dragee*	1 Sweet/4g	17	0.6	472	10	68.3	17.9	2.5
Balla Stixx, Strawberry, Haribo*	1 Stick/25g	93	0.9	373	2.7	82	3.6	0
Big Purple One, Quality Street, Nestle*	1 Sweet/39g	191	9.9	490	4.7	60.5	25.5	0.7
Blackcurrant & Liquorice, M&S*	1 Sweet/8g	32	0.3	400	0.6	89	4.3	0
Blackcurrant Liquorice, Dark, Glacier, Fox's*	1 Sweet/5g	18	0	360	0	90.1	0	0
Blueberry, Bliss, Candy Kittens*	1 Sweet/6g	20	0	335	0.8	81	0.1	0
Boiled, Rosey Apples, Crillys*	8 Sweets/25g	100	0	398	0.1	98.9	0.2	0.2
Boiled, Spiced Pumpkin, Uncle Joe's*	1 Sweet/6g	23	0	387	0	96.4	0.2	0.1
Bon Bons, Raspberry, Tesco*	1 Serving/25g	103	1.5	411	0.1	89.3	5.9	0.5
Butter Candies, Original, Werther's*	1 Sweet/5g	21	0.4	424	0.1	85.7	8.9	0.1
Butter Mintoes, Dominion, Aldi*	3 Sweets/22g	93	1.7	418	0.5	87	7.8	0.5

S

SWEETS

Item	Measure INFO/WEIGHT	per Measure KCAL	FAT	KCAL	PROT	CARB	FAT	FIBRE
Butterscotch, Sugar Free, Morrisons*	1 Sweet/3g	9	0.2	295	0.2	90.4	8.1	0
Candy Cane, Average	**1 Cane/13g**	**50**	**0**	**386**	**0**	**96**	**0**	**0.2**
Candy Corn, Brachs*	19 Pieces/39g	140	0	359	0	92.3	0	0
Candy Floss, Asda*	1 Tub/75g	292	0	390	0	100	0	0
Chew	**1oz/28g**	**107**	**1.6**	**381**	**1**	**87**	**5.6**	**1**
Chew Bars, Great British Puds, Swizzles*	1 Sweet/18g	64	1.1	355	0.1	74	6.1	0
Chewits, Sour Apple, Xtreme, Chewits*	1 Pack/34g	133	1	391	0	86	3	0
Chewitts, Blackcurrant	**1 Pack/33g**	**125**	**0.9**	**378**	**0.3**	**86.9**	**2.7**	**0**
Chews, Just Fruit, Fruit-tella*	1 Serving/43g	170	2.8	400	0.9	79.5	6.5	0
Chews, Sour, Infernal, Chupa Chups*	1 Sweet/8g	32	0.5	397	0.9	82	5.9	0
Chews, Spearmint, Victoria, Aldi*	1 Sweet/10g	40	0.8	405	0.3	83.8	7.6	0
Chews, Strawberry Mix, Starburst*	1 Sweet/4g	15	0.3	401	0	83.9	7.3	0
Chewy, Vimto*	1 Pack/30g	115	0.9	384	0	88	3	0
Choco & Mint, Mentos*	1 Pack/38g	156	3.2	410	2.8	79	8.5	0
Chocolate Caramels, Milk, Tesco*	1 Sweet/3g	15	0.5	444	2.7	72.1	16.1	0.1
Chocolate Eclairs, Cadbury*	1 Sweet/8g	36	1.4	455	4.5	68.9	17.9	0
Chocolate Eclairs, Co-Op*	1 Sweet/8g	38	1.6	480	3	71	20	0.6
Chocolate Eclairs, Holland & Barrett*	1 Sweet/6g	18	0.7	306	1.8	81.9	11.3	1.4
Chocolate Limes, Pascall*	1 Sweet/8g	27	0.2	333	0.3	77.2	2.5	0
Chocolate Limes, Poundland*	1 Sweet/5g	21	0.2	414	0.5	95.5	3.3	0
Chocolate Limes, Tesco*	1 Sweet/8g	33	0.3	408	0.7	93.7	3.3	0.5
Cola Bottles, Barratt*	1 Sweet/10g	34	0	337	1.3	82	0.4	0.1
Cola Bottles, Dominion, Aldi*	1 Serving/25g	85	0.1	339	0.5	84	0.5	0.5
Cola Bottles, Fizzy, M&S*	1 Pack/200g	650	0	325	6.4	75	0	0
Cola Bottles, Giant, Morrisons*	1 Pack/140g	469	0.1	335	8.9	74.3	0.1	0.6
Cola Sherbets, Sugar Free, Dominion, Aldi*	2 Sweets/10g	23	0	238	0.5	96	0.5	0.5
Crazy Roxx, Maoam, Haribo*	1 Serving/25g	96	1.2	386	0.9	84	4.9	0
Creamy Strawberry, Sugar Free, Dominion, Aldi*	1 Sweet/4g	11	0.2	266	0.5	87	6.2	0
DipDab, Softies, Barratt*	1 Bag/160g	557	0.3	348	0.4	86.2	0.2	0
Dolly Mix, Bassett's*	1 Bag/45g	171	1.4	380	3	85.1	3.1	0.4
Dolly Mixtures, M&S*	1 Pack/115g	431	1.6	375	1.8	89.2	1.4	0
Dolly Mixtures, Sainsbury's*	1 Serving/10g	40	0.2	401	1.4	94.4	1.9	0.1
Dolly Mixtures, Smart Price, Asda*	1 Sweet/3g	11	0	380	0.5	91	1.6	0
Dolly Mixtures, Tesco*	1 Pack/100g	376	1.5	376	1.6	88.9	1.5	0
Double Lolly, Swizzels Matlow*	1 Lolly/10g	41	0.3	407	0	92.4	3.4	0
Double Lolly, Swizzle*	1 Lolly/10g	41	0.3	411	0	93.7	3.4	0
Dragibus, Haribo*	1 Serving/25g	94	0.1	375	0	93	0.5	0
Drops, Lemon & Orange, M&S*	1 Pack42g	97	0	230	0	61	0	0
Drumstick, Matlow's*	1 Pack/40g	164	2.2	409	0.4	88.3	5.5	0
Drumstick, Squashies, Sour Cherry & Apple, Swizzels*	1 Serving/30g	105	0.1	349	3.4	82	0.2	0
Eclair, Assortment, M&S*	1 Sweet/7g	32	1.4	474	2.7	69.2	20.6	0.5
Edinburgh Rock, Gardiners of Scotland*	1 Piece/2g	8	0	380	0.1	94.4	0.3	0.8
Eton Mess, Candy Kittens*	1 Sweet/6g	20	0	340	1.4	82	0.2	0
Fizzy Belts, Multi Coloured, Dominion, Aldi*	1/3 Pack/25g	24	0.1	94	0.9	28.7	0.5	0.5
Fizzy Cola Gums, WW*	½ Pack/40g	68	0	170	6.7	20.3	0	49.4
Fizzy Dummies, Barratt*	1 Pack/200g	688	0	344	0	84.4	0	0
Fizzy Fangs, Co-Op*	3 Sweets/20g	70	0.1	350	0.5	87	0.5	0.8
Fizzy Fish, Maynards*	4 Sweets/26g	92	0	352	0.1	87	0.1	0
Fizzy Fruits, Lidl*	5 Sweets/19g	63	0	330	3.9	78.4	0.1	0.5
Fizzy Lances, Strawberry, Sweet Corner, Lidl*	1/3 Pack/25g	94	0.6	375	2.8	85.3	2.2	1.2
Fizzy Mix, Candy King*	1 Serving/20g	66	0	328	5.4	76.4	0	0
Fizzy Mix, Tesco*	½ Bag/50g	166	0	332	5.2	75.2	0	0
Fizzy Multicolour Belts, Tesco*	5 Belts/25g	92	0.5	370	2.5	85	1.9	1.4

SWEETS

INFO/WEIGHT	Measure	per Measure KCAL	FAT	Nutrition Values per 100g / 100ml KCAL	PROT	CARB	FAT	FIBRE
Fizzy Pop, M&S*	1 Sweet/4g	14	0	352	0.1	88.7	0.5	0.5
Flumps, Bassett's*	1 Serving/5g	16	0	325	4	77	0	0
Foamy Mushrooms, Chewy, Asda*	1 Sweet/2.6g	9	0	347	4.2	82	0.2	0
Forest Fruit Drops, Simpkins*	1 Sweet/5g	20	0	403	0	98	0	0
Fruit Chews, Crestiplus*	1 Sweet/7g	27	0.3	412	1.1	90	5.1	0
Fruit Gums & Jellies	*1 Tube/33g*	*107*	*0*	*324*	*6.5*	*79.5*	*0*	*0*
Fruit Kingpins, Sweet Corner, Lidl*	1 Serving/20g	77	0.7	384	0.1	87	3.6	0.5
Fruit Pastilles, Sweet Corner, Lidl*	11 Sweets/40g	133	0	333	4	77.6	0.1	3.4
Fruit Pastilles, Taveners*	5 Sweets/28g	97	0.1	345	4.1	80.9	0.4	0.6
Fruit Twists, Assorted, Bebeto*	1 Pack/250g	952	3.5	381	2.1	91	1.4	0
Fruity Chews, Percy Pig, M&S*	¼ Bag/38g	129	0.1	344	0.5	84.4	0.2	1.1
Fruity Chews, Starburst*	1 Sweet/8g	34	0.6	404	0	83.4	7.4	0
Fruity Frogs, Rowntree's*	1 Serving/40g	128	0.1	321	4.7	74.5	0.2	0
Go Bananas, & Monkeys, M&S*	1 Bag/70g	264	0.1	377	2.9	91.3	0.1	0.5
Gummie, Zoo Mix, Katja*	1 Sweet/9g	30	0	333	1.1	81	0.2	0
Gummy Bears	*10 Bears/25g*	*80*	*0*	*320*	*8*	*76*	*0*	*0*
Gummy Mix, Dominion, Aldi*	1 Serving/25g	84	0.1	338	0.5	84	0.5	0.5
Gummy Mix, Tesco*	1 Pack/100g	327	0.1	327	5.9	75.7	0.1	0
Gummy Worms	*10 Worms/74g*	*286*	*0*	*386*	*0*	*98.9*	*0*	*98.9*
Happy Cola Zing, Haribo*	1 Pack/25g	96	1	384	1.8	85	4.2	0
Henry Hippo, Sweet Corner, Lidl*	1 Serving/25g	88	0.1	350	0.8	86.1	0.2	0.5
Ice Cream Sundae, Asda*	1 Sweet/2g	9	0	387	4.9	70	0.5	0.5
Jellies, Fruit, Ringtons*	4 Jellies/44g	150	0.2	341	0.1	84	0.4	0.7
Jellies, Very Berry, Rowntrees*	1 Sweet/4g	12	0	326	5	74.8	0.2	0.1
Jelly Beans, Lucozade*	1 Pack/30g	111	0	370	0	92	0	0
Jelly Beans, Tesco*	¼ Bag/63g	243	0.2	385	0.1	94.5	0.3	0.3
Jelly Bunnies, Bassetts, Maynards*	4 Sweets/26g	87	0	330	3.5	78	0.1	0
Jelly Tots, Rowntree's*	1 Pack/42g	145	0	346	0.1	86.5	0	0
Juicy Chews, Fruit-tella*	1 Piece/6g	24	0.4	400	0.8	83	6.8	0
Kingpins, Sweet Corner, Lidl*	1 Serving/50g	192	1.8	383	0.1	87	3.6	0.5
Kisses, Hershey*	1 Sweet/5g	28	1.6	561	7	59	32	0
Laces, Apple Flavour, Tesco*	5 Laces/15g	52	0.5	347	3.6	74.8	3.2	2.1
Laces, Strawberry, Sainsbury's*	1 Serving/25g	94	1.2	377	3.3	76.3	4.6	0.1
Laces, Strawberry, Tesco*	1 Serving/75g	260	2.4	347	3.6	74.8	3.2	2.1
Lances, Strawberry Flavour, Fizzy, Tesco*	½ Pack/50g	177	1.3	354	2.8	79.8	2.6	1.8
Lemon, Drops, Cool, Trebor*	1 Sweet/2g	5	0	237	0.1	96	0.1	0
Licorice Love, Tweek*	½ Pack/40g	68	0.1	170	7.1	18	0.3	55
Licorice, Sugar Free, Dominion, Aldi*	1 Serving/25g	56	0.1	224	0.5	77	0.5	1.6
Liquorice Gums, WW*	1 Pack/35g	88	0.1	250	5.7	48.8	0.4	14.1
Liquorice, Boiled, Sugar Free, Sula*	1 Sweet/3g	7	0	227	0.2	93	0	0.2
Liquorice, Catherine Wheels, M&S*	1 Wheel/19g	61	0.2	321	4.2	72.2	1.1	2.8
Liquorice, Gums, Lion*	1 Sweet/4g	14	0	351	8.5	77.7	0.6	0.7
Lovehearts, Swizzels*	1 Sweet/2g	7	0	359	0.7	88.2	0	0
Mango Vanilla, Lakrids*	1 Sweet/8g	42	2.3	527	4	62	29	0
Maoam Stripes, Haribo*	1 Chew/7g	27	0.4	384	1.2	81.7	6.1	0.3
Maoam, Maomixx, Haribo*	1 Sweets/25g	98	1.6	394	1	84	6.4	0
Maynards Sours, Bassett's*	1 Pack/52g	169	0	325	6.1	75	0	0
Mentos, Fruit, Mentos*	1 Sweet/3g	12	0.1	388	0	92	1.9	0
Midget Gems, Co-Op*	12 Sweets/28g	100	0.1	356	0.5	89	0.5	0.5
Midget Gems, Maynards*	12 Sweets/24g	78	0	325	7.4	73	0.2	0
Midget Gems, Sweet Corner, Lidl*	12 Sweets/28g	83	0.1	300	3.6	76.1	0.4	1.8
Midget Gems, Value, Tesco*	1 Serving/40g	130	0.1	324	4.5	76.1	0.2	0
Milk Chocolate Eclairs, Sainsbury's*	1 Sweet/8g	33	1.1	442	2.1	75.7	14.5	0.5

SWEETS

	Measure INFO/WEIGHT	per Measure KCAL	FAT	KCAL	PROT	CARB	FAT	FIBRE
Milk Chocolate Eclairs, Value, Tesco*	1 Bag/200g	918	32.6	459	2.6	75.2	16.3	1
Milk Duds, Hershey*	13 Pieces/33g	170	6	510	3	84	18	0
Milk Teeth, Barratt*	1 Serving/20g	64	0	318	3.9	75.6	0	0
Mini Macs, CBY, Asda*	1 Pack/200g	437	13.1	218	1	38.8	6.6	0
Mini Marti, Mushrooms, Asda*	1 Sweet/3g	10	0	340	3.8	81.1	0.1	0
Minions, Haribo*	½ Pack/35g	120	0.2	342	6.6	77	0.5	0
Minis, Starburst*	1 Serving/49g	198	2.9	404	0	87	5.9	0
Mint Balls, Uncle Joe's*	1 Sweet/6g	24	0	393	0	97	0.5	0
Mint Humbugs, Crillys Sweets*	1 Sweet/8g	32	0.1	402	0.1	98.7	0.7	0.1
Mint Humbugs, Dominion, Aldi*	1 Sweet/8g	33	0.2	407	0.5	95	2.7	0.5
Mint Humbugs, Sugar Free, Morrisons*	1 Sweet/3g	9	0.2	287	0.3	92.5	7	0
Mint Humbugs, Sugar Free, Sula*	1 Sweet/3g	8	0.2	280	0.2	87.1	7.7	0
Mint Humbugs, Toffee Centre, Crawford & Tilley*	1 Serving/20g	77	0.2	383	0.2	93	1.2	0
Mint imperial , Dominion, Aldi*	1 Serving/20g	78	0.1	389	0.5	96	0.5	0.5
Myles the Meerkat, Fruit Jellies, Spar*	1 Pack/60g	202	0.1	337	0.1	83.8	0.1	0.2
Mystery Swirl, Laffy Taffy*	1 Rope/23g	80	1.5	349	0	78.6	6.6	0
Nerds, Grape & Strawberry, Wonka*	1 Serving/30g	120	0	400	0	93.3	0	0
Nougat, Caramel, Soft, Lonka*	1 Cube/11g	45	1.1	409	2.3	78	9.6	0
Paradise Fruits, Dominion, Aldi*	1 Sweet/6g	23	0	382	0	95.5	0	0
Parma Violets, Swizzlers*	1 Sm Tube/10g	41	0.3	414	0	94.9	3.3	0
Party Size, Haribo*	1 Pack/25g	86	0.1	343	6.7	78	0.5	0
Pear Drops, Free From Fellows*	1 Sweet/4g	11	0	273	0	97	0	0
Pencils, Strawberry, Co-Op*	2 Pencils/16g	59	0.5	369	3.1	87.5	3.1	3.1
Percy Pig & Pals, Soft, M&S*	1 Sweet/8g	30	0	344	5.8	80	0.1	0
Percy Pig, 1/3 Less Sugar, M&S*	1 Percy/9g	29	0	320	1	72.5	0.4	11
Pic 'n' Mix, Woolworths*	1 Serving/180g	750	6	417	0	96.7	3.3	0
Pick & Mix, Cup, Asda*	1 Cup/160g	554	1.1	346	3.2	82	0.7	0.6
Pizza, Gummi, Gummy zone*	1 Pack/23g	80	0.1	347	5.8	81	0.5	0.5
Pomegranate Hearts, Biona Organic*	1 Pack/75g	238	0.2	317	0.1	78	0.2	2.3
Rainbow Twists, Haribo*	1 Pack/70g	234	1.8	334	0.5	80	2.5	0
Randoms, 30% Less Sugar, Rowntree's*	9 Sweets/35g	106	0	299	5	63	0.1	13
Randoms, Juicers, Rowntree's*	5 Sweets/25g	80	0	322	4.4	75.9	0.1	0.1
Randoms, Rowntree's*	1 Pack/50g	164	0.2	328	4.9	75.7	0.3	0.6
Randoms, Sours, Rowntree's*	1 Serving/20g	67	0	334	4	77.3	0	0
Raspberry Flavour Mushrooms, Tesco*	1 Serving/25g	90	0.3	359	3.8	83	1.2	0.6
Refreshers, Candyland, Barratt*	1 Tube/34g	129	0.5	380	0	89.1	1.4	0
Refreshers, Softies, Mini, Barratt*	1 Bag/30g	107	0.2	358	3.2	85	0.6	0.5
Refreshers, Strawberry, Soft Chew, Swizzels*	1 Sweet/5g	44	0.7	873	0.2	185.1	13.3	0
Rhubarb & Custard, Sainsbury's*	1 Sweet/8g	28	0	351	0.1	87.7	0	0
Rhubarb & Custard, One Pounders*	1 Sweet/10g	36	0.1	362	0	88	0.6	0
Rhubarb & Custards, Tesco*	1 Sweet/8g	32	0	395	0.1	98.2	0.1	0.5
Rotella, Haribo*	1 Sweet/8g	26	0.1	325	0.5	78	1.6	0
Rowntree's*	1 Tube/49g	170	0.1	344	4.8	81.3	0.2	0
Sherbert Lemons, M&S*	1 Serving/20g	76	0	380	0	93.9	0	0
Sherbet Lemons, Bassett's*	1 Sweet/7g	25	0	375	0	93.9	0	0
Sherbet Pip, Old Sam's Sweet Shoppe*	12 Pips/9g	35	0.1	394	0.5	95	1.6	0.5
Shockers, Orange Sherbet, Tango*	1 Bar/11g	41	0.4	371	0	79	3.9	0
Shrimps & Bananas, Sainsbury's*	½ Pack/50g	188	0	376	2.5	91.3	0.1	0.5
Shrimps, & Bananas, Barratt*	1 Serving/25g	94	0.1	376	2.9	90.5	0.3	0.5
Shrimps, & Bananas, Tesco*	1 Pack/80g	299	0.2	374	2.8	90.1	0.2	0.6
Snakes, Super Sour, Fizzy, Asda*	½ Pack/20g	70	0.1	350	5.4	82	0.5	0.5
Soft Foams, Sweet Corner, Lidl*	1 Serving/10g	20	0	199	0.4	83.7	0	0
Soft Fruits, Trebor*	1 Roll/45g	165	0	367	0	90.9	0	0

	Measure INFO/WEIGHT	per Measure KCAL	FAT	Nutrition Values per 100g / 100ml KCAL	PROT	CARB	FAT	FIBRE
SWEETS								
Soft Gums, Sugar Free, Morrisons*	1 Serving/25g	55	0.1	219	0.5	81.8	0.4	0
Soft Jellies, Scary Jellies, Maynards*	1 Pack/17g	54	0	321	3.1	76	0.2	0
Sour Kingpins, Sweet Corner, Lidl*	1 Serving/20g	78	0.9	388	0.1	84.5	4.5	0.5
Sour Snakes, Gelatine Free, Fruitella*	1 Bag/120g	409	0	341	0	84	0	0
Sour Sparks, Haribo*	1 Serving/30g	100	0.2	334	0.5	82	0.5	0
Sour Watermelon, Candy Kittens*	1 Serving/25g	85	0	341	0.8	83	0.1	0
Spiders, Trolli*	1 Sweet/13g	43	0	333	5.3	77	0.1	0
Spogs, Average	**1 Sweet/4g**	**13**	**0**	**332**	**3.9**	**79**	**0.1**	**0**
Squashies, Drumsticks, Raspberry & Milk, Swizzels*	¼ Pack/40g	142	0.1	355	3.4	83.9	0.2	0
Squidglets, Haribo*	1 Sweet/3g	11	0	339	4.5	79	0.5	0
Squidgy Babies, Haribo*	1 Serving/25g	86	0.1	346	5.7	80	0.5	0
Squish'ems, Randoms, Rowntrees*	5 Sweets/20g	68	0	334	4.8	77	0.1	0
Strawberry & Cream, Sugar Free, Sula*	1 Sweet/3g	9	0.2	267	0.2	90.5	5.4	0
Strawberry Laces, Asda*	1 Pack/40g	145	1	363	3.3	81	2.4	2.6
Strawberry Straws, Fizzy, Sainsburys*	1 Straw/8g	30	0.2	373	2.8	85	2.2	1.2
Strawberry Trunks, Bebito*	1 Stick/15g	57	0.2	381	2.1	90	1.4	0
Strawberry, Wild, Candy Kittens*	1 Sweet/6g	20	0	334	0.8	81	0.1	0
Sugar Free, Sula*	1 Sweet/3g	7	0	231	0	96.1	0	0
Summer Fruits, 30% Less Sugar, Fruit-tella*	1 Sweet/4g	14	0.2	350	1.6	69	5.6	0
Super Party Mix, Sweet Corner, Lidl*	1 Pack/25g	83	0.5	332	5.2	76	2	2
Tangfastics, Mini, Haribo*	1 Pack/16g	55	0.1	346	6.6	80	0.5	0
Tangfastics, Stixx, Haribo*	1 Stick/25g	95	0.8	381	1.3	87	3.3	0
Teeth & Lips, Dominion, Aldi*	1 Serving/25g	85	0.1	341	0.5	84	0.5	0.5
Terrific Turtles, Haribo*	1 Serving/30g	104	0.2	345	5.8	79	0.5	0
Tic Tac, Cool Cherry, Ferrero*	1 Pack/18g	69	0.1	382	0.2	92.2	0.7	0
Tooty Frooties, Rowntree's*	1 Bag/28g	111	1	397	0.1	91.5	3.5	0
Treacle Toffee, Buchanan's*	1 Sweet/8g	32	1.4	404	1.8	62	17	0
Twists, Hawaiian Punch, Kenny's*	4 Twists/27g	80	0	296	3.7	77.8	0	0
Twizzlers, Strawberry, Hershey*	1 Twizzler/11g	40	0.2	353	2.9	79.4	1.5	0
Very Cherry, Candy Kittens*	1 Serving/25g	84	0	338	0.4	82	0.1	0
Wendy the Worm, Veggie, Dominion, Aldi*	1 Sweet/13g	44	0.1	339	0.5	85	0.5	0.7
Wine Gummies, Matlow, Swizzels*	1 Pack/16g	52	0	324	0	58.7	0	0
Wine Gums, Free From Fellows*	1 Sweet/6g	12	0	217	0	81	0.3	0
Yo Yo's, All Flavours, 100% Fruit, We Are Bear*	1 Roll/10g	28	0	275	1.9	63.4	0.2	12
SWORDFISH								
Grilled, Average	**1oz/28g**	**39**	**1.5**	**139**	**22.9**	**0**	**5.2**	**0**
Raw, Average	**1oz/28g**	**42**	**2**	**149**	**21.1**	**0**	**7.2**	**0**
SYRUP								
Black Forest, Premium, Monin*	1 Serving/30ml	100	0	334	0	82	0	0
Brown Rice, Biona Organic*	1 Tbsp/15g	47	0.1	316	0.5	79	0.5	0.5
Butterscotch, Monin*	1 Serving/30ml	100	0	333	0	80	0	0
Caramel, for Coffee, Lyle's*	2 Tsps/10ml	33	0	329	0	83	0	0
Caramel, Sugar Free, Monin*	1 Serving/30ml	0	0	0	0	13.3	0	0
Caramel, Sweet Freedom*	1 Tsp/5g	14	0	277	0	70	0	5.3
Chocolate Caramel, Zero Calorie, Active Foods, Bulk*	1 Tbsp/15g	1	0	6	0	0.4	0	1.2
Chocolate Mint, Monin*	1 Serving/30ml	100	0	333	0	80	0	0
Cinnamon, Monin*	1 Serving/30ml	100	0	333	0	80	0	0
Cinnamon, Sweet Freedom*	1 Tsp/5g	14	0	283	0	71	0	5
Dropsiroop, Meenk*	1 Tsp/5g	13	0	260	0	66.2	0	0
Fire, Gold, Sukrin*	1 Serving	600	0	2000	0	8	0	69
French Vanilla, Simply*	1 Tbsp/15ml	40	0	265	0	65	0	0
Gingerbread, Monin*	1 Serving/30ml	90	0	300	0	76.7	0	0
Gingerbread, Sugar Free, Monin*	1 Serving/20g	3	0	14	0	0.6	0	0

S

SYRUP

INFO/WEIGHT	Measure	per Measure KCAL	FAT	Nutrition Values per 100g / 100ml KCAL	PROT	CARB	FAT	FIBRE
Gold, Sukrin*	1 Serving/30g	45	0	149	0	21	0	49
Golden, Average	**1 Tbsp/20g**	**61**	**0**	**304**	**0.4**	**78.2**	**0**	**0**
Golden, Zero Calorie, The Skinny Food Co.*	1 Tbsp/15ml	1	0	4	0	0.2	0	1.1
Hazelnut, Monin*	1 Serving/30ml	90	0	300	0	73.3	0	0
Inulin, Chocolate, A Spoonful of Fibre, Troo*	1 Serving/15g	27	0.3	182	2	9.3	2	59.3
Maple, Average	**1 Tbsp/20g**	**52**	**0**	**262**	**0**	**67.2**	**0.2**	**0**
Maple, Skinny Syrup, Zero Calorie, The Skinny Food Co.*	1 Tbsp/15ml	1	0	4	0	0.2	0	1.1
Organic Rice Malt, Clearspring*	2 Tbsp/42g	133	0.2	316	1.5	76.8	0.4	0
Passion Fruit, Premium, Monin*	1 Serving/30ml	103	0	343	0	84.9	0	0
Passionfruit, Tasti*	1 Tbsp/15ml	28	0.2	188	1	46.1	1	0
Stem Ginger, Average	**1 Tbsp/15ml**	**45**	**0**	**300**	**0**	**76.7**	**0**	**0**
Sugar	**1 Tbsp/20g**	**64**	**0**	**319**	**0**	**83.9**	**0**	**0**
Sweet like Syrup, with Maple, Good Good*	1 Tbsp/15g	24	0	160	0	5	0	70
Vanilla, Monin*	1 Shot/35ml	119	0	340	0	84.4	0	0
Vanilla, Tate & Lyle*	1 Tbsp/15ml	52	0	348	0	87	0	0

	Measure INFO/WEIGHT	per Measure KCAL	FAT	Nutrition Values per 100g / 100ml KCAL	PROT	CARB	FAT	FIBRE
TABLET								
Scottish, Lee's*	1 Bar/60g	223	1.5	371	0.6	86.5	2.5	0.1
Vanilla, Victor James*	1 Pack/100g	415	11.1	415	3	75.8	11.1	0.5
Walnut, Victor James*	1 Bar/100g	434	14.6	434	4.3	71.4	14.6	0.5
TABOULEH								
Average	*1oz/28g*	*33*	*1.3*	*119*	*2.6*	*17.2*	*4.6*	*0*
Chickpea, Lemony, Warm, Box Ingredients Only, Gousto*	1 Serving/394g	469	4.7	119	4.6	23	1.2	5.8
Lamb, Lemony, Warm, Box Ingredients Only, Gousto*	1 Serving/359g	589	22.3	164	9.6	19	6.2	4.4
TACO KIT								
Crispy Chicken, Soft, Stand 'N' Stuff, Old El Paso*	1 Taco/44g	100	1.5	227	7	41.1	3.4	2.5
Enchilada, Open, Stand 'N' Stuff, Old El Paso *	1 Enchilada/50g	102	2	204	5.5	34.7	4	3.4
Garlic & Paprika, Crunchy, As Sold, Old El Paso *	1 Taco/26g	77	3.6	296	3.8	37.3	13.8	2.7
Mexican, Street Food, Wahaca*	½ Pack/205g	441	7.2	215	5.8	40.9	3.5	3.2
TACO SHELLS								
Corn, Crunchy, Old El Paso*	1 Taco/13g	66	3.5	509	5.4	59.2	27	3.6
TAGINE								
Aubergine, Spiced, Allplants*	1 Pack/380g	429	9.5	113	3.8	17	2.5	3.1
Beef, Slow Cooked, Cook*	1 Serving/325g	462	15.6	142	13.5	11.2	4.8	1.3
Butternut, with Giant Couscous, Shake That Weight*	1 Pack/275g	231	6.9	84	7.1	7.2	2.5	2.2
Chicken, Aromatic, Fodmap, Field & Flower*	1 Serving/380g	414	20.9	109	5.7	8.2	5.5	1.8
Chicken, Moroccan, with British Spelt One Pot, Aldi*	1 Pot/380g	346	6.5	91	4	14	1.7	2.8
Chickpea, Jane Plan*	1 Pack/300g	135	4.2	45	1.5	6.7	1.4	1.6
Lamb, & Couscous, Finest, Tesco*	1 Pack/422g	570	16	135	7.2	17.1	3.8	1.8
Lamb, Moroccan Style with Couscous, M&S*	1 Pack/400g	340	5.6	85	8.9	8.3	1.4	1.6
Lamb, Slow Cooked, M&S*	½ Pack/234g	290	9.1	124	15.6	5.8	3.9	1.6
Moroccan Inspired, The Happy Pear*	1 Pack/400g	288	4.4	72	2.1	12	1.1	2.6
Moroccan, Quorn*	1 Pack/376g	361	4.1	96	4.7	15.2	1.1	3.3
Moroccan, Veggie Bowl, Birds Eye*	1 Serving/380g	433	11.4	114	4.9	15	3	3.3
TAGLIATELLE								
Chicken, & Mushroom, BFY, M&S*	1 Pack/370g	407	8.9	110	8.1	13	2.4	1.8
Dry, Average	*1 Serving/100g*	*356*	*1.8*	*356*	*12.6*	*72.4*	*1.8*	*1*
Egg, Dry, Average	*1 Serving/75g*	*272*	*2.5*	*362*	*14.2*	*68.8*	*3.3*	*2.3*
Egg, Fresh, Dry, Average	*1 Serving/125g*	*345*	*3.5*	*276*	*10.6*	*53*	*2.8*	*2.1*
Fresh, Dry, Average	*1 Serving/75g*	*211*	*2*	*281*	*11.4*	*53.3*	*2.6*	*2.6*
Ham, & Mushroom, Counted, Morrisons*	1 Pack/323g	284	7.1	88	4.1	12.5	2.2	1
Ham, & Mushroom, Creamy, Meal for One, M&S*	1 Pack/400g	564	20.4	141	7.4	15.8	5.1	1.1
Lamb Ragu, Slow Cooked, Finest, Tesco*	1 Pack/400g	560	19.2	140	8.5	14.9	4.8	1.1
Verdi, Fresh, Average	*1 Serving/125g*	*171*	*1.8*	*137*	*5.5*	*25.5*	*1.5*	*1.8*
TAHINI PASTE								
Average	*1 Tbsp/15g*	*97*	*8.9*	*649*	*23*	*8.1*	*59.3*	*8.1*
Dark, Meridian Foods*	1 Serving/10g	61	6	608	18.2	0.9	60	7.9
TANGERINES								
Fresh, Raw	*1 Sm/50g*	*18*	*0*	*35*	*0.9*	*8*	*0.1*	*1.3*
Fresh, Raw, Weighed with Peel, Average	*1 Med/70g*	*13*	*0.1*	*18*	*0.5*	*4.2*	*0.1*	*0.7*
TANGO*								
Cherry, Britvic*	1 Bottle/500ml	55	0	11	0	2.4	0	0
Dark Berry, Sugar Free, Britvic*	1 Can/330ml	13	0	4	0	0	0	0
Orange, Britvic*	1 Can/330ml	63	0	19	0.1	4.4	0	0
Orange, Sugar Free, Britvic*	1 Can/330ml	13	0	4	0	0	0	0
Strawberry & Watermelon, Sugar Free, Britvic*	1 Can/330ml	10	0	3	0	0	0	0
Tropical, Sugar Free, Britvic*	1 Can/330ml	13	0	4	0	0.5	0	0
TAPENADE								
Green Olive, Lemon, & Coriander, Waitrose*	1 Tsp/5g	12	1.2	245	1.2	3.3	24.7	2.1
Olive, Black, Antipasti, Belazu*	1 Serving/25g	105	10.8	420	1.9	3.6	43	4.9

T

	Measure INFO/WEIGHT	per Measure KCAL	FAT	Nutrition Values per 100g / 100ml KCAL	PROT	CARB	FAT	FIBRE
TAPENADE								
Olive, Black, M&S*	¼ Jar/33g	122	12.8	374	1.2	0.1	39.5	6.8
Olive, Black, Specially Selected, Aldi*	1 Tbsp/20g	46	4.6	231	1.4	2.7	23	4.4
Olive, Green, Belazu*	1 Serving/25g	66	6.8	265	0.9	2.7	27.2	2.2
Olive, Kalamata, Sainsbury's*	1 Serving/25g	63	6.6	253	1.6	1.4	26.2	2.8
TAPIOCA								
Creamed, Ambrosia*	½ Can/213g	159	3.4	75	2.6	12.6	1.6	0.2
Raw	**1oz/28g**	**101**	**0**	**359**	**0.4**	**95**	**0.1**	**0.4**
TARAMASALATA								
Average	**1 Tbsp/30g**	**143**	**14.4**	**478**	**4.2**	**7.9**	**47.9**	**1.1**
Smoked, Co-Op*	¼ Pack/42g	199	20.2	474	3.1	7.6	48	0.6
TARRAGON								
Dried, Ground	**1 Tsp/2g**	**5**	**0.1**	**295**	**22.8**	**42.8**	**7.2**	**0**
Fresh, Average	**1 Tbsp/3.8g**	**2**	**0**	**49**	**3.4**	**6.3**	**1.1**	**0**
TART								
Almond, & Blueberry, Bakery in Store, M&S*	1 Tart/90g	335	17	372	5.6	43.3	18.9	1.1
Apple & Custard, Asda*	1 Tart/84g	227	11	270	3.1	35	13.1	0.1
Apple, & Salted Caramel, Tesco*	1 Slice/83g	222	7.9	267	3.1	41.5	9.5	1.9
Apple, Danish, No.1, Waitrose*	1/6 Tart/87g	148	5.4	171	2.5	25.5	6.2	1.4
Apple, Frangipane, TTD, Sainsbury's*	1/6 Tart/72g	230	11.7	320	4.3	38.4	16.2	1.9
Bakewell, Average	**1 Tart/50g**	**228**	**14.8**	**456**	**6.3**	**43.5**	**29.7**	**1.9**
Bakewell, Lemon, Average	**1 Tart/46g**	**206**	**9.7**	**447**	**3.7**	**60.9**	**21.1**	**0.9**
Balsamic Onion, & Vintage Cheddar, Waitrose*	1 Tart/400g	1096	66.8	274	8.6	21.9	16.7	1.2
Blackcurrant, Sundae, Tesco*	1 Tart/55g	240	11	436	3	60	19.9	2.2
Caramel, Salted, & Chocolate, Waitrose*	1/12 Tart/79g	349	18.5	443	5.1	52.2	23.5	1.2
Caramelised Onion, & Goats Cheese, M&S*	1 Tart/600g	405	27	68	1.3	4.7	4.5	0
Cheese, & Asparagus, Oven Baked, Asda*	1 Tart/100g	271	17	271	7.9	20	17	1.8
Cherry Bakewell, Sainsbury's*	1 Tart/45g	191	7.3	425	3.6	65.6	16.3	0.6
Chocolate, Co-Op*	1 Tart/22g	102	6.8	465	4	42	31	0.7
Chorizo, Cheddar, & Mixed Pepper, Sainsbury's*	1 Tart/150g	384	27.4	256	7.2	15.2	18.3	1.2
Coconut, & Raspberry, Holly Lane, Aldi*	1 Tart/48g	191	8.2	397	4.4	56	17	3.3
Courgette, & Pecorino, Finest, Tesco*	¼ Tart/100g	302	21.6	302	5.8	20.5	21.6	1.3
Custard, Individual, Average	**1 Tart/94g**	**260**	**13.6**	**277**	**6.3**	**32.4**	**14.5**	**1.2**
Custard, Portuguese, Tesco*	1 Tart/55g	160	7.2	290	4.4	38.4	13	1
Danish, Apple, & Caramel, Finest, Tesco*	¼ Tart/100g	272	10.8	272	3.6	39.3	10.8	1.8
Date, Pecan & Almond, Sticky, Sainsbury's*	1/8 Tart/75g	298	10.3	397	5	63.5	13.7	1.7
Egg Custard, Asda*	1 Tart/80g	215	10.4	269	9	29	13	1.2
Egg Custard, Free Range, Sainsbury's*	1 Tart/81g	223	9.5	276	6.6	35.7	11.7	0.7
Egg Custard, Twin Pack, Tesco*	1 Tart/86g	244	10.6	284	6.8	35.9	12.3	1.3
Feta Cheese & Spinach, Puff Pastry, Tesco*	1 Tart/108g	306	19.2	283	7.1	23.5	17.8	0.9
Jam, Average	**1 Slice/90g**	**342**	**13.4**	**380**	**3.3**	**62**	**14.9**	**1.6**
Lemon Curd, Asda*	1 Tart/30g	121	4.5	402	2.8	64	15	2.2
Lemon Curd, Tesco*	1 Tart/30g	128	4.7	428	3.4	67	15.8	2
Lemon, & Raspberry, Finest, Tesco*	1 Tart/120g	360	16.8	300	5.2	38.4	14	2.9
Lemon, Cook*	1 Tart/110g	397	24.4	361	5.4	34.5	22.2	0
Lemon, M&S*	1/6 Tart/50g	208	14.6	415	5	32.7	29.3	0.9
Lemon, Mini, The Best, Morrisons*	1 Tart/20g	77	3.1	383	5.1	54.6	15.7	1
Lemon, Sicilian, No.1, Waitrose*	1/8 Tart/66g	257	16.4	390	3.4	37.8	24.9	0.6
Lemon, Waitrose*	1 Slice/50g	218	12.8	437	3.6	47.4	25.7	0.8
Lemon, Zesty, Tesco*	1/6 Tart/64g	260	15.5	405	5.3	41	24.2	0.7
Millionaires, Finest, Tesco*	1 Tart/75g	364	19.2	485	5.3	57.7	25.6	1.5
Mixed Fruit, Fresh, Waitrose*	1 Tart/129g	351	17.4	272	4.2	32.8	13.5	1.5
Passion Fruit, & Raspberry, Finest, Tesco*	1 Slice/75g	286	14.6	382	4.3	47.1	19.5	0.7
Pecan, Free From, Sainsbury's*	1 Tart/50g	239	13.2	477	4.7	54.4	26.4	1.7

	Measure INFO/WEIGHT	per Measure		Nutrition Values per 100g / 100ml				
		KCAL	FAT	KCAL	PROT	CARB	FAT	FIBRE
TART								
Pineapple, Individual, Waitrose*	1 Tart/54g	216	6.1	400	2.2	77.2	11.3	0.5
Portobello Mushroom, & Spinach, Creamy, Asda*	1 Tart/165g	471	30	285	6.7	23.6	18.2	1.6
Portuguese, Aldi*	1 Tart/55g	159	7.1	290	4.4	38	13	1
Rhubarb, & Custard, Crumble, Deluxe, Lidl*	1 Slice/90g	297	14	330	4.3	42.2	15.6	2
Strawberry, & Fresh Cream, Finest, Tesco*	1 Tart/129g	350	19.1	271	3.3	31.1	14.8	1.2
Strawberry, & White Chocolate, Tesco*	1 Tart/80g	318	15.2	398	4.1	52.1	19	1
Strawberry, British Cream, Asda*	1 Tart/127g	348	17.8	274	3.6	33	14	0.6
Strawberry, Custard, Asda*	1 Tart/100g	335	15	335	3.1	47	15	0
Strawberry, Fresh, M&S*	1 Tart/120g	305	18.4	255	3.1	26.4	15.4	2.4
Tomato, & Mascarpone, Cherry, Asda*	1 Tart/160g	290	18	181	4.4	15.6	11.2	1.1
Treacle, Average	**1 Serving/125g**	**460**	**17.6**	**368**	**3.7**	**60.4**	**14.1**	**1.1**
Treacle, with Custard	**1 Serving/251g**	**586**	**23.5**	**233**	**3.1**	**36.1**	**9.4**	**0.8**
Vegetable & Feta, Deli, M&S*	½ Tart/115g	315	18.4	274	5	20	16	6
Vegetable, Roasted, Finest, Tesco*	¼ Tart/113g	213	10.4	188	2.9	22.5	9.2	2.1
Vegetable, Spiced, Finest, Tesco*	¼ Tart/100g	225	11.5	225	4.3	23.7	11.5	4.7
Victoria Sponge, Holly Lane, Aldi*	1 Tart/43g	177	7.4	412	4.2	59.3	17.2	1.2
TARTE								
Au Chocolat, Seriously Chocolatey, Waitrose*	1/6 Tarte/70g	348	22.8	497	6	43.8	32.6	2.6
Au Citron, Frozen, TTD, Sainsbury's*	1/6 Tarte/80g	232	13.4	290	4.7	40.7	16.8	7.7
Au Citron, Waitrose*	1 Tarte/100g	325	18.1	325	4.9	35.7	18.1	1
Bacon, Leek & Roquefort, Bistro, Waitrose*	¼ Tarte/100g	277	18.2	277	8.4	19.8	18.2	0.6
Mixed Berry, Crumble, Frozen, Waitrose*	1/6 Tarte/76g	224	8.3	296	3.3	44.8	11	2.2
Tatin, 1, Waitrose*	1 Tarte/50g	106	4.6	212	1.9	29.9	9.1	1.6
TEA								
Assam, Blended, TTD, Sainsbury's*	1 Serving/2g	0	0	0	0	0	0	0
Blackberry & Nettle, Twinings*	1 Mug/250ml	5	0	2	0	0.3	0	0
Chai, Latte, Spiced, Drink Me*	1 Sachet/15g	68	2.3	452	7.6	70.5	15.3	1.2
Chai, Twinings*	1 Mug/200ml	2	0	1	0.1	0	0	0
Choco, Yogi Tea*	1 Mug/200ml	8	0	4	0	1	0	0
Cleanse, Pukka Herbs*	1 Teabag/5g	0	0	0	0	0	0	0
Coconut, Infusion, Cuppanut*	1 Serving/215ml	15	1.5	7	0.1	0.1	0.7	0
Cranberry & Elderflower, Boost, Tetley*	1 Mug/225ml	5	0	2	0.1	0.6	0	0
Cranberry, & Blood Orange, Twinings*	1 Cup/250ml	5	0	2	0	0	0	0
Damask, Rose, Chinese, Choi Time*	1 Mug/500ml	0	0.3	0	0	0	0.1	0
Decaf, Tetley*	1 Mug/100ml	1	0	1	0	0.3	0	0
Earl Grey, Infusion with Water, Average	**1 Mug/250ml**	**2**	**0**	**1**	**0**	**0.2**	**0**	**0**
Fennel, Three, Pukka Herbs*	1 Serving/200ml	8	0	4	0	0	0	0
Fruit Or Herbal, Made with Water, Twinings*	1 Mug/200ml	8	0	4	0	1	0	0
Fruit, Twinings*	1 Mug/227ml	4	0	2	0	0.4	0	0
Ginger, Lemon, & Turmeric, Good Earth*	1 Serving/200ml	5	0	2	0	0	0	0
Green, Brown Rice, Dong suh*	1 Teabag/5g	0	0	0	0	0	0	0
Green, Chocolate Coconut, Twinings*	1 Serving/200ml	2	0	1	0	0	0	0
Green, Ice, with Lemon, Zero Sugar, Lipton*	1 Serving/250ml	2	0	1	0	0	0	0
Green, Matcha, Twinings*	1 Mug/250ml	2	0	1	0	0	0	0
Green, Pure, Tetley*	1 Mug/250ml	2	0	1	0	0.3	0	0
Green, Rooibos, Naturally Caffeine Free, Tick Tock*	1 Mug/250ml	0	0	0	0	0	0	0
Green, with Jasmine, Twinings*	1 Mug/100ml	1	0	1	0	0.2	0	0
Green, with Lemon, Knightsbridge, Lidl*	1 Mug/200ml	1	0	0	0	0	0	0
Ice, with Lemon, Lipton*	1 Bottle/325ml	91	0	28	0	6.9	0	0
Ice, with Peach, Lipton*	1 Bottle/500ml	140	0	28	0	6.8	0	0
Latte, Chai, Instant, Sainsbury's*	3 Spoons/30g	22	0.6	73	3.9	9.7	2	0.5
Lemon, & Ginger, Lipton*	1 Cup/200ml	8	0	4	0.5	0.5	0	0
Lemon, & Ginger, Lazy Days, Tea Pigs*	1 Mug/200ml	2	0	1	0	0	0	0

T

	Measure INFO/WEIGHT	per Measure KCAL	FAT	Nutrition Values per 100g / 100ml KCAL	PROT	CARB	FAT	FIBRE
TEA								
Lemon, & Orange, Taylor's of Harrogate*	1 Cup/250ml	5	0	2	0	0.3	0	0
Lemon, Ginger, & Manuka Honey, Pukka Herbs*	1 Mug/200ml	6	0	3	0	0	0	0
Lemon, Iced, Diet, Nestea*	1 Glass/250ml	3	0	1	0	0	0	0
Lemon, Instant, Original, Lift*	2 Tsp/7g	23	0	324	1.4	79.6	0	0
Lemon, Instant, Tesco*	1 Serving/7g	23	0	326	1	80.5	0	0
Made with 1% Milk, Average	**1 Mug/250ml**	**12**	**0.2**	**5**	**0.4**	**0.8**	**0.1**	**0**
Made with Water	**1 Mug/227ml**	**0**	**0**	**0**	**0.1**	**0**	**0**	**0**
Made with Water with Semi-Skimmed Milk, Average	**1 Mug/200ml**	**14**	**0.4**	**7**	**0.5**	**0.7**	**0.2**	**0**
Made with Water with Skimmed Milk, Average	**1 Mug/270ml**	**16**	**0.5**	**6**	**0.5**	**0.7**	**0.2**	**0**
Made with Water with Whole Milk, Average	**1 Mug/200ml**	**16**	**0.8**	**8**	**0.4**	**0.5**	**0.4**	**0**
Mango, Pineapple. with Ginseng, Twinning *	1 Serving/200ml	2	0	1	0	0.2	0	0
Nettle & Sweet Fennel, Twinings*	1 Mug/200ml	4	0	2	0	0.3	0	0
Oolong, Average	**1 Mug/200ml**	**5**	**0.2**	**2**	**0.1**	**0.2**	**0.1**	**0.2**
Peppermint, Made with Water, Average	**1 Mug/200ml**	**3**	**0**	**2**	**0**	**0.2**	**0**	**0**
Raspberry & Cranberry, T of Life, Tetley*	1 Mug/100ml	36	0	36	0	9	0	0
Raspberry Leaf, Organic, Heath & Heather*	1 Mug/200ml	4	0	2	0	0.5	0	0
Red Berries, Brewed, PG Tips*	1 Mug/200ml	5	0	2	0	0.6	0	0
Red Bush, Made with Water, Tetley*	1 Mug/250ml	2	0	1	0	0.1	0	0
Redbush, Pure, Tetley*	1 Serving/200ml	2	0	1	0.1	0.1	0	0
Sleep, Herbal Infusion, Brewed, Twinings*	1 Mug/200ml	4	0	2	0	0.3	0	0
Strawberry Lemonade, Cold Infuse, Twinings*	1 Mug/200ml	4	0	2	0	0	0	0
Super Fruits, Blueberry, & Rasberry, Boost, Tetley*	1 Mug/250ml	5	0	2	0.1	0.6	0	0
Turmeric, Orange, & Star Anise, Superblends, Twinings*	1 Mug/200ml	2	0	1	0	0.5	0	0
Very Berry, Caffeine Free, Knightsbridge, Lidl*	1 Cup/200ml	4	0	2	0	0	0	0.8
TEACAKES								
Average	**1 Teacake/60g**	**178**	**4.5**	**296**	**8**	**52.5**	**7.5**	**0**
Black Forest, Co-Op*	1 Teacake/22g	94	3.6	427	4.6	63.6	16.4	2.3
Chocolate, & Orange, M&S*	1 Teacake/18g	80	3.1	445	5.4	66.4	17.1	2.1
Fruited, Free From, Waitrose*	1 Teacake/67g	176	2.4	263	3	50.9	3.6	7.5
Jam, Lees*	1 Teacake/19g	82	2.9	443	4.2	69.8	15.8	2.5
Large, Sainsbury's*	1 Teacake/73g	212	3.6	291	7.6	52.4	4.9	3.4
Mallow, Strawberry, Huntley & Palmers*	1 Teacake/15g	67	2.9	449	5.5	61	19.2	5.1
Marshmallow, Merry Mallows, Jacob's*	1 Teacake/17g	71	2.7	429	4.6	65	16	1.9
Marshmallow, Milk Chocolate, Tunnock's*	1 Teacake/24g	106	4.6	440	4.9	61.9	19.2	2.4
Mini Bites, M&S*	1 Bite/6g	29	1.2	484	3.2	72.6	20.3	2.1
Salted Caramel, M&S*	1 Teacake/18g	80	3.2	448	5.3	65.3	17.9	1.4
Toasted, Average	**1 Teacake/60g**	**197**	**5**	**329**	**8.9**	**58.3**	**8.3**	**0**
Wagon Wheel, Burton's*	1 Teacake/15g	66	2.6	440	3.3	66	17.3	2
with Orange Filling, M&S*	1 Teacake/20g	80	2.8	410	4.5	66.6	14.2	0.9
TEMPEH								
Average	**1 Avg Serving/70g**	**116**	**4.5**	**166**	**20.7**	**6.4**	**6.4**	**4.3**
Barbecue, Slices, Oasis*	1 Serving/30g	58	4.2	193	12.4	2.9	14	0
Curry Flavoured, Pieces, Plant Power*	½ Pack/90g	331	27	368	21	3.5	30	7.7
Sweet Chilli, Pieces, Tiba*	1 Serving/67g	191	8	285	25	13	12	6.5
TEQUILA								
Average	**1 Pub Shot/35ml**	**78**	**0**	**224**	**0**	**0**	**0**	**0**
Clean T, Non-Alcoholic, 0.5%, Clean Co.*	1 Serve/50ml	12	0	24	0	5	0	0
TERRINE								
Crab, & King Prawn, M&S*	1 Pack/120g	244	17.6	203	8.9	8.6	14.7	0.1
Ham Hock, M&S*	1 Slice/70g	98	4.1	140	22.5	0.1	5.8	0.5
Raspberry Jelly, Plant Kitchen, M&S*	¼ Pack/137g	81	0.3	59	0.5	13.5	0.2	0.7
Salmon & King Prawn, Waitrose*	1 Serving/75g	98	4	130	19.3	1.3	5.3	0
Salmon, Pate, Sainsbury's*	1 Terrine/50g	116	9.7	233	11.8	2.5	19.4	0.5

T

	Measure INFO/WEIGHT	per Measure KCAL	FAT	Nutrition Values per 100g / 100ml KCAL	PROT	CARB	FAT	FIBRE
TERRINE								
Salmon, Scottish, M&S*	1 Terrine/58g	116	8.3	200	14	3.7	14.3	0.5
Vegetable, Waitrose *	1 Serving/60g	86	5.1	143	3.5	11.7	8.4	3.7
THYME								
Dried, Average	**1 Tsp/1g**	**3**	**0.1**	**276**	**9.1**	**45.3**	**7.4**	**0**
Fresh, Average	**1 Tsp/1g**	**1**	**0**	**95**	**3**	**15.1**	**2.5**	**0**
TIA MARIA								
Original	**1 Pub Shot/35ml**	**105**	**0**	**300**	**0**	**0**	**0**	**0**
TIC TAC								
Extra Strong Mint, Ferrero*	2 Tic Tacs/1g	4	0	381	0	95.2	0	0
Fresh Mint, Ferrero*	2 Tic Tacs/1g	4	0	390	0	97.5	0	0
Lime & Orange, Ferrero*	2 Tic Tacs/1g	4	0	386	0	95.5	0	0
TIKKA MASALA								
Cauliflower, Fire Roasted, Bol*	1 Serving/405g	413	15	102	3.5	12.3	3.7	2.5
Cheeky, Wicked Kitchen, Tesco*	1 Pack/353g	487	15.2	138	5.9	17.6	4.3	3
Chicken, & Rice, Ready Meal, Healthy Range, Average	**1 Serving/400g**	**390**	**6.4**	**98**	**6.6**	**14.3**	**1.6**	**1.1**
Chicken, Frozen, Asda*	1 Pack/390g	581	13.3	149	6.7	22	3.4	1.1
Chicken, Hot, Sainsbury's*	1 Pack/400g	604	37.2	151	13.2	3.6	9.3	1.5
Chicken, Hot, Takeaway, Tesco*	½ Pack/194g	244	13.9	126	9	5.3	7.2	2
Chicken, Slow Cooked, British, Sainsburys*	½ Pack/225g	367	20	163	17.6	3	8.9	0.6
Chicken, with Pllau Rice, Meal for 1, Sainsbury's*	1 Pack/366g	512	20.1	140	6.4	15.4	5.5	1.6
Chicken, with Pilau Rice, What's Cooking?, Lidl*	1 Pack/400g	452	15.2	113	6.2	13	3.8	1.1
Chicken, with Rice, Free From, Sainsbury's*	1 Pack/375g	435	12.8	116	7.2	12.5	3.4	3.1
Chickenless, Plant Kitchen, M&S*	½ Pack/200g	272	17.2	136	5.9	8.1	8.6	1.4
Meal Kit, Pataks*	½ Pack/157g	221	15.7	141	2.4	7.8	10	0
Paneer & Potato, Heat & Enjoy, Tesco*	½ Pack/212g	343	25.4	162	4.9	7.8	12	1.7
Paneer, Co-Op*	1 Pack/400g	320	12.4	80	4.5	7.5	3.1	2.1
Tantalizing, Quorn*	1 Pack/373g	414	8.8	111	4	17.2	2.4	2.2
Tasty Bite*	1 Serving/142g	126	6	89	2.7	7.8	4.2	4.4
Vegetarian, Chef's Selection, Quorn*	½ Pack/170g	274	17	161	6	10	10	3.5
TILAPIA								
Raw, Average	**100g**	**95**	**1**	**95**	**20**	**0**	**1**	**0**
Roasted, Spiced, with Tomatoes, & Lentils, Hello Fresh*	1 Serving/483g	261	3	54	7	4.3	0.6	0
TIME OUT								
Break Pack, Cadbury*	1 Serving/20g	108	6.3	530	6.2	58.3	30.7	0
Chocolate Fingers, Cadbury*	2 Fingers/35g	186	10.6	530	7.1	57.3	30.3	1.1
Timeout, Cadbury*	1 Bar/21g	111	6	524	6.7	60	28.3	2.1
TIRAMISU								
Asda*	1 Pot/100g	252	11	252	4.3	34	11	0.5
Classic, Individual, Sainsbury's*	1 Pot/100g	242	9.9	242	3.8	30.6	9.9	1.2
Classic, Sainsbury's*	1 Serving/84g	209	8.5	250	4.2	31.7	10.2	1.1
Co-Op*	1/6 Pack/83g	218	7.6	263	4.1	37	9.2	0.6
Dessert Menu, Aldi*	¼ Pack/125g	340	15	272	4.3	32	12	1.4
Dine in Dessert, M&S*	½ Dessert/145g	515	36.7	355	2.6	28.8	25.3	0.7
Envia*	1 Pot/80g	243	12.9	304	3.2	33	16.1	0
Family Size, Tesco*	1 Serving/125g	356	18.1	285	4.3	34.5	14.5	4.3
Lemon, Aldi*	1 Pot/100g	228	7.8	228	3.7	33	7.8	1.2
Limoncello, Dessert Menu, Aldi*	1 Pot/100g	228	7.8	228	3.7	33	7.8	1.2
Morrisons*	1 Pot/90g	248	9.9	276	4	38	11	0
Raspberry, Bonta Divina*	1 Pot/100g	227	8.7	227	3.6	30.7	8.7	1.4
Single Size, Tesco*	1 Pot/100g	290	12.9	290	3.8	35.1	12.9	4.5
Waitrose*	1 Pot/90g	221	11.2	246	6.4	27.2	12.4	0
TOAD IN THE HOLE								
Average	**1 Serving/231g**	**640**	**40.2**	**277**	**11.9**	**19.5**	**17.4**	**1.1**

T

	Measure INFO/WEIGHT	per Measure KCAL	FAT	Nutrition Values per 100g / 100ml KCAL	PROT	CARB	FAT	FIBRE
TOASTIE								
All Day Breakfast, M&S*	1 Toastie/174g	375	13.8	215	11.2	25	7.9	1.7
Cheese & Pickle, M&S*	1 Toastie/136g	320	9.1	235	10.4	33.5	6.7	2.6
Cheese & Onion, Ginsters*	1 Toastie/122g	330	12.3	269	10.9	33.1	10	1.5
Cheese, & Tomato , Real Wrap Co.*	1 Toastie/164g	364	11.8	222	10.2	28.4	7.2	0
Cheese, Three, Heat to Eat, Tesco*	1 Pack/161g	454	19.3	282	13.7	28.9	12	1.7
Ham & Cheese, White Bread	**1 Toastie/150g**	**409**	**14.9**	**273**	**14.5**	**31.3**	**9.9**	**0.9**
TOFFEE APPLE								
Average	**1 Apple/141g**	**188**	**3**	**133**	**1.2**	**29.2**	**2.1**	**2.3**
TOFFEE CRISP								
Biscuit, Nestle*	1 Biscuit/19g	99	5.3	519	3.9	62.3	27.8	1.4
Bitesize, Nestle*	1 Serving/20g	101	5.4	518	3.8	63	27.6	1.3
TOFFEES								
Assorted, Bassett's*	1 Toffee/8g	35	1.1	434	3.8	73.1	14	0
Assorted, Sainsbury's*	1 Toffee/8g	37	1.3	457	2.2	76.5	15.8	0.2
Butter, Smart Price, Asda*	1 Toffee/8g	37	1.3	440	1.3	75	15	0
Chewy, Werther's*	1 Toffee/5g	22	0.8	436	3.5	71.3	15.2	0.1
Dairy, Sainsbury's*	1 Toffee/8g	38	1.7	471	2.5	65.3	21.3	4.1
Dairy, Waitrose*	1 Toffee/8g	37	1.1	458	2	80.2	14.3	0.5
Dark Chocolate, Riesen*	1 Toffee/30g	135	5.5	449	4.1	66.3	18.3	0
Devon Butter, Thorntons*	1 Toffee/9g	40	1.5	444	1.7	72.2	16.7	0
English Butter, Co-Op*	1 Toffee/8g	38	1.6	470	2	71	20	0
Everyday Value, Tesco*	1 Toffee/8g	34	1.1	450	2.1	77.3	14.8	0.3
Liquorice, Thorntons*	1 Bag/100g	506	29.4	506	1.9	58.8	29.4	0
Mixed, Average	**1oz/28g**	**119**	**5.2**	**426**	**2.2**	**66.7**	**18.6**	**0**
Original, Cartwright & Butler*	1 Toffee/8g	36	1	445	1.5	80	13	0.5
Original, Thorntons*	1 Bag/100g	514	30.1	514	1.8	59.3	30.1	0
TOFU								
Average	**1 Pack/250g**	**297**	**16.5**	**119**	**13.4**	**1.4**	**6.6**	**0.1**
Basilico, Taifun*	1 Serving/100g	198	13	198	18	1.7	13	0
Bites, Smoked BBQ, Crispy, The Tofoo Co.*	½ Pack/113g	269	12.4	238	14.1	19.8	11	1.9
Deep Fried, Tofu King*	½ Pack/115g	384	31.3	334	21.2	0.7	27.2	0
Extra Firm, Nasoya*	1/5 Pack/91g	130	7	143	15.4	2.2	7.7	2.2
Firm, Hacendado*	1 Block/275g	302	19	110	11.1	0.9	6.9	0.5
Fried, Average	**1oz/28g**	**75**	**4**	**268**	**28.6**	**9.3**	**14.1**	**0**
Marinated, Clearspot*	½ Pack/95g	143	7.9	151	16.1	2.6	8.3	0.8
Marinated, Vemondo, Lidl*	1 Block/180g	254	15.8	141	13	2.5	8.8	0
Organic, Block, Cauldron Foods*	½ Pack/198g	234	14.1	118	12.6	1	7.1	1.9
Pieces, Asian Spiced, SoFine *	½ Pack/90g	178	12.5	198	15.3	1	13.9	2.3
Pieces, Marinated, Organic, Cauldron Foods*	1 Serving/80g	186	13.6	232	18	1	17	2.7
Puffs, Sunrise*	1 Pack/104g	312	22.1	300	20	6.2	21.2	0
Silken, Firm, Mori-Nu*	1 Pack/349g	195	9.1	56	7.1	0.6	2.6	0
Smoked, Firm, Average	**1 Avg Serving/75g**	**115**	**6.5**	**153**	**17.4**	**1.4**	**8.7**	**0.2**
Sticky, with Pilaf Rice, & Mango Chutney, Hello Fresh*	1 Serving/617g	586	12.3	95	4	15	2	3
Super Firm, Organic, Plant Kitchen, M&S*	1 Pack/300g	369	19.8	123	15	0.3	6.6	1.1
Super Firm, So Organic, Sainsbury's*	1/3 Pack/100g	118	6.8	118	11.9	1.8	6.8	1.1
Sweet Chilli, Spicy, Bites, Cooked, The Tofoo Co.*	½ Pack/113g	356	16.6	316	12.9	31.8	14.7	2.3
Teriyaki, Organic, Cauldron Foods*	½ Pack/80g	168	12	210	16	2.8	15	2.1
Teriyaki, Organic, The Tofoo Co.*	1/3 Pack/70g	109	5.5	156	15.6	5.9	7.8	0.5
Teriyaki, Sticky, Plant Kitchen, M&S*	1 Pack/360g	464	14	129	5.9	16.7	3.9	1.5
with Pesto, Soyami*	1 Serving/100g	226	16	226	20	1	16	0.9
TOMATILLOS								
Raw	**1 Med/34g**	**11**	**0.3**	**32**	**1**	**5.8**	**1**	**1.9**

T

	Measure INFO/WEIGHT	per Measure KCAL	FAT	Nutrition Values per 100g / 100ml KCAL	PROT	CARB	FAT	FIBRE
TOMATO PASTE								
Average	*1 Tbsp/20g*	*19*	*0*	*96*	*5*	*19.2*	*0.2*	*1.5*
Sun Dried, Average	*1 Hpd Tsp/10g*	*38*	*3.5*	*385*	*3.2*	*13.8*	*35.2*	*0*
TOMATO PUREE								
Average	*1 Tbsp/15g*	*11*	*0*	*76*	*4.5*	*14.1*	*0.2*	*2.3*
Double Concentrate, Average	*1 Tbsp/15g*	*13*	*0*	*85*	*4.9*	*14.9*	*0.2*	*3.6*
Garlic, Double Concentrate, Morrisons*	1 Tbsp/15g	13	0	86	3.9	14.9	0.3	3.8
Tomato & Garlic, GIA*	1 Tbsp/15g	14	0.1	91	3.3	17.6	0.4	0
TOMATOES								
Cherry, Average	*1 Tomato/15g*	*3*	*0*	*18*	*0.7*	*3*	*0.3*	*0.5*
Cherry, Marinated, with Italian Mozzarella, The Deli, Aldi*	½ Pack/75g	186	17.2	248	8.4	2.3	23	1.3
Cherry, on the Vine, Average	*1 Serving/80g*	*15*	*0.3*	*18*	*0.7*	*3.1*	*0.3*	*1.2*
Chopped, Canned, Branded Average	*1 Serving/130g*	*27*	*0.2*	*21*	*1.1*	*3.8*	*0.1*	*0.8*
Chopped, Italian, Average	*½ Can/200g*	*47*	*0.2*	*23*	*1.3*	*4.4*	*0.1*	*0.9*
Chopped, with Garlic, Average	*½ Can/200g*	*43*	*0.3*	*21*	*1.2*	*3.8*	*0.1*	*0.8*
Chopped, with Herbs, Average	*½ Can/200g*	*42*	*0.3*	*21*	*1.1*	*3.8*	*0.1*	*0.8*
Fresh, Raw, Average	*1 Med/123g*	*22*	*0.2*	*18*	*0.9*	*3.9*	*0.2*	*1.2*
Fried in Blended Oil	*1 Med/85g*	*77*	*6.5*	*91*	*0.7*	*5*	*7.7*	*1.3*
Grilled, Average	*1 Med/85g*	*17*	*0.3*	*20*	*0.8*	*3.5*	*0.3*	*1.5*
Heritage, Jewel, TTD, Sainsbury's*	1 Pack/250g	62	1.2	25	1.1	3.4	0.5	1.2
Marinated, with Garlic & Oregano, The Deli, Aldi*	½ Pack/75g	68	3.5	90	2.8	7.8	4.7	2.7
Marmonde, Raw, Waitrose*	1 Tomato/120g	24	0.4	20	0.7	3.1	0.3	1
Plum, Baby, Average	*1 Serving/50g*	*9*	*0.2*	*18*	*1.5*	*2.3*	*0.3*	*1*
Plum, in Tomato Juice, Average	*1 Can/400g*	*71*	*0.4*	*18*	*1*	*3.3*	*0.1*	*0.7*
Plum, in Tomato Juice, Premium, Average	*1 Can/400g*	*93*	*1.2*	*23*	*1.3*	*3.8*	*0.3*	*0.7*
Pome Dei Moro, Waitrose*	1 Serving/80g	16	0.2	20	0.7	3.1	0.3	1.2
Pomodorino, TTD, Sainsbury's*	1 Tomato/8g	2	0	25	1.1	3.4	0.5	1.2
Ripened on the Vine, Average	*1 Med/123g*	*22*	*0.4*	*18*	*0.7*	*3.1*	*0.3*	*0.7*
Santini, M&S*	1 Serving/80g	16	0.2	20	0.7	3.1	0.3	1
Stuffed with Rice Based Filling, Average	*1oz/28g*	*59*	*3.8*	*212*	*2.1*	*22.2*	*13.4*	*1.1*
Sun Dried in Oil	*100g*	*301*	*24.8*	*301*	*5.8*	*13.5*	*24.8*	*7*
Sun Dried, Average	*3 Pieces/20g*	*43*	*3.2*	*214*	*4.7*	*13*	*15.9*	*3.3*
TONGUE								
Lunch, Average	*1oz/28g*	*51*	*3*	*181*	*20.1*	*1.8*	*10.6*	*0*
Ox, British, Waitrose*	1 Slice/32g	68	4.9	213	17	1.7	15.4	0
Ox, Deli Counter, Sainsbury's*	1 Serving/100g	195	13.3	195	18.3	0.5	13.3	0.1
Pork, Lunch, Carvery Slices, Morrisons*	1 Slice/25g	45	2.7	179	18.9	1.6	10.6	0.9
Pork, Lunch, Slices, Iceland*	1 Pack/80g	184	12	230	22.4	0.9	15	1
Slices, Average	*1oz/28g*	*56*	*3.9*	*201*	*18.7*	*0*	*14*	*0*
TONIC WATER								
Average	*1 Glass/250ml*	*82*	*0*	*33*	*0*	*8.8*	*0*	*0*
Clementine, Refreshingly Light, Fever-Tree*	1 Serving/250ml	48	0	19	0	4.7	0	0
Cucumber, Light, Fever-Tree*	1 Serving/250ml	48	0	19	0	4.8	0	0
Diet, Asda*	1 Glass/200ml	2	0	1	0	0	0	0
Indian, Low Calorie, Vive, Aldi*	1 Glass/250ml	3	0	1	0	0	0	0
Indian, Premium, Fever-Tree*	1 Can/150ml	42	0	28	0	7.1	0	0
Indian, Schweppes*	1 Glass/250ml	55	0	22	0	5.1	0	0
Indian, Slimline, Schweppes*	1 Serving/188ml	3	0	2	0.4	0	0	0
Lemon, Sicilian, Fever-Tree*	1 Bottle/200ml	70	0	35	0	8.7	0	0
Light, Refreshingly, Fever-Tree*	1 Can/150ml	22	0	15	0	3.8	0	0
Low Calorie, Tesco*	1 Glass/200ml	4	0	2	0	0.5	0	0
Mediterranean, Refreshingly Light, Fever-Tree*	1 Serving/250ml	48	0	19	0	4.8	0	0
Pink Rhubarb, Light, The Best, Morrisons*	1 Serving/200ml	4	0	2	0	0	0	0
Schweppes*	1 Can/237ml	80	0	34	0	8.9	0	0

T

	Measure INFO/WEIGHT	per Measure KCAL	FAT	Nutrition Values per 100g / 100ml KCAL	PROT	CARB	FAT	FIBRE
TOPIC								
Mars*	1 Bar/47g	234	12.3	498	6.2	59.6	26.2	1.7
TORTE								
Cherry Bakewell, No.1, Waitrose*	1 Slice/85g	252	12.6	297	4.5	36.2	14.8	0.5
Chocolate Fondant, Gu*	1 Slice/62g	264	18.9	423	5.7	32	30.2	1.8
Chocolate, Luxury, Kirstys*	1 Slice/83g	301	18.3	363	3	36.4	22.1	3.4
Chocolate, Plant Kitchen, M&S*	1 Torte/70g	312	21.1	445	4.5	37.4	30.1	3.3
Chocolate, Tesco*	1 Slice/50g	126	6	251	3.6	32.3	11.9	1
Lemon & Mango, Waitrose*	1 Slice/80g	142	2.4	177	3.9	33.6	3	0.6
TORTELLINI								
Arrabbiata, Spicy, Morrisons*	½ Pack/210g	489	13.6	233	7.3	35.4	6.5	2.1
Cheese, & Ham, Italiano, Tesco*	½ Pack/150g	396	12.3	264	12.8	34.8	8.2	3
Cheese, Four, Inspired Cuisine, Aldi*	½ Pack/202g	396	8.1	196	8.7	30	4	1.8
Ham, & Cheese, Fresh, Asda*	½ Pack/150g	255	9	170	6	23	6	1.7
Mushroom, Asda*	1 Serving/125g	218	5.2	174	6	28	4.2	2.3
Pepperoni, Spicy, Asda*	½ Pack/150g	252	6	168	7	26	4	0
Sausage, & Ham, Italiano, Tesco*	1 Pack/300g	816	27.9	272	13.1	34	9.3	3.7
Spinach, & Ricotta, Italian, Asda*	½ Pack/150g	189	3.6	126	5	21	2.4	0.6
Spinach, & Ricotta, Italian, Morrisons*	½ Pack/210g	286	5.9	136	4.9	22.1	2.8	1.5
Tomato, & Mozzarella, Fresh, Sainsbury's*	½ Pack/150g	291	12	194	7.5	23	8	3.4
TORTELLONI								
al Fungi, Porcini, Fresh, Bertagni*	½ Pack/125g	322	9.6	258	9.2	38	7.7	0
Arrabiata, Sainsbury's*	½ Pack/210g	407	11.8	194	7.1	28.8	5.6	2.6
Aubergine, Parmigiana, Rana La Famiglia*	½ Pack/175g	374	11.9	214	8.1	29	6.8	2.4
Beef, & Red Wine, Sainsbury's*	½ Pack/150g	256	5.8	171	7.4	25.9	3.9	1.7
Butternut Squash, Jamie Oliver*	½ Pack/125g	224	4.6	179	5.4	30	3.7	2.2
Cheese, & Smoked Ham, As Consumed, Tesco*	½ Pack/270g	535	17.3	198	8.4	25.8	6.4	1.8
Cheese, & Tomato, Cucina, Aldi*	1 Pack/250g	555	12	222	8.1	36	4.8	2
Cheese, & Tomato, Italian, Cooked, Asda*	½ Pack/209g	454	13.4	217	7.9	31	6.4	2.1
Cheese, & Tomato, Tesco*	½ Pack/195g	404	10.3	207	8.2	30	5.3	3
Chicken & Bacon, As Consumed, Italiano, Tesco*	½ Pack/280g	567	14	202	6.8	30.7	5	3.7
Chicken, & Bacon, Inspired Cuisine, Aldi*	½ Pack/150g	370	13.8	247	8	32	9.2	1.8
Chicken, & Bacon, Italian, Cooked, Morrisons*	½ Pack/210g	399	8.2	190	6.8	31	3.9	2.1
Chicken, & Prosciutto, Buitoni*	1 Serving/109g	330	9	302	14.7	42.2	8.2	1.8
Chorizo, Smoky, Fresh, Sainsbury's*	½ Pack/203g	398	12.8	196	8.5	25.6	6.3	1.5
Ham & Cheese, Italian Cuisine, Aldi*	½ Pack/150g	340	10.2	227	9.3	31	6.8	1.6
Ham, & Cheese, Cooked, Morrisons*	½ Pack/210g	389	9.5	185	7.5	27.9	4.5	1.6
Mushroom, Porcini, & Ricotta, Chef Select, Lidl*	½ Pack/125g	278	6.8	222	11.2	31.3	5.4	1.5
Parmegiano Reggiano, Specially Selected, Aldi*	½ Pack/168g	352	12.1	209	7.6	28	7.2	1.3
Spinach & Ricotta, Cooked, Sainsbury's*	½ Pack/203g	368	11.6	181	6.5	24.8	5.7	2.4
Spinach, & Ricotta Cheese, Co-Op*	½ Pack/126g	315	6.3	250	10	41	5	4
Spinach, & Ricotta, Fresh, Waitrose*	½ Pack/150g	239	5.3	159	6.3	24.4	3.5	2.5
Spinach, & Ricotta, Chef Select, Lidl*	1 Serving/125g	288	11.9	230	9.5	24.4	9.5	4.6
Spinach, & Ricotta, Cooked, HFC, Tesco*	½ Pack/175g	326	5.8	186	6.1	31.5	3.3	3.2
Tomato, Mozzarella, & Basil , Dell'ugo*	½ Pack/150g	249	4.5	166	7.4	26.6	3	1.8
Wild Mushroom, Italian, Sainsbury's*	½ Pack/150g	309	12.3	206	7.7	25.4	8.2	2.3
TORTIGLIONI								
Beef Ragu, No.1, Waitrose*	1 Pack/373g	656	17.9	176	11.4	20.8	4.8	1.8
Dry, Average	**1 Serving/75g**	**266**	**1.4**	**355**	**12.5**	**72.2**	**1.9**	**2.1**
Tomato, & Mascarpone, TTD, Sainsbury's*	1 Pack/378g	506	18.5	134	3.9	17.8	4.9	1.7
TORTILLA								
Chorizo, & Roasted Vegetables, Morrisons*	1 Tortilla/130g	238	15.2	183	9.1	10	11.7	1
Chorizo, & Serrano, Tesco*	½ Tortilla/250g	405	24.5	162	6	11.9	9.8	1.2
Mozzarella, & Cherry Tomato, M&S*	¼ Serving/90g	151	9.8	168	6.6	9.7	10.9	2.5

T

	Measure INFO/WEIGHT	per Measure KCAL	FAT	Nutrition Values per 100g / 100ml KCAL	PROT	CARB	FAT	FIBRE
TORTILLA								
Potato, & Onion, Vegan, Ready to Eat, Squeaky Bean*	½ Pack/125g	170	5.9	136	3.9	18	4.7	3.4
Red Pepper & Chorizo, Slices, Waitrose*	1 Slice/113g	180	10.3	160	10	8.6	9.2	1.6
Red Pepper, Roasted, & Spicy Chorizo, Atlantica*	¼ Pack/125g	207	16.8	165	9.6	11.3	13.4	1.5
Roasted Onion, & Potato, M&S*	1 Tortilla/220g	297	12.1	135	5.9	13.5	5.5	3.7
Spanish Style, Vegan, Poeto*	¼ Tortilla /125g	190	8.4	152	3.4	19	6.7	0
Vegetable, Roasted, Mediterranean, M&S*	½ Pack/110g	138	5.9	125	6.9	11.1	5.4	2.3
with Chickpeas, & Onions, Vegan, Vemondo, Lidl*	¼ Tortilla/125g	190	8.4	152	3.4	19	6.7	1
TORTILLA CHIPS								
Chorizo & Red Pepper, M&S*	1 Serving/25g	122	5	487	5.9	68.2	20.2	4.3
Cool Flavour, BGTY, Sainsbury's*	1 Pack/22g	94	2.7	425	7.1	71.4	12.3	4.5
Cool Flavour, Sainsbury's*	1 Serving/50g	232	9.4	463	5.7	68.1	18.7	3.7
Cool Original, Snaktastic, Lidl*	1 Serving/25g	116	5.3	466	5.9	60.6	21.2	4.5
Cool, Tesco*	1 Serving/40g	202	10	505	6.1	62.6	25	2.7
Lime Salsa, Tortilla Scoops, M&S*	1 Serving/30g	147	6.9	491	5.7	61.9	23.1	6.1
Nachips, Original, Old El Paso*	1 Serving/50g	250	13.4	500	6.2	56.4	26.7	4.7
Plain	**1 Serving/100g**	**486**	**21.1**	**486**	**6.8**	**62**	**21.1**	**4.2**
Rainbow, Sainsbury's*	1 Pack/20g	96	4.3	479	5.5	62.1	21.5	7.6
Sweet Potato, M&S*	½ Bag/75g	375	19.1	500	7.1	57.4	25.5	6.3
Tomatillo Salsa, Manomasa*	1 Serving/25g	127	6.8	507	6.8	54.9	27.4	7
Turkey, & Stuffing, Free From, Tesco*	½ Pack/75g	370	16.9	494	6.2	65.2	22.5	2.9
Vegan Cheese, Plant Menu, Aldi*	1 Serving/40g	193	8.8	482	6.1	64	22	4.9
Veggie, Lightly Salted, Co-Op*	1 Serving/33g	165	8.3	499	5.9	60	25	4.8
with Guacamole	**1 Serving/100g**	**515**	**30.8**	**515**	**6**	**53**	**30.8**	**6.3**
TREACLE								
Black, Average	**1 Tbsp/20g**	**51**	**0**	**257**	**1.2**	**67.2**	**0**	**0**
TRIFLE								
Average	**1 Serving/170g**	**272**	**10.7**	**160**	**3.6**	**22.3**	**6.3**	**0.5**
Berry, Mixed, Waitrose*	1 Pot/120g	200	13	167	2.2	15	10.8	0.7
Chocolate, Milbona, Lidl*	1 Pot/90g	202	12.8	224	4.4	19	14.2	1.1
Fruit Cocktail, Individual, M&S*	1 Pot/135g	205	9.2	150	2.7	19.3	6.7	0.7
Fruit Cocktail, Individual, Tesco*	1 Pot/113g	175	8.8	155	1.7	19.6	7.8	0.6
Fruit, Cocktail, Morrisons*	1 Pot/135g	167	7.2	124	1.7	17	5.3	0.8
Peach & Zabaglione, COU, M&S*	1 Glass/130g	150	3	115	2.8	20.6	2.3	0.8
Raspberry & Sherry, Waitrose*	1 Pot/120g	223	14.3	186	2.5	16.9	11.9	0.7
Raspberry, Large, Tesco*	¼ Pack/150g	207	10.2	138	1.8	17.1	6.8	0.6
Raspberry, Pot, Sainsbury's*	1 Pot/125g	181	7.6	145	2.1	19.9	6.1	1.3
Raspberry, Tesco*	1 Pot/145g	188	8.8	130	1.7	16.8	6.1	0.6
Sticky Toffee, The Best, Morrisons*	1/6 Trifle/150g	368	13.8	245	3.4	37	9.2	0.5
Strawberry Jelly, M&S*	1 Pot/135g	167	6.5	124	2.6	17.2	4.8	0.6
Strawberry, Aldi*	1/3 Trifle/153g	193	8	126	1.9	18	5.2	0.7
Strawberry, Aldi*	1 Pack/600g	852	43.8	142	2	17	7.3	0.5
Strawberry, Co-Op*	1 Pot/125g	146	5.5	117	1.7	17	4.4	0.7
Strawberry, Everyday Value, Tesco*	¼ Trifle/118g	157	6.4	133	1.4	18.5	5.4	2.4
Strawberry, Individual, Morrisons*	1 Pot/135g	173	7.3	128	1.7	17.7	5.4	0.9
Strawberry, Individual, Pots, Tesco*	1 Pot/135g	174	6.1	129	1.8	20	4.5	0.6
Strawberry, Individual, Sainsbury's*	1 Pot/125g	168	8.2	134	2.1	16.2	6.6	0.6
Strawberry, Individual, Waitrose*	1 Pot/150g	206	8.6	137	1.8	19.7	5.7	1
Strawberry, Low Fat, COU, M&S*	1 Pot/140g	148	3.5	106	2.9	17.6	2.5	0.8
Strawberry, Milbona, Lidl*	1 Trifle/125g	196	11.2	157	1.9	16.8	9	0
Strawberry, Tesco*	¼ Pack/150g	213	10.8	142	1.7	17.2	7.2	0.6
TRIPE								
& Onions, Stewed	**1oz/28g**	**26**	**0.8**	**93**	**8.3**	**9.5**	**2.7**	**0.7**
Ox, Real Lancashire*	1 Serving/100g	36	0.7	36	7.2	0.1	0.7	0

T

	Measure INFO/WEIGHT	per Measure KCAL	FAT	Nutrition Values per 100g / 100ml KCAL	PROT	CARB	FAT	FIBRE
TROUT								
Brown, Steamed, Average	**1 Serving/120g**	**162**	**5.4**	**135**	**23.5**	**0**	**4.5**	**0**
Fillets, Loch, Scottish, M&S*	1 Fillet/110g	226	13.2	205	24.2	0	12	0
Fillets, Loch, Scottish, Skin On, Aldi*	1 Fillet/95g	192	10.5	202	26	0.5	11	0.5
Fillets, with Juniper Berries, Ocean Sea, Lidl*	1 Serving/63g	87	3.5	138	22	0	5.5	0
Hot Smoked, Loch, M&S*	1 Pack/160g	314	18.6	196	22.5	0.4	11.6	0.6
Rainbow, Grilled, Average	**1 Serving/120g**	**162**	**6.5**	**135**	**21.5**	**0**	**5.4**	**0**
Rainbow, Raw, Average	**1oz/28g**	**33**	**1.3**	**118**	**19.1**	**0**	**4.7**	**0**
Rainbow, Smoked, Average	**1 Pack/135g**	**190**	**7.6**	**140**	**21.7**	**0.8**	**5.6**	**0**
Raw, Average	**1 Serving/120g**	**159**	**6.5**	**132**	**20.6**	**0**	**5.4**	**0**
Smoked, Average	**2 Fillets/135g**	**187**	**7.1**	**138**	**22.7**	**0.3**	**5.2**	**0.1**
TUNA								
Albacore, Wild, Canned, Wild Planet*	½ Can/60g	90	3.5	150	21.7	0	5.8	0
Bluefin, Cooked, Dry Heat, Average	**1 Serving/100g**	**184**	**6.3**	**184**	**29.9**	**0**	**6.3**	**0**
Chilli, & Garlic, Fusions, Fishmonger, Aldi*	1 Can/80g	142	7.4	177	21	2.5	9.2	0.5
Chunks, in Brine, Average, Drained	**1 Can/130g**	**141**	**0.7**	**108**	**25.9**	**0**	**0.5**	**0**
Chunks, in Brine, Drained, Average	**1 Can/130g**	**141**	**0.7**	**108**	**25.9**	**0**	**0.5**	**0**
Chunks, in Spring Water, Average, Drained	**1 Sm Can/56g**	**60**	**0.4**	**108**	**25.4**	**0**	**0.6**	**0.1**
Chunks, in Sunflower Oil, Average, Drained	**1 Can/138g**	**260**	**12.6**	**188**	**26.5**	**0**	**9.2**	**0**
Chunks, Skipjack, in Brine, Average	**1 Can/138g**	**141**	**0.8**	**102**	**24.3**	**0**	**0.6**	**0**
Flakes, in Brine, Average	**1oz/28g**	**29**	**0.2**	**104**	**24.8**	**0**	**0.6**	**0**
Flakes, in Coronation Dressing, Sainsbury's*	1 Can/80g	72	0.4	90	15	5.7	0.5	1.2
Flakes, Indian Spiced, Infusions, John West*	1 Tub/80g	168	9.6	210	24	1.5	12	0.1
Flakes, Sundried Tomato, Infusions, John West*	1 Tub/80g	157	8	196	24	2.2	10	0.1
in Mayonnaise, Corentin Kermeur*	1 Tin/135g	243	20.2	180	8.1	2.9	15	0
in Water, Average	**1 Serving/120g**	**126**	**1**	**105**	**24**	**0.1**	**0.8**	**0**
Lemon, & Thyme, Fusions, Drained, Fishmonger, Aldi*	1 Tin/80g	170	11.2	212	20	1.9	14	0.5
Lime & Black Pepper, John West*	1 Serving/85g	134	7	158	18	2	8.2	2.1
Lunch, French Style, Watersons*	1 Pack/200g	208	3.6	104	9.2	11.9	1.8	0
Lunch, Mediterranean Style, Watersons*	1 Pack/200g	190	3.2	95	9.6	9.7	1.6	0
Soy, & Ginger, Fusions, Fishmonger, Aldi*	1 Can/80g	152	8	190	21	3.2	10	0.5
Steak, in Spring Water, Drained, M&S*	1 Tin/80g	79	0.5	99	23.5	0.5	0.6	0
Steaks, in Brine, Average	**1 Sm Can/99g**	**106**	**0.5**	**107**	**25.6**	**0**	**0.6**	**0**
Steaks, in Olive Oil, Average	**1 Serving/111g**	**211**	**10.7**	**190**	**25.8**	**0**	**9.6**	**0**
Steaks, in Sunflower Oil, Average	**1 Can/150g**	**269**	**12.6**	**179**	**26**	**0**	**8.4**	**0**
Steaks, Raw, Average	**1 Serving/140g**	**179**	**2.7**	**128**	**27.6**	**0.1**	**1.9**	**0.2**
Steaks, Skipjack, in Brine, Average	**½ Can/75g**	**73**	**0.4**	**98**	**23.2**	**0**	**0.6**	**0**
Yellowfin, Cooked, Dry Heat, Average	**1 Serving/100g**	**139**	**1.2**	**139**	**30**	**0**	**1.2**	**0**
TURBOT								
Grilled	**1oz/28g**	**34**	**1**	**122**	**22.7**	**0**	**3.5**	**0**
Raw	**1oz/28g**	**27**	**0.8**	**95**	**17.7**	**0**	**2.7**	**0**
TURKEY								
& Stuffing, Sliced, Asda*	1 Slice/40g	50	0.9	124	22	3.3	2.3	1
Breast, Butter Basted, Average	**1 Serving/75g**	**110**	**3.6**	**146**	**23.7**	**1.9**	**4.9**	**0.4**
Breast, Diced, Healthy Range, Average	**1oz/28g**	**30**	**0.4**	**108**	**23.8**	**0**	**1.3**	**0**
Breast, Honey Roast, Sliced, Average	**1 Serving/50g**	**57**	**0.7**	**114**	**24**	**1.6**	**1.4**	**0.2**
Breast, Joint, Bacon Wrapped, Iceland*	1 Serving/100g	146	4.8	146	24.9	0.7	4.8	0.5
Breast, Joint, Raw, Average	**1 Serving/125g**	**134**	**2.6**	**108**	**21.3**	**0.7**	**2.1**	**0.6**
Breast, Raw, Average	**1oz/28g**	**33**	**0.6**	**117**	**24.1**	**0.5**	**2**	**0.1**
Breast, Roasted, Average	**1oz/28g**	**37**	**0.9**	**131**	**24.6**	**0.7**	**3.3**	**0.1**
Breast, Roll, Cooked, Average	**1 Slice/10g**	**9**	**0.1**	**92**	**17.6**	**3.5**	**0.8**	**0**
Breast, Slices, Cooked, Average	**1 Slice/20g**	**23**	**0.3**	**114**	**24**	**1.2**	**1.4**	**0.3**
Breast, Smoked, Sliced, Average	**1 Slice/20g**	**23**	**0.4**	**113**	**23.4**	**0.7**	**2**	**0**
Breast, Steaks, in Crumbs, Average	**1 Steak/76g**	**217**	**14.1**	**286**	**13.7**	**16.4**	**18.5**	**0.2**

INFO/WEIGHT	Measure	per Measure KCAL	FAT	Nutrition Values per 100g / 100ml KCAL	PROT	CARB	FAT	FIBRE
TURKEY								
Breast, Steaks, Raw, Average	1oz/28g	30	0.3	107	24.3	0	1.1	0
Breast, Strips, for Stir Fry, Average	1 Serving/175g	205	2.7	117	25.6	0.1	1.6	0
Dark Meat, Raw, Average	1oz/28g	29	0.7	104	20.4	0	2.5	0
Leg, Dark Meat, Raw , Average, Weighed with Bone	1 Serving/100g	73	1.8	73	14.3	0	1.8	0
Light Meat, Raw, Average	1oz/28g	29	0.2	105	24.4	0	0.8	0
Light Meat, Roasted	1 Cup/140g	163	3.3	116	22.1	0	2.4	0
Mince, Average	1oz/28g	45	2	161	23.9	0	7.2	0
Mince, Lean, Healthy Range, Average	1oz/28g	33	1.1	118	20.3	0	4.1	0
Rashers, Average	1 Rasher/26g	26	0.4	101	19.1	2.3	1.6	0
Rashers, Smoked, Average	1 Serving/75g	76	1.4	101	19.8	1.5	1.8	0
Roast, Meat & Skin, Average	1oz/28g	48	1.8	171	28	0	6.5	0
Roast, Meat Only, Average	1 Serving/100g	157	3.2	157	29.9	0	3.2	0
Strips, Stir-Fried, Average	1oz/28g	46	1.3	164	31	0	4.5	0
Thigh, Diced, Average	1oz/28g	33	1.2	117	19.6	0	4.3	0
Thigh, Joint, Bone In, As Sold, Tesco*	1 Serving/125g	175	9	140	18.1	0.5	7.2	0.5
Wafer Thin, Honey Roast, Average	1 Slice/10g	11	0.2	109	19.2	4.2	1.7	0.2
TURKEY DINNER								
& Ham, Irish Classics, Tesco*	1 Pack/500g	481	12.5	96	7.3	10.4	2.5	1.6
Homestyle, Cooked, Kershaws*	1 Pack/400g	256	4	64	2.9	10.1	1	1.7
Roast, Asda*	1 Pack/400g	344	6.4	86	7	11	1.6	2
Roast, Meal for One, M&S*	1 Pack/435g	492	17.8	113	8.1	9.6	4.1	2.4
Roast, Sainsbury's*	1 Pack/450g	354	9	79	6.8	8.4	2	1.9
TURKEY HAM								
Average	1 Serving/75g	81	2.9	108	15.6	2.8	3.9	0
TURKISH DELIGHT								
Fry's*	1 Bar/51g	185	3.4	363	1.2	74	6.7	1.2
Ginger, Shah Baba*	1 Piece/13g	48	0.1	381	1.5	89.7	0.9	0
Milk Chocolate, M&S*	1 Pack/55g	220	4.7	400	1.6	79	8.5	0
Rose, & Lemon, Sainsbury's*	2 Pieces/34g	117	0.2	343	0.5	85.5	0.5	0.5
TURMERIC								
Powder	1 Tsp/3g	11	0.3	354	7.8	58.2	9.9	0
TURNIP								
Boiled, Average	1oz/28g	3	0.1	12	0.6	2	0.2	1.9
Greens, Seasoned, Allen's*	½ Cup/25g	5	0	21	1.7	4.2	0	1.7
Raw, Unprepared, Average	1oz/28g	5	0.1	17	0.7	3.5	0.2	1.8
TURNOVER								
Apple, Bramley, & Cream, Sainsbury's*	1 Turnover/74g	244	14.9	330	4.3	31.6	20.2	2.3
Apple, Bramley, & Cream, Waitrose*	1 Turnover/82g	254	15	309	4.1	31	18.3	2.3
Apple, Co-Op*	1 Turnover/77g	308	20.8	400	4	35	27	1
Apple, Puff Pastry, Bakery, Tesco*	1 Turnover/83g	263	13	317	4.3	38.6	15.7	1.8
Raspberry, Fresh Cream, Asda*	1 Turnover/100g	411	23	411	6	45	23	2.1
Raspberry, Fresh Cream, Tesco*	1 Turnover/74g	244	15.6	330	4.4	29.9	21.1	1.6
Raspberry, with Cream, Sainsbury's*	1 Turnover/65g	222	13.1	342	4.5	34.7	20.2	1.7
TWIGLETS								
Original, Jacob's*	1 Sm Bag/25g	104	3	414	13.3	57.3	12	11.5
TWIRL								
Cadbury*	1 Finger/22g	118	6.8	535	7.6	56	30.9	0.8
Treat Size, Cadbury*	1 Bar/21g	115	6.6	535	7.6	56	30.9	0.8
TWIX								
'Xtra, Mars*	1 Pack/85g	416	20.1	490	4.7	65.5	23.7	1.5
40g, Mars*	1 Finger/20g	99	4.8	493	4.4	65	24	0
Fun Size, Mars*	1 Bar/20g	99	4.8	495	4.5	64.6	24	1.5
Salted Caramel, Mars*	1 Bar/23g	113	5.5	491	4.3	65	24	0

T

	Measure INFO/WEIGHT	per Measure KCAL	FAT	Nutrition Values per 100g / 100ml KCAL	PROT	CARB	FAT	FIBRE
TWIX								
Standard, Mars*	1 Pack/58g	284	13.7	490	4.7	65.5	23.7	1.5
Top, Mars*	1 Bar/28g	143	7.8	511	5.2	60.2	27.7	0
White, Fingers, Mars*	1 Bar/23g	115	5.8	502	4.8	64	25	0
White, Mars*	1 Pack/46g	231	11.5	502	4.8	64	25	0
TZATZIKI								
Average	**1 Tbsp/15g**	**11**	**0.8**	**76**	**3.4**	**3.4**	**5.5**	**0.2**

T

	Measure INFO/WEIGHT	per Measure KCAL	FAT	Nutrition Values per 100g / 100ml KCAL	PROT	CARB	FAT	FIBRE
VANILLA EXTRACT								
Average	**1 Tbsp/13g**	**37**	**0**	**288**	**0.1**	**12.6**	**0.1**	**0**
VEAL								
Chop, Loin, Raw, Weighed with Bone, Average	**1 Chop/195g**	**317**	**17.8**	**163**	**18.9**	**0**	**9.1**	**0**
Escalope, Fried, Average	**1oz/28g**	**55**	**1.9**	**196**	**33.7**	**0**	**6.8**	**0**
Mince, Raw, Average	**1oz/28g**	**40**	**2**	**144**	**20.3**	**0**	**7**	**0**
Shoulder, Lean Only, Roasted, Average	**1oz/28g**	**35**	**1.3**	**125**	**19.9**	**0**	**4.4**	**0**
Sirloin, Lean & Fat, Roasted, Average	**1oz/28g**	**43**	**2.2**	**152**	**18.9**	**0**	**7.8**	**0**
Sirloin, Lean Only, Roasted, Average	**1oz/28g**	**33**	**1.2**	**118**	**18.4**	**0**	**4.4**	**0**
Steak, Osso Bucco, Rose, M&S*	1 Steak/250g	262	5.7	105	21	0.1	2.3	0
with Madeira Sauce, Slow Cooked, Waitrose*	½ Pack/161g	196	7.6	122	19	0.9	4.7	0
VEGAN								
Festive Wreath, Plant Kitchen, M&S*	¼ Pack/180g	432	29.9	240	7.1	10.9	16.6	9.1
Fillets, Quorn*	1 Fillet/63g	58	0.4	92	14.2	3.5	0.6	7.8
Mexican, Ready Meal, Lazy Vegan*	1 Pack/350g	434	15	124	7.7	12	4.3	3.3
Pieces, Vegan, Quorn*	¼ Pack/70g	79	2	113	15.3	3.9	2.8	5.3
Seitan Pieces, Ginger & Soy Marinated, Biona Organic*	1 Serving/100g	92	0.4	92	18.3	3.9	0.4	0.3
Seitan, Original, Alberts*	1 Slice/66g	92	0.5	139	26.6	6	0.7	0
Steak, Sizzle, Gro, Co-Op*	1 Serving/100g	158	4.9	158	12	14	4.9	5.3
Steak, with Garlic Melt, Plant Chef, Tesco*	1 Steak/171g	398	18.3	233	16.9	15.3	10.7	3.6
Veggie, Balls, Waitrose*	4 Balls/80g	118	3.9	148	8.5	15.1	4.9	5.3
VEGEMITE								
Australian, Kraft*	1 Tsp/5g	9	0	173	23.5	19.7	0	0
VEGETABLE CHIPS								
Cassava, Average	**1oz/28g**	**99**	**0.1**	**353**	**1.8**	**91.4**	**0.4**	**4**
Oven Cooked, Aunt Bessie's*	1 Serving/125g	205	11.9	164	2.2	14	9.5	5.8
VEGETABLE FINGERS								
Crispy, Birds Eye*	2 Fingers/60g	107	4.8	179	3.2	23.5	8	2.3
Crispy, Gro, Co-Op*	1 Finger/28g	57	2.3	202	3.9	26	8.3	3.2
Oven Baked, Plant Based, Asda*	2 Fingers/53g	123	4.6	234	4.4	32	8.8	4.2
Plant Chef, Tesco*	3 Fingers/75g	154	6.4	206	4.1	26.4	8.6	3.3
Plant Menu, Aldi*	3 Fingers/85g	211	9.4	248	5.2	29	11	4.8
Sainsbury's*	3 Fingers/79g	191	8.4	243	4.6	30	10.7	4.1
Tesco*	1 Finger/25g	52	2.2	206	4.1	26.4	8.6	3.3
VEGETABLE MEDLEY								
Broccoli, Carrot, & Brussel Sprout, Nature's Pick, Aldi*	1 Serving/80g	27	0.8	34	2.3	4	1	2.5
Broccoli, Romanesco, Peas, & Spinach, Birds Eye*	1 Bag/150g	76	0.8	51	4	5.4	0.5	4.3
Buttery, Asda*	½ Pack/143g	86	4.1	60	2.3	4.5	2.9	3.2
Cauliflower, & Broccoli, Florets, Oaklands, Lidl*	1 Serving/80g	23	0.6	29	2.6	3.2	0.7	2.4
Chargrilled, Waitrose*	1 Serving/100g	77	3	77	2.5	8.3	3	3.3
Colourful, Waitrose*	½ Pack/171g	60	0.9	35	1.9	5.1	0.5	1.6
Country Mix, As Sold, Morrisons*	1 Serving/80g	30	0.1	37	2.5	4.7	0.1	3.5
Five, Tesco*	¼ Pack/115g	45	0.6	39	1.9	5.1	0.5	3.4
Floret, & Carrot, Mix, Boiled, Iceland*	1 Serving/80g	9	0.2	11	0.7	1.4	0.2	0.8
Four Seasons, Aldi*	1 Serving/80g	38	0.7	48	3.1	5.6	0.9	2.6
Frozen, M&S*	1 Pack/500g	175	4	35	3.4	3.9	0.8	3.1
Green Grocers, Lidl*	1 Serving/80g	22	0.4	28	1.6	2.8	0.5	2.7
Green, Microwaved, Extra Special, Asda*	½ Pack/74g	53	3.1	72	3.1	2.8	4.2	5.1
Green, Peas, Broccoli, & Kale, with Salted Butter, Tesco*	½ Pack/125g	105	4.6	84	5.2	3.1	3.7	8.5
Green, with Bouillon Butter, Co-Op*	1 Serving/80g	54	2.4	67	3.5	4.8	3	3.2
Grilled, Essential, Waitrose*	1 Serving/81g	38	0.2	47	1.8	8.1	0.3	2.4
Hearty Farmhouse Mix, SteamFresh, Birds Eye*	1 Bag/135g	46	0.8	34	1.8	4.2	0.6	2.5
Medley, Tender, Green, Sainsbury's*	1 Pack/160g	62	0.8	39	2.9	4.3	0.5	3.6
Mixed, Special, Sainsbury's*	1 Serving/80g	48	0.9	60	3.5	7	1.1	4

V

	INFO/WEIGHT		KCAL	FAT	KCAL	PROT	CARB	FAT	FIBRE
VEGETABLE MEDLEY									
Mixed, Tesco*	½ Pack/112g		46	0.6	41	2.3	4.9	0.5	3.8
Potatoes, Green Beans, & Peas, with Dressing, Tesco*	½ Pack/175g		156	2.8	89	2.7	14.9	1.6	2.4
Roasted, Waitrose*	½ Pack/200g		282	15.6	141	1.2	16.4	7.8	3.7
Runner Bean, & Mixed Veg Selection, M&S*	½ Pouch/100g		36	0.5	36	2.9	3.1	0.5	3.6
Seasonal, Morrisons*	1 Pot/200g		66	0.4	33	0.9	6.5	0.2	1.1
Tender, Ready to Cook, Tesco*	1 Serving/80g		27	0.2	34	2.9	3.5	0.3	2.7
with Parsley Butter, 1141, Wiltshire Farm Foods*	1 Serving/110g		97	7.8	88	1.8	3.4	7.1	0
VEGETABLES									
Carrot, Cauliflower, & Broccoli, Fresh, Mixed, Tesco*	1 Pack/370g		148	1.5	40	1.6	5.9	0.4	3.4
Greens, Boiled, Sklavenitis*	½ Pack/200g		262	25.2	131	1.4	1.4	12.6	6.1
Grilled, Frozen, Sainsbury's*	1 Serving/80g		42	2.9	52	1.2	3.8	3.6	1.5
Mediterranean Style, Roast, Nature's Pick, Aldi*	½ Pack/200g		114	6.4	57	1.2	5.2	3.2	1.5
Mediterranean, Chunky, Cooked, Sainsbury's*	¼ Pack/119g		56	2	47	1.1	5.9	1.7	2
Mediterranean, Roasting, Waitrose*	½ Pack/200g		96	4.6	48	1.4	4.9	2.3	1.4
Mediterranean, Roasting, with Dressing, M&S*	¼ Pack/165g		58	1.5	35	1	4.7	0.9	2.1
Peas, Spinach, Spring Greens, & Samphire, M&S*	½ Pack/105g		85	4.4	81	3.8	4.7	4.2	4.6
Peppers, Mixed, Stir Fry, Tesco*	1 Pack/320g		173	9	54	1.6	4.4	2.8	2.4
Roasted, & Pasta, M&S*	½ Pack/157g		295	15.9	188	7.2	16	10.1	2
Roasting, with Rosemary, & Thyme, Tesco*	1 Serving/100g		119	3.1	119	1.3	18	3.1	7
Root, Mashed, Microwaved, Growers Selection, Asda*	½ Pack/200g		116	4.4	58	0.7	7.2	2.2	2.7
Root, Rainbow, Collection, M&S*	½ Pack/176g		67	2.5	38	0.7	3.9	1.4	3.6
Root, Roasted, Extra Special, Asda*	½ Pack/205g		160	3.1	78	1.1	15	1.5	6
Root, Roasted, Ready to Roast, Mash Direct*	1 Pack/350g		200	7.4	57	0.8	5.8	2.1	5.9
Selection, Roasted, COU, M&S*	1 Pack/250g		88	2	35	1.2	6.1	0.8	0.6
Stir Fry, Frozen, Sainsbury's*	1 Serving/80g		19	0.2	24	1.3	3.9	0.3	2
Stir Fry, Oriental, Nature's Pick, Aldi*	1 Pack/300g		123	1.5	41	1.8	6.8	0.5	2
VEGETABLES MIXED									
Baby Corn, & Vegetable Selection, Eat Well, M&S*	½ Pack/100g		38	0.5	38	2.3	4.5	0.5	3.3
Baby Courgette, & Mixed Veg Selection, M&S*	½ Pack/100g		29	0.4	29	2	3.3	0.4	2.3
Broccoli, Peas & Green Beans, Mixed, Co-Op*	1 Serving/80g		36	0.3	45	4.8	3.8	0.4	3.6
Carrot, Cauliflower & Broccoli, Mixed, Waitrose*	1 Serving/80g		32	0.5	40	2.4	4.9	0.6	2.9
Carrot, Cauliflower & Broccoli, Prepared, Mixed, Co-Op*	1 Pack/250g		100	1.5	40	2.4	5	0.6	2.7
Carrot, Cauliflower, & Broccoli, Steam Bags, Aldi*	1 Bag/160g		54	1	34	1.6	4.6	0.6	2
Carrots, Peas, Green Beans & Sweetcorn, Mixed, Tesco*	1 Serving/80g		47	0.8	58	3.3	6.9	1	4.3
Carrots, Peas, Green Beans, & Sweetcorn, Morrisons*	1 Serving/80g		40	0.2	50	2.5	7.5	0.3	3.9
Casserole with Baby Potatoes, Fresh, Mixed, M&S*	½ Pack/350g		140	1	40	1.2	7.8	0.3	2.1
Casserole, Mixed, Tesco*	1 Serving/80g		35	0.2	44	1	7.9	0.3	2.6
Farmhouse, Mixed, Frozen, Boiled in Salted Water, Tesco*	1 Serving/80g		41	0.7	51	3.2	5.7	0.9	3.5
Italian Style, Seasoned, Frozen, Freshona, Lidl*	¼ Pack/188g		90	5.6	48	1.6	2.8	3	1.9
Mediterranean Style, Oven Cooked, Fire Pit, Tesco*	1 Serving/91g		66	2.9	73	1.8	8.3	3.2	2
Mediterranean, Chargrilled, Frozen, Sainsbury's*	1 Serving/80g		81	1.6	101	2.9	15.7	2	4.3
Mediterranean, Roasting, Cooked, Tesco*	½ Pack/200g		56	0.4	28	1	5.2	0.2	0.9
Mediterranean, Tray, Oven Baked, Asda*	½ Pack/133g		57	1.5	43	1.4	6	1.1	1.4
Mix, Steamer, Love Life, Waitrose*	1 Bag/160g		83	1.8	52	2.8	7.7	1.1	2.8
Mixed, Freshly Frozen, Iceland*	1 Serving/100g		54	0.8	54	3.3	8.3	0.8	3.7
Mixed, Frozen, Cooked, Sainsbury's*	1 Serving/80g		45	0.6	56	2.9	7.5	0.7	4
Mixed, Layered, Classics, M&S*	½ Pack/160g		112	6.2	70	1.2	7.3	3.9	1.2
Peas & Carrots, Buttery & Tender, Mixed, Tesco*	½ Pack/150g		138	6.1	92	3.7	7.9	4.1	4.5
Peas, Cabbage, & Tenderstem, Layers, Waitrose*	1/3 Pack/83g		85	4.2	103	6.2	6.2	5	4
Peas, Carrots, & Sweetcorn, Pepper & Butter, Tesco*	½ Pack/178g		128	4.4	72	2.8	7.6	2.5	3.9
Roasting, Selection, Sweet & Colourful, Waitrose*	½ Pack/300g		147	3	49	1	7.5	1	2.8
Root, Diced, Tesco*	1/3 Pack/240g		120	0.7	50	0.6	9.3	0.3	3.6
Stir Fry, Peppers, Mixed, Nature's Pick, Aldi*	1 Serving/80g		27	0.4	34	1.7	5	0.5	1.8

	Measure INFO/WEIGHT	per Measure KCAL	FAT	Nutrition Values per 100g / 100ml KCAL	PROT	CARB	FAT	FIBRE
VEGETABLES MIXED								
Tenderstem, & Mixed Vegetables, Tesco*	½ Pack/80g	54	0.6	34	2.1	4.2	0.4	2.6
VEGETARIAN								
Chunks, Pulled, Pea Protein, Vegini*	1 Pack/140g	308	14	220	26	4.2	10	4.5
Galette, Vegetale, le Bistrot, Sojasun*	1 Galette/90g	189	8	210	17	13	8.9	5
Roast, Nut & Date, with Gravy, Asda*	1 Serving/196g	300	12.7	153	4.7	16.1	6.5	5.5
Schnitzel, Breaded, Tivall*	1 Schnitzel/100g	202	9.5	202	16	11	9.5	4
Schnitzel, Cheese, Jumbo Lekker Veggie*	1 Schnitzel/100g	229	10.2	229	10.1	23.9	10.2	0.7
Slices, Peppered , Tofurky*	5 Slices/52g	100	3.5	192	25	9.6	6.7	1.9
Slices, Sage & Onion, VBites Foods Ltd*	1 Slice/10g	23	1.4	234	21.3	5.2	14.1	0.6
Slices, Sage & Onion, Vegi Deli, The Redwood Co*	1 Slice/10g	23	1.4	233	21.4	5	14.1	0.5
Steak, Beef Style, Quorn*	1 Steak/86g	126	4.5	146	16	5.3	5.2	6.9
Steak, Soya, & Wheat, Barbecue, Cereal*	1 Veg Steak/80g	160	7.7	200	19	6.3	9.6	6.2
Steak, Vivera*	1 Steak/100g	195	10	195	18	6.3	10	4.6
Strips, BBQ, Quorn*	½ Pack/140g	183	4.1	131	14.3	8.4	2.9	6.8
Strips, Sweet, & Smoky, Quorn*	3 Strips/92g	171	3.3	186	10.6	25.1	3.6	5.5
VEGETARIAN MINCE								
Beef, Ground, Plant Based, Beyond Meat*	¼ Pack/113g	260	18	230	17.7	4.4	15.9	1.8
Beefless, Alt*	¼ Pack/90g	140	3.9	156	24	2.1	4.4	5.6
Frozen, Plant Chef, Tesco*	1/6 Pack/70g	88	1.2	126	17.1	9.9	1.7	1.4
Meat Free, As Sold, The Meatless Farm Co*	1 Pack/400g	796	40.8	199	19.3	7.8	10.2	4.9
Meat Free, Improved Recipe, Frozen Sainsbury's*	1 Serving/77g	131	3.9	170	18.6	11.7	5	2
Meat Free, No Beef, As Sold, Richmond*	¼ Pack/84g	161	5.3	192	22	10	6.3	3.5
Moving Mountains*	½ Pack/130g	318	22.1	245	16	5.6	17	5.3
Mushroom, Meat Free, Bolognese, Aldi*	½ Pack/85g	56	3.7	66	2.5	3.3	4.4	1.6
No Beef, As Sold, Plant Pioneers, Sainsbury's*	½ Pack/110g	182	8.5	165	10.8	10.6	7.7	5.2
No Meat, Plant Kitchen, M&S*	½ Pack/90g	110	2.9	122	16.1	4.3	3.2	5.7
Pea Protein, Fry's*	1 Serving/100g	127	1.6	127	24	5	1.6	0.5
Plant Based, Tender, Gro, Co-Op*	1 Serving/125g	168	4.4	134	20	1.4	3.5	7.5
Plant Based, Without Meat, Lidl*	½ Pack/138g	308	19.9	224	17.9	4.8	14.5	3.7
Simply, Garden Gourmet*	1 Serving/80g	119	2.4	149	19.3	6.9	3	8.8
Vegan, Meat Free, Ocado*	¼ Pack/128g	115	0.6	90	15	3.7	0.5	5.8
Vegan, Plant, Vivera*	1 Pack/220g	277	1.3	126	20	7.2	0.6	5.8
Vegemince, Fried, Linda McCartney*	1/6 Pack/70g	119	3	171	19.9	11.7	4.3	3.2
Vegemince, Realeat*	1 Serving/125g	218	12.5	174	18	3	10	3
Vegetarian, Mince, Frozen & Chilled, Quorn*	1 Serving/87g	80	1.5	92	13	2.3	1.7	7.5
VENISON								
Grill Steak, Average	**1 Steak/150g**	**178**	**3.8**	**119**	**19**	**5**	**2.5**	**1**
in Red Wine & Port, Average	**1oz/28g**	**21**	**0.7**	**76**	**9.8**	**3.5**	**2.6**	**0.4**
Minced, Cooked, Average	**1 Serving/100g**	**187**	**8.2**	**187**	**26.4**	**0**	**8.2**	**0**
Minced, Raw, Average	**1 Serving/100g**	**157**	**7.1**	**157**	**21.8**	**0**	**7.1**	**0**
Raw, Haunch, Meat Only, Average	**1 Serving/100g**	**103**	**1.6**	**103**	**22.2**	**0**	**1.6**	**0**
Roasted, Average	**1oz/28g**	**46**	**0.7**	**165**	**35.6**	**0**	**2.5**	**0**
Steak, Raw, Average	**1oz/28g**	**30**	**0.5**	**108**	**22.8**	**0**	**1.9**	**0**
VERMICELLI								
Dry	**1oz/28g**	**99**	**0.1**	**355**	**8.7**	**78.3**	**0.4**	**0**
Egg, Cooked, Average	**1 Serving/185g**	**239**	**2.6**	**129**	**5**	**24**	**1.4**	**1**
VERMOUTH								
Alcohol Free, Versin*	1 Serve/50ml	32	0	64	0	16	0	0
Dry	**1 Shot/50ml**	**54**	**0**	**109**	**0.1**	**3**	**0**	**0**
Sweet	**1 Shot/50ml**	**76**	**0**	**151**	**0**	**15.9**	**0**	**0**
VIMTO*								
Cordial, No Added Sugar, Undiluted, Vimto*	1 Serving/50ml	2	0	4	0	0.7	0	0
Grape, Blackcurrant & Raspberry Drink, Fizzy, Vimto*	1 Can/330ml	147	0	44	0	11	0	0

V

	Measure INFO/WEIGHT	per Measure KCAL	FAT	Nutrition Values per 100g / 100ml KCAL	PROT	CARB	FAT	FIBRE
VIMTO*								
Mango, Strawberry & Pineapple, Remix, Diluted, Vimto*	1 Serving/200ml	4	0	2	0	0.2	0	0
Raspberry, Orange & Passionfruit, Remix, Diluted, Vimto*	1 Serving/200ml	4	0	2	0	0.2	0	0
VINAIGRETTE								
Balsamic Vinegar & Pistachio, Finest, Tesco*	1 Tbsp/15ml	56	5.9	370	0.2	2.8	39.2	0
Balsamic, Hellmann's*	1 Tbsp/15ml	12	0.4	82	0.1	9.6	2.7	0.6
Balsamic, Specially Selected, Aldi*	1 Tbsp/15ml	44	3.9	293	0.5	15	26	0.5
Classic, Mellow Yellow, Farrington's*	1 Tbsp/15ml	92	9.9	614	1.1	3.9	66.1	0
Fat free vinaigrette , Bramwells, Aldi*	1 Tbsp/15ml	9	0.1	59	0.5	13.8	0.5	0.5
Fat Free, Hellmann's*	1 Tbsp/15ml	8	0.1	48	0.5	11	0.5	0
French Style, Finest, Tesco*	1 Tbsp/15ml	93	9.8	620	0.6	6.3	65.3	0.2
Garlic, & Chives, Fat Free, Hellmann's*	1 Tbsp/15ml	5	0.1	36	0.5	7.7	0.5	0
Light, Dressing, Asda*	1 Tbsp/15ml	6	0.1	38	0.5	7.2	0.6	1.7
Olive Oil & Lemon, Amoy*	1 Tbsp/15ml	38	3.6	250	0.3	3	24	0
PB, Waitrose*	1 Tbsp/15ml	13	0.1	89	0.4	20.9	0.4	0.5
Rhubarb, & Vinegar, The Little Herb Farm*	1 Tbsp/15ml	21	0	139	0.3	33.9	0	0.5
Shallot, & Red Wine, Maille*	1 Serving/30ml	103	10.5	344	0.5	5	35	0
VINDALOO								
Chicken, Average	**1 Serving/410g**	**787**	**51.2**	**192**	**18.5**	**2.6**	**12.5**	**0.3**
Chicken, Takeaway, Iceland*	1 Pack/351g	548	31.9	156	10.8	6.1	9.1	3
Volcanic, Takeaway, Morrisons*	½ Pack/175g	205	9.8	117	10.7	5.1	5.6	2
VINE LEAVES								
Stuffed with Rice	**1oz/28g**	**73**	**5**	**262**	**2.8**	**23.8**	**18**	**0**
VINEGAR								
Balsamic, Average	**1 Tsp/5ml**	**6**	**0**	**115**	**0.9**	**26**	**0**	**0**
Balsamic, with Garilc, Heinz*	1 Serving/15ml	12	0.6	82	0.4	10.3	4.3	0
Cider	**1 Tbsp/15ml**	**2**	**0**	**14**	**0**	**5.9**	**0**	**0**
Malt, Average	**1 Tbsp/15g**	**1**	**0**	**4**	**0.4**	**0.6**	**0**	**0**
Red Wine, Average	**1 Tbsp/15ml**	**3**	**0**	**19**	**0**	**0.3**	**0**	**0**
Rice Wine, Tesco*	1 Tbsp/15ml	2	0.1	11	0.1	1.2	0.5	0.5
Rice, Japanese, Yutaka*	1 Serving/15ml	4	0.1	24	0.5	5.8	0.5	0.5
VODKA								
& Diet Coke, Average	**1 Serving/150ml**	**68**	**0**	**45**	**0**	**0**	**0**	**0**
& Tonic, Ready Mixed, M&S*	1 Can/250ml	202	0	81	0	6.3	0	0
37.5% Volume	**1 Pub Shot/35ml**	**72**	**0**	**207**	**0**	**0**	**0**	**0**
40% Volume	**1 Pub Shot/35ml**	**78**	**0**	**222**	**0**	**0**	**0**	**0**
Clean V, Non-Alcoholic, 0.5%, Clean Co.*	1 Serve/50ml	10	0	20	0	4.1	0	0
Rhubarb, Average	**1 Single/25ml**	**57**	**0**	**229**	**0**	**0**	**0**	**0**
Smirnoff & Cranberry, Premixed, Canned, Diageo*	1 Can/250ml	175	0	70	0	8.5	0	0
Smirnoff & Diet Cola, Premixed, Canned, Diageo*	1 Can/250ml	100	0	40	0	0	0	0
Smirnoff & Schweppes Tonic, Premixed, Canned, Diageo*	1 Can/250ml	158	0	63	0	6.4	0	0
Vanilla, Absolut*	1 Shot/25ml	55	0	221	0	0	0	0
VOL AU VENTS								
Deluxe, Lidl*	1 Pastry/7g	40	2.8	567	7.8	41.5	40.7	1.5
Mushroom, Sainsbury's*	1 Serving/14g	49	3.1	350	6.9	30.8	22.1	1.4
Seafood, Party, Youngs*	1 Serving/17g	60	4.2	354	8.3	26	24.8	1

V

	Measure INFO/WEIGHT	per Measure KCAL	FAT	Nutrition Values per 100g / 100ml KCAL	PROT	CARB	FAT	FIBRE
WAFERS								
Caramel, Dark Chocolate, Tunnock's*	1 Wafer/30g	148	7.6	492	5.2	60.7	25.4	0
Caramel, Log, Tunnock's*	1 Wafer/32g	150	6.7	468	4.2	65.7	21	3.4
Caramel, Tunnock's*	1 Wafer/30g	134	5.2	448	3.6	69.2	17.4	2.5
Chocolate, Sugar Free, Gullon*	1 Wafer/9g	39	2	434	4.4	68	22	3.4
for Ice Cream, Askeys*	1 Wafer/2g	6	0	388	11.4	79	2.9	0
WAFFLES								
Belgian, Sugar, Aldi*	1 Waffle/55g	249	12.6	452	5.7	54	23	2
Belgian, TTD, Sainsbury's*	1 Waffle/25g	122	7.3	490	6	50.6	29.3	1.2
Caramel, Asda*	1 Waffle/8g	37	1.8	459	3.3	62	22	1.1
Caramel, M&S*	1 Waffle/33g	154	6.2	473	3.3	71.7	18.9	1.2
Choco-Sugar, Waffle Amour*	1 Waffle/60g	287	16.3	478	5.9	51.3	27.1	0
Chocolate, Toastie, McVitie's*	1 Waffle/25g	114	6.3	458	6.7	50.3	25.2	2.6
Classic, Frozen, Hello Morning, Birds Eye*	1 Waffle/30g	97	4.3	319	7	40	14	2.6
Filled, Chocolate & Hazelnut, Village Bakery, Aldi*	1 Waffle/34g	169	9.9	497	6.2	52.9	29.1	1.5
Stroop, Caramel, Mini, Daelmans*	1 Waffle/7g	29	1.1	421	3.5	65	16	1.5
Stroopwafel, Caramel, Daelmans*	1 Wafel/29g	131	6.1	452	3	62	21	1.5
Sugar, Rowan Hill Bakery, Lidl*	1 Waffle/55g	246	12.7	447	6.2	53	23	1.7
Sweet, American Style, Sainsbury's*	1 Waffle/35g	160	8.9	457	7.2	50.6	25.3	1.1
Toasting, McVitie's*	1 Waffle/25g	115	6.3	461	5.7	52.6	25.5	0.8
WAGON WHEEL								
Jammie, Burton's*	1 Biscuit/40g	168	5.6	420	5.1	67.7	14.1	1.9
WALNUT WHIP								
Classic, M&S*	1 Whip/28g	144	8.1	515	6.8	55.8	28.9	2
Nestle*	1 Whip/35g	173	8.8	494	5.3	61.3	25.2	0.7
WALNUTS								
Average	**1 Nut/7g**	**48**	**4.8**	**688**	**14.7**	**3.3**	**68.5**	**3.5**
Halves, Average	**1 Half/3g**	**23**	**2.3**	**669**	**17.4**	**6.3**	**65**	**4.7**
Pickled, in Malt Vinegar, Drained, Opies*	1 Walnut/25g	23	0	92	0.8	23	0	3.4
WASABI								
Paste, Ready Mixed, Japanese, Yutaka*	1 Tsp/5g	14	0.4	286	2.7	53	7	0
WATER								
Apple, & Raspberry, Sparkling, Spring, Tesco*	1 Glass/330ml	7	0	2	0	0.5	0	0
Apple, & Strawberry, Flavoured, Morrisons*	1 Serving/200ml	3	0	2	0.2	0.1	0	0
Cherry, & Plum, Flavoured, Asda*	1 Serving/250ml	2	0	1	0	0.5	0	0
Citrus, Apple, & Mint, Protein, Vieve*	1 Bottle/500ml	85	0	17	4	0	0	0
Coconut, Sparkling, Natural, Coco fusion 100*	1 Can/250ml	60	0	24	0	5.9	0	0
Coconut, with Kefir, Canned, Remedy*	1 Can/250ml	5	1.2	2	0.5	1.6	0.5	0.5
Elderflower, Presse, Sparkling, M&S*	1 Bottle/330ml	99	0.3	30	0.1	7.4	0.1	0.5
Lemon & Lime, Flavoured, Sparkling, Spring, Sainsbury's*	1 Glass/250ml	4	0.2	2	0.1	0.1	0.1	0.1
Lemon & Lime, Sugar Free, Touch of Fruit, Volvic*	1 Bottle/150ml	2	0	1	0	0	0	0
Lemon & Lime, Sparkling, M&S*	1 Bottle/500ml	15	0	3	0	0.4	0	0
Mineral Or Tap	**1 Glass/200ml**	**0**	**0**	**0**	**0**	**0**	**0**	**0**
Peach, & Raspberry, Still, M&S*	1 Bottle/500ml	10	0	2	0	0	0	0
Peach, & Passion Fruit, Sparkling, Tesco*	1 Glass/250ml	5	0	2	0	0.3	0	0
Peach, & Raspberry, Protein, Vieve*	1 Bottle/500ml	90	0	18	4	0	0	0
Sparkling, Lemon & Lime, Aquaroma*	1 Glass/250ml	2	0	1	0	0	0	0
Sparkling, San Pellegrino*	1 Glass/200ml	0	0	0	0	0	0	0
Sparkling, Smart Price, Asda*	1 Glass/300ml	0	0	0	0	0	0	0
Sparkling, Triple Berry, Ugly Brands Inc*	1 Can/330ml	3	0	1	0	0	0	0
Sparkling, with Touch of Raspberry, Dash*	1 Can/330ml	0	0	0	0	0	0	0
Still, Highland Spring*	1 Bottle/750ml	0	0	0	0	0	0	0
Strawberry, & Guava, Still, M&S*	1 Glass/250ml	5	0	2	0	0.1	0	0
Strawberry, & Kiwi, Still, Sainsbury's*	1 Serving/200ml	8	0	4	1	0	0	0

W

	Measure INFO/WEIGHT	per Measure KCAL	FAT	Nutrition Values per 100g / 100ml KCAL	PROT	CARB	FAT	FIBRE
WATER								
Strawberry, Sparkling, Spring, Tesco*	1 Bottle/1000g	20	0	2	0	0.2	0	0
Strawberry, Sugar Free, Touch of Fruit, Volvic*	1 Bottle/500ml	7	0	1	0	0.1	0	0
WATER CHESTNUTS								
Raw, Average	**1oz/28g**	**8**	**0**	**29**	**0.8**	**6.6**	**0**	**0.1**
WATERCRESS								
Raw, Trimmed, Average	**1 Sprig/2.5g**	**1**	**0**	**22**	**3**	**0.4**	**1**	**1.5**
WATERMELON								
Flesh Only, Average	**1 Serving/250g**	**75**	**0.8**	**30**	**0.4**	**7**	**0.3**	**0.4**
Raw	**1 Wedge/286g**	**48**	**0.6**	**17**	**0.3**	**3.7**	**0.2**	**0.3**
Raw, Weighed with Skin, Average	**1 Wedge/286g**	**49**	**0.5**	**17**	**0.2**	**4**	**0.2**	**0.2**
WELLINGTON								
Beef, Christmas, M&S*	1 Serving/150g	315	13.4	210	13.6	18	8.9	1.5
Beef, Fillet, Deluxe, Lidl*	1 Wellington/297g	659	35.3	222	8.8	19.4	11.9	1.2
Beetroot, Vegan, Waitrose*	1 Wellington/187g	411	23.2	220	4.2	21.5	12.4	2.6
Lentil, & Spinach, Easy to Cook, Waitrose*	1 Wellington/180g	499	26.5	277	5.5	29.6	14.7	2.2
Mushroom, Creamy, The Best, Morrisons*	1 Wellington/169g	439	27.9	260	5.8	20.8	16.5	2.6
Mushroom, M&S*	½ Pack/305g	805	52.8	264	4.8	21	17.3	2.3
Portabello Mushroom, Vegetarian, Tesco*	¼ Pack/117g	268	12.2	229	5.1	27.6	10.4	2
WHEAT BRAN								
Average	**1 Tbsp/7g**	**14**	**0.4**	**206**	**14.1**	**26.8**	**5.5**	**36.4**
WHISKY								
& Cola, Premixed, White Label, 500ml, Jim Beam*	1 Bottle /500ml	254	0	51	0	4.5	0	0
37.5% Volume	**1 Pub Shot/35ml**	**72**	**0**	**207**	**0**	**0**	**0**	**0**
40% Volume	**1 Pub Shot/35ml**	**78**	**0**	**222**	**0**	**0**	**0**	**0**
Scots, 37.5% Volume	**1 Pub Shot/35ml**	**72**	**0**	**207**	**0**	**0**	**0**	**0**
Scots, 40% Volume	**1 Pub Shot/35ml**	**78**	**0**	**224**	**0**	**0**	**0**	**0**
Tennessee Apple, 35%, Jack Daniel's*	1 Pub Shot/35ml	86	0	245	0	0	0	0
Tennessee Fire, 35%, Jack Daniel's*	1 Pub Shot/35ml	86	0	245	0	0	0	0
Tennessee Honey, 35%, Jack Daniel's*	1 Pub Shot/35ml	86	0	245	0	13.3	0	0
WHITE PUDDING								
Average	**1oz/28g**	**126**	**8.9**	**450**	**7**	**36.3**	**31.8**	**0**
WHITEBAIT								
in Flour, Fried	**1oz/28g**	**147**	**13.3**	**525**	**19.5**	**5.3**	**47.5**	**0.2**
Raw, Average	**1 Serving/100g**	**172**	**11**	**172**	**18.3**	**0**	**11**	**0**
WHITING								
in Crumbs, Fried in Blended Oil	**1 Serving/180g**	**344**	**18.5**	**191**	**18.1**	**7**	**10.3**	**0.2**
Raw	**1oz/28g**	**23**	**0.2**	**81**	**18.7**	**0**	**0.7**	**0**
Steamed	**1 Serving/85g**	**78**	**0.8**	**92**	**20.9**	**0**	**0.9**	**0**
WIENER SCHNITZEL								
Average	**1oz/28g**	**62**	**2.8**	**223**	**20.9**	**13.1**	**10**	**0.4**
WINE								
0% Alcohol, Freixenet*	1 Glass/125ml	31	0	25	0	6	0	0
Cava Rosado, Tesco*	1 Glass/125ml	139	0	111	0	0	0	0
Fruit, Average	**1 Glass/125ml**	**115**	**0**	**92**	**0**	**5.5**	**0**	**0**
Madeira, Henriques & Henriques*	1 Glass/125ml	162	0	130	0	0	0	0
Mead, Average	**1 Glass/125ml**	**193**	**0**	**155**	**0**	**17.4**	**0**	**0**
Mulled, Homemade, Average	**1 Glass/125ml**	**245**	**0**	**196**	**0.1**	**25.2**	**0**	**0**
Nosecco , Alcohol Free, Asda*	1 Glass/125ml	35	0.6	28	0.5	7	0.5	0
Nozecco, Sparkling, Non Alcoholic, Nozeco*	1 Sm Glass/125ml	25	0.1	20	0.1	5	0.1	0
Original, Lambrini*	1 Glass/125ml	88	0	70	0	0	0	0
Red, Amarone, Average*	**1 Glass/125ml**	**120**	**0**	**96**	**0.1**	**3**	**0**	**0**
Red, Australian, 13.5%, 19 Crimes*	1 Glass/125ml	110	0	88	0	0	0	0
Red, Average	**1 Glass/125ml**	**104**	**0**	**83**	**0**	**2**	**0**	**0**

W

WINE	Measure INFO/WEIGHT	per Measure KCAL	FAT	Nutrition Values per 100g / 100ml KCAL	PROT	CARB	FAT	FIBRE
Red, Beaujolais Villages, Louis Jadot*	1 Glass/125ml	156	0	125	0	4	0	0
Red, Burgundy, 12.9% Abv, Average	*1 Glass/125ml*	*110*	*0*	*88*	*0.1*	*3.7*	*0*	*0*
Red, Cabernet Sauvignon, 13.1% Abv, Average	*1 Glass/125ml*	*105*	*0*	*84*	*0.1*	*2.6*	*0*	*0*
Red, Cabernet Sauvignon, Alcohol Free, Lindemans*	1 Glass/125ml	21	0	17	0	3.5	0	0
Red, Cabernet Tempranillo, Low Alcohol, Tesco*	1 Glass/125ml	78	0	62	0	14.7	0	0
Red, Claret, 12.8% Abv, Average	*1 Glass/125ml*	*105*	*0*	*84*	*0.1*	*3*	*0*	*0*
Red, De-Alcoholised, 0.0%, Sangre De Toro*	1 Glass/125ml	29	0	23	0	3.5	0	0
Red, Gamay, 12.3% Abv, Average	*1 Glass/125ml*	*99*	*0*	*79*	*0.1*	*2.4*	*0*	*0*
Red, Garnacha Syrah, De-Alcoholised, Natureo, Torres*	1 Glass/125ml	29	0	23	0	3.5	0	0
Red, Merlot, 13.3% Abv, Average	*1 Glass/125ml*	*105*	*0*	*84*	*0.1*	*2.5*	*0*	*0*
Red, Merlot, Alcohol Free, Vintense*	1 Glass/125ml	21	0	17	0	3.9	0	0
Red, Merlot, Red Grape, Alcohol Free, M&S*	1 Glass/125ml	55	0.1	44	0.2	10.7	0.1	0.1
Red, Non Alcoholic, Ame*	1 Glass/125ml	42	0	34	0	5.7	0	0
Red, Petit Sirah, 13.5% Abv, Average	*1 Glass/125ml*	*108*	*0*	*86*	*0.1*	*2.7*	*0*	*0*
Red, Pinot Noir, 13% Abv, Average	*1 Glass/125ml*	*104*	*0*	*83*	*0.1*	*2.3*	*0*	*0*
Red, Sangiovese, 13.6% Abv, Average	*1 Glass/125ml*	*109*	*0*	*87*	*0.1*	*2.6*	*0*	*0*
Red, Shiraz, 10.8%, Fair Trade, Co-Op*	1 Glass/125ml	96	0	77	0	0	0	0
Red, Shiraz, Alcohol Free, Zero, McGuigan*	1 Glass/125ml	36	0.2	29	0.3	7	0.2	0
Red, Shiraz, Grapevine, Aldi*	1 Glass/125ml	94	0	75	0	1	0	0
Red, Shiraz, Sumika, M&S*	1 Glass/125ml	65	0	52	0	0	0	0
Red, Shiraz, Unvined, Alcohol Removed, Jacob's Creek*	1 Glass/150ml	25	0	17	0	3.7	0	0
Red, Syrah, 13.1% Abv, Average	*1 Glass/125ml*	*105*	*0*	*84*	*0.1*	*2.6*	*0*	*0*
Red, Zinfandel, 13.9% Abv, Average	*1 Glass/125ml*	*111*	*0*	*89*	*0.1*	*2.9*	*0*	*0*
Rose, Alcohol Free, Eisberg*	1 Glass/125ml	32	0	26	0	5.9	0	0
Rose, Dealcoholised, Delight, McGuigan*	1 Glass/125ml	34	0.1	27	0.2	6	0.1	0
Rose, Fizzero, Sparkling, Zero Alcohol, M&S*	1 Glass/125ml	28	0	22	0	5.2	0	0
Rose, Garnacha, Low Alcohol, Tesco*	1 Glass/125ml	78	0	62	0	14.7	0	0
Rose, Medium, Average	*1 Glass/125ml*	*98*	*0*	*79*	*0*	*2.1*	*0*	*0*
Rose, Muscat, Non Alcoholic, Co-Op*	1 Glass/125ml	55	0	44	0	11	0	0
Rose, Sparkling, Average	*1 Glass/125ml*	*102*	*0*	*82*	*0*	*2.5*	*0*	*0*
Rose, The Pink Chill, Co-Op*	1 Glass/125ml	85	0	68	0	0	0	0
Rose, White Grenache, Blossom Hill*	1 Glass/125ml	105	0	84	0	3.2	0	0
Rose, White Zinfandel, Barefoot*	1 Glass/125ml	74	0	60	0	0	0	0
Rose, White Zinfandel, Ernest & Julio Gallo*	1 Glass/125ml	101	0	81	0.2	2.7	0	0
Sangria, Average	*1 Glass/125ml*	*95*	*0*	*76*	*0.1*	*9.9*	*0*	*0.1*
Summer Berry, Fruit Fusion, Three Mills*	1 Glass/125ml	60	0	48	0	0	0	0
Vie, Rose, Low Alcohol, Blossom Hill*	1 Glass/125ml	66	0	53	0	3.9	0	0
White, Average	*1 Glass/125ml*	*95*	*0*	*76*	*0*	*2.4*	*0*	*0*
White, Chablis, Las Terrasse*	1 Glass/125ml	102	0	82	0	0	0	0
White, Chardonnay, 0.5% ABV, Artis*	1 Glass/125ml	25	0.6	20	0.5	4.4	0.5	0
White, Chardonnay, Alcohol Free, Vintense*	1 Glass/125ml	22	0	18	0	4.1	0	0
White, Chardonnay, Alcohol Removed, Fre*	1 Glass/125ml	33	0	26	0	7.5	0	0
White, Chenin Blanc, 12% Abv, Average	*1 Glass/125ml*	*101*	*0*	*81*	*0.1*	*3.3*	*0*	*0*
White, Cotes De Gascogne Blanc, Tesco*	1 Glass/125ml	80	0	64	0	0.3	0	0
White, De-Alcoholised, 0.0%, Sangre De Toro*	1 Glass/125ml	25	0	20	0	3.6	0	0
White, Dry, Average	*1 Glass/125ml*	*88*	*0*	*70*	*0.1*	*0.6*	*0*	*0*
White, Fume Blanc, 13.1% Abv, Average	*1 Glass/125ml*	*104*	*0*	*83*	*0.1*	*2.3*	*0*	*0*
White, Gewurztraminer, 12.6% Abv, Average	*1 Glass/125ml*	*102*	*0*	*82*	*0.1*	*2.6*	*0*	*0*
White, Late Harvest, 10.6% Abv, Average	*1 Glass/125ml*	*141*	*0*	*113*	*0.1*	*13.4*	*0*	*0*
White, Medium, Average	*1 Glass/125ml*	*92*	*0*	*74*	*0.1*	*3*	*0*	*0*
White, Moscato, Blanco, Low Alcohol, 5.5%, Lidl*	1 Glass/125ml	62	0	50	0	0	0	0
White, Muller-Thurgau, 11.3% Abv, Average	*1 Glass/125ml*	*96*	*0*	*77*	*0.1*	*3.5*	*0*	*0*
White, Muscat, 0% Alcohol, Natureo, Torres*	1 Glass/125ml	32	0	26	0	4.5	0	0

W

	Measure INFO/WEIGHT	per Measure KCAL	FAT	Nutrition Values per 100g / 100ml KCAL	PROT	CARB	FAT	FIBRE
WINE								
White, Muscat, 11% Abv, Average	**1 Glass/125ml**	**104**	**0**	**83**	**0.1**	**5.2**	**0**	**0**
White, Pinot Blanc, 13.3% Abv, Average	**1 Glass/125ml**	**102**	**0**	**82**	**0.1**	**0**	**0**	**0**
White, Pinot Grigio, 11.5%, Yellow Tail*	1 Glass/125ml	95	0	76	0	0.5	0	0
White, Pinot Grigio, 13.4% Abv, Average	**1 Glass/125ml**	**105**	**0**	**84**	**0.1**	**2.1**	**0**	**0**
White, Pinot Grigio, Cataratto, 11.5%, 789 Di Mondelli*	1 Glass/125ml	84	0	67	0	0	0	0
White, Retsina, Kourtaki*	1 Glass/125ml	94	0	75	0	0	0	0
White, Riesling, 11.9% Abv, Average	**1 Glass/125ml**	**101**	**0**	**81**	**0.1**	**3.7**	**0**	**0**
White, Sauvignon Blanc, 13.1% Abv, Average	**1 Glass/125ml**	**102**	**0**	**82**	**0.1**	**2**	**0**	**0**
White, Sauvignon Blanc, Alcohol Free, Vintense*	1 Glass/125ml	20	0	16	0	4.5	0	0
White, Sauvignon Blanc, Dealcoholised, Tesco*	1 Glass/125ml	41	0	33	0.7	9.9	0	0
White, Sauvignon Blanc, Low Alcohol, Tesco*	1 Glass/125ml	66	0	53	0	12.6	0	0
White, Sauvignon Blanc, New Zealand, 12%, Tesco*	1 Glass/125ml	88	0	70	0	0	0	0
White, Sauvignon, Alcohol Free, Eisberg*	1 Glass/125ml	28	0	22	0	4.9	0	0
White, Semillon, 12.5% Abv, Average	**1 Glass/125ml**	**104**	**0**	**83**	**0.1**	**3.1**	**0**	**0**
White, Sparkling, Alcohol Free, Zero, McGuigan*	1 Glass/125ml	41	0.2	33	0.1	8	0.2	0
White, Sparkling, Average	**1 Glass/125ml**	**92**	**0**	**74**	**0.3**	**5.1**	**0**	**0**
White, Sparkling, ICE Edition, J.P.Chenet*	1 Glass/125ml	92	0	74	0	0	0	0
White, Sparkling, Low Alcohol, Tesco*	1 Glass/125ml	39	0	31	0	10.2	0	0
White, Sparkling, Zero Sugar, Slim Wine*	1 Serving/125ml	69	0	55	0	0	0	0
White, Sweet, Average	**1 Glass/125ml**	**118**	**0**	**94**	**0.2**	**5.9**	**0**	**0**
WINE GUMS								
Average	**1 Sweet/6g**	**19**	**0**	**315**	**5**	**73.4**	**0.2**	**0.1**
Haribo*	1 Pack/175g	609	0.4	348	0.1	86.4	0.2	0.4
Maynards*	4 Sweets/24g	79	0	329	4.8	76	0.2	0
Tangy, Maynards*	1 Serving/30g	100	0.1	334	4.3	78	0.2	0
WISPA								
Cadbury*	1 Bar/40g	220	13.6	550	7.3	52.5	34	1
Gold, Cadbury*	1 Bar/52g	265	15.1	510	5.3	56	29	0.7
WOTSITS								
Baked, Really Cheesy, Walkers*	1 Pack/17g	82	5.3	494	5.4	46.2	31.9	0.2
Flamin Hot, Giants, Walkers*	1 Serving/30g	160	9.3	533	5.7	57.4	31	1.7
Flaming Hot, Wotsits*	1 Bag/16g	85	4.8	534	5.5	60	30	1.1
Really Cheesy, Big Eat, Walkers*	1 Bag/36g	197	11.9	547	5.5	56	33	1.1
Really Cheesy, Giant, Walkers*	1 Serving/30g	165	9.8	549	4.9	55.2	32.7	1.7
Sizzling Steak, Wotsits*	1 Bag/14g	69	3.3	511	6.7	65.6	24.3	1.7
WRAP								
BBQ Chicken, One Stop*	1 Pack/154g	339	7.2	220	12	31.6	4.7	1.7
Bean, & Sweet Potato, Mexican Style, M&S*	1 Pack/238g	450	15	189	5	26.9	6.3	2.2
Bean, Spicy, with Cheese, Tesco*	1 Pack/198g	423	15.8	213	7.6	25.8	8	3.9
Bean, Three, Mexican Style, Sainsbury's*	1 Pack/190g	435	12.2	229	5.8	35.5	6.4	3.3
Biriyani, Sweet Potato, Plant Kitchen, M&S*	1 Pack/221g	396	12.8	179	5.2	24.6	5.8	4
Breakfast Scramble, Amy's kitchen *	1 Pack/100g	287	13	287	10	31	13	3
Buffalo Chicken, Tesco*	1 Pack/181g	370	10.2	204	11.8	26	5.6	1
Caesar, Plant Chef, Tesco*	1 Pack/169g	383	17.6	226	7.7	24	10.4	3
Cauliflower, Coronation, Plant Chef, Tesco*	1 Pack/220g	426	20.5	194	4	22	9.3	3
Chicken Katsu, Tesco*	1 Pack/190g	450	16.9	237	9.5	29	8.9	1.3
Chicken, & Bacon, Caesar, COU, M&S*	1 Pack/205g	607	31	296	13.3	26	15.1	1.3
Chicken, BBQ, & Coleslaw, Tesco*	1 Pack/221g	417	12.6	189	9.2	24.4	5.7	1.5
Chicken, BBQ, No Mayo, Tesco*	1 Pack/154g	353	8.6	229	12.2	31.7	5.6	1.7
Chicken, BBQ, On the Go, Sainsbury's*	1 Pack/199g	418	8.6	210	11.5	30.7	4.3	1.2
Chicken, BBQ, Shapers, Boots*	1 Pack/156g	278	4.5	178	11	26	2.9	1.8
Chicken, Cajun, Tesco*	1 Pack/175g	310	10	177	6.3	24.6	5.7	1.1
Chicken, Coronation , Waitrose*	1 Pack/164g	283	8.3	173	10.1	21.3	5.1	2.2

W

WRAP

INFO/WEIGHT	Measure	per Measure KCAL	FAT	Nutrition Values per 100g / 100ml KCAL	PROT	CARB	FAT	FIBRE
Chicken, Fajita, GF, Made Without Wheat, M&S*	1 Pack/210g	323	12.4	154	9.3	12.3	5.9	7.2
Chicken, Fajita, M&S*	1 Pack/213g	394	15.1	185	8.8	20.1	7.1	2.5
Chicken, Fajita, Morrisons*	1 Pack/214g	430	16.5	201	9.5	22.5	7.7	1.9
Chicken, Fajita, PB, Waitrose*	1 Pack/218g	368	5.7	169	10.5	26	2.6	1.9
Chicken, Fillets, with Cheese, & Bacon, Asda*	1 Pack/164g	366	21.3	223	25	1.4	13	0
Chicken, Jerk, Tesco*	1 Pack/218g	473	16.1	217	9.4	26.2	7.4	4
Chicken, Korma, Rainbow, Co-Op*	1 Pack/198g	348	8.5	176	8.6	24	4.3	2.4
Chicken, Lemon, & Garlic, Tesco*	1 Pack/185g	411	14.6	222	10.1	27.2	7.9	1.1
Chicken, M&S*	1 Pack/247g	530	24.9	215	8.2	23.4	10.1	1.6
Chicken, Mexican Style, Co-Op*	1 Pack/163g	367	14.7	225	11	26	9	3
Chicken, Peanut Satay, Tesco*	1 Pack/192g	455	17.1	237	12.8	25.5	8.9	1.9
Chicken, Piri Piri, Aldi*	1 Pack/168g	324	10.6	193	9.3	24	6.3	1.6
Chicken, Salad, Roast, Sainsbury's*	1 Pack/214g	443	19.9	207	10	20.9	9.3	2.5
Chicken, Southern Fried, CBY, Asda*	1 Pack/210g	452	17	215	7.1	27	8.1	2.7
Chicken, Sweet Chilli , Sainsbury's*	1 Pack/209g	434	11.5	208	8.5	30.1	5.5	1.8
Chicken, Sweet Chilli, Tesco*	1 Pack/175g	317	6.7	181	9.6	26.4	3.8	1.7
Chicken, Tikka, Average	**1 Wrap/200g**	**403**	**15.1**	**202**	**9.5**	**23.6**	**7.6**	**4.4**
Chicken, Tikka, with Onion Bhaji, Tesco*	1 Pack/192g	435	15.9	227	10.3	26.6	8.3	2.2
Duck, Hoisin, GF, M&S*	1 Pack/183g	285	6	156	10.2	17.5	3.3	7.6
Duck, Hoisin, M&S*	1 Pack/225g	405	8.3	180	8.4	27.7	3.7	1.5
Duck, Hoisin, No Mayo, Tesco*	1 Pack/178g	361	10	203	9.8	27.7	5.6	1.2
Falafel, & Houmous, Plant Chef, Tesco*	1 Pack/200g	442	13.6	221	5.6	32.2	6.8	4.5
Falafel, & Spinach, Aldi*	1 Pack/207g	486	24.8	235	6.7	25	12	2.9
Falafel, & Spinach, No Mayo, M&S*	1 Pack/227g	499	20	220	5.9	27.8	8.8	2.8
Ham, Smoked, & Mozzarella, Co-Op*	1 Pack/204g	483	16.3	237	10	30	8	1.3
Hoisin Duck, No Mayo, M&S*	1 Pack/217g	447	15	206	9.8	25.4	6.9	1.5
Hoisin, No Duck, Plant Kitchen, M&S*	1 Pack/200g	418	9.6	209	9.9	30	4.8	3.3
Hoisin, Plant Chef, Tesco*	1 Pack/175g	387	6.8	221	11	34.8	3.9	1.4
Mozzarella, & Pesto, M&S*	1 Pack/243g	559	27.9	230	7.8	23	11.5	1.7
Pork, Gochujang, Tesco*	1 Pack/173g	384	13.7	222	9.7	27.3	7.9	1.5
Smokehouse No Chicken, Plant Kitchen, M&S*	1 Pack/248g	498	15.6	201	7	29.7	6.3	3
Snack Day, Lidl*	1 Wrap/62g	196	4.3	316	9.3	52.4	7	0
Soft Cheese, & Spinach, to Go*	1 Pack/250g	278	6.7	111	4.5	17.4	2.7	0
Southern Fried Chicken, Morrisons*	1 Pack/199g	414	13.3	208	7.1	28.8	6.7	2
Sriracha, Egg, & Chorizo, Waitrose*	1 Pack/212g	415	14.8	196	7.8	24	7	2.7
Sushi, Tuna & Avocado, Eat Well, M&S*	1 Wrap/118g	212	6.9	180	5.9	25.2	5.9	1.4
Sweet Chilli Chicken, Triple, Eat & Go, Aldi*	1 Pack/276g	587	16.8	213	11	28	6.1	1.5
Teriyaki Chicken, On The Go, Tesco*	1 Pack/185g	340	6.1	184	8.9	29.1	3.3	1.3
Turkey, Bacon, & Cranberry, COU, M&S*	1 Pack/144g	230	2.2	160	9.6	27.1	1.5	2.3
Turkey, Feast, Sainsbury's*	1 Pack/212g	502	18.2	237	11.3	27.6	8.6	1.8
Vegetable, Roasted, & Pesto, Plant Chef, Tesco*	1 Pack/168g	351	15.1	209	3.8	26.5	9	3.5

	INFO/WEIGHT	KCAL	FAT	KCAL	PROT	CARB	FAT	FIBRE
YAM								
Baked	**1oz/28g**	**43**	**0.1**	**153**	**2.1**	**37.5**	**0.4**	**1.7**
Boiled, Average	**1oz/28g**	**37**	**0.1**	**133**	**1.7**	**33**	**0.3**	**1.4**
YEAST								
Extract	**1 Tsp/9g**	**16**	**0**	**180**	**40.7**	**3.5**	**0.4**	**0**
Extract, Reduced Salt, Sainsbury's*	1 Tsp/4g	10	0	246	41.2	17.6	0.5	4.3
Flakes, Nutritional, Nooch!, Bosh*	1 Tbsp/15g	50	0.6	334	51	13	3.7	22
Flakes, Nutritional, Whole Food Earth*	1 Tbsp/5g	17	0.2	341	53	34.8	5	21
Fresh, Average	**1 Serving/30g**	**32**	**0.6**	**105**	**8.4**	**18**	**1.9**	**0**
Quick, Doves Farm*	1 Serving/8g	28	0.5	355	43.5	19	5.7	27
YOGHURT								
0% Fat, Active, Brooklea, Aldi*	1 Pot/125g	59	0.6	47	4.2	7.3	0.5	0.5
0% Fat, Envia*	1 Pot/125g	45	0.1	36	4.3	4.5	0.1	0
3.8% Fat, Alnatura Bioland*	1 Pot/150g	111	5.7	74	4.2	5	3.8	0.1
Activia, Danone*	1 Pot/132g	125	4.2	94	3.5	12.8	3.2	2
All Flavours, Smooth, Ski, Nestle*	1 Pot/120g	100	3.1	83	3.3	11.6	2.6	0
Apple, & Pear, Low Fat, Sainsbury's*	1 Pot/125g	115	1.9	92	4.3	15.2	1.5	0.2
Apricot, Bio Activia, Danone*	1 Pot/125g	121	4	97	3.7	13.3	3.2	1.7
Apricot, Fat Free, Weight Watchers*	1 Pot/110g	45	0.1	41	4	5	0.1	0.2
Apricot, Low Fat, Brooklea, Aldi*	1 Pot/125g	99	1	79	2.8	15.1	0.8	0
Apricot, Low Fat, Sainsbury's*	1 Pot/124g	108	1.6	87	4.2	14.3	1.3	0.5
Apricot, Low Fat, Tesco*	1 Pot/125g	112	2.2	90	4.3	14.1	1.8	0
Apricot, Rich & Creamy, Rowan Glen*	1 Pot/85g	151	8.2	178	6.2	16.6	9.6	0.1
Banana, & Custard, Smooth, Mullerlight, Muller*	1 Pot/175g	94	0.2	54	4.1	8.6	0.1	0.6
Banana, & Custard, Milbona, Lidl*	1 Pot/165g	99	0.2	60	4.4	10	0.1	0.5
Banana, & Peanut Butter, Skyr, Light & Free, Danone*	1 Pot/150g	82	0.8	55	9.1	4.4	0.5	0
Banana, Choco Flakes, Crunch Corner, Muller*	1 Pot/130g	177	6.2	136	4.5	18	4.8	0
Banana, Fat Free, Light, Sainsbury's*	1 Pot/100g	54	0.5	54	5.2	7.5	0.5	0.5
Banana, Longley Farm*	1 Pot/150g	178	8.4	119	4.3	13.7	5.6	0
Banana, Low Fat, Average	**1 Serving/100g**	**98**	**1.4**	**98**	**4.6**	**16.7**	**1.4**	**0.1**
Banoffee, Snackpot, Activia, Danone*	1 Pot/155g	116	0.2	75	5	13.3	0.1	0.3
Berry, Five, Greek Style, Reduced Fat, M&S*	1 Pot/205g	322	17	157	6.7	12.6	8.3	2.5
Berry, Lite, Hansells Foods*	1 Serving/222g	151	0.2	68	5.1	11.8	0.1	0
Bianco, Intero, Vipiteno*	1 Serving/150g	111	6.3	74	3.7	5.5	4.2	0
Black Cherry, Low Fat, Live, M&S*	1 Serving/100g	81	1	81	3.8	14.1	1	0
Black Cherry, West Country, Extra Special, Asda*	1 Pot/150g	200	10.2	133	2.8	15	6.8	0.5
Black Cherry, West Country, TTD, Sainsbury's*	1 Pot/150g	186	9.3	124	3	13.7	6.2	0.5
Blackberry, Soya, Alpro*	1 Pot/125g	94	2.4	75	3.6	9.7	1.9	1.1
Blackcurrant, & Elderflower, Soya, Alpro*	1 Pot/125g	92	2.4	74	3.6	9.5	1.9	1.1
Blackcurrant, Garden Fruits, Low Fat, Tesco*	1 Pot/125g	120	2.4	95	3.8	15.1	1.9	0.3
Blackcurrant, Greek Style, Tims Dairy*	1 Serving/50g	72	4.2	144	4.6	12.5	8.5	0.2
Blackcurrant, Live, Little Town Dairy*	1 Pot/85g	93	3.7	109	4.5	13.4	4.4	0.5
Blackcurrant, Soya, Go On, Alpro*	1 Pot/150g	122	4.2	81	5.1	7.5	2.8	2
Blueberry, & Blackcurrant, Layered, Deluxe, Lidl*	1 Pot/150g	254	14.8	169	2.3	17.3	9.9	0.5
Blueberry, Barry*	1 Pot/250g	225	6.8	90	3.3	12	2.7	0
Blueberry, Cream Top, Rachel's Organic*	1 Pot/150g	188	10.4	125	3.4	12.1	6.9	0
Blueberry, Fruit Corner, Muller*	1 Pot/150g	156	5.7	104	3.8	12.9	3.8	0.4
Blueberry, Greek Style, Alpro*	1 Pot/150g	123	4	82	4.7	8.6	2.7	1.7
Blueberry, Greek Style, Fat Free, Deluxe, Lidl*	1 Serving/150g	120	0.2	80	7.5	11	0.1	0
Blueberry, Icelandic Style, Isey Skyr*	1 Pot/180g	157	0.4	87	9.7	12	0.2	0
Blueberry, Icelandic Style, Skyr, Brooklea, Aldi*	1 Pot/150g	122	0.8	81	7.7	12	0.5	0.5
Blueberry, Light & Free, Danone*	1 Pot/115g	54	0.1	47	4.4	6.8	0.1	0.3
Blueberry, Protein, Arla*	1 Pot/200g	140	0.4	70	10	6.5	0.2	0
Blueberry, Skyr, Milbona, Lidl*	½ Pot/175g	100	0.4	57	8.9	4.6	0.2	0

Y

YOGHURT

INFO/WEIGHT	Measure	per Measure KCAL	per Measure FAT	Nutrition Values per 100g / 100ml KCAL	PROT	CARB	FAT	FIBRE
Blueberry, Soya, Alpro*	1 Pot/125g	91	2.5	73	3.6	9.4	2	1.2
Blueberry, SoYummy, Aldi*	1 Serving/150g	111	2	74	3.5	11.5	1.3	0
Breakfast, Exante Diet*	1 Pack/200g	741	24.4	370	31.5	31.5	12.2	6.8
Cafe Vanille, Isey Skyr*	1 Serving/170g	126	3.6	74	9.6	4.2	2.1	0
Caramel, Indulgent Layered, Specially Selected, Aldi*	1 Pot/150g	276	16.5	184	2.3	19	11	1.4
Caramel, Salted, Cheesecake, Greek, Whipped, Muller*	1 Pot/100g	180	7.9	180	4.2	21.8	7.9	0
Caramel, Salted, Greek Style, Luxury, Oykos, Danone*	1 Pot/110g	172	9.2	157	2.7	17.6	8.4	0
Caramelised Apple, Easiyo*	1 Serving/222g	222	8.7	100	3.7	12.5	3.9	0
Cereals, Fibre, Bio Activia, Danone*	1 Pot/120g	119	4.1	99	3.7	13.5	3.4	3
Champagne Rhubarb, Irish Yogurts*	1 Pot/125g	88	3.9	70	4.4	6.3	3.1	0.5
Champagne, Clonakilty*	1 Serving/100g	87	1.9	87	4.3	13	1.9	0.5
Cherry, Bio, Gut Health, Activia*	1 Pot/115g	58	0	50	4.6	7.4	0	0
Cherry, Biopot, Onken*	1 Serving/150g	153	4	102	3.8	14	2.7	0
Cherry, Black, & Cream, The Best, Morrisons*	1 Pot/150g	218	9.4	146	3.2	19	6.3	0
Cherry, Black, Average	**1 Serving/100g**	**96**	**2.2**	**96**	**3.4**	**16.5**	**2.2**	**0.1**
Cherry, Black, Low Fat, Average	**1 Serving/100g**	**69**	**0.6**	**69**	**3.8**	**12.2**	**0.6**	**0.3**
Cherry, Fat Free, Mullerlight, Muller*	1 Pot/160g	85	0.8	53	4.9	7.4	0.5	0
Cherry, Greek Style, Layered, Brooklea, Aldi*	1 Pot/125g	89	0.6	71	5.7	11	0.5	0.5
Cherry, Greek Style, Layers, Mullerlight, Muller*	1 Pot/120g	61	0.6	51	4.7	7.3	0.5	0
Cherry, Greek Style, Light & Free, Danone*	1 Pot/115g	55	0.1	48	4.3	7.4	0.1	0.1
Cherry, Light, Fat Free, Muller*	1 Pot/175g	88	0.2	50	3.9	7.9	0.1	0.2
Cherry, Low Fat, Brooklea, Aldi*	1/3 Pot/150g	135	3.4	90	4.1	13	2.3	0.5
Cherry, Luscious, Intensely Creamy, Activia, Danone*	1 Pot/110g	109	3.3	99	5	12.8	3	0.2
Cherry, Luscious, Rachel's Organic*	1 Pot/150g	176	8.6	117	3.5	13	5.7	0
Cherry, Mascarpone Style, Bliss, Muller*	1 Pack/110g	131	5.3	119	3.1	15	4.8	0
Cherry, Red, Fruit Corner, Muller*	1 Pot/143g	157	5.6	110	4.3	13.8	3.9	0.5
Cherry, Soya, Alpro*	1 Pot/125g	91	2.5	73	3.6	9.4	2	1.2
Chocolate Orange, Protein, Arla*	1 Pot/200g	150	1.4	75	10	7.6	0.7	0
Coconut, & Vanilla, Greek Style, Fat Free, Brooklea, Aldi*	1 Pot/125g	74	0.6	59	5.9	7.6	0.5	0.5
Coconut, Dairy Free, Erity*	1 Serving/50g	104	10.8	208	2.1	1.6	21.5	2.5
Coconut, Dairy Free, V-Love, Migros*	1 Pot/150g	158	15	105	1	2.7	10	0.5
Coconut, Dairy Free, Yoplait*	1 Pot/100g	95	3.9	95	0.5	14	3.9	0
Coconut, Greek Style, Brooklea, Aldi*	1 Serving/150g	212	12.9	141	3.7	12	8.6	0.5
Coconut, Greek Style, Milbona, Lidl*	1 Pot/150g	236	14.7	157	3.9	13	9.8	0.5
Coconut, Light & Fit, Danone*	1 Yogurt/80g	43	0	53	8	6	0	0
Coconut, Low Fat, Tesco*	1 Serving/150g	150	4	100	5	13.8	2.7	0.1
Coconut, Natural, The Coconut Collaborative*	1 Serving/100g	115	10	115	1.2	6.8	10	0.7
Coconut, Protein, Arla*	1 Pot/200g	144	1	72	10	6.2	0.5	0
Creamy, 5% Fat, Skyr, Arla*	1 Serving/150g	153	7.5	102	9.6	3.9	5	0
Fat Free, Activia, Danone*	1 Pot/120g	107	3.4	89	3.9	11.8	2.8	0
Fat Free, Smooth, Milbona, Lidl*	1 Pot/175g	88	0.2	50	4.4	7.3	0.1	0.1
Fig, Bio, Activia, Danone*	1 Pot/125g	124	4.2	99	3.6	13.4	3.4	0.2
Framboise, Siggi's, Skyr*	1 Pot/140g	123	2.7	88	8.9	8.9	1.9	0
French, Set, Low Fat, Iceland*	1 Pot/125g	100	1.5	80	3.6	13.6	1.2	0
Fruit, Low Fat, Average	**1 Pot/125g**	**112**	**0.9**	**90**	**4.1**	**17.9**	**0.7**	**0**
Fudge, Deluxe, Lidl*	1 Pot/150g	226	11	151	3.1	17.9	7.3	0.5
Fudge, Devonshire Style, Finest, Tesco*	1 Pot/150g	206	9.2	137	4	16.4	6.1	0.4
Gin & Tonic, Inspired, Mullerlight, Muller*	1 Pot/160g	72	0.7	45	4.4	6	0.5	0
Ginger, Greek Style, Bio, Live, Rachel's Organic*	1 Serving/100g	137	7.4	137	3.2	14.4	7.4	0
Gingerbread, Mullerlight, Muller*	1 Pot/160g	80	0.8	50	4.8	6.7	0.5	0
Goats Whole Milk	**1 Carton/150g**	**94**	**5.7**	**63**	**3.5**	**3.9**	**3.8**	**0**
Gooseberry, & Elderflower, Fragrant, Creamy, Waitrose*	1 Pot/150g	188	9.9	125	2.6	13.8	6.6	0.5
Gooseberry, & Elderflower, West Country, M&S*	1 Pot/150g	190	10.2	127	3	13.5	6.8	0

YOGHURT

INFO/WEIGHT	Measure	per Measure		Nutrition Values per 100g / 100ml				
		KCAL	FAT	KCAL	PROT	CARB	FAT	FIBRE
Gooseberry, Low Fat, Average	**1 Serving/100g**	**90**	**1.4**	**90**	**4.5**	**14.5**	**1.4**	**0.2**
Gourmet, Live, Deluxe, Lidl*	1 Serving/150g	206	8.4	137	5	16.4	5.6	0.5
Greek Style, 0% Fat, Eat Well, M&S*	1 Pot/200g	116	0.4	58	10.1	3.4	0.2	1.1
Greek Style, Dairy & Soya Free, Thick & Creamy, Koko*	¼ Pot/100g	113	9.6	113	1.1	5.7	9.6	0.1
Greek Style, Fat Free, Brooklea, Aldi*	1 Serving/150g	100	0.8	67	7	9.2	0.5	0.5
Greek Style, Fat Free, Iceland*	1/5 Pot/100g	70	0.4	70	6.2	10.3	0.4	0.7
Greek Style, Fat Free, Morrisons*	¼ Pot/125g	68	0.2	54	6.7	6.3	0.2	0
Greek Style, Free From, Tesco*	¼ Pot/100g	54	3.3	54	5.8	0	3.3	0.7
Greek Style, Full Fat, Asda*	1 Serving/75g	94	7	125	5.1	4.9	9.4	0
Greek Style, Honey, Easiyo*	1 Serving/250g	250	9.8	100	3.6	12.5	3.9	0
Greek Style, Honey, Tims Dairy*	1 Tub/175g	262	15	150	4.7	13.6	8.6	0.1
Greek Style, Layered, Light, Brooklea, Aldi*	1 Pot/125g	69	0.6	55	5.7	7.5	0.5	0.5
Greek Style, Low Fat, Fresh, Easiyo*	1 Bowl/200g	140	2.6	70	5.7	8.5	1.3	0
Greek Style, Low Fat, Milbona, Lidl*	1 Serving/150g	88	3	59	6	4	2	0
Greek Style, with Honey, Brooklea, Aldi*	1/3 Pot/150g	206	11	137	3.3	15	7.3	0.5
Greek Style, with Honey, Milbona, Lidl*	1 Serving/150g	204	10.6	136	3.1	14.6	7.1	0.5
Greek Style, with Honey, Tesco*	1 Pot/100g	144	8	144	4.2	13.7	8	0
Greek, 0% Fat, Strained, Authentic, Total, Fage*	1 Pot/170g	92	0	54	10.3	3	0	0
Greek, 0% Fat, with Honey, Total, Fage*	1 Pot/170g	180	0	106	8.3	18	0	0
Greek, 10% Fat, Brooklea, Aldi*	1/5 Pot/100g	123	10	123	6.4	3.7	10	0
Greek, 2% Fat, Strained, Authentic, Total, Fage*	1 Pot/170g	119	3.4	70	9.9	3	2	0
Greek, Authentic, 0% Fat, Milbona, Lidl*	1 Serving/150g	84	0	56	9	4.8	0	0
Greek, Authentic, Fat Free, TTD, Sainsbury's*	¼ Pot/125g	81	0.6	65	9.9	6	0.5	0.5
Greek, Authentic, Natural, Strained, Waitrose*	1 Serving/125g	164	12.8	131	5.9	3.7	10.2	0.3
Greek, Authentic, TTD, Sainsbury's*	1 Serving/100g	137	10.7	137	6	4.1	10.7	0
Greek, Creamy, Authentic, Milbona, Lidl*	1 Serving/100g	132	10	132	6	4.5	10	0
Greek, Natural, Strained, Fat Free, No.1, Waitrose*	1 Serving/125g	81	0.6	65	9.6	5.5	0.5	0.5
Greek, with Blueberries, Total 0%, Total, Fage*	1 Serving/150g	123	0	82	8.3	12.3	0	0
Hazelnut, Longley Farm*	1 Pot/150g	201	8.5	134	5.5	16	5.7	0
Hazelnut, Low Fat, Deliciously Nutty, Waitrose*	1 Pot/150g	153	4.2	102	6.1	12.9	2.8	0.5
Honey, Greek Style, 0% Fat, Tesco*	1/3 Pot/150g	122	0.3	81	6.8	13.1	0.2	0
Honey, Greek Style, Hansell*	1 Serving/222g	233	9.5	105	4.1	12.3	4.3	0
Honey, Greek Style, Morrisons*	1/3 Pot/150g	236	14.3	157	4.1	13.5	9.5	0.7
Honey, Greek Style, Strained, 0% Fat, Liberte, Yoplait*	1 Pot/100g	92	0.1	92	7.7	14.1	0.1	0.1
Kefir, Greek Style, Coconut, Tims Dairy*	1 Serving/150g	226	15.2	151	4.8	10.6	10.1	0.4
Kefir, Greek Style, Natural, Tims Dairy*	1 Serving/100g	130	10	130	5.5	4.7	10	0
Kefir, Natural, Fermented, Milbona, Lidl*	1/3 Pot/150g	110	3	73	4.7	8.8	2	0.5
Kefir, Natural, Organic, Yeo Valley*	1 Pot/350g	224	7.4	64	4.7	6.4	2.1	0
Kefir, Raspberry, Spoonable, M&S*	¼ Pot/88g	63	1.5	72	4.3	9.6	1.7	0.4
Kefir, Strawberry, Organic, Yeo Valley*	½ Pot/175g	138	3.3	79	4.2	11.1	1.9	0
Kefir, Vanilla, Morrisons*	1 Pot/151g	122	3	81	3.8	11.7	2	0.5
Kiwi, Bio, Activia, Danone*	1 Pot/125g	122	4.2	98	3.6	12.9	3.4	0.3
Kiwi, Mixed Fruit, Activia, Danone*	1 Pot/120g	109	3.5	91	3.9	12.2	2.9	0
Kvarg, Nestle*	1 Serving/150g	82	0.3	55	10	3.4	0.2	0
Kvarg, Vanilla, Protein, Lindahls, Nestle*	1 Pot/150g	81	0.3	54	10	3.5	0.2	0
Lactose Free, Sainsbury's*	1 Serving/100g	108	7.2	108	5.3	5.6	7.2	0.5
Layered, Brooklea, Aldi*	1 Pot/125g	69	0.6	55	5.5	7.7	0.5	0.5
Lemon Curd, Luxury, Extra Special, Asda*	1 Pot/150g	242	13.2	161	3.2	17	8.8	0.5
Lemon Curd, Whole Milk, Yeo Valley*	1 Pot/120g	149	5.3	124	4.7	16.3	4.4	0
Lemon, Greek Style, Fat Free, Brooklea, Aldi*	1 Pot/125g	71	0.6	57	5.8	8	0.5	0.5
Lemon, Greek Style, Fat Free, Country Farm, Lidl*	¼ Pot/250g	152	1	61	6.1	8.4	0.4	0.5
Lemon, Greek Style, Fat Free, Muller*	1 Pot/120g	72	0.2	60	6.3	7.5	0.2	0
Lemon, Greek Style, Light & Free, Danone*	1 Pot/115g	53	0.1	46	4.5	6.8	0.1	0

Y

YOGHURT

INFO/WEIGHT	Measure	per Measure KCAL	FAT	Nutrition Values per 100g / 100ml KCAL	PROT	CARB	FAT	FIBRE
Lemon, Greek Style, Light, Fat Free, Milbona, Lidl*	1 Serving/150g	87	0.3	58	5.8	8	0.2	0.5
Lemon, Greek Style, Whipped, Bliss Corner, Muller*	1 Pot/110g	177	6.5	161	4	22.2	5.9	0
Lemon, Italian Inspired, Light, Amore, Muller*	1 Pot/130g	78	0.6	60	8.5	6.4	0.5	0
Lemon, Lavish, Greek Style, Light & Free, Danone*	1 Pot/115g	56	0.1	49	4.9	7.1	0.1	0.1
Lemon, Luscious, Greek Style, Mullerlight, Muller*	1 Sm Pot/120g	72	0.7	60	6.3	7.5	0.6	0
Lemon, Sicilain, The Best, Morrisons*	1 Pot/150g	235	12.1	157	3.4	17.5	8.1	0
Lemon, Sicilian, Deluxe, Lidl*	1 Pot/150g	197	9.8	131	3	15	6.5	0.3
Lemon, Soya, Free From, Asda*	1 Pot/100g	77	2	77	3.7	11	2	0.5
Mandarin, Fat Free, Mullerlight, Muller*	1 Pot/175g	95	0.2	54	4.2	8.5	0.1	0
Mandarin, Llaeth Y Llan, Village Dairy*	1 Pot/125g	130	3.5	104	5.6	14.3	2.8	0.1
Mango, & Honey, Kefir, M&S*	1 Pack/140g	98	2.4	70	3.8	9.9	1.7	0.5
Mango, & Passion Fruit, Cream Top, Rachel's Organic*	1 Pot/150g	192	10.4	128	3.4	13	6.9	0
Mango, & Passion Fruit, Finest, Tesco*	1 Pot/150g	166	7.6	111	3.8	12.3	5.1	0.2
Mango, & Passion Fruit, Low Fat, Morrisons *	1 Pot/125g	96	1.4	77	4.5	12.2	1.1	0.4
Mango, & Passion Fruit, Skyr, M&S*	1 Serving/75g	62	0.3	83	10.3	9.3	0.4	0.5
Mango, & Vanilla, Layered, Indulgent, Aldi*	1 Pot/150g	224	14.1	149	3.3	14	9.4	1.5
Mango, Bio, Activia, Danone*	1 Pot/125g	124	4.2	99	3.5	13.5	3.4	0.2
Mango, Carrot, Banana, Simply Fruit & Veg, Danone*	1 Pot/110g	78	2.8	71	4.3	7.6	2.5	0
Mango, Papaya, & Passion Fruit, Bio, Morrisons*	1 Serving/150g	156	5.1	104	3.1	14.9	3.4	0.5
Mango, Papaya, & Passion Fruit, Onken*	1 Serving/150g	144	4	96	3.8	13	2.7	0.2
Mango, Prebiotic, Gut-Loving, Bio & Me*	1 Serving/150g	129	4.8	86	4.9	8.5	3.2	1.8
Mango, Soya, Go On, Alpro*	1 Pot/150g	129	4.2	86	5	9.1	2.8	1.3
Mango, TruBlend, Fage*	1 Pot/150g	111	2.4	74	8	4.8	1.6	0
Milky Bar, Mixup, Nestle*	1 Pot/65g	98	3.8	150	4.5	18.5	5.9	0
Mixed Yellow Fruit, Sainsbury's*	1 Pot/125g	104	1.5	83	3.9	14	1.2	0.5
Muesli, Bircher Style, M&S*	1 Pot/190g	230	5.9	121	5.4	17	3.1	1.6
Muesli, Bircher, Summer Berry, M&S*	1 Pot/195g	277	13.1	142	3.7	15	6.7	3.4
Natural, 5% Fat, Icelandic Style, Skyr, Arla*	1/3 Pot/150g	153	7.5	102	9.6	3.9	5	0
Natural, Bifidus, Migros*	1 Pot/150g	110	5.2	73	5.4	4.8	3.5	1.1
Natural, Bio Activia, Individual Pots, Danone*	1 Pot/125g	86	4.2	69	4.2	5.5	3.4	0
Natural, Bio Live, Low Fat, Organic, Waitrose*	1/4 Pot/125g	81	1.2	65	5.8	8.3	1	0
Natural, Bio Set, Low Fat, Sainsbury's*	1 Pot/150g	78	2.2	52	3.9	5.7	1.5	0
Natural, Bio, Lancashire Farm*	3 Dstsps/40g	32	1.4	80	5.2	7	3.5	0.5
Natural, Biopot, Onken*	1 Serving/125g	82	4.4	66	4.5	4.1	3.5	0
Natural, Coconut, The Coconut Collective*	1 Serving/150g	188	15	125	1.2	6.8	10	0.7
Natural, Cypriot Style, Live, Thick Set, Tims Dairy*	1 Serving/100g	87	5	87	4.8	6	5	0
Natural, Fat Free, Lancashire Farm Dairies*	1 Serving/100g	48	0.1	48	5	7.3	0.1	0.9
Natural, Fat Free, Llaeth Y Llan, Village Dairy*	1 Serving/100g	57	0.2	57	5.7	7.9	0.2	0.1
Natural, Fat Free, Morrisons*	1 Serving/100g	47	0.2	47	5	6.4	0.2	0
Natural, Fat Free, Onken*	1 Serving/150g	63	0	42	5.6	3.1	0	0
Natural, Greek Style, Average	*1 Serving/100g*	*138*	*10.6*	*138*	*4.7*	*6.1*	*10.6*	*0*
Natural, Greek Style, Low Fat, Average	*1 Serving/100g*	*77*	*2.7*	*77*	*6.1*	*7.3*	*2.7*	*0.2*
Natural, Icelandic Style, Strained, Fat Free, Skyr, Arla*	1 Serving/150g	98	0.3	65	11	4	0.2	0
Natural, Isey Skyr*	1 Serving/170g	104	0.3	61	11	3.7	0.2	0
Natural, Kefir, Gut Health*	1/3 Pot/150g	94	3	63	5.1	6.1	2	0
Natural, Kefir, Nourish, Morrisons*	1/2 Tub/175g	133	7.2	76	5.1	4.3	4.1	0.5
Natural, Kerned, Super Thick, 0% Fat, Yeo Valley*	1 Serving/113g	64	0.6	57	10	3.5	0.5	0
Natural, Kerned, Super Thick, 5% Fat, Yeo Valley*	1 Serving/150g	142	7.5	95	9	3.5	5	0
Natural, Live, 0% Fat, Eat Well, M&S*	1 Serving/125g	68	0.2	54	5.6	7.5	0.2	0.5
Natural, Live, with Raspberries, Katy Rodgers*	1/4 Pot/123g	127	5.5	104	4.5	10.1	4.5	0.5
Natural, Live, with Strawberries, Glenilen Farm*	1 Serving/100g	84	2	84	3.7	11.4	2	0
Natural, Low Fat, Average	*1 Med Pot/125g*	*75*	*1.6*	*60*	*5.4*	*7*	*1.3*	*0*
Natural, Probiotic, Organic, Yeo Valley*	1 Pot/120g	98	5.4	82	5.1	5.6	4.5	0

Y

YOGHURT

INFO/WEIGHT	Measure	per Measure KCAL	FAT	Nutrition Values per 100g / 100ml KCAL	PROT	CARB	FAT	FIBRE
Natural, Sainsbury's*	1 Serving/100g	81	3.8	81	5.1	6.5	3.8	0.5
Natural, Scottish, Mccallums*	1 Serving/150g	116	4.8	78	4.9	7.2	3.2	0
Natural, Simplesmente, Pingo Doce*	1 Pot/125g	62	1.9	50	3.9	5.2	1.5	0
Natural, with Honey, Greek Style, Sainsbury's*	1 Sm Pot/125g	174	9.8	139	3.7	13.4	7.8	0.5
Oat Based, Light & Free, Danone*	1 Serving/150g	69	0.6	46	0.6	9.6	0.4	0
Oat-Gurt, Plain, Oatly*	¼ Pot/100g	84	3.5	84	1.5	11	3.5	1
Orange, & Pink Grapefruit, Finest, Tesco*	1 Pot/150g	162	7.8	108	4	11.2	5.2	0.4
Orange, Sprinkled with Dark Chocolate, Light, Muller*	1 Pot/165g	91	0.8	55	4.3	7.4	0.5	0.1
Passion Fruit, Greek Style, Luxury, Oykos, Danone*	1 Pot/110g	159	9	144	2.7	14.6	8.2	0.2
Passion Fruit, Soya, Go On, Alpro*	1 Pot/150g	126	4.4	84	5.2	8.5	2.9	1.4
Peach, & Apricot, Fruit Corner, Muller*	1 Pot/150g	160	5.7	107	3.9	13.5	3.8	0.5
Peach, & Cream, Intensely Creamy, Activia, Danone*	1 Pot/120g	118	3.6	98	4.8	13	3	0.3
Peach, & Mango, Thick & Creamy, Waitrose*	1 Pot/125g	136	3.1	109	3.7	17.8	2.5	0.3
Peach, & Passion Fruit, Fat Free, Milbona, Lidl*	1 Pot/180g	122	0.7	68	12.4	3.5	0.4	0.5
Peach, & Pineapple, Fat Free, Mullerlight, Muller*	1 Pot/175g	89	0.2	51	4.3	7.7	0.1	0.2
Peach, & Mango, Ann Forshaw's*	1 Pot/150g	196	8.8	131	4.1	15.4	5.9	0
Peach, & Nectarine, Low Fat, Super Fruity, M&S*	1 Pot/150g	104	1.7	69	3.9	10.5	1.1	0.8
Peach, & Pear, Soya, No Bits, Alpro*	1 Pot/125g	99	2.5	79	3.7	10.7	2	1
Peach, 0% Fat, No Added Sugar, Activia *	1 Pot/120g	60	0.1	50	4.8	7.4	0.1	0
Peach, Bio, Activia, Fat Free, Danone*	1 Pot/125g	71	0.1	57	4.7	9.3	0.1	1
Peach, Greek Style, Luxury, Oykos, Danone*	1 Pot/110g	154	8.9	140	3.1	13.4	8.1	0.3
Peach, Jogobella, Zott*	1 Pot/400g	364	10.8	91	3.5	12.2	2.7	0
Peach, Low Fat, Average	**1 Serving/100g**	**86**	**1.1**	**86**	**4.5**	**14.6**	**1.1**	**0.2**
Peach, Melba, Low Fat, Average	**1 Serving/100g**	**75**	**0.7**	**75**	**2.6**	**14.5**	**0.7**	**0**
Pear, & Blackcurrant, M&S*	1 Pot/150g	183	9.6	122	2.8	12.9	6.4	0.8
Pear, Fat Free, Milbona, Lidl*	1 Pot/125g	104	0.1	83	3.9	15.8	0.1	0.5
Pear, Irish, 0% Fat, Duneen, Aldi*	1 Carton/125g	66	0.6	53	4.7	7.5	0.5	0.5
Pineapple, & Peach, Fruity, Mullerlight, Muller*	1 Pot/175g	89	0.2	51	4.2	7.7	0.1	0.2
Pineapple, Fat Free, Milbona, Lidl*	1 Pot/125g	104	0.1	83	3.9	15.8	0.1	0.5
Plain, Coconut, Dairy Free, Just Free, Lidl*	1 Pot/125g	85	4.4	68	0.5	8.4	3.5	0.2
Plain, Greek Style, Alpro*	1 Serving/50g	34	1.6	68	5.8	2.6	3.3	1.5
Plain, Greek Style, Fat Free, M&S*	1 Pot/150g	84	0.6	56	8.3	4.9	0.4	0.6
Plain, Low Fat, Average	**1 Serving/100g**	**63**	**1.6**	**63**	**5.2**	**7**	**1.6**	**0**
Plain, Skyr, Fat Free, Siggis*	1 Serving/150g	81	0	54	10	6	0	0
Plain, Skyr, Lidl*	1 Pack/150g	93	0.3	62	11	4	0.2	0
Plain, Soya, Average	**1oz/28g**	**20**	**1.2**	**72**	**5**	**3.9**	**4.2**	**0**
Plain, Whole Milk, Average	**1oz/28g**	**22**	**0.8**	**79**	**5.7**	**7.8**	**3**	**0**
Plain, with Almond, Soya, Alpro*	1 Tbsp/20g	11	0.6	54	3.9	2.3	2.8	1.1
Plain, with Coconut, Soya, Alpro*	1 Tbsp/20g	11	0.6	55	3.9	2.3	3	0.8
Pomegranate, Soya, Alpro*	1 Pot/125g	92	2.4	74	3.6	9.5	1.9	1.1
Pouring, Court Lodge Organic*	1 Serving/125g	91	5.9	73	3	4.7	4.7	0
Protein Isolate, Soy, Vanilla, Myprotein*	1 Scoop/30g	100	0.4	333	81	4.8	1.4	0
Protein Pouch, On The Go, Brooklea, Aldi*	1 Pouch/200g	148	0.9	74	12.5	5	0.4	0.4
Proviact, Milbona, Lidl*	1 Pot/125g	59	0.1	47	3.1	8.2	0.1	0.5
Prune, Bio, Activia, Danone*	1 Pot/125g	122	4.1	98	3.6	13.1	3.3	0.8
Prune, Live, M&S*	1 Pack/159g	254	6.5	160	5.4	24.4	4.1	1.7
Quark, Plain, Muller*	1 Pot/150g	176	9.2	117	7.1	8.3	6.1	0
Quark, Strawberry, Muller*	1 Pot/150g	186	7.2	124	5.5	13.7	4.8	0
Quark, Vanilla, Muller*	1 Pot/150g	186	7.4	124	6.4	13.4	4.9	0
Raspberry, & Cranberry, Fat Free, Milbona, Lidl*	1 Pot/174g	87	0.2	50	4.2	7.8	0.1	0.5
Raspberry, & Cranberry, Fat Free, Mullerlight, Muller*	1 Pot/175g	91	0.2	52	4.3	7.8	0.1	0.5
Raspberry, & Cream, The Best, Morrisons*	1 Pot/150g	205	9.7	137	3.2	16.2	6.5	0.3
Raspberry, & Apple, No Added Sugar, Alpro*	½ Pot/200g	116	3.8	58	3.6	4.8	1.9	1.3

Y

YOGHURT	Measure INFO/WEIGHT	per Measure KCAL	FAT	Nutrition Values per 100g / 100ml KCAL	PROT	CARB	FAT	FIBRE
Raspberry, & Cranberry, Soya, Alpro*	1 Pot/125g	94	2.4	75	3.6	9.7	1.9	1.1
Raspberry, Active, Brooklea, Aldi*	1 Pot/125g	59	0.6	47	4.2	6.8	0.5	0.6
Raspberry, Fat Free, Average	*1 Serving/100g*	*64*	*0.1*	*64*	*4.9*	*11*	*0.1*	*1.7*
Raspberry, Greek Style, Bio-Live, Rachel's Organic*	1 Serving/150g	194	10.6	129	3.1	13.1	7.1	0
Raspberry, Greek Style, Brooklea, Aldi*	1 Pot/150g	124	0.8	83	8.3	12	0.5	0.5
Raspberry, Greek Style, Easiyo*	1 Serving/180g	198	6.7	110	3.9	15.3	3.7	0
Raspberry, Greek Style, Light, Fat Free, Brooklea, Aldi*	1 Pot/125g	72	0.6	58	5.8	8.2	0.5	0.5
Raspberry, Greek Style, Oykos, Danone*	1 Serving/110g	156	9	142	2.7	13.9	8.2	0.5
Raspberry, Greek Style, Tim's Dairy*	1 Pot/125g	179	10.5	143	4.6	12.4	8.4	0.4
Raspberry, High Protein, Fat Free, Milbona, Lidl*	1 Pot/180g	223	0.7	124	12.6	3.4	0.4	0.5
Raspberry, Intensely Creamy, Juicy, Activia, Danone*	1 Pot/110g	109	3.3	99	4.8	12.7	3	0.6
Raspberry, Low Fat, Average	*1 Serving/100g*	*83*	*1.1*	*83*	*4.1*	*14.1*	*1.1*	*0.8*
Raspberry, Organic, Yeo Valley*	1 Pot/150g	152	5.8	101	4.2	12.3	3.9	0.4
Raspberry, Pouring, Icelandic Style, Skyr, Arla*	1 Serving/150g	96	0.8	64	6	9.1	0.5	0.1
Raspberry, Protein, Arla*	1 Pot/200g	126	0.4	63	10	5.6	0.2	0
Raspberry, Protein, Brooklea, Aldi*	1 Pouch/200g	148	1	74	12	5	0.5	0.5
Raspberry, Protein, Milbona, Lidl*	1 Pot/180g	124	0.7	69	12.6	3.4	0.4	0.5
Raspberry, Protein, Thick, Eat Well, M&S*	1 Pot/200g	154	0.4	77	11.7	6.9	0.2	0.5
Raspberry, Razzle, Greek Style, Light & Free, Danone*	1 Pot/115g	58	0.1	50	4.3	7.5	0.1	1.1
Raspberry, River Cottage*	1 Jar/160g	85	3.1	53	2.6	7.6	1.9	0.1
Raspberry, Simply, Danone*	1 Pot/110g	79	2.8	72	4.3	7.6	2.5	0
Raspberry, Skyr, Icelandic, Siggi's*	1 Pot/150g	108	0	72	10	7.7	0	0
Raspberry, Skyr, Light & Free, Danone*	1 Pot/150g	81	0.8	54	9.2	3.7	0.5	0
Raspberry, Skyr, Milbona, Lidl*	½ Pot/175g	100	0.4	57	8.9	4.6	0.2	0.5
Raspberry, Squidgy Pouches, Brooklea, Aldi*	1 Pouch/80g	67	2.3	84	3.4	11	2.9	0.5
Raspberry, Summer Fruits, Benecol*	1 Pot/120g	90	2	75	0.2	9.7	1.7	3.7
Raspberry, Summer, Biopot, Onken*	1/5 Pot/90g	91	2.4	101	3.8	15	2.7	0.6
Rhubarb, & Vanilla, Greek Style, Fat Free, Asda*	1 Pot/125g	60	0.6	48	5.8	5.3	0.5	0.6
Rhubarb, Champagne, Scottish, Deluxe, Lidl*	1 Pot/150g	198	9.3	132	4	14.7	6.2	0.5
Rhubarb, Crumble, Inspired, Mullerlight, Muller*	1 Pot/172g	86	0.2	50	4.1	7.5	0.1	0
Rhubarb, Fruity, Mullerlight, Muller*	1 Pot/175g	91	0.2	52	4.2	7.9	0.1	0
Rhubarb, Layer, Bonne Maman*	1 Pot/125g	134	5.1	107	2.3	15	4.1	0.6
Rhubarb, Live, Thick & Creamy, Manor Farm*	1 Pot/128g	166	9.3	130	5	13.4	7.3	0
Rhubarb, Longley Farm*	1 Pot/150g	165	5.6	110	4.9	14.3	3.7	0
Rhubarb, Low Fat, Average	*1 Serving/100g*	*83*	*1.2*	*83*	*4.6*	*13.3*	*1.2*	*0.2*
Rhubarb, Spiced, Thick & Creamy, COU, M&S*	1 Pot/170g	68	0.2	40	4.3	5.8	0.1	0.5
Rhubarb, SuperValu*	1 Jar/140g	161	8.1	115	3.4	12	5.8	0
Rhubarb, Timperley, TTD, Sainsbury's*	1 Pot/150g	170	9.9	113	3.2	10.1	6.6	0.5
Rhubarb, West Country, Finest, Tesco*	1 Pot/150g	147	6.8	98	3.5	10.9	4.5	0
Roasted Hazelnut, Low Fat, Super Nutty, M&S*	1 Pot/150g	153	4.2	102	6.1	12.9	2.8	0.4
Roasted Hazelnut, West Country, Luxury, M&S*	1 Pot/150g	236	13.6	157	3.5	15.2	9.1	0.5
Salted Caramel, Protein, Arla*	1 Pot/200g	146	1.2	73	10	7.5	0.6	0
Salted Caramel, The Best, Morrisons*	1 Pot/150g	225	11.4	150	4	16.3	7.6	0.4
Salted Caramel, Thick & Creamy, Live, Nomadic*	1 Pot/160g	181	6.7	113	5.4	13.4	4.2	0.5
Skyr, Apple, Baked, Isey Skyr*	1 Serving/75g	40	0.2	54	9	4.1	0.2	0
Skyr, Icelandic, Raspberry Granola, Corner, Muller*	1 Pot/180g	256	11.9	142	7.4	12.2	6.6	0
Skyr, Mango & Passion Fruit, Fat Free, Tesco*	1 Pot/150g	114	0	76	8.5	10.2	0	0.4
Skyr, Natural, Icelandic Style, M&S*	1/3 Pot/150g	99	0.2	66	12.2	3.7	0.1	0.5
Skyr, Natural, Migros*	1 Pot/170g	104	0.2	61	11	4	0.1	0
Skyr, Raspberry, & White Chocolate, Sainsbury's*	1 Pot/150g	106	0.8	71	9.2	7.6	0.5	0.5
Skyr, Raspberry, Fat Free, Tesco*	1 Pot/150g	110	0	73	8.3	9.7	0	0.4
Smooth Strawberry, Mullerlight, Muller*	1 Pot/100g	49	0.5	49	4.9	6.5	0.5	0
Smooth Toffee, Fat Free, Mullerlight, Muller*	1 Pot/160g	78	0.8	49	4.8	6.6	0.5	0

YOGHURT

INFO/WEIGHT	Measure	per Measure KCAL	FAT	Nutrition Values per 100g / 100ml KCAL	PROT	CARB	FAT	FIBRE
Soya, Blueberry, Pot, Actileaf, Aldi*	1 Serving/125g	99	3	79	3.7	10	2.4	0.6
Soya, Mercadona*	1 Pot/125g	54	3.4	43	4.6	0	2.7	0
Soya, Natural, SoYummy, Aldi*	1 Serving/100g	48	1.5	48	4.2	4.2	1.5	0
Soya, Plain, No Sugars, Alpro*	1 Tbsp/30g	13	0.7	42	4	0	2.3	0.9
Soya, Strawberry Flavoured, Asda*	1 Pot/100g	75	2.1	75	3.8	10	2.1	0.5
Soya, Woolworths*	1 Pot/150g	115	2.6	77	1.8	13.3	1.7	2.5
Stracciatella, Kvarg, Lindahls, Nestle*	1 Pot/151g	95	0.9	63	11	3.4	0.6	0
Strained, 2% Fat, Olympos*	1 Serving/200g	140	4	70	9	4	2	0
Strained, Fat Free, The Dorset Dairy Co*	1 Serving/150g	82	0.8	55	8.5	4.2	0.5	0
Strawberry Cheesecake Inspired, Crunch, Mullerlight*	1 Pot/107g	98	2	92	4.6	13.5	1.9	0
Strawberry, & Acai, Skyr, Light, Muller*	1 Pot/150g	90	0.8	60	9.5	4.3	0.5	0
Strawberry, & Cream, Finest, Tesco*	1 Pot/150g	206	10.4	137	3.4	15.4	6.9	0.5
Strawberry, & Cream, Scottish, Deluxe, Lidl*	1 Pot/150g	198	9	132	4.1	15.1	6	0.5
Strawberry, & Vanilla, Double Up, Munch Bunch, Nestle*	1 Pot/86g	85	2.3	99	6.1	12.6	2.7	0
Strawberry, & Banana, Soya, No Bits, Alpro*	1 Pot/125g	99	2.5	79	3.7	10.7	2	1
Strawberry, & Raspberry, Greek Style, High Protein, Alpro*	1 Pot/150g	123	4	82	4.7	8.8	2.7	1.5
Strawberry, Active, Brooklea, Aldi*	1 Pot/125g	118	3.9	94	3	13	3.1	0.5
Strawberry, Active, Fat Free, Optifit, Aldi*	1 Pot/125g	54	0.5	43	3	7.1	0.4	0.4
Strawberry, Activia, Danone*	1 Pot/120g	107	3.4	89	3.9	11.8	2.8	0
Strawberry, Benecol*	1 Pot/120g	85	2.3	71	3.8	9.6	1.9	0
Strawberry, Bio, Activia, Danone*	1 Pot/125g	124	4.1	99	3.6	13.6	3.3	0.2
Strawberry, Breakfast Crunch, Corner, Muller*	1 Pot/135g	163	3.5	121	5.5	0	2.6	0
Strawberry, Creamy, Milbona, Lidl*	1 Pot/150g	204	11.1	136	3.1	14	7.4	0.5
Strawberry, Fat Free, Average	**1 Serving/100g**	**66**	**0.1**	**66**	**4.9**	**11.1**	**0.1**	**0.6**
Strawberry, Greek Style, 0% Fat, Liberte, Yoplait*	1 Pot/100g	79	0.2	79	8	11	0.2	0.4
Strawberry, Greek Style, Almarai*	1 Pot/150g	220	10.6	147	5.7	15.2	7.1	0
Strawberry, Greek Style, Bio Live, Activia, Danone*	1 Pot/110g	109	3.3	99	5	12.9	3	0.2
Strawberry, Greek Style, Fat Free, Brooklea, Aldi*	1 Pot/125g	72	0.3	57	4.9	8.8	0.2	0.2
Strawberry, Greek Style, Fat Free, Milbona, Lidl*	1 Pot/125g	78	0.6	62	5.9	8.4	0.5	0.5
Strawberry, Greek Style, Fat Free, Morrisons*	1 Pot/125g	64	0.2	51	4.8	7.5	0.2	0.1
Strawberry, Greek Style, Fruitopolis, Mullerlight, Muller*	1 Pot/130g	84	0.1	65	4.8	10.8	0.1	0
Strawberry, Greek Style, Light & Free, Danone*	1 Pot/115g	55	0.1	48	4	6.9	0.1	1.9
Strawberry, Greek Style, Luxury, Oykos, Danone*	1 Pot/110g	159	8.9	145	3.2	14.6	8.1	0.3
Strawberry, Greek Style, Milbona, Lidl*	1 Pot/125g	160	7.8	128	2.4	15.5	6.2	0.5
Strawberry, Greek Style, Whipped, Bliss, Corner, Muller*	1 Pot/110g	142	6.5	129	4.1	14.3	5.9	0
Strawberry, Greek, Brooklea, Aldi*	1 Pot/150g	118	0.8	79	8.3	11	0.5	0.5
Strawberry, Greek, Lactose Free, Morrisons *	1 Pot/150g	100	1.8	67	6.1	7.7	1.2	0.7
Strawberry, Gut Health, Activia, Danone*	1 Pot/115g	104	3.2	90	3.9	12	2.8	0
Strawberry, Icelandic Style, Strained, Fat Free, Skyr, Arla*	1 Pot/150g	109	0.7	73	9.6	7.4	0.5	0.1
Strawberry, Irish, Coolree Creamery*	1 Pot/125g	121	4.2	97	5.3	11	3.4	0.5
Strawberry, Jogobella, Zott*	1 Serving/125g	112	3.4	90	3.5	12	2.7	0
Strawberry, Jogurtpur Erdbeer, Emmi*	1 Becher/150g	147	4.2	98	4.5	13	2.8	0
Strawberry, Lactose Free, Lactofree, Arla*	1 Pot/125g	126	3.2	101	3.5	15.9	2.6	0.4
Strawberry, Layer, Bonne Maman*	1 Pot/125g	139	5.1	111	2.3	16	4.1	0.4
Strawberry, Liberte, Yoplait*	1 Yogurt/100g	81	0.1	81	7.8	11.1	0.1	0
Strawberry, Live, 0% Fat, Irish, Clonakilty*	1 Pot/125g	50	0.2	40	3.8	5.7	0.2	0.5
Strawberry, Low Fat, Average	**1 Serving/100g**	**81**	**1**	**81**	**4.5**	**13.6**	**1**	**0.2**
Strawberry, Milbona, Lidl*	1 Pot/175g	175	5.2	100	3	15	3	0
Strawberry, Mullerlight, Muller*	1 Pot/160g	83	0.8	52	4.9	7	0.5	0
Strawberry, Naked, Good to Go, Onken*	1 Pack/100g	88	2.8	88	4	11	2.8	0
Strawberry, Organic, Bio Live, Yeo Valley*	1 Serving/150g	147	6	98	4.5	10.9	4	0
Strawberry, Probiotic, Organic, Yeo Valley*	1 Pot/125g	125	5	100	4.4	11.7	4	0.1
Strawberry, Protein 20g, Arla*	1 Pot/200g	140	0.4	70	10	6.5	0.2	0

Y

YOGHURT

INFO/WEIGHT	Measure	per Measure KCAL	FAT	Nutrition Values per 100g / 100ml KCAL	PROT	CARB	FAT	FIBRE
Strawberry, Protein, Grahams*	1 Pot/190g	148	0.8	78	11.4	7.2	0.4	0
Strawberry, Protein, Pouch, Aldi*	1 Pouch/200g	144	1	72	12	4.7	0.5	0.5
Strawberry, Protein, Thick, M&S*	1 Pot/200g	154	0.4	77	11.7	6.9	0.2	0.5
Strawberry, Rice, Low Fat, Muller*	1 Pot/180g	193	4.1	107	3.2	18.4	2.3	0.4
Strawberry, Shortcake, Crunch Corner, Muller*	1 Pot/130g	192	7.3	148	4.5	19.3	5.6	0.1
Strawberry, Skyr, High Protein, Isey Skyr*	1 Pot/170g	143	0.3	84	9.2	11	0.2	0
Strawberry, Skyr, Icelandic Style, Eat Well, M&S*	1 Pot/150g	123	0.6	82	10.2	9.2	0.4	0.5
Strawberry, Soya, Alpro*	¼ Pot/125g	92	2.4	74	3.6	9.4	1.9	1
Strawberry, Split Pot, Asda*	1 Pot/151g	134	3.6	89	3	14	2.4	0.5
Strawberry, Summer Fruits, Benecol*	1 Pot/120g	90	2	75	0.2	9.7	1.7	3.7
Strawberry, Thick & Creamy, Brooklea, Aldi*	1 Pot/150g	206	11.1	137	3.1	14	7.4	0.5
Strawberry, Thick & Creamy, Golden Acre*	1 Pot/150g	219	11.7	146	2.3	16.5	7.8	0.5
Strawberry, Thick & Creamy, Lichfields*	1 Pot/125g	174	9.2	139	2.7	15	7.4	0.7
Strawberry, TruBlend, Fage*	1 Cup/150g	114	2.4	76	8	4.8	1.6	0
Strawberry, West Cork Made, Dunnes Stores*	1 Pot/70g	62	2.1	89	4.3	12	3	0
Strawberry, Yoplait*	1 Pack/125g	112	2.9	90	3.3	13	2.3	0.2
Strawberry, Zero Fat, Yoplait*	1 Pot/125g	56	0.1	45	4.5	5.6	0.1	0.2
Sweet Shop Inspired, Mullerlight, Muller*	1 Yoghurt/160g	78	0.8	49	4.8	6.5	0.5	0
Taillefine aux Fruits, Danone*	1 Pot/125g	58	0.1	46	4.5	6.7	0.1	0
Toffee, Creamfields*	1 Pot/125g	86	1.2	69	2	13	1	0
Toffee, Greek Style, Fat Free, Light, Asda*	1 Pot/125g	68	0.6	54	5.7	7	0.5	0.5
Toffee, Low Fat, Deliciously Silky, Waitrose*	1 Pot/151g	143	3	95	4.6	14.5	2	0.5
Toffee, Smooth, Milbona, Lidl*	1 Pot/175g	105	0.4	60	4.5	9.7	0.2	0.5
Toffee, Smooth, Mullerlight, Muller*	1 Pot/120g	73	1.3	61	6.3	8.5	1.1	0
Toffee, Tempting, Greek Style, Muller Light *	1 Pot/120g	84	0.1	70	6.3	10.1	0.1	0
Tropical, Granola, Duo, Brooklea, Aldi*	1 Pot/135g	177	6.2	131	3.6	18.5	4.6	0.8
Unsweetened, Easiyo*	1 Serving/200g	101	0.3	50	5.1	7	0.2	0
Unsweetened, Greek Style, Hansells Foods*	1 Serving/200g	214	13.2	107	6.6	6.9	6.6	0
Vanilla, & Chocolate Sprinkles, Fat Free, Milbona, Lidl*	1 Pot/175g	93	0.9	53	3.9	7.6	0.5	0.1
Vanilla, & Granola, Low Fat, Activia, Danone*	1 Pot/165g	185	3.3	112	5.3	18.2	2	1.8
Vanilla, & Salted Caramel, Skyr, Light & Fit, Danone*	1 Pot/150g	80	0.8	53	9.3	3.7	0.5	0
Vanilla, & Salted Caramel, Skyr, Light & Free, Danone*	1 Pot/150g	80	0.8	53	9.3	3.7	0.5	0
Vanilla, Average	**1 Serving/120g**	**100**	**5.4**	**83**	**4.5**	**12.4**	**4.5**	**0.8**
Vanilla, Bio Live, Luscious, Organic, Rachel's Organic*	1 Serving/150g	164	8.1	109	3.3	11.8	5.4	0
Vanilla, Choco Balls, Crunch Corner, Snack Size, Muller*	1 Pot/85g	118	4.1	139	3.8	20.2	4.8	0
Vanilla, Fat Free, Onken*	½ Pot/225g	166	0.2	74	4.4	12.6	0.1	0.3
Vanilla, Greek Style, 0% Fat, COU, M&S*	1 Pot/140g	81	0.3	58	6.8	7.2	0.2	0.5
Vanilla, Greek Style, Light & Free, Danone*	1 Pot/115g	58	0.1	50	4.5	6.8	0.1	2
Vanilla, Greek, Lactose Free, Morrisons*	1 Pot/150g	105	0.9	70	5.6	10.5	0.6	0
Vanilla, Isey Skyr*	1 Pot/170g	94	0.3	55	9.7	3.5	0.2	0
Vanilla, Junior, Fage*	1 Pot/100g	92	3.9	92	7.2	7	3.9	0
Vanilla, Light, Brooklea, Aldi*	1 Pot/160g	74	0.8	46	4.5	7	0.5	0
Vanilla, Light, Fat Free, Milbona, Lidl*	1 Serving/165g	92	0	56	4.7	8.9	0	0
Vanilla, Madagascan, West Country, TTD, Sainsbury's*	1 Pot/150g	197	11.8	132	3.1	11.9	7.9	0.5
Vanilla, No Added Sugar, 0% Fat, Gut Health, Activia*	1 Pot/115g	60	0	52	4.9	6.9	0	0
Vanilla, Pouring, Icelandic Style, Skyr, Arla*	1 Serving/150g	92	0.8	61	6.3	8.1	0.5	0
Vanilla, Protein, Milbona, Lidl*	1 Pot/180g	121	0.7	67	12.5	3	0.4	0.5
Vanilla, Smooth, Light, Fat Free, Mullerlight, Muller*	1 Pot/175g	88	0.2	50	4.3	7.2	0.1	0
Vanilla, Soya, Alpro*	1 Sm Pot/125g	82	2.8	66	3.7	7.5	2.2	0.9
Vanilla, SoYummy, Aldi*	1 Serving/150g	106	2	71	3.5	10.9	1.3	0
Vanilla, TruBlend, Fage*	1 Pot/150g	111	2.4	74	8	4.1	1.6	0
Vanilla, Vibe, Light & Free, Danone*	1 Pot/115g	61	0.1	53	4.9	7.1	0.1	0
Vanilla, with Oreo Pieces, Muller*	1 Pot/120g	186	7.1	155	3.5	21.3	5.9	0

	Measure INFO/WEIGHT	per Measure KCAL	FAT	Nutrition Values per 100g / 100ml KCAL	PROT	CARB	FAT	FIBRE

YOGHURT

	Measure INFO/WEIGHT	KCAL	FAT	KCAL	PROT	CARB	FAT	FIBRE
White Chocolate, Greek Style, Light & Free, Danone*	1 Pot/115g	59	0.1	51	4.5	7.1	0.1	1.7
Whole Milk, County Farm *	1 Serving/100g	81	4	81	4.7	6.3	4	0.5
with Apricot Layer, Bonne Maman*	1 Pot/125g	140	5.1	112	2.4	16	4.1	0.5
with Biscuit, Split Pot, Brooklea, Aldi*	1 Pot/135g	262	10.7	194	4	26	7.9	0
with Raspberry Layer, Bonne Maman*	1 Pot/125g	136	5.1	109	2.4	15	4.1	1

YOGHURT DRINK

	Measure INFO/WEIGHT	KCAL	FAT	KCAL	PROT	CARB	FAT	FIBRE
Actimel, Blueberry, Danone*	1 Bottle/100ml	74	1.5	74	2.6	11.8	1.5	0.5
Aktifit, Probiotic, Peach Flavour, Emmi*	1 Pot/65ml	47	0.8	73	2.5	12	1.3	0
Average	**1fl oz/30ml**	**19**	**0**	**62**	**3.1**	**13.1**	**0**	**0**
Blueberry, & Blackcurrant, Skyr, Arla*	1 Bottle/350ml	214	0.7	61	5.8	8.1	0.2	0
Blueberry, Cholesterol Lowering, Tesco*	1 Bottle/100ml	49	1.5	49	2.5	6.2	1.5	0.1
Blueberry, Cholesterol Reducing, Morrisons*	1 Bottle/100ml	36	1.1	36	2.7	3.9	1.1	0.1
Cholesterol Lowering, Asda*	1 Bottle/100ml	76	1.4	76	2.9	13	1.4	1
Fat Free, Brooklea, Aldi*	1 Bottle/100ml	26	0.2	26	2.1	4.2	0.2	0.2
Fruit, Mixed, Actimel, Danone*	1 Bottle/100ml	88	1.5	88	2.7	16	1.5	0
Lemon, 0% Fat, No Added Sugar, Actimel, Danone*	1 Bottle/100ml	27	0.1	27	2.6	3.2	0.1	0.2
Light, Benecol*	1 Bottle/68ml	40	1.4	60	2.8	7.3	2.1	0.1
Light, Yakult*	1 Bottle/65ml	27	0	42	1.4	10.2	0	1.8
Multi Fruit, Actimel, Danone*	1 Bottle/100ml	85	1.5	85	2.7	14.4	1.5	0.1
Multi Fruit, Immune Support, Sainsbury's*	1 Bottle/100ml	32	0.5	32	2.7	4	0.5	0.5
Multifruit, Brooklea, Aldi*	1 Bottle/100ml	71	1.3	71	2.5	12	1.3	0.5
Original, 0.1% Fat, Actimel, Danone*	1 Bottle/100ml	27	0.1	27	2.7	3	0.1	0.2
Original, Cholesterol Lowering, Sainsbury's*	1 Bottle/100ml	36	1.1	36	2.7	3.4	1.1	0.5
Original, Cholesterol Reducing, Tesco*	1 Bottle/100ml	51	1.6	51	2.7	6.1	1.6	0.8
Original, No Added Sugar, Benecol*	1 Bottle/68ml	32	1.4	47	2.8	4.3	2	0
Peach, & Apricot, Benecol*	1 Bottle/68ml	33	1.4	49	2.9	4.8	2	0
Strawberry, Actimel, Danone*	1 Bottle/100ml	74	1.5	74	2.9	11.5	1.5	0
Strawberry, Benecol*	1 Bottle/68ml	38	1.4	56	3.2	6.2	2	0
Strawberry, Cholesterol Lowering, Brooklea, Aldi*	1 Bottle/100ml	37	1.2	37	2.4	3.9	1.2	0.6
Strawberry, Cholesterol Lowering, Milbona, Lidl*	1 Bottle/100ml	53	1.4	53	3.3	6.6	1.4	0
Strawberry, Cholesterol Lowering, Sainsbury's*	1 Bottle/100ml	37	1.2	37	2.4	3.9	1.2	0.6
Strawberry, Cholesterol Reducing, Morrisons*	1 Bottle/100ml	36	1.2	36	2.4	3.9	1.2	0.1
Strawberry, Cholesterol Reducing, Tesco*	1 Bottle/100ml	46	1.7	46	2.7	4.7	1.7	0.8
Strawberry, Fat Free, Actimel, Danone*	1 Bottle/100ml	27	0.1	27	2.6	3.2	0.1	0.2
Yakult*	1 Bottle/65ml	43	0.1	66	1.3	14.7	0.1	0

YORKIE

	Measure INFO/WEIGHT	KCAL	FAT	KCAL	PROT	CARB	FAT	FIBRE
Original, Nestle*	1 Bar/55g	302	17.4	546	6.2	57.9	31.5	1.9
Raisin & Biscuit, Duo, Nestle*	1 Bar/33g	165	8.3	505	6.2	60.2	25.4	2
Raisin & Biscuit, Nestle*	1 Bar/44g	223	11.2	505	6.2	60.2	25.4	2

YORKSHIRE PUDDING

	Measure INFO/WEIGHT	KCAL	FAT	KCAL	PROT	CARB	FAT	FIBRE
Average	**1 Pudding/30g**	**62**	**3**	**208**	**6.6**	**24.7**	**9.9**	**0.9**
Batters, in Foils, Ready to Bake, Frozen, Aunt Bessie's*	1 Pudding/17g	47	1.8	276	9.1	32.6	10.8	1.4
Beef Dripping, Cooked, Specially Selected, Aldi*	1 Pudding/44g	129	5.7	293	9.4	32	13	3
Beef Dripping, Oven Baked, Extra Special, Asda*	1 Pudding/46g	132	5.1	287	9.2	3.6	11	3
Beef Dripping, Oven Baked, Luxury, Iceland*	1 Yorkshire/44g	122	5.3	276	10.1	30.8	12	2.4
Beef Filled, Inspired Cuisine, Aldi*	1 Pack/381g	587	25.2	154	6.8	16	6.6	1.7
Beef Filled, Microwaved, Iceland*	1 Yorkshire/311g	351	5.3	113	5.5	18	1.7	2.2
Beef, Mini, Waitrose*	1 Pudding/14g	33	1.3	234	13.5	23.2	9.4	1.3
Carvery, Aunt Bessie's*	1 Pudding/57g	140	4.2	244	9.1	34	7.3	3.3
Chicken Filled, Inspired Cuisine, Aldi*	1 Pudding/400g	600	21.2	150	8.7	16	5.3	1.8
Chicken, with Potatoes, Stuffing, & Chipolatas, M&S*	1 Serving/365g	646	31.4	177	9.5	14.7	8.6	1.2
Extra Large, Aunt Bessie's*	1 Yorkshire/42g	113	3.6	266	8.2	39	8.4	1.5
Frozen, Oven Baked, Tesco*	1 Pudding/27g	79	2.8	294	11.9	36.2	10.4	4.2

Y

	Measure INFO/WEIGHT	per Measure KCAL	FAT	Nutrition Values per 100g / 100ml KCAL	PROT	CARB	FAT	FIBRE
YORKSHIRE PUDDING								
Frozen, Ovenbaked, Iceland*	1 Pudding/20g	53	1.8	262	7.4	36.8	8.8	3.1
Frozen, Waitrose*	1 Yorkshire Pudding/16g	36	1.1	225	8.5	31.5		6.9
2.2								
Giant, Aunt Bessie's*	1 Pudding/97g	260	7.5	269	8.6	42	7.8	2.6
Large, Co-Op*	1 Pudding/42g	110	2.8	262	10.7	38.1	6.7	3.1
Mini, Farmfoods*	1 Pudding/3g	8	0.2	281	9.6	43.2	7.7	1.9
Original, Golden, As Consumed, Aunt Bessie's*	1 Pudding/19g	53	1.6	279	8.4	41.6	8.4	2.6
Sainsbury's*	1 Pudding/41g	108	2.7	264	10.7	38.9	6.6	3.1
Stamford St. Food Company, Sainsbury's*	2 Yorkshires/29g	83	2.4	285	9	42.1	8.3	2.8
YULE LOG								
Chocolate, Belgian, Finest, Tesco*	1 Slice/93g	294	14.6	316	4.7	38.2	15.7	1.8
Chocolate, Festive Food To Order, Tesco *	1 Serving/76g	261	11.1	343	5.7	46.4	14.6	1.8
Chocolate, Frozen, Tesco*	1 Slice/80g	251	14.6	315	7.5	28.8	18.3	2.3
Chocolate, Sainsbury's*	1 Slice/35g	153	7.7	432	5	51.6	21.8	4.6
Chocolate, Tesco*	1 Slice/30g	133	6.7	439	5.3	52.6	22.2	3.6
Mini, M&S*	1 Cake/36g	165	8.4	460	5.7	56.9	23.3	1.1

ALL BAR ONE

BEEF
Steak, & Frites	1089
Steak, Ribeye, 8oz, with Peppercorn Sauce, & Fries	1069

BEETROOT
Carpaccio	313

BREAD
Rustic, with Olive Oil	711

BREAKFAST
Vegan	745
Vegetarian	801
Vegetarian, Sm Appetites	499

BREAKFAST - FULL ENGLISH
& Toasted Sourdough	1098
with Spinach & Potato Hash, & Toasted Sourdough	1419
Sausage, Egg, Beans, & Toast, Sm Appetites	629

BREAKFAST - POT
Chorizo, Egg	610
Egg, Protein	725

BREAKFAST - PROTEIN POWER UP
Salmon, Egg, Avocado, & Grapefruit, with Salad	372

BREAKFAST - SHAKSHUKA
Standard	589
with Avocado	1017
with Halloumi	1017
with Sourdough	748
with Streaky Bacon	702

BREAKFAST CEREAL
Bircher, Blueberry	528

BROWNIES
Chocolate, with Bourbon Vanilla Ice Cream	582
Chocolate, with Vanilla Ice Cream, Sm Appetites	389

BRUSCHETTA
Avocado, & Tomato, Crushed	545

BURGERS
Beef, Bacon & Cheese	921
Beef, Classic	543
Beef, Dirty	914
Beef, Sliders, Sm Appetites	445
Beef, The Californian	1267
Beef, The French	1166
Beef, The Hipster	1243
Beef, The Skinny	549
Beef, The Smoky	1399
Beef, The Spanish	1205
Beef, The Wagyu	1403
Chicken, Grilled, Classic	496

BURGERS VEGAN
Plant Based	755

BURGERS VEGETARIAN
Tomato, Beetroot, & Mozzarella	905
Tomato, Beetroot, & Mozzarella, The Californian	1205
Tomato, Beetroot, & Mozzarella, The French	1104
Tomato, Beetroot, & Mozzarella, The Hipster	1181

ALL BAR ONE

BURGERS VEGETARIAN
Tomato, Beetroot, & Mozzarella, The Skinny	487
Tomato, Beetroot, & Mozzarella, The Smoky	1337
Tomato, Beetroot, & Mozzarella, The Spanish	1144

BURRITO
Chicken	776
Chicken, with Fries	1179
Chicken, with House Salad	967

CAKE
Chocolate, Mascarpone, & Orange, Mousse	250
Raspberry, & Pistachio, Traybake	150

CHEESECAKE
Biscoff, with Banana, & Caramel	849
Lemon, Sicilian, with Blueberry Compote, Baked	558

CHICKEN
Katsu, Main	702
Piri Piri, Half	450
Piri Piri, Half, with Fries	853
Piri Piri, Half, with House Salad	641
Karaage, Sticky, Bites	477
Schnitzel, with Fries, & Garlic Cream	694
Skewers, Teriyaki, Ginger	335
Wings, BBQ	586
Wings, Buttermilk	657

CROISSANT
with Butter, & Jam	661

DOUGHNUTS
Churros	582

DUMPLINGS
Duck, Crispy	400

EGGS
Benedict, Standard	750
Benedict, with Avocado	1178
Florentine, Standard	748
Florentine, with Avocado	1176
Poached, with Mushrooms, on Toasted Sourdough	461
Royale, Standard	824
Royale, with Avocado	1252
Scrambled, & Salmon, on Toasted Sourdough	722

FISH
Cod, & Mushy Peas, & Tartare Sauce, Sm Appetites	301
Goujons, with Aioli	349
Goujons, with Tartare Sauce, Sm Appetites	278

FISH & CHIPS
Main	758

FISH CAKES
Haddock, Smoked, & Mustard	291
Haddock, Smoked, & Mustard, with Fries	694
Haddock, Smoked, & Mustard, with House Salad	482

FLATBREAD
Garlic, Stonebaked	1054
Houmous, & Kale	615

ALL BAR ONE

FRIES
Halloumi, Standard	460
Potato, Standard	399
Potato, Sm Appetites	177
Potato, with Parmesan, Truffle Oil, & Rosemary	482
Potato, with Smoked Paprika & Saffron Aioli	482
Trio, Standard	1125

FRUIT
Strawberries, & Bananas, Fresh, Sm Appetites	253

HASH
Potato, Spinach, & Onion, Pan Fried	582

HOUMOUS
Duo	715

ICE CREAM
Trio	318
Vanilla, 2 Scoops, Sm Appetites	244

KEBAB
Chorizo, & Halloumi, Skewers	601

LAMB
Kibbeh	553

LASAGNE
Plant Based	747

MACARONI CHEESE
Main	430

MEATBALLS
Lamb, Spiced	499

MELT
Chicken, BBQ, Bacon, & Cheese	774

MEZZE
Little, Sm Appetites	738

MUFFIN
Blueberry	547
Blueberry Cheesecake	463
Carrot Cake	459
Chocolate, Triple	505
Lemon, & White Chocolate	462

NACHOS
Original	997
Vegan	831
with BBQ Pulled Pork	1425

NOODLES
Pad Thai	606
Pad Thai, Little, Sm Appetites	313
Pad Thai, with Chicken Breast	808
Pad Thai, with Pan Fried King Prawns	703
Pad Thai, with Sliced Beef Fillet	775

PAIN AU CHOCOLAT
Pastry	425

PANCAKES - BUTTERMILK
with Maple Syrup, Banana, & Berries	491
with Maple Syrup, & Smoked Bacon	568

PASTRY
Spinach & Feta, Bourek	303

ALL BAR ONE

PIE
Pecan, Bourbon, with Cinnamon Ice Cream	540

PLATTER
Deli Board, Sharing, Whole Board	1826
Grazing Board, Sharing, Whole Board	2170
Mezze Board, Sharing, Whole Board	2016

POTATOES
Patatas Bravas	283

PRAWN CRACKERS
Portion	58

PRAWNS
King, Pan Fried, Add On	104
King, Pan Fried	292

QUESADILLA
Chicken	514
Lentil, & Chickpea	460

RIBS
BBQ, Smoked	1494

RICE
Miso, Bowl	474
Miso, Bowl, with Chicken Breast	670
Miso, Bowl, with Pan Fried King Prawns	585
Miso, Bowl, with Sliced Beef Fillet	726
Steamed, Sm Appetites	179

ROLL
Bacon, Sour Cream, Chilli Tomato Jam, & Coriander	716

SALAD
Chicken, & Avocado, Chargrilled	905
Chicken, & Avocado, Chargrilled, Sm Appetites	427
Duck, Crispy	568
Feta, Beetroot, & Walnut	509
Feta, Carrot, & Quinoa	626
House	202
Rocket, & Parmesan	234
Side	202
Small Appetites	96
Superfood	440
Superfood, with Chicken Breast	634
Superfood, with Garlic & Lemon Marinated Halloumi	634
Superfood, with Pan Fried King Prawns	654

SANDWICH
Bacon, with Sliced Tomatoes, & Tomato Sauce	670
Chicken, Grilled, Focaccia	610
Club	1454
Sausage	939
Sausage, Veggie	685
Steak, Fillet	606

SAUCE
Katsu Curry	156

SAUSAGE
Cocktail, Maple Glazed	572

SORBET
Raspberry, 2 Scoops, Sm Appetites	255

	KCAL
ALL BAR ONE	
SORBET	
Raspberry	546
SOUP	
Tomato, Vegetable, & Quinoa	122
SQUID	
Calamari, Salt & Pepper	404
TACO	
Chilli Non Carne	503
TOAST	
Sourdough, with Avocado, & Feta	732
TORTE	
Chocolate, Salted Caramel, with Hazelnut Ice Cream	535
TORTILLA	
Huevos Rancheros	585
VEGETABLES	
Tempura	351
WAFFLES	
Belgian, with Maple Syrup, Fruit, & Yoghurt	1028
WRAP	
Fish Finger	534

	KCAL
ASK ITALIAN	
ANTIPASTO	
The Mixed One, Classico	6479
ARANCINI	
Spinach & Ricotta, with Tomato Dip	387
BEEF	
in Chianti Sauce, Slow Cooked	876
BREAD	
Garlic	588
Garlic, with Mozzarella	784
Rosemary, & Olive Oil	499
BREADSTICKS	
& Tomato, Dip, Little Tums, Kids Menu	159
BROCCOLI	
Side, Kids Menu	13
BRUSCHETTA	
BLANK	365
CALZONE	
Con Carne Piccante	970
Goats Cheese, & Spinach	991
Pollo	899
CANNELLONI	
Sausage, Ragu, Baked, with Creme Fraiche	658
CARBONARA	
Asparagus & Pancetta, Fresca	882
Asparagus & Pancetta, Light, with Salad	541
Linguine	814
CHEESE	
Fonduta, with Dough Sticks	864
CHEESECAKE	
Honeycomb. with Vanilla Gelato	719
Passion Fruit, & Raspberry	481
CHICKEN	
with Tomato Dip, & Garlic Mayo, Lecca-Lecca	675
Pollo, Milanese	753
Pollo, Milanese, with Chips	1009
CHIPS	
Garlic, & Cheese, Side	892
with Mayo, Side	863
COURGETTE	
Zucchine Fritti	328
DESSERT	
Chocolate Etna	851
Gelato, Warm Cookie, & Salted Caramel	968
Gelato Gondola, Salted Caramel	516
DESSERT PIZZA	
Chocolate, Kids Menu	160
DESSERT RAVIOLI	
Rhubarb & Custard	445
DOUGH BALLS	
Cheese, Fontal, & Chilli	711
Plain	550
FETTUCCINE	
Bolognese	692

ASK ITALIAN

FETTUCCINE
Con Melanzane, Vegan	843
Con Verdure, Vegan	1042

FRIES
Sweet Potato, Rosemary	300

FRUIT MIX
Kids Menu	14

GIRASOLE
Spinach, & Ricotta	743

GNOCCHI
Chocolate, Baked	473

ICE CREAM
Gelato, Chocolate, 3 Scoops	268
Gelato, Hazelnut, 3 Scoops	332
Gelato, Salted Caramel, 3 Scoops	308
Gelato, Vanilla, 3 Scoops	283

ICE LOLLY
Apple, & Raspberry, Kids Menu	43
Orange, & Apple, Kids Menu	45

LASAGNE
Beef, & Pork, Ragu	717
Grande	1021

LINGUINE
Seafood, Con Frutti Di Mare	828

MEATBALLS
Pork, & Beef, Picante, in Spicy, Tomato Sauce	718

MUSHROOMS
Al Forno	540

OLIVES
Italian	204

PANNA COTTA
Portion	191

PASTA
Crab & Ricotta, Half Moon	692
in Tomato Sauce, Little Tums, Kids Menu	201
King Prawn, & Crayfish, Fresca	708
Sausage, & Truffle Infused Olive Oil, Fresca	940
with Butter, Little Tums, Kids Menu	245

PASTA SAUCE
Bolognese, Choose Your Favourite, Kids Menu	137
Cheese, Choose Your Favourite, Kids Menu	217
Tomato, Choose Your Favourite, Kids Menu	109

PENNE
Arrabiata	759
Arrabiata, with Chicken	869
Beef, Meatballs, Ragu, Mozzarella, Manzo Piccante	718
Chicken, Al Pollo Della Casa	842
Plain, Choose Your Favourite, Kids Menu	346

PIZZA
Caprina, Light, Prima (Pizza Only)	382
Caprina, Prima	863
Fiorentina, Two Egg, Prima	903
Margherita, Classic	733

ASK ITALIAN

PIZZA
Margherita, Four Cheese	738
Margherita, Vegan, Prima	535
Pollo E Funghi, Classic	764
Pollo Picante Con Pancetta, Light, Prima	435
Pollo Picante Con Pancetta, Prima	914
Salami, Misti, Prima	1011
Salsiccia, Sausage, Spicy, Prima	1116
Stromboli, Classic	881
Super Green, Prima	691
Verdure, Classic	793

PIZZA TOPPING
Cheese, Extra, Top Your Own, Kids Menu	158
Chicken, Top Your Own, Kids Menu	44
Ham, Top Your Own, Kids Menu	34
Mushrooms, Top Your Own, Kids Menu	14
Olives, Black, Top Your Own, Kids Menu	13
Pepperoni, Top Your Own, Kids Menu	93
Red Peppers, Roasted, Top Your Own, Kids Menu	8

PORK
Belly, Porchetta	1143

PRAWNS
King, Butterfly, Light	114
King, Butterfly, on Italian Bread	416

PROFITEROLES
Ice Cream, Chocolate Sauce	325

RAVIOLI
Beef, & Chianti	728
Ravioli, Four Cheese, & Beef Ragu	571

RISOTTO
Con Pollo E Funghi	818

SALAD
Caesar, Chicken, Kale	571

SALAD
Cheese, Burrata, Tomatoes, Rocket, Caprese	303
Insalata Di Pollo E Pancetta	743
Mixed, Side	18
Rainbow, Side	66
Rainbow, Vegan	243
Side, Kids Menu	44

SEA BASS
Al Forno	465

SNACKS
Nibbles, Spicy	167

SORBET
Sorbetti, Mango, 3 Scoops	154
Sorbetti, Raspberry, 3 Scoops	196

SOUFFLE
Cheese, Twice Baked	376

SPAGHETTI
Al Pomodoro	672
Lentil, Ragu, Vegan	849
Pomodoro, Vegan	765

	KCAL
ASK ITALIAN	
SQUID	
Calamari, Breaded	476
SUNDAE	
Ice Cream, Chocolate, Make Your Own, Kids Menu	89
Ice Cream, Vanilla, Make Your Own, Kids Menu	94
TAGLIATELLE	
Pesto, Genovese, Purple	926
Pesto, Genovese, Purple, Light, with Salad	486
TART	
Chocolate, & Blood Orange	310
Pear	333
TIRAMISU	
Portion	419
TOMATOES	
Plum, Side, Kids Menu	4
TOPPING	
Grapes, Make Your Own Sundae	8
Marshmallow & Sprinkles, Make your Own Sundae	25
Meringue, Plain, Make Your Own Sundae,	40
Strawberries, Make Your Own Sundae	8
White Chocolate Swirl, Make Your Own Sundae	55
TORTELLINI	
Cheese, & Vegetable, Dip & Tip	281
VEGETABLES	
Sticks, with Bread, & Dip, Kids Menu	175
WHITEBAIT	
Breaded	683

	KCAL
BEEFEATER RESTAURANT	
BEANS	
Baked, in Tomato Sauce, Side, Kids Menu	51
BBQ, Spiced, Side	157
BEEF	
Duo	1437
Slow Cooked, Kids, Sunday Lunch Menu	697
Slow Cooked, Sunday Lunch Menu	1351
Steak, & Frites	686
Steak, & Frites, Daytime Saver	629
Steak, Fillet, 8oz, & Chips	813
Steak, Fillet, 8oz, & Chips, & Salad	831
Steak, Fillet, 8oz, & Side Salad	461
Steak, Fillet, 8oz, with Veg Medley	505
Steak, Flat Iron, 6oz, & Chips	747
Steak, Flat Iron, 6oz, & Chips, & Salad	765
Steak, Flat Iron, 6oz, & Side Salad	395
Steak, Flat Iron, 6oz, with Veg Medley	439
Steak, Porterhouse, 18oz, & Chips	1503
Steak, Porterhouse, 18oz, & Chips, & Salad	1521
Steak, Porterhouse, 18oz, & Side Salad	1151
Steak, Porterhouse, 18oz, with Veg Medley	1197
Steak, Rib-eye, 10oz, & Chips	988
Steak, Rib-eye, 10oz, & Chips, & Salad	993
Steak, Rib-eye, 10oz, & Side Salad	624
Steak, Rib-eye, 10oz, with Veg Medley	668
Steak, Ribs, & Prawn, Combo	1720
Steak, Rump, 10oz, & Chips	941
Steak, Rump, 10oz, & Chips, & Salad	966
Steak, Rump, 10oz, with Veg Medley	651
Steak, Rump. 10oz, & Side Salad	595
Steak, Sirloin, 8oz, & Chips	802
Steak, Sirloin, 8oz, & Chips, & Salad	808
Steak, Sirloin, 8oz, & Salad	437
Steak, Sirloin, 8oz, with Veg Medley	482
Steak, with Chips, Kids Menu	461
BREAD	
Brown, Buttered, Extra	257
Flatbread, Garlic, & Dips	912
Flatbread, Garlic, Strips	1013
Garlic	218
Garlic, Kids Menu	112
White, Buttered, Extra	254
BROWNIES	
Chocolate	555
Chocolate, Daytime Saver Menu	555
BURGERS	
Beef, Bacon & Cheese, Triple	1697
Beef, Kids Menu	587
Steak, Daytime Saver Menu	863
Steak, Double, Daytime Saver Menu	1152
Steak, with Cheese & Bacon, Daytime Saver Menu	1080
Beef, Bacon & Cheese, Double	1530
Steak, with Cheese & Bacon	1187

BEEFEATER RESTAURANT

BURGERS

Chicken, Tabasco, Crispy	1059
Steak, Smoky BBQ, Summer BBQ Specials	1463

BURGERS VEGAN

with BBQ Pulled Soya	938

BURGERS VEGETARIAN

Main	910

CAKE

Trio of Sponges, with Custard	695

CAULIFLOWER CHEESE

Sunday Lunch Menu	283

CHEESE

Halloumi, Battered, & Chips, Daytime Saver Menu	983

CHEESECAKE

Vanilla, Baked	675

CHICKEN

BBQ, with Half Rack Of Ribs	1025
BBQ, with Whole Rack Of Ribs	1432
Breast, Kids, Sunday Lunch Menu	453
Breast, Plain	693
Breast, Smoky Paprika, Grilled	729
Breast, Smoky Paprika, Grilled, Daytime Saver Menu	578
Escalope, Breast, Breaded	1309
Goujons, Buttermilk, Summer BBQ Specials	742
Half, Roasted, Sunday Lunch Menu	1486
Melt, BBQ Sauce, Grilled	858
Poppin, with Chips, & Beans, Kids Menu	400
Wings, with BBQ, Spicy, 3, Side	160
Wings, with BBQ, Crispy, 5	260
Wings, with BBQ, Crispy, 8	401
Wings, with Piri Piri, Crispy, 5	252
Wings, with Piri Piri, Crispy, 8	394
Wings, with Piri Piri, Spicy, 3, Side	153

CHIPS

Cheesy, & Gravy	726
Side, Kids Menu	187
Triple Cooked, Side	418
Triple Cooked, Spicy, Side	420

COD

Bites, Breaded, Kids Menu	517

CORN

Cob, Mini, Side	61
Cob, Mini, Side, Kids Menu	29

CRUMBLE

Apple, Toffee, Salted	596

DESSERT

Caramel Apple Betty, with Custard	496
Caramel Apple Betty, with Ice Cream	462
Caramel Apple Betty, with Pouring Cream	531
Caramel Apple Betty, with Whipped Cream	455
Chocolate Challenge, Mini, Kids Menu	342
Mississippi Mud Pie	991

BEEFEATER RESTAURANT

DOUGHNUTS

Mini, Kids Menu	249

FISH & CHIPS

Beer Battered, Daytime Saver Menu	886

BEEFEATER RESTAURANT

FRIES

Potato, Skinny, Side	328
Potato, Skinny, Spicy, Side	329

FROZEN YOGHURT

Strawberry	235
Strawberry, Kids Menu	197

FRUIT SALAD

Mixed, Kids Menu	49

GAMMON

Blackened, with Egg, Daytime Saver Menu	751
Blackened, with Pineapple, Daytime Saver Menu	729
Steak, Blackened, in Spicy Rub	1034
Steak, Chargrilled, with Egg & Pineapple	1026
Steak, with Egg, Daytime Saver Menu	746
Steak, with Pineapple, Daytime Saver Menu	723

HADDOCK - BEER BATTERED

with Chips, Ultimate, Daytime Saver Menu	920
with Chips & Mushy Peas	958
with Chips & Peas	920

ICE CREAM

Vanilla, with Caramel Sauce, Kids Menu	254
Vanilla, with Chocolate Sauce, Kids Menu	253
Vanilla, with Raspberry Sauce, Kids Menu	253
with Chocolate Sauce	279
with Chocolate Sauce, Sunday Lunch Menu	275

KEBAB

Pork & Beef, Kofta, Grilled	444

LAMB

Rump, Minted, Grilled	720
Rump, Sunday Lunch Menu	1270

LASAGNE

Beef & Pork, with Chips, Daytime Saver	872
Beef & Pork, with Salad, Daytime Saver	595
Sweet Potato & Feta, with Chips	975
Sweet Potato & Feta, with Chips, Daytime Saver	937
Sweet Potato & Feta, with Salad	697
Sweet Potato & Feta, with Salad, Daytime Saver	659

LINGUINE

Roast Vegetable, in Tomato Sauce	563
Roast Vegetable, In Tomato Sauce, with Chicken	718
Roast Vegetable, in Tomato Sauce, with Salmon	1010

MACARONI CHEESE

Daytime Saver Menu	888

MAKHANI

Chicken, Daytime Saver Menu	998

MEATBALLS

Arrabiata, Linguine	821

BEEFEATER RESTAURANT

MIXED GRILL

	KCAL
Rump Steak, Chicken Breast, Gammon, Sausage	1741
Flat Iron Steak, Chicken Breast, Gammon, Sausage	1498
Sirloin Steak, Chicken Breast, Gammon, Sausage	1583

MUSHROOMS

Crispy, Flat Cap, in Breadcrumbs	489

NACHOS

with Cheesy Yoghurt Dip, Kids Menu	235

ONION RINGS

Beer Battered, Crispy, Side	221

PASTA

Penne, in Tomato Sauce, Kids Menu	347

PATE

Duck, with Ciabatta	430

PEAS

Side, Kids Menu	47

PIE

Banoffee	701
Beef, & Cheddar, with Mash & Gravy	1397
Chicken & Ham, Daytime Saver Menu	1114

PLATTER

The Beefeater, Sharing	700
The Beefeater, with Ribs, Sharing	904

POTATO MASH

Side, Kids Menu	131

POTATOES

Crushed, Garlic, Side	344
Dauphinoise, Sunday Lunch Menu	320
Dippers, With Cheese, & Bacon, Loaded	587
Dippers, with Cheese, Loaded	492
Dippers, with Cheese, Sharing	1262
Dippers, with Cheese & Spring Onion, Loaded	517
Jacket, Side	438

PRAWN COCKTAIL

Classic, with Ciabatta	340

PRAWNS

Garlic, with Ciabatta	371
King, Garlic, 3, Side	151

PROFITEROLES

Main Menu	465
Daytime Saver Menu	465

PUDDING

Apple Crisp	299

RIBS - BBQ

Sticky, Summer BBQ Specials	451
Half Rack, & Chips, Daytime Saver Menu	946
Sticky Bourbon, Grill	1320

RISOTTO

Chicken, & Mushroom, Creamy	833
Chicken, & Mushroom, Daytime Saver Menu	831
Mushroom, Creamy	678
Mushroom, Daytime Saver Menu	676

BEEFEATER RESTAURANT

SALAD

	KCAL
BLT, with Egg, Daytime Saver Menu	328
Caesar, Chicken, Goujons, Summer BBQ Specials	986
Caesar, Chicken, Grilled, Daytime Saver Menu	463
Caesar, Salmon, Blackened, Summer BBQ Specials	1076
Caesar, Summer BBQ Specials	421
Chicken, Jerk, Mango, Summer BBQ Specials	323
Chunky Slaw, Side	149
Greek, Crunchy, Side	173
Halloumi, Jerk, Mango, Summer BBQ Specials	421
Mixed, Large, Side	68
Mixed Bean	604
Salmon, Jerk, Mango, Summer BBQ Specials	621
Side, Kids Menu	6
Steak, with Pear	778

SALMON

Grilled	1014

SANDWICH

Chicken Goujons, Buttermilk, Daytime Saver Menu	1054
Steak, Open, with Fries, Daytime Saver Menu	986

SAUCE

Bearnaise, Steak Sauces	135
Beef, Rich, Steak Sauces	42
Cheddar, Pulled Ham, & Mushroom, Steak Sauces	98
Peppercorn, Triple, Steak Sauces	41
Prawn & Lobster, Steak Sauces	67

SAUSAGE & MASH

Bangers, Kids Menu	391
Main	902
Quorn	729
Vegetarian, Bangers, Kids Menu	361

SEA BASS

Oven Baked, with Crunchy Greek Salad	451

SORBET

Lemon Curd	242

SOUP

Tomato	351

SPAGHETTI BOLOGNESE

Kids Menu	345

SPINACH

Creamy, Side	123

SUNDAE

Cookie Dough	694
Funny Face, Kids Menu	265
Rocky Road	688

TRIFLE

Strawberry, Pimms, Summer BBQ Specials	699

VEGETABLES

Medley, Side	112
Sticks, Side, Kids Menu	28
Sticks, with Yoghurt Dip	51

WAFFLES

Apple, Salted, Toffee, Summer BBQ Specials	881

BEEFEATER RESTAURANT

WELLINGTON
Vegetable, Sunday Lunch Menu	1646

WRAP
Chicken Breast, Cheese, Vegetables, Kids Menu	540
Quorn Sausage, Cheese, Vegetables, Kids Menu	540
Salmon, Cheese, Vegetables, Kids Menu	605

YOGHURT
Strawberry, Kids Menu	127

BELLA ITALIA

ANTIPASTI
Board, Starter	806

ARANCINI
Starter	477

BEANS
Green, Side	42

BEEF - STEAK
Sirloin, with Chips	1453
Sirloin, with Salad	525

BOLOGNESE
Penne, GF	756
Penne, GF, Vegan	944
Spaghetti	688
Spaghetti, Vegan	668

BREAD
Pane Bella	801

BROWNIES
Chocolate	396

BRUSCHETTA
GF, with Tomatoes, & Red Onion, Starter	343
with Tomatoes, & Red Onion, Starter	674

BURGERS
Americano, GF	664
Bean, Cannellini, No Sides	593
Beef, Black Angus, No Sides	664
Chicken, Pollo, No Sides	659
Vegan, No Sides	472

CALZONE
Carne	1102
Diavola	1162
Verdure, Pesto	1312

CARBONARA
Main	792
GF	1035

CHEESE
Goats, Extra	120
Mozzarella, Carrozza, Starter	849

CHEESECAKE
Strawberry	675

CHICKEN
Breast, Grilled, with Fries	1284
Breast, Grilled, with Salad	356
Breast, Grilled, with Salad, GF	737
Extra	168
Half, Barbecue, Fries, Onion Rings, & Coleslaw	1579
Half, Piri Piri, Fries, Onion Rings, & Coleslaw	1634
Half, Sweet & Sour, Fries, Onion Rings, & Coleslaw	3019
Pollo, Lenticchie, Lighter	335
Pollo Funghi	681
Pollo Milanese	848

CHICKEN
Wings, Barbecue	372
Wings, Piri Piri	434

BELLA ITALIA

	KCAL
CHICKEN	
Wings, Sweet & Sour	469
COLESLAW	
Side	109
DESSERT	
Cookie Dough, Al Forno	867
Cookie Dough, Vegan, Al Forno	864
Dolcetti, Sharing	956
DOUGH BALLS	
Bites, with Basil Pesto	520
Bites, with Garlic & Rosemary Dip	473
DOUGHNUTS	
with Chocolate Sauce, Mini	516
FLATBREAD	
GF, with Caramelised Onion, Vegan	915
GF, with Garlic Butter	677
GF, with Mozzarella, & Garlic Butter	867
GF, with Pomodoro, & Pesto	611
GF, with Sausage, 'Nduja, & Mozzarella	657
with Garlic Butter	723
with Mozzarella, & Garlic Butter	907
with Onion, Caramelised, & Mozzarella	976
with Pomodoro, & Pesto	732
with Sausage, 'Nduja, & Mozzarella	808
FRIES	
Potato, Side	1116
Potato, Side	458
Sweet Potato, Side	335
ICE CREAM	
Bubblegum	292
Cherry, Amarena	347
Chocolate Chip	305
Hazelnut	291
Honeycomb	335
Limoncello	209
Mint Chocolate Chip	332
Raspberry	118
Strawberry	205
Vanilla	258
LASAGNE	
Traditional, Al Forno	836
MEATBALLS	
Pork, & Beef, Polpette, Starter	511
Vegan, GF, Polpette, Starter	316
Vegan, Polpette, Starter	454
MUSHROOMS	
Funghi, Arrosto, GF, Starter	332
Funghi, Arrosto, Starter	440
OLIVES	
Sicilain	196
ONION RINGS	
Side	667

BELLA ITALIA

	KCAL
PANNA COTTA	
Coconut	378
PASTA	
Bolognese Spirali, Lighter	283
Cacio E Pepe	1193
Cacio E Pepe, GF	1476
Calabrese	774
Calabrese, GF	1388
Carne Festa, Al Forno	1029
Gamberoni Spirali, Lighter	259
Lenticchie Spirali, Lighter	299
Marco Polo	1006
Marco Polo, GF	1070
Marco Polo, Vegan, & GF	1093
Marco Polo, Vegan	1002
Penne, Pomodoro, GF	423
Pollo Alla Crema, Al Forno	1043
Pollo Pesto	1037
Pollo Pesto, GF	1205
Pollo Pesto, Vegan, & GF	1089
Pollo Pesto, Vegan	1318
Pomodoro Rustica	574
PIZZA	
Campagna, Standard	869
Campagna, GF	1029
Campagna, Ripiena Crust	1461
Campagna, Roma	869
Carne Mista, Standard	1006
Carne Mista, GF	1171
Carne Mista, Ripiena Crust	1541
Carne Mista, Roma	1006
Cotto, Standard	801
Cotto, GF	873
Cotto, Ripiena Crust	1233
Cotto, Roma	801
Diavola Forte, Standard	1255
Diavola Forte, GF	1523
Diavola Forte, Ripiena Crust	1871
Diavola Forte, Roma	1255
Funghi Luganica, Standard	1404
Funghi Luganica, GF	1454
Funghi Luganica, Ripiena Crust	1788
Funghi Luganica, Roma	1435
Gamberoni, Standard	895
Gamberoni, GF	1065
Gamberoni, Ripiena Crust	1289
Gamberoni, Roma	910
Margherita, Standard	764
Margherita, GF	911
Margherita, Ripiena Crust	1187
Margherita, Roma	764
Vegan Cheese, Standard	931
Milli Colori, Lighter	525

BELLA ITALIA
PIZZA

	KCAL
Parma Bufala, Standard	1039
Parma Bufala, GF	1334
Parma Bufala, Ripiena Crust	1388
Parma Bufala, Roma	1110
Pepperoni Piccante, Standard	963
Pepperoni Piccante, Roma	963
Pepperoni Piccante, GF	1065
Pepperoni Piccante, Ripiena Crust	1408
Pollo, Barbecue, Standard	979
Pollo, Barbecue, GF	1167
Pollo, Barbecue, Ripiena Crust	1596
Pollo, Barbecue, Roma	979
Pollo, Sapori, Lighter	533
Pollo, Vesuvio, Standard	924
Pollo, Vesuvio, GF	1144
Pollo, Vesuvio, Ripiena Crust	1311
Pollo, Vesuvio, Roma	924
Margherita, Queen, Standard	1085
Margherita, Queen, GF	989
Margherita, Queen, Ripiena Crust	1514
Margherita, Queen, Roma	1085
Barbecue, Vegan, Standard	930
Barbecue, Vegan, GF	987
Barbecue, Vegan, Roma	930

PIZZA BASE

Create Your Own	832
GF, Create Your Own	726
Ripiena, Create Your Own	1328
Roma, Create Your Own	844
Vegan, GF, Create Your Own	935

PIZZA TOPPING

Black Olives	30
Chicken	358
Cotto Ham	112
Goats Cheese	155
Green Chilli	4
Mozzarella, Buffalo	106
Mushrooms, Garlic	48
Pancetta	68
Pepperoni	127
Red Onion	42
Roast Peppers	55
Rocket	1
Salami	64
Sausage, 'Nduja	146
Sausage, Luganica	101
Spinach	6
Spring Onion	12
Tuna	66

POTATOES

New, Crushed, with Spring Onions, Side	249

BELLA ITALIA
PRAWNS

	KCAL
King, Gamberi, GF, Starter	332
King, Gamberi, Starter	303

RIBS - RACK, BARBECUE

& Chicken, Half, with Coleslaw, Onion Rings, & Fries	1391
Slow Roasted, with Coleslaw, Onion Rings, & Fries	1609

RIBS - RACK, PIRI PIRI

& Chicken, Half, with Coleslaw, Onion Rings, & Fries	1352
Slow Roasted, with Coleslaw, Onion Rings, & Fries	1532

RIBS - RACK, SWEET & SOUR

& Chicken, Half, with Coleslaw, Onion Rings, & Fries	2932
Slow Roasted, with Coleslaw, Onion Rings, & Fries	3028

RIGATONI

Funghi Crema	654
Funghi Crema, GF	896

RISOTTO

Pescatore	570
Pollo Funghi	620
Verdura	560

SALAD

Insalata Caesar	432
Insalata Caesar, with Pollo, & Pancetta	561
Insalata Caprese, Starter	339
Insalata di Verona	875
Insalata Giardiniera	265
Insalata Parma Bufala	655
Mixed, Side	98
Side	188

SALMON

Extra	342
Salmone Al Forno	906
Salmone Al Forno, GF	946

SAUCE

Garlic Butter, Steak Sauce	65
Mushroom, Creamy, Steak Sauce	226
Peppercorn, Steak Sauce	83

SOUP

Seasonal, GF, Starter	294
Seasonal, Starter	410

SPAGHETTI

Gamberoni, Arrabiata	692
Gamberoni, Arrabiata, GF	526
Marinara	653
Marinara, GF	965

SPAGHETTI & MEATBALLS

Polpette American, Vegan, & GF	727
Polpette American, Vegan	797
Polpette Americano	760

SQUID

Calamari, Starter	282

SUNDAE

Banoffee	1192
Rocky Road	1023

BELLA ITALIA

TAGLIATELLE

	KCAL
Capra	906
Capra, GF	908

TIRAMISU

Portion	463

TOPPING

Banana	79
Biscuits, Amaretti	45
Chocolate Tagliatelle	40
Ice Cream Cone, Crushed	39
Marshmallows	33
Popping Candy	59
Sprinkles	41
Whipped Cream	92

VEGETABLES

Mediterranean, Roasted, Side	65

BILL'S

ASPARAGUS

	KCAL
& Baby Spinach, Side	154

BEEF - STEAK

Flat Iron	694
Minute, with Chips, & Egg, & Garlic Butter	968
no Chips, Kids	359
Ribeye, 14oz	650
Sirloin, 10oz	617
with Chips, Kids	534

BREAD

& Houmous, For 2	392
Basket, without Butters, Whole Basket	956
Focaccia, for Soup	130
Focaccia, with Houmous, & Olives	392
Garlic, & Herb, Flatbread, ½ Bread	290
Sourdough, Rosemary, Pea Houmous, & Garlic	632
Sourdough, Rosemary & Garlic, Grilled, & Eggs	960
Stone Baked, with Balsamic, & Olive Oil, For 2	264
Tortilla, Corn, Spiced, with Guacamole	516
Tortilla, Corn, Spiced, without Guacamole	441

BREAKFAST

Eggs, Baked, with Spicy Beans, & Chorizo	444
Eggs, Baked, Spicy Beans, & Chorizo, & Flatbread	564
Full English, Brunch, with Toast	1317
Full English, with Toast	887
Full English, Veggie, with Toast	807
Garden, No Hollandaise	707
Garden, Plate, No Hollandaise	951
Kids	558
Vegan, Full	626

BREAKFAST CEREAL

Porridge, Oat	600

BROCCOLI

Long Stem, Side	179

BROWNIES

Chocolate, Warm, no Ice Cream	569
Chocolate, Warm, no Ice Cream, Kids	218
Chocolate, Warm, with Ice Cream	676
Chocolate, Warm, with Ice Cream, Kids	325

BUNS

Bacon, Breakfast	667
Sausage, Cumberland, Breakfast	563

BURGERS

Chicken, Buttermilk, no Chipotle Mayo	592
Chicken, Buttermilk, with Chipotle Mayo	822
Chicken, Fillet, Kids	365
Halloumi, with Lime Mayo	939
Halloumi	684
Hamburger	696
Hamburger, with Mayo, Kids	372
Lamb, no Tzatziki	804
Lamb, with Tzatziki	833
Naked, with Salad, & Tzatziki, no Bun	525

BILL'S

CAKE
Carrot, no Whipped Cream	198
Carrot, with Whipped Cream	312
Victoria Sponge	598

CAULIFLOWER CHEESE
for Two, ½ Portion	119

CHEESE
Halloumi, Sticks, Crispy, no Lemon Garlic Mayo	578

CHEESECAKE
Banana, & Honeycomb	827

CHICKEN
Half, Paprika, Garlic, & Chilli, with Fries	1302
Milanese, with Salad	738
Paillard	596
Pan Fried, with Wild Mushrooms	705
Skewers, Devilled	452
Skewers, Mojo Marinated, no Dressing	1057
Skewers, Mojo Marinated, with Dressing	1154

CHOCOLATES
Truffles, Salted Caramel, 3 Truffles	168

COD - BEER BATTERED
with Pea Puree, Tartare Sauce, & Fries	1123

CRAB CAKES
Baked, with Tartare Sauce	567
Baked, without Tartare Sauce	417
with Egg, & Asparagus	655

CREME BRULEE
Coconut, & Orange Rice	344

CRUMBLE
Apple, & Salted Caramel	613

CURRY
Chicken, Thai Green, with Rice	734

CURRY
Chicken, Thai Green, without Rice	507

DESSERT
Chocolate Bombe, Meltin	937
Eton Mess, Mango, & Passion Fruit	477

DHAL - AUBERGINE
Lentil, & Chickpea, Roasted	543
Lentil, & Chickpea, Roasted, with Flatbread	695

DOUGHNUTS
Cinnamon, Mini, no Sauce	483
Cinnamon, Mini, Salted Caramel & Chocolate Sauce	649
Strawberry Dusted, Warm	711

DUMPLINGS
Chicken, Sesame, with Chutney	336
Pork, Sesame, Golden Fried, with Dipping Sauce	451

EGGS
Benedict, with Hollandaise	468
Benedict, without Hollandaise	244
Florentine, with Hollandaise	680
Florentine, without Hollandaise	456
on Toast, Kids	337

BILL'S

EGGS
Royale, with Hollandaise	534
Royale, without Hollandaise	310
Scrambled, on Toast	731
Scrambled, on Toast, with Bacon	745
Scrambled, on Toast, with Salmon	698

FISH FINGERS
Cod, Kids	271

FRIES
Potato, Kids, Side	175
Potato, Side	349
Sweet Potato, Side	510

FRUIT
Strawberries, & Banana, no Sauce, Kids	93
Strawberries, & Banana, Chocolate Sauce, Kids	198

GNOCCHI
Diablo	928

ICE CREAM
Vanilla, Kids	107

KALE
Sauteed	104

MACARONI CHEESE
Kids	429
with Focaccia	1290
with Mushroom, & Leek	1167
with Side Salad, & Dressing	1269
with Side Salad, No Dressing	1172
without Sides	1160

MASH
Potato, Side	194

MAYONNAISE
Chipotle	216
Truffle, Side	347

MERINGUE
Eton Mess, Lemon	847

MEZZE
Halloumi, & Houmous, for 4	377
Sharing, for 4, ¼ Mezze	429
Veggie, Sharing, for 4, ¼ Mezze	343

MOUSSE
Chocolate, & Hazelnut, Kids	202

MUSHROOMS
Garlic, Sauteed, Chestnut	180

NUTS
Spiced, & Roasted Corn, For 2	303

OLIVES
Green, Giant, Gordal	161

OMELETTE
Summer	488

PANCAKES - BUTTERMILK
Kids	375
with Bacon, & Syrup, 3 Stack	803
with Bacon, & Syrup, 5 Stack	1271

BILL'S

PANCAKES - BUTTERMILK

with Banana, Berries, with Syrup, 3 Stack	542
with Banana, Berries, with Syrup, 5 Stack	845

PATE

Chicken Liver, Oak Smoked, Parfait, with Toast	809
Chicken Liver, Oak Smoked, Parfait, without Toast	528

PIE

Fish	794

RIBS

BBQ, Kids	305
Main	791

RISOTTO

Crab, & Courgette	620

SALAD

Caesar, Chicken, without Dressing	627
Chicken, with Turmeric, & Freekeh	1292
Feta, Crispy, & Watermelon	425
Glow Bowl	1133
Halloumi, Grilled, & Pesto Toast, with Dressing	706
Halloumi, Grilled, with Dressing	548
Halloumi, Grilled, no Dressing	356
Halloumi, Grilled, & Pesto Toast, no Dressing	514
Kale, Chickpea, & Miso, Houmous	755
Mixed, no Dressing	24
Mixed, with Dressing	121
Rainbow, Side	137
Salmon, Seared	728
Summer	695
Summer, with Flatbread	815

SANDWICH

Bacon, Kids	512
Fish Finger	884
Sausage, Kids	482

SAUCE

Bearnaise, for Steak	158
Garlic Butter, for Steak	193
Hollandaise	224
Mushroom, for Steak	69
Peppercorn, for Steak	46

SAUSAGE

Cumberland, Kids	427
Cumberland, Mini, Glazed	294

SCONE

Cream Tea, No Clotted Cream	552
Cream Tea, with Clotted Cream	728
with Jam, & Clotted Cream, Warm	709
with Jam, Warm	562

SEA BASS

Pan Fried, with Rosti	523

SOUP

Pea, & Watercress, without Focaccia	161
Salad, & Half Sandwich	676
Tomato, Roasted, with Cream	209

BILL'S

SOUP

Tomato, Roasted, with Cream & Pesto Toast	367
Tomato, Roasted, with Pesto Toast	250
Tomato, Roasted, without Cream & Pesto Toast	92

SQUID

Calamari, Crispy, with lemon Garlic Mayonnaise	624
Calamari, Crispy, without lemon Garlic Mayonnaise	369

SUNDAE

Granola, Breakfast	467
Banoffee, Melting	658
Ice Cream, Vanilla, Kids	292

TART

Ricotta, Red Pepper, & Cheddar, no Dressing	664
Ricotta, Red Pepper, & Cheddar, with Dressing	761

TEACAKES

Toasted, no Butter	267
Toasted, with Butter	527

TOAST

& Butter, Bloomer	356
with Avocado, & Bacon	687
with Avocado, & Poached Eggs	426
with Avocado, & Salmon	640
with Avocado	497
with Beans, Kids	219
with Butter, Kids	180

TOASTIE

Ham, & Cheese, Kids	478

TORTILLA CHIPS

Corn, Crispy, Kids	247
Spiced, For 2	258

WELLINGTON

Carrot, & Cashew Nut	715

YOGHURT

Strawberries, Banana, & Honey, Kids	108

BREWERS FAYRE

BACON
	KCAL
Back, Rasher, Breakfast	165

BEANS
Baked, Breakfast	91
Baked, in Tomato Sauce, Side, Kids Menu	51

BEEF
Steak, Rib-eye, with Hollandaise Sauce	1250
Steak, Rib-eye, with Peppercorn Sauce	1199
Steak, Rump, Grilled	874
Steak, Sirloin, Grilled	886
Steak, & Eggs	1041
Yorkshire, Wrap, with Chips, & Gravy	1129

BHAJI
Sweet Potato	58

BITES
Hog Roast, with Apple Sauce	263
Mac 'N' Cheese	442

BREAD
Flatbread, Garlic	312
Flatbread, Garlic, with Cheese	379
Garlic, Kids Menu	110
Garlic, Side, Kids Menu	106
Garlic, with Cheese, Side	318

BROWNIES
Chocolate, with Ice Cream	755

BUBBLE & SQUEAK
Side	348

BURGERS
Chicken, Breaded, The South Western	925
Beef, Bash Street, Kids Menu	697
Beef, Black & Blue, with Chips	1328
Beef, Cheese, & Mushroom	988
Beef, Cheese, & Mushroom, Double	1308
Beef, Extra	327
Beef, Ultimate, with Chips	1741
Chicken, Extra	211
Cluck 'N' Ale, with Chips	1517
Cluck 'N' Ale, with Sweet Potato Fries	1564
Halloumi, Heaven, with Chips	1136
Halloumi Heaven, with Sweet Potato Fries	1069
The New Yorker	1139
Vegan, with Chips	899

BURRITO
Bowl, with Salad	555
Chicken, Bowl	710

CAKE
Chocolate, & Orange, Mousse, Mini	220
Chocolate, Fudge, Luxury	810

CAULIFLOWER CHEESE
Side	281

CHEESE
& Bacon, Extra	115
Brie, Breaded, Bites	326

BREWERS FAYRE

CHEESE
	KCAL
Halloumi, & Chips, with Mushy Peas	1035
Halloumi, & Chips, with Peas	997
Mozzarella, Sticks, Side	330

CHEESECAKE
Raspberry, & Prosecco	502
Vanilla, with Blackcurrant & Prosecco Compote	375

CHICKEN
& Ribs, Combo, Full Rack, Chips, Coleslaw, Salad	1628
& Ribs, Combo, Half Rack, Chips, Coleslaw, & Salad	1248
Bites, Breaded, Kids Menu	525
Bites, Buffalo, Poppin	246
Breast, Garlic, Breaded	1326
Breast, Smoky Paprika, Grilled	430
Smothered, BBQ Sauce,	914
Smothered, BBQ Sauce, Double Up	1271
Smothered, BBQ Sauce, with Mac 'N' Cheese	1213
Buttermilk, & Cheesy Nachos	750
Katsu Curry	1037
Combo	1344
Forestiere, with Crushed Potatoes, & Green Beans	441
Goujons, Combo Feast	1849
Goujons, with Chicken Wings, Combo Feast	2269
Goujons, Southern Fried	406
Half, Roasted, Lemon & Thyme, with Chips	1600
Half, Roasted, with Chips	799
Half, Roasted, BBQ, with Chips	436
Stuffed, Mozzarella, with Bacon, & Chips	886
Stuffed, Mozzarella, with Bacon, & Roast Potatoes	746
Skewers, Honey & Mustard	212
Skewers, Jerk	292
Wings, Buffalo	463
Tikka, with Rice	851

CHILLI
Bean, Three, with Rice, & Tortilla Chips	537
Beef, Mexican, with Rice	716

CHIPS
Side	363
Smothered, Creamy Cheese Sauce, Side	551
Smothered, Curry Sauce, Side	467
Smothered, Gravy, Side	436

COD
Bites, Breaded, Kids Menu	642
Loin, Baked, with Ratatouille, & Roast Potatoes	447

COLESLAW
Side	138
Side, Kids Menu	40

CORN
Cob, Mini, Side, Kids Menu	29

CRUMBLE
Apple, Toffee, Salted	670

DESSERT
Caramel Apple Betty	496

BREWERS FAYRE

DESSERT
Chocolate, Mini, Mash Up, Kids Menu	344
Dirty Mud Pie	995
Fondue, Chocolate Fudge, Sharing	854

DIP
Dessicated Coconut	158

DOUGHNUTS
Cinnamon	547

EGGS
Breakfast	311

EMPANADAS
Cheese	401

FISH & CHIPS
with Mushy Peas	939
with Peas	901

FISH CAKES
Single	126

FRIES
Furious, Side	409
Tiger, Side	381

FROZEN YOGHURT
Strawberry	274

FRUIT SALAD
Kids Menu	49

GAMMON - STEAK
With Egg, Grilled	903
with Egg & Pineapple, Grilled	833
with Pineapple, Grilled	764

HADDOCK - BATTERED
with Chips & Mushy Peas, Atlantic, Giant	1093
with Chips & Peas, Atlantic, Giant	1055

HOT DOG
The Big Bad Dog, Kids Menu	612

ICE CREAM
Vanilla, with Caramel Sauce, Kids Menu	259
Vanilla, with Chocolate Sauce, Kids Menu	256
Vanilla, with Raspberry Sauce, Kids Menu	256

LAMB
Shank, Slow Cooked, in Gravy	760

LASAGNE
Beef & Pork, Main	580
Beef & Pork, with Side Salad	713
Sweet Potato & Feta, with Side Salad	744

MEATBALLS
Chicken, Tikka	261

MIXED GRILL
Flat Iron Steak, Gammon, Chicken, & Sausage	1412
Mediterranean	1355
Mediterranean, with Rice	1199
Rump Steak, Gammon, Chicken, & Sausage	1485
Ultimate, Summer	1781
Ultimate, Summer, with Prawns	1983

BREWERS FAYRE

MOUSSE
Lemon	730
Lemon, Mini	151

MUSHROOMS
Closed Cup, Breakfast, Brewers Fayre*	169
Garlic, & Herb, Breaded	303

NACHOS
with Cheesy Yoghurt Dip, Kids Menu	230

ONION RINGS
Battered, Side	467

PASTA
in Tomato Sauce, Kids Menu	344
Mac 'N' Cheese, Side	301
Mac 'N' Cheese, with Garlic Bread, & Salad	896
Penne, Tomato, & Roasted Vegetable, with Chicken	731

PATE
Chicken Liver, with Toast	388

PEAS
Side, Kids Menu	47

PEPPERS
Jalapeno, Cheesy, Poppers, Side	378

PIE
Apple, with Custard	316
Beef, & Stout, with Mash, Beans, & Gravy	1171
Chicken, & Chorizo, Creamy Sauce	516
Fish	747
Lemon Meringue, with Cream	606

PIZZA
Chocolate, Kids Menu	375

PLATTER
Chip Shop	1327

POPPADOMS
Single	32

POTATO DIPPERS
Crispy	483
Loaded, Sharing	526
Spicy Cheese Sauce, Loaded, Sharing	494

PRAWN COCKTAIL
Starter	369

PRAWNS
Crispy, with Garlic Mayo	488
King, Tempura, with Sweet Chilli	475

PROFITEROLES
with Salted Caramel Sauce	422

PUDDING
Beef, & Doom Bar Ale	1300
Bread & Butter, Summer Berry	587
Jaffa, Sharing	1034
Sticky Toffee, with Custard	753
Sticky Toffee	719

QUICHE
Cheese, Three, Crustless	572

BREWERS FAYRE

RIBS - RACK
Full, BBQ	1297
Full, in Whisky Glaze	1160

SALAD
Caesar, Chicken & Bacon	536
Chicken, & Bacon, Grilled	434
Chicken, Coronation	549
Cobb, Brewers	567
Mixed, Side	51
Ploughmans	480
Prawn, Sweet Chilli, Battered	718
Salmon	384

SALMON
Baked, with Hollandaise Sauce	727

SAMOSAS
Vegetable	191

SANDWICH
Chicken, Strips, Spicy, Brown Bread	688
Chicken, Strips, Spicy, White Bread	682
Fish, Goujons, Brown Bread	682
Fish, Goujons, White Bread	676
Ham & Cheese, Brown Bread	630
Ham & Cheese, White Bread	624
Prawn, Brown Bread	589
Prawn, White Bread	583

SAUCE
Blue Cheese	39
Hollandaise	81
Peppercorn	29
Tennessee Whisky Glaze, Jack Daniels	89

SAUSAGE
Egg, & Chips	1012
Pork, Battered	159
Premium, Breakfast	137
Vegetarian, Egg, & Chips	858

SAUSAGES & MASH
Bangers, Kids Menu	391
Vegetarian, Bangers, Kids Menu	364

SCAMPI
Wholetail, Breaded, with Mushy Peas	868
Wholetail, Breaded, with Peas	830

SOUP
Tomato	251

SPAGHETTI BOLOGNESE
Beano-ese, Kids Menu	320

SUNDAE
Choc-A-Block, Caramel, Cadbury	583
Choc-a-block, Cadbury	639
Funny Face, Kids Menu	268
Oreo	919
Salted Caramel, Brownie, & Popcorn	714

TOAST
with Creamy Mushrooms	210

BREWERS FAYRE

TOMATOES
Grilled, Halved, Breakfast	28

TRIFLE
Strawberry Pimms	634

VEGETABLES
Green, Medley, Side	112
Sticks, & Cucumber Yoghurt Dip, Kids Menu	49
Sticks, Side, Kids Menu	28

WAFFLES - BELGIAN
with Chocolate Honeycomb Ice Cream	497
with Salted Caramel Ice Cream	468

WRAP
Chicken, Build Your Own, Kids Menu	491
Salmon, Build Your Own, Kids Menu	495
Sausage, Quorn, Build Your Own, Kids Menu	491

YORKSHIRE PUDDING
with Sausage & Mash, Giant	1329
with Sausage & Mash, Vegetarian, Ultimate	1093

BURGER KING

BITES
Cheese, Chilli, 6	302

BURGERS
Bacon, Double Cheese, XL	905
Bacon King	1064
Veggie Bean	668
Cheeseburger. Bacon, Double	431
Cheeseburger, Kids	282
Chicken, Royale, Bacon, & Cheese	703
Chicken, Royale, with Cheese	671
Chicken Royale	596
Crispy Chicken	605
Halloumi Bacon King	704
Halloumi King	616
Hamburger, Kids	244
Steakhouse	748
Veggie, Kids	289
Whopper	635
Whopper, Double	881

CHICKEN
Fries	212
Fries, Jalapeno	218
Nuggets, 6	249
Nuggets, Kids	166

FRIES
Reg	282

ONION RINGS
Reg, 5	300

CAFFE NERO

BARS
Chocolate, Dark, & Hazelnut	196

BEANS
Protein Mix, Savoury	121

BISCUITS
Biscotti, Almond	147
Stem Ginger	133

BREAKFAST CEREAL
Porridge, with Semi Skimmed Milk, no Topping	234
Porridge, with Skimmed Milk, no Topping	210
Porridge, with Soya Milk, no Topping	232

BROWNIES
Chocolate, Belgian	241
Chocolate, Caramel & Sea Salt	257
Chocolate, GF	252

CAKE
Banana & Walnut Loaf	345
Billionaires	514
Cappuccino, Coffee, & Caramel	444
Cappuccino, Individual	553
Carrot	541
Chocolate Fudge	420
Ginger Spiced, Vegan, Loaf	321
Lemon Drizzle, Loaf	372
Raspberry, & Coconut, Slice	248
Raspberry & Amaretti, Crumble	338

CHEESECAKE
Lemon, Sicilian	343
Salted Caramel, & Chocolate, Vegan	350

CHOCOLATE
Coins	109
Milk, Stracciatella	200

COFFEE - AMERICANO
Grande	23
Iced	15
Regular	15

COFFEE - CAPPUCCINO
Coconut Milk, Grande	88
Coconut Milk, Regular	50
Iced	24
Oat Milk, Grande	106
Oat Milk, Regular	64
Semi Skimmed, Grande	107
Semi Skimmed, Regular	65
Skimmed Milk, Grande	83
Skimmed Milk, Regular	52
Soya Milk, Grande	97
Soya Milk, Regular	59

COFFEE - CORTADO
Standard	49

COFFEE - ESPRESSO
Single	7
Con Panna	56

CAFFE NERO

COFFEE - ESPRESSO

Tonic, Original	52
Tonic, Ultimate	95

COFFEE - FLAT WHITE

Whole Milk	95

COFFEE - LATTE

Coconut Milk, Grande	86
Coconut Milk, Regular	49
Gingerbread, Coconut Milk, Grande	148
Gingerbread, Coconut Milk, Regular	90
Gingerbread, Oat Milk, Grande	110
Gingerbread, Oat Milk, Regular	110
Gingerbread, Semi Skimmed, Grande	352
Gingerbread, Semi Skimmed, Regular	280
Gingerbread, Skimmed Milk, Grande	323
Gingerbread, Skimmed Milk, Regular	263
Gingerbread, Soya Milk, Grande	175
Gingerbread, Soya Milk, Regular	105
Gingerbread, Whole Milk, Grande	391
Gingerbread, Whole Milk, Regular	301
Iced, Coconut	142
Iced, Semi Skimmed	155
Oat Milk, Grande	123
Oat Milk, Regular	70
Caramel, Salted, Coconut Milk, Grande	155
Caramel, Salted, Coconut Milk, Regular	95
Caramel, Salted, Oat Milk, Grande	191
Caramel, Salted, Oat Milk, Regular	116
Caramel, Salted, Semi Skimmed, Grande	191
Caramel, Salted, Semi Skimmed, Regular	116
Caramel, Salted, Skimmed Milk, Grande	160
Caramel, Salted, Soya Milk, Grande	183
Caramel, Salted, Soya Milk, Regular	111
Caramel, Salted, Whole Milk, Grande	233
Caramel, Salted, Whole Milk, Regular	140
Semi Skimmed, Grande	131
Semi Skimmed, Regular	72
Skimmed Milk, Grande	97
Skimmed Milk, Regular	55
Soya Milk, Grande	115
Soya Milk, Regular	66

COFFEE - MACCHIATTO

Standard	9

COFFEE - MOCHA

Coconut Milk, Grande	171
Coconut Milk, Regular	117
Oat Milk, Grande	188
Oat Milk, Regular	131
Semi Skimmed, Grande Milk	363
Semi Skimmed, Regular	305
Skimmed Milk, Grande	339
Skimmed Milk, Regular	292
Soya Milk, Grande	179

CAFFE NERO

COFFEE - MOCHA

Soya Milk, Regular	126
White Chocolate, Coconut Milk	368
White Chocolate, Oat Milk	405
White Chocolate, Semi Skimmed milk	397
White Chocolate, Skimmed milk	365
White Chocolate, Soya Milk	384

COFFEE BEANS

Chocolate Coated	133

CONSERVE

Raspberry	72
Strawberry	72

COOKIES

Caramel, Chocolate	330
Chocolate, Belgian	314
Oat & Raisin	301

CREAM

Clotted	234
Whipped, for Coffee	171

CRISPS

Mature Cheddar, & Red Onion, Kettle	202
Sea Salt, Kettle	205
Sea Salt & Balsamic Vinegar, Kettle	201

CROISSANT

Almond	343
Apricot	251
Butter	219
Ham, & Mature Cheddar	325
Raspberry, Vegan	296

DRIED FRUIT & NUTS

Mix	192

FLAPJACK

Fruit, Vegan	315

FRUIT

Rolls, Bear Yo Yo's	54

FRUIT SALAD

Seasonal	106

GINGERBREAD

Man, Ginnie	289
Man, Gino	289

HONEY

Topping, for Porridge	97

HOT CHOCOLATE

Coconut Milk, Grande	260
Coconut Milk, Reg	164
Milano, Standard	458
Mint, Coconut Milk, Grande	327
Mint, Coconut Milk, Reg	214
Mint, Oat Milk, Grande	362
Mint, Oat Milk, Reg	236
Mint, Semi Skimmed, Grande	532
Mint, Semi Skimmed, Reg	406
Mint, Skimmed Milk, Grande	502

CAFFE NERO

HOT CHOCOLATE

Mint, Skimmed Milk, Reg	387
Mint, Soya Milk, Grande	355
Mint, Soya Milk, Reg	231
Mint, Whole Milk, Grande	573
Mint, Whole Milk, Reg	431
Oat Milk, Grande	298
Oat Milk, Reg	186
Roasted Hazelnut, Coconut Milk, Grande	323
Roasted Hazelnut, Coconut Milk, Reg	207
Roasted Hazelnut, Oat Milk, Grande	362
Roasted Hazelnut, Oat Milk, Reg	229
Roasted Hazelnut, Semi Skimmed, Grande	532
Roasted Hazelnut, Semi Skimmed, Reg	399
Roasted Hazelnut, Skimmed Milk, Grande	499
Roasted Hazelnut, Skimmed Milk, Reg	380
Roasted Hazelnut, Soya Milk, Grande	354
Roasted Hazelnut, Soya Milk, Reg	224
Roasted Hazelnut, Whole Milk, Grande	575
Roasted Hazelnut, Whole Milk, Reg	424
Semi Skimmed Milk, Grande	524
Semi Skimmed Milk, Reg	398
Skimmed Milk, Grande	484
Skimmed Milk, Reg	374
Soya Milk, Grande	290
Soya Milk, Reg	182

JUICE

Mango & Passionfruit, Booster	196
Raspberry & Peach, Booster	220

LEMONADE

Garden Mint	96

MARSHMALLOWS

for Hot Chocolate	20

MILK SHAKE

Frappe, Belgian Chocolate	215
Frappe Creme, Espresso & Caramel	503
Frappe, Latte, Semi Skimmed Milk	229
Frappe Creme, Salted Caramel & Pistachio	480
Frappe, Strawberry, Semi Skimmed	245
Frappe, Strawberry, Soya Milk	234
Frappe Creme, Triple Belgian Chocolate	435
Frappe, Vanilla, Semi Skimmed	240
Frappe, Vanilla, Soya Milk	230

MUFFIN

Blueberry	376
Chocolate Filled	448
Cranberry, Seeds, & Oat	387
Lemon, with Lemon Curd Filling	398

PAIN AU CHOCOLAT

Single	268

PAIN AU RAISIN

Single	296

CAFFE NERO

PANINI

Brie, Bacon, & Cranberry	536
Festive Feast, Vegan	436
Ham, & Mozzarella	414
Mozzarella, & Tomato	480
Tuna Melt	513
Turkey Feast	490

PARCELS

Tomato, & Caramelised Onion, with Mozzarella	374
Vegetables, Roasted, & Spanish Chorizo	390

PASTRY

Chocolate Twist	280
Cinnamon Swirl	350

PIE

Mince, Star Topped	354

POPCORN

Sea Salt	87
Sweet & Salty	114

RICE CAKES

Chocolate	81

ROULADE

Black Forest, Luxury	414

SALAD

Chicken, & Mozzarella, Italian Style	246
Falafel, & Houmous	305

SANDWICH

Bacon, Coffee Cured, Ciabatta, Roll	348
BLT, Classic	496
Chicken Salad, Chargrilled	441
Egg Mayonnaise, Free Range	449
Sausage, Ciabatta Roll	413
Tuna, Red Pepper, & Rocket	333

SAUSAGE ROLL

Pork, & Pancetta	467
Vegetable, Vegan	354

SCONE

Fruit, Sultana	287

SHORTBREAD

Caramel, with Belgian Chocolate	377
Crunchy, All Butter	264

SYRUP

Vanilla	97

TEA

Black, & Peach	84
Chai Latte, Coconut Milk	188
Chai Latte, Oat Milk	230
Chai Latte, Semi Skimmed Milk	232
Chai Latte, Skimmed Milk	195
Chai Latte, Soya Milk	216
Green, & Mango	76

TEACAKES

Rich Fruit, Toasted, with Butter	272

CAFFE NERO

TOASTIE

Mozzarella, & Roasted Tomato, Melt, Tostati	406
Mushroom, & Mascarpone, Melt, Tostati	388
Pigs in Blankets, Melt, Tostati	588
Tomato, Roasted, & Pesto, Tostati	362

WAFFLES

Caramel	332

YOGHURT

Raspberry	249

COOPLANDS

BAKE

Chicken	386
Lamb, & Mint	418
Steak	409

BISCUITS

Ginger, Teddy	181
Melting Moment	234
Oaty	227
Parkin	152
Shortbread, Bunny	221

BREAD

Baguette	250
Baguette, Sandwich Choice	250
Country Grain, Batch Loaf	72
Multiseed, Loaves	75
Roll, Scotch	263
Roll, Scotch, Sandwich Choice	171
Roll, Scotch, Wholemeal	166
Roll, Scotch, Wholemeal, Sandwich Choice	166
Roll, Wholemeal, Large	261
Rolls, Bridge, White, Large	179
Rolls, Bridge, White, Small	121
Rolls, Bridge, Wholemeal	166
Rolls, Country Grain	208
Rolls, Country Grain, Sandwich Choice	208
Rolls, Dinner	121
Rolls, Dinner	119
Rolls, White, Large	289
Rolls, White, Large, Sandwich Choice	289
White, Loaves, Large	90
White, Loaves, Small	70
Wholemeal, Loaves, Large	79
Wholemeal, Loaves, Small	62

BREAKFAST

Porridge, Pots	266

BROWNIE

Chocolate	393

BUNS

Iced, Chocolate	218
Iced, White	207

CAKE

Almond Tart	302
Bakewell Slice	537
Bakewell Tart	330
Caramel Crispie	195
Cookie Monster	455
Cornflake Nest	279
Cream Roll	1228
Cream Slice	397
Currant Square	390
Date Square	324
Devonshire Split	438
Freesale, Celebration	233

COOPLANDS

CAKE

Fruit, Celebration	448
Ginger Square	202
Iced Finger	236
Jam Tart	279
Lemon Tart	290
Maids of Honour	285
Sponge, Celebration	221
Sponge, Chocolate, Mini	326
Sponge, Cream	246
Sponge, Cream, Mini	296
Strawberry Tart	307
Vanilla Slice	332
Yum Yum	252

DANISH PASTRY

Chocolate, Toffee	581

DESSERT

Peach Melba	276

DOUGHNUT

Cream	314
Jam	206
Toffee	292

FLAN

Summer Fruit	465

FLAPJACK

Chocolate	374

MARGERINE

Large, Sandwich Choice	34
Reg, Sandwich Choice	20

MERINGUE

Nuts	283

MUFFIN

Chocolate Filled	404

PASTRY

Bacon, & Cheese, Wrap	428
Breakfast Roll	340
Cheese Straw	93

PASTY

Apple	281
Cheese & Onion	402
Corned Beef, & Potato	380
Sausage, Cheese & Beans	509
Traditional	437

PIE

Apple	233
Mince, & Onion	585
Mince, Sweet	233
Steak	588

PIZZA

Cheese & Tomato	234
Pepperoni	266

QUICHE

Cheese & Bacon	422

COOPLANDS

QUICHE

Cheese & Onion	401
Cheese & Onion	597

SALAD

Ham & Egg	398
Roast Chicken, & Bacon	396

SANDWICH

Beef & Onion, Baguette	402
Beef & Onion, Country Grain Roll	318
Beef & Onion, Lge White Roll	496
Beef & Onion, Lge Wholemeal Roll	469
Beef & Onion, White Roll	279
Beef & Onion, Wholemeal Roll	261
Cheese Ploughmans, Baguette	499
Cheese Ploughmans, Country Grain Roll	378
Cheese Ploughmans, Lge White Roll	554
Cheese Ploughmans, Lge Wholemeal Roll	526
Cheese Ploughmans, White Roll	391
Cheese Ploughmans, Wholemeal Roll	362
Cheese Salad, Scotch Roll	398
Cheese Savoury Salad, Baguette	778
Cheese Savoury Salad, Country Grain Roll	556
Cheese Savoury Salad, Lge White Roll	834
Cheese Savoury Salad, Lge Wholemeal Roll	789
Cheese Savoury Salad, White Roll	536
Cheese Savoury Salad, Wholemeal Roll	515
Chicken & Bacon Mayo, Baguette	522
Chicken & Bacon Mayo, Country Grain Roll	389
Chicken & Bacon Mayo, Lge White Roll	559
Chicken & Bacon Mayo, Lge Wholemeal Roll	531
Chicken & Bacon Mayo, White Roll	359
Chicken & Bacon Mayo, Wholemeal Roll	335
Chicken Mayo Salad, Lge White Roll	549
Chicken Salad, Baguette	380
Chicken Salad, Country Grain Roll	287
Chicken Salad, Lge White Roll	417
Chicken Salad, Lge Wholemeal Roll	389
Chicken Salad, White Roll	248
Chicken Salad, Wholemeal Roll	232
Chicken Tikka, Baguette	513
Chicken Tikka, Country Grain Roll	426
Chicken Tikka, Lge White Roll	550
Chicken Tikka, Lge Wholemeal Roll	522
Chicken Tikka, White Roll	344
Chicken Tikka, Wholemeal Roll	328
Corned Beef, Tomato, & Onion, Baguette	457
Corned Beef, Tomato, & Onion, Country Grain Roll	344
Corned Beef, Tomato, & Onion, Lge White Roll	499
Corned Beef, Tomato, & Onion, Lge Wholemeal Roll	472
Corned Beef, Tomato, & Onion, White Roll	309
Corned Beef, Tomato, & Onion, Wholemeal Roll	292
Egg Mayonnaise, in White Roll	322
Ham, in White Roll	257

COOPLANDS

SANDWICH

Ham & Cheese, Baguette	499
Ham & Cheese, Country Grain Roll	402
Ham & Cheese, Lge White Roll	579
Ham & Cheese, Lge Wholemeal Roll	549
Ham & Cheese, White Roll	364
Ham & Cheese, Wholemeal Roll	347
Ham & Pease Pudding, in White Roll	283
Ham Salad, in Lge White Roll	429
Ham Salad, in White Roll	261
Seafood Cocktail, Baguette	683
Seafood Cocktail, Country Grain Roll	495
Seafood Cocktail, Lge White Roll	740
Seafood Cocktail, Lge Wholemeal Roll	694
Seafood Cocktail, White Roll	466
Seafood Cocktail, Wholemeal Roll	440
Sweet Chilli Chicken Salad, Baguette	380
Sweet Chilli Chicken Salad, Country Grain Roll	323
Sweet Chilli Chicken Salad, Lge White Roll	417
Sweet Chilli Chicken Salad, Lge Wholemeal Roll	389
Sweet Chilli Chicken Salad, White Roll	285
Sweet Chilli Chicken Salad, Wholemeal Roll	269
Tuna & Sweetcorn Salad, Baguette	468
Tuna & Sweetcorn Salad, Country Grain Roll	352
Tuna & Sweetcorn Salad, Lge White Roll	509
Tuna & Sweetcorn Salad, Lge Wholemeal Roll	479
Tuna & Sweetcorn Salad, White Roll	314
Tuna & Sweetcorn Salad, Wholemeal Roll	299
Tuna Salad, Baguette	365
Tuna Salad, Country Grain Roll	284
Tuna Salad, Lge White Roll	407
Tuna Salad, Lge Wholemeal Roll	379
Tuna Salad, White Roll	245
Tuna Salad, Wholemeal Roll	229
Turkey Salad, Baguette	369
Turkey Salad, Country Grain Roll	284
Turkey Salad, Lge White Roll	408
Turkey Salad, Lge Wholemeal Roll	381
Turkey Salad, White Roll	251
Turkey Salad, Wholemeal Roll	232

SANDWICH FILLING

Bacon, Large, Sandwich Choice	170
Bacon, Reg, Sandwich Choice	113
Beef, Sliced, Large, Sandwich Choice	122
Beef, Sliced, Reg, Sandwich Choice	82
Cheese, Grated, Large, Sandwich Choice	305
Cheese, Grated, Reg, Sandwich Choice	203
Cheese, Savoury, Large, Sandwich Choice	487
Cheese, Savoury, Reg, Sandwich Choice	325
Cheeze, Vegan, Large, Sandwich Choice	128
Cheeze, Vegan, Reg, Sandwich Choice	86
Chicken, & Bacon Mayo, Large, Sandwich Choice	239
Chicken, & Bacon Mayo, Reg, Sandwich Choice	159

COOPLANDS

SANDWICH FILLING

Chicken, Roast, Large, Sandwich Choice	79
Chicken, Roast, Reg, Sandwich Choice	53
Chicken Mayo, Large, Sandwich Choice	214
Chicken Mayo, Reg, Sandwich Choice	142
Chicken Tikka, Large, Sandwich Choice	239
Chicken Tikka, Reg, Sandwich Choice	159
Chopped Tomato, Large, Sandwich Choice	18
Chopped Tomato, Reg, Sandwich Choice	12
Egg Mayo, Large, Sandwich Choice	196
Egg Mayo, Reg, Sandwich Choice	130
Ham, Sliced, Large, Sandwich Choice	98
Ham, Sliced, Reg, Sandwich Choice	65
Mushrooms, Large, Sandwich Choice	46
Mushrooms, Reg, Sandwich Choice	29
Salad, Large, Sandwich Choice	5
Salad, Reg, Sandwich Choice	8
Sausage, Large, Sandwich Choice	346
Sausage, Reg, Sandwich Choice	259
Tuna, & Sweetcorn, Large, Sandwich Choice	176
Tuna, & Sweetcorn, Reg, Sandwich Choice	118
Turkey, Sliced, Large, Sandwich Choice	80
Turkey, Sliced, Reg, Sandwich Choice	54

SAUCE

BBQ, Sandwich Choice	20
Brown, Sandwich Choice	16
Caesar Dressing, Sandwich Choice	45
English Mustard, Sandwich Choice	10
Mayonnaise, Light, Sandwich Choice	40
Mayonnaise, Sandwich Choice	109
Onion Relish, Sandwich Choice	31
Pease Pudding, Sandwich Choice	21
Pickle, Sandwich Choice	24
Prawn, Sandwich Choice	44
Salad Cream, Sandwich Choice	44
Sweet Chilli, Sandwich Choice	28
Tomato Ketchup, Sandwich Choice	15

SAUSAGE ROLL

Baked	187

SCONE

Cheese	299
Cream	421
Sultana	269

SHORTBREAD

Caramel	262

TART

Curd, Large	305
Curd, Small	324
Egg Custard, Large	187
Egg Custard, Small	220

TEACAKES

Plain	218
Iced	250

COSTA

BISCUITS

Biscotti, Italian	155
Bourbon, Giant	322
Chocolate, Triple	253
Custard Cream, Giant	322
Fruit, & Oat	228
Ginger, Stem	234
Gingerbread, Walking Cat	235
Gingerbread, Walking Dog	228
Gingerbread, Walking Vampire	233

BITES

Flapjack, Chocolate	69
Mallow, Millionaire	85

BREAKFAST

Bacon, Smoked, Soft Bap	414
Box, Veggie	302
Porridge, Pot	294
Porridge, Wholegrain, Pot	223
Sausage, Pork, Soft Bap	628
Vegan Bac'n, Bap	360

BROWNIES

Chocolate, Belgian	309
Salted Caramel	398
Terrys Chocolate Orange	334

BUNS

Brioche, Cinnamon	337

CAKE

Apple & Caramel, Loaf	343
Banana, & Pecan, Loaf	325
Carrot, & Walnut	576
Chocolate, & Hazelnut, Rich, Shimmer	578
Chocolate, Tiffin	402
Chocolate, Ultimate, Slice, BOSH!	425
Christmas	320
Ginger, Jamaican, Loaf	412
Golden Caramel, & Chocolate	590
Lemon, Drizzle, Loaf	368
Lemon & Blueberry	524
Lime & Coconut, Loaf	491
Raspberry & Almond, Traybake	452
Rocky Road	421

CHILLI

Vegan, Rice, Pot	291

CHOCOLATE

After Eight	37
Coins	380
Dark, Bar	178
Flake, Extras	43
Milk, Bar	176
Milk, Medal	125
Terrys Chocolate Orange, Segsations	41
The Purple One	48

COSTA

COFFEE - AMERICANO

Large	23
Medium	18
Medium, Iced	42
Medium, Iced, Takeaway	42
Mini, Takeaway	6
Small	12
Small, Iced	25
Small, Iced, Takeaway	25

COFFEE - BABYCCINO

Coconut Milk	30
Oat Milk	55
Semi Skimmed Milk	41
Skimmed Milk	29
Soya Milk	38
Whole Milk	59

COFFEE - CAPPUCCINO

Almond Milk, Large	103
Almond Milk, Medium	93
Almond Milk, Mini, Takeaway	50
Almond Milk, Small	74
Coconut Milk, Large	130
Coconut Milk, Medium	118
Coconut Milk, Mini, Takeaway	64
Coconut Milk, Small	94
Oat Milk, Large	214
Oat Milk, Medium	197
Oat Milk, Mini, Takeaway	106
Oat Milk, Small	157
Semi Skimmed Milk, Large	169
Semi Skimmed Milk, Medium	155
Semi Skimmed Milk, Mini, Takeaway	83
Semi Skimmed Milk, Small	123
Shaken, Almond Milk, Iced, Medium	67
Shaken, Almond Milk, Iced, Small	48
Shaken, Coconut Milk, Iced, Medium	76
Shaken, Coconut Milk, Iced, Small	56
Shaken, Oat Milk, Iced, Medium	102
Shaken, Oat Milk, Iced, Small	83
Shaken, Skimmed Milk, Iced, Medium	75
Shaken, Skimmed Milk, Iced, Small	55
Shaken, Soya Milk, Iced, Medium	84
Shaken, Soya Milk, Iced, Small	65
Shaken, Whole Milk, Iced, Medium	107
Shaken, Whole Milk, Iced, Small	88
Skimmed Milk, Large	127
Skimmed Milk, Medium	116
Skimmed Milk, Mini, Takeaway	62
Skimmed Milk, Small	92
Soya Milk, Large	157
Soya Milk, Medium	144
Soya Milk, Mini, Takeaway	77
Soya Milk, Small	114

COSTA

COFFEE - CAPPUCCINO

Whole Milk, Large	229
Whole Milk, Medium	211
Whole Milk, Mini, Takeaway	113
Whole Milk, Small	168

COFFEE - COLD BREW

Black, Medium	8
Black, Small	6
White, Almond Milk, Medium	22
White, Almond Milk, Small	20
White, Coconut Milk, Medium	27
White, Coconut Milk, Small	24
White, Oat Milk, Medium	41
White, Oat Milk, Small	38
White, Semi Skimmed Milk, Medium	33
White, Cold Brew, Semi Skimmed Milk, Small	31
White, Skimmed Milk, Medium	26
White, Skimmed Milk, Small	24
White, Soya Milk, Medium	31
White, Soya Milk, Small	29
White, Whole Milk, Medium	43
White, Whole Milk, Small	41
with Whipped Milk, Medium	24
with Whipped Milk, Small	22

COFFEE - CORTADO

Almond Milk	37
Almond Milk, Iced	41
Almond Milk, Takeaway	46
Caramel, Almond Milk	54
Caramel, Almond Milk, Takeaway	62
Caramel, Coconut Milk	74
Caramel, Coconut Milk, Takeaway	88
Caramel, Oat Milk	96
Caramel, Oat Milk, Takeaway	115
Caramel, Semi Skimmed Milk	79
Caramel, Semi Skimmed Milk, Takeaway	94
Caramel, Skimmed Milk	63
Caramel, Skimmed Milk, Takeaway	73
Caramel, Soya Milk	74
Caramel, Soya Milk, Takeaway	88
Caramel, Whole Milk	101
Caramel, Whole Milk, Takeaway	122
Coconut Milk	49
Coconut Milk, Iced	49
Coconut Milk, Takeaway	60
Oat Milk	84
Oat Milk, Iced	73
Oat Milk, Takeaway	105
Semi Skimmed Milk	65
Semi Skimmed Milk, Iced	60
Semi Skimmed Milk, Takeaway	81
Skimmed Milk	47
Skimmed Milk, Iced	48

COSTA

COFFEE - CORTADO

Skimmed Milk, Takeaway	59
Soya Milk	60
Soya Milk, Iced	57
Soya Milk, Takeaway	75
Whole Milk	90
Whole Milk, Iced	77
Whole Milk, Takeaway	113

COFFEE - ESPRESSO

Character Roast, Double	12
Character Roast, Single	6
con Pana, Double	145
con Pana, Single	139
Decaff, Double	6
Decaff, Single	3
Iced, Double	38
Iced, Single	19
Mocha Italia, Double	12
Mocha Italia, Single	6
Ristretto, Double	12
Ristretto, Single	6
Macchaito, Almond Milk, Double	16
Macchaito, Almond Milk, Single	8
Macchaito, Coconut Milk, Double	18
Macchaito, Coconut Milk, Single	9
Macchaito, Oat Milk, Double	24
Macchaito, Oat Milk, Single	12
Macchaito, Semi Skimmed Milk, Double	21
Macchaito, Semi Skimmed Milk, Single	10
Macchaito, Skimmed Milk, Double	18
Macchaito, Skimmed Milk, Single	9
Macchaito, Soya Milk, Double	20
Macchaito, Soya Milk, Single	10
Macchaito, Whole Milk, Double	25
Macchaito, Whole Milk, Single	12

COFFEE - FILTER

Premium, Large	17
Premium, Medium	13
Premium, Small	10

COFFEE - FLAT BLACK

Mini, Takeaway	14
Small	11

COFFEE - FLAT WHITE

Almond Milk, Iced	60
Almond Milk, Mini, Takeaway	54
Almond Milk, Small	76
Coconut Milk, Iced	71
Coconut Milk, Mini, Takeaway	70
Coconut Milk, Small	100
Oat Milk, Iced	104
Oat Milk, Mini, Takeaway	117
Oat Milk, Small	176
Semi Skimmed Milk, Iced	86

COSTA

COFFEE - FLAT WHITE

Semi Skimmed Milk, Mini, Takeaway	92
Semi Skimmed Milk, Small	135
Skimmed Milk, Iced	70
Skimmed Milk, Mini, Takeaway	68
Skimmed Milk, Small	98
Soya Milk, Iced	82
Soya Milk, Mini, Takeaway	85
Soya Milk, Small	125
Whole Milk, Iced	110
Whole Milk, Mini, Takeaway	126
Whole Milk, Small	189

COFFEE - LATTE

Almond Milk, Iced, Medium	94
Almond Milk, Iced, Small	67
Almond Milk, Large	112
Almond Milk, Large, Takeaway	117
Almond Milk, Medium	84
Almond Milk, Medium, Takeaway	84
Almond Milk, Mini, Takeaway	49
Almond Milk, Small	53
Almond Milk, Small, Takeaway	63
Coconut Milk, Large	147
Coconut Milk, Large, Takeaway	155
Coconut Milk, Medium	112
Coconut Milk, Medium, Iced	114
Coconut Milk, Medium, Takeaway	112
Coconut Milk, Mini, Takeaway	65
Coconut Milk, Small	70
Coconut Milk, Small, Iced	83
Coconut Milk, Small, Takeaway	83
Gingerbread, Almond Milk, Medium	212
Gingerbread, Almond Milk, Small	183
Gingerbread, Coconut Milk, Medium	234
Gingerbread, Coconut Milk, Small	196
Gingerbread, Oat Milk, Medium	302
Gingerbread, Oat Milk, Small	237
Gingerbread, Semi Skimmed Milk, Medium	266
Gingerbread, Semi Skimmed Milk, Small	215
Gingerbread, Skimmed Milk, Medium	231
Gingerbread, Skimmed Milk, Small	194
Gingerbread, Soya Milk, Medium	256
Gingerbread, Soya Milk, Small	209
Gingerbread, Whole Milk, Medium	314
Gingerbread, Whole Milk, Small	245
Oat Milk, Iced, Medium	179
Oat Milk, Iced, Small	132
Oat Milk, Large	257
Oat Milk, Large, Takeaway	271
Oat Milk, Medium	197
Oat Milk, Medium, Takeaway	197
Oat Milk, Mini, Takeaway	116
Oat Milk, Small	125

COSTA

COFFEE - LATTE

Oat Milk, Small, Takeaway	143
Semi Skimmed Milk, Iced, Medium	144
Semi Skimmed Milk, Iced, Small	106
Semi Skimmed Milk, Large	198
Semi Skimmed Milk, Large, Takeaway	209
Semi Skimmed Milk, Medium	151
Semi Skimmed Milk, Medium, Takeaway	151
Semi Skimmed Milk, Mini, Takeaway	89
Semi Skimmed Milk, Small	96
Semi Skimmed Milk, Small, Takeaway	111
Skimmed Milk, Large	143
Skimmed Milk, Large, Takeaway	151
Skimmed Milk, Medium	109
Skimmed Milk, Medium, Iced	112
Skimmed Milk, Medium, Takeaway	109
Skimmed Milk, Mini, Takeaway	63
Skimmed Milk, Small	68
Skimmed Milk, Small, Iced	81
Skimmed Milk, Small, Takeaway	81
Soya Milk, Large	182
Soya Milk, Large, Takeaway	192
Soya Milk, Medium	139
Soya Milk, Medium, Iced	135
Soya Milk, Medium, Takeaway	139
Soya Milk, Mini, Takeaway	81
Soya Milk, Small	88
Soya Milk, Small, Iced	99
Soya Milk, Small, Takeaway	102
Whole Milk, Large	276
Whole Milk, Large, Takeaway	292
Whole Milk, Medium	212
Whole Milk, Medium, Iced	190
Whole Milk, Medium, Takeaway	212
Whole Milk, Mini, Takeaway	125
Whole Milk, Small	135
Whole Milk, Small, Iced	141
Whole Milk, Small, Takeaway	154

COFFEE - MOCHA

Almond Milk, Large	207
Almond Milk, Medium	172
Almond Milk, Medium, Iced	134
Almond Milk, Mini, Takeaway	93
Almond Milk, Small	131
Almond Milk, Small, Iced	99
Coconut Milk, Medium	193
Coconut Milk, Medium, Iced	149
Coconut Milk, Mini, Takeaway	105
Coconut Milk, Small	149
Coconut Milk, Small, Iced	111
Oat Milk, Large	308
Oat Milk, Medium	256
Oat Milk, Medium, Iced	195

COSTA
COFFEE - MOCHA

Oat Milk, Mini, Takeaway	140
Oat Milk, Small	204
Oat Milk, Small, Iced	146
Semi Skimmed Milk, Large	267
Semi Skimmed Milk, Medium	222
Semi Skimmed Milk, Medium, Iced	171
Semi Skimmed Milk, Mini, Takeaway	121
Semi Skimmed Milk, Small	174
Semi Skimmed Milk, Small, Iced	127
Skimmed Milk, Large	229
Skimmed Milk, Medium	191
Skimmed Milk, Medium, Iced	148
Skimmed Milk, Mini, Takeaway	103
Skimmed Milk, Small	147
Skimmed Milk, Small, Iced	109
Soya Milk, Large	256
Soya Milk, Medium	213
Soya Milk, Medium, Iced	164
Soya Milk, Mini, Takeaway	116
Soya Milk, Small	166
Soya Milk, Small, Iced	122
Whole Milk, Large	321
Whole Milk, Medium	268
Whole Milk, Medium, Iced	204
Whole Milk, Mini, Takeaway	147
Whole Milk, Small	214
Whole Milk, Small, Iced	152

COOKIES

Belgian Chocolate, All Butter	349
Gingerbread Latte, Vegan	371

CREAM

Whipping, Extras	133

CROISSANT

Almond	318
Butter	247

FLAPJACK

Fruit & Nut	341
Fruity	246
Jammy	220
Salted Caramel, Loaded	292

FLATBREAD

Cheddar, & Black Pepper	195

FROSTINO

Belgian Chocolate, Almond Milk, Medium	344
Belgian Chocolate, Almond Milk, Small	292
Belgian Chocolate, Coconut Milk, Medium	358
Belgian Chocolate, Coconut Milk, Small	303
Belgian Chocolate, Oat Milk, Medium	403
Belgian Chocolate, Oat Milk, Small	338
Belgian Chocolate, Semi Skimmed Milk, Medium	379
Belgian Chocolate, Semi Skimmed Milk, Small	320
Belgian Chocolate, Skimmed Milk, Medium	356

COSTA
FROSTINO

Belgian Chocolate, Skimmed Milk, Small	302
Belgian Chocolate, Soya Milk, Medium	372
Belgian Chocolate, Soya Milk, Small	315
Belgian Chocolate, Whole Milk, Medium	411
Belgian Chocolate, Whole Milk, Small	345
Coffee, Almond Milk, Medium	107
Coffee, Almond Milk, Medium, Takeaway	109
Coffee, Almond Milk, Small	76
Coffee, Almond Milk, Small, Takeaway	77
Coffee, Coconut Milk, Medium	116
Coffee, Coconut Milk, Medium, Takeaway	119
Coffee, Coconut Milk, Small	85
Coffee, Coconut Milk, Small, Takeaway	86
Coffee, Oat Milk, Medium	144
Coffee, Oat Milk, Medium, Takeaway	150
Coffee, Oat Milk, Small	111
Coffee, Oat Milk, Small, Takeaway	114
Coffee, Semi Skimmed Milk, Medium	129
Coffee, Semi Skimmed Milk, Medium, Takeaway	133
Coffee, Semi Skimmed Milk, Small	97
Coffee, Semi Skimmed Milk, Small, Takeaway	99
Coffee, Skimmed Milk, Medium	115
Coffee, Skimmed Milk, Medium, Takeaway	118
Coffee, Skimmed Milk, Small	84
Coffee, Skimmed Milk, Small, Takeaway	85
Coffee, Soya Milk, Medium	125
Coffee, Soya Milk, Medium, Takeaway	129
Coffee, Soya Milk, Small	93
Coffee, Soya Milk, Small, Takeaway	95
Coffee, Whole Milk, Medium	149
Coffee, Whole Milk, Medium, Takeaway	155
Coffee, Whole Milk, Small	116
Coffee, Whole Milk, Small, Takeaway	119
Mint Choc Chip, Almond Milk, Medium	383
Mint Choc Chip, Almond Milk, Small	314
Mint Choc Chip, Coconut Milk, Medium	397
Mint Choc Chip, Coconut Milk, Small	325
Mint Choc Chip, Oat Milk, Medium	442
Mint Choc Chip, Oat Milk, Small	360
Mint Choc Chip, Semi Skimmed Milk, Medium	418
Mint Choc Chip, Semi Skimmed Milk, Small	342
Mint Choc Chip, Skimmed Milk, Medium	396
Mint Choc Chip, Skimmed Milk, Small	324
Mint Choc Chip, Soya Milk, Medium	412
Mint Choc Chip, Soya Milk, Small	337
Mint Choc Chip, Whole Milk, Medium	450
Mint Choc Chip, Whole Milk, Small	367
Salted Caramel, Almond Milk, Medium	331
Salted Caramel, Almond Milk, Small	285
Salted Caramel, Coconut Milk, Medium	345
Salted Caramel, Coconut Milk, Small	296
Salted Caramel, Oat Milk, Medium	390

COSTA
FROSTINO

Salted Caramel, Oat Milk, Small	331
Salted Caramel, Semi Skimmed Milk, Medium	366
Salted Caramel, Semi Skimmed Milk, Small	313
Salted Caramel, Skimmed Milk, Medium	344
Salted Caramel, Skimmed Milk, Small	295
Salted Caramel, Soya Milk, Medium	360
Salted Caramel, Soya Milk, Small	308
Salted Caramel, Whole Milk, Medium	398
Salted Caramel, Whole Milk, Small	338
Strawberry, Almond Milk, Medium	347
Strawberry, Almond Milk, Medium, Takeaway	349
Strawberry, Almond Milk, Small	295
Strawberry, Almond Milk, Small, Takeaway	296
Strawberry, Coconut Milk, Medium	361
Strawberry, Coconut Milk, Medium, Takeaway	365
Strawberry, Coconut Milk, Small	306
Strawberry, Coconut Milk, Small, Takeaway	308
Strawberry, Oat Milk, Medium	406
Strawberry, Oat Milk, Medium, Takeaway	412
Strawberry, Oat Milk, Small	341
Strawberry, Oat Milk, Small, Takeaway	344
Strawberry, Semi Skimmed Milk, Medium	382
Strawberry, Semi Skimmed Milk, Medium, Takeaway	387
Strawberry, Semi Skimmed Milk, Small	322
Strawberry, Semi Skimmed Milk, Small, Takeaway	325
Strawberry, Skimmed Milk, Medium	360
Strawberry, Skimmed Milk, Medium, Takeaway	363
Strawberry, Skimmed Milk, Small	305
Strawberry, Skimmed Milk, Small, Takeaway	306
Strawberry, Soya Milk, Medium	376
Strawberry, Soya Milk, Medium, Takeaway	380
Strawberry, Soya Milk, Small	317
Strawberry, Soya Milk, Small, Takeaway	319
Strawberry, Whole Milk, Medium	414
Strawberry, Whole Milk, Medium, Takeaway	421
Strawberry, Whole Milk, Small	347
Strawberry, Whole Milk, Small, Takeaway	351

FRUIT

Apple, & Grapes, Pot	62
Melon Medley, Pot	48

FRUIT COOLERS

Mango & Passion Fruit, Medium	165
Mango & Passion Fruit, Small	125
Mango & Passion Fruit, Small, Takeaway	125
Red Summer Berries, Medium	220
Red Summer Berries, Small	167
Red Summer Berries, Small, Takeaway	167

HOT CHOCOLATE

Almond Milk, Large	302
Almond Milk, Large, Takeaway	324
Almond Milk, Medium	215
Almond Milk, Medium, Takeaway	234

COSTA
HOT CHOCOLATE

Almond Milk, Mini, Takeaway	135
Almond Milk, Small	127
Almond Milk, Small, Takeaway	160
Babyccino, with Flake, Coconut Milk	97
Babyccino, with Flake, Oat Milk	120
Babyccino, with Flake, Semi Skimmed Milk	108
Babyccino, with Flake, Skimmed Milk	96
Babyccino, with Flake, Soya Milk	104
Babyccino, with Flake, Whole Milk	124
Babyccino, with Marshmallow, Coconut Milk	74
Babyccino, with Marshmallow, Oat Milk	98
Babyccino, with Marshmallow, Semi Skimmed Milk	85
Babyccino, with Marshmallow, Skimmed Milk	73
Babyccino, with Marshmallow, Soya Milk	82
Babyccino, with Marshmallow, Whole Milk	102
Black Forest, Almond Milk, Medium	299
Black Forest, Almond Milk, Medium, Takeaway	319
Black Forest, Almond Milk, Small	237
Black Forest, Almond Milk, Small, Takeaway	260
Black Forest, Coconut Milk, Medium	318
Black Forest, Coconut Milk, Medium, Takeaway	340
Black Forest, Coconut Milk, Small	250
Black Forest, Coconut Milk, Small, Takeaway	276
Black Forest, Oat Milk, Medium	378
Black Forest, Oat Milk, Medium, Takeaway	408
Black Forest, Oat Milk, Small	290
Black Forest, Oat Milk, Small, Takeaway	329
Black Forest, Semi Skimmed Milk, Medium	346
Black Forest, Semi Skimmed Milk, Small	268
Black Forest, Semi Skimmed Milk, Small, Takeaway	301
Black Forest, Skimmed Milk, Medium	316
Black Forest, Skimmed Milk, Medium, Takeaway	338
Black Forest, Skimmed Milk, Small	248
Black Forest, Skimmed Milk, Small, Takeaway	275
Black Forest, Soya Milk, Medium	338
Black Forest, Soya Milk, Medium, Takeaway	362
Black Forest, Soya Milk, Small	263
Black Forest, Soya Milk, Small, Takeaway	293
Black Forest, Whole Milk, Medium	388
Black Forest, Whole Milk, Medium, Takeaway	420
Black Forest, Whole Milk, Small	297
Black Forest, Whole Milk, Small, Takeaway	338
Coconut Milk, Large	339
Coconut Milk, Large, Takeaway	364
Coconut Milk, Medium	244
Coconut Milk, Medium, Takeaway	265
Coconut Milk, Mini, Takeaway	154
Coconut Milk, Small	146
Coconut Milk, Small, Takeaway	185
Oat Milk, Large	455
Oat Milk, Large, Takeaway	487
Oat Milk, Medium	334

COSTA
HOT CHOCOLATE

Oat Milk, Medium, Takeaway	363
Oat Milk, Mini, Takeaway	211
Oat Milk, Small	206
Oat Milk, Small, Takeaway	261
Semi Skimmed Milk, Large	393
Semi Skimmed Milk, Large, Takeaway	421
Semi Skimmed Milk, Medium	286
Semi Skimmed Milk, Medium, Takeaway	311
Semi Skimmed Milk, Mini, Takeaway	181
Semi Skimmed Milk, Small	174
Semi Skimmed Milk, Small, Takeaway	220
Skimmed Milk, Large	335
Skimmed Milk, Large, Takeaway	359
Skimmed Milk, Medium	241
Skimmed Milk, Medium, Takeaway	262
Skimmed Milk, Mini, Takeaway	152
Skimmed Milk, Small	144
Skimmed Milk, Small, Takeaway	182
Soya Milk, Large	376
Soya Milk, Large, Takeaway	403
Soya Milk, Medium	273
Soya Milk, Medium, Takeaway	297
Soya Milk, Mini, Takeaway	172
Soya Milk, Small	165
Soya Milk, Small, Takeaway	209
White, Almond Milk, Large	248
White, Almond Milk, Large, Takeaway	248
White, Almond Milk, Medium	208
White, Almond Milk, Medium, Takeaway	208
White, Almond Milk, Mini, Takeaway	120
White, Almond Milk, Small	149
White, Almond Milk, Small, Takeaway	161
White, Coconut Milk, Large	284
White, Coconut Milk, Large, Takeaway	284
White, Coconut Milk, Medium	239
White, Coconut Milk, Medium, Takeaway	239
White, Coconut Milk, Mini, Takeaway	140
White, Coconut Milk, Small	169
White, Coconut Milk, Small, Takeaway	186
White, Oat Milk, Large	396
White, Oat Milk, Large, Takeaway	396
White, Oat Milk, Medium	337
White, Oat Milk, Medium, Takeaway	337
White, Oat Milk, Mini, Takeaway	203
White, Oat Milk, Small	232
White, Oat Milk, Small, Takeaway	263
White, Semi Skimmed Milk, Large	336
White, Semi Skimmed Milk, Large, Takeaway	336
White, Semi Skimmed Milk, Medium	285
White, Semi Skimmed Milk, Medium, Takeaway	285
White, Semi Skimmed Milk, Mini, Takeaway	169
White, Semi Skimmed Milk, Small	198

COSTA
HOT CHOCOLATE

White, Semi Skimmed Milk, Small, Takeaway	221
White, Skimmed Milk, Large	280
White, Skimmed Milk, Large, Takeaway	280
White, Skimmed Milk, Medium	236
White, Skimmed Milk, Medium, Takeaway	236
White, Skimmed Milk, Mini, Takeaway	138
White, Skimmed Milk, Small	167
White, Skimmed Milk, Small, Takeaway	183
White, Soya Milk, Large	320
White, Soya Milk, Large, Takeaway	320
White, Soya Milk, Medium	271
White, Soya Milk, Medium, Takeaway	271
White, Soya Milk, Mini, Takeaway	160
White, Soya Milk, Small	189
White, Soya Milk, Small, Takeaway	210
White, Whole Milk, Large	416
White, Whole Milk, Large, Takeaway	416
White, Whole Milk, Medium	355
White, Whole Milk, Medium, Takeaway	355
White, Whole Milk, Mini, Takeaway	214
White, Whole Milk, Small	243
White, Whole Milk, Small, Takeaway	276
Whole Milk, Large	475
Whole Milk, Large, Takeaway	510
Whole Milk, Medium	350
Whole Milk, Medium, Takeaway	381
Whole Milk, Mini, Takeaway	222
Whole Milk, Small	216
Whole Milk, Small, Takeaway	275

MARSHMALLOWS

Extras	20

MILK DRINK

Chocolate, Almond Milk, Medium, Iced	199
Chocolate, Almond Milk, Medium, Iced, Takeaway	207
Chocolate, Almond Milk, Small, Iced	143
Chocolate, Almond Milk, Small, Iced, Takeaway	145
Chocolate, Coconut Milk, Medium, Iced	220
Chocolate, Coconut Milk, Medium, Iced, Takeaway	231
Chocolate, Coconut Milk, Small, Iced	161
Chocolate, Coconut Milk, Small, Iced, Takeaway	164
Chocolate, Oat Milk, Medium, Iced	286
Chocolate, Oat Milk, Medium, Iced, Takeaway	307
Chocolate, Oat Milk, Small, Iced	217
Chocolate, Oat Milk, Small, Iced, Takeaway	223
Chocolate, Semi Skimmed Milk, Medium, Iced	250
Chocolate, Semi Skimmed Milk, Small, Iced	187
Chocolate, Skimmed Milk, Medium, Iced	250
Chocolate, Skimmed Milk, Medium, Iced, Takeaway	266
Chocolate, Skimmed Milk, Small, Iced	159
Chocolate, Skimmed Milk, Small, Iced, Takeaway	162
Chocolate, Soya Milk, Medium, Iced	241
Chocolate, Soya Milk, Medium, Iced, Takeaway	256

COSTA

MILK DRINK

Chocolate, Soya Milk, Small, Iced	179
Chocolate, Soya Milk, Small, Iced, Takeaway	183
Chocolate, Whole Milk, Medium, Iced	297
Chocolate, Whole Milk, Medium, Iced, Takeaway	320
Chocolate, Whole Milk, Small, Iced	227
Chocolate, Whole Milk, Small, Iced, Takeaway	233

MUFFIN

Blueberry	407
Caramel, with Munchies	384
Chocolate, Celebration	462
Chocolate, with Kit Kat	372
Gingerbread	390
Lemon, Sicilian	387
Lotus Biscoff	76
Strawberries & Cream	418

PAIN AU RAISIN

Pastry	304

PANETTONE

Chocolate Chip	407
Fruited	377

PANINI

Brie, Maple Bacon, & Cranberry	502
Mozzarella, & Tomato, Stonebaked	525
Steak, & Onion Gravy, Stonebaked	386
Tuna, Melt, Stonebaked	462
Vegan BBQ Chick'N	426

PASTRY

Chocolate, Twist	301
Danish, Caramel & Pecan	304

PIE

Mince, All Butter	329

RAISINS

Chocolate, Milk	161

SALAD

Chicken & Sweetcorn, Pot	523
Tomato, & Mozzarella, Pot	370

SANDWICH

Chicken, Bacon, & Cheddar, Club	484
Chicken, Roast	335
Egg Mayo, Free Range	316
Ham, British, Simply	141
Mature Cheddar, Simply	210
Ploughmans, Cheddar	387
Triple Selection	514

SAUCE

Belgian Chocolate	19
Caramel Chocolate	21
Cherry	6
Irish Coffee	10
Salted Caramel	14
Strawberry	20
White Chocolate	29

COSTA

SAUSAGE ROLL

Pork, & Bramley Apple	400

SHORTBREAD

All Butter, Bites, Mini	53
Chocolate Chunk, Milk	349
Jammy	238
Millionaire's	396
Millionaire's, GF	276

SHORTCAKE

Mallow Pumpkin	291

SNACKS

Rice Snacks, Sweet Chilli	103

SYRUP

Caramel	11
Caramel, Sugar Free	1
Chai	13
Gingerbread, Sugar Free	1
Golden Caramel	12
Gomme	13
Mint Flavour	11
Orange	10
Roasted Hazelnut	11
Roasted Hazelnut, Sugar Free	1
Spiced Toffee	11
Vanilla	13
Vanilla, Sugar Free	1

TART

Bakewell, Cherry, Mini	241
Bakewell	389
Custard, Portugese, Pastel De Nata	169
Lemon Curd	331
Mince	342

TEA

Chai Latte, Almond Milk, Large	175
Chai Latte, Almond Milk, Large, Takeaway	175
Chai Latte, Almond Milk, Medium	138
Chai Latte, Almond Milk, Medium, Iced	90
Chai Latte, Almond Milk, Medium, Iced, Takeaway	93
Chai Latte, Almond Milk, Medium, Takeaway	138
Chai Latte, Almond Milk, Mini, Takeaway	82
Chai Latte, Almond Milk, Small	95
Chai Latte, Almond Milk, Small, Iced	69
Chai Latte, Almond Milk, Small, Iced, Takeaway	70
Chai Latte, Almond Milk, Small, Takeaway	107
Chai Latte, Coconut Milk, Large	216
Chai Latte, Coconut Milk, Large, Takeaway	216
Chai Latte, Coconut Milk, Medium	170
Chai Latte, Coconut Milk, Medium, Iced	105
Chai Latte, Coconut Milk, Medium, Iced, Takeaway	108
Chai Latte, Coconut Milk, Medium, Takeaway	170
Chai Latte, Coconut Milk, Mini, Takeaway	103
Chai Latte, Coconut Milk, Small	116
Chai Latte, Coconut Milk, Small, Iced	80

COSTA

TEA

Chai Latte, Coconut Milk, Small, Iced, Takeaway	82
Chai Latte, Coconut Milk, Small, Takeaway	132
Chai Latte, Oat Milk, Large	342
Chai Latte, Oat Milk, Large, Takeaway	342
Chai Latte, Oat Milk, Medium	268
Chai Latte, Oat Milk, Medium, Iced	150
Chai Latte, Oat Milk, Medium, Iced, Takeaway	156
Chai Latte, Oat Milk, Medium, Takeaway	268
Chai Latte, Oat Milk, Mini, Takeaway	166
Chai Latte, Oat Milk, Small	179
Chai Latte, Oat Milk, Small, Iced	115
Chai Latte, Oat Milk, Small, Iced, Takeaway	118
Chai Latte, Oat Milk, Small, Takeaway	209
Chai Latte, Semi Skimmed Milk, Large	274
Chai Latte, Semi Skimmed Milk, Large, Takeaway	274
Chai Latte, Semi Skimmed Milk, Medium	215
Chai Latte, Semi Skimmed Milk, Medium, Iced	126
Chai Latte, Semi Skimmed Milk, Medium, Takeaway	215
Chai Latte, Semi Skimmed Milk, Mini, Takeaway	132
Chai Latte, Semi Skimmed Milk, Small	145
Chai Latte, Semi Skimmed Milk, Small, Iced	97
Chai Latte, Semi Skimmed Milk, Small, Takeaway	168
Chai Latte, Skimmed Milk, Large	211
Chai Latte, Skimmed Milk, Large, Takeaway	211
Chai Latte, Skimmed Milk, Medium	166
Chai Latte, Skimmed Milk, Medium, Iced	103
Chai Latte, Skimmed Milk, Medium, Iced, Takeaway	106
Chai Latte, Skimmed Milk, Medium, Takeaway	166
Chai Latte, Skimmed Milk, Mini, Takeaway	100
Chai Latte, Skimmed Milk, Small	113
Chai Latte, Skimmed Milk, Small, Iced	79
Chai Latte, Skimmed Milk, Small, Iced, Takeaway	81
Chai Latte, Skimmed Milk, Small, Takeaway	129
Chai Latte, Soya Milk, Large	256
Chai Latte, Soya Milk, Large, Takeaway	256
Chai Latte, Soya Milk, Medium	201
Chai Latte, Soya Milk, Medium, Iced	119
Chai Latte, Soya Milk, Medium, Iced, Takeaway	123
Chai Latte, Soya Milk, Medium, Takeaway	201
Chai Latte, Soya Milk, Mini, Takeaway	123
Chai Latte, Soya Milk, Small	136
Chai Latte, Soya Milk, Small, Iced	92
Chai Latte, Soya Milk, Small, Iced, Takeaway	94
Chai Latte, Soya Milk, Small, Takeaway	157
Chai Latte, Whole Milk, Large	364
Chai Latte, Whole Milk, Large, Takeaway	364
Chai Latte, Whole Milk, Medium	285
Chai Latte, Whole Milk, Medium, Iced	158
Chai Latte, Whole Milk, Medium, Iced, Takeaway	164
Chai Latte, Whole Milk, Medium, Takeaway	285
Chai Latte, Whole Milk, Mini, Takeaway	177
Chai Latte, Whole Milk, Small	190

COSTA

TEA

Chai Latte, Whole Milk, Small, Iced	122
Chai Latte, Whole Milk, Small, Iced, Takeaway	125
Chai Latte, Whole Milk, Small, Takeaway	223
Earl Grey	3
English Breakfast	1
English Breakfast, Decaff	3
Fruit Infusion	2
Green, Jasmine	1
Green, Pure	3
Iced, Peach, Medium	87
Iced, Peach, Medium, Takeaway	87
Iced, Peach, Small	67
Iced, Peach, Small, Takeaway	67
Iced, Strawberry, Infusion, Medium	88
Iced, Strawberry, Infusion, Medium, Takeaway	88
Iced, Strawberry, Infusion, Small	67
Iced, Strawberry, Infusion, Small, Takeaway	67
Mint Infusion	3

TEACAKES

Fruited	295

TOAST

Brown, Seeded, No Butter	356
White, No Butter	257

TOASTIE

Cheddar, & Tomato, Slow Roasted	463
Chicken, British, & Mushroom	358
Ham, & Cheese	354
Ham, Wiltshire, & Mature Cheddar	434
Heinz Beanz, & Cheese	340
Sausage, & Caramelised Onion	478
Three Cheese, & Chutney	465
Vegan Smoky Ham, & Cheeze	352

TOPPING

Caramel Vermicelli	20
Chocolate Chip Pieces	51
Golden Twinkle Sprinkle	2
Shimmer Curls	10
Strawberry Sprinkle	3

WAFFLES

Caramel	363

WRAP

Breakfast, Ultimate	603
Chicken, Fajita, Roast	406

YOGHURT

Natural, Greek Style, with Mango & Passionfruit	122
Natural, Greek Style, with Mixed Berry Compote	118

DOMINO'S PIZZA

BREAD
Garlic, Dippers	238
Garlic, Pizza	307

CHICKEN
Chick 'n' Mix	386
Kickers, 7	366
Kickers, Combo Box	188
Pop'n, Standard Portion	239
Strippers, 7	540
Strippers, Combo Box	222
Wings, 7	510
Wings, Combo Box	200
Wings, Red Hot, Franks, 7	552
Wings, Spicy BBQ, 7	502

COLESLAW
BLANK	145

COOKIES
BLANK	182

DESSERT
Cinni Dippers	198

DIP
BBQ	47
Garlic & Herb	169
Honey & Mystard	109
Red Hot, Franks	6
Salsa, Tangy	42
Sweet Chilli	54

DOUGH BALLS
Twisted, with Ham	341
Twisted, with Pepperoni	373

FRIES
BLANK	139
Sweet Potato	176

MILK SHAKE
Chocolate, ThickShakes	416
Strawberry, ThickShakes	396
Vanilla, ThickShakes	371

NACHOS
no Jalapenos	253
with Jalapenos	253

NUGGETS
Vegan, 14	1072
Vegan, 7	536
Vegan, Combo Box	198

PIZZA - ABSOLUTE BANGER
Classic Crust, Large	656

PIZZA - AMERICAN HOT
Classic Crust, Large	626
Classic Crust, Medium	567
Classic Crust, Personal	588
Classic Crust, Small	1044
Double Decadence, Large	724
Double Decadence, Medium	675

DOMINO'S PIZZA

PIZZA - AMERICAN HOT
Italian Style Crust, Large	519
Italian Style Crust, Medium	458
Italian Style Crust, Small	915
Stuffed Crust, Large	673
Stuffed Crust, Medium	656
Thin & Crispy Crust Crust, Large	481
Thin & Crispy Crust Crust, Medium	452

PIZZA - AMERICANO
Classic Crust, Large	703
Classic Crust, Medium	643
Classic Crust, Small	1098
Italian Style Crust, Large	606
Italian Style Crust, Medium	658
Italian Style Crust, Small	952
Stuffed Crust, Large	820
Stuffed Crust, Medium	755
Thin & Crispy Crust Crust, Large	537
Thin & Crispy Crust Crust, Medium	495

PIZZA - BACON DOUBLE CHEESE
Classic Crust, Large	657
Classic Crust, Medium	585
Classic Crust, Personal	629
Classic Crust, Small	1064
Italian Style Crust, Large	547
Italian Style Crust, Medium	477
Italian Style Crust, Small	934
Stuffed Crust, Large	704
Stuffed Crust, Medium	674
Thin & Crispy Crust, Large	511
Thin & Crispy Crust, Medium	471

PIZZA - BUFFALO CHICKEN
Classic Crust, Large	576
Classic Crust, Medium	509
Classic Crust, Personal	541
Classic Crust, Small	924
Italian Style Crust, Large	466
Italian Style Crust, Medium	401
Italian Style Crust, Small	794
Stuffed Crust, Large	688
Stuffed Crust, Medium	598
Thin & Crispy Crust, Large	430
Thin & Crispy Crust, Medium	395

PIZZA - CHEESE & TOMATO
Classic Crust, Large	582
Classic Crust, Medium	515
Classic Crust, Personal	526
Classic Crust, Small	922
GF Crust, Small	716
Italian Style Crust, Large	471
Italian Style Crust, Medium	406
Italian Style Crust, Small	776
Stuffed Crust, Large	628

DOMINO'S PIZZA
PIZZA - CHEESE & TOMATO
Stuffed Crust, Medium	604
Thin & Crispy Crust, Large	435
Thin & Crispy Crust, Medium	400

PIZZA - CHICKEN FEAST
Classic Crust, Large	595
Classic Crust, Medium	531
Classic Crust, Personal	557
Classic Crust, Small	955
Double Decadence, Large	702
Italian Style Crust, Lge	485
Italian Style Crust, Medium	422
Italian Style Crust, Small	825
Stuffed Crust, Large	642
Stuffed Crust, Medium	620
Thin & Crispy Crust, Large	449
Thin & Crispy Crust, Medium	416

PIZZA - CHOCOLATE
Lotta, Dessert	208

PIZZA - DELUXE
Classic Crust, Large	623
Classic Crust, Medium	563
Classic Crust, Personal	581
Classic Crust, Small	1033
Italian Style Crust, Large	514
Italian Style Crust, Medium	455
Italian Style Crust, Small	904
Stuffed Crust, Large	670
Stuffed Crust, Medium	652
Thin & Crispy Crust, Large	478
Thin & Crispy Crust, Medium	460

PIZZA - FAMRHOUSE
Stuffed Crust, Large	599
Stuffed Crust, Medium	581
Classic Crust, Large	552
Classic Crust, Medium	493
Classic Crust, Personal	522
Classic Crust, Small	894
Italian Style Crust, Large	443
Italian Style Crust, Medium	384
Italian Style Crust, Small	763
Thin & Crispy Crust, Large	408
Thin & Crispy Crust, Medium	378

PIZZA - FOUR VEGI
Classic Crust, Large	539
Classic Crust, Medium	479
Classic Crust, Personal	515
Classic Crust, Small	867
Italian Style Crust, Large	429
Italian Style Crust, Medium	370
Italian Style Crust, Small	737
Stuffed Crust, Large	586
Stuffed Crust, Medium	568

DOMINO'S PIZZA
PIZZA - FOUR VEGI
Thin & Crispy Crust, Large	393
Thin & Crispy Crust, Medium	365

PIZZA - FULL HOUSE
Classic Crust, Large	633
Classic Crust, Medium	568
Classic Crust, Personal	623
Classic Crust, Small	1043
Italian Style Crust, Large	523
Italian Style Crust, Medium	459
Italian Style Crust, Small	913
Stuffed Crust, Large	680
Stuffed Crust, Medium	657
Thin & Crispy Crust, Large	487
Thin & Crispy Crust, Medium	454

PIZZA - HAM & PINEAPPLE
Classic Crust, Large	551
Classic Crust, Medium	492
Classic Crust, Personal	522
Classic Crust, Small	893
Italian Style Crust, Large	442
Italian Style Crust, Medium	383
Italian Style Crust, Small	763
Stuffed Crust, Large	599
Stuffed Crust, Medium	581
Thin & Crispy Crust, Large	406
Thin & Crispy Crust, Medium	377

PIZZA - HAWAIIAN
Classic Crust, Large	556
Classic Crust, Medium	496
Classic Crust, Personal	526
Classic Crust, Small	900
Double Decadence, Large	670
Double Decadence, Medium	627
Italian Style Crust, Large	446
Italian Style Crust, Medium	387
Italian Style Crust, Small	770
Stuffed Crust, Large	603
Stuffed Crust, Medium	585
Thin & Crispy Crust, Large	410
Thin & Crispy Crust, Medium	381

PIZZA - HOT & SPICY
Classic Crust, Large	724
Classic Crust, Medium	655
Classic Crust, Personal	720
Classic Crust, Small	1200
Italian Style Crust, Large	615
Italian Style Crust, Medium	547
Italian Style Crust, Small	1070
Stuffed Crust, Large	604
Stuffed Crust, Medium	581
Thin & Crispy Crust, Large	411
Thin & Crispy Crust, Medium	378

DOMINO'S PIZZA
PIZZA - HOUSE SPECIAL
Tandoori, Classic Crust, Large	724
Tandoori, Classic Crust, Medium	655
Tandoori, Classic Crust, Personal	720
Tandoori, Classic Crust, Small	1200
Tandoori, Italian Style Crust, Large	615
Tandoori, Italian Style Crust, Medium	547
Tandoori, Italian Style Crust, Small	1070
Tandoori, Stuffed Crust, Large	772
Tandoori, Stuffed Crust, Medium	744
Tandoori, Thin & Crispy, Large	579
Tandoori, Thin & Crispy, Medium	541

PIZZA - MEAT LOVERS
Classic Crust, Large	676
Classic Crust, Medium	612
Classic Crust, Personal	637
Classic Crust, Small	1135
Italian Style Crust, Large	567
Italian Style Crust, Medium	503
Italian Style Crust, Small	1005
Stuffed Crust, Large	723
Stuffed Crust, Medium	700
Thin & Crispy Crust, Large	530
Thin & Crispy Crust, Medium	497

PIZZA - MEATEOR
Classic Crust, Large	747
Classic Crust, Medium	685
Classic Crust, Personal	779
Classic Crust, Small	1187
Italian Style Crust, Large	700
Italian Style Crust, Medium	650
Italian Style Crust, Small	1042
Stuffed Crust, Large	865
Stuffed Crust, Medium	798
Thin & Crispy Crust, Large	581
Thin & Crispy Crust, Medium	537

PIZZA - MEATILICIOUS
Classic Crust, Large	648
Classic Crust, Medium	585
Classic Crust, Personal	664
Classic Crust, Small	1084
Italian Style Crust, Large	539
Italian Style Crust, Medium	476
Italian Style Crust, Small	954
Stuffed Crust, Large	696
Stuffed Crust, Medium	673
Thin & Crispy Crust, Large	496
Thin & Crispy Crust, Medium	470

PIZZA - MEATZZA
Classic Crust, Large	664
Classic Crust, Medium	600
Classic Crust, Personal	612
Classic Crust, Small	1108

DOMINO'S PIZZA
PIZZA - MEATZZA
Italian Style Crust, Large	554
Italian Style Crust, Medium	492
Italian Style Crust, Small	979
Stuffed Crust, Large	710
Stuffed Crust, Medium	690
Thin & Crispy Crust, Large	518
Thin & Crispy Crust, Medium	486

PIZZA - MEXICAN HOT
Classic Crust, Large	658
Classic Crust, Medium	591
Classic Crust, Personal	590
Classic Crust, Small	1074
Italian Style Crust, Large	548
Italian Style Crust, Medium	482
Italian Style Crust, Small	944
Stuffed Crust, Large	705
Stuffed Crust, Medium	680
Thin & Crispy Crust, Large	512
Thin & Crispy Crust, Medium	477

PIZZA - MIGHTY MEATY
Classic Crust, Large	674
Classic Crust, Medium	610
Classic Crust, Personal	621
Classic Crust, Small	1124
Italian Style Crust, Large	565
Italian Style Crust, Medium	501
Italian Style Crust, Small	994
Stuffed Crust, Large	721
Stuffed Crust, Medium	698
Thin & Crispy Crust, Large	529
Thin & Crispy Crust, Medium	495

PIZZA - MIXED GRILL
Classic Crust, Large	638
Classic Crust, Medium	577
Classic Crust, Personal	624
Classic Crust, Small	1069
Italian Style Crust, Large	529
Italian Style Crust, Medium	468
Italian Style Crust, Small	940
Stuffed Crust, Large	685
Stuffed Crust, Medium	665
Thin & Crispy Crust, Large	493
Thin & Crispy Crust, Medium	462

PIZZA - NEW YORKER
Classic Crust, Large	644
Classic Crust, Medium	582
Classic Crust, Personal	610
Classic Crust, Small	1081
GF Crust, Small	569
Italian Style Crust, Large	534
Italian Style Crust, Medium	474
Italian Style Crust, Small	951

DOMINO'S PIZZA

PIZZA - NEW YORKER

Stuffed Crust, Large	691
Stuffed Crust, Medium	671
Thin & Crispy Crust, Large	498
Thin & Crispy Crust, Medium	468

PIZZA - PEPPERONI PASSION

Classic Crust, Large	721
Classic Crust, Medium	655
Classic Crust, Personal	678
Classic Crust, Small	1215
GF Crust, Small	828
Italian Style Crust, Large	611
Italian Style Crust, Medium	546
Italian Style Crust, Small	1085
Stuffed Crust, Large	768
Stuffed Crust, Medium	743
Thin & Crispy Crust, Large	575
Thin & Crispy Crust, Medium	540

PIZZA - RANCH BBQ

Classic Crust, Large	730
Classic Crust, Medium	661
Classic Crust, Personal	680
Classic Crust, Small	1128
Italian Style Crust, Large	633
Italian Style Crust, Medium	677
Italian Style Crust, Small	982
Stuffed Crust, Large	848
Stuffed Crust, Medium	773
Thin & Crispy Crust, Large	564
Thin & Crispy Crust, Medium	513

PIZZA - SCRUMMY

Classic Crust, Large	728
Classic Crust, Medium	662
Classic Crust, Personal	737
Classic Crust, Small	1225
Italian Style Crust, Large	619
Italian Style Crust, Medium	553
Italian Style Crust, Small	1095
Stuffed Crust, Large	775
Stuffed Crust, Medium	750
Thin & Crispy Crust, Large	583
Thin & Crispy Crust, Medium	547

PIZZA - SIZZLER

Classic Crust, Large	662
Classic Crust, Medium	584
Classic Crust, Personal	606
Classic Crust, Small	1335
Italian Style Crust, Large	553
Italian Style Crust, Medium	479
Italian Style Crust, Small	922
Stuffed Crust, Large	726
Stuffed Crust, Medium	696

DOMINO'S PIZZA

PIZZA - SIZZLER

Thin & Crispy Crust, Large	490
Thin & Crispy Crust, Medium	461

PIZZA - TANDOORI HOT

Classic Crust, Large	555
Classic Crust, Medium	492
Classic Crust, Personal	522
Classic Crust, Small	889
Double Decadence, Large	825
Italian Style Crust, Large	445
Italian Style Crust, Medium	383
Italian Style Crust, Small	759
Stuffed Crust, Large	602
Stuffed Crust, Medium	581
Thin & Crispy Crust, Large	409
Thin & Crispy Crust, Medium	378

PIZZA - TANDOORI SIZZLER

Classic Crust, Large	551
Classic Crust, Medium	488
Classic Crust, Personal	519
Classic Crust, Small	883
Italian Style Crust, Large	442
Italian Style Crust, Medium	379
Italian Style Crust, Small	754
Stuffed Crust, Large	598
Stuffed Crust, Medium	576
Thin & Crispy Crust, Large	406
Thin & Crispy Crust, Medium	373

PIZZA - TEXAS BBQ

Classic Crust, Large	633
Classic Crust, Medium	571
Classic Crust, Personal	622
Classic Crust, Small	957
GF Crust, Small	608
Italian Style Crust, Large	587
Italian Style Crust, Medium	536
Italian Style Crust, Small	811
Stuffed Crust, Large	751
Stuffed Crust, Medium	684
Thin & Crispy Crust, Large	468
Thin & Crispy Crust, Medium	427

PIZZA - THE CHEESEBURGER

Classic Crust, Large	635
Classic Crust, Medium	564
Classic Crust, Personal	587
Classic Crust, Small	1023
Italian Style Crust, Large	525
Italian Style Crust, Medium	455
Italian Style Crust, Small	893
Stuffed Crust, Large	682
Stuffed Crust, Medium	652
Thin & Crispy Crust, Large	489
Thin & Crispy Crust, Medium	449

DOMINO'S PIZZA

PIZZA - THE CHICK-AINT

	KCAL
Vegan, Italian Style, Large	632
Vegan, Medium	586

PIZZA - THE MEATFIELDER

Classic Crust, Large	718
Classic Crust, Medium	652
Classic Crust, Personal	729
Classic Crust, Small	1205
Italian Style Crust, Large	609
Italian Style Crust, Medium	548
Italian Style Crust, Small	1076
Stuffed Crust, Large	955
Stuffed Crust, Medium	741
Thin & Crispy Crust, Large	573
Thin & Crispy Crust, Medium	538

PIZZA - TUNA SUPREME

Classic Crust, Large	573
Classic Crust, Medium	503
Classic Crust, Personal	536
Classic Crust, Small	915
Italian Style Crust, Large	464
Italian Style Crust, Medium	394
Italian Style Crust, Small	786
Stuffed Crust, Large	620
Stuffed Crust, Medium	591
Thin & Crispy Crust, Large	428
Thin & Crispy Crust, Medium	388

PIZZA - VEG-A-ROMA

Classic Crust, Large	570
Classic Crust, Medium	493
Classic Crust, Personal	541
Classic Crust, Small	1158
Italian Style Crust, Large	461
Italian Style Crust, Medium	388
Italian Style Crust, Small	745
Stuffed Crust, Large	634
Stuffed Crust, Medium	605
Thin & Crispy Crust, Large	398
Thin & Crispy Crust, Medium	370

PIZZA - VEGI CLASSIC

Classic Crust, Large	528
Classic Crust, Medium	467
Classic Crust, Personal	499
Classic Crust, Small	843
Italian Style Crust, Large	418
Italian Style Crust, Medium	358
Italian Style Crust, Small	714
Stuffed Crust, Large	575
Stuffed Crust, Medium	555
Thin & Crispy Crust, Large	382
Thin & Crispy Crust, Medium	352

PIZZA - VEGI SIZZLER

Classic Crust, Large	525

DOMINO'S PIZZA

PIZZA - VEGI SIZZLER

	KCAL
Classic Crust, Medium	464
Classic Crust, Personal	497
Classic Crust, Small	840
Fiery, Classic Crust, Large	523
Fiery, Classic Crust, Medium	464
Fiery, Classic Crust, Personal	496
Fiery, Classic Crust, Small	8379
Fiery, Double Decadence, Large	638
Fiery, Double Decadence, Medium	590
Fiery, Italian Style Crust, Large	414
Fiery, Italian Style Crust, Medium	355
Fiery, Italian Style Crust, Small	708
Fiery, Stuffed Crust, Large	570
Fiery, Stuffed Crust, Medium	552
Fiery, Thin & Crispy Crust, Large	378
Fiery, Thin & Crispy Crust, Medium	349
Italian Style Crust, Large	415
Italian Style Crust, Medium	356
Italian Style Crust, Small	710
Stuffed Crust, Large	572
Stuffed Crust, Medium	553
Thin & Crispy Crust, Large	379
Thin & Crispy Crust, Medium	350

PIZZA - VEGI SUPREME

Classic Crust, Large	539
Classic Crust, Medium	477
Classic Crust, Personal	508
Classic Crust, Small	862
GF Crust, Small	515
Italian Style Crust, Large	429
Italian Style Crust, Medium	368
Italian Style Crust, Small	732
Stuffed Crust, Large	586
Stuffed Crust, Medium	566
Thin & Crispy Crust, Large	393
Thin & Crispy, Medium	367
Vegan, Italian Style, Large	446
Vegan, Medium	514

PIZZA - VEGI VOLCANO

Classic Crust, Large	621
Classic Crust, Medium	539
Classic Crust, Personal	572
Classic Crust, Small	1228
Italian Style Crust, Large	512
Thin & Crispy, Large	449

SPICES

Chilli Flakes	4

WRAP

Test	700
Texas BBQ, Wrapzz	420
Vegi Supreme, Wrapzz	303

FARMHOUSE INNS

BACON

Cheese, & BBQ Sauce, Hunters, Steak Topper	440
Extra	106

BEANS

BBQ, Combo Feast	127
Extra	129

BEEF

Steak, Rib-eye, 9oz, Naked	771
Steak, Rib-eye, 9oz, with Sides	1597
Steak, Rump, 4oz, Extra	144
Steak, Rump, 8oz, Naked	415
Steak, Rump, 8oz, with Sides	1241
Steak, Sirloin, 8oz, Naked	474
Steak, Sirloin, 8oz, with Sides	1300

BHAJI

Onion, Extra	361

BREAD

Ciabatta, Garlic, Cheesy	655
Ciabatta, Garlic, Sides	450
Garlic, Combo Feast	225
Malted, & Butter, Sides	337
White, & Butter, Sides	374

BREAKFAST

All Day, with Malted Bread	1696
All Day, with White Bread	1733

BURGERS - BEEF

Patty Only, Extra	357

BURGERS - BEEF - SIGNATURE CARVERY

Double Up, with Chips, & Coleslaw	2118
with Chips, & Coleslaw	1761

BURGERS - BEEF, FARMHOUSE BBQ

Mac Stack, Double Up, with Chips, & Coleslaw	2307
Mac Stack, with Chips, & Coleslaw	1950

BURGERS - BEEF, GIANT

The Farm, with Chips, & Coleslaw	2252

BURGERS - CHEESEBURGER

Double Up, with Chips, & Coleslaw	1751
Smoked Bacon, Double Up, with Chips, & Coleslaw	1816
Smoked Bacon, with Chips, & Coleslaw	1459
with Chips, & Coleslaw	1394

BURGERS - CHICKEN

Bombay Bird, Double Up, with Chips, & Coleslaw	2481
Bombay Bird, with Chips, & Coleslaw	2121
Dirty Hunters, Double Up, with Chips, & Coleslaw	2071
Dirty Hunters, with Chips, & Coleslaw	1749
Tex Mex, Double Up, with Chips, & Coleslaw	2192
Tex Mex, with Chips, & Coleslaw	1870

BURGERS - CHICKPEA & RED PEPPER

Double Up, with Chips, & Coleslaw	1550
with Chips, & Coleslaw	1366

CHEESE

Extra	165
Parmigiana, Topper	151

FARMHOUSE INNS

CHICKEN

Breast, Curried, Skewer	1092
Breast, Extra	89
Breast, Kebab, Skewer, Combo Feast	189
Breast, Kebab, Skewer, Extra	189
Fillets, Roast, Combo Feast	179
Goujons, Southern Fried, with BBQ Dip	596
Hunters	1401
Medley, Crispy, no Sauce	1739
Smothered	1850
Southern Fried, Curried, Skewer	1325
Southern Fried, Extra	322
Southern Fried, Skewer, Combo Feast	422
Southern Fried, Skewer, Extra	422
Strips, Fully Loaded	1601
Strips, Louisiana, Combo Feast	280
Wings, Combo Feast	538
Wings, no Sauce	1015

CHIPS

Combo Feast	655
Curry Sauce, Topped, Side	796
Hunters, Topped, Side	1023
Side	655

COD

Battered, with Chips, & Garden Peas, Large	1685
Battered, with Chips, & Mushy Peas, Large	1736

COLESLAW

Combo Feast	306
Sides	205

CORN

Cob, Combo Feast	161
Cob, Side	161

EGGS

Fried, 2, Steak Topper	240
Fried, Extra	120

FISH

Battered, Atlantic, with Chips, & Mushy Peas	1817
Battered, Atlantic, with Chips, & Peas	1766

FISH & CHIPS

Chip Shop Supper	2330

GAMMON - STEAK

4oz, Extra	198
Naked	486
Naked, with Egg, & Pineapple	672
Naked, with Fried Egg	726
Naked, with Pineapple	618
with Chips, & Peas	1302

GRAVY

Chip Shop Supper	42
Extra	42

GRILLS

Mixed, Farmhouse	2202

FARMHOUSE INNS

GUACAMOLE
	KCAL
Portion	93

HAM
Hand Carved, & Eggs, with Chips, & Peas	1126

HASH BROWNS
Extra	78

JACKET POTATO
with Baked Beans	431
with Cheese, & Baked Beans	510
with Mozzarella, & Cheddar Cheese	424
with Tuna Mayonnaise	483

LAMB
Shank, Minted, with Mash, & Veg	1213

LASAGNE
Beef, Naked	584
Beef, with Chips, & Garlic Bread	1381

MACARONI CHEESE
Combo Feast	232
Luxury	778

MAYONNAISE
Garlic	190

MUSHROOMS
Button, Breaded, Garlic, with Garlic Mayonnaise	655
Button, Sides	283

NACHOS
Cheesy, Big	888

ONION RINGS
Combo Feast	327
Sides	654

PATE
Chicken, Liver, with Bread, Onion Chutney, & Salad	474

PEAS
Garden, Chip Shop Supper	56
Mushy, Chip Shop Supper	107

PIE
Beef & Ale, Slow Cooked, No Sides	1184
Beef & Ale, Slow Cooked, with Chips	1839
Beef & Ale, Slow Cooked, with Mashed Potato	1436
Chicken & Mushroom, No Sides	1215
Chicken & Mushroom, with Chips	1870
Chicken & Mushroom, with Mashed Potato	1467

PLATTER
Chicken, Sharer	2459

RIBS
Rack, Mini, Extra	204

SALAD
Chicken, & Bacon, Hot	884
Chicken, Skewer	467
Side, Combo Feast	45
Side	45

SALMON
Fillet, Scottish, Grilled	431
Fillet, Scottish, Grilled, with Hollandaise Sauce	538

FARMHOUSE INNS

SALSA
	KCAL
Portion	56

SANDWICH
Carvery, Bap	1149
Cheese & Chutney, Ciabatta Roll	1042
Cheese & Chutney, Floured Bap	1027
Chicken, Bacon, Tomato, Melt, Ciabatta Roll	1180
Chicken, Bacon Tomato, Melt, Floured Bap	1165
Chicken Goujons, & Mayo, Ciabatta Roll	1318
Chicken Goujons, & Mayo, Floured Bap	1303
Hunters Chicken, Melt, Ciabatta Roll	1170
Hunters Chicken, Melt, Floured Bap	1155
Fish Fingers, & Tartare Sauce, Ciabatta Roll	1148
Fish Fingers, & Tartare Sauce, Floured Bap	1133
Tuna, Melt, Ciabatta Roll	989
Tuna, Melt, Floured Bap	974

SAUCE
BBQ, Texan	144
Char Sui, Combo Feast	195
Char Sui, for Chicken Wings	130
Curry, Chip Shop Supper	141
Diane	425
Peppercorn	101
Piri Piri, Combo Feast	30
Piri Piri	40
Piri Piri, for Chicken Wings	20
Sour Cream	165
Sweet Chilli	131

SAUSAGE
Extra	181
Pigs in Blanket, Extra	209

SAUSAGE & MASH
Main	1447

SCAMPI
Wholetail, Breaded	1251
Wholetail, Breaded, Naked	550

TART
Vegetable, no Sides	483
Vegetable, with Chips	1138
Vegetable, with Mashed Potato	735

TIKKA MASALA - CHICKEN
no Sides	1100
with Chips	1755
with Pilau Rice, & Chips	1699
with Pilau Rice	1534

YORKSHIRE PUDDING
& Pigs in Blanket, Extra	309
Extra	100
Giant, Extra	490
Wrap, All The Meats, Giant	1604
Wrap, Beef, & Horseradish, Giant	1684
Wrap, Turkey, & Cranberry, Giant	1611

FIVE GUYS

BACON
Rashers, 2	78

BANANA
Milkshake Mix-in	148

BISCUITS
Oreo, Pieces, Milkshake Mix-in	62

BUNS
Burger	238
Hot Dog	215

BURGERS
Beef, Patty Only	195

CHOCOLATE
Milkshake Mix-in	201

COFFEE
Milkshake Mix-in	5

CREAM
Whipped, Milkshake Mix-in	88

EGGS
Extra	119

FRIES
Large	1491
Little	694
Reg	1019

HOT DOG
Sausage Only	192

MILK
Malted, Mlkshake Mix-in	59

MILK SHAKE
Base, No Mix-in	714

PEANUT BUTTER
Milkshake Mix-in	348

SEASONING MIX
Cajun, for Fries	20

SPREAD
Lotus Biscoff, Milkshake Mix-in	145

STRAWBERRIES
Milkshake Mix-in	94

SUGAR
Caramel, Salted, Milkshake Mix-in	113

TOPPING
BBQ Sauce	20
Brown Sauce, HP	10
Cheese, Slice	64
Hot Sauce	2
Jalapeno Peppers	1
Lettuce	3
Mayonnaise	113
Mushrooms, Grilled	12
Mustard	4
Onions	9
Onions, Grilled	11
Peppers, Green	2
Pickles	2

Relish	15
Tomato Ketchup	14
Tomatoes	6

GOURMET BURGER KITCHEN

BITES
Falafel	272

BURGERS
Beef, Avo Bacon	837
Beef, Blue Cheese Gorgonzola	829
Beef, Blue Cheese Sauce	975
Beef, Cheese & Bacon, GBK, American Cheese	904
Beef, Cheese & Bacon, GBK, Cheddar	910
Beef, Classic	705
Beef, Classic, with American Cheese	826
Beef, Classic, with Cheddar	828
Beef, Rocket Man	900
Beef, Taxidriver	1416
Beef, The Mighty	1328
Chicken, Classic, Chargrilled	588
Chicken, Classic, Panko	644
Chicken, Hey Pesto, Chargrilled	951
Chicken, Hey Pesto, Panko	1007
Chicken, Satay, Chargrilled	784
Chicken, Satay, Panko	841

BURGERS VEGETARIAN
Californian	639
Cluck Free	569
Falafel	327
The Beyond, & Cheese	678
The Beyond	656
Vegan, Classic	429

CHEESE
Halloumi, Bites	458

CHICKEN
Tenders, Fresh	895

COLESLAW
Homeslaw, GBK	325

DRINK
Franklin & Sons, Orange & Grapefruit	96
Franklin & Sons, Rhubarb Lemonade	69
Strawberry & Elderflower, Fizz	95

FRIES
Chunky, Skin On, Hei Hei	333
Chunky, Skin On, Rosemary	334
Skinny, Hei Hei	645
Skinny, Rosemary	646
Sweet Potato	555
Truffle Cheese	468

ICE CREAM
Chocolate, Vegan	426
Double Chocolate, Belgian, Yeo Valley	627
Madagascan Vanilla, Yeo Valley	507
Sea-Salted Caramel, Yeo Valley	561
Strawberry, Yeo Valley	513

MILK SHAKE
Double Chocolate, Belgian	633
Oreo	606

GOURMET BURGER KITCHEN

MILK SHAKE
Peanut Butter	634
Sea-Salted Caramel	567
Strawberry	519
Vanilla, Madagascan	513

ONION RINGS
Homemade	555

SALAD
Green, Simple	87

SAUCE
Baconnaise	193
BBQ	38
Burger	82
Habanero Jam, Hot	44
Mayo, Blue Cheese	179
Mayo, Chipotle	149
Mayo, Garlic	171
Mayo, Harissa, Vegan	131
Mayo, House	173
Mayo, Sriracha	182
Pesto, Basil	168
Raita	12
Relish, Cajun	61
Relish	38
Satay	110

GREGGS

BAGUETTE

	KCAL
Bacon, & Omelette, Breakfast	553
Bacon, & Sausage, Breakfast	589
Bacon, Breakfast	505
Cheese, Cheddar, Mature, & Salad	477
Chicken, Mexican	524
Chicken, Roast, & Bacon, Club	492
Chicken, Roast, & Stuffing	526
Chicken, Southern Fried	593
Chicken, Tandoori	503
Chicken Mayonnaise, Roast	497
Ham, & Cheese	526
Ham, Honey Roast, & Salad	437
Omelette, Breakfast	511
Sausage, & Omelette, Breakfast	615
Sausage, Breakfast	586
Steak & Cheese	519
Tuna, Crunch	454
Vegan Ham, & Cheeze	467

BAKE

Cheese, & Onion	437
Chicken	422
Steak	408
Vegetable	425

BISCUITS

Chocolate, Star	192
Gingerbread, Man	173
Jammy Heart	273
Shortbread, Chocolate Caramel	293

BREAKFAST CEREAL

Porridge, Apple & Cinnamon, Gluten Free	232
Porridge, Golden Syrup, Gluten Free	244
Porridge, Simply Creamy, Gluten Free	210

BROWNIES

Chocolate, Triple, Gluten Free	98

BUNS

Belgian	390

CAKE

Raspberry, & Almond, Baked, Mini	69

CHERRYADE

Sparkling, No Added Sugar	20

CHICKEN

Bites, Spicy BBQ	290
Goujons, Southern Fried	394

COFFEE

Americano, Lrg	11
Americano, Reg	9
Black, Decaf, Lrg	7
Black, Decaf, Reg	6
Capuccino, Lrg	114
Cappuccino, Reg	94
Flat White	71
Latte, Caramel, Lrg	248

GREGGS

COFFEE

	KCAL
Latte, Caramel, Reg	223
Latte, Lrg	133
Latte, Pumpkin Spice, Lrg	253
Latte, Pumpkin Spice, Reg	228
Latte, Reg	111
Latte, Vanilla, Lrg	248
Latte, Vanilla, Reg	223
Mocha, Lrg	300
Mocha, Reg	233
White, Lrg	45
White, Reg	34

COOKIES

Chocolate, Milk	358
Chocolate, Triple	347
Chocolate, White	360

CRISPS

Cheese Puffs	201
Mature Cheddar & Onion	198
Salt & Vinegar, Crunchy Sticks	175
Sea Salt, & Cider Vinegar	194
Thai Sweet Chilli	203
Tortilla, Chilli	193

CROISSANT

All Butter	306
Almond	332

DOUGHNUTS

Caramel Custard	290
Chocolate, Triple	330
Cream, Finger	355
Glazed, Ring	195
Iced, Ring	236
Jam	236
Pink, Jammie	316
Sugar Strand	228
Yum Yum	323

DRIED FRUIT

Mix, Chocolate, & Yoghurt Coated	128

DRINK

Mango & Pineapple, Sparkling, No Added Sugar	15

ECLAIR

Cream	344

FRUIT

Medley	82
Tropical, Pot	108

HASH BROWNS

2	151

HOT CHOCOLATE

Lrg	281
Reg	219

JUICE

Apple, Fairtrade, 150ml Bottle	71
Orange, Fairtrade, 150ml Bottle	69

GREGGS

LEMONADE
Cloudy, Sparkling, 500ml Bottle	15
Raspberry, Sparkling, 500ml Bottle	10

MELT
Sausage, Bean, & Cheese	453
Sausage, Bean, & Cheese, Vegan	427

MUFFIN
Chocolate, Triple	462
Sticky Toffee	382

NUTS
Naked, Mixed	157

PAIN AU CHOCOLAT
Pastry	308

PASTA SALAD
Chicken, & Bacon	460
Feta, & Tomato	380
Mexican Chicken, Spicy	440
Tuna, Crunch	375

PASTRY
Wrap, Bacon & Cheese	385

PASTY
Beef, & Vegetable	459

PIE
Mince, Savoury	417

PIZZA
Margherita	552
Pepperoni	617

POPCORN
Sweet & Salty	118

POTATO WEDGES
Southern Fried	278

ROLL
Bacon, & Omelette, Breakfast	378
Bacon, & Sausage, Breakfast	414
Bacon, Breakfast	330
Cheese, & Onion, Salad, Sub	451
Cheese	196
Chicken, Roast, & Salad	342
Ham	172
Ham, Honey Roast, & Egg, Salad	329
Ham, Honey Roast, & Egg Salad, Sub	346
Omelette, Breakfast	382
Sausage, & Omelette, Breakfast	418
Sausage, Breakfast	391
Sausage, Vegan, Breakfast	411
Tuna Mayonnaise	333

SANDWICH
Chicken, Chargrill, Oval Bite	412
Chicken, Mexican, Oval Bite	462
Egg Mayonnaise, Free Range	369
Ploughmans, Cheddar Cheese, Mature, Oval Bite	474
Tuna Mayonnaise, & Cucumber	351

GREGGS

SAUSAGE ROLL
Freshly Baked	328
Vegan	309

SNACKS
BBQ, Smoky, Crunch	104

SOUP
Chicken, & Red Pepper, Spicy	120
Tomato, Cream of	216

TEA
English Breakfast, Lrg	12
English Breakfast, Reg	9
Green, Reg	0
Peppermint, Reg	0

TOASTIE
Cheese, Cheddar, & Chutney	462
Chicken, BBQ, & Bacon	503
Ham, & Cheddar Cheese	462

WRAP
Chicken, & Bacon, Caesar	522
Chicken, Mexican	464
Chicken, Spicy BBQ, & Bacon	570
Mexican Bean, & Sweet Potato	452

HARVESTER RESTAURANT

AVOCADO

Smashed, Build Your Own Breakfast	349

BACON

Back, Build Your Own Breakfast	83
Extra	94

BEANS

Baked, Extra	63
Baked, Heinz, Build Your Own Breakfast	63
Baked, Side, Kids Menu	51

BEEF - BRISKET

Hickory Smoked, with Mash, & Veg	1001

BEEF - STEAK, FILLET

8oz, for Mixed Grill	287
8oz, with Fries, Mushroom, Tomato, & Onion Rings	432

BEEF - STEAK, RUMP

4oz, Build Your Own Breakfast	224
4oz, Extra, Breakfast	224
4oz, for Mixed Grill	164
4oz, Kids Menu	164
8oz, & Fries, Mushroom, Tomato, & Onion Rings	475
8oz, for Mixed Grill	329

BEEF - STEAK, SIRLOIN

10oz, Ancho Chilli	970
10oz, for Mixed Grill	521
10oz, with Fries, Mushroom, Tomato, & Onion Rings	666

BISCUITS

Oreo, Crumb, Extra	145
Oreo, Extra	93

BITES

Quorn, Southern Fried, Kids Menu	199
Quorn, Southern Fried, Starter	327

BLACK PUDDING

Build Your Own Breakfast	81
Extra	81

BREAD

Garlic, Cheesy, Side	354
Garlic, Cheesy, Tapas	633
Garlic, Side	165
Garlic, Tapas	331

BREAKFAST

Signature, Kids, No Egg	300
The Classic, No Egg	838
The Vegan	1002
The Vegan, Kids	310
The Veggie, No Egg	572
The Veggies, Kids, No Egg	378

BROCCOLI

Tenderstem, Chargrilled, Side	37
Tenderstem, Chargrilled, Side, Kids Menu	28

BROWNIES - CHOCOLATE

Belgian, with Chocolate Sauce, & Ice Cream	673
with Chocolate Sauce, Belgian, Mini	287

HARVESTER RESTAURANT

BURGERS

Bean, Beyond, Vegan	666
Bean, Patty, Extra	241
Beef, Mini, Kids Menu	330
Beef, Patty, Extra	391
Beef, The Classic	971
Chicken, Mini, Kids Menu	213
Chicken, Southern Fried, Extra	438
Chicken, The Classic	731
Vegan, Plant Based, Moving Mountains, Extra	302
The Big One	1808
The Cowboy	993
Vegan, The Purist	1432
The True Blue	1099

CAKE

Chocolate, Fudge, Chocolate Sauce, & Ice Cream	922

CAULIFLOWER

Buffalo, with Garlic Mayo, Starter	470

CHEESE

Halloumi, Battered, & Chips, No Peas	877
Halloumi, Extra	179
Monterey Jack, Extra	65
Stilton, Long Clawson, Extra	164

CHEESE ALTERNATIVE

Mature, Slice, Violife, Extra	57

CHEESECAKE

Vanilla, Baked	622
Vanilla, Baked, Mini	260

CHICKEN - BBQ

Breast, Grilled, Kids Menu	298
BBQ	833

CHICKEN - BURGER

Breast, Extra	176

CHICKEN - BUTTERMILK

Fried, Kids Menu	253
Tenders, Fried, Starter	395

CHICKEN - CAJUN

Breast, Extra	176

CHICKEN - CAJUN, SURF & TURF

Rump Steak, Prawns, Corn, Apple & Fennel Slaw	723

CHICKEN - CARIBBEAN

with Golden Rice & Beans, Grilled Pineapple	469

CHICKEN - GRILLED

Breast, Kids Menu	176
Breast, with Jacket Potato, Simply	282

CHICKEN - ROTISSERIE

Half	510
Half, Jerk, Grilled, with Coconut Rice, & Beans	1065
Half, with Half Rack Ribs, Combo	931
Quarter, Extra	200
Quarter, Kids Menu	359
Quarter, Triple, Combo	715
Quarter, with Ribs, Original Combo	732

HARVESTER RESTAURANT

CHICKEN - SKEWERS
with Chorizo, Churrasco	964

CHICKEN - STRIPS
Kids Menu, Sm Bites	88

CHICKEN - VEGETARIAN
Quorn, Stack, BBQ	697

CHICKEN - WINGS
Sticky, Tapas	296
with BBQ, Sticky	530

CHILLI
Beef, Chipotle, Pulled	328
Non Carne, Kids Menu	545
Non Carne, Vegan, for Nachos	136
Non Carne, with Rice	542

CHIPS - TRIPLE COOKED
Chunky, Nashville Hot, Side	484
Chunky, Sage & Onion, Side	500
Chunky, Side	484
Chunky, Side, Kids Menu	218

COD
Fillet, Battered, Kids Menu	308
& Chips, with Mushy Peas	688
& Chips, with Peas	675

CORN
Buttered, Side	207
Cobette, Side, Kids Menu	58

CREAM
Fluffy, Extra	103

CURRY
Vegetable, Thai Green	628

CUSTARD
Extra	90

DESSERT
Cherry Blizzard	534
Chocolate Orange, Slice	329
Mini Combo, Brownie, Blackcurrant, & Cheesecake	751

EGGS
Benedict, Portion	668
Fried, Free Range, Build Your Own Breakfast	130
Fried, Free Range, Extra	85
Mediterranean, Portion	599
Poached, Free Range, Build Your Own Breakfast	86
Scrambled, Free Range, Build Your Own Breakfast	108
Scrambled, on Toast, Kids Menu, Sm Bites	265

FISH CAKES
Salmon, with Watercress, Melting Middle	638

FISH FINGERS
Kids Menu	220
Kids Menu, Sm Bites	166

FRIES
Halloumi, with Green Devil Sauce	427
Sweet Potato, Side	503
Sweet Potato, Side, Kids Menu	201

HARVESTER RESTAURANT

FRITTERS - SWEETCORN
Smoked Cheddar, & Chilli, Build Your Own Breakfast	135
Spicy, with Avocado, & Eggs	614

FRUIT SALAD
Tutti Frutti, with Strawberry Yoghurt, Kids Menu	107

GAMMON - STEAK
7oz, No Topping	611
7oz, Double Up	1076
7oz, Double Up, with Egg, & Pineapple	1189
7oz, Double Up, with Egg	1161
7oz, Double Up, with Pineapple	1103
7oz, Egg, & Pineapple	724
7oz, for Mixed Grill	273
7oz, with Egg	696
7oz, with Pineapple	638

GRAVY
Chicken, Specialty, Extra	29

HASH
Potato, & Spinach	334

HASH BROWNS
Build Your Own Breakfast	91

HOUMOUS
Build Your Own Breakfast	844

ICE CREAM
Extra	101
Non Dairy, Extra	223

JELLY
Peach, Fruitypot, Kids Menu	72

LAMB
Shank, Moroccan Style	1197

MACARONI CHEESE
Bites, with Smokey Ketchup	428
Cauliflower, Kids Menu	313
Extra	279
Side	279

MIXED GRILL
Excludes Steak	961
Ultimate, Excludes Steak	1999
The Pitmaster	3389

MOUSSAKA
Feta, & Butternut Squash	654

MOUSSE
Blackcurrant	295
Blackcurrant, Kids Menu	164
Blackcurrant, Mini	164

MUSHROOMS
Breaded, with Garlic Mayo Dip, Starter	501
Flat, Build Your Own Breakfast	12
Garlic, Oven Baked, with Garlic Bread, Starter	272

NACHOS
Starter	529
Vegan, Starter	523

HARVESTER RESTAURANT

ONION RINGS
Side	487

PANCAKES
Buttermilk, & Bacon, with Syrup	752
Buttermilk, with Fruit, & Syrup, Kids	192
Buttermilk, with Fruit, & Syrup	623
Butttermilk, Side	106

PASTA
In Tomato Sauce, Kids Menu, Sm Bites	237
Spinach, & Ricotto, in Tomato & Basil Sauce	831

PEAS
Chilli & Garlic, Kickin', Side	124
Garden, Side	60
Mushy, Side	73
Side, Kids Menu	60

PIE
Cherry, Sugar Dusted	563
Cookies, & Cream	315
Fish, Cheddar Mash Topped	440

PORK
Bell, Glazed, with Hash Potatoes, Mac & Cheese	1646
Pulled, BBQ, Extra	239
Pulled, BBQ, for Nachos	239

POTATOES
Skins, Cheese, & Bacon, Tapas	407
Skins, Cheese, Tapas	313
Jacket, Side	273
Jacket, Side, Kids Menu	273
Jacket, with Sour Cream, Side	348
Mashed, Side	212
Mash, Side, Kids Menu	94

PRAWNS
Crackerjack, with Green Devil Sauce, Starter	293
Garlic, King, & Chilli, Extra	172
Garlic, King, & Chilli Butter, with Garlic Bread, Starter	358

RIBS - FULL RACK
Jerk BBQ, with Chicken Wings, Corn, Slaw, & Chips	1828
Jerk BBQ, with Chips, Slaw, & Corn	1516
Slow Cooked, BBQ Sauce, with Chips, Slaw, & Corn	1000

RIBS - HALF RACK
BBQ, Extra	403
Kids Menu	348

RIBS - KILO
Kiln Smoked, Bourbon Sauce	509

RICE
Chicken, Katsu, Bowl	505
Golden, & Beans, Side	229
Vegetable, Sunshine, Kids Menu	190

SALAD
Feel Good	307
Feel Good, with Cajun Chicken	503
Feel Good, with Chicken Breast	483
Feel Good, with Quorn Fillets, Cajun	850

HARVESTER RESTAURANT

SALAD
Feel Good, with Salmon	699
Feel Good, with Steak, Rump, 8oz	644
Feel Good, with Tofu Skewers, Peri Peri	544

SALMON
Grilled, Spiked Sticky, with Golden Rice, & Beans	674
Grilled, Kids Menu	218

SANDWICH
Steak	591

SAUCE
Caribbean Curry, Steak Sauce	250
Chasseur, Steak Sauce	30
Chocolate, Belgian, Dessert	58
Chocolate, Belgian, Dessert, Kids Menu	29
Craft Ale, Bacon, & Mushroom, Steak Sauce	67
Katsu, Steak Sauce	92
Peppercorn, Steak Sauce	46
Raspberry, Dessert	57
Salted Caramel, Dessert	51
Strawberry, Dessert	57
Toffee, Fudge, Dessert	64
Toffee, Fudge, Dessert, Kids Menu	32

SAUSAGE
& Yorkie, Kids Menu	275
& Yorkie, Kids Menu, Sm Bites	192
Pork, Build Your Own Breakfast	217
Pork, Extra	217
Pork, Cheddar, Jalapeno, with BBQ Sauce	452
Vegan	80
Vegetarian, & Yorkie, Kids Menu	265
Vegetarian, & Yorkie, Kids Menu, Sm Bites	185

SCAMPI
Extra	139
Wholetail, Whitby, Excluding Peas	425

SEA BASS
Grilled, Meal, Simply	518

SOUP
Tomato, & Basil	193

SPINACH
Build Your Own Breakfast	12

SPONGE PUDDING
Lemon	493
Treacle	941

SQUID
Calamari, Strips, with Garlic Mayo, Starter	278

SUNDAE
Best	255
Best, Kids Menu	239
Best, Vegan	673
Best, Vegan, Kids Menu	448
Blueberry, Eton Mess	530
Build Your Own, Kids Menu	453
Caramel, Salted, Rocky Road	618

HARVESTER RESTAURANT

SUNDAE
	KCAL
Chocolate, Brownie, Rocky Horror	683
Chocolate, Brownie, Rocky Horror, Kids Menu	446
Passion Fruit, & White Chocolate	678
Strawberry Cheesecake	619

TAGINE
Aubergine, & Red Lentil	1077

TART
Camembert, & Cherry Tomato, Puff Pastry	635

TOFU
Skewers, Peri Peri	641

TOMATOES
Build Your Own Breakfast	6

TOPPING
Cheese, Stilton, & Bacon	352

VEGETABLES
Steamed, Side	77
Steamed, Side, Kids Menu	46
Sticks, Side, Kids Menu	44

WAFFLES
Belgian, Extra	390
Chicken, Buttermilk Fried, & Bacon, with Syrup	1323

WRAP
Chicken, Breast, Cajun, Grilled	467
Chicken, Breast, Grilled	448
Chicken, Build Your Own, Kids Menu	415
Chicken, Buttermilk Fried	525
Halloumi	629
Quorn, Fillet, Cajun	390
Quorn, Southern Fried	475

HUNGRY HORSE

BACON
	KCAL
Streaky, Side, Extra	66

BAGUETTE
Cheesy Melt	755
Chicken, Club	889
Chicken, Mayo, Southern Fried	663
Fish Fingers, & Mayo	661

BEANS
Baked, Jacket Potato Topping	73
Baked, Side, Extra	73

BEEF
Dinner, Roast, Sunday	967
Rump Steak, 12oz, Big Plate Specials	1344
Rump Steak, 12oz, Naked, Big Plate Specials	520
Rump Steak, 12oz, Side, Extra	435
Rump Steak, 4oz	821
Rump Steak, 4oz, Naked	230
Rump Steak, 8oz	966
Rump Steak, 8oz, Mix it Up, Big Plate Specials	289
Rump Steak, 8oz, Naked	375
Sirloin Steak, 9oz, Big Plate Specials	1304
Sirloin Steak, 9oz, Naked, Big Plate Specials	480
Steak, Smothered, 8oz, Sizzler, Big Plate Specials	1364
Dinner, Sunday Roast, Big Plate Specials	1597
Dinner, Sunday Roasts, Kids	523

BHAJI
Onion, Extra Portion	541

BREAD
Baguette, ½, & Butter, Extra	197
Brown, & Butter, Side	337
Garlic, Ciabatta, Cheesy	522
Garlic, Ciabatta	358
Naan, Extra	345
White, & Butter, Side	374
Wrap, Tortilla, Soft, Mix it Up, Big Plate Specials	329

BREAKFAST
All Day, Big Plate Specials	1561
Full English, Classics	845

BURGERS
Beef, & Chicken, Quadzilla	2768
Beef, Bacon, & Egg, Sunny Stacker	1308
Beef, Bacon, Chicken, & Pulled Pork, Carni-Four	2368
Beef, Classic, Double	1527
Beef, Classic	1170
Beef, Double Daddy	2219
Beef, Extra Patty	357
Beef, Sizzler, Combo, Big Plate Specials	2412
Beef, Smokin' Jack	1539
Beef, with Cheese, & Bacon, Double	1619
Beef, with Cheese, & Bacon	1262
Beef, with Cheese, Double	1553
Beef, with Cheese	1196
Chicken, Bombay Bird	1828

HUNGRY HORSE

BURGERS

Chicken, Extra Fillet	290
Chicken, Southern Fried, Double	1534
Chicken, Southern Fried, Extra Patty	360
Chicken, Southern Fried	1174
Veggie, Chinese, Double	1251
Veggie, Chinese	1021
Veggie, Hoisin, Extra Patty	185

BUTTER

Portion	29

CAKE

Chocolate, Fudge, Warm	905

CHEESE

Grated, Side, Extra	165
Halloumi, Battered, & Chips	1183
Halloumi, Battered, & Chips, with Baked Beans	1256
Halloumi, Battered, & Chips, with Garden Peas	1263
Halloumi, Battered, & Chips, with Mushy Peas	1303
Halloumi, Battered, & Chips, with Salad	1195
Halloumi, Battered, Mix It Up, Big Plate Specials	764
Halloumi, Extra	800
Halloumi, Fingers	886
Mozzarella, Mature Cheddar, Jacket Potato Topping	165

CHEESECAKE

Millionaires	593

CHICKEN

Breast, Extra Portion	179
Skewers, Breast, Kebab, Mix It Up, Big Plate Special	378

CHICKEN

Roast, Breast, Sunday, Kids Menu	508
Skewers, Breast, Extra	189
Crispy, Jumbo, with Curry Sauce, Big Plate Specials	1709
Roast, Fillet, Sunday	864
Roast, Fillet, Sunday, Big Plate Special	1436
Fingers, Battered, Mix it Up, Big Plate Specials	660
Fingers, Battered, Plain, Starter	607
New Yorker, & Salad, Live Well	449
New Yorker, Big Plate Specials	1721
New Yorker, Classics	1168
Parmigiana, Big Plate Specials	1179
Roast, Half, Flattened, Mix it Up, Big Plate Special	304
Skewers, Southern Fried, Mix It Up, Big Plate Special	844
Skewers, Southern Fried, Extra	422
Wings, Plain, Starter	766
Wings, with Caribbean Dressing, Starter	916
Wings, with Caribbean Dressing, Starter	757
Wings, with Char Sui Sauce, Starter	929
Wings, with Char Sui Sauce, Starter	770
Wings, with Fajita Seasoning, Starter	801
Wings, with Fajita Seasoning, Starter	642
Wings, with Garlic & Parmesan Sauce, Starter	965
Wings, with Garlic & Parmesan Sauce, Starter	806
Wings, with Hot Sauce, Starter	834

HUNGRY HORSE

CHICKEN

Wings, with Hot Sauce, Starter	675
Wings, with Lemon & Pepper Sauce, Starter	959
Wings, with Lemon & Pepper Sauce, Starter	800
Wings, with Piri Piri Hot Sauce, Starter	791
Wings, with Piri Piri Hot Sauce, Starter	632
Wings, with Texan BBQ Sauce, Starter	856
Wings, with Texan BBQ Sauce, Starter	697

CHILLI

Con Carne, Jacket Potato Topping	162

CHIPS

Cheesy, Side	583
Mix it Up, Big Plate Specials	574
Side	418

COD & CHIPS

Jumbo, No Sides Big Plate Specials	1605
Jumbo, with Baked Beans, Big Plate Specials	1678
Jumbo, with Garden Peas, Big Plate Specials	1665
Jumbo, with Mushy Peas, Big Plate Specials	1725
Jumbo, with Salad, Big Plate Specials	1617

COLESLAW

Jacket Potato Topping	75
Mix it Up, Big Plate Specials	100
Side	75

CORN

Cobs, Mini, Mix it Up, Big Plate Specials	39
on the Cob, Side	72

CRUMBLE

Apple	515

CURRY

Chickpea, & Sweet Potato, Big Plate Specials	2247
Chickpea, & Sweet Potato, Classics	691

CUSTARD

Extra	89

DESSERT

Piecaken, Black Forest	967
Piecaken, Black Forest, Vegan	1024

DRESSING

Caribbean, Mix It Up, Big Plate Specials	300

EGGS

Fried, Side, Extra	118

FISH & CHIPS

Vegan, Fillets, No Sides, Classics	696
Vegan, Fillets, with Baked Beans, Classics	769
Vegan, Fillets, with Garden Peas, Classics	756
Vegan, Fillets, with Mushy Peas, Classics	816
Vegan, Fillets, with Salad, Classics	708
No Sides, Classics	1337
Battered, with Baked Beans, Classics	1410
Battered, with Garden Peas, Classics	1397
Battered, with Mushy Peas, Classics	1457
Battered, with Salad, Classics	1349

HUNGRY HORSE

FRIES

Dirty, Mac & Bacon, Side	910
Dirty, Mac & Cheese, Side	778
Dirty, Nacho Cheese, & Bacon, Side	760
Dirty, Pizza Topper, Side	691
Dirty, Tikka, Side	1034
Mix it Up, Big Plate Specials	546
Side	546
Sweet Potato, Side	410

GAMMON

Grilled, 15oz, Big Plate Specials	1503
Grilled, 5oz, Classics	782
Grilled, 5oz, Mix It Up, Big Plate Specials	498

ICE CREAM

Bubblegum, Extra	120
Chocolate, Extra	99
Vanilla, Extra	97

LASAGNE

& Salad, Live Well	543
Beef, Classics	687

MACARONI CHEESE

Classics	756
Side	281

MAYONNAISE

Muddy, Extra	286

MIXED GRILL

Full Monty, Big Plate Special	1878
Mini	1308

MUSHROOMS

Breaded, Garlic	686
Side, Extra	57

NACHOS

Muchos Nachos Grande	1101

ONION RINGS

5, Side	389
Horseshoe Stacker, 20, ½	892
Mix it Up, Big Plate Specials	311

PASTA

Deli, Live Well	401
Deli, with Halloumi, Live Well	600
Deli, with Roast Chicken, Live Well	580
Deli, with Rump Steak, Live Well	545
Deli, with Salmon Fillet, Live Well	771

PEAS

Mushy, Side, Extra	120
Side, Extra	60

PIE

Steak & Ale, No Sides	1111
Steak & Ale, with Chips	1529
Steak & Ale, with Mash	1360
Chicken & Mushroom, Woodland, No Sides	1142
Chicken & Mushroom, Woodland, with Chips	1560
Chicken & Mushroom, Woodland, with Mash	1391

HUNGRY HORSE

PINEAPPLE

Slice, Side, Extra	14

PIZZA

Margherita, Classics	903
Meat Feast, Classics	1229
Pepperoni, Classics	1067

PLATTER

Ultimate, Big Combo, Starter	2568

POPPADOMS

& Chutney, Extra Portion	190

POTATOES

Jacket, Mix it Up, Big Plate Specials	194
Jacket, Plain, Add Toppings Seperately	259
Jacket, Plain, Side	194
Mashed, Side, Extra	249
Roast, Extra	335

RICE

Dirty, Mix it Up, Big Plate Specials	191

ROULADE - RED CABBAGE & APPLE

Sunday Roast, Vegetarian, Big Plate Specials	1750
Sunday Roast, Vegetarian	950
Sunday Roast, Vegetarian, Kids	687

SALAD

Classic, Live Well	58
Classic, with Halloumi, Live Well	254
Classic, with Roast Chicken, Live Well	233
Classic, with Rump Steak, Live Well	198
Classic, with Salmon Fillet, Live Well	424
Dressed, Side	33
Side, Mix It Up, Big Plate Specials	49

SALMON

Fillet, Mix It Up, Big Plate Specials	370

SANDWICH

Chicken, Crispy, Big Plate Specials	2531
Chicken, Southern Fried, Steak, Big Plate Specials	2472
Halloumi, Big Plate Specials	3060

SAUCE

BBQ, Texan, Extra	90
BBQ, Texan, Mix it Up, Big Plate Specials	180
BBQ, with Jack Daniels, Steak Sauce	146
Char Sui, Mix It Up, Big Plate Specials	325
Curry	141
Garlic, & Parmesan, Mix it Up, Big Plate Specials	199
Hot, Mix it Up, Big Plate Specials	68
Lemon, & Pepper, Mix It Up, Big Plate Specials	386
Lemon, & Garlic, Steak Sauce	160
Parmigiana, Extra	35
Peppercorn, Steak Sauce	52
Piri Piri, Extra	25
Piri Piri, Hot, Mix it Up, Big Plate Specials	50
Sour Cream	103
Sweet Chilli	82

	KCAL			KCAL

HUNGRY HORSE

SAUSAGE
Side, Extra	348

SAUSAGE & MASH
Vegetarian, Quorn*, Classics	541

SCAMPI
Breaded, Wholetail, & Salad, Live Well	481
Breaded, Wholetail, No Sides, Classics	939
Breaded, Wholetail, with Baked Beans, Classics	1012
Breaded, Wholetail, with Garden Peas, Classics	999
Breaded, Wholetail, with Mushy Peas, Classics	1059
Breaded, Wholetail, with Salad, Classics	951
Jumbo, No Sides, Big Plate Specials	1310
Jumbo, with Baked Beans, Big Plate Specials	1383
Jumbo, with Garden Peas, Big Plate Specials	1370
Jumbo, with Mushy Peas, Big Plate Specials	1430
Jumbo, with Salad, Big Plate Specials	1322

SOUP
Tomato, Roasted	283
Tomato, Roasted, Vegan	171

SPICES
Fajita Seasoning, Mix It Up, Big Plate Specials	52

SPONGE PUDDING
Syrup	665

SUNDAE
Candymania, Big, The Ultimate	1853
Candymania	841
Trifle-tastic	412

TIKKA MASALA
Chicken, Big Plate Specials	2366
Chicken, Classics	810

TOMATOES
Side, Extra	8

TOPPING
Hot, Steak Topper	71
New Yorker, Steak Topper	177
Sunny, Steak Topper	235
Surf, Steak Topper	172

WRAP
Cheesy Melt	646
Chicken, Club	780
Chicken, Mayo, Southern Fried	554
Fish Fingers, & Mayo	552

YORKSHIRE PUDDING
Extra	100

ITSU

BARS
Brownie, Cocoa Butter	185
Chocolate, Pie, Raw	167
Coconut, Crushed, & Chocolate	293
Pecan, Cashew, & Date, Glazed	184

BEANS
Edamame, Chocolate Coated	152
Edamame	192

BROWNIES
Cocoa Butter, with Caramelised Miso	185

BUNS
Bao, Duck, Hoisin	294
Bao, Spicy Veg	262

CHICKEN
Katsu, Klean, Rice Bowl	574
Korean, Rice Bowl, Spicy	556
Teriyaki, Rice Bowl	596
Thai, Rice Bowl	765

CHOCOLATE
Bar, Crushed Coconut, & Matcha	293
Pie, with Pink Himalayan Salt, Raw	167

DESSERT
Mochi, Chocolate Ganache	230
Mochi, Mango Cheesecake	208
Salted Caramel, Pot, The Coconut Collaborative	127

DUMPLINGS - GYOZA
Beef, Korean BBQ	352
Chicken, & Spring Onion	251
Chicken, Frozen	157
King Prawn	216
Vegetable, Fusion	240
Veggie, Steamed	192

FRUIT SALAD
Cup	76

JERKY
Beef Twerky	97

JUICE
Orange, Press	118
Veg Press	113

JUICE DRINK
Ginger, Detox, Zinger, Super Tonic	56
Goji, Mandarin, & Lime, Super Tonic	33

KOMBUCHA
Ginger, & Lemon	27
Original	26
Passionfruit	28

MOUSSE
Chocolate	248

NOODLES
Udon, Chicken, Chargrilled	507
Udon, Chicken, Chilli	559
Udon, I'thai, Stir Fry Style	669
Udon, with Gyoza, Veggie	496

ITSU

PEAS
Dried, Wasabi	111

PRAWN CRACKERS
Peking Duck	96
Salt, & Vinegar	98
Wasabi, Mild	95

PUDDING
Lemon Zinger	234
White Chocolate Dream	293

RICE CAKES
Chocolate, Dark	85
Chocolate, Milk	83
Yoghurt	80

SALAD
Chicken, Sesame, No Dressing	369
Chicken, Teriyaki, On a Bed, No Dressing	471
Salmon, Poke, On a Bed, No Dressing	541
Salmon, Teriyaki, On a Bed, No Dressing	501
Sushi, Japanese	203
Tofu, No Meat Mondays, No Dressing	406

SEAWEED
Crispy Thins, Korean BBQ	23
Crispy Thins, Sea Salt Flavour	24
Crispy Thins, Sweet Soy & Sea Salt Flavour	22
Crispy Thins, Wasabi Flavour	22

SMOOTHIE
Raw Fruitifix, Beauty	258
Raw Veg, Beauty	232

SOUP
Chicken Noodle	293
Coconut, with Veggie Meatballs	506
Miso	36
Miso, Noodle, Detox	177
Paste, Miso, Chilli, Easy	31

SUSHI
Avocado, Baby, Rolls	259
California Rolls	292
Festival	517
Health & Happiness, Box	575
Itsu Classics	616
Salmon, & Avo, Dragon Roll	422
Salmon, Avocado, Rolls	287
Salmon, Full House	636
Salmon	299
Salmon, Sashimi	240
Salmon, Super, Light	402
Tuna, Line Caught, Bento	333
Tuna, Spicy, Dragon Roll	373
Veggie, Collection	588
Veggie, Dragon Roll	358

WATER
Ginger, Low	65
Lemon, Low	66

ITSU

WATER
Zen, Cucumber, & Mint	3
Zen, Peach, & Lychee	4

J D WETHERSPOON

APPLES
Slices, Kids Menu	43

AVOCADO
Side or Add On	84

BACON
Maple Cured, & American Style Cheese, Extra	168
Maple Cured, & Cheddar Cheese, Extra	170
Maple Cured, Extra	86
Rashers, Extra or Add On	103

BANANA
Extra or Add On	105

BEANS
Baked, Extra or Add On	126
Baked, No Added Sugar, Kids Menu	63
Baked, on Toast, White	543
Baked, on Toast, White, Small	240
Baked, on Toast, Wholewheat	546
Baked, on Toast, Wholewheat Small	242

BEEF - STEAK, RUMP
10oz, Eggs, & Chips, Sunday Brunch	1225
10oz, with Chips, & Cheese & Leek Sauce	1426
10oz, with Chips, & Peppercorn Sauce	1413
10oz, with Chips, & Jack Daniels Honey Glaze	1413
10oz, with Chips, & Whisky Sauce	1406
10oz, with Chips	1086
10oz, with Jacket Potato, & Cheese & Leek Sauce	1129
10oz, with Jacket Potato, & Peppercorn Sauce	1116
10oz, with Jacket Potato, & Jack Daniels Glaze	1115
10oz, with Jacket Potato, & Whisky Sauce	1108
10oz, with Jacket Potato	789
10oz, with Rainbow Quinoa Salad	668
10oz, with Side Salad	558

BEEF - STEAK, SIRLOIN
8oz, Eggs, & Chips, Sunday Brunch	1199
8oz, with Chips, & Cheese & Leek Sauce	1395
8oz, with Chips, & Peppercorn Sauce	1382
8oz, with Chips, & Jack Daniels Honey Glaze	1382
8oz, with Chips, & Whisky Sauce	1375
8oz, with Chips	1055
8oz, with Jacket Potato, & Cheese & Leek Sauce	1120
8oz, with Jacket Potato, & Peppercorn Sauce	1085
8oz, with Jacket Potato, & Jack Daniels Honey Glaze	1085
8oz, with Jacket Potato, & Whisky Sauce	1100
8oz, with Jacket Potato	758
8oz, with Rainbow Quinoa Salad	638
8oz, with Side Salad	527

BHAJI
Onion, 2, Curry Club	330

BITES
Macaroni Cheese, with Salsa, Side or Add On	276

BLACK PUDDING
Extra or Add On	352

J D WETHERSPOON

BLUEBERRIES
Extra or Add On	17

BOLOGNESE
Spaghetti, Kids Menu	285

BREAD
Naan, Garlic	281
Naan, Plain	224
Two Slices, & Butter, Extra or Add On	191
Two Slices, & Lurpak Spreadable	442

BREAKFAST
All Day, Brunch, Pub Classics	1238
All Day, Brunch, Small, Pub Classics	678
All Day, Brunch, Vegetarian, Pub Classics	1175
All Day, Brunch, Vegetarian, Small, Pub Classics	709
American	1368
American, Small	684
Freedom	447
Large	1420
Small	460
Traditional	819
Vegan	879
Vegetarian	932
Vegetarian, Large	1357
Vegetarian, Small	374

BREAKFAST CEREAL
Porridge, Moma	250

BROWNIES
Chocolate, with Ice Cream, Warm	797
Chocolate, with Ice Cream, Warm, Mini	424

BURGERS - BEEF
6oz, Extra	346
6oz Classic	1171
BBQ, with Chips, & Onion Rings	1679
Caledonian, with Chips, & Onion Rings	1758
Empire State, with Chips, & Onion Rings	1949
Tennessee, with Chips, & Onion Rings	1585
Ultimate, with Chips, & Onion Rings	1703

BURGERS - CHICKEN, BUTTERMILK
BBQ, with Chips, & Onion Rings	1683
Breaded, Fried	1175
Tennessee, with Chips, & Onion Rings	1590
with Brie, & Chilli Jam, with Chips, & Onion Rings	1616

BURGERS - CHICKEN, GRILLED
Breast, BBQ, with Chips, & Onion Rings	1539
Breast	1031
Breast, Skinny	453
Breast, Tennessee, with Chips, & Onion Rings	1446
with Brie, & Chilli Jam, with Chips, & Onion Rings	1472

BURGERS - VEGAN
Beyond, Meat Free	1112
Beyond, Meat Free, Patty, Extra or Add On	287
Gourmet, with Chips, & Onion Rings	1464

J D WETHERSPOON

BURGERS - VEGETABLE

	KCAL
Breaded	1082
Breaded, Patty, Extra or Add On	257
with Brie, & Chilli Jam, with Chips, & Onion Rings	1523

CARROTS

Bag, Kids Menu	30

CHEESE

American, Burger Topping	82
Brie, Extra or Add On	150
Cheddar, Burger Topping	83
Halloumi, Grilled, Extra or Add On	477

CHICKEN - BREAST

Bites, 5, with Sticky Soy Sauce, Extra or Add On	251
Buttermilk Fried, Extra or Add On	350
Grilled, Extra or Add On	206
Grilled, Kids Menu	206

CHICKEN - GRILLED, & RIBS

Half Rack, BBQ, with Onion Rings, & Chips	1721
Half Rack, BBQ, with Onion Rings, & Jacket Potato	1446

CHICKEN - MELT, BBQ

with Peas, Tomato, & Mushrooms, Chips	1146
with Peas, Tomato, & Mushrooms, Jacket Potato	871

CHICKEN - NUGGETS

Breast, Kids Menu	155
Quorn*, Kids Menu	238

CHICKEN - STRIPS, SOUTHERN FRIED

with Smoky Chipotle Mayo, Sm Plates	653
& Chips, Small	625
with Jack Daniels Honey Glaze, Extra or Add On	406
with Jack Daniels Honey Glaze, & Chips	1225

CHICKEN - WINGS

5, with Sriracha Hot Sauce, Extra or Add On	588
Sriracha Hot Sauce, & Blue Cheese Dip, Sm Plates	1289

CHICKEN - WINGS, & RIBS

Half Rack, BBQ, with Onion Rings, & Chips	2020
Half Rack, BBQ, with Onion Rings, & Jacket Potato	1745

CHILLI

Beef, Burger Topping	178
Beef, Rice, Tortilla Chips, & Sour Cream	780
Five Bean, Burger Topping	119
Five Bean, with Rice, & Tortilla Chips, Pub Classics	587
Five Bean, with Rice, Kids Menu	322
Vegan, Smoky, with Rice, Kids Menu	342

CHIPS

Bowl, Side	955
Bowl, with Curry Sauce, Side	1073
Kids Menu	326
Side	597

CHIPS - TOPPED

Curry Sauce, Chip Shop Style, Sm Plates	1073
Loaded, Cheese, Bacon, & Sour Cream, Sm Plates	1281

COD

Battered, Kids Menu	376

J D WETHERSPOON

CORN

	KCAL
Cob, Mini, Kids Menu	55
Cobs, Mini, Two, Extra or Add on	101

CRUMBLE

Apple, Bramley, with Ice Cream	633

CUCUMBER

Sticks, & Tomato Wedges, Kids Menu	12

CURRY - CAULIFLOWER & SPINACH MANGALOREAN

with Chips, Simple	1069
with Pilau Rice, Naan Bread, & Poppadoms	944
with Pilau Rice, Simple	672

CURRY - FLAMING DRAGON

Chicken, Curry Club	918

CURRY - PRAWN & FISH SRI LANKAN

with Rice, Naan Bread, & Poppadoms	1233

CURRY - SWEET POTATO, CHICKPEA & SPINACH

Curry Club	878

DESSERT

Cookie Dough Sandwich, & Ice Cream, Warm	705

DIP

Garlic & Herb, Extra	177

EGGS - BENEDICT

Standard	519
Miners	760
with Mushroom	484

EGGS - FRIED

Extra	72

EGGS - POACHED

Extra or Add On	63

EGGS - SCRAMBLED

Extra or Add On	167
on Toast	533
on Toast, Wholemeal	536

FISH & CHIPS

Cod, Fillet, Battered, & Mushy Peas	1384
Cod, Fillet, Battered, & Peas	1312
Cod, Fillet, Battered, & Mushy Peas, Small	827
Cod, Fillet, Battered, & Peas, Small	758
Haddock, Fillet, Battered, & Mushy Peas	1357
Haddock, Fillet, Battered, & Mushy Peas, Small	815
Haddock, Fillet, Battered, & Peas	1288
Haddock, Fillet, Battered, & Peas, Small	746

FRIES

Halloumi, Side or Add On	475
Halloumi, with Sweet Chilli Sauce, Sm Plates	475

FRUIT

Fresh, & Ice Cream	304
Fresh, Breakfast	178

GAMMON

10oz, with Egg, & Chips	1310
10oz, with Egg, & Jacket Potato	1035
5oz, with Egg, & Chips	1048
5oz, with Egg, & Jacket Potato	773

J D WETHERSPOON

GARLIC BREAD
Pizza, 11"	707
Pizza, 11", Sm Plates	707
Pizza, 8", Side	354
Pizza, with Cheese, 11"	853
Pizza, with Cheese, 8", Side	427

HADDOCK
Battered, Kids Menu	364

HAGGIS
Scottish, Neeps, & Tatties, Pub Classics	923

HAM
& Egg, Wiltshire Cured, Kids Menu	125
Egg, & Chips, Wiltshire Cured, Pub Classics	847
Egg, & Chips, Wiltshire Cured, Small, Pub Classics	453

HASH BROWNS
Two, Extra or Add On	216

HONEY
Extra or Add On	92

ICE CREAM
Vanilla, Extra or Add On	125
Vanilla, with Raspberry Sauce, Pot, Childrens	119
Vegan, Extra or Add On	162

JACKET POTATO
Plain, Kids Menu	225
with Beans, & Salad, Deli Deals	483
with Beans, Kids Menu	288
with Cheese, & Salad	531
with Five Bean Chilli, & Salad	413
with Five Bean Chilli, Kids Menu	344
with Roasted Vegetables, & Salad	374
with Roasted Vegetables, Kids Menu	305
with Smoky Vegan Chilli, Kids Menu	364
with Tuna Mayo, & Salad, Deli Deals	532

JALFREZI
Chicken, Curry Club	908

JAM
Smoky Chilli, Burger Topping	41
Strawberry, Extra or Add On	76

KORMA
Chicken, Curry Club	1066

LASAGNE
Beef, British, with Dressed Side Salad	756
Vegetable, Mediterranean, with Dressed Side Salad	603

MADRAS
Beef, Curry Club	1077

MARMALADE
Extra or Add On	75

MIXED GRILL
with Chips	1454
with Chips, Large	1949
with Jacket Potato	1179
with Jacket Potato, Large	1674

J D WETHERSPOON

MUFFIN
Breakfast	499
Egg, & Bacon, Breakfast	331
Egg, & Cheese, Breakfast	279
Egg, & Sausage, Breakfast	448

MUSHROOMS
Extra or Add On	126

NACHOS
Sm Plates	627

ONION RINGS
Six, Extra or Add On	255
Twelve, Side	510

PANCAKES - AMERICAN
Small, with Maple Flavour Syrup	295
Small, with Maple Flavour Syrup, & Bacon	338
with Ice Cream, Mini	420
with Bacon, & Maple Flavour Syrup, Breakfast	676
Maple Flavour Syrup, & Ice Cream	715
Maple Flavour Syrup, Breakfast	590

PANINI
Chicken, Bacon, & Cheese, BBQ, Deli Deals	637
Brie, Bacon, & Smoky Chilli Jam, Deli Deals	624
Cheese, & Tomato, Deli Deals	587
Ham, & Cheese, Wiltshire Cured, Deli Deals	552
Tuna, Cheese, & Mayo, Melt, Deli Deals	731

PASTA
Alfredo	645
Tomato, & Mascarpone, Kids Menu	243

PEAS
Extra or Add On	110
Mushy, Side	248

PIZZA
Chicken, BBQ, 11"	1103
Chicken, BBQ, 8"	559
Ham & Mushroom, 11"	1002
Ham & Cheese, Kids Menu	420
Ham & Mushroom, 8"	501
Hawaiian, 11"	1033
Hawaiian, 8"	516
Hawaiian, Kids Menu	443
Margherita, 11"	931
Margherita, 8"	466
Margherita, Kids Menu	392
Meat Feast, Spicy, 11"	1227
Meat Feast, Spicy, 8", Sm Plates	622
Pepperoni, 11"	1186
Pepperoni, 8"	593
Vegetable, Roasted, 11"	1024
Vegetable, Roasted, 8"	512
Vegetable, Roasted, Kids Menu	432
Vegetable, Roasted, Vegan, 11"	710
Vegetable, Roasted, Vegan, 8", Sm Plates	355
Vegetable, Roasted, Vegan, Kids Menu	348

J D WETHERSPOON

PIZZA TOPPING

Avocado, Half	84
Bacon, Maple Cured	86
BBQ Sauce	69
Chicken, Breast	103
Chillies, Sliced	7
Ham	56
Mozzarella	169
Mushrooms	8
Onion, Red	10
Pepperoni	128
Pineapple	24
Tomato, Slices	13
Vegetables, Roasted	80

POPPADOMS

Side	95

POTATO

Rosti, Two, Extra or Add On	165

POTATOES

Mashed, Kids Menu	134

PRAWNS

King, Spicy Coated, with Sweet Chilli Sauce	474

PUDDING - STEAK & KIDNEY

with Chips, Peas, & Gravy, Pub Classics	1261

RIBS - PORK, BBQ

Half Rack, Extra or Add on	581
Half Rack, with Onion Rings, Sm Plates	836
with Coleslaw, Onions Rings, & Chips	2013
with Coleslaw, Onions Rings, & Jacket Potato	1738

RICE

Mexican, Side	203
Pilau, Side	225

RISOTTO

Mushroom, Creamy, Pub Classics	470

ROGAN JOSH

Lamb, Curry Club	980

SALAD

Chicken, Pulled, Avocado, & Bacon	444
Quinoa, Rainbow	407
Quinoa, Side or Add on	179
Quinoa, with Grilled Halloumi, & Kale Dressing	823
Side	72

SAMOSAS

Vegetable, 2, Curry Club	209

SANDWICH

Bacon, Butty, White	509
Bacon Butty, Wholewheat	512
Sausage, Butty, Quorn* White	605
Sausage, Butty, White	691
Sausage, Butty, Wholewheat	694
Sausage, Quorn*, Butty, Wholewheat	608

SAUCE

BBQ, Burger Topping	83

J D WETHERSPOON

SAUCE

Bearnaise, Beef Dripping	123
Chocolate, Belgian, Extra or Add On	58
Curry, Chip Shop Style	118
Honey Glaze, Jack Daniels	73
Peppercorn, Creamy	74
Toffee, Extra or Add On	72

SAUSAGE

Extra or Add On	168
Pork, Kids Menu	336
Quorn, Vegan, Extra or Add On	125
Quorn, Vegan, Kids Menu	251

SCAMPI - BREADED

Extra or Add On	222
Kids Menu	205
Whitby, with Chips, & Mushy Peas	1037
Whitby, with Chips, & Mushy Peas, Small	655
Whitby, with Chips, & Peas	971
Whitby, with Chips, & Peas, Small	588

SCONE

Potato, Extra or Add On	80

STRAWBERRIES

Extra or Add On	14

SYRUP

Maple Flavoured, Extra or Add On	97

TART

Chocolate, & Salted Caramel	855

TIKKA MASALA - CHICKEN

with Chips, Simple	1291
with Pilau Rice, Naan Bread, Poppadoms	1166
with Pilau Rice, Simple	895

TOAST

& Preserves, Marmalade, White	458
& Preserves, Marmalade, Wholewheat	461
& Preserves	459
& Preserves, Strawberry Jam, Wholewheat	461

TOMATOES

Halves, Grilled, Extra or Add On	16

VEGETABLES

Roasted, Extra	80
Roasted, Kids Menu	80
Roasted, Side	120
Tomatoes, Mushrooms, & Peas, Extra or Add On	126

VINDALOO

Chicken, Curry Club	920

WRAP

Breakfast	721
Breakfast, Vegetarian	861
Chicken, & Avocado, with Mayonnaise	688
Chicken, Breast, Pulled, & Sweet Chilli Sauce	478
Chicken, Southern Fried, Smokey Chipotle May	637
Halloumi, Grilled, with Sweet Chilli Sauce	698

	KCAL

JOE & THE JUICE

BITES
Cacao, Raw	60
Hazelnut, Raw	70

BREAKFAST
Bowl, Acai, 2.0	450
Bowl, Spirulina	485

BROWNIES
Chocolate	235

CAKE
Banana Bread	290
Carrot	250

COFFEE
Americano, Iced	0
Cappuccino	140
Cold Brew, Nitro	16
Cortado, Purple, 8oz	75
Cup of Joe	0
Espresso	0
Flat White, 8oz	75
Latte, Iced	220
Latte, Oat, Nitro	143
Latte, Pink, 16oz	260
Latte, Yellow, 12oz	145
Macchiato, Grey, 4oz	45

DRINK
Shot, Ginger	25
Shot, Turmeric	35

JUICE
Energizer	235
Fibre Active	380
Go Away Doc	235
Green Haven	230
Green Shield	180
Green Tonic	60
Hell Of A Nerve	235
Herb Tonic	255
Iron Man	225
Joes AMG	235
Joes Green Mile	240
Joes Identity	85
Pick Me Up	217
Prince of Green	93
Sex Me Up	250
Sports Juice	215
Stress Down	210
Young Blood	235

MILK SHAKE
Avo	500
Blue Magic, Vegan	400
Cheeta	420
Choco	390
Coffee	250
Green Gains, Vegan	435

JOE & THE JUICE

MILK SHAKE
Power	400
Re-Build 2.0, Vegan	515
Red Supreme, Vegan	478

MUFFIN
Blueberry	245
Choco	315

SALAD
Bowl, Green, Tuna	600
Bowl, Green, Vegan	545

SANDWICH
Avocado	485
Joes Club	430
Serrano	490
Spicy Tuna	415
Tunacado	460
Turkey	420
Vavo, Avocado, Vegan	433

SNACKS
Power Shake Ball	135

TEA
English Breakfast	0
Green, Rhubarb	0
Green Mandarin	0
Vanilla Rooibos	0
White Temple	0

WATER
Sparkling	0
Still	0

KFC

BEANS

Baked, BBQ, Large	250
Baked, BBQ, Reg	105

BITES

Sweet Chilli	355

BURGERS

BBQ Bacon, Tower, 1 PC, Box Meal	1245
BBQ Bacon, Tower, 2 Hot Wings, Box Meal	1170
BBQ Bacon, Tower	690
BBQ Bacon, Tower, Meal	925
Chicken, Big Daddy, Box Meal	1260
Chicken, Big Daddy, Burger Only	685
Double Down, Box Meal	1145
Double Down, Burger Only	575
Double Down, Meal	825
Chicken Fillet, Bacon & Cheese	585
Chicken Fillet, Box Meal	1045
Chicken Fillet, Burger Only	475
Chicken Fillet, Meal	720
Chicken Fillet, Mini	290
Chicken Fillet, Tower	620
Chicken Fillet, Tower, Meal	870
Chicken, Kids	265
Chicken, Meal, Kids	455
Chicken Zinger, Box Meal	945
Chicken Zinger, Burger Only	450
Chicken Zinger, Meal	700
Chicken Zinger, Stacker, Box Meal	1280
Chicken Zinger, Stacker	780
Chicken Zinger, Stacker, Meal	1030
Chicken Zinger, Tower	595
Chicken Zinger, Tower, Meal	845
Trilogy, Box Meal, with Lipton	1200
Trilogy, Box Meal, with Pepsi Max	1145
Vegan, Burger Only	450

CHICKEN

Allstars, BBQ, Meal	685
Allstars, Flamin', Meal	720
Boneless, 3 Piece, Dips Meal	705
Boneless, 4 Piece, Dips Meal	835
Boneless, Banquet, Box Meal	920
Boneless, Feast, Dipping, 12 Piece	910
Boneless, Feast, Dipping, 8 Piece	780
Bucket, Bargain, 10 Piece	850
Bucket, Bargain, 14 Piece	1090
Bucket, Bargain, 6 Piece	610
Bucket, Mighty, For One	1155
Bucket, Party, 14 Piece	1225
Colonel, 2 Piece, Meal	730
Colonel, 3 Piece, Meal	970
Colonel, 4 Piece, Meal	1210
Drumstick, Original Recipe	170
Family Feast, 10 Piece	930

KFC

CHICKEN

Family Feast, 6 Piece	690
Fillet, Mini	130
Fillet, Mini, Snackbox	475
Fillet, Original Redcipe	220
Fillet, Zinger	200
Fillets, Mini, 10	655
Keel, Original recipe	265
Megabox, with Gravy	930
Original Recipe, Mini Fillet, Meal, Kids	345
Original Recipe, Snackbox	585
Popcorn, Large	465
Popcorn, Meal	535
Popcorn, Meal, Kids	330
Popcorn, Meal, Large	710
Popcorn, Reg	285
Popcorn, Small	135
Popcorn, Snackbox	480
Rib, Original Recipe	325
Thigh, Original Recipe	285
Variety, 2 Piece, Meal	1025
Variety, 3 Piece, Meal	1265
Wicked Variety, 10 Piece	1145
Wicked Variety, 6 Piece	905
Wing, Original Recipe	175
Wings, Hot, 6, Meal	740
Wings, Hot	85
Wings, Hot, Snackbox	510

COFFEE

Americano, Black, Reg	15
Americano, White, Reg	80
Cafe Mocha, Reg	180
Cappuccino, Reg	125
Espresso, Single	10
Latte, Caramel, Reg	195
Latte, Reg	140
Latte, Vanilla, Reg	195

COLA

Pepsi*, Diet or Max, Kids	5
Pepsi*, Diet or Max, Large	15
Pepsi*, Diet or Max, Reg	10
Pepsi*, Kids	100
Pepsi*, Large	180
Pepsi*, Max Cherry, Kids	5
Pepsi*, Max Cherry, Large	10
Pepsi*, Max Cherry, Reg	5
Pepsi*, Reg	130

COLESLAW

Large	320
Reg	160

COOKIES

Chocolate, Milk	325
Chocolate, White	335

KFC

CORN

Cobette	85
Cobette, Lge Portion	165

DESSERT

Krushems, Malteser	225
Krushems, Milky Bar	325
Krushems, Oreo	280
Krushems, Salted Caramel, Soft Serve	375

FRIES

Large	345
Reg	250

GRAVY

Large	110
Reg	45

HOT CHOCOLATE

Reg	180

JUICE

Orange, Tropicana*	120

JUICE DRINK

Apple, & Blackcurrant, Robinsons*, Kids	5
Apple, & Blackcurrant, Robinsons*, Reg	5
Blackcurrant, & Apple, Fruit Shoot	10
Club Orange*, Kids	125
Club Orange*, Large	230
Club Orange*, Reg	160
Club Orange*, Zero, Kids	10
Club Orange*, Zero, Large	15
Club Orange*, Zero, Reg	10
Orange, Fruit Shoot	10

LEMONADE

7up*, Free, Kids	5
7up*, Free, Large	10
7up*, Free, Reg	5

MUFFIN

Chocolate	555
Lemon	470

ONION RINGS

Side	400

PINEAPPLE

Sticks	30

POTATOES

Mashed	110

RICE

Chicken, Fillet, Ricebox	490
Chicken, Fillet, Ricebox, Meal	740
Chicken, Fillet, Ricebox, with Sugar Free Drink	500
Chicken, Zinger, Ricebox	480
Chicken, Zinger, Ricebox, Meal	725
Chicken, Zinger, Ricebox, with Sugar Free Drink	480
Southern	210
Veggie, Ricebox	365
Veggie, Ricebox, Meal	615
Veggie, Ricebox, with Sugar Free Drink	365

KFC

SALAD

Chicken, Fillet	370
Chicken, Fillet, Meal	620
Chicken, Fillet, with Sugar Free Drink	375
Chicken, Zinger	350
Chicken, Zinger, Meal	600
Chicken, Zinger, with Sugar Free Drink	350
Garden, Side	75
Veggie	235
Veggie, Meal	485
Veggie, with Sugar Free Drink	235

SAUCE

BBQ, Kentucky Smoky, Dip Pot	50
Curry, Large	175
Curry, Reg	75
Hot, Original, Dip Pot	40
HP, BBQ, Heinz, Sachet	15
HP, Brown, Heinz, Sachet	15
Ketchup, Heinz, Sachet	10
Mayo, Garlic Buttermilk, Dip Pot	110
Mayonnaise, Light, Heinz, Sachet	30
Supercharger, Spicy, Dip Pot	150
Sweet Chilli, Sticky, Dip Pot	75
Tomato Sauce, Real, Dip Pot	40

SUNDAE

Cherry	220
Cherry, Mini	145
Chocolate	230
Chocolate, Mini	150

TANGO*

Orange, Large	80
Orange, Reg	60

TEA

Iced, Lipton*, Kids	20
Iced, Lipton*, Large	60
Iced, Lipton*, Reg	45

WRAP

Chicken, BBQ	300
Chicken, Flamin'	335
Chicken, Twister, Kentucky Mayo, Box Meal	965
Chicken, Twister, Kentucky Mayo	500
Chicken, Twister, Kentucky Mayo, Meal	750
Chicken, Twister, Nashville Hot, Box Meal	950
Chicken, Twister, Nashville Hot	490
Chicken, Twister, Nashville Hot, Meal	735
Chicken, Twister, Smoky BBQ, Box Meal	935
Chicken, Twister, Smoky BBQ	475
Chicken, Twister, Smoky BBQ, Meal	725
Chicken, Twister, Sweet Chilli, Box Meal	945
Chicken, Twister, Sweet Chilli	485
Chicken, Twister, Sweet Chilli, Meal	735

YOGHURT

Much Bunch	100

KRISPY KREME

COFFEE

Americano, Black, 12oz	34
Americano, Black, 16oz	46
Cappuccino, 12oz	111
Cappuccino, 16oz	133
Flat White, 8oz	88
Latte, 12oz	132
Latte, 16oz	169
Mocha, 12oz	192
Mocha, 16oz	247

DOUGHNUTS

Apple Pie	296
Bites	138
Caramel, Iced, Ring	257
Chocolate, Double, Duoghnut	485
Chocolate, White, Dreamcake	405
Chocolate Dreamcake	351
Chocolate Iced, Custard Filled	289
Chocolate Iced, Ring	237
Chocolate Iced, with Sprinkles	262
Chocolate Praline, Cheesecake, Duoghnut	384
Glazed, Lemon Filled	290
Glazed, Original	200
Glazed, with a Creme Filling	371
Lemon Meringue	346
Lotus Biscoff	396
Nutty Chocolatta	379
Raspberry, Glazed	324
Reese's Peanut Butter	395
Salted Caramel, Cheesecake	367
Strawberries & Kreme	326
Strawberry Gloss	244
Vimto, Shimmer	389

HOT CHOCOLATE

12oz	234
16oz	359

ICE CREAM

Solo	240
with Caramel Sauce, & Shortbread	319
with Caramel Sauce, Shortbread, & Bites	453
with Caramel Sauce, Shortbread, & Doughnut	369
with Chocolate Sauce, & Shortbread	313
with Chocolate Sauce, Shortbread, & Bites	448
with Chocolate Sauce, Shortbread, & Doughnut	363

MILK SHAKE

Chocolate Kreme	515
Lotus Biscoff	521
Strawberries, & Kreme	515

LEON RESTAURANTS

BARS

Paleon, Bits in Between	332

BEANS

Brazilian, Black	412

BITES

Mac & Cheeze, Aioli	323

BREAKFAST

Beans, Saucy, Pot	157
Egg, & Beans, Pot	155
Full English, Pot	398
Halloumi, Mushroom, Egg, Pot	340
Sausage, & Beans, Pot, Kids	201
Shakshuka	305
The Big Breakfast Box	590
The Halloumi Breakfast Box	464

BREAKFAST CEREAL

Porridge, Banana & Chocolate	207
Porridge, Banana & Cinnamon, Dairy Free	299
Porridge, Banana & Cinnamon, Organic Dairy Milk	367
Porridge, Black Forest	442
Porridge, Ruby Red, Organic Dairy Milk	337

BROWNIES

Better, Bits in Between	415

BURGERS

Chicken, Chargrilled, GF	470
Chicken, Chargrilled	432
Chicken, Korean, GF	466
Chicken, Korean	399
Vegan, LOVe, GF	589
Vegan, LOVe	546
Vegan, Sweet n' Smoky Carolina, GF	579
Vegan, Sweet n' Smoky Carolina	547

CHEESE

Halloumi Fingers, & Rice, Box, Kids	357

CHICKEN

& Rice, Kids	290
Aioli, Box	590
Chargrilled, Mezze	141
Chilli, Box	608
Nuggets, GFC, & Fries, Kids	474
Nuggets, GF, GFC	371
Satay, Box	582

COFFEE

Americano, Iced	1
Americano	1
Cappucino	121
Filter	6
Flat White	102
Latte, Iced	224
Latte	179
Mocha	383

COLESLAW

Slaw, Fresh, Sides	131

LEON RESTAURANTS

COOKIES
Chocolate Chip, Bits in Between	274
Double Chocolate, Bits in Between	294
Peacn, Maple, & Oat, Vegan, Bits in Between	200

CURRY
Masala, Lentil	562

FRIES
Baked	268
Cheezy, Loaded	528

HASH BROWNS
Breakfast	159

HOT CHOCOLATE
Regular	415

JUICE DRINK
Raspberry, & Acai	77

KOMBUCHA
Ginger, LA	66

LEMONADE
Fresh	106

MEATBALLS
Meatless, Vegan	566

MUFFIN
Bacon, & Egg, Breakfast	422
Bacon, Breakfast	338
Breakfast Stack	506
Egg, Kids, Breakfast	300
Salmon & Egg, Breakfast	440
Salmon & Egg, GF, Breakfast	523
Sausage, Vegan, Breakfast	322
Smashed Avocado, & Halloumi, Breakfast	433
Smashed Avocado, & Halloumi, GF, Breakfast	502

SALAD
Warm, with Grilled Aubergine	291
Warm, with Paprika Chicken	397

SHORTBREAD
Billionaire's, Vegan, Bits in Between	160

SMOOTHIE
Acai Berry	130
Clean Green Shake	175
Mango, & Coconut	150

SWEETCORN
Ribs, with Truffle, & Cheese	175

TART
Custard, Pastel de Nata, Raspberry, Bits in Between	215
Lemon Ginger Crunch, Bits in Between	327

TEA
White, & Peach	50

TOAST
Sourdough, with Butter	328

WRAP
Fish Finger, Hot	715
Halloumi, Grilled	656

LOCH FYNE

BEANS
Edamame, with Ginger, & Chilli	189

BEEF
Steak, Ribeye, with Chimichurri Sauce	1703

BREAD
Basket, with Balsamic Oil	797
Garlic, Starter, Kids	349

BURGERS - BEEF
Chargrilled, Pancetta, Cheese, & Burger Sauce	1669
Gruyere Cheese, No Sides, Kids	459

BUTTER
Garlic, Fish Bar	188
Garlic	188
Harissa, Fish Bar	207
Harissa	208
Lobster, Fish Bar	131
Lobster	132
Paprika, Smoked, & Sunblush Tomato, Fish Bar	192
Paprika, Smoked, & Sunblush Tomato	192
Salted	221

CABBAGE
Savoy, Shallot, & Chestnuts, Fish Bar	257
Savoy, Shallot, & Chestnuts	257
Savoy, Shallot, & Chestnuts, Side, Kids	128

CARROTS
Rainbow, with Harissa Butter, Fish Bar	109
Rainbow, with Harissa Butter	126

CHEESE
Plate, Scottish	595

CHIPS
Twice Cooked, Fish Bar	526
Twice Cooked	526

COD
Fillet, Panko Crusted, No Sides, Kids	380
Fillet, Roasted, Pancetta, & Red Wine Lentils	883
Grilled, Line Caught, Fish Bar	325
Pan Fried, Line Caught, Fish Bar	399
Steamed, Line Caught, Fish Bar	319

CREME BRULEE
Dessert	621

CRUDITES
Starter, Kids	166

CRUMBLE
Plum, Granola, Baked	691

CURRY
Cauliflower, & Squash, Goan, Spiced	460
Malabar, King Prawn, Kids	303
Seafood, Goan	565

DESSERT
Chocolate, Fondant	568

DUCK
Smoked, Gressingham, Fig, & Goats Cheese	241

LOCH FYNE

FISH

	KCAL
Megrim, Whole, Grilled, Fish Bar	415
Megrim, Whole, Pan Fried, Fish Bar	490
Megrim, Whole, Steamed, Fish Bar	415

FISH & CHIPS

Cod, Battered	1620
Haddock, Battered	1373
Haddock, Takeaway	1437
Portion	1624

FISH CAKES

Haddock, No Sides, Kids	407
Haddock, Smoked, with Mustard Leeks	733

FRIES

French, Fish Bar	616
French	560
French, Side, Kids	420
Halloumi, with Chimichurri	743

FRUIT

Plate, Kids	34

GNOCCHI

Spinach, Mushroom, Cheese, Leek, & Artichoke	1114

HADDOCK

Smoked, Poached	643

ICE CREAM

Amaretti Amaretto, Luxury	136
Chocolate Split, Luxury	129
Mint Chocolate, Luxury	122
Strawberry, Luxury	82
Vanilla, 3 Scoops, Luxury	305
Vanilla, Luxury	110
Vanilla, Vegan, Luxury	102
Walnut, Luxury	130

ICE LOLLY

Apple, Organic, Kids	17
Rainbow, Organic, Kids	18
Tropical, Organic, Kids	20

KETCHUP

Portion	20

LANGOUSTINE

Grilled, with Romesco Sauce, Premium	823

LINGUINE

Pomodoro, Kids	234
Prawn, & Chilli	729

LOBSTER

Thermidor, Whole, with Basmiti Rice	688
Thermidor, Whole, with French Fries	1211

MACKEREL - FILLET, CURED

Red Cabbage, & Apple, with Honey Mustard, Main	474
Red Cabbage, & Apple, with Honey Mustard, Starter	346

MACKEREL - WHOLE

Grilled, Fish Bar	849
Pan Fried, Fish Bar	923
Steamed, Fish Bar	849

LOCH FYNE

MAYONNAISE

	KCAL
Portion	113

MONKFISH

Roast, Smoked Pancetta, & Red Wine Lentils	1033

MUSSELS

Scottish, Rope Grown, Main	1186
Scottish, Rope Grown, Starter	375

OIL

& Balsamic Vinegar	323
Chilli, Roasted, Fish Bar	114
Chilli, Roasted	152

OLIVES

Nocellara	186

OYSTERS

Fyne Vinegar, 1	62
Fyne Vinegar, 12	674
Fyne Vinegar, 3	173
Fyne Vinegar, 6	339
My First Oyster	61
Soy & Ginger, 1	68
Soy & Ginger, 12	680
Soy & Ginger, 3	179
Soy & Ginger, 6	345
Wasabi & Cucumber, 1	71
Wasabi & Cucumber, 12	683
Wasabi & Cucumber, 3	182
Wasabi & Cucumber, 6	348

PAKORA

Samphire, & Sweet Potato, with Date Chutney	404

PEAS

Mushy	68

PEPPERS

Padron, with Smoked Sea Salt	199

PETIT POIS

Side, Kids	29

PIE

Apple, No Ice Cream	314

PLATTER

Shellfish, with Lobster, & Crab	1420

PORK

Belly, Black Pudding Mash, Spinach, & Apple Puree	748

POTATOES

Dauphinoise, Fish Bar	615
Dauphinoise	615
Mashed, Creamed, with Chives, Fish Bar	248
Mashed, Creamed, with Chives	248
Mashed, Side, Kids	74
New, Sauteed, Fish Bar	191
New, Sauteed	191
New, with Butter, Fish Bar	238
New, with Butter	239
New, with Butter, Side, Kids	119

LOCH FYNE

PRAWNS
Karagee, with Soy & Ginger Sauce	325
King, Chilli & Garlic, Pan Fried	857

PUDDING
Sticky Toffee, with Tablet Ice Cream	1194

SALAD - GREEN
Side	126

SALAD - WARM WINTER
Puy Lentil & Red Pepper Dressing, Main	603
Puy Lentil & Red Pepper Dressing, Starter	311

SALMON
Fillet, No Sides, Kids	199
Grilled, Scottish, Fish Bar	536
Pan Fried, Scottish, Fish Bar	611
Smoked, Plate, Classic	337
Steamed, Scottish, Fish Bar	536

SALSA
Verde	176

SAMPHIRE
with Lemon, Fish Bar	11
with Lemon	11

SAUCE
Chimichurri, Fish Bar	114
Chimichurri	114
Cream Anglaise	62
Pesto, Wild Garlic	54
Pesto, Wild Garlic	54
Soy, & Ginger, Fish Bar	23
Soy, & Ginger	23

SAUSAGE
Chorizo, in Parsley & White Wine	393

SAUSAGE ROLL
Mini	244

SCALLOPS
with Chickpea, & Nduja Stew	311

SCOTCH EGG
Haggis, Curried Potato Cream, & Turnip	773

SEA BASS
Fillet, No Sides, Kids	250
Whole, Grilled, Fish Bar	596
Whole, Pan Fried, Fish Bar	670
Whole, Steamed, Fish Bar	593

SEA BREAM
Gilt Head, Grilled, Fish Bar	274
Gilt Head, Pan Fried, Fish Bar	311
Gilt Head, Steamed, Fish Bar	274

SEAFOOD
Clams, Cockles, & Chorizo, on Sourdough	353
Grill	1003

SORBET
Lemon, Luxury	62
Pear, Luxury	63
Raspberry, Luxury	65

LOCH FYNE

SOUP
Fish	468

SPINACH
Buttered, Fish Bar	50
Buttered	50

SQUID
Salt & Pepper	490

SUNDAE
Popcorn	564

SWEET POTATO
Wedges, Side, Kids	283

TART
Squash. & Ricotta, with Beetroot	140

TORTELLONI
Beetroot, & Ricotta, Goats Cheese Cream, Main	566
Beetroot, & Ricotta, Goats Cheese Cream, Starter	321
Crab, Devonshire, with Lemon Oil	731
Crab, Devonshire, with Lemon Oil, Premium	712

TRIFLE
Black Forest	788

TUNA
Chargrilled, Fish Bar	396
Grilled, Fish Bar	392
Pan Fried, Fish Bar	433

TURBOT
Whole, Grilled, Fish Bar	604
Whole, Pan Fried, Fish Bar	589
Whole, Steamed, Fish Bar	604

VEGETABLES
Sticks, Side, Kids	166

MCDONALD'S

BROWNIES
	KCAL
Chocolate	273

BURGERS
Big Mac, Double	694
Big Mac	508
Big Tasty, with Bacon	850
Cheeseburger, Bacon, Double	495
Cheeseburger, Double	445
Cheeseburger	301
Cheeseburger, Triple	588
Chicken Legend, with BBQ Sauce	484
Chicken Legend, with Cool Mayo	529
Chicken Legend, with Hot & Spicy Mayo	519
Filet-O-Fish	329
Hamburger	250
Mayo Chicken, Bacon	370
Mayo Chicken	319
McChicken Sandwich	388
McPlant	429
Quarter Pounder, Double, with Cheese	750
Quarter Pounder, with Cheese	518
Vegetable, Deluxe	380

CARROTS
Sticks	34

CHEESE
Mozzarella, Dippers	256

CHICKEN
McNuggets, 6 Pieces	259
McNuggets, 9 Pieces	388
McNuggets, Sharebox, 20	863
Selects, 3 Pieces	359
Selects, 5 Pieces	599

COFFEE
Black, Large	8
Black, Reg	6
Cappuccino, Large	128
Cappuccino, Reg	97
Flat White, Semi Skimmed Milk	86
Frappe, Caramel, Iced, Large	399
Frappe, Caramel, Iced, Reg	319
Latte, Iced	102
Latte, Large	197
Latte, Reg	145
Latte, Salted Caramel, Large	206
Latte, Salted Caramel, Reg	164
Latte, Toffee, Large	232
Latte, Toffee, Reg	187
White, Large	74
White, Reg	54

COLA
Coca-Cola, Diet, Large	2
Coca-Cola, Diet, Medium	1
Coca-Cola, Diet, Small	1

MCDONALD'S

COLA
	KCAL
Coke, Zero, Large	2
Coke, Zero, Medium	1
Coke, Zero, Small	1

COOKIES
Triple Chocolate	320

DOUGHNUTS
Millionaires	250
Sugar	195

FANTA
Orange, Large	95
Orange, Medium	76
Orange, Small	48

FLATBREAD
Cheesy, Bacon	278

FRIES
French, Large	444
French, Medium	337
French, Small	237

FRUIT
Bag, Apple & Grape	46

FRUIT SHOOT
Apple & Blackcurrant, Robinsons	10

HAPPY MEAL
Cheeseburger, Meal	472
Chicken Nuggets, 4 Piece, Meal	344
Fish Fingers, Meal	365
Hamburger, Meal	421
Veggie Dippers, 2 Pieces, Meal	331

HASH BROWNS
Portion	127

HOT CHOCOLATE
Large	231
Reg	173

ICE CREAM CONE
with Flake	185

JUICE DRINK
Oasis, Large	83
Oasis, Medium	67
Oasis, Small	42

LEMONADE
Sprite, Zero, Large	5
Sprite, Zero, Medium	4
Sprite, Zero, Small	3
Strawberry, Frozen, Large	255
Strawberry, Frozen, Reg	201

MCFLURRY
Crunchie, Cadbury	347
Crunchie, Cadbury, Mini	173
Maltesers	266
Maltesers, Mini	133
Oreo	258
Oreo, Mini	129

MCDONALD'S

MCFLURRY
Smarties	273
Smarties, Mini	137

MCMUFFIN
Bacon, & Egg, Double	376
Bacon, & Egg	335
Egg, & Cheese	295
Sausage, & Egg, Double	551
Sausage, & Egg	423

MILK
Organic	125

MILK SHAKE
Banana, Large	459
Banana, Medium	357
Banana, Small	188
Chocolate, Large	468
Chocolate, Medium	364
Chocolate, Small	192
Strawberry, Large	458
Strawberry, Medium	356
Strawberry, Small	188
Vanilla, Large	469
Vanilla, Medium	366
Vanilla, Small	192

MUFFIN
Mixed Berry	298
with Jam	214

PANCAKE
& Syrup	477
& Sausage, with Syrup	612

PIE
Apple, Hot	243

POTATO WEDGES
Nacho Cheese, 15 Piece, Sharebox	924
Nacho Cheese, 5 Piece	495

ROLL
Bacon, with Brown Sauce	336
Bacon, with Tomato Ketchup	332
Breakfast, with Brown Sauce	500
Breakfast, with Ketchup	496

SALAD
Chicken, Crispy, & Bacon	311
Chicken, Crispy	261
Side	15

SMOOTHIE
Mango & Pineapple, Iced, Large	241
Mango & Pineapple, Iced, Reg	187

TEA
with Milk, Large	12
with Milk, Reg	6

VEGETARIAN
Dippers, 2 Pieces	160
Dippers, 4 Pieces	321

MCDONALD'S

WRAP
The BBQ & Bacon Chicken One, Crispy	500
The Sweet Chilli Chicken One, Crispy	474
The Veggie One, Spicy	363

NANDO'S

AVOCADO
Extra	85
Salad Extra	170

BREAD
Garlic, Kids Menu	218
Garlic, Large, Side	698
Garlic, Reg, Side	349
Pitta, Toasted, with Butter, Extra	246

BROCCOLI
Long Stem, Large, Side	48
Long Stem, Reg, Side	24
Long Stem, Side, Kids Menu	12

BROWNIES
Salted Caramel	389

BURGERS
Beanie, Peri Peri, Extra Hot	593
Beanie, Peri Peri, Hot	552
Beanie, Peri Peri, Lemon & Herb	521
Beanie, Peri Peri, Mango & Lime	534
Beanie, Peri Peri, Medium	531
Beanie, Plain	511
Chicken, Breast, Peri-Peri, Extra Hot	469
Chicken, Breast, Peri-Peri, Hot	428
Chicken, Breast, Peri-Peri, Lemon & Herb	397
Chicken, Breast, Peri-Peri, Mango & Lime	410
Chicken, Breast, Peri-Peri, Medium	407
Chicken, Breast, Plain, Kids Menu	296
Chicken, Breast, Plain	387
Chicken, Butterfly, Peri Peri, Extra Hot	663
Chicken, Butterfly, Peri Peri, Hot	622
Chicken, Butterfly, Peri Peri, Lemon & Herb	591
Chicken, Butterfly, Peri Peri, Mango & Lime	604
Chicken, Butterfly, Peri Peri, Medium	601
Chicken, Butterfly, Plain	581
Chicken, Double, Peri Peri, Extra Hot	607
Chicken, Double, Peri Peri, Hot	566
Chicken, Double, Peri Peri, Lemon & Herb	535
Chicken, Double, Peri Peri, Mango & Lime	548
Chicken, Double, Peri Peri, Medium	545
Chicken, Double, Plain	525
Chicken, Sunset, Peri Peri, Extra Hot	680
Chicken, Sunset, Peri Peri, Hot	639
Chicken, Sunset, Peri Peri, Lemon & Herb	608
Chicken, Sunset, Peri Peri, Mango & Lime	621
Chicken, Sunset, Peri Peri, Medium	618
Chicken, Sunset, Plain	598
Mushroom & Halloumi, Peri Peri, Extra Hot	743
Mushroom & Halloumi, Peri Peri, Hot	702
Mushroom & Halloumi, Peri Peri, Lemon & Herb	671
Mushroom & Halloumi, Peri Peri, Mango & Lime	684
Mushroom & Halloumi, Peri Peri, Medium	681
Mushroom & Halloumi, Plain	661
Supergreen, Peri Peri, Extra Hot	487

NANDO'S

BURGERS
Supergreen, Peri Peri, Hot	446
Supergreen, Peri Peri, Lemon & Herb	415
Supergreen, Peri Peri, Mango & Lime	428
Supergreen, Peri Peri, Medium	425
Supergreen, Plain	405
Sweet Potato & Butternut, Kids Menu	333
Sweet Potato & Butternut, Pattie Only, Kids Menu	219
Sweet Potato & Butternut, Peri Peri, Extra Hot	511
Sweet Potato & Butternut, Peri Peri, Hot	470
Sweet Potato & Butternut, Peri Peri, Lemon & Herb	439
Sweet Potato & Butternut, Peri Peri, Mango & Lime	452
Sweet Potato & Butternut, Peri Peri, Medium	449
Sweet Potato & Butternut, Plain	429

CAKE
Carrot	737
Choc-A-Lot	582

CHEESE
Feta, Extra	138
Halloumi, Grilled, Extra	177
Halloumi, Sticks, & Dip	441

CHEESECAKE
Caramel, Gooey	415
White Chocolate, & Raspberrry	446

CHICKEN
Breast, Fillet, Peri-Peri, Extra Hot	220
Breast, Fillet, Peri-Peri, Hot	179
Breast, Fillet, Peri-Peri, Lemon & Herb	148
Breast, Fillet, Peri-Peri, Mango & Lime	161
Breast, Fillet, Peri-Peri, Med	158
Breast, Fillet, Plain, Salad Extra	138
Breast, Fillet, Plain, Kids Menu	138
Butterfly, Crispy, Peri Peri, Extra Hot	414
Butterfly, Crispy, Peri Peri, Hot	373
Butterfly, Crispy, Peri Peri, Lemon & Herb	342
Butterfly, Crispy, Peri Peri, Mango & Lime	355
Butterfly, Cripsy, Peri Peri, Medium	352
Butterfly, Crispy, Plain	332
Half, Peri-Peri, Extra Hot	650
Half, Peri-Peri, Hot	609
Half, Peri-Peri, Lemon & Herb	578
Half, Peri-Peri, Mango & Lime	591
Half, Peri-Peri, Medium	588
Half, Plain	568
Breast, Quarter, Peri-Peri, Extra Hot	405
Breast, Quarter, Peri-Peri, Hot	364
Breast, Quarter, Peri-Peri, Lemon & Herb	333
Breast, Quarter, Peri-Peri, Mango & Lime	346
Breast, Quarter, Peri-Peri, Medium	343
Breast, Quarter, Plain	323
Leg, Quarter, Peri-Peri, Extra Hot	327
Leg, Quarter, Peri-Peri, Hot	286
Leg, Quarter, Peri-Peri, Lemon & Herb	255

NANDO'S

CHICKEN

Leg, Quarter, Peri-Peri, Mango & Lime	268
Leg, Quarter, Peri-Peri, Medium	265
Leg, Quarter, Plain	245
Thighs, Deboned, Peri-Peri, Extra Hot	637
Thighs, Deboned, Peri-Peri, Hot	596
Thighs, Deboned, Peri-Peri, Lemon & Herb	565
Thighs, Deboned, Peri-Peri, Mango & Lime	578
Thighs, Deboned, Peri-Peri, Medium	575
Thighs, Deboned, Plain	555
Thighs, 2, Salad Extra, Peri Peri, Extra Hot	359
Thighs, 2, Salad Extra, Peri Peri, Hot	318
Thighs, 2, Salad Extra, Peri Peri, Lemon & Herb	287
Thighs, 2, Salad Extra, Peri Peri, Mango & Lime	300
Thighs, 2, Salad Extra, Peri Peri, Medium	297
Thighs, 2, Salad Extra, Plain	277
Whole, Peri-Peri, Extra Hot	1218
Whole, Peri-Peri, Hot	1177
Whole, Peri-Peri, Lemon & Herb	1146
Whole, Peri-Peri, Mango & Lime	1159
Whole, Peri-Peri, Medium	1156
Whole, Plain	1136
Wings, Peri-Peri, Extra Hot, 10	868
Wings, Peri-Peri, Extra Hot, 3	318
Wings, Peri-Peri, Extra Hot, 5	475
Wings, Peri-Peri, Hot, 10	827
Wings, Peri-Peri, Hot, 3	277
Wings, Peri-Peri, Hot, 5	434
Wings, Peri-Peri, Lemon & Herb, 10	796
Wings, Peri-Peri, Lemon & Herb, 3	246
Wings, Peri-Peri, Lemon & Herb, 5	403
Wings, Peri-Peri, Mango & Lime, 10	809
Wings, Peri-Peri, Mango & Lime, 3	259
Wings, Peri-Peri, Mango & Lime, 5	416
Wings, Peri-Peri, Medium, 10	806
Wings, Peri-Peri, Medium, 3	256
Wings, Peri-Peri, Medium, 5	413
Wings, Plain, 10	786
Wings, Plain, Kids Menu, 3	236
Wings, Plain, 3	236
Wings, Plain, 5	393

CHIPS

Kids Menu	336
Large, Side	1256
Peri Salted, Large, Side	1260
Peri Salted, Reg, Side	467
Reg, Side	465

COFFEE

Americano	0
Cappuccino	73
Espresso	0
Latte	63

NANDO'S

COLESLAW

Large, Side	526
Reg, Side	263

CORDIAL

Green, Kids Menu	26

CORN

Cob, Kids Menu	72
Cob, Large, Side	288
Cob, Reg, Side	144

DIP

Red Pepper, & Chilli, with Pitta	464

FROZEN YOGHURT

Chocolate	79
Mango	71
Strawberry	70

HOT CHOCOLATE

BLANK	291

HOUMOUS

Peri Drizzle, & Pitta	819
Salad Extra	204

ICE CREAM

Chocolate	145
Coconut	157
Mango	99
Vanilla, Kids Menu	158
Vanilla	161

ICE LOLLY

Chilly Billy	30

JUICE

Apple, Pressed	134
Orange	118

JUICE DRINK

Mango Quencher	120

LEMONADE

Cloudy	143

MASH

Creamy, Large, Side	496
Creamy, Reg, Side	248

MILK

Organic, Kids Menu	113

MUSHROOMS

Portabello, Extra	105

NUTS

Peri-Peri	793

OLIVES

Mixed, Spicy	138

PEAS

Macho, Large, Side	283
Macho, Reg, Side	141

PEPPER

Chargrilled, Extra	39

PINEAPPLE

Slice, Grilled, Extra	37

NANDO'S

RELISH

Chilli, Jam, Extra	149

RICE

Spicy, Large, Side	492
Spicy, Reg, Side	246

ROLL - CHICKEN, LIVERS

Portuguese, Peri Peri, Extra Hot	622
Portuguese, Peri Peri, Hot	581
Portuguese, Peri Peri, Lemon & Herb	550
Portuguese, Peri Peri, Mango & Lime	563
Portuguese, Peri Peri, Medium	560
Portuguese, Plain	540

ROLL - STEAK, FILLET

Prego, Peri Peri, Extra Hot	487
Prego, Peri Peri, Hot	446
Prego, Peri Peri, Lemon & Herb	415
Prego, Peri Peri, Mango & Lime	428
Prego, Peri Peri, Medium	425
Prego, Plain	405

SALAD - CAESAR

Side	285
with Chicken Breast, Peri Peri, Extra Hot	504
with Chicken Breast, Peri Peri, Hot	463
with Chicken Breast, Peri Peri, Lemon & Herb	432
with Chicken Breast, Peri Peri, Mango & Lime	445
with Chicken Breast, Peri Peri, Med	442
with Chicken Breast, Plain	422

SALAD - GRAINS N GREENS

Side, Kids Menu	104
Large, Side	356
Side	189
with Chicken Breast, Peri Peri, Extra Hot	409
with Chicken Breast, Peri Peri, Hot	368
with Chicken Breast, Peri Peri, Lemon & Herb	337
with Chicken Breast, Peri Peri, Mango & Lime	350
with Chicken Breast, Peri Peri, Medium	347
with Chicken Breast, Plain	327

SALAD - HOUSE

Side	126
with Chicken Breast, Peri Peri, Extra Hot	345
with Chicken Breast, Peri Peri, Hot	304
with Chicken Breast, Peri Peri, Lemon & Herb	273
with Chicken Breast, Peri Peri, Mango & Lime	286
with Chicken Breast, Peri Peri, Medium	283
with Chicken Breast, Plain	263

SALAD - MIXED LEAF

Reg, Side	13
with Chicken Breast, Peri Peri, Extra Hot	244
with Chicken Breast, Peri Peri, Hot	203
with Chicken Breast, Peri Peri, Lemon & Herb	172
with Chicken Breast, Peri Peri, Mango & Lime	185
with Chicken Breast, Peri Peri, Medium	182
with Chicken Breast, Plain	162

NANDO'S

SANDWICH - PITTA

Beanie, Pitta, Peri Peri, Extra Hot	602
Beanie, Pitta, Peri Peri, Hot	561
Beanie, Peri Peri, Lemon & Herb	530
Beanie, Peri Peri, Mango & Lime	543
Beanie, Peri Peri, Medium	540
Beanie, Plain	520
Chicken, Breast, Peri-Peri, Extra Hot	478
Chicken, Breast, Peri-Peri, Hot	437
Chicken, Breast, Peri-Peri, Lemon & Herb	406
Chicken, Breast, Peri-Peri, Mango & Lime	419
Chicken, Breast, Peri-Peri, Medium	416
Chicken, Breast, Plain	396
Chicken, Double, Peri Peri, Extra Hot	616
Chicken, Double, Peri Peri, Hot	575
Chicken, Double, Peri Peri, Lemon & Herb	544
Chicken, Double, Peri Peri, Mango & Lime	557
Chicken, Double, Peri Peri, Medium	554
Chicken, Double, Plain	534
Chicken, Thigh, Fino, Peri Peri, Extra Hot	838
Chicken, Thigh, Fino, Peri Peri, Hot	797
Chicken, Thigh, Fino, Peri Peri, Lemon & Herb	766
Chicken, Thigh, Fino, Peri Peri, Mango & Lime	779
Chicken, Thigh, Fino, Peri Peri, Medium	776
Chicken, Thigh, Fino, Plain	756
Mushroom & Halloumi, Peri Peri, Extra Hot	727
Mushroom & Halloumi, Peri Peri, Hot	686
Mushroom & Halloumi, Peri Peri, Lemon & Herb	655
Mushroom & Halloumi, Peri Peri, Mango & Lime	668
Mushroom & Halloumi, Peri Peri, Medium	665
Mushroom & Halloumi, Plain	645
Steak, Fillet, & Veg, Peri Peri, Extra Hot	531
Steak, Fillet, & Veg, Peri Peri, Hot	490
Steak, Fillet, & Veg, Peri Peri, Lemon & Herb	459
Steak, Fillet, & Veg, Peri Peri, Mango & Lime	472
Steak, Fillet, & Veg, Peri Peri, Medium	469
Steak, Fillet, & Veg, Plain	449
Supergreen, Peri Peri, Extra Hot	536
Supergreen, Peri Peri, Hot	495
Supergreen, Peri Peri, Lemon & Herb	464
Supergreen, Peri Peri, Mango & Lime	477
Supergreen, Peri Peri, Medium	474
Supergreen, Plain	454
Sweet Potato & Butternut, Peri Peri, Extra Hot	560
Sweet Potato & Butternut, Peri Peri, Hot	519
Sweet Potato & Butternut, Peri Peri, Lemon Herb	488
Sweet Potato & Butternut, Peri Peri, Mango Lime	501
Sweet Potato & Butternut, Peri Peri, Medium	498
Sweet Potato & Butternut, Plain	478

SAUCE

Peri Peri Drizzle, Side	97
Perinaise, Condiments	159

NANDO'S

SPINACH

Saucy, Large, Side	195
Saucy, Reg, Side	98

STEW

Cataplana, Veggie	515

SWEET POTATO

& Butternut Squash, Fino Side	174
& Butternut Squash, Side, Kids Menu	71
Mash, Fino Side	97
Mash, Kids Menu	48

TART

Custard, Naughty Natas	169

TEA

Infusions, All Flavours	0
Organic, Everyday	23
Rubro, Iced	57

TOMATOES

Kids Menu	13

VEGETABLES

Chargrilled, Fino Side	93

WRAP

Beanie, Peri Peri, Extra Hot	736
Beanie, Peri Peri, Hot	695
Beanie, Peri Peri, Lemon & Herb	664
Beanie, Peri Peri, Mango & Lime	677
Beanie, Peri Peri, Medium	674
Beanie, Plain	654
Chicken, Breast, Peri-Peri, Extra Hot	613
Chicken, Breast, Peri-Peri, Hot	572
Chicken, Breast, Peri-Peri, Lemon & Herb	541
Chicken, Breast, Peri-Peri, Mango & Lime	554
Chicken, Breast, Peri-Peri, Medium	551
Chicken, Breast, Plain	531
Chicken, Double, Peri Peri, Extra Hot	750
Chicken, Double, Peri Peri, Hot	709
Chicken, Double, Peri Peri, Lemon & Herb	678
Chicken, Double, Peri Peri, Mango & Lime	691
Chicken, Double, Peri Peri, Medium	688
Chicken, Double, Plain	668
Chicken, Mozam, Grilled, Peri Peri, Extra Hot	546
Chicken, Mozam, Grilled, Peri Peri, Hot	505
Chicken, Mozam, Grilled, Peri Peri, Lemon & Herb	474
Chicken, Mozam, Grilled, Peri Peri, Mango & Lime	487
Chicken, Mozam, Grilled, Peri Peri, Medium	484
Chicken, Mozam, Grilled, Plain	464
Mushroom & Halloumi, Peri-Peri, Extra Hot	802
Mushroom & Halloumi, Peri-Peri, Hot	761
Mushroom & Halloumi, Peri-Peri, Lemon & Herb	730
Mushroom & Halloumi, Peri-Peri, Mango & Lime	743
Mushroom & Halloumi, Peri-Peri, Medium	740
Mushroom & Halloumi, Plain	720
Steak, Fillet, & Veg, Peri Peri, Extra Hot	623
Steak, Fillet, & Veg, Peri Peri, Hot	582

NANDO'S

WRAP

Steak, Fillet, & Veg, Peri Peri, Lemon & Herb	551
Steak, Fillet, & Veg, Peri Peri, Mango & Lime	564
Steak, Fillet, & Veg, Peri Peri, Medium	561
Steak, Fillet, & Veg, Plain	541
Supergreen, Peri Peri, Extra Hot	670
Supergreen, Peri Peri, Hot	629
Supergreen, Peri Peri, Lemon & Herb	598
Sipergreen, Peri Peri, Mango & Lime	611
Supergreen, Peri Peri, Medium	608
Supergreen, Plain	588
Sweet Potato & Butternut, Peri Peri, Extra Hot	694
Sweet Potato & Butternut, Peri Peri, Hot	653
Sweet Potato & Butternut, Peri Peri, Lemon & Herb	622
Sweet Potato & Butternut, Peri Peri, Mango & Lime	635
Sweet Potato & Butternut, Peri Peri, Medium	632
Sweet Potato & Butternut, Plain	612

PIZZA EXPRESS

BITES
Halloumi	351

BOLOGNESE
Penne, Al Forno	674
Penne, Piccolo	353

BREAD
Garlic	280
Garlic, Vegan	345
Garlic, with Mozzarella	356
Garlic, with Vegan Mozzarella	330

BROWNIES
Chocolate, Dolcetti	206
Chocolate, Piccolo	206
Chocolate, with Ice Cream	519

BRUSCHETTA
Originale	362

CAKE
Carrot, Vegan, Dolcetti	336
Chocolate, Fudge	312

CALZONE
'Nduja	1196
Verdure	906

CANNELLONI
Spinach, & Ricotta, Al Forno	705

CHEESE
Mascarpone, Side	118

CHEESECAKE
Raspberry, Honeycomb, Cream, Slice	578
Lotus Biscoff, Dolcetti	319
Vanilla, Reduced Fat & Sugar	384
White Chocolate & Raspberry	440

CHICKEN
Wings, Lemon & Herb	556

CHIPS
Polenta	454

COULIS
Fruit, Side	25

CREAM
Side	139

DESSERT
Chocolate Fondant, with Vanilla Ice Cream	657

DIP
Trio, Vegan	270

DOUGH BALLS
Doppio	828
GF, with Garlic Butter	370
Piccolo	115
Plain	396
Sticks, Side	263
Vegan	336
with Balsamic Vinegar, & Olive Oil, Piccolo	153
with Garlic Butter, & Salad, Piccolo	233
with Butter, Piccolo	54

PIZZA EXPRESS

DOUGH BALLS
with Houmous, & Salad, Piccolo	193
with Houmous, Piccolo	130
without Butter	230

DRESSING
Caesar	157
Honey & Mustard	196
House, Classic	191
House, Light	135

FIGS
Caffe Reale, Dolcetti	208

ICE CREAM
Chocolate, & Chocolate Straw, Coppa Gelato	246
Caramel, Salted, & Chocolate Straw, Coppa Gelato	287
Strawberry, & Chocolate Straw, Coppa Gelato	211
Vanilla, & Chocolate Straw, Coppa Gelato	247
Vanilla, Gelato, Side	114

ICE LOLLY
Fruit, Organic, Pip	18
Rainbow, Organic, Pip	20

JUICE DRINK
Apple, & Pear, Cawston	54
Apple, & Summer Berries, Cawston	50

LASAGNE
Classica, Al Forno	712

OLIVES
Marinate	137

PENNE
Bianca, Piccolo	355
Napoletana, Piccolo	284

PESTO
Pollo, Al Forno, GF	1082

PIZZA
American, Classic	978
American hot, Romana	1010
American, Piccolo	482
American Hot, Leggera, Wholemeal	548
Barbacoa, Leggera, Wholemeal	547
Barbacoa, Romana	1118
Calbrese, Classic	1275
Diavolo, Leggera, Wholemeal	556
Diavolo, Romana	1167
Fiorentina, Classic	942
Giardiniera, Vegan, Classic	843
Giardiniera, Vegan, Leggera, Wholemeal	556
Giardiniera, Vegan, Romana	970
La Reine, Classic	898
La Reine, Leggera, Wholemeal	498
La Reine, Piccolo	437
Margherita, Bufala, Romana	1152
Margherita, Classic	834
Margherita, Vegan, Classic	711
Margherita, Leggera, Wholemeal	440

PIZZA EXPRESS

PIZZA

Margherita, Vegan, Leggera, Wholemeal	452
Margherita, Piccolo	435
Mezze, Leggera, Wholemeal	522
Mezze, Vegan, Romana	932
Padana, Leggera, Wholemeal	587
Padana, Vegan, Leggera, Wholemeal	560
Padana, Romana	1108
Padana, Vegan, Romana	911
Pollo, Ad Astra, Leggera, Wholemeal	599
Pollo, Ad Astra, Romana	1145
Pollo, Forza, Leggera, Wholemeal	578
Pollo, Forza, Romana	1253
Pollo, Piccolo, Classic	458
Sloppy Giuseppe, Classic	897
Sloppy Giuseppe, Leggera, Wholemeal	490
Veneziana, Classic	938
Veneziana, Vegan, Classic	815
Veneziana, Leggera, Wholemeal	517
Veneziana, Vegan, Leggera, Wholemeal	544

PRAWNS

King, Garlic	289

PROFITEROLES

Salted Caramel, Dolcetti	257

SALAD

Mixed, Side, no Dressiing	74
Mixed, Side, with House Dressing	202
Mozzarella, & Tomato, Buffalo	336
Nicoise, no Dressing	366
Nicoise, with Dressing, & Dough Sticks	820
Nicoise, with Dressing	558
Pollo, no Dressing	502
Pollo, with Dough Balls, Piccolo	283
Pollo, with Dressing, & Dough Sticks	954
Pollo, with Dressing	693
Pollo, with Polenta Chips, Piccolo	265
Rucola	140
Side, Piccolo	16
Superfood, Leggera	171
Superfood, Leggera, with Dressing	424

SORBET

Coconut, Coppa Gelato	201
Raspberry, Leggera	122

SQUID

Calamari	504

SUNDAE

Ic Cream, with Chocolate Sauce, Piccolo	149
Ice Cream, with Fruit Sauce, Piccolo	131

TIRAMISU

Classic	412

TOMATOES

Roasted	67

PIZZA HUT

APPLES

Salad Station	10

BACON

Bits, Salad Station	104

BEETROOT

Diced, Salad Station	10

BITES

Cheesy	469
Cinnamon, Hot	472
Cinnamon, Kids	248
Hot Dog	404

BOLOGNESE

Spaghetti, Little Boss	198

BREAD

Garlic	511
Garlic, with Mozzarella	689

BREADSTICKS

Salad Station	245

BROWNIES

Chocolate, Hot	600
Chocolate, Kids	394

CARROTS

Shredded, Salad Station	10

CHEESE TRIANGLES

Fried	425
Oven Baked	396

CHEESECAKE

Chocolate, Honeycomb	639
I Can't Believe It's Not	513
Strawberries, & Cream	537

CHICKEN

Bites	397
Breaded, & Fries, Fried, Big Boss	619
Breaded, & Fries, Fried, Little Boss	548
Breaded, & Fries, Oven Baked, Big Boss	472
Breaded, & Fries, Oven Baked, Little Boss	400
Breaded, & Seasoned Fries, Fried, Big Boss	704
Breaded, & Seasoned Fries, Fried, Little Boss	563
Breaded, & Seasoned Fries, Oven Baked, Big Boss	533
Breaded, & Seasoned Fries, Oven Baked, Little Boss	421
Melt, BBQ Americano	396
Melt, Garlic Mushroom	447
Melt, Naked	246
Melt, Pepperoni	423
Nuggets, Southern Fried	248
Wings	379

CHOCOLATE

Beans, Ice Cream Factory	460
Chips, Ice Cream Factory	516
Toffee, Crunch, Ice Cream Factory	465
Tricolor, Pieces, Ice Cream Factory	542

PIZZA HUT

COLESLAW
Salad Station	38

COOKIES
Dough, Chocolate Chip, Hot	651
Dough, S'mores, Hot	691
Dough, Salted Caramel, Hot	631

CORN
Cob, 3, Side	203
Cob, 5, Side	328
Cob, Mini, Side	328

CROUTONS
Salad Station	85

CUCUMBER
Salad Station	2

DIP
BBQ	35
Blue Cheese, Salad Station	75
Garlic Sauce	89
Sour Cream, & Chive, Dressing	102

DRESSING
French, Low Fat, Salad Station	15
Olive Oil, & Balsamic Vinegar, Salad Station	124
Ranch, Salad Station	79
Thousand Island, Salad Station	54

FLATBREAD
BBQ Steak, & Chicken	535
Chicken Delight	440
Ham, & Garlic Mushroom	459
Tuna, & Sweetcorn	457
Virtuous Veg	375
Virtuous Veg, Vegan	332

FRIES
Cheesy, Fried, Side	854
Cheesy, Oven Baked, Side	680
Fried, Side	673
Oven Baked, Side	355
Seasoned, Fried, Side	702
Seasoned, Oven Baked, Side	384
Sweet Potato, Side	772

ICE CREAM
Vanilla, Ice Cream Factory, Kids	192
Vanilla, Ice Cream Factory	329

ICE CREAM FLOAT
Cream Soda, Black Cherry	300
Cream Soda	300

ICE LOLLY
Orange	69

KETCHUP
Portion	99

LASAGNE
Beef	790
Beef, with Garlic Bread, Big Boss	523

PIZZA HUT

LETTUCE
Mix, Salad Station	2

MACARONI CHEESE
Big Boss	412
Portion	824
with Chicken, Pulled	867
with Garlic Mushrooms	894

MAYONNAISE
Garlic, Salad Station	92
Light, Salad Station	77

MILK SHAKE
Chocoholic, Kids	273
Chocoholic	622
Oreo, Kids	309
Oreo	775
Salted Caramel, Kids	328
Salted Caramel	679
Strawberry, Kids	287
Strawberry	698
Vanilla, Kids	263
Vanilla	581

OIL
Garlic, & Chilli, Salad Station	180

ONION RINGS
Fried, Side	236
Oven Baked, Side	154

ONIONS
Crispy, Salad Station	125
Red, Salad Station	7

PASTA
Cheesy, Little Boss	385

PASTA BAKE
Cheese, 4, & Spinach, Buffet	245
Marinara, Buffet	273

PASTA SAUCE
Cheese, Buffet	128
Marinara, Buffet	87

PENNE
Buffet	265

PEPPERS
Jalapeno, Poppers, Fried	438
Jalapeno, Poppers, Oven Baked	354
Jalapeno, Salad Station	2
Mixed, Salad Station	3

PIZZA - ALL ABOUT MUSHROOMS
Cheesy Bites Crust	2224
Deep Pan, Large	2072
Deep Pan, Reg	1014
GF	918
Stuffed Crust, Individual	1224
Stuffed Crust, Large	2224
Thin Crust, Individual	894
Thin Crust, Large	1472

PIZZA HUT

PIZZA - ALL ABOUT MUSHROOMS

Vegan, Deep Pan, Large	1979
Vegan, Deep Pan, Reg	964
Vegan, GF	959
Vegan, Thin Crust, Individual	827
Vegan, Thin Crust, Large	1378

PIZZA - BBQ AMERICANO

Cheesy Bites Crust	2584
Deep Pan, Large	2432
Deep Pan, Reg	1158
GF	1068
Stuffed Crust, Individual	1374
Stuffed Crust, Large	2584
Thin Crust, Individual	1038
Thin Crust, Large	1840

PIZZA - BBQ JACK 'N' CHEESE

Cheesy Bites Crust	2296
Deep Pan, Large	2144
Deep Pan, Reg	1038
GF	942
Stuffed Crust, Individual	1248
Stuffed Crust, Large	2296
Thin Crust, Individual	912
Thin Crust, Large	1536

PIZZA - CHICKEN SUPREME

Cheesy Bites Crust	2344
Deep Pan, Large	2192
Deep Pan, Reg	1050
GF	954
Stuffed Crust, Individual	1260
Stuffed Crust, Large	2344
Thin Crust, Individual	930
Thin Crust, Large	1592

PIZZA - HAWAIIAN

Cheesy Bites Crust	2216
Deep Pan, Large	2072
Deep Pan, Reg	1008
GF	912
Stuffed Crust, Individual	1212
Stuffed Crust, Large	2216
Thin Crust, Individual	888
Thin Crust, Large	1472

PIZZA - HOT 'N' SPICY

Chicken, Cheesy Bites Crust	2408
Chicken, Deep Pan, Large	2256
Chicken, Deep Pan, Reg	1092
Chicken, GF	996
Chicken, Stuffed Crust, Individual	1302
Chicken, Stuffed Crust, Large	2408
Chicken, Thin Crust, Individual	972
Chicken, Thin Crust, Large	1656
Veg, Cheesy Bites Crust	2296
Veg, Deep Pan, Large	2152

PIZZA HUT

PIZZA - HOT 'N' SPICY

Veg, Deep Pan, Reg	1050
Veg, GF	954
Veg, Stuffed Crust, Individual	1260
Veg, Stuffed Crust, Large	2296
Veg, Thin Crust, Individual	924
Veg, Thin Crust, Large	1536
Vegan, Deep Pan, Large	1976
Vegan, Deep Pan, Reg	966
Vegan, GF	870
Vegan, Thin Crust, Individual	840
Vegan, Thin Crust, Large	1368

PIZZA - JACK N CH**SE

Vegan, Deep Pan, Large	2058
Vegan, Deep Pan, Reg	994
Vegan, GF	984
Vegan, Thin Crust, Individual	873
Vegan, Thin Crust, Large	1457

PIZZA - MARGHERITA

Cheesy Bites Crust	2280
Deep Pan, Big Boss	453
Deep Pan, Large	2128
Deep Pan, Little Boss	423
Deep Pan, Reg	1038
GF, Big Boss	433
GF, Little Boss	412
GF	942
Stuffed Crust, Individual	1248
Stuffed Crust, Large	2280
Thin Crust, Big Boss	374
Thin Crust, Individual	918
Thin Crust, Large	1528
Thin Crust, Little Boss	327
Vegan, Deep Pan, Large	2163
Vegan, Deep Pan, Reg	1056
Vegan, GF	958
Vegan, Thin Crust, Individual	935
Vegan, Thin Crust, Large	1563

PIZZA - MEAT FEAST

Cheesy Bites Crust	2528
Deep Pan, Large	2376
Deep Pan, Reg	1140
Epic, Cheesy Bites Crust	2592
Epic, Deep Pan, Large	2448
Epic, Deep Pan, Reg	1188
Epic, GF	1170
Epic, Stuffed Crust, Individual	1398
Epic, Stuffed Crust, Large	2592
Epic, Thin Crust, Individual	1068
Epic, Thin Crust, Large	1848
GF	1044
Stuffed Crust, Individual	1350
Stuffed Crust, Large	2528

PIZZA HUT

PIZZA - MEAT FEAST

Thin Crust, Individual	1020
Thin Crust, Large	1776

PIZZA - NEW YORK HOT DOG

Cheesy Bites Crust	2720
Deep Pan, Large	2568
Deep Pan, Reg	1248
GF	1152
Stuffed Crust, Individual	1458
Stuffed Crust, Large	2720
Thin Crust, Individual	1128
Thin Crust, Large	1968

PIZZA - PEPPERONI

Cheesy Bites Crust	2384
Deep Pan, Large	2232
Deep Pan, Reg	1092
Epic, Cheesy Bites Crust	2760
Epic, Deep Pan, Large	2616
Epic, Deep Pan, Reg	1266
Epic, GF	1170
Epic, Stuffed Crust, Individual	1476
Epic, Stuffed Crust, Large	2760
Epic, Thin Crust, Individual	1146
Epic, Thin Crust, Large	2008
GF	996
Stuffed Crust, Individual	1296
Stuffed Crust, Large	2384
Thin Crust, Individual	972
Thin Crust, Large	1632

PIZZA - PHILLY CHEESE STEAK

Cheesy Bites Crust	3000
Deep Pan, Large	2848
Deep Pan, Reg	1392
GF	1302
Stuffed Crust, Individual	1602
Stuffed Crust, Large	3000
Thin Crust, Individual	1278
Thin Crust, Large	2248

PIZZA - SUPREME

Deep Pan, Large	2440
Deep Pan, Reg	1158
GF	1068
Stuffed Crust, Individual	1368
Stuffed Crust, Large	2600
Thin Crust, Individual	1038
Thin Crust, Large	1840

PIZZA - TEXAS MEAT MELTDOWN

Cheesy Bites Crust	2880
Deep Pan, Large	2728
Deep Pan, Reg	1308
GF	1014
Stuffed Crust, Individual	1524
Stuffed Crust, Large	2880

PIZZA HUT

PIZZA - TEXAS MEAT MELTDOWN

Thin Crust, Individual	1188
Thin Crust, Large	2256

PIZZA - THE G.O.A.T

Cheesy Bites Crust	2456
Deep Pan, Large	2312
Deep Pan, Reg	1134
GF	1032
Stuffed Crust, Individual	1338
Stuffed Crust, Large	2456
Thin Crust, Individual	1002
Thin Crust, Large	1696

PIZZA - VEGGIE

Cheesy Bites Crust	2184
Deep Pan, Large	2032
Deep Pan, Reg	984
Epic, Cheesy Bites Crust	2320
Epic, Deep Pan, Large	2176
Epic, Deep Pan, Reg	1062
Epic, GF	966
Epic, Stuffed Crust, Individual	1272
Epic, Stuffed Crust, Large	2320
Epic, Thin Crust, Individual	942
Epic, Thin Crust, Large	1568
GF	888
Stuffed Crust, Individual	1194
Stuffed Crust, Large	2184
Thin Crust, Individual	864
Thin Crust, Large	1432
Vegan, Deep Pan, Large	1932
Vegan, Deep Pan, Reg	933
Vegan, GF	929
Vegan, Thin Crust, Individual	812
Vegan, Thin Crust, Large	1332

PIZZA -SUPREME

Cheesy Bites Crust	2600

PIZZA TOPPING

Chicken	20
Ham	13
Pepperoni	34
Peppers	2
Pineapple	21
Sweetcorn	15
Tuna	14

POTATO SALAD

Salad Station	27

RIBS

Pork, BBQ	582
Pork, Rack, All American	787

ROLLS

Jack 'N' Roll, Vegan	305

SALSA

Salad Station	12

	KCAL
PIZZA HUT	
SAUCE	
BBQ	119
Chocolate, Ice Cream Factory, Kids	32
Chocolate, Ice Cream Factory	59
Hot & Spicy	65
Hut House Seasoning	322
Raspberry, Ice Cream Factory	263
Sweet Chilli	175
SULTANAS	
Salad Station	55
SWEETCORN	
Salad Station	15
TOMATOES	
Cherry, Salad Station	3
TOPPING	
Gold Crunch, Ice Cream Factory	681
Lemon Crunch, Ice Cream Factory	382
Sprinkles, Ice Cream Factory	421
Strawberry Crunch, Ice Cream Factory	382
TORTILLA CHIPS	
Salad Station	96
VINEGAR	
Sarsons	21
WRAP	
Chicken, & Cheese, Little Boss	535
Chicken, & Sweetcorn, Little Boss	426
Chicken, Big Boss	396
Tuna, & Cheese	350
Tuna, & Sweetcorn	245
Tuna	210

	KCAL
PRET A MANGER	
ALMONDS	
Chocolate, Dark	217
BAGUETTE	
Avo, Olives, & Toms	511
Cheddar, & Pickle, Posh	620
Chicken Caesar, & Bacon	592
Chicken Katsu, Naked	529
BAGUETTE	
Egg, & Avo, Breakfast	395
Egg, & Bacon, Breakfast	358
Eggless Mayo & Cress, Vegan	620
Ham, Wiltshire Cured, & Greve	615
Jambon-Beurre	354
Losange, Stone Baked, for Soup	188
Prosciutto, Italian	536
Salmon, & Egg, Breakfast	358
Tuna Mayo, & Cucumber, Pole & Line Caught	560
BARS	
Choc	348
Chocolate Brownie	291
Love	325
Nut	248
Popcorn	171
BISCUITS	
Gingerbread	197
BITES	
Chocolatey Coconut	208
Protein Ball, Almond Butter	159
BREAD	
Focaccia, Firecracker Chicken, Toasted	490
BREAKFAST	
Bircher Muesli	309
Bowl, Acai, & Almond Butter	349
Bowl, Five Berry	347
Bowl, Mango, & Banana, Sunshine	253
BREAKFAST CEREAL	
Bircher Muesli, Supermarket	369
Porridge, No Topping	216
BURRITO	
Chicken & Chilli	521
CHEESECAKE	
Lemon	321
CHOCOLATE	
Dark, with Sea Salt	136
Milk	145
CHOCOLATES	
Truffles, Hazelnut	146
COFFEE	
Americano, Iced	1
Americano	0
Cappuccino	92
Cold Brew	10
Espresso	0

PRET A MANGER

COFFEE

	KCAL
Filter	3
Flat White	80
Latte, Iced	120
Latte	118
Latte, Pumpkin Spice	167
Macchiato	5
Mocha, Iced	185
Mocha	185

COOKIES

Chocolate, Dark, & Almond Butter	377
Chocolate Chunk	370
Fruit, Oat, & Spelt	347
Pecan, & Caramel	391

CORN CAKES

Dark Chocolate	239

CRISPS

Chilli, Bean, & Seed, Tortilla Chips	199
Mature Cheddar, & Red Onion	200
Sea Salt, & Cider Vinegar	196
Sea Salt	203
Smoked Chipotle	203
Vegetable	202

CROISSANT

Almond	374
Chocolate	350
French Butter	291
Ham, Cheese, Tomato, & Bacon	338
Mozzarella, & Tomato	322
Very Berry	299

DESSERT

Chocolate Moose	306

DRIED FRUIT

Mango	119

ENCHILADAS

Chicken, Spicy, Bake	646
Vegan Chilli	571

FLATBREAD

Chicken, Pesto, & Rocket	569
Falafel, Avo, & Chipotle	478
Mexican Avocado	482

FRUIT

Mango & Lime, Pot	92
Melon, & Blueberry Pot	38

FRUIT & NUT MIX

with Chocolate Covered Raisins	177

FRUIT SALAD

Pot	111
Superfruit Salad, Pot	109

GINGER BEER

Pure Pret	129

HOT CHOCOLATE

Iced, Coconut	260

PRET A MANGER

HOT CHOCOLATE

	KCAL
Iced	256
Iced, Soya	230
Semi Skimmed Milk	256

JUICE

Apple	120
Daily Greens	144
Orange, Large	168
Orange	105

JUICE DRINK

Apple Fizz, Sparkling, Pure	112
Cranberry, & Raspberry, Still, Pure Pret	175
Ginger Shot	55
Grape & Elderflower, Sparkling, Pure Pret	109
Green Tea, & Peach, Still	104
Hot Shot	47
Lemon, & Ginger, Still	93
Mango, & Passion Fruit, Still	111
Roots & Fruits	147
Vitamin Volcano	137

KOMBUCHA

Ginger	43

LEMONADE

Rhubarb, Pure Pret	118

MACARONI CHEESE

Kale, & Cauliflower	549
Prosciutto	586

MEATBALLS

Meatless, Protein Pot	246

MILK

Babyccino, with Chocolate Sprinkles	14
Cold, for Kids	94

MILK SHAKE

Chocolate	439
Frappe, Classic	251

MUFFIN

Double Berry	441

PAIN AU RAISIN

Pastry	394

PASTRY

Cinnamon Danish	489

POPCORN

Sea Salt	143
Sweet, & Salt	163

ROLL

Bacon, & Egg	410
Bacon	455
Ham, & Egg, Breakfast	405
Sausage, & Egg	408
Veggie	332

SALAD

Chicken, Italian, Chef's, without Dressing	612
Chicken, Tamari & Ginger, Bowl	329

PRET A MANGER

SALAD

Egg, & Spinach, Protein Pot	104
Houmous, & Falafel, Mezze, no Dressing	451
Houmous, & Falafel, Mezze, With Dressing	712
Roasted Chickpea, Mozzarella, & Pesto, Bowl	547
Salmon, & Mango, Bowl	358
Salmon, Smoked, Protein Box	496
Tuna, Nicoise, with Dressing	455

SALAD DRESSING

French, Large	294

SANDWICH

Cheese, Kids	399
Chicken, Avocado, & Basil	464
Christmas Lunch	531
Egg Mayo, Free-Range	347
Ham, & Cheese	522
Ham, Kids	290
Houmous, & Roasted Peppers, Open	503
Smashed Avo, Open	293
Smoked Salmon, & Soft Cheese, Open	303
Smoked Salmon, Scottish	405
Super Club, Classic	511
Tuna & Cucumber	385

SAUSAGE ROLL

Baked	376

SHORTBREAD

Biscuit	419

SMOOTHIE

Berry Blast	239
Mango, & Pineapple	209
Mango	143
Strawberry, & Banana	211

SOUP

Chicken, Broccoli, & Brown Rice	85
Chicken, Broccoli, & Brown Rice, Side	51
Chicken, Katsu	208
Chicken, Katsu, Side	124
Chicken, Laksa	291
Chicken, Laksa, Side	176
Chicken Pot Pie, EAT	280
Chicken Pot Pie, EAT, Side	169
Mushroom, Risotto	116
Mushroom, Risotto, Side	69
Pea, & Mint	246
Pea, & Mint, Side	146
Tomato, Souper	207
Tomato, Souper, Side	123
Vegetable, Red Thai	184
Vegetable, Red Thai, Side	110

TEA

Ceylon, Breakfast	14
Earl Grey	14
Green, Tropical	0

PRET A MANGER

TEA

Latte, Chai, Organic	218
Latte, Matcha	205
Latte, Turmeric	198
Peppermint, Peace	0

TOASTIE

Cheese, Classic	610
Ham, Cheese, & Mustard	605
Tuna Melt	572

TOPPING

Soup, Pot Pie	91

WRAP

Avocado, & Herb Salad	506
Falafel, & Halloumi, Hot	624
Hoisin Duck Salad	449
Houmous, & Chipotle	469
Meatless Meatball, Hot	510
Ragu, & Red Pepper, Vegan, Hot	420
Swedish Meatball, Hot	661

PREZZO

ANTIPASTI
Meats, Cured, Sharers	979

BITES
Pizza, Sharers	860
Pizza, Spicy, Sharers	860
Pizza, Spicy, Starter	356
Pizza, Starter	356

BOLOGNESE
Spaghetti	589
Spaghetti, with King Prawns	564

BREAD
Garlic, Pizza, Large, Sharers	892
Garlic, Starter	271
Garlic, with Balsamic Onions, & Mozzarella, Starter	520
Garlic, with Mozzarella, Starter	386

BROCCOLI
Tenderstem, & Cauliflower	88

BROWNIE
Chocolate, Dome	467

BRUSCHETTA
Tomato, Starter	415

BURGER
Calabrese, with Fries	1382

CALZONE
Spicy Carne	898
Tre Carni	930

CARBONARA
Spaghetti, Chicken, Al Forno	1033
Spaghetti	662

CHEESE
Mozzarella, Breaded, Starter	561

CHEESECAKE
Honeycomb Smash, Mini	219
Honeycomb Smash	500
Vanilla, with Caramel Sauce, Mini	203
Vanilla, with Raspberries, Mini	242

CHICKEN
Breast, Chargrilled, with Mushrooms	384

DESSERT
Affogato	320

FLATBREAD
Sharers	849

FRIES
House, Side	582
Truffle Oil Infused, Side	671

HOUMOUS
Italian, Starter	667

ICE CREAM
Chocolate	194
Strawberry	171
Vanilla	171

LASAGNE
Traditional, Al Forno	687

PREZZO

MEATBALLS
Giant, Starter	453

MUSHROOMS
Stuffed, Baked, Starter	395

OLIVES
Marinated	102

PANNA COTTA
with Fruit Compote, Mini	126
with Fruit Compote	375

PASTA - PENNE
Alla Rusticana	756
Arrabbiata	501
Aubergine	554
Goats Cheese, Al Forno	1033
Gorgonzola	633
Pancetta, Pea, & Mushroom, Light	492
Pesto & Pea	681
Prawn, Spicy, & Basil Pesto, Light	506
Salmon, Oak Smoked	840

PASTRY
Cannoli, Mini	282

PIZZA
Chicken, & Roasted Pepper, Large	1111
Chicken, & Roasted Pepper, Reg	923
Chicken, Primavera, Light	524
Fiorentina, Large	1016
Fiorentina, Reg	699
Goats Cheese, & Aubergine, Light	554
Goats Cheese, & Red Pepper, Large	1053
Goats Cheese, & Red Pepper, Reg	910
Margherita, Large	837
Margherita, Reg	705
Margherita, Royale, Premium	979
Garlic Mushroom, Large	725
Garlic Mushroom, Reg	595
Pepperoni, Posh, Premium	1242
Tre Gusti, Large	1339
Tre Gusti, Reg	929
Tropicana, Large	1018
Tropicana, Reg	783
Vesuvio, Large	1052
Vesuvio, Reg	872

PRAWNS
King, Starter	406

PUDDING
Sticky Toffee	631

RAVIOLI
Lobster, & Crab	510

RISOTTO
Chicken, & Asparagus	787
Mushroom	725
Prawn, King, & Salmon	471

PREZZO

SALAD
Caesar, Chicken, no Garlic Bread	737
Caprese, Starter	241
Chicken, Bacon & Avocado, no Garlic Bread	512
Lentil, Beetroot, & Butternut, no Garlic Bread	321
Mix, Side	103
Rocket, with Italian Cheese, Side	93

SALMON
Fillet, Roast, with Vegetables	483

SEA BASS
with Vegetables, & Pesto	506

SORBET
Raspberry	13

SPAGHETTI & MEATBALLS
Al Forno	903

SQUID
Calamari, Starter	702

TART
Chocolate, Salted Caramel	599

TIRAMISU
Portion	323

SLIM CHICKENS

APPLE SAUCE
Sides	40

BUTTER
Whipped, Scoop	106

CHEESECAKE
Oreo, Jar	574
Peanut Butter Cup, Jar	802
Pecan Pie, Jar	618
Pumpkin, Jar	548
Strawberry, Jar	393
Strawberry, Platter, Large	3308
Strawberry, Platter, Small	1654

CHICKEN
Tenders, Fried, 1	95
Tenders, Grilled, 1	56
Wings, Plain, 1	56

CHIPS
Ranch, Lge Crowd, Sides	5464
Ranch, Reg, Sides	449
Ranch, Sm Crowd, Sides	2732

COLESLAW
Large, Sides	705
Large Crowd, Sides	3762
Reg, Sides	235
Small Crowd, Sides	1881

COOKIE
Bliss	360
Chocolate Chip, Hope's	190
Chocolate Chip	187
White Chocolate, Macadamia, Hope's	196

FRENCH FRIES
Large, Sides	1367
Reg, Sides	470

MACARONI CHEESE
Large, Sides	1333
Large Crowd, Sides	7107
Reg, Sides	444
Small Crowd, Sides	3554

MUSHROOMS
Fried, Large, Sides	762
Fried, Reg, Sides	476

OKRA
Fried, Large, Sides	535
Fried, Reg, Sides	335

PICKLES
Fried, Large, Sides	667
Fried, Reg, Sides	476

POTATO SALAD
Large, Sides	900
Large Crowd, Sides	4800
Reg, Sides	300
Small Crowd, Sides	2400

SLIM CHICKENS

PUDDING

Chocolate Brownie, Jar	697
Chocolate Brownie, Platter, Large	5677
Chocolate Brownie, Platter, Small	2869

SALAD

Reg, No Dressing, Sides	65
Slim, with Fried Tenders	499
Slim, with Grilled Tenders	380
Spring Salad Tray, Lge Crowd	1494
Spring Salad Tray, Sm Crowd	825

SALAD DRESSING

Balsamic	90
Lite Italian	60
Raspberry Vinaigrette	195

SANDWICH

Chicken, Buffalo Ranch	685
Chicken, Cayenne Ranch	655
Chicken, Club	746
Chicken, Crispy	589

SAUCE

BBQ, Large	324
BBQ	81
Blue Cheese, Large	1080
Blue Cheese	270
Buffalo, Large	480
Buffalo	75
Cayenne Ranch, Large	653
Cayenne Ranch	163
Garlic Parmesan, Large	600
Garlic Parmesan	150
Gravy, Large	113
Gravy	57
Honey BBQ, Large	337
Honey BBQ	90
Honey Mustard, Large	755
Honey Mustard	195
Hot, Large	180
Hot	45
Inferno, Large	162
Inferno	30
Korean BBQ, Large	420
Korean BBQ	105
Mango Habanero, Large	300
Mango Habanero	75
Ranch, Lge	653
Ranch	163
Slim, Large	686
Slim	210
Spicy BBQ, Large	324
Spicy BBQ	81
Sriracha Garlic, Large	240
Sriracha Garlic	60
Sweet Red Chilli, Large	1080

SLIM CHICKENS

SAUCE

Sweet Red Chilli	120

SYRUP

Topping	300

TOAST

Texas, Buttered, Sides	104

WAFFLE

1	327

WRAP

Chicken, Tender, Fried, Buffalo	629
Chicken, Tender, Fried	596
Chicken, Tender, Grilled, Buffalo	549
Chicken, Tender, Grilled	516
Smokey Cheddar, with Fried Tender	693
Smokey Cheddar, with Grilled Tender	614

STARBUCKS

ALMONDS
Smoked	305

BANANA
Fairtrade	109

BARS
Granola	346
Peanut, & Cashew	209

BISCOTTI
Almond	201

BISCUIT
Ginger	133

BREAD
Banana	374
Ciabatta, Cheese, & Marmite, Mini	352

BREAKFAST CEREAL
Oatmeal, 5 Grain	225
Oatmeal, Classic	234

BROWNIES
Chocolate	334

CAKE
Carrot, Loaf	390
Lemon, Loaf	397

CHOCOLATE
Coin, Milk	120
Dark, Bar, 40g	221
Milk, Bar, 40g	223
Peanut Butter Cup	196

COFFEE - AMERICANO
Grande	16
Short	5
Tall	11
Venti	22

COFFEE - BLONDE LATTE
Vanilla, Almond Milk, Grande	137
Vanilla, Almond Milk, Short	58
Vanilla, Almond Milk, Tall	103
Vanilla, Almond Milk, Venti	180
Vanilla, Coconut Milk, Grande	204
Vanilla, Coconut Milk, Short	89
Vanilla, Coconut Milk, Tall	155
Vanilla, Coconut Milk, Venti	267
Vanilla, Oat Milk, Grande	248
Vanilla, Oat Milk, Short	110
Vanilla, Oat Milk, Tall	189
Vanilla, Oat Milk, Venti	323
Vanilla, Original Nut Blend, Grande	191
Vanilla, Original Nut Blend, Short	83
Vanilla, Original Nut Blend, Tall	145
Vanilla, Original Nut Blend, Venti	250
Vanilla, Semi Skimmed Milk, Grande	226
Vanilla, Semi Skimmed Milk, Short	99
Vanilla, Semi Skimmed Milk, Tall	171
Vanilla, Semi Skimmed Milk, Venti	294

STARBUCKS

COFFEE - BLONDE LATTE
Vanilla, Skimmed Milk, Grande	173
Vanilla, Skimmed Milk, Short	75
Vanilla, Skimmed Milk, Tall	131
Vanilla, Skimmed Milk, Venti	227
Vanilla, Soya Milk Milk, Grande	195
Vanilla, Soya Milk Milk, Short	85
Vanilla, Soya Milk Milk, Tall	147
Vanilla, Soya Milk Milk, Venti	254
Vanilla, Whole Milk, Grande	274
Vanilla, Whole Milk, Short	122
Vanilla, Whole Milk, Tall	209
Vanilla, Whole Milk, Venti	357

COFFEE - CAPPUCCINO
Almond Milk, Grande	74
Almond Milk, Short	35
Almond Milk, Tall	67
Almond Milk, Venti	104
Coconut Milk, Grande	127
Coconut Milk, Short	60
Coconut Milk, Tall	114
Coconut Milk, Venti	177
Oat Milk, Grande	161
Oat Milk, Short	76
Oat Milk, Tall	144
Oat Milk, Venti	225
Original Nut Blend, Grande	117
Original Nut Blend, Short	55
Original Nut Blend, Tall	105
Original Nut Blend, Venti	163
Semi Skimmed Milk, Grande	143
Semi Skimmed Milk, Short	68
Semi Skimmed Milk, Tall	129
Semi Skimmed Milk, Venti	201
Skimmed Milk, Grande	103
Skimmed Milk, Short	49
Skimmed Milk, Tall	93
Skimmed Milk, Venti	144
Soya Milk, Grande	119
Soya Milk, Short	56
Soya Milk, Tall	107
Soya Milk, Venti	167
Whole Milk, Grande	181
Whole Milk, Short	85
Whole Milk, Tall	163
Whole Milk, Venti	253

COFFEE - COLD BREW
Grande	1
Tall	1
Venti	1
Almond Milk, Grande	53
Almond Milk, Tall	40
Almond Milk, Venti	63

STARBUCKS

COFFEE - COLD BREW

	KCAL
Coconut Milk, Grande	97
Coconut Milk, Tall	73
Coconut Milk, Venti	115
Oat Milk, Grande	125
Oat Milk, Tall	95
Oat Milk, Venti	148
Original Nut Blend, Grande	89
Original Nut Blend, Tall	67
Original Nut Blend, Venti	105
Semi Skimmed Milk, Grande	110
Semi Skimmed Milk, Tall	83
Semi Skimmed Milk, Venti	130
Skimmed Milk, Grande	77
Skimmed Milk, Tall	58
Skimmed Milk, Venti	91
Soya Milk, Grande	91
Soya Milk, Tall	69
Soya Milk, Venti	107
Whole Milk, Grande	142
Whole Milk, Tall	108
Whole Milk, Venti	168

COFFEE - CORTADO

	KCAL
Almond Milk	34
Coconut Milk	53
Oat Milk	65
Original Nut Blend	49
Semi Skimmed Milk	59
Skimmed Milk	44
Soya Milk	50
Whole Milk	72

COFFEE - ESPRESSO

	KCAL
Con Panna, Doppio	80
Con Panna, Solo	64
Doppio	11
Macchiato, Almond Milk, Doppio	15
Macchiato, Almond Milk, Solo	7
Macchiato, Coconut Milk, Doppio	18
Macchiato, Coconut Milk, Solo	8
Macchiato, Oat Milk, Doppio	23
Macchiato, Oat Milk, Solo	8
Macchiato, Original Nut Blend, Doppio	17
Macchiato, Original Nut Blend, Solo	7
Macchiato, Semi Skimmed Milk, Doppio	19
Macchiato, Semi Skimmed Milk, Solo	7
Macchiato, Skimmed Milk, Doppio	16
Macchiato, Skimmed Milk, Solo	7
Macchiato, Soya Milk, Doppio	17
Macchiato, Soya Milk, Solo	8
Macchiato, Whole Milk, Doppio	21
Macchiato, Whole Milk, Solo	9
Solo	6

STARBUCKS

COFFEE - FILTER

	KCAL
Grande	3
Short	2
Tall	2
Venti	4

COFFEE - FLAT WHITE

	KCAL
Almond Milk, Short	47
Coconut Milk, Short	77
Oat Milk, Short	97
Original Nut Blend, Short	71
Semi Skimmed Milk, Short	87
Skimmed Milk, Short	63
Soya Milk, Short	73
Whole Milk, Short	108

COFFEE - ICED

	KCAL
DoubleShot, 10oz	26
DoubleShot, Vanilla, 10oz	97

COFFEE - ICED, AMERICANO

	KCAL
Grande	16
Tall	11
Venti	22

COFFEE - ICED, BLONDE LATTE

	KCAL
Vanilla, Almond Milk, Grande	65
Vanilla, Almond Milk, Tall	54
Vanilla, Almond Milk, Venti	78
Vanilla, Coconut Milk, Grande	111
Vanilla, Coconut Milk, Tall	90
Vanilla, Coconut Milk, Venti	130
Vanilla, Oat Milk, Grande	140
Vanilla, Oat Milk, Tall	114
Vanilla, Oat Milk, Venti	163
Vanilla, Semi Skimmed, Grande	125
Vanilla, Semi Skimmed, Tall	102
Vanilla, Semi Skimmed, Venti	146
Vanilla, Skimmed Milk, Grande	90
Vanilla, Skimmed Milk, Tall	74
Vanilla, Skimmed Milk, Venti	106
Vanilla, Soya Milk Milk, Grande	104
Vanilla, Soya Milk Milk, Tall	85
Vanilla, Soya Milk Milk, Venti	122
Vanilla, Whole Milk, Grande	158
Vanilla, Whole Milk, Tall	128
Vanilla, Whole Milk, Venti	183

COFFEE - ICED, CAPPUCCINO

	KCAL
Almond Milk, Grande	70
Almond Milk, Tall	58
Almond Milk, Venti	83
Coconut Milk, Grande	120
Coconut Milk, Tall	98
Coconut Milk, Venti	139
Oat Milk, Grande	152
Oat Milk, Tall	123
Oat Milk, Venti	175

STARBUCKS
COFFEE - ICED, CAPPUCCINO

Original Nut Blend, Grande	110
Original Nut Blend, Tall	90
Original Nut Blend, Venti	128
Semi Skimmed Milk, Grande	136
Semi Skimmed Milk, Tall	110
Semi Skimmed Milk, Venti	156
Skimmed Milk, Grande	97
Skimmed Milk, Tall	80
Skimmed Milk, Venti	113
Soya Milk, Grande	113
Soya Milk, Tall	92
Soya Milk, Venti	131
Whole Milk, Grande	171
Whole Milk, Tall	138
Whole Milk, Venti	196

COFFEE - ICED, LATTE

Almond Milk, Grande	65
Almond Milk, Tall	54
Almond Milk, Venti	78
Coconut Milk, Grande	111
Coconut Milk, Tall	90
Coconut Milk, Venti	130
Matcha Tea, Almond Milk, Grande	68
Matcha Tea, Almond Milk, Tall	53
Matcha Tea, Almond Milk, Venti	80
Matcha Tea, Coconut Milk, Grande	114
Matcha Tea, Coconut Milk, Tall	89
Matcha Tea, Coconut Milk, Venti	132
Matcha Tea, Oat Milk, Grande	143
Matcha Tea, Oat Milk, Tall	112
Matcha Tea, Oat Milk, Venti	165
Matcha Tea, Original Nut Blend, Grande	105
Matcha Tea, Original Nut Blend, Tall	82
Matcha Tea, Original Nut Blend, Venti	122
Matcha Tea, Semi Skimmed Milk, Grande	128
Matcha Tea, Semi Skimmed Milk, Tall	100
Matcha Tea, Semi Skimmed Milk, Venti	148
Matcha Tea, Skimmed Milk, Grande	93
Matcha Tea, Skimmed Milk, Tall	72
Matcha Tea, Skimmed Milk, Venti	108
Matcha Tea, Soya Milk, Grande	107
Matcha Tea, Soya Milk, Tall	83
Matcha Tea, Soya Milk, Venti	124
Matcha Tea, Whole Milk, Grande	161
Matcha Tea, Whole Milk, Tall	126
Matcha Tea, Whole Milk, Venti	185
Oat Milk, Grande	140
Oat Milk, Tall	114
Oat Milk, Venti	163
Original Nut Blend, Grande	102
Original Nut Blend, Tall	83
Original Nut Blend, Venti	120

STARBUCKS
COFFEE - ICED, LATTE

Semi Skimmed Milk, Grande	125
Semi Skimmed Milk, Tall	102
Semi Skimmed Milk, Venti	146
Skimmed Milk, Grande	90
Skimmed Milk, Tall	74
Skimmed Milk, Venti	106
Soya Milk, Grande	104
Soya Milk, Tall	85
Soya Milk, Venti	122
Whole Milk, Grande	158
Whole Milk, Tall	128
Whole Milk, Venti	183

COFFEE - ICED, MACCHIATO

Caramel Cloud, Grande	179
Caramel Cloud, Tall	139
Caramel Cloud, Venti	196
Caramel, Almond Milk, Grande	140
Caramel, Almond Milk, Tall	110
Caramel, Almond Milk, Venti	171
Caramel, Coconut Milk, Grande	182
Caramel, Coconut Milk, Tall	144
Caramel, Coconut Milk, Venti	219
Caramel, Oat Milk, Grande	212
Caramel, Oat Milk, Tall	167
Caramel, Oat Milk, Venti	252
Caramel, Original Nut Blend, Grande	173
Caramel, Original Nut Blend, Tall	137
Caramel, Original Nut Blend, Venti	209
Caramel, Semi Skimmed, Grande	199
Caramel, Semi Skimmed, Tall	157
Caramel, Semi Skimmed, Venti	239
Caramel, Skimmed Milk, Grande	164
Caramel, Skimmed Milk, Tall	129
Caramel, Skimmed Milk, Venti	199
Caramel, Soya Milk, Grande	178
Caramel, Soya Milk, Tall	141
Caramel, Soya Milk, Venti	215
Caramel, Whole Milk, Grande	232
Caramel, Whole Milk, Tall	183
Caramel, Whole Milk, Venti	276

COFFEE - LATTE

Almond Milk, Grande	92
Almond Milk, Short	43
Almond Milk, Tall	74
Almond Milk, Venti	121
Coconut Milk, Grande	158
Coconut Milk, Short	75
Coconut Milk, Tall	126
Coconut Milk, Venti	207
Macchiato, Almond Milk, Grande	78
Macchiato, Almond Milk, Short	34
Macchiato, Almond Milk, Tall	78

STARBUCKS
COFFEE - LATTE

	KCAL
Macchiato, Almond Milk, Venti	102
Macchiato, Coconut Milk, Grande	139
Macchiato, Coconut Milk, Short	65
Macchiato, Coconut Milk, Tall	112
Macchiato, Coconut Milk, Venti	169
Macchiato, Oat Milk, Grande	177
Macchiato, Oat Milk, Short	82
Macchiato, Oat Milk, Tall	142
Macchiato, Oat Milk, Venti	214
Macchiato, Original Nut Blend, Grande	128
Macchiato, Original Nut Blend, Short	59
Macchiato, Original Nut Blend, Tall	103
Macchiato, Original Nut Blend, Venti	156
Macchiato, Semi Skimmed Milk, Grande	132
Macchiato, Semi Skimmed Milk, Short	66
Macchiato, Semi Skimmed Milk, Tall	110
Macchiato, Semi Skimmed Milk, Venti	184
Macchiato, Skimmed Milk, Grande	94
Macchiato, Skimmed Milk, Short	47
Macchiato, Skimmed Milk, Tall	79
Macchiato, Skimmed Milk, Venti	133
Macchiato, Soya Milk, Grande	110
Macchiato, Soya Milk, Short	55
Macchiato, Soya Milk, Tall	92
Macchiato, Soya Milk, Venti	154
Macchiato, Whole Milk, Grande	166
Macchiato, Whole Milk, Short	83
Macchiato, Whole Milk, Tall	138
Macchiato, Whole Milk, Venti	232
Oat Milk, Grande	202
Oat Milk, Short	95
Oat Milk, Tall	160
Oat Milk, Venti	264
Original Nut Blend, Grande	146
Original Nut Blend, Short	69
Original Nut Blend, Tall	116
Original Nut Blend, Venti	191
Semi Skimmed Milk, Grande	180
Semi Skimmed Milk, Short	85
Semi Skimmed Milk, Tall	143
Semi Skimmed Milk, Venti	235
Skimmed Milk, Grande	128
Skimmed Milk, Short	60
Skimmed Milk, Tall	102
Skimmed Milk, Venti	168
Soya Milk, Grande	149
Soya Milk, Short	70
Soya Milk, Tall	119
Soya Milk, Venti	195
Vanilla, Almond Milk, Grande	164
Vanilla, Almond Milk, Short	79
Vanilla, Almond Milk, Tall	127

STARBUCKS
COFFEE - LATTE

	KCAL
Vanilla, Almond Milk, Venti	210
Vanilla, Coconut Milk, Grande	230
Vanilla, Coconut Milk, Short	110
Vanilla, Coconut Milk, Tall	179
Vanilla, Coconut Milk, Venti	296
Vanilla, Cold Brew, Grande	182
Vanilla, Cold Brew, Tall	137
Vanilla, Cold Brew, Venti	220
Vanilla, Oat Milk, Grande	164
Vanilla, Oat Milk, Short	131
Vanilla, Oat Milk, Tall	213
Vanilla, Oat Milk, Venti	210
Vanilla, Original Nut Blend, Grande	217
Vanilla, Original Nut Blend, Short	104
Vanilla, Original Nut Blend, Tall	169
Vanilla, Original Nut Blend, Venti	279
Vanilla, Semi Skimmed Milk, Grande	253
Vanilla, Semi Skimmed Milk, Short	121
Vanilla, Semi Skimmed Milk, Tall	196
Vanilla, Semi Skimmed Milk, Venti	324
Vanilla, Skimmed Milk, Grande	201
Vanilla, Skimmed Milk, Short	96
Vanilla, Skimmed Milk, Tall	155
Vanilla, Skimmed Milk, Venti	257
Vanilla, Soya Milk Milk, Grande	222
Vanilla, Soya Milk Milk, Short	106
Vanilla, Soya Milk Milk, Tall	172
Vanilla, Soya Milk Milk, Venti	284
Vanilla, Whole Milk, Grande	301
Vanilla, Whole Milk, Short	143
Vanilla, Whole Milk, Tall	233
Vanilla, Whole Milk, Venti	386
Whole Milk, Grande	228
Whole Milk, Short	108
Whole Milk, Tall	181
Whole Milk, Venti	298

COFFEE - MACCHIATO

	KCAL
Caramel, Almond Milk, Grande	155
Caramel, Almond Milk, Short	74
Caramel, Almond Milk, Tall	122
Caramel, Almond Milk, Venti	193
Caramel, Coconut Milk, Grande	210
Caramel, Coconut Milk, Short	100
Caramel, Coconut Milk, Tall	165
Caramel, Coconut Milk, Venti	259
Caramel, Oat Milk, Grande	248
Caramel, Oat Milk, Short	118
Caramel, Oat Milk, Tall	195
Caramel, Oat Milk, Venti	304
Caramel, Original Nut Blend, Grande	199
Caramel, Original Nut Blend, Short	95
Caramel, Original Nut Blend, Tall	157

STARBUCKS

COFFEE - MACCHIATO

Caramel, Original Nut Blend, Venti	245
Caramel, Semi Skimmed Milk, Grande	229
Caramel, Semi Skimmed Milk, Short	109
Caramel, Semi Skimmed Milk, Tall	180
Caramel, Semi Skimmed Milk, Venti	281
Caramel, Skimmed Milk, Grande	187
Caramel, Skimmed Milk, Short	89
Caramel, Skimmed Milk, Tall	146
Caramel, Skimmed Milk, Venti	231
Caramel, Soya Milk, Grande	205
Caramel, Soya Milk, Short	97
Caramel, Soya Milk, Tall	161
Caramel, Soya Milk, Venti	253
Caramel, Whole Milk, Grande	273
Caramel, Whole Milk, Short	129
Caramel, Whole Milk, Tall	215
Caramel, Whole Milk, Venti	335

COFFEE - MISTO

Almond Milk, Grande	48
Almond Milk, Short	24
Almond Milk, Tall	33
Almond Milk, Venti	64
Coconut Milk, Grande	86
Coconut Milk, Short	44
Coconut Milk, Tall	59
Coconut Milk, Venti	115
Oat Milk, Grande	111
Oat Milk, Short	56
Oat Milk, Tall	76
Oat Milk, Venti	149
Original Nut Blend, Grande	79
Original Nut Blend, Short	40
Original Nut Blend, Tall	54
Original Nut Blend, Venti	105
Semi Skimmed Milk, Grande	98
Semi Skimmed Milk, Short	50
Semi Skimmed Milk, Tall	67
Semi Skimmed Milk, Venti	132
Skimmed Milk, Grande	69
Skimmed Milk, Short	35
Skimmed Milk, Tall	47
Skimmed Milk, Venti	92
Soya Milk, Grande	81
Soya Milk, Short	41
Soya Milk, Tall	55
Soya Milk, Venti	108
Whole Milk, Grande	126
Whole Milk, Short	64
Whole Milk, Tall	86
Whole Milk, Venti	169

COFFEE - MOCHA

Almond Milk, Grande	225

STARBUCKS

COFFEE - MOCHA

Almond Milk, Short	128
Almond Milk, Tall	179
Almond Milk, Venti	256
Coconut Milk, Grande	263
Coconut Milk, Short	143
Coconut Milk, Tall	206
Coconut Milk, Venti	300
Oat Milk, Grande	333
Oat Milk, Short	174
Oat Milk, Tall	257
Oat Milk, Venti	383
Original Nut Blend, Grande	296
Original Nut Blend, Short	159
Original Nut Blend, Tall	231
Original Nut Blend, Venti	341
Semi Skimmed Milk, Grande	283
Semi Skimmed Milk, Short	151
Semi Skimmed Milk, Tall	220
Semi Skimmed Milk, Venti	322
Skimmed Milk, Grande	249
Skimmed Milk, Short	137
Skimmed Milk, Tall	196
Skimmed Milk, Venti	283
Soya Milk, Grande	263
Soya Milk, Short	143
Soya Milk, Tall	205
Soya Milk, Venti	299
Whole Milk, Grande	315
Whole Milk, Short	163
Whole Milk, Tall	242
Whole Milk, Venti	359
White Choc, Almond Milk, Grande	350
White Choc, Almond Milk, Short	188
White Choc, Almond Milk, Tall	276
White Choc, Almond Milk, Venti	426
White Choc, Coconut Milk, Grande	388
White Choc, Coconut Milk, Short	204
White Choc, Coconut Milk, Tall	306
White Choc, Coconut Milk, Venti	479
White Choc, Oat Milk, Grande	466
White Choc, Oat Milk, Short	235
White Choc, Oat Milk, Tall	369
White Choc, Oat Milk, Venti	588
White Choc, Original Nut Blend, Grande	388
White Choc, Original Nut Blend, Short	204
White Choc, Original Nut Blend, Tall	307
White Choc, Original Nut Blend, Venti	479
White Choc, Semi Skimmed Milk, Grande	408
White Choc, Semi Skimmed Milk, Short	212
White Choc, Semi Skimmed Milk, Tall	322
White Choc, Semi Skimmed Milk, Venti	507
White Choc, Skimmed Milk, Grande	374

STARBUCKS
COFFEE - MOCHA

White Choc, Skimmed Milk, Short	198
White Choc, Skimmed Milk, Tall	295
White Choc, Skimmed Milk, Venti	459
White Choc, Soya Milk, Grande	387
White Choc, Soya Milk, Short	203
White Choc, Soya Milk, Tall	306
White Choc, Soya Milk, Venti	478
White Choc, Whole Milk, Grande	440
White Choc, Whole Milk, Short	225
White Choc, Whole Milk, Tall	347
White Choc, Whole Milk, Venti	551

COFFEE - NITRO

Cappuccino, Skimmed Milk, 10oz	21
Cappuccino, Skimmed Milk, Grande	35
Cappuccino, Skimmed Milk, Tall	26
Cappuccino, Skimmed Milk, Venti	45
Cold Brew, Grande	2
Cold Brew, Mini	1
Cold Brew, Tall	1
Cold Brew, Venti	2
Latte, Grande	101
Latte, Mini	53
Latte, Tall	75
Latte, Venti	131

COOKIES

Chocolate, Milk, Chunk	361
Gingerbread, Iced, Bearista	183
Gingerbread, Iced, Latte	234
Straw	90

CRISPS

Kettle, Lightly Salted	205
Kettle, Mature Cheddar, & Red Onion	202
Kettle, Sea Salt, & Balsamic Vinegar	201
Kettle, Sweet Chilli, & Sour	202

CROISSANT

Almond	341
Butter	259
Ham & Cheese	463

DRINK

Refresha, Acai, Grande	86
Refresha, Acai, Tall	63
Refresha, Acai, Venti	108
Refresha, Cool Lime, Grande	80
Refresha, Cool Lime, Tall	61
Refresha, Cool Lime, Venti	100
Refresha, Pink Coconut, Grande	139
Refresha, Pink Coconut, Tall	104
Refresha, Pink Coconut, Venti	175

FRAPPUCCINO - ESPRESSO

No Whip, Almond Milk, Grande	129
No Whip, Almond Milk, Mini	65
No Whip, Almond Milk, Tall	90

STARBUCKS
FRAPPUCCINO - ESPRESSO

No Whip, Almond Milk, Venti	160
No Whip, Coconut Milk, Grande	147
No Whip, Coconut Milk, Mini	75
No Whip, Coconut Milk, Tall	104
No Whip, Coconut Milk, Venti	179
No Whip, Oat Milk, Grande	159
No Whip, Oat Milk, Mini	82
No Whip, Oat Milk, Tall	113
No Whip, Oat Milk, Venti	192
No Whip, Original Nut Blend, Grande	144
No Whip, Original Nut Blend, Mini	74
No Whip, Original Nut Blend, Tall	102
No Whip, Original Nut Blend, Venti	176
No Whip, Semi Skimmed Milk, Grande	153
No Whip, Semi Skimmed Milk, Mini	79
No Whip, Semi Skimmed Milk, Tall	109
No Whip, Semi Skimmed Milk, Venti	186
No Whip, Skimmed Milk, Grande	139
No Whip, Skimmed Milk, Mini	71
No Whip, Skimmed Milk, Tall	98
No Whip, Skimmed Milk, Venti	170
No Whip, Soya Milk, Grande	145
No Whip, Soya Milk, Mini	74
No Whip, Soya Milk, Tall	102
No Whip, Soya Milk, Venti	177
No Whip, Whole Milk, Grande	166
No Whip, Whole Milk, Mini	86
No Whip, Whole Milk, Tall	119
No Whip, Whole Milk, Venti	200

FRAPPUCCINO - JAVA CHIP

Whipped Cream, Almond Milk, Grande	357
Whipped Cream, Almond Milk, Mini	185
Whipped Cream, Almond Milk, Tall	256
Whipped Cream, Almond Milk, Venti	415
Whipped Cream, Coconut Milk, Grande	386
Whipped Cream, Coconut Milk, Mini	200
Whipped Cream, Coconut Milk, Tall	278
Whipped Cream, Coconut Milk, Venti	449
Whipped Cream, Oat Milk, Grande	398
Whipped Cream, Oat Milk, Mini	207
Whipped Cream, Oat Milk, Tall	288
Whipped Cream, Oat Milk, Venti	462
Whipped Cream, Semi Skimmed, Grande	382
Whipped Cream, Semi Skimmed, Mini	198
Whipped Cream, Semi Skimmed, Tall	276
Whipped Cream, Semi Skimmed, Venti	442
Whipped Cream, Skimmed Milk, Grande	367
Whipped Cream, Skimmed Milk, Mini	190
Whipped Cream, Skimmed Milk, Tall	264
Whipped Cream, Skimmed Milk, Venti	426
Whipped Cream, Soya Milk, Grande	373
Whipped Cream, Soya Milk, Mini	194

STARBUCKS

FRAPPUCCINO - JAVA CHIP

Whipped Cream, Soya Milk, Tall	269
Whipped Cream, Soya Milk, Venti	432
Whipped Cream, Whole Milk, Grande	395
Whipped Cream, Whole Milk, Mini	206
Whipped Cream, Whole Milk, Tall	286
Whipped Cream, Whole Milk, Venti	457

FRAPPUCCINO - MOCHA

Whipped Cream, Almond Milk, Grande	276
Whipped Cream, Almond Milk, Mini	148
Whipped Cream, Almond Milk, Tall	202
Whipped Cream, Almond Milk, Venti	323
Whipped Cream, Coconut Milk, Grande	295
Whipped Cream, Coconut Milk, Mini	159
Whipped Cream, Coconut Milk, Tall	218
Whipped Cream, Coconut Milk, Venti	345
Whipped Cream, Oat Milk, Grande	315
Whipped Cream, Oat Milk, Mini	170
Whipped Cream, Oat Milk, Tall	233
Whipped Cream, Oat Milk, Venti	370
Whipped Cream, Original Nut Blend, Grande	300
Whipped Cream, Original Nut Blend, Mini	161
Whipped Cream, Original Nut Blend, Tall	221
Whipped Cream, Original Nut Blend, Venti	352
Whipped Cream, Semi Skimmed, Grande	299
Whipped Cream, Semi Skimmed, Mini	161
Whipped Cream, Semi Skimmed, Tall	221
Whipped Cream, Semi Skimmed, Venti	350
Whipped Cream, Skimmed Milk, Grande	286
Whipped Cream, Skimmed Milk, Mini	154
Whipped Cream, Skimmed Milk, Tall	210
Whipped Cream, Skimmed Milk, Venti	334
Whipped Cream, Soya Milk, Grande	291
Whipped Cream, Soya Milk, Mini	157
Whipped Cream, Soya Milk, Tall	214
Whipped Cream, Soya Milk, Venti	340
Whipped Cream, Whole Milk, Grande	312
Whipped Cream, Whole Milk, Mini	169
Whipped Cream, Whole Milk, Tall	232
Whipped Cream, Whole Milk, Venti	364

HOT CHOCOLATE - CARAMEL

Whipped Cream, Almond Milk, Grande	486
Whipped Cream, Almond Milk, Short	302
Whipped Cream, Almond Milk, Tall	361
Whipped Cream, Almond Milk, Venti	633
Whipped Cream, Coconut Milk, Grande	522
Whipped Cream, Coconut Milk, Short	322
Whipped Cream, Coconut Milk, Tall	384
Whipped Cream, Coconut Milk, Venti	680
Whipped Cream, Oat Milk, Grande	546
Whipped Cream, Oat Milk, Short	335
Whipped Cream, Oat Milk, Tall	399
Whipped Cream, Oat Milk, Venti	711

STARBUCKS

HOT CHOCOLATE - CARAMEL

Whipped Cream, Original Nut, Grande	515
Whipped Cream, Original Nut, Short	318
Whipped Cream, Original Nut, Tall	380
Whipped Cream, Original Nut, Venti	671
Whipped Cream, Semi Skimmed, Grande	534
Whipped Cream, Semi Skimmed, Short	328
Whipped Cream, Semi Skimmed, Tall	392
Whipped Cream, Semi Skimmed, Venti	695
Whipped Cream, Skimmed Milk, Grande	506
Whipped Cream, Skimmed Milk, Short	313
Whipped Cream, Skimmed Milk, Tall	374
Whipped Cream, Skimmed Milk, Venti	659
Whipped Cream, Soya Milk, Grande	517
Whipped Cream, Soya Milk, Short	319
Whipped Cream, Soya Milk, Tall	381
Whipped Cream, Soya Milk, Venti	674
Whipped Cream, Whole Milk, Grande	560
Whipped Cream, Whole Milk, Short	343
Whipped Cream, Whole Milk, Tall	408
Whipped Cream, Whole Milk, Venti	729

HOT CHOCOLATE - CLASSIC

Whipped Cream, Almond Milk, Grande	221
Whipped Cream, Almond Milk, Short	127
Whipped Cream, Almond Milk, Tall	181
Whipped Cream, Almond Milk, Venti	263
Whipped Cream, Coconut Milk, Grande	301
Whipped Cream, Coconut Milk, Short	162
Whipped Cream, Coconut Milk, Tall	245
Whipped Cream, Coconut Milk, Venti	369
Whipped Cream, Oat Milk, Grande	332
Whipped Cream, Oat Milk, Short	175
Whipped Cream, Oat Milk, Tall	271
Whipped Cream, Oat Milk, Venti	411
Whipped Cream, Original Nut, Grande	292
Whipped Cream, Original Nut, Short	159
Whipped Cream, Original Nut, Tall	238
Whipped Cream, Original Nut, Venti	356
Whipped Cream, Semi Skimmed, Grande	284
Whipped Cream, Semi Skimmed, Short	152
Whipped Cream, Semi Skimmed, Tall	234
Whipped Cream, Semi Skimmed, Venti	350
Whipped Cream, Skimmed Milk, Grande	247
Whipped Cream, Skimmed Milk, Short	137
Whipped Cream, Skimmed Milk, Tall	203
Whipped Cream, Skimmed Milk, Venti	299
Whipped Cream, Soya Milk, Grande	262
Whipped Cream, Soya Milk, Short	143
Whipped Cream, Soya Milk, Tall	215
Whipped Cream, Soya Milk, Venti	319
Whipped Cream, Whole Milk, Grande	318
Whipped Cream, Whole Milk, Short	167
Whipped Cream, Whole Milk, Tall	262

STARBUCKS

HOT CHOCOLATE - CLASSIC

Whipped Cream, Whole Milk, Venti	397

HOT CHOCOLATE - HAZELNUT

Whipped Cream, Almond Milk, Grande	464
Whipped Cream, Almond Milk, Short	285
Whipped Cream, Almond Milk, Tall	341
Whipped Cream, Almond Milk, Venti	609
Whipped Cream, Coconut Milk, Grande	500
Whipped Cream, Coconut Milk, Short	305
Whipped Cream, Coconut Milk, Tall	365
Whipped Cream, Coconut Milk, Venti	656
Whipped Cream, Oat Milk, Grande	524
Whipped Cream, Oat Milk, Tall	380
Whipped Cream, Semi Skimmed, Tall	372
Whipped Cream, Whole Milk, Venti	705
Whipped Cream, Oat Milk, Short	318
Whipped Cream, Oat Milk, Venti	687
Whipped Cream, Semi Skimmed, Grande	512
Whipped Cream, Semi Skimmed, Short	311
Whipped Cream, Semi Skimmed, Venti	671
Whipped Cream, Skimmed Milk, Grande	484
Whipped Cream, Skimmed Milk, Short	295
Whipped Cream, Skimmed Milk, Tall	354
Whipped Cream, Skimmed Milk, Venti	634
Whipped Cream, Soya Milk, Grande	495
Whipped Cream, Soya Milk, Short	302
Whipped Cream, Soya Milk, Tall	361
Whipped Cream, Soya Milk, Venti	649
Whipped Cream, Whole Milk, Grande	538
Whipped Cream, Whole Milk, Short	325
Whipped Cream, Whole Milk, Tall	389

HOT CHOCOLATE - SIGNATURE

Whipped Cream, Almond Milk, Grande	383
Whipped Cream, Almond Milk, Short	242
Whipped Cream, Almond Milk, Tall	280
Whipped Cream, Almond Milk, Venti	509
Whipped Cream, Coconut Milk, Grande	415
Whipped Cream, Coconut Milk, Short	259
Whipped Cream, Coconut Milk, Tall	300
Whipped Cream, Coconut Milk, Venti	550
Whipped Cream, Oat Milk, Grande	479
Whipped Cream, Oat Milk, Short	294
Whipped Cream, Oat Milk, Tall	341
Whipped Cream, Oat Milk, Venti	634
Whipped Cream, Semi Skimmed, Grande	431
Whipped Cream, Semi Skimmed, Short	268
Whipped Cream, Semi Skimmed, Tall	310
Whipped Cream, Semi Skimmed, Venti	571
Whipped Cream, Skimmed Milk, Grande	403
Whipped Cream, Skimmed Milk, Short	253
Whipped Cream, Skimmed Milk, Tall	292
Whipped Cream, Skimmed Milk, Venti	535
Whipped Cream, Soya Milk, Grande	414

STARBUCKS

HOT CHOCOLATE - SIGNATURE

Whipped Cream, Soya Milk, Short	259
Whipped Cream, Soya Milk, Tall	299
Whipped Cream, Soya Milk, Venti	550
Whipped Cream, Whole Milk, Grande	457
Whipped Cream, Whole Milk, Short	282
Whipped Cream, Whole Milk, Tall	327
Whipped Cream, Whole Milk, Venti	605

MUFFIN

Blueberry	414
Chocolate, Triple	468
Lemon	428

NUT MIX

Almonds, Cashews, Cranberries, & Raisins	233

PAIN AU CHOCOLAT

Pastry	314

PANINI

Ham, & Cheese, GF	349
Ham, & Cheese	446
Tomato, & Mozzarella	442
Tuna Melt	450

PASTRY

Cinnamon Swirl	479
Twist, Chocolate	274

ROLL

Bacon, Smoked	334

SANDWICH

Beyond Meat, Breakfast	425
Breakfast, Signature	401
Egg Mayonnaise, Free Range	499
Sausage	513

SHORTBREAD

Chocolate Caramel	390
Chocolate Chunk, Fairtrade	445
Biscuit	271

TEA - CHAI

Grande	0
Latte, Almond Milk, Grande	186
Latte, Almond Milk, Short	92
Latte, Almond Milk, Tall	143
Latte, Almond Milk, Venti	241
Latte, Coconut Milk, Grande	227
Latte, Coconut Milk, Short	111
Latte, Coconut Milk, Tall	175
Latte, Coconut Milk, Venti	297
Latte, Oat Milk, Grande	253
Latte, Oat Milk, Short	124
Latte, Oat Milk, Tall	195
Latte, Oat Milk, Venti	333
Latte, Original Nut Blend, Grande	219
Latte, Original Nut Blend, Short	108
Latte, Original Nut Blend, Tall	168
Latte, Original Nut Blend, Venti	286

STARBUCKS

TEA - CHAI

Latte, Semi Skimmed Milk, Grande	239
Latte, Semi Skimmed Milk, Short	117
Latte, Semi Skimmed Milk, Tall	185
Latte, Semi Skimmed Milk, Venti	315
Latte, Skimmed Milk, Grande	208
Latte, Skimmed Milk, Short	103
Latte, Skimmed Milk, Tall	160
Latte, Skimmed Milk, Venti	271
Latte, Soya Milk, Grande	220
Latte, Soya Milk, Short	109
Latte, Soya Milk, Tall	170
Latte, Soya Milk, Venti	289
Latte, Whole Milk, Grande	268
Latte, Whole Milk, Short	131
Latte, Whole Milk, Tall	208
Latte, Whole Milk, Venti	355
Short	0
Tall	0
Venti	0

TEA - CHAMOMILE

Grande	0
Short	0
Tall	0
Venti	0

TEA - EARL GREY

Grande	0
Short	0
Tall	0
Venti	0

TEA - EMPEROR'S CLOUD & MIST

Short	0
Grande	0
Tall	0
Venti	0

TEA - ENGLISH BREAKFAST

Grande	0
Short	0
Tall	0
Venti	0

TEA - HIBISCUS

Grande	0
Short	0
Tall	0
Venti	0

TEA - ICED, BLACK

Black, Grande	0
Black, Tall	0
Black, Venti	0

TEA - ICED, CHAI

Latte, Almond Milk, Grande	109
Latte, Almond Milk, Tall	84
Latte, Almond Milk, Venti	141

STARBUCKS

TEA - ICED, CHAI

Latte, Coconut Milk, Grande	143
Latte, Coconut Milk, Tall	111
Latte, Coconut Milk, Venti	186
Latte, Oat Milk, Grande	164
Latte, Oat Milk, Tall	129
Latte, Oat Milk, Venti	215
Latte, Original Nut Blend, Grande	136
Latte, Original Nut Blend, Tall	106
Latte, Original Nut Blend, Venti	177
Latte, Semi Skimmed Milk, Grande	153
Latte, Semi Skimmed Milk, Tall	120
Latte, Semi Skimmed Milk, Venti	200
Latte, Skimmed Milk, Grande	127
Latte, Skimmed Milk, Tall	99
Latte, Skimmed Milk, Venti	165
Latte, Soya Milk, Grande	138
Latte, Soya Milk, Tall	107
Latte, Soya Milk, Venti	180
Latte, Whole Milk, Grande	177
Latte, Whole Milk, Tall	139
Latte, Whole Milk, Venti	233

TEA - ICED, GREEN

Grande	0
Tall	0
Venti	0

TEA - ICED, HIBISCUS

Shaken, Grande	0
Shaken, Tall	0
Shaken, Venti	0

TEA - ICED, JASMINE PEARLS

Grande	0
Short	0
Tall	0
Venti	0

TEA - ICED, LEMON

Grande	74
Tall	54
Venti	94

TEA - ICED, LEMONADE

Black Tea, Shaken, Grande	46
Black Tea, Shaken, Tall	35
Black Tea, Shaken, Venti	56
Green Tea, Shaken, Grande	46
Green Tea, Shaken, Tall	35
Green Tea, Shaken, Venti	56

TEA - ICED, PEACH

Grande	75
Tall	54
Venti	95

TEA - MATCHA

Latte, Almond Milk, Grande	96
Latte, Almond Milk, Short	45

STARBUCKS
TEA - MATCHA

Latte, Almond Milk, Tall	73
Latte, Almond Milk, Venti	125
Latte, Coconut Milk, Grande	164
Latte, Coconut Milk, Short	79
Latte, Coconut Milk, Tall	127
Latte, Coconut Milk, Venti	214
Latte, Oat Milk, Grande	208
Latte, Oat Milk, Short	100
Latte, Oat Milk, Tall	161
Latte, Oat Milk, Venti	272
Latte, Original Nut Blend, Grande	151
Latte, Original Nut Blend, Short	72
Latte, Original Nut Blend, Tall	116
Latte, Original Nut Blend, Venti	197
Latte, Semi Skimmed Milk, Grande	186
Latte, Semi Skimmed Milk, Short	89
Latte, Semi Skimmed Milk, Tall	144
Latte, Semi Skimmed Milk, Venti	242
Latte, Skimmed Milk, Grande	133
Latte, Skimmed Milk, Short	63
Latte, Skimmed Milk, Tall	102
Latte, Skimmed Milk, Venti	174
Latte, Soya Milk, Grande	154
Latte, Soya Milk, Short	74
Latte, Soya Milk, Tall	119
Latte, Soya Milk, Venti	201
Latte, Whole Milk, Grande	235
Latte, Whole Milk, Short	113
Latte, Whole Milk, Tall	182
Latte, Whole Milk, Venti	306

TEA - MINT BLEND

Grande	0
Short	0
Tall	0
Venti	0

TEA - MINT CITRUS

Green Tea, Grande	0
Green Tea, Short	0
Green Tea, Tall	0
Green Tea, Venti	0

TEA - YOUTHBERRY

Grande	0
Short	0
Tall	0
Venti	0

TOAST

Fruit, Luxury	452

TOASTIE

Cheese, Five	386
Ham, Hickory, & Cheese	487

WAFFLES

Caramel, Duos	176

STARBUCKS
WAFFLES

Caramel, Mini	144

YOGHURT

Berry Crunch, Pot	262

SUBWAY

BREAD
Garlic, Cheesy, Sides	400

COOKIES
Chocolate Chunk	214
Double Chocolate	210
Oatmeal Raisin	195
Rainbow Candy Chip	215
Vegan, Double Chocolate	220
White Chip Macadamia Nut	215

DOUGHNUTS
Chocolate	270
Sugared	217

HASH BROWNS
& Bacon, Super SubStack, Add On	113
Sides	153
SubStack, Add On	77

MEATBALLS
Bowl, Sides	290
Meatless, Bowl Sides	212

MUFFIN
Cadburys Caramel	480
Nutella	481
Oreo	485

NACHOS
Flamin' Hot, with Salsa, Cheese, & Jalapenos, Sides	441
Doritos, with Salsa, Cheese, & Jalapenos, Sides	425

SALAD
B.L.T., without Dressing	112
Cheesy Pepperoni, without Dressing	214
Chicken, & Bacon, with Cheese, without Dressing	242
Chicken, Breast, without Dressing	123
Chicken, Pizziola, without Dressing	265
Chicken, Rotisserie-Style, without Dressing	147
Chicken, Teriyaki, without Dressing	141
Chicken, Thai, without Dressing	153
Chicken Tikka, without Dressing	127
Ham, without Dressing	106
Italian B.M.T., without Dressing	218
Meatball, Marinara, without Dressing	314
Meatless Meatball Marinara, without Dressing	222
Mega Meat, without Dressing	434
Plant Patty, without Dressing	189
Spicy Italian, without Dressing	281
Steak, & Cheese, without Dressing	175
Subway Melt, with Cheese, without Dressing	190
T.L.C, without Dressing	147
Tuna, without Dressing	182
Tuna Nicoise, without Dressing	244
Turkey Breast, & Ham, without Dressing	110
Turkey Breast, without Dressing	94
Veggie Delite, without Dressing	38

SANDWICH
Cheese, Toasted, Bite, Roll, Sides	151

SUBWAY

SANDWICH
Ham, & Cheese, Toasted, Bite, Roll, Sides	117
Steak, & Cheese, Toasted, Bite, Roll, Sides	102
Tuna Melt, Toasted, Bite, Roll, Sides	131

SAUCE
Barbecue	39
Chilli, Hot	48
Chilli, Sweet	46
Chipotle Southwest	90
Deli Mustard	23
Honey Mustard	32
Ketchup	22
Mayonnaise, Lite	50
Ranch	43
Sriracha	27
Sweet Onion	34

SAUSAGE
Pigs in Blankets, Hot Pot	191

SUB
Bacon, 9 Grain Multi-Seed, Breakfast	370
Bacon, 9 Grain Wheat, Breakfast	285
Bacon, Egg, & Cheese, 9 Grain Multi-Seed, Breakfast	378
Bacon, Egg, & Cheese, 9 Grain Wheat, Breakfast	339
Bacon, Egg, & Cheese, GF Bread, Breakfast	390
Bacon, Egg, & Cheese, Hearty Italian, Breakfast	313
Bacon, Egg, & Cheese, Herbs & Cheese, Breakfast	317
Bacon, Egg, & Cheese, Italian White, Breakfast	284
Bacon, GF Bread, Standard	382
Bacon, Hearty Italian, Breakfast	305
Bacon, Italian Herbs & Cheese, Breakfast	309
Bacon, Italian White, Breakfast	276
Cheesy Pepperoni, 9 Grain Multi-Seed	386
Cheesy Pepperoni, 9 Grain Wheat	302
Cheesy Pepperoni, GF Bread	399
Cheesy Pepperoni, Hearty Italian	322
Cheesy Pepperoni, Italian Herbs & Cheese	326
Cheesy Pepperoni, Italian White	292
Chicken, Teriyaki, Italian Herbs & Cheese	240
Chicken, Teriyaki, Italian White	207
Chicken, Tikka, Hearty Italian	325
Chicken, Tikka, Italian Herbs & Cheese	330
Chicken, Tikka, Italian White	296
Chicken & Bacon, 9 Grain Multi-Seed	423
Chicken & Bacon, 9 Grain Wheat	338
Chicken & Bacon, GF Bread	435
Chicken & Bacon, Hearty Italian	358
Chicken & Bacon, Italian Herbs & Cheese	363
Chicken & Bacon, Italian White	329
Chicken Teriyaki, 9 Grain Multi-Seed	301
Chicken Teriyaki, 9 Grain Wheat	216
Chicken Teriyaki, GF Bread	313
Chicken Teriyaki, Hearty Italian	236
Chicken Tikka, 9 Grain Multi-Seed	390

SUBWAY
SUB

	KCAL
Chicken Tikka, 9 Grain Wheat	306
Chicken Tikka, GF	402
Egg, & Cheese, 9 Grain Multi-Seed, Breakfast	343
Egg, & Cheese, 9 Grain Wheat, Breakfast	259
Egg, & Cheese, GF Bread, Breakfast	355
Egg, & Cheese, Hearty Italian, Breakfast	278
Egg, & Cheese, Italian Herbs & Cheese, Breakfast	283
Egg, & Cheese, Italian White, Breakfast	249
Ham, 9 Grain Multi-Seed	369
Ham, 9 Grain Wheat	285
Ham, GF Bread	381
Ham, Hearty Italian	304
Ham, Italian Herbs & Cheese	309
Ham, Italian White	275
Italian BMT, 9 Grain Multi-Seed	481
Italian BMT, 9 Grain Wheat	396
Italian BMT, GF Bread	493
Italian BMT, Hearty Italian	416
Italian BMT, Italian Herbs & Cheese	420
Italian BMT, Italian White	387
Meatball Marinara, 9 Grain Multi-Seed	576
Meatball Marinara, 9 Grain Wheat	492
Meatball Marinara, GF Bread	588
Meatball Marinara, Hearty Italian	511
Meatball Marinara, Italian Herbs & Cheese	516
Meatball Marinara, Italian White	482
Meatless Meatball Marinara, 9 Grain Multi-Seed	329
Meatless Meatball Marinara, 9 Grain Wheat	400
Meatless Meatball Marinara, GF Bread	341
Meatless Meatball Marinara, Hearty Italian	264
Meatless Meatball Marinara, Italian Herbs & Cheese	269
Meatless Meatball Marinara, Italian White	235
Mega Meat, 9 Grain Multi-Seed	697
Mega Meat, 9 Grain Wheat	612
Mega Meat, GF Bread	709
Mega Meat, Hearty Italian	632
Mega Meat, Italian Herbs & Cheese	636
Mega Meat, Italian White Bread, Standard	603
Mega Melt, 9 Grain Multi-Seed, Breakfast	555
Mega Melt, 9 Grain Wheat, Breakfast	470
Mega Melt, GF Bread, Breakfast	567
Mega Melt, Hearty Italian, Breakfast	490
Mega Melt, Italian Herbs & Cheese, Breakfast	494
Mega Melt, Italian White, Breakfast	461
Plant Patty, 9 Grain Multi-Seed	301
Plant Patty, 9 Grain Wheat	368
Plant Patty, GF Bread	313
Plant Patty, Hearty Italian	236
Plant Patty, Italian Herbs & Cheese	240
Plant Patty, Italian White	207
Roast Chicken Breast, 9 Grain Multi-Seed	386
Roast Chicken Breast, 9 Grain Wheat	301

SUBWAY
SUB

	KCAL
Roast Chicken Breast, GF Bread	398
Roast Chicken Breast, Hearty Italian	321
Roast Chicken Breast, Italian Herbs & Cheese	326
Roast Chicken Breast, Italian White	292
Sausage, 9 Grain Multi-Seed, Breakfast	478
Sausage, 9 Grain Wheat, Breakfast	393
Sausage, Egg, & Cheese, 9 Grain Multi-Seed	582
Sausage, Egg, & Cheese, 9 Grain Wheat	498
Sausage, Egg, & Cheese, GF Bread	594
Sausage, Egg, & Cheese, Hearty Italian	517
Sausage, Egg, & Cheese, Italian Herbs & Cheese	522
Sausage, Egg, & Cheese, Italian White	488
Sausage, GF Bread, Breakfast	490
Sausage, Hearty Italian, Breakfast	413
Sausage, Italian Herbs & Cheese, Breakfast	417
Sausage, Italian White, Breakfast	384
Spicy Italian, 9 Grain Multi-Seed	544
Spicy Italian, 9 Grain Wheat	459
Spicy Italian, GF Bread	556
Spicy Italian, Hearty Italian	479
Spicy Italian, Italian Herbs & Cheese	483
Spicy Italian, Italian White	450
Steak & Cheese, 9 Grain Multi-Seed	437
Steak & Cheese, 9 Grain Wheat	352
Steak & Cheese, GF Bread	449
Steak & Cheese, Hearty Italian	372
Steak & Cheese, Italian Herbs & Cheese	376
Steak & Cheese, Italian White	343
T.L.C., 9 Grain Wheat	216
T.L.C., GF Bread	313
T.L.C., Hearty Italian	236
T.L.C., Italian Herbs & Cheese	240
T.L.C., Italian White	207
Tiger Pig, Standard	416
Tuna, 9 Grain Multi-Seed	445
Tuna, 9 Grain Wheat	360
Tuna, GF Bread	457
Tuna, Hearty Italian	380
Tuna, Italian Herbs & Cheese	384
Tuna, Italian White	351
Turkey Breast, 9 Grain Multi-Seed	357
Turkey Breast, 9 Grain Wheat	273
Turkey Breast, GF Bread	369
Turkey Breast, Hearty Italian	292
Turkey Breast, Italian Herbs & Cheese	297
Turkey Breast, Italian White	263
Turkey Breast & Ham, 9 Grain Multi-Seed	372
Turkey Breast & Ham, 9 Grain Wheat	288
Turkey Breast & Ham, GF Bread	385
Turkey Breast & Ham, Hearty Italian	308
Turkey Breast & Ham, Italian Herbs & Cheese	312
Turkey Breast & Ham, Italian White	278

SUBWAY

SUB

Veggie Delite, 9 Grain Multi-Seed	301
Veggie Delite, 9 Grain Wheat	216
Veggie Delite, GF Bread	313
Veggie Delite, Hearty Italian	236
Veggie Delite, Italian Herbs & Cheese	240
Veggie Delite, Italian White	207

WRAP

B.L.T., Standard	305
Bacon, Breakfast	300
Bacon, Omelette, & Cheese, Breakfast	354
Bacon, Poached Egg, & Cheese, Breakfast	370
Cheesy Pepperoni, Standard	407
Chicken, & Bacon, Standard	398
Chicken, Breast, Standard	316
Chicken, Rotisserie-Style, Standard	340
Chicken, Teriyaki, Standard	334
Chicken, Tikka, Standard	321
Ham, Standard	300
Italian B.M.T, Standard	411
Meatless Meatball Marinara, Standard	415
Mega Meat, Standard	627
Mega Melt, with Omelette, Breakfast	531
Mega Melt, with Poached Egg, Breakfast	547
Nacho Chicken, Standard	401
Omelette, & Cheese, Breakfast	319
Plant Patty, Standard	382
Poached Egg, & Cheese, Breakfast	336
Sausage, & Bacon, Breakfast	443
Sausage, Breakfast	408
Sausage, Omelette, & Cheese, Breakfast	496
Sausage, Poached Egg, & Cheese, Breakfast	513
Spicy Italian, Standard	474
Steak & Cheese, Standard	367
Subway Melt, Standard	382
T.L.C., Standard	340
Tiger Pig, Standard	422
Tuna, Standard	375
Turkey Breast, & Ham, Standard	303
Turkey Breast, Standard	288
Veggie Delite, Standard	231

TABLE TABLE

BACON

Back, Cooked, Breakfast	49

BAGEL

Cinnamon, & Raisin, Breakfast	293

BEANS

Baked, in Tomato Sauce, Breakfast	91

BEEF

Roast, Dinner, Kids Menu	671
Steak, Rib-eye, 10oz	1033
Steak, Rump, 8oz, with Chips	835
Steak, Rump, 8oz, with Salad	550
Steak, Rump, 8oz, with Skinny Fries, Value Menu	675
Steak, Sirloin, 8oz, & Prawns, King, Surf & Turf	1108
Steak, Sirloin, 8oz, with Chips	847
Steak, Sirloin, 8oz, with Salad	563
Roast, Topside, Dinner	1398

BLACK PUDDING

Slice, Breakfast	122

BREAD

Garlic, Flatbread, Side	306
Garlic, Flatbread, with BBQ Dip	492
Garlic, Flatbread, with Cheese, Side	456
Garlic, Flatbread, with Tomato Dip	496
Garlic, Side, Kids Menu	109
Garlic, Starter, Kids Menu	112

BROCCOLI

Tenderstem, Side	139

BROWNIES

Chocolate, Triple	666
Chocolate, Warm, Value Menu	523

BUBBLE & SQUEAK

Breakfast	169

BURGERS

Beef, with Chips, Kids Menu	619
Chicken, & Avocado	1121
Chicken, with Jacket Potato, & Beans	453
Lamb, & Feta	1015
Mac & Cheese	1380
Mac & Cheese, Value Menu	822
Sloppy Joe	1073
Steak, with Cheese, & Bacon, Double Stack	1308
Steak, with Cheese, Double Stack	1245
Steak, with Cheese, Value Menu	952
Surf & Turf	1471

BUTTER

Salted, Portion, Breakfast	48

CAKE

Chocolate, Fudge, Sensation	810
Lemon, Drizzle	144

CAULIFLOWER CHEESE

Sunday Roast	283

CHEESE

Camembert, Baked, Starter	622

TABLE TABLE

CHEESECAKE

Baked	551
Strawberry, Mini	223

CHICKEN

Breast, Pancetta, Wrapped, & Mozzarella Stuffed	947
Breast, Topped, Bacon & Cheese, with Chips	747
Breast, Topped, Bacon & Cheese, with Jacket Potato	760
Escalope	1357
Forestiere	713
Goujons, Buttermilk, & Rosemary, Starter	407
Half, Roast, Dinner	1458
Paprika, Value Menu	525
Poppin, with Chips, & Beans, Kids Menu	394
Roast, Kids Menu	581
Wings, BBQ, Starter	304

CHIPS

Side, Kids Menu	181
Side	363

COD

Bites, Breaded, Kids Menu	507

CORN

Cob, Side, Kids Menu	79

CROISSANT

Breakfast	161

CRUMBLE

Apple, Bramley, & Blackberry	633

CRUMPETS

Sourdough, Breakfast	91

CURRY

Chicken, Kids Menu	444
Chicken, Makhani	934

DOUGHNUTS

Mini, Kids Menu	203

DRIED FRUIT MIX

Breakfast	308

EGGS

Boiled, Single, Breakfast	82
Fried, Single, Breakfast	108
Poached, Single, Breakfast	79
Scrambled, Breakfast	269

FISH & CHIPS

Battered, with Peas, Value Menu	909
Haddock, Hand Battered, with Peas, Value Menu	1087

FRIES

Dirty, Side	516
Halloumi, Side	586
Skinny Cut, Side	328
Sweet Potato, Side	290
Tiger, Side	353

FRUIT SALAD

Breakfast	49
Kids Menu	49

TABLE TABLE

GAMMON

Steak, with Chips, & Egg, Value Menu	769
Steak, with Chips, & Eggs	877
Steak, with Chips, & Pineapple	953
Steak, with Chips, & Pineapple, Value Menu	699
Steak, with Chips, Egg, & Pineapple	807
Steak, with Jacket Potato, & Eggs	890
Steak, with Jacket Potato, & Pineapple	751
Steak, with Jacket Potato, Egg, & Pineapple	820

HADDOCK

Beer Battered, & Chips, with Mushy Peas	1125
Beer Battered, & Chips, with Peas	1087

HAM

Egg, & Chips, Dayime Value Menu	857

HASH BROWNS

Single, Breakfast	94

HONEY

Breakfast	65

ICE CREAM

Dairy, with Caramel Sauce	277
Dairy, with Chocolate Sauce	276
Dairy, with Raspberry Sauce	273
Vanilla, with Caramel Sauce, Kids Menu	199
Vanilla, with Chocolate Sauce, Kids Menu	199
Vanilla, with Raspberry Sauce, Kids Menu	197

JAM

Strawberry, Breakfast	33

LAMB

Rump	631

LASAGNE

Beef, & Pork, Value Menu	577
Beef, Luxury	949
Sweet Potato, & Feta	704
Sweet Potato, & Feta, Value Menu	608

MEATBALLS

Chicken, Kids Menu	177

MIXED GRILL

Table Table	1205
Table Table, with Rump Steak, 8oz	1355

MUFFIN

Blueberry, Breakfast	114

MUSHROOMS

Breaded, Garlic & Herb	314
with Butter, Breakfast	161

NACHOS

Loaded, Sharing	1175
Loaded, Starter	614

OMELETTE

Breakfast	404

ONION RINGS

Battered, Beer, Side	210

PAIN AU CHOCOLAT

Mini, Breakfast	172

TABLE TABLE

PAIN AU RAISIN
Mini, Breakfast	128

PANCAKE
Kids Menu	218
Reduced Sugar, Breakfast	96

PASTA
Penne, Tomato Sauce, Kids Menu	359
Tomato, with Chicken Meatballs	525

PATE
Chicken, & Pork, Starter	392

PAVLOVA
Mixed Berry	137

PEAS
Side, Kids Menu	47

PIE
Apple, Caramel, with Custard, Value Menu	475
Beef, & Doom Bar	1175
Chicken, & Mushroom	1121
Chicken, & Chorizo	551
Chicken, & Ham, Value Menu	1061
Cottage, Luxury	710
Fake, & Ale, Vegan, Sunday Roast	1708
Fake, & Ale, Vegan	837
Fish, Luxury	765

PLATTER
Fish & Chip Shop	1240
Sharing	2102
Sharing, with Chicken Wings	2285

PORK
Roast, Kids Menu	761

PORK DINNER
Loin, Roast	1508

POTATOES
Dippers, with Cheese, & Bacon, Starter	401
Jacket, Mini, Side, Kids Menu	155
Jacket, with Cheese, & Beans, Value Menu	758
Mashed, Side, Kids Menu	131

PRAWN COCKTAIL
Classic, Starter	462

PUDDING
Chocolate, Fondant, Warm	578
Sticky Toffee	720

RIBS
Whole Rack, & Smoky Paprika Chicken	1380
½ Rack, & Smoky Paprika Chicken	988

RICE
Brown, Side, Kids Menu	192

SALAD
Bacon, & Blue Cheese	387
Chicken, Grilled	233
Halloumi, Grilled	360
Mixed, Side, Kids Menu	23
Mixed, Side	39

TABLE TABLE

SANDWICH
Chicken, & Bacon, Club, Open, Value Menu	835

SAUCE
Bearnaise	122
Diane	73
Peppercorn, Creamy	29

SAUSAGE
Breakfast	114
Quorn*, Breakfast	78

SAUSAGE & MASH
Bangers, Kids Menu	402
Vegetarian, Bangers, Kids Menu	354

SCAMPI
Breaded, & Chips, with Mushy Peas	828
Breaded, & Chips, with Peas	790

SORBET
Coconut	233

SOUP
Broccoli	255
Carrot, & Coriander	261
Leek, & Potato	312
Mushroom, Cream Of	291

SPAGHETTI BOLOGNAISE
Kids Menu	322

SPREAD
Sunflower, Portion, Breakfast	43

SQUID
Calamari, with Sweet Chilli, Starter	438

SUNDAE
Chocolate, Churros	748
Chocolate, with Kit Kat	526
Chocolate Browne, Mini, Value Menu	277
Funny Face, Kids Menu	196

SYRUP
Maple, Breakfastr	62

TART
Lemon	450

TOAST
GF, Breakfast	84
Malted, Breakfast	92
White, Breakfast	92

TOMATOES
Half, Breakfast	9

TORTE
Chocolate, Greek Yoghurt, Mini	295

VEGETABLES
Green, Side	112
Sticks, Side, Kids Menu	26
Sticks, Starter, Kids Menu	48

YOGHURT
Greek Style	87
Strawberry, Frozen, Kids Menu	142
Strawberry, Kids Menu	115

TABLE TABLE

YOGHURT
	KCAL
Strawberry	115
Vanilla	96

THE REAL GREEK FOOD COMPANY LTD

ASPARAGUS
	KCAL
Grilled, Hot Meze	140

CHEESE
Halloumi, Grilled, Hot Meze	151
Halloumi, Skewers, Hot Meze	118
Halloumi, Skewers, Kids Menu	118

CHICK PEAS
Revithia, Cold Meze	286

CHICKEN
Skewers, Hot Meze	177
Skewers, Kids Menu	88

CHIPS
Side	528

COD
Salt, Hot Meze	346

CRUDITES
Cold Meze	37

DESSERT
Watermelon, Sweet & Salty	124
Yoghurt, Greek with Raspberries	223

DIP
Aioli, Parsley	176
Dip, Selection	589
Mayonnaise, Lemon, Preserved	279
Melitzanasalata, Cold Meze	236
Relish, Chilli, Smoked	42
Relish, Sun-Dried Tomato & Roast Red Pepper	92

DOLMADES
Cold Meze	254

FLATBREAD
Greek, Cold Meze	615
Greek, with Olive & Dukkah, Nibbles	538

HOUMOUS
Cold Meze	298

LAMB
Cutlets, Hot Meze	881
Kefte, Hot Meze	344
Skewers, Hot Meze	255

NUTS
Mixed, Athenian, Nibbles	479

OCTOPUS
Grilled, Hot Meze	447

OLIVES
Nibbles	317

PARCELS
Tiropitakia, Filo Pastry, Hot Meze	416

PORK
Skewers, Hot Meze	281

POTATOES
New, in Olive Oil & Lemon Juice, Hot Meze	293

RICE
Saffron, Hot Meze	406

THE REAL GREEK FOOD COMPANY LTD

SALAD
	KCAL
Cos	42
Tabouleh, Cold Meze	117
Watermelon, Mint & Feta, Cold Meze	102

SARDINES
Grilled, Hot Meze	619

SOUVLAKI
Lamb, Kefte	730
Lamb	607
Pork	633
Souvlaki, Halloumi & Vegetable	451

SQUID
Kalamari, Grilled, Hot Meze	286

TARAMASALATA
Cold Meze	913

TZATZIKI
Cold Meze	163

TIM HORTONS

BAGEL
	KCAL
Breakfast Sandwich, Grilled, with Bacon	321
Breakfast Sandwich, Grilled, with Sausage	402
Cinnamon Raisin, with Butter	324
Cinnamon Raisin, with Cream Cheese	357
Everything, with Butter	312
Everything, with Cream Cheese	345
Plain, with Butter	301
Plain, with Cream Cheese	334

BARS
Rocky Road, Traybake	380
Shortbread, Caramel, Traybake	349

BREAKFAST CEREAL
Porridge	237
Porridge, with Mixed Berries	246

BURGERS
Veggie, Moving Mountains	514

CAKE
Chocolate, & Hazelnut	600

CHICKEN
Tenders, 3	236
Tenders, 5	394
Tenders, Timmies Minis	158

COFFEE
Cappuccino, Iced, Large	399
Cappuccino, Iced, Medium	305
Cappuccino, Iced, Small	211
Cappuccino, Large	140
Cappuccino, Iced, Light, Large	202
Cappuccino, Iced, Light, Medium	152
Cappuccino, Iced, Light, Small	101
Cappuccino, Medium	110
Cappuccino, Small	75
Cappuccino, Iced, Supreme, Large	490
Cappuccino, Iced, Supreme, Medium	395
Cappuccino, Iced, Small	302
Cappuccino, Iced, with Caramel, Large	616
Cappuccino, Iced, with Caramel, Medium	479
Cappuccino, Iced, with Caramel, Small	344
Cappuccino, Iced, with Chocolate Syrup, Large	604
Cappuccino, Iced, with Chocolate Syrup, Medium	472
Cappuccino, Iced, with Chocolate Syrup, Small	340
Cappuccino, Iced, with Oreo, Large	566
Cappuccino, Iced, Supreme, with Oreo, Medium	444
Cappuccino, Iced, Supreme, with Oreo, Small	322
Dark Roast, Large	5
Dark Roast, Medium	4
Decaf, Large	5
Decaf, Medium	4
Decaf, Small	3
Espresso, Single	1
Flat White, Medium	121
Latte, Chai, Large	270

TIM HORTONS

COFFEE

Latte, Chai, Medium	214
Latte, Chai, Small	158
Latte, Chocolate, Large	279
Latte, Chocolate, Medium	210
Latte, Chocolate, Small	137
Latte, Iced, Large	134
Latte, Iced, Medium	99
Latte, Iced, Small	65
Latte, Large	164
Latte, Medium	134
Latte, Small	99
Latte, Vanilla, French, Large	384
Latte, Vanilla, French, Medium	329
Latte, Vanilla, French, Small	274
Mocha, Large	378
Mocha, Medium	324
Mocha, Small	270
Original Blend, Large	5
Original, Medium	4
Original Blend, Small	3
Dark Roast, Small	3

COOKIES

Chocolate, Chunk, Double	232
Chocolate, Chunk, Triple	239
Chocolate, Chunk, White	239

CROISSANT

Single	231

DOUGHNUTS

Apple, Fritter	319
Apple, Fritter, Timbit	41
Boston Cream	239
Chocolate, Birthday Cake, Timbit	94
Chocolate, Dip	234
Chocolate, Doughnut	287
Chocolate, Filled, Timbit	64
Chocolate, Glazed, Timbit	80
Glazed, Old Fashioned	298
Honey, Dip, Timbit	48
Honey Cruller	260
Honey Cruller, Timbit	60
Maple, Canadian	242
Maple, Dip	233
Maple, Moose	313
Strawberry, Filled, Timbit	54
Strawberry, Vanilla	270
Valentines	289
Vanilla, Dip	276

HASH BROWNS

Portion	79

HOT CHOCOLATE

Frozen, Large	539
Frozen, Medium	391

TIM HORTONS

HOT CHOCOLATE

Frozen, Small	254
Large	377
Medium	323
Small	269
White, Frozen, Large	619
White, Frozen, Medium	466
White, Frozen, Small	332
White, Praline, Frozen, Large	579
White, Praline, Frozen, Medium	402
White, Praline, Frozen, Small	342

JUICE DRINK

Mango, & Passionfruit, Fruit Cooler, Large	263
Mango, & Passionfruit, Fruit Cooler, Medium	198
Mango, & Passionfruit, Fruit Cooler, Small	136
Raspberry, Fruit Cooler, Large	255
Raspberry, Fruit Cooler, Medium	185
Raspberry, Fruit Cooler, Small	136

LEMONADE

Frozen	178
Original, Large	260
Original, Medium	200
Original, Small	120

MILK

Whole, Timmies Minis	365

MUFFIN

Bacon, Double, Egg, & Cheese	346
Bacon, Egg, & Cheese	301
Bacon	198
Blueberry	366
Chocolate, Chip	452
Chocolate, Lava	456
Egg, & Cheese	257
Sausage, Double, Egg, & Cheese	507
Sausage, Egg, & Cheese	382
Sausage	225
Sausage, Vegetarian, Egg, & Cheese	416

PANCAKE

Bacon, & Maple, Meal	505
Bacon, & Maple	426
Chocolate, & Hazelnut	577
Maple, Caramel, & White Chocolate	481
Maple Syrup, Meal	447
Maple Syrup	368
Nutella, Meal	467
Nutella	388
Red Berry, & White Chocolate	407

PANINI

Chicken, & Mozzarella	506
Meatball	608
Mozzarella, & Tomato	431

POTATO WEDGES

Portion	260

TIM HORTONS

ROLL
Bacon	587

SANDWICH
Chicken, Crispy	590
Ham, Timmies Minis	136
Meatless Chicken, Crispy	569
Tuna, Timmies Minis	160

SMOOTHIE
Strawberry, Banana, Large	332
Strawberry, Banana, Medium	249
Strawberry, Banana, Small	175

SOUP
Tomato, & Basil, Vegan	110

TEA
Freshly Brewed, Large	0
Freshly Brewed, Medium	0
Freshly Brewed, Small	0
Speciality, Large	0
Speciality, Medium	0
Speciality, Small	0

TEACAKES
Toasted	265

TOAST
Plain	218
with Butter	325
with Jam	266

TOASTIE
Cheese, & Bacon, Melt	559
Cheese, & Ham, Melt	339
Cheese, Grilled, Melt	487
Cheese, Melt, Timmies Minis	158
Ham, & Cheese, Melt, Timmies Minis	190
Ham, Melt, Timmies Minis	156
Tuna, & Cheese, Melt	380

WRAP
Breakfast, Big	743
Breakfast, Big, Vegetarian, Moving Mountains	725
Breakfast, Original	589
Breakfast, Vegetarian, Moving Mountains	572
Chicken, Crispy, & Bacon	645
Chicken, Crispy	460
Chicken, Grilled, & Bacon	525
Chicken, Grilled	340
Chicken, Timmies Minis	251
Meatball	449
Tuna	340
Vegan, Moving Mountains	365
Veggie, Chipotle, Moving Mountains	367

YOGHURT
& Granola, Rachels	227

TOBY CARVERY

BAKE
Leek, Crumble, Carvery	103
Potato, & Carrot, Carvery	121
Potato, & Leek, Carvery	120
Potato, & Parsnip, Carvery	145
Potato, & Squash, Carvery	123
Tomato, Crumble, Carvery	118

BEANS
Baked, Breakfast	77
Baked, Side, Kids Menu	76
Green, Carvery	44
Romano, Carvery	63

BEEF
Deck Veg Garnish	65
Roast, Carvery	274

BREAD
Brown, Sandwich Choice	405
Ciabatta, Sanwich Choice	311
Ciabatta, with Lurpak	337
Garlic, Ciabatta	363
Garlic, Ciabatta, with Cheese	488
Garlic, Kids Menu	182
White, Bap, Sandwich Choice	342
White, Sandwich Choice	438
Wholemeal, Bap, Sandwich Choice	264

BREAKFAST
Kids, Vegetarian	1330
Toby Carvery	1838
Toby Carvery, Vegetarian	1330

BREAKFAST CEREAL
Porridge, Breakfast	243

BROCCOLI
Carvery	51

BROWNIES
Chocolate, Pieces, Mini	352

BUBBLE & SQUEAK
Carvery	88

BURGERS
Chicken, Kids Menu	340

CABBAGE
Red, Carvery	63
Seasonal, Carvery	241

CAKE
Birthday	587
Black Forest Square	863
Chocolate, Fudge	567
Mousse, Chocolate, & Orange	319
Salted Caramel, Sticky, Giant	869

CARROTS
Carvery	31

CAULIFLOWER CHEESE
Carvery	55

TOBY CARVERY

CHEESE
Camembert, Baked, for Two	897

CHEESECAKE
Vanilla, Baked	772

CHICKEN
Nuggets, Kids Menu	190
Strips, Southern Fried, Spicy, with BBQ Sauce	302

CHICKEN DINNER
Baby's, Heinz, Kids Menu	123

CHOCOLATE
Flake, Extra	44

COOKIES
Chocolate Chip, Sundae Topping	256

CORN
Cob, Mini, Carvery	51

COURGETTE
Lemon & Thyme, Roasted, Carvery	39

CREAM
Whipped, for Desserts	148

CRUMBLE
Apple, Blackberry, & Redcurrant, Mini	285
Apple, Blackberry, & Redcurrant	402

CUSTARD
for Desserts	90
Soya, Vegan, for Desserts	81

DESSERT
Eton Mess	2315

DUMPLINGS
in Onion Gravy, Carvery	469

EGGS
Fried, Free Range, Breakfast	157
Scrambled, Breakfast	181

FRUIT COMPOTE
Apple, with Cinnamon, Porridge Topping	33
Toffee, Apple, & Banana, Porridge Topping	82

GAMMON
Deck Veg Garnish	57
Pomegranate Glaze, Carvery	196

GATEAU
Black Forest	863

GRAVY
Breakfast	54
Classic, Carvery	23
Vegan, Carvery	36
Vegetarian, Carvery	317

HASH
Potato, Cheese, & Onion, Breakfast	102

HASH BROWNS
Breakfast	166

HOUMOUS
with Veg, & Bread	474
with Veg, Vegan	374

TOBY CARVERY

ICE CREAM
for Desserts	105
Kids Menu	176
No Sauce	209

ICE LOLLY
Pip Organic, Kids Menu	20

LAMB
Deck Veg Garnish	215
Roast, Carvery	214

LEEKS
Carvery	30

MACARONI CHEESE
Carvery	99
Kids Menu	150

MARSHMALLOWS
Sundae Topping	50

MASH
Colcannon, Carvery	92

MUSHROOMS
Garlic	251
Roasted, Breakfast	461

MUSTARD
English, Carvery	194
Wholegrain, Carvery	213

ONIONS
in Gravy, Carvery	61

PARCELS
Broccoli, & Brie	492

PARSNIP
Honey Roast, Carvery	162

PASTA
Tomato, & Meatballs, Kids Menu	316

PEAS
Carvery	82

PETIT POIS
Ala Creme, Carvery	97

PIE
Allotment	352
Apple	246
Mushroom, & Ale, Roast	761

PLATTER
Taster	1708
Tobys Ultimate, Sharing	2734
Vegetarian, Sharing	1950

PORK
Deck Veg Garnish	78
Roast, Apple & Sage Glaze, Carvery	230

PORK CRACKLING
Cravery	669

POTATOES
Mashed, Carvery	103
Mashed, Cheesy, Carvery	149
Roast, Beef Dripping, Carvery	111

TOBY CARVERY

POTATOES
Roast, Bowl, Side	229
Roast, Carvery	94
Roast, Loaded	350

PRAWN COCKTAIL
King, with Bread	417
King, with Wholemeal Bread, Mini, Kids Menu	300

PUDDING
Arctic Roll, with Whipped Cream	418
Three Little	1226

SALAD
House	107
Topping, Cheddar Cheese	311
Topping, Prawns	387

SANDWICH FILLING
Beef, Mushroom, & Chutney, Add Bread	912
Cheese, & Chutney, Add Bread	304
Gammon, Camembert, & Cranberry, Add Bread	894
Hunters Gammon, Add Bread	643
Pork, Roast, Add Bread	521
Prawn, King, Add Bread	332
Turkey, Roast, Club, add Bread	497

SAUCE
Apple, Carvery	103
Bread, Carvery	443
Chocolate, Belgian	58
Cranberry, Carvery	148
Horseradish, Carvery	178
Lemon, Sicillian	55
Mint, Carvery	124
Parsley, Carvery	467
Strawberry	57
Toffee, Devon Cream	64

SAUSAGE
& Giant Yorkshire Pudding, Kids Menu	327
Pigs, In Blankets, Mini	531
Pigs in Blankets, Apple & Sage Glazed, Sharer	494
Pigs in Blankets, Pomegranate Glazed, Sharer	487
Pigs in Blankets, Glazed, Sharer	587
Pigs in Blankets, Maple Glazed, Sharer	517
Pork, British, Breakfast	217
Quorn, Breakfast	128
Quorn*, & Giant Yorkshire Pudding, Kids Menu	292

SAUSAGE ROLL
Squashage, Salad Topping	507
Vegan, with Gravy	542

SEA BASS
Steamed	362

SORBET
Trio	453

SOUP
Small, Side	58
Tomato, with Wholemeal Bread, Kids Menu	226

TOBY CARVERY

SPINACH
Creamed, Carvery	41

SPONGE
Apricot, with Custard	405
Cherry, with Custard	398
Rhubarb, with Custard	410
Rolo Toffee, with Custard	509
Strawberry, with Custard	407
Treacle	526

SPROUTS
Carvery	65

STRAWBERRIES
& Cream	200
& Ice Cream	164

STUFFING
Sage, & Cranberry, Carvery	340
Sage, & Onion, Carvery	204

SUNDAE
Banoffee	955
Chocolate Heaven, Kids Menu	364
Cookie Dough	473
Honeycomb Dream	397
Ice Cream, Make Your Own, Kids Menu	158

SUNDAE TOPPING
Banana, Make Your Own, Kids Menu	72
Chocolate Chip Cookie, Make Your Own, Kids Menu	256
Fruit Salad Crunch, Make Your Own, Kids Menu	40
Honeycomb Pieces, Make Your Own, Kids Menu	59
Marshmallows, Make Your Own, Kids Menu	50
Meringue, Make Your Own, Kids Menu	25
Strawberries, Make Your Own, Kids Menu	20

SWEDE
Carvery	188

SWEETS
Bear Yo Yo's, Strawberry, Kids Menu	56

TOAD IN THE HOLE
Veggie	1091

TOAST
White, Breakfast	451

TOMATOES
Plum, Breakfast	15

TURKEY
Deck Veg Garnish	88
Roast, Carvery	118

VEGETABLES
Greens, Leek, Cabbage, & Peas, Carvery	64
Sticks, Side, Kids Menu	25
Sticks, wih Houmous Dip, Kids Menu	201

WAFERS
Extra	8

YORKSHIRE PUDDING
& Gravy, Side	168
Breakfast	381

TOBY CARVERY

	KCAL
YORKSHIRE PUDDING	
Carvery	224
Sandwich Choice	328
Stuffed, Beef	313

	KCAL
BAKE - SLOW ROASTED TOMATO	
& Almond, with Roast Potatoes, & Veg	1170
BEANS	
Baked, Side, Childrens	80
BEEF - STEAK SIRLOIN, 8OZ	
Triple Cooked Chips, Onion Rings, Roasted Tomato	966
BEEF - STEAK, FILLET, 7OZ	
Triple Cooked Chips, Onion Rings, Roasted Tomato	798
BEEF - STEAK, RIBEYE, 10OZ	
Triple Cooked Chips, Onion Rings, Roasted Tomato	963
BEEF - STEAK, RUMP, 8OZ	
Triple Cooked Chips, Onion Rings, Roasted Tomato	927
BEEF BOURGUIGNON	
Porcini, with Mash, Carrots, & Dumplings	432
BEEF DINNER, SIRLOIN	
Yorkshire Pudding, Roast Potatoes, Veg, & Gravy	1598
BEEF DINNER, TRIO	
Turkey, & Pork, Roast Potatoes, Veg, & Gravy	1379
BITES	
Black Pudding	417
Black Pudding, Yorkshire	367
Yorkshire Pudding	299
BREAD	
Garlic, Side, Childrens	373
BREAD & BUTTER PUDDING	
Marmalade, with Custard	642
BROWNIES - CHOCOLATE	
Belgian, Chocolate Sauce, & Irish Liqueur Ice Cream	832
with Vanilla Ice Cream, Childrens	553
BURGERS	
Beef, Chargrilled, Dirty	1324
Beef, Chargrilled, with Mayo, Relish, & Onion Rings	734
Beef, no Sides, Children's	173
Beef, Prime, Dirty	933
Beef, Prime, with Mayo, Relish, & Onion Rings	343
Beef, Wagyu, with Salsa, Mayo, & Onion Rings	1460
Chicken, no Sides, Childrens	328
Chickpea, & Aubergine, Spiced	447
Plant Based, Moving Mountanis, with Side Salad	601
CAULIFLOWER	
Roasted, Spiced, with Couscous, & Coconut Sauce	1104
CAULIFLOWER CHEESE	
Portion	222
CHEESE	
Camembert, Garlic & Rosemary, Baked	1035
Cheeseboard, with Biscuits, Grapes, & Chutney	1122
CHEESECAKE	
Blackcurrant, & Prosecco	471
Caramel, Biscuit, Vegan, with Banana	777
Vanilla, Baked	414
CHICKEN	
Hunters, with Bacon, & Tomato Sauce, & Chips	1478
Hunters, with Gammon, Chips, & BBq Sauce	1430

VINTAGE INNS

CHICKEN
Wings, Southern Fried	599

CHIPS
Side, Childrens	698
Triple Cooked	499

COD
Battered, Fillet, no Sides, Childrens	290
Loin, & Chorizo Roasted Potatoes	572
Loin, & Tomatoes, Heirloom	330

CREME BRULEE
Apricot, with Biscuits	416

CRUMBLE
Winter Fruit, Spiced, with Custard	557
Winter Fruit, Spiced, with Soya Custard	572

DESSERT
Eton Mess	372

FISH & CHIPS - COD, BATTERED
Chips, Mushy Peas, & Tartare Sauce, Lunch Bites	963
Chips, Mushy Peas, & Tartare Sauce	1330

FISH CAKES - LOBSTER
with Bouillabaisse, Broccoli, & Potatoes, Lunch Bites	441
with Bouillabaisse, Broccoli, & Potatoes	602

FLATBREAD - GARLIC BUTTER
with Cheese, Stonebaked, Sharers & Grazing	864

FRIES
Skin On, Side, Childrens	539
Sweet Potato, Side, Childrens	293
Sweet Potato	377

GAMMON
Steak, 4oz, with Eggs, & Chips, Lunch Bites	765
Steak, 8oz, with Eggs, & Chips	1262

ICE CREAM
Chocolate, Childrens	355
Chocolate, Double	315
Irish Cream Liqueur	255
Vanilla, Childrens	278
Vanilla Pod	122

ICE LOLLY
Tropical Fruit, Childrens	20

JELLY
Peach, Childrens	144

KEBAB
Lamb Kofta, with Tzatziki, & Dressed Slaw, Starter	340

LAMB - DINNER, RUMP
Yorkshire Pudding, Roast Potatoes, Veg, & Gravy	1758

LAMB - DUO
Rump, & Shepherd's Pie, Veg, & Red Wine Jus	1204

LAMB - RACK
Roasted, with Veg, & Spiced Potatoes	1142

LASAGNE
Beef, & Red Wine	583
Beef, no Sides, Children's	349

VINTAGE INNS

MUSHROOMS - GARLIC, BAKED
& Cheese, Steak Add On	109
& Cheddar Sauce, with Rustic Bread, Starter	296

OLIVES
Mixed, Marinated in Garlic & Red Pepper	184

ONION RINGS
Homemade	86

PASTA
Tomato, Childrens	238

PATE
Duo, with Rustic Bread, Starter	432

PEAS
Side, Childrens	45

PIE - APPLE, BRAMLEY
with Custard, & Vanilla Pod Ice Cream	754

PIE - CHICKEN & MUSHROOM
with Mash, Roasted Carrots, & Veg	942

PIE - LEMON MERINGUE
Portion	393

PIE - STEAK & ALE
with Mash, Seasonal Veg, & a Jug of Gravy	1004

PIZZA
Chicken, Spicy Cajun, Stonebaked	1288
Four Cheese, Stonebaked	1209
Margherita, Childrens	577
Margherita, Stonebaked	963
Meat Feast, Stonebaked	1404
Vegetable, Roasted, with Pesto, Stonebaked	1134

PLATTER
Mezze, Sharers & Grazing	1293
Pudding, Tasting	2391
Sticky, Sharers & Grazing	2200

PORK - BELLY, ROAST
Yorkshire Pudding, Roast Potatoes, Veg, & Gravy	1703

PORK - BELLY, SLOW COOKED
with Mash, Crackling & Veg	1365

POTATOES
Baby, Side, Childrens	77
Mashed, Side, Children's	141
Roast	482

PRAWN COCKTAIL
with Lobster, with Rustic Bread, Starter	751

PRAWNS
Garlic, Steak Add On	209
Tempura, with Rice Cracker, & Soy, Lime & Chilli Dip	475

PUDDING
Sticky Toffee, with Butterscotch Sauce, & Custard	356

RIBS
Pork, Caramelised Sticky, with Mango Salsa	466

RICE
Sunshine, Side, Childrens	190

RISOTTO
Mushroom, Wild	1045

VINTAGE INNS

RISOTTO
Mushroom, Wild, with Chicken	1243
Mushroom, Wild, with Halloumi	1443
Mushroom, Wild, with Salmon	1871
Seafood, with Roasted Tomatoes	1097

ROLLS
Squashsage & Mushroom, Vegan	409

SALAD
Super Green	135

SALAD - CAESAR
with Chicken, & Garlic Flatbread	1201
with Garlic Flatbread	710
with Halloumi, & Garlic Flatbread	1050
with Salmon, & Garlic Flatbread	1141

SALAD - DUCK
Aromatic	337

SALAD - SIDE
Childrens	46

SALAD - WHEATBERRY, APPLE & CRANBERRY
Main	1223
with Chicken, Lunch Bites	1212
with Chicken	1459
with Halloumi, Lunch Bites	1064
with Halloumi	1311
with Lamb Koftas, Lunch Bites	890
with Lamb Koftas	1137
with Salmon, Lunch Bites	1078
with Salmon	1753

SALMON
Pesto Crusted, & Mascarpone, Broccoli, Butter Sauce	1107

SANDWICH
Beef, Brisket, on Sourdough, no Chips	729
Beef, Roast, on a Rustic Roll, no Chips	1086
Chicken, & Camembert, Hot, on Foccacia, no Chips	769
Fish Finger, Cod, on a Rustic Roll, no Chips	578
Ham, & Cheddar, Melt, on Sourdough, no Chips	733

SAUCE
Bearnaise, Steak Sauce	210
Beef Dripping, Steak Sauce	162
Peppercorn, Steak Sauce	46

SAUSAGE
Pork, with Gravy, no Sides, Childrens	278

SCALLOPS
Extra	47
Black Pudding, Minted Pea Puree, Bacon, Starter	731

SEA BASS
with Pancetta Veloute, Broccoli, & Mash	754

SOUP
Broccoli, & Stilton	213
Pea, Mint, & Ham	302
Pea & Mint	204

SQUID - CALAMARI
Salt, Pepper, Chorizo, & Chipotle Chilli Mayo, Starter	476

VINTAGE INNS

STUFFING
Lemon & Thyme, Bacon Wrapped, Extra	385

TART
Carrot, & Apricot Chutney, & Salad, & Baby Potatoes	1078

TURKEY DINNER
Yorkshire Pudding, Roast Potatoes, Veg, & Gravy	1408

VEGETABLES
Skewer, no Sides, Childrens	83
Sticks, Side, Childrens	38

WRAP
Jackfruit, Smoky, with Side Salad, Vegan	233
Jackfruit, Smoky, without Chips	215

YORKSHIRE PUDDING
Extra	99
Roast Potatoes, Veg, & Gravy, No Meat, Childrens	660
Roast Potatoes, Veg, & Gravy, No Meat	660

WAGAMAMA

BANANA
Katsu, with Salted Caramel Ice Cream	247

BEANS
Edamame, with Chilli	255
Edamame, with Salt	247

BEEF
Teriyaki, & Rice, Donburi	881

BROCCOLI
& Bok Choi, Wok-Fried, Greens	177

BUNS
Beef, Korean BBQ, & Red Onion, Steamed, Hirata	306
Mushroom, Mixed, Steamed, Hirata	338
Pork, Belly, & Panko Apple, Steamed, Hirata	391

CAKE
Chocolate, Caramel, Smoked, with Vanilla Ice Cream	518
Chocolate Orange, with Miso Caramel Ice Cream	567

CAULIFLOWER
Bang Bang	472

CHEESECAKE
Salted Caramel	383
White Chocolate, & Matcha	510
White Chocolate, & Ginger	449

CHICKEN
Grilled, Katsu, Naked	607
Grilled, Katsu, with Amai Sauce, Mini, Kids Menu	402
Grilled, Katsu, with Curry Sauce, Mini, Kids Menu	426
Katsu, with Amai Sauce, Mini, Kids Menu	453
Katsu, with Curry Sauce, Mini, Kids Menu	477
Skewers, Teriyaki, Yakitori	266
Teriyaki, & Rice, Donburi	777

CHILLI
Side	2

CURRY
Chicken, Firecracker, & White Rice	1185
Chicken, Raisukaree, & White Rice	1123
Chicken Katsu, & Sticky Rice	1079
Chicken Katsu, Hot, & Sticky Rice	1121
Prawn, Firecracker, & White Rice	1067
Prawn, Raisukaree, & White Rice	1035
Tofu, Firecracker, & White Rice	1208
Tofu, Raisukaree, & White Rice	1167
Vegatsu, Hot, Seitan, Panko Crusted, with Sticky Rice	1200
Vegatsu, Seitan, Panko Crusted, with Sticky Rice	1110
Yasai Katsu, & Sticky Rice	1110
Yasai Katsu, Hot, & Sticky Rice	1197

CURRY - YASAI, VEGETABLE
& Sticky Rice, Katsu, Amai Sauce, Mini, Kids Menu	369
& Sticky Rice, Katsu, Curry Sauce, Mini, Kids Menu	393

DUCK
Grilled, Teriyaki, with Rice, Donburi	1399
Vegan, No Duck, with Brown Rice, Donburi	460

DUMPLINGS
Chicken, Steamed, Gyoza	223

WAGAMAMA

DUMPLINGS
Duck, Fried, Gyoza	373
Pork, Pulled, Steamed, Gyoza	231
Prawn, Fried, Gyoza	231
Yasai, Steamed, Gyoza	221

EGGS
Tea Stained, Side	95

FISH
Bites, Crispy, with Amai Sauce, Mini, Kids Menu	565
Bites, Crispy, with Curry Sauce, Mini, Kids Menu	588

ICE CREAM
Chocolate, & Orange Blossom	294
Coconut, Reika	432
Coffee, Vietnamese	337
Miso Caramel	419
Strawberry, & Yuzu	325
Vanilla, Pod, Kids Menu	136

ICE LOLLY
Blackcurrant, & Apple, Little Ko Pop	30
Mango, & Apple, Little Ko Pop	34

JUICE
Apple, & Orange, Mini, Kids Menu	87
Apple, Mini, Kids Menu	68
Blueberry, Spice	164
High-Five	211
Nourish-Mint	155
Orange, Mini, Kids Menu	73
Orange	110
Positive	234
Power	170
Tropical	152
Up-Beet	150

KIMCHI
Side	15

LEMONADE
Cloudy	0

MILK
Mini, Kids Menu	109

NOODLES - KIDS
Chicken, Grilled, Mini	450
Chicken, Grilled, Mini	400
Chicken, Mini	410
Fish, Grilled, Mini	380
Tofu, & Vegetable, Rice Noodles, Ramen, Mini	306
Tofu, & Vegetable, Thin Noodles, Ramen, Mini	328
Tofu, & Vegetable, Udon Noodles, Mini	954
Tofu, & Vegetable, Rice Noodles, Mini	338
Tofu, & Vegetable, Thin Noodles, Mini	402
Tofu, & Vegetable, Yaki Soba, Udon, Mini	259

NOODLES - RAMEN
Beef, Brisket, Tantanmen	690
Beef, Steak, Chilli	681
Chicken, Grilled, Chilli	606

WAGAMAMA

NOODLES - RAMEN

	KCAL
Chicken, Grilled	499
Cod, Miso Glazed	668
Pork, Belly, Shirodashi	725
Prawn, Chilli,& Kimchee	533
Tofu, Kare Burosu	489

NOODLES - SOBA

Plain, Side	398

NOODLES - TEPPANYAKI

Vegetable, Yasai Yaki Soba	790
Beef, Steak, Teriyaki, Soba	899
Chicken, & Prawn, Pad-Thai	801
Chicken, & Prawn, Yaki Soba	824
Chicken, & Prawn, Yaki Udon	650
Chicken, Ginger, Udon	678
Cod, Mokutan Soba	829
Salmon, Teriyaki, Soba	882
Tofu, & Vegetable, Pad-Thai	849

PICKLE

Japanese, Side	4

PRAWNS

Ebi Katsu, Crispy, Fried, with Chilli Garlic Sauce	281
Skewers, Lollipop, Kushiyaki	140

RIBS

Vegan, Sticky	306

RICE

Brown, Side	501
Steamed, Side	480
Sticky, Side	492

SALAD

Chicken, Teriyaki, Hiyashi Bowl	510
Duck, Teriyaki, Shredded, Hiyashi Bowl	743
Mixed Vegetable, Miso, Hiyashi Bowl	391
Salmon, Harusame	389
Tofu, Harusame	320

SORBET

Pink Guava, & Passion Fruit	166

SOUP

Miso, & Japanese Pickles, Side	35

SQUID

Balls, Tama	344
Chilli	586
Vegan, Chilli	575

STIR FRY

Avant Gard'n, Vegan	567
Chicken, Cha Han, Mini, Kids	403
Chicken, Shu's 'Shiok', Kokoro Bowl	570
Tofu, Cha Han, Yasai, Mini, Kids	395
Tofu, Cha Han, Yasai, Vegan, Mini, Kids	352

TART

Yuzu, & Lemon	305

TEA

Ginger & Lemongrass	0

WAGAMAMA

TEA

	KCAL
Green	0
Jasmine, Flowering	0
Mint, Fresh	0
Peach, Iced	0

TUNA

Steak, Nuoc Cham, Seared	468

VEGETABLES

Tempura	384

WIMPY

BACON
Slice	65

BEANS
Baked, Heinz, Extra	69

BREAKFAST
All Day	832
Country	359
Hashbrown	396
Sunrise	340
The Great Wimpy	758

BROWNIES
Chocolate	639

BURGERS
Bender, in a Bun, with Cheese	527
Fish Finger	577
Hamburger	392
Kingsize	823
Mega	789

BURGERS - BEAN
Spicy, & Slaw, Stack, Vegetarian	673
Spicy, Vegetarian	557

BURGERS - CHEESEBURGER
Double	647
Original	433
Junior, with Beans, Kids	477
Junior, with Chips, Kids	601
Junior, with Salad, Kids	422

BURGERS - CHICKEN
Fillet, Firecracker Sauce	498
Fillet, with BBQ Sauce	503
Fillet, with Wimpy Mayo	527
Gourmet	510

BURGERS - HALFPOUNDER
Original	876
with Bacon & Cheese	861

BURGERS - JUNIOR
with Beans, Kids	436
with Chips, Kids	560
with Salad, Kids	381

BURGERS - QUARTERPOUNDER
Club	736
Patty Only	264
Smoky BBQ	693
with Cheese, Original	613
with Mushroom	646
with Bacon & Cheese	597

BURGERS - QUORN
Southern Fried, Spicy, Vegetarian	506

CHEESE
Mozzarella, Melts, 6	390
Slices, Extras	41

CHICKEN
Platter, Gourmet	645

WIMPY

CHICKEN
Strips, & Chips	685
Strips, with Beans, Kids	310
Strips, with Chips, Kids	433
Strips, with Salad, Kids	254
Wings, Coated, with BBQ Sauce	477
Wings, Coated, with Firecracker Sauce	466

CHIPS
Large	333
Reg	267
Sweet Potato, Large	340
Sweet Potato, Reg	269

CHOCOLATE
Flake, for Sundae	45

COFFEE - AMERICANO
Black, Large	5
Black, Reg	3
with Milk, Large	26
with Milk, Reg	16

COFFEE - CAPPUCCINO
Large	109
Reg	81

COFFEE - ESPRESSO
Large	5
Reg	3

COFFEE - LATTE
Large	139
Reg	111

COFFEE - MOCHA
Large	248
Reg	183

COFFEE - SHOT
Extra	3

COLA
Pepsi, Diet, Kids	2
Pepsi, Diet, Large	3
Pepsi, Diet, Reg	2
Pepsi, Large	181
Pepsi, Max, Kids	1
Pepsi, Max, Large	2
Pepsi, Max, Reg	2
Pepsi, Reg	143

COLESLAW
Extra	171

CREAM
Extra, for Desserts	70
Extra, for Drinks	39

DESSERT
Brown Derby with Dairy Ice Cream	436

DRESSING
Caesar	219
French	60
Wimpy Mayo	199

WIMPY

EGGS

	KCAL
Fried, Extra	90
Fried, on Toast, White	458
Scrambled, Extra	65
Scrambled, on Toast, White	409

FISH

Bites, with Beans, Kids	255
Bites, with Chips, Kids	379
Bites, with Salad, Kids	200

FISH & CHIPS

Cod	705

GRILLS

International	1024
Wimpy	803

HASH BROWNS

Extra	98

HOT CHOCOLATE

without Cream, Large	281
without Cream, Reg	224

ICE CREAM

Extra	95

ICE CREAM FLOAT

7 Up	99
Pepsi, Diet	96
Pepsi	183
Pepsi Max	96
Tango Orange	97

JAM

Extra	48

JELLY

Orange, Pot, Kids	3
Strawberry, Pot, Kids	5

JUICE

Apple, Kids	122
Apple, Large	206
Apple, Reg	163
Orange, Kids	120
Orange, Large	202
Orange, Reg	160

LEMONADE

7 Up, Free, Kids	5
7 Up, Free, Large	9
7 Up, Free, Reg	7

MARMALADE

Extra	49

MILK

Kids	125
Large	211
Reg	167

MILK SHAKE - BANANA

Thick, Kids	187
Thick, Large	300
Thick, Reg	244

WIMPY

MILK SHAKE - CHOCO TOFFEE POPCORN

	KCAL
Thick, Reg	425

MILK SHAKE - CHOCOLATE

Thick, Kids	189
Thick, Large	303
Thick, Reg	246

MILK SHAKE - CHOCOLATE PEPPERMINT

Thick, Reg	365

MILK SHAKE - LIME

Thick, Kids	152
Thick, Large	243
Thick, Reg	197

MILK SHAKE - STRAWBERRY

Thick, Kids	187
Thick, Large	299
Thick, Reg	243

MILK SHAKE - VANILLA

Thick, Kids	151
Thick, Large	241
Thick, Reg	196

MUFFIN

Bacon, & Egg	347
Bacon, & Hasbrown	445
Hashbrown	380
Sausage, & Egg	380
Sausage, & Hashbrown	478

MUSHROOMS

Extra	110

ONION RINGS

8	317
CheesO, 4	481

PANCAKE

& Ice Cream, no Toppings, Kids	178
& Ice Cream, no Toppings	344

PEAS

Extras	86

PEPPER

Jalapeno, Burger Extras	1

POTATO FILLING

Bacon	65
Beans, Baked, Heinz	79
Cheese, Grated	189
Coleslaw	194
Mushrooms	137

POTATOES

Baked, Jacket, Half, with Beans, Kids	297
Baked, Jacket, Half, with Cheese, Kids	347
Baked, Jacket, Half, with Chips, Kids	421
Baked, Jacket, Half, with Salad, Kids	241
Baked, Jacket, Plain, with Butter	516
Jacket, with Butter, & Salad, add Fillings Seperately	523

SALAD

Chicken, Breaded, no Dressing	360

WIMPY

SALAD

Chicken, Gourmet, no Dressing	317
Junior, Side, Kids	8
Mixed, Side	67
Quorn, Southern Fried, Spicy, no Dressing	320

SAUCE

BBQ	41
Chocolate, for Sundae	81
Firecracker	29
Ketchup	29
Mango, for Sundae	25
Maple Flavoured, for Sundae	86
Special	114
Strawberry, for Sundae	80
Summer Fruits, for Sundae	38
Toffee Fudge, for Sundae	91
Mayo	100

SAUSAGE

Bender, with Egg & Chips, Grill	628
Patty, Extra	98
Pork, Bender	271
Pork, Breakfast	130
with Beans, Kids	322
with Chips, Kids	446
with Egg & Chips, Grill	615
with Salad, Kids	267

SMOOTHIE

Mango, Iced	181
Summer Fruits, Iced	274

SQUASH

Apple, & Blackcurrant, Kids	4
Orange, Kids	3

SUNDAE

Brownie	591
Ice Cream, No Toppings, Kids	95
Ice Cream, No Toppings	159
Knickerbocker Glory	372

TANGO*

Orange, Free, Kids	3
Orange, Free, Large	4
Orange, Free, Reg	3

TEA

Black, Large	1
Black, Reg	1
Herbal, Large	3
Herbal, Reg	2
with Milk, Large	22
with Milk, Reg	14

TEACAKES

Toasted, with Butter	295

TOAST

White, with Butter	279

WIMPY

TOASTIE

Cheese, & Red Onion, White	391
Cheese, & Tomato, White	386
Cheese, with Beans, White, Kids	400
Cheese, with Chips, White, Kids	521
Cheese, with Salad, White, Kids	345
Chicken, BBQ, White	523
Ham, & Cheese, White	436

TOPPING

Flake, Crushed, for Drinks	45
Fruit Cocktail, for Sundae	18
Fudge, Pieces, Mini	40
Marshmallows, Mini, for Drinks	32
Marshmallows, Mini, for Sundae	32
Strawberries, for Sundae	10

TORTE

Apple, no Toppings	245

VEGETABLES

Sticks, Carrot, & Cucumber, Kids	24

WAFFLES

Eskimo, no Toppings	663

YO! SUSHI

AUBERGINE

Fried, in Garlic, Ginger, Sesame, & Soy, Harusame	108

BEANS

Edamame, Side	134

BEEF

Tataki	96

BEEF TERIYAKI

Large	940
Standard	329

BROCCOLI

Tenderstem, & Sesame	135

BROWNIES

Chocolate	363

BURGERS

Chicken, Katsu	476
Chicken, Teriyaki	286
Mushroom, Teriyaki	228

CAULIFLOWER

Pepper, Spicy	146

CHEESECAKE

Japanese	195

CHICKEN

Fried, Japanese	382
Fried, Korean	386

CHICKEN TERIYAKI

Large	837
Standard	272

DESSERT

Mochi, Chocolate	236
Mochi, Strawberry Cheesecake	188
Platter	605

DOUGH BALLS

Takoyaki	276

DUMPLINGS - GYOZA

Chicken, 5	206
Chicken	140
Prawn, 5	220
Prawn	148
Vegetable, 5	193
Vegetable	132

FRIES

YO!	400

FRUIT

Fresh, Plate	61

KATSU

Chicken, Curry, with Rice, Large	936
Chicken, Curry, with Rice	522
Chicken	225
Prawn, Curry, with Rice, Large	757
Prawn, Curry, with Rice	432
Prawn	173
Pumpkin, Curry, with Rice, Large	789
Pumpkin, Curry, with Rice	434

YO! SUSHI

KATSU

Pumpkin	152
Tofu, Curry, with Rice, Large	794
Tofu, Curry, with Rice	451
Tofu	154

MOUSSE

Chocolate, Pot	246

NOODLES

Side	187

NOODLES - RAMEN

Chicken, Curry, Large	758
Chicken, Curry	416
Seafood, Spicy, Large	466
Seafood, Spicy	269
Shitake, Large	377
Shitake	225

NOODLES - YAKISOBA

Chicken	264
Vegetable	202

PAK CHOI

& Garlic, Stir Fried	86

PANCAKE

Dorayaki	130

RICE

Brown, Side	198
Chicken, Fried	347
Salmon, Fried	348
Vegetable, Fried	343
White, Side	303

SALAD

Chicken, & Tangerine	148
Leaf, Side	35

SEAWEED

Kaiso	175

YO! SUSHI

SHRIMP

Popcorn	355

SOUP

Miso	53

SQUID

Pepper, Spicy	207

SUSHI

Aubergine, Glazed, Nigiri	74
Avocado, Maki	204
Avocado, Nigiri	110
Beef, Seared, Nigiri	108
Chicken, & Avocado, Roll, Platter	656
Chicken, & Avocado, Roll	215
Chicken, Katsu, Spicy, Roll, Platter	423
Chicken, Katsu, Spicy, Roll	145
Cucumber, Maki	150
Duck, Aromatic, Roll	218
Mixed, Maki, Plate	196

YO! SUSHI

SUSHI

	KCAL
Mixed, Nigiri, Platter	312
Prawn, & Tuna, Blossom, Roll	209
Prawn, Panko Nigiri	121
Prawn, Star, Roll	240
Salmon, & Avocado, Dynamite, Roll	200
Salmon, & Avocado, Temaki, Hand Roll	164
Salmon, Aburi, Nigiri	112
Salmon, Beetroot Cured, Sashimi	111
Salmon, Cream Cheese, & Cucumber, Ginza, Roll	215
Salmon, Dragon, Roll	212
Salmon, Kickin', Roll, Platter	615
Salmon, Kickin', Roll	212
Salmon, Maki	189
Salmon, Nigiri	99
Salmon, Ponzu Salsa, Sashimi	104
Salmon, Sashimi	112
Salmon, Selection, Platter	572
Salmon, YO! Roll	163
Salmon Roll, Crispy	192
Surimi, & Avocado, Californian, Crunchy, Roll, Platter	693
Surimi, & Avocado, Californian, Crunchy, Roll	285
Surimi, & Avocado, Temaki, Californian Roll	233
Tuna, Coriander Seared, Sashimi	94
Tuna, Maki	178
Tuna, Mayo, Roll	127
Tuna, Nigiri	90
Tuna, Sashimi	86
Vegetable, Yasai, Roll, Platter	510
Vegetable, Yasai, Roll	170
Vegetable, Yasai, Temaki, Hand Roll	145

Useful Resources

Weight Loss
Weight Loss Resources is home to the UK's largest calorie and nutrition database along with diaries, tools and expert advice for weight loss and health.
Tel: 01733 345592 Email: helpteam@weightlossresources.co.uk
Website: www.weightlossresources.co.uk

Products to Help You Keep Track
From food diaries to weight graphs and calorie counted recipe books visit the wlr shop.
Tel: 01733 345592 Email: helpteam@weightlossresources.co.uk
Website: www.weightlossresources.co.uk/shop

Dietary Advice
The British Dietetic Association has helpful food fact leaflets and information on how to contact a registered dietitian.
Tel: 0121 200 8080 Email: info@bda.uk.com
Website: www.bda.uk.com

Healthy Eating
The British Nutrition Foundation has lots of in depth scientifically based nutritional information, knowledge and advice on healthy eating for all ages.
Tel: 0207 7557 7930 Email: postbox@nutrition.org.uk
Website: www.nutrition.org.uk

Healthy Heart
The British Heart Foundation provides advice and information for all on all heart aspects from being healthy, to living with heart conditions, research and fundraising.
Tel: 0207 554 000 Email: via their website
Website: www.bhf.org.uk

Cancer Research
Cancer Research UK is the leading UK charity dedicated to research, education and fundraising for all forms of cancer.
Tel: 0300 123 1022 Email: via their website

Website: www.cancerresearchuk.org

Diabetes Advice
Diabetes UK is the leading charity working for people with diabetes.
Their mission is to improve the lives of people with diabetes and to
work towards a future without diabetes
Tel : 0345 123 2399 Email: info@diabetes.org.uk
Website: www.diabetes.org.uk

Beating Bowel Cancer
Beating Bowel Cancer is a leading UK charity for bowel cancer
patients, working to raise awareness of symptoms, promote early
diagnosis and encourage open access to treatment choice for
those affected by bowel cancer.Tel: 08450 719301 Email: nurse@
beatingbowelcancer.org
Website: www.beatingbowelcancer.org

Safety and Standards
The Food Standards Agency is an independent watchdog, set up to
protect the public's health and consumer interests in relation to
food.Tel: 0207 276 8829 Email: helpline@foodstandards.gsi.gov.uk
Website: www.food.gov.uk

Feedback

If you have any comments or suggestions about The Calorie, Carb & Fat
Bible, or would like further information on Weight Loss Resources, please
call, email, or write to us:

Tel:	01733 345592
Email:	helpteam@weightlossresources.co.uk
Address:	Rebecca Walton,
	Weight Loss Resources Ltd,
	2C Flag Business Exchange,
	Vicarage Farm Road,
	Peterborough,
	PE1 5TX.

Reviews for The Calorie Carb & Fat Bible

'What a brilliant book. I know I'll be sinking my teeth into it.'
GMTV Nutritionist Amanda Ursell, BSc RD

'To help you make low-cal choices everyday, invest in a copy.'
ZEST magazine

'There is no doubt that the food listings are extremely helpful for anyone wishing to control their calorie intake in order to lose pounds or maintain a healthy weight.'
Women's Fitness magazine

'Useful if you don't want to exclude any overall food groups.'
Easy Living magazine

'Quite simply an astonishing achievement by the authors.'
Evening Post, Nottingham

'The book gives you all the basic information so you can work out your daily calorie needs.'
Woman magazine

'This is a welcome resource in view of the 'national epidemic of obesity.'

Bryony Philip, Bowel Cancer UK

'The authors seem to understand the problems of slimming.'

Dr John Campion

'Jam-packed with info on dieting, and full to bursting point with the calorie, carbohydrate and fat values of thousands of different foods, it's the perfect weight loss tool.'

Evening Express, Aberdeen

'Excellent resource tool - used by myself in my role as a Practice Nurse.'

Pam Boal, Sunderland

'I recently bought your book called the Calorie, Carb & Fat Bible and would love to tell you what a brilliant book it is. I have recently started a weight management programme and I honestly don't know where I'd be without your book. It has helped me a lot and given me some really good advice.'

Rachel Mitchell

About Weight Loss Resources

If you want to lose weight in a healthy, sustainable way, you'll find all the tools and support you need at wlr. Available on your phone, tablet, or PC.

HERE'S THE HIGHLIGHTS:

- Track calories: how many you need, how many you've consumed and burned, and how many you have left

- New Visual Food Diary, a more relaxed way to track. Enables you to reflect on choices and gain insights about your relationship with food

- The best kept online UK food database

- 1000s of recipes and meal ideas that you can add to your online diary and adapt to suit yourself

- Create and calorie count your own recipes and diet plans

- Set a weight loss goal, see how many calories you need to get there, and the date you can expect to reach it

- Fantastic support from our knowledgeable Helpteam, available 7 days a week

You can take a free trial at www.weightlossresources.co.uk or give us a call on 01733 345592